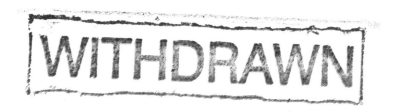

ANTICANCER
DRUG
DEVELOPMENT

ANTICANCER DRUG DEVELOPMENT

Edited by

Bruce C. Baguley

Auckland Cancer Society Research Centre

The University of Auckland

Auckland, New Zealand

David J. Kerr

Institute for Cancer Medicine

University of Oxford

Oxford, United Kingdom

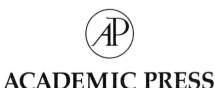

ACADEMIC PRESS

A Division of Harcourt, Inc.

San Diego   San Francisco   New York   Boston   London   Sydney   Tokyo

Academic Press
A division of Harcourt, Inc.
525 B Street, Suite 1900, San Diego, California 92101-4495, USA
http://www.academicpress.com

Academic Press
Harcourt Place, 32 Jamestown Road, London NW1 7BY, UK
http://www.academicpress.com

Library of Congress Catalog Card Number: 2001090931

International Standard Book Number: 0-12-072651-3

PRINTED IN THE UNITED STATES OF AMERICA
01   02   03   04   05   06   EB   9   8   7   6   5   4   3   2   1

CONTENTS

CHAPTER 10

STRUCTURE-BASED DRUG DESIGN AND ITS CONTRIBUTIONS TO CANCER CHEMOTHERAPY

Robert C. Jackson

CHAPTER 11

THE CONTRIBUTION OF SYNTHETIC ORGANIC CHEMISTRY TO ANTICANCER DRUG DEVELOPMENT

William A. Denny

CHAPTER 12

BIOSYNTHETIC PRODUCTS FOR ANTICANCER DRUG DESIGN AND TREATMENT: THE BRYOSTATINS

George R. Pettit, Cherry L. Herald, and Fiona Hogan

CHAPTER 13

DNA-ENCODED PEPTIDE LIBRARIES AND DRUG DISCOVERY

Sachdev S. Sidhu and Gregory A. Weiss

CHAPTER 14

MECHANISM-BASED HIGH-THROUGHPUT SCREENING FOR NOVEL ANTICANCER DRUG DISCOVERY

Wynne Aherne, Michelle Garrett, Ted McDonald, and Paul Workman

CHAPTER 15

TUMOR CELL CULTURES IN DRUG DEVELOPMENT

Bruce C. Baguley, Kevin O. Hicks,
and William R. Wilson

CHAPTER 16

SCREENING USING ANIMAL SYSTEMS

Angelika M. Burger and Heinz-Herbert Fiebig

CHAPTER 17

RELEVANCE OF PRECLINICAL PHARMACOLOGY AND TOXICOLOGY TO PHASE I TRIAL EXTRAPOLATION TECHNIQUES: RELEVANCE OF ANIMAL TOXICOLOGY

Joseph E. Tomaszewski, Adaline C. Smith,
Joseph M. Covey, Susan J. Donohue, Julie K. Rhie,
and Karen M. Schweikart

CHAPTER 18

CLINICAL TRIAL DESIGN: INCORPORATION OF PHARMACOKINETIC, PHARMACODYNAMIC, AND PHARMACOGENETIC PRINCIPLES

Alex Sparreboom, Walter J. Loos,
Maja J. A. de Jonge, and Jaap Verweij

CHAPTER 19

TUMOR IMAGING APPLICATIONS IN THE TESTING OF NEW DRUGS
Eric Ofori Aboagye, Azeem Saleem, and
Patricia M. Price

CHAPTER 20

MECHANISTIC APPROACHES TO PHASE I CLINICAL TRIALS
David R. Ferry and David J. Kerr

CONTRIBUTORS

Numbers in parentheses indicate page numbers on which authors' contributions begin.

Eric Ofori Aboagye (353) Cancer Research Campaign, Imperial College School of Medicine, Hammersmith Hospital, London W12 0NN, United Kingdom

Wynne Aherne (249) Cancer Research Campaign Centre for Cancer Therapeutics, Institute of Cancer Research, Sutton, Surrey SM2 5NG, United Kingdom

Bruce C. Baguley (1, 269) Auckland Cancer Society Research Centre, The University of Auckland, Auckland 1000, New Zealand

Alex Bridges (31) Pfizer Global Research and Development, Ann Arbor, Michigan 48105

Angelika M. Burger (285) Tumor Biology Centre, University of Freiburg, D-79110 Freiburg, Germany

Jian Cao (91) School of Medicine, State University of New York at Stony Brook, Stony Brook, New York 11794

Joseph M. Covey (301) Division of Cancer Treatment and Diagnosis, National Cancer Institute, National Institutes of Health, Rockville, Maryland 20892

Thomas Davis (157) Oncology, Medarex, Annandale, New Jersey 08801

Stuart Decker (31) Pfizer Global Research and Development, Ann Arbor, Michigan 48105

Maja J. A. de Jonge (329) Department of Medical Oncology, Rotterdam Cancer Institute, 3075 EA Rotterdam, The Netherlands

William A. Denny (187) Auckland Cancer Society Research Centre, Faculty of Medical and Health Sciences, University of Auckland, Auckland 1000, New Zealand

Susan J. Donohue (301) Division of Cancer Treatment and Diagnosis, National Cancer Institute, National Institutes of Health, Rockville, Maryland 20892

Nathalie Droin (55) INSERM U517, Faculty of Medicine, 21000 Dijon, France

Patrick Ducoroy (55) INSERM U517, Faculty of Medicine, 21000 Dijon, France

David Ferry (371) Department of Oncology, New Cross Hospital, Wolverhampton, West Midlands WV10 0QP, United Kingdom

Heinz-Herbert Fiebig (285) Tumor Biology Centre, University of Freiburg, D-79110 Freiburg, Germany

Rodolphe Filomenko (55) INSERM U517, Faculty of Medicine, 21000 Dijon, France

David W. Fry (31) Pfizer Global Research and Development, Ann Arbor, Michigan 48105

Michelle Garrett (249) Cancer Research Campaign Centre for Cancer Therapeutics, Institute of Cancer Research, Sutton, Surrey SM2 5NG, United Kingdom

Cherry L. Herald (203) Cancer Research Institute, Arizona State University, Tempe, Arizona 85287

Kevin O. Hicks (269) Auckland Cancer Society Research Centre, The University of Auckland, Auckland 1000, New Zealand

Fiona Hogan (203) Cancer Research Institute, Arizona State University, Tempe, Arizona 85287

Robert C. Jackson (171) Cyclacel Limited, Dundee DD1 5JJ, United Kingdom

David J. Kerr (371) Institute for Cancer Medicine, University of Oxford, 0X2 6HE, United Kingdom

Kurt W. Kohn (13) Laboratory of Molecular Pharmacology, Center for Cancer Research, National Institutes of Health, Bethesda, Maryland 20892

Elianne Koop (123) Laboratory of Medical Oncology, Division of Medical Oncology, University Medical Centre Utrecht, 3584 CX Utrecht, The Netherlands

Alan Kraker (31) Pfizer Global Research and Development, Ann Arbor, Michigan 48105

W. R. Leopold (31) Pfizer Global Research and Development, Ann Arbor, Michigan 48105

Walter J. Loos (329) Department of Medical Oncology, Rotterdam Cancer Institute, 3075 EA Rotterdam, The Netherlands

Ted McDonald (249) Cancer Research Campaign Centre for Cancer Therapeutics, Institute of Cancer Research, Sutton, Surrey SM2 5NG, United Kingdom

Christopher J. Molloy (91) 3-Dimensional Pharmaceuticals, Inc., Exton, Pennsylvania 19341

Ion Niculescu-Duvac (137) Cancer Research Campaign Centre for Cancer Therapeutics, Institute of Cancer Research, Sutton, Surrey SM2 5NG, United Kingdom

George R. Pettit (203) Cancer Research Institute, Arizona State University, Tempe, Arizona 85287

Stephanie Plenchette (55) INSERM U517, Faculty of Medicine, 21000 Dijon, France

Yves Pommier (13) Laboratory of Molecular Pharmacology, Center for Cancer Research, National Institutes of Health, Bethesda, Maryland 20892

Patricia M. Price (353) Cancer Research Campaign, Imperial College School of Medicine, Hammersmith Hospital, London W12 0NN, United Kingdom

Cédric Rebe (55) INSERM U517, Faculty of Medicine, 21000 Dijon, France

Julie K. Rhie (301) Division of Cancer Treatment and Diagnosis, National Cancer Institute, National Institutes of Health, Rockville, Maryland 20892

Azeem Saleem (353) Cancer Research Campaign, Imperial College School of Medicine, Hammersmith Hospital, London W12 0NN, United Kingdom

Karen M. Schweikart (301) Division of Cancer Treatment and Diagnosis, National Cancer Institute, National Institutes of Health, Rockville, Maryland 20892

Judith Sebolt-Leopold (31) Pfizer Global Research and Development, Ann Arbor, Michigan 48105

Sachdev Sidhu (237) Department of Protein Engineering, Genentech, Inc., South San Francisco, California 94080

Adaline C. Smith (301) Division of Cancer Treatment and Diagnosis, National Cancer Institute, National Institutes of Health, Rockville, Maryland 20892

Eric Solary (55) INSERM U517, Faculty of Medicine, 21000 Dijon, France; and Hematology Unit, CHU le Bocage, BP1542, 21034 Dijon, France

Olivier Sordet (55) INSERM U517, Faculty of Medicine, 21000 Dijon, France

Alex Sparreboom (329) Department of Medical Oncology, Rotterdam Cancer Institute, 3075 EA Rotterdam, The Netherlands

Caroline J. Springer (137) Cancer Research Campaign Centre for Cancer Therapeutics, Institute of Cancer Research, Sutton, Surrey SM2 5NG, United Kingdom

Mario Sznol (157) Clinical Affairs, Vion Pharmaceuticals, New Haven, Connecticut 06511

Joseph Tomaszewski (301) Division of Cancer Treatment and Diagnosis, National Cancer Institute, National Institutes of Health, Rockville, Maryland 20892

Akihiro Tomida (77) Institute of Molecular and Cellular Biosciences, University of Tokyo, Tokyo 113-0032, Japan

Takashi Tsuruo (77) Institute of Molecular and Cellular Biosciences, University of Tokyo, Tokyo 113-0032, Japan

Jaap Verweij (329) Department of Medical Oncology, Rotterdam Cancer Institute, 3075 EA Rotterdam, The Netherlands

Emile E. Voest (123) Laboratory of Medical Oncology, Division of Medical Oncology, University Medical Centre Utrecht, 3584 CX Utrecht, The Netherlands

Gregory A. Weiss (237) Department of Protein Engineering, Genentech, Inc., South San Francisco, California 94080

William R. Wilson (269) Auckland Cancer Society Research Centre, The University of Auckland, Auckland 1000, New Zealand

Paul Workman (249) Cancer Research Campaign Centre for Cancer Therapeutics, Institute of Cancer Research, Sutton, Surrey SM2 5NG, United Kingdom

Anne Wotawa (55) INSERM U517, Faculty of Medicine, 21000 Dijon, France

Qiang Yu (13) Laboratory of Molecular Pharmacology, Center for Cancer Research, National Institutes of Health, Bethesda, Maryland 20892

Stanley Zucker (91) Department of Veterans Affairs Medical Center, Northport, New York 11768

PREFACE

The development of more effective drugs for treating patients with cancer has been a major human endeavor over the past 50 years, and the 21st century now promises some dramatic new directions. While improvements in surgery and radiotherapy have had a major impact on cancer treatment, the concept of systemic chemotherapy, specific for cancer cells and free of major side effects, remains a critical goal for the future. The issues underlying the achievement of this goal are complex, extending from an understanding of how cancer growth is controlled, through the technology of drug synthesis and testing, to the multifactorial requirements for clinical trial. For anyone working in any single area of anticancer drug development, it is important to have an overview of the whole process.

This book aims to provide such an overview. The opening chapters discuss possible targets for drug design, including the cell division cycle, growth signal transduction, apoptosis induction, and the manifold interactions between tumor cells and host tissues. Succeeding chapters then consider techniques of identifying new potential drugs, including molecular modeling, chemical synthesis, and screening. The concluding chapters detail the required steps that any new potential anticancer agent must go through before it can be considered for routine clinical treatment. In each of these areas, a number of eminently qualified contributors have provided commentaries. Inevitably there are areas of overlap, but these have been retained because they reflect the interdependence of different areas of research.

We hope that this book will provide a useful commentary, including both overviews and specific detail, on this vital but fascinating subject. We also hope that it will stimulate original thought and further encourage those from both scientific and medical backgrounds who are committed to improving the outlook of cancer patients worldwide.

Acknowledgments

This book represents the results of a considerable amount of work by many talented contributors. As editors we thank all of these contributors for their enthusiasm and patience. We thank our research colleagues for providing advice when needed and the staff of Academic Press for their support over many months. B.C.B particularly acknowledges the support of the Auckland Division of the Cancer Society of New Zealand, and through them the members of the public who have donated money for cancer research.

Bruce C. Baguley
David J. Kerr

CHAPTER 1

A BRIEF HISTORY OF CANCER CHEMOTHERAPY

Bruce C. Baguley

Auckland Cancer Society Research Centre

The University of Auckland

Auckland, New Zealand

Summary

Clinical cancer chemotherapy in the 20th century has been dominated by the development of genotoxic drugs, initiated by the discovery of the anticancer properties of nitrogen mustard and the folic acid analogue aminopterin in the 1940s. The development of inbred strains of mice in the early part of the 20th century led to the use of transplantable tumors for the screening of very large numbers of compounds, both natural and synthetic, for experimental antitumor activity. Such screening led to the identification of clinically useful drugs at a rate of approximately one every 2 years. New targets for cytotoxicity were identified in this program, including tubulin and DNA topoisomerases I and II. The huge expansion in our basic knowledge of cancer has facilitated the development of two new anticancer strategies: the inhibition of specific cellular growth pathways and the inhibition of growth of cancer as a tissue. One of the most important principles to emerge is that loss of growth control of cancer cells is mechanistically associated with an increased tendency to undergo programmed cell death, or apoptosis. Thus, cancer growth is a balance between cell birth and cell death. The balance is maintained not only by the genetic status of the cancer cell but by interactions with host cells and extracellular matrix components in the tumor environment. The identification of estrogen as a factor for stimulating the growth led to antiestrogens as therapeutic agents and, more recently, to antagonists of growth factor receptor-mediated pathways. The early use of bacterial toxins in cancer treatment has led to strategies based on host–tumor interactions, such as antiangiogenic and immune approaches. Current research has underlined the enormous complexity not only of growth and death control systems within the tumor cell but of interactions of tumor cells with vascular endothelial, immune, and other cells in cancer tissue. The challenge of future development of low-molecular-weight anticancer drugs is to apply knowledge gained in basic studies to develop new strategies.

1. Introduction

It is difficult to assign a date to the beginning of the treatment of cancer with drugs because herbal and other preparations have been used for cancer treatment since antiquity. However, the 1890s, a decade that represents an extraordinarily creative period in painting, music, literature, and technology, encompassed discoveries that were to set the scene for developments in cancer treatment in the 20th century. The discovery of penetrating radiation, or x-rays, by Roentgen in Germany in 1895 was complemented 3 years later by the discovery of radium by Marie and Pierre Curie. The discovery of ionizing radiation led not only to radiotherapy as form of cancer treatment but eventually to the development of anticancer drugs that mimicked the effect of radiation by damaging DNA. The discovery by George Beatson, working in Scotland in 1896, that the growth of a breast cancer could be halted by removal of the ovaries indicated that the growth of cancer cells in the body could be influenced by external factors. This provided the basis for cancer treatment strategies that changed the regulation of cancer cell growth. The demonstration by William Coley in 1898 that the administration to cancer patients of a bacterial extract, sterilized by passage through a porcelain filter, caused regressions in lymphoma and sarcoma indicated that activation of the body's defense systems might provide a strategy for cancer treatment. Each of these three advances lent weight to the bold assumption, made by Paul Ehrlich and others in the early part of the 20th century, that low-molecular-weight drugs might be used in the management of cancer as well as infectious diseases. This chapter considers each of these three approaches in turn.

2. Genotoxic (Cytotoxic) Therapy

The first practical anticancer drugs were discovered accidentally. One such discovery was an outcome of war, stemming from the finding that sulfur mustard gas, used as a toxic vesicant in the First World War, caused myelosuppression. Although gas warfare was not employed in the Second World War, a considerable stock of mustard gas canisters was maintained in the Mediterranean area. An accident in the Italian port of Bari, involving leakage of one of these canisters, rekindled interest in the myelosuppressive effect of nitrogen mustard, leading to clinical trials in lymphoma patients (Karnofsky *et al.,* 1948; Kohn, 1996).

The identification of vitamins as small low-molecular-weight enzyme cofactors was an important biochemical achievement in the early part of the 20th century. The structural elucidation and crystallization of folic acid in 1946 led, as with other isolated vitamins, to studies on its effect on the course of a number of diseases. Unexpectedly, administration to leukemia patients of folic acid and its glutamylated derivatives resulted in an increase in tumor growth. While the use of low-folate diets in the management of leukemia was investigated, the development of the folic acid analogue aminopterin provided a significant advance in the management of childhood acute leukemia (Farber *et al.,* 1948; Bertino, 1979).

The link between these two disparate types of drugs and their biological activity was found to be related to their damaging effect on DNA. Although Friedrich Miescher had characterized DNA as a substance in 1862, the informational complexity and significance to life of DNA was not appreciated until the 1940s. The elucidation in 1953 by James Watson and Francis Crick of the double-helical structure of DNA had a singular impact on strategies of anticancer drug development. The cancer chemotherapeutic agent nitrogen mus-

tard was found to react chemically with DNA (Kohn *et al.,* 1966). Studies on aminopterin indicated that it interrupted DNA biosynthesis and in so doing caused DNA damage. The next two decades brought a massive development of new drugs that affected the integrity of the cell's genetic material, with approximately one new drug entering widespread clinical use every 2 years. Many of these drugs, which revolutionized the treatment of many types of cancer, are shown in Figure 1.

A. Development of *in Vivo* Cancer Screening Systems

Developments in chromatography and analytical chemistry in the first half of the 20th century allowed compounds of defined structure to be isolated from a variety of plants, animals, and microorganisms (see Chapter 12). The evolution of synthetic organic chemistry over this time provided anticancer drugs in addition to antimicrobial and other medicinal drugs (see Chapter 11). It was quickly realized that it would be impossible to test such a large number of compounds in cancer patients and that some type of model tumor system was required. Transplantable animal cancers became accepted as the best basis for the screening of such drugs. This was made possible by the availability of inbred mouse strains, which had their beginnings in the early part of the 20th century. Three inbred strains of particular importance to anticancer drug screening—DBA, BALB/c, and C57BL—were introduced in 1909, 1916, and 1921, respectively. Spontaneous or carcinogen-induced tumors in these strains could be transplanted from one inbred mouse to another, allowing repeated testing of potential anticancer drugs (Stock, 1954). A detailed description of the role of animal testing in drug development is provided in Chapter 16. In the 1950s and 1960s, most testing programs used the transplantable L1210 and P388 murine leukemia models for primary screening and transplantable solid tumors for more advanced testing (Goldin *et al.,* 1981). The discovery of the athymic "nude" mouse, which had lost its ability to mount a cell-mediated immune response, allowed the testing of new drugs against human tumor material growing as xenografts in such mice (Rygaard and Povlsen, 1969).

B. Mitotic Poisons

Many of the early drugs that were screened for anticancer activity were derived from natural products. The plant product colchicine, isolated from the autumn crocus, was one of the first of these to demonstrate activity against experimental murine tumor models. It was found to induce arrest of cultured cells in mitosis and demonstrated a new mode of induction of genomic damage: that of disturbing the correct distribution of genetic material into daughter cells at mitosis. Colchicine, although useful at lower doses for the treatment

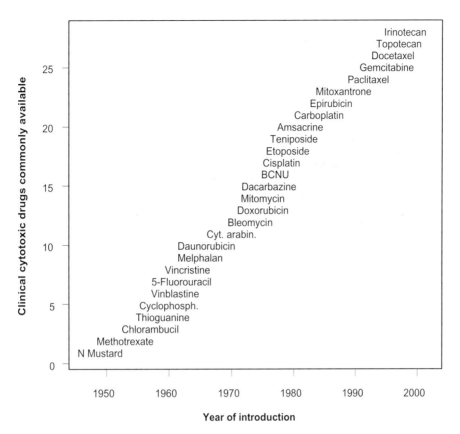

FIGURE 1 Chronology for the development of some of the anticancer drugs currently in use today. The abbreviations are N mustard (nitrogen mustard), cyt. arabin. (cytosine arabinoside), and BCNU (bischloroethylnitrosourea).

of gout, proved too toxic for use as an anticancer drug, and early attention focused on the *Vinca* alkaloids from the periwinkle plant (Johnson *et al.*, 1963). Two such alkaloids, vincristine and vinblastine, had a major impact on the early treatment of patients with malignancy (Rowinsky and Donehower, 1991). The protein tubulin was identified as the target for colchicine and the *Vinca* alkaloids (reviewed by Uppuluri *et al.*, 1993) and is the subject of considerable anticancer drug research. The broadening of the spectrum of tumor types susceptible to spindle poisons resulted from the discovery of the taxane class of compounds. Paclitaxel, discovered as a component of some *Taxus* species (Wani *et al.*, 1971), escaped detailed investigation until it was found to have a novel biochemical action distinct from that of the *Vinca* alkaloids, involving promotion rather than inhibition of microtubule assembly (Schiff *et al.*, 1979). Paclitaxel (Rowinsky *et al.*, 1990) and docetaxel (Bissery *et al.*, 1991) have a prominent place in cancer therapy today.

C. DNA-Reactive Drugs

Nitrogen mustard was the basis for the synthesis of a large series of clinically useful derivatives, including melphalan and cyclophosphamide, all found to exert their antitumor effects by alkylation of DNA. Natural products also yielded a number of clinically useful compounds that reacted chemically with DNA, such as mitomycin C (Whittington and Close, 1970), and bleomycin, which required the presence of oxygen and ferric ions to react (Crooke and Bradner, 1976). A particularly important development in DNA-reactive drugs came with the discovery of cisplatin, which had its origins in the chance observation that bacterial growth was inhibited around one of the platinum electrodes of an electrophoresis apparatus containing ammonium chloride in the buffer (Rosenberg *et al.*, 1965). Platination of DNA became a new mode of DNA damage induction and formed the basis for developing new analogues of cisplatin with reduced host toxicity.

D. Inhibitors of DNA Replication

A consequence of the elucidation of the structure of DNA was the rational design of analogues of the DNA bases, which were hypothesized to exert their anticancer activity by disruption of DNA replication. These included the thymine analogue 5-fluorouracil (Heidelberger *et al.*, 1957) and the purine analogues 6-mercaptopurine and 8-azaguanine (Hitchings and Elion, 1954). The cytotoxic effects of aminopterin and methotrexate were traced to their inhibition, through their effect on the enzyme dihydrofolate reductase, of the conversion of deoxyuridine monophosphate to thymidine monophosphate. The phenomenon of "thymineless death," whereby bacteria unable to synthesize the DNA base thymine died in its absence, was found to have a parallel in mammalian cells and shaped the rationale for the development of the antimetabolite class of drugs. As the individual enzymes responsible for DNA replication were identified it became clear that the successful operation of the DNA replicase complex relied on a constant supply of the triphosphate precursors of DNA and that interruption of this supply resulted in damage to newly synthesized DNA. Natural products also played a role in the development of anticancer drugs acting on DNA replication. Arabinose nucleosides from the sponge *Cryptothethya* were found to have experimental antitumor activity, and one of them, the antimetabolite cytosine arabinoside, has found extensive use in the treatment of persons with leukemia (Ellison *et al.*, 1968). The testing of chemical analogues of cytosine arabinoside led more recently to drugs such as gemcitabine, which has activity against carcinoma (Plunkett *et al.*, 1996).

E. DNA Topology as a Target for Drug Development

In the 1960s, two logical problems concerning DNA structure became evident. The first was that the unwinding of DNA associated with DNA replication appeared to be thermodynamically impossible in the time frame involved, since the average chromosome would have tens of millions of helical twists. The second, familiar to anyone who has tried to untangle a fishing line, was that the separation of daughter DNA strands produced by DNA replication, prior to cell division, was thermodynamically impossible. Closed circular duplex DNA in some bacterial and mammalian viruses provided smaller molecular weight models for the study of these problems. Such DNA was found to exist in several distinct forms, each with the same sequence but with a different number of helical twists, and these were called topoisomers, based on topology (the branch of mathematics dealing with such differences in shape). In 1976, a new ATP-requiring enzyme, DNA gyrase, with the property of being able to change the topology of closed circular duplex DNA, was discovered in bacterial cells (Gellert *et al.*, 1976). DNA gyrase was found to have an essential role in DNA replication, and because it could pass one strand of DNA through another, it elegantly solved the problems of how DNA could be rapidly unwound during replication and how the daughter DNA strands could be separated after replication. Subsequent studies of mammalian cells demonstrated two main classes of enzymes. The first, topoisomerase I, changed DNA topology by breaking and rejoining a single DNA strand (Been and Champoux, 1980). The second, topoisomerase II, with some of the characteristics of bacterial gyrase, broke both strands of one double-stranded DNA to allow passage of a second double-helical strand through the breakage point (Miller *et al.*, 1981).

The discovery of the DNA topoisomerases also solved a problem concerning the activity of a number of natural products with anticancer activity that caused DNA damage but did not appear to react chemically. Actinomycin D, identified from *Streptomyces* cultures, found extensive early clinical use particularly in pediatric tumors (Farber *et al.*, 1960) and was found to bind DNA by intercalating its polycyclic chromophore between the base pairs of the DNA double helix (Müller and Crothers, 1968). It was of great biochemical interest because of its potent inhibition of RNA synthesis, but this did not appear to explain its antitumor activity. Subsequently, two anthracycline derivatives, daunorubicin and doxorubicin, were also found to bind DNA by intercalation of their chromophores, but their effects on RNA synthesis were less than those of actinomycin D. The clinical activity of daunorubicin was generally confined to hematologic malignancies but that of doxorubicin was broader (Arcamone, 1985). The synthetic compound amsacrine, which had clinical activity against acute leukemia (Arlin, 1989), bound DNA by intercalation of its acridine chromophore (Wilson *et al.*, 1981) but had little or no effect on RNA synthesis. Both amsacrine and doxorubicin were found to induce covalent links between DNA and proteins (Zwelling *et al.*, 1981), and subsequent work demonstrated that this protein was in fact the enzyme topoisomerase II (Nelson *et al.*, 1984). The drugs acted as poisons of this enzyme, subverting its normal function to one of inducing DNA damage.

A parallel development in plant natural product research provided podophyllotoxin analogues derived from the mandrake root (Stahelin and Von Wartburg, 1991). Podophyllotoxin itself, like colchicine, bound to tubulin, but some semisynthetic glycosidic derivatives, termed epipodophyllotoxins, were found to have superior experimental antitumor activity to podophyllotoxin itself. Etoposide, first tested clinically in 1971, was found to be useful against a variety of malignancies (Issell and Crooke, 1979). Investigation of the action of etoposide and of the related drug teniposide revealed that they had reduced binding to tubulin but induced DNA damage and poisoned the enzyme topoisomerase II. The plant product camptothecin, which did not bind DNA and previously had no known function, was found to be a specific poison for topoisomerase I (Hsiang *et al.*, 1985). Water-soluble analogues of camptothecin, such as topotecan and irinotecan, have clinical potential, and topoisomerase I is now an established tumor target (Pommier, 1993).

F. The Search for Selectivity

While the selectivity of radiotherapy was progressively increased by localization of the radiation field to specific areas of tumor growth, the selectivity of cytotoxic therapy was dependent on particular properties of cancer tissue. The use of microbial models gave rise to the important concept that alkylating drugs killed cells in an exponential fashion, with a certain percentage of the cell population killed with each dose (Pittillo *et al.*, 1965). For some drugs, cytotoxicity was found to be maximal at a particular phase of the cell cycle. Skipper and colleagues (Skipper, 1967) used animal models to select administration schedules with optimal cytotoxicity for the cell-cycle-selective agents, and drug combination schedules that allowed optimal intensity of treatment. The spacing between treatments and the rate of appearance of resistant populations could make the difference between success and failure of treatment (Carl, 1989). Such reasoning was applied with success to hematologic malignancies, which often had a high rate of cell division, but was less successful in the management of solid tumors.

Another basis for selectivity was to exploit an enzyme or drug transport mechanism that was present to a different extent in tumor and normal cells. Many antimetabolites were found to exert their selectivity by such mechanisms. Topoisomerase enzymes provided a particularly good example of such selectivity since high cellular activity, which tended to occur in rapidly dividing cell populations, was associated with greater sensitivity to topoisomerase-directed anticancer drugs (Pommier, 1993). More recently, selectivity has been generated by the development of prodrugs, which have no cytotoxicity until an enzyme or other agent activates them. Initially, naturally occurring cellular enzymes, such as nitroreductases, were considered as candidates for activating prodrugs, but more recently the concept of introducing a different activating enzyme by means of a localizing antibody or gene therapy has been investigated. These concepts are discussed in Chapters 8 and 11.

3. Growth Control Pathways

While cytotoxic agents dominated the development of clinical cancer chemotherapy, the alternative approach of altering the signals that determine cancer growth was not forgotten. The demonstration by Beatson in 1896 of the role of the ovary in the progression of some types of breast cancer raised the question of whether the growth of all cancer types might be controlled by circulating hormones. Subsequent surgical studies showed that, apart from the case of prostate cancer, removal of endocrine glands was generally ineffective in cancer treatment. It was another 30 years before estrogen, one of the main hormones accounting for Beatson's result, was identified (Frank *et al.*, 1925), but the biochemical pathways linking steroid hormones to cell growth stimulation remained a mystery. During the 1960s and 1970s, studies of cultured cells, both normal and tumor, indicated that a diverse

series of polypeptide growth factors were essential for cell growth, many specific for certain tissue types (reviewed by James and Bradshaw, 1984). An understanding of the action of such factors first required the elucidation of the molecular mechanism of regulation DNA replication and cell division.

A. The Cell Cycle Clock

One of the most fascinating questions posed by dividing normal and cancer cells was the nature of the molecular clock that instructed the cell as to when it would replicate its DNA and when it would divide. Early studies of cancer tissue identified mitotic cells by their morphology and DNA-synthesizing (S-phase) cells by their uptake of tritium-labeled thymidine, and these phases were found to be separated by periods of cell enlargement, termed G_1 and G_2 phase (reviewed by Tannock, 1978). The first clues to the nature of the oscillator that ran the molecular clock were provided by the discovery in developing sea urchin eggs of a protein termed *cyclin*. The cellular concentration of this protein increased up to the time of cell division and then abruptly decreased (Evans *et al.*, 1983). Studies of the division of fertilized frog eggs also indicated the presence of a cyclin, the synthesis of which was necessary to cell division (Cross *et al.*, 1989). A second component of the clock was identified from two lines of research, one using frog embryos and one using yeast mutants (Cross *et al.*, 1989). A specific enzyme, termed a cyclin-dependent kinase (cdk), was found both to associate physically with a cyclin and to be activated by it, providing a link between the oscillator and the actuator. Several distinct cdk's and cyclins were found to be present in mammalian cells. A third component of the clock mechanism was a protease (in the form of a proteasome) that was responsible for the degradation of the cyclin and thus the resetting of the clock (Glotzer *et al.*, 1991; King *et al.*, 1996). In the general scheme of the cell cycle (Fig. 2), the multiple functions required for cell division and DNA replication are exquisitely coordinated by cdk's 1 and 2, respectively, each activated at the appropriate time by specific associated cyclins. The cell cycle time for human tumors varies from around 2 days to several weeks (Wilson *et al.*, 1988).

B. Stopping and Starting the Cell Cycle Clock

While the majority of the body's cells are in a nondividing state, certain cells, such as blood cell precursors in the bone marrow and epithelial cells in the gut, are capable of dividing rapidly. Some mechanism must therefore regulate the passage of cells from a quiescent state to a dividing state. Most early studies utilized cultured fibroblasts to investigate this process. Time-lapse studies (Smith and Martin, 1973) indicated that the commitment to DNA replication and mitosis was determined by a stochastic (random) mechanism, and a

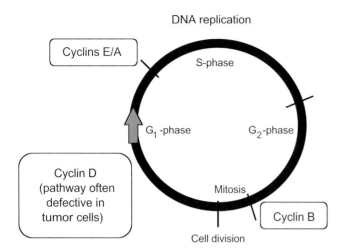

FIGURE 2 The cell cycle clock, with two key alternating processes: DNA replication and cell division. The timing of these processes is controlled primarily by oscillations (one per cell cycle) in the cellular levels of cyclin E/A and cyclin B, respectively. Activation of these processes is controlled by cyclin-dependent kinases 2 and 1, respectively. Normal cells have a further control on the decision to enter the cell cycle, timed by cyclin D and activated by cyclin-dependent kinases 4/6. This control system is deficient in cancer cells.

"restriction point" in the G_1 phase of the cell cycle was defined (Pardee, 1974), past which cells were irreversibly committed. A clear requirement was established for the presence of external polypeptide growth factors to allow passage of cells past the restriction point. Such factors were found to interact with membrane-bound surface receptors on target cells, and by the end of the 1970s it was established that at least some of these receptors, including that for epidermal growth factor, became phosphorylated as a consequence of growth factor engagement (Carpenter *et al.*, 1979). Internal cellular proteins were also phosphorylated in response to growth factors, but the identification of the complex linkages between growth factor receptors and commitment to DNA replication and cell division required new findings.

A major step forward in the identification of the pathway for initiation of cell growth had its origins in Peyton Rous's study of cancer-causing viruses in birds, mice, and rats in the early part of the 20th century (Rous, 1983). In 1983, the extraordinary finding was made that a gene in a tumor-transforming virus of simian apes was similar or identical to that specifying a known growth factor for cultured cells (Doolittle *et al.*, 1983; Waterfield *et al.*, 1983). Subsequent work defined a variety of genes that could be transmitted by retroviruses to the tissue of a variety of birds and animals, causing a tumorigenic change. As the functions of these corresponding gene products were elucidated, it was found that they mapped to biochemical pathways linking the binding of growth factors to the commitment of cells to DNA replication and cell division.

The above work led to identification not only of a network of regulatory proteins but also of new cyclins (D-cyclins) and cdk's (4 and 6) that control the passage of the cell from a quiescent phase into the cell cycle. The retinoblastoma protein and the transcription factors E2F and c-myc were also implicated in a complex control system that resulted in the up-regulation of the E and A cyclins and subsequent initiation of DNA replication.

As the elements of this control system were identified, it also became clear that the function of one or more of these elements was defective in cancer. For instance, many human cancers were found to be associated with a mutated *ras* oncogene such that the cells behaved as though they were being continuously stimulated by growth factors (Pronk and Bos, 1994). Furthermore, many cancer cells lacked the proper function of proteins, such as the retinoblastoma protein, that regulated entry into S phase (Herwig and Strauss, 1997).

C. Programmed Cell Death

In 1972, a pivotal hypothesis was advanced that cell death was, like progress through the cell cycle, a product of precise cellular programming (Kerr *et al.*, 1972). This hypothesis was to have a profound effect not only in explaining the loss of cells during the development of the embryo but in advancing our understanding of cancer growth. Apoptosis was found to be an energy-dependent process whereby a cell was converted to fragments that could be absorbed by surrounding tissue without the initiation of an inflammatory response (Wyllie, 1993). The molecular mechanisms of apoptosis are described in Chapter 4.

In a multicellular organism, loss of a single cell is generally unimportant. On the other hand, loss of growth control in a single cell could lead, in the absence of any protective mechanism, to unrestricted and catastrophic growth. The body appears to have a protective mechanism to ensure that any such cells losing growth control are eliminated. The mechanistic links are not yet fully defined, but transcription factors such as E2F and c-myc, which are involved in driving cells into the cell cycle, are also involved in driving cells into apoptosis (Evan and Littlewood, 1998; King and Cidlowski, 1998). Thus, cancer growth is a balance between cell birth and cell death, each initiated by the same pathway (Fig. 3). Cancer cells (as well as normal cells) can be prevented from undergoing apoptosis by so-called survival factors (Evan and Littlewood, 1998), such as insulin-like growth factor 1 (Juin *et al.*, 1999) and cell–matrix interactions (Meredith *et al.*, 1993).

D. The Cell Cycle Calendar

The pioneering studies of Hayflick showed that when human fibroblasts were cultured, they would die after a certain

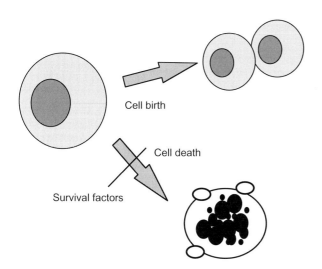

FIGURE 3 The balance of cell birth and death in a tumor cell population. In human tumors there is a high rate of turnover such that the overall doubling time of tumor tissue is generally considerably longer than the cell cycle time of the tumor cells. The rate of cell death is controlled to some extent by external factors called survival factors.

number of generations by a process called senescence (Hayflick and Moorhead, 1961; Hayflick, 1965). The number of generations of doublings, typically 60–80 for fetal cells, progressively reduced as the age of the donor of the fibroblasts increased, suggesting that some kind of calendar was running during the lifetime of an individual cell. More recently, evidence for a slightly different calendar mechanism has been obtained in breast epithelial cells (Romanov *et al.,* 2001).

Tumor cells in culture, in contrast to normal cells, appeared to grow indefinitely, suggesting that the lack of a functioning calendar may be a common characteristic (Goldstein, 1990). An understanding of the mechanism behind the calendar was provided by research on the question of how a linear chromosome could be replicated. Characterization of the DNA replication machinery indicated that DNA polymerase had to start from a priming strand, either DNA or RNA, bound to a DNA strand in a duplex conformation (Lingner *et al.,* 1995). Thus, DNA polymerase could not replicate the ends of chromosomes, and with each successive round of DNA replication the chromosomes would become progressively shorter. The solution to this "end-replication" problem was provided by the discovery of the enzyme telomerase, which added repetitive sequences to the ends or telomeres of chromosomes (Morin, 1989). Normal tissues, unlike embryonic tissues, generally lack telomerase activity. Thus, loss of telomeric DNA sequences might provide a mechanism to ensure that cells that mutate to allow inappropriate cell division, even if not killed directly by apoptosis, die as a result of telomeric DNA loss. It appears that the acquisition of an active telomerase is a very common feature of cancer tissue (Kim *et al.,* 1994).

E. Therapeutic Possibilities

One of the earliest therapeutic successes in cell growth control was the discovery of triphenylethylene derivatives that antagonized the effects of estrogens (Ward, 1973). These so-called antiestrogens revolutionized the management of some types of breast cancer. The basis for the antitumor action of antiestrogens is complex and multifactorial. Estrogen was found to bind to an internal protein that acted as a transcription factor (McKnight *et al.,* 1975), and further work indicated that the products of transcription had multiple effects on target cells, including changes in the expression of growth factor receptors (Curtis *et al.,* 1996). Thus, one possible mechanism of action of the antiestrogens is to decrease the action of survival factors and thus increase the rate of cell death.

More recently, research suggesting that cancer growth represents a balance between cell birth and cell death suggested new approaches. Thus, either a drug-induced decrease in cell birth rate or an increase in cell death rate might result in tumor regression. Low-molecular-weight drugs have been developed that either reduce the progress of cells through the cell cycle, thereby decreasing the cell birth rate, or increase the rate of apoptosis. One important consequence of this research was the finding that cytotoxic drugs, discussed in earlier sections of this chapter, could increase the rate of apoptosis. Cisplatin was one of the first cytotoxic drugs demonstrated to induce cultured cells to undergo apoptosis (Barry *et al.,* 1990). Damaged DNA appears to activate specific enzymes, such as Ataxia Telangiectasia Mutated (ATM) kinase, which in turn initiate the series of steps leading to apoptosis (Meyn, 1995). This topic is further discussed in Chapters 2–4.

The reinstatement of cancer cell mortality constitutes another possible therapeutic approach to cancer treatment. If the "calendar" could be reactivated, such as by inactivation of telomerase activity, cancer cells might once again have a finite lifetime. The design of therapies aimed at inhibiting telomerase activity is still at an early stage and has not been reviewed specifically in this volume. However, a number of excellent reviews can be found (Neidle and Kelland, 1999; Perry and Jenkins Thomas, 1999).

4. Host–Tumor Interactions

Cancer cells do not exist as isolated units but as components of a tissue containing both host and tumor cells. Host cells not only provide, through the vascular endothelium, the precursors of cancer cell growth but also secrete factors that have profound effects on the life and death of tumor cells. The early finding that a mixture of bacterial exotoxins and endotoxins present in "Coley's toxins" were effective in some types of cancer, particularly lymphomas and sarcomas (reviewed by Wieman and Starnes, 1994), prepared the way for both vascular and immune approaches to the treatment of patients with cancer (Pardoll, 1993). Early studies of the action of bacterial lipopolysaccharides in mice led to the discovery of their induced effects on tumor capillaries, leading to vascular collapse and tumor necrosis (Algire *et al.*, 1947). Based on these results, a variety of clinical studies using nonspecific immune stimulants such as *Corynebacterium parvum* and bacillus Calmette-Guérin were instituted (reviewed by Mathé *et al.*, 1973). In the 1960s, polypeptides were identified that stimulated the proliferation of various types of blood cells (Metcalf, 1971). This was followed by the identification of cytokines that mediated the communication between cells in the immune system and other types of cells. One of these cytokines, a protein termed tumor necrosis factor (TNF), was found to mediate the effects of bacterial toxins (Carswell *et al.*, 1975), acting on capillaries to increase their permeability and induce their collapse (Watanabe *et al.*, 1988). Thus, a new approach to drug development became identified in which host cells rather than tumor cells were targeted, leading ultimately to increased tumor cell death. Some of the pathways involved in the complex interactions are shown in Figure 4.

A. Low-Molecular-Weight Inducers of Tumor Necrosis

One of the first reports on the antitumor activity of colchicine described the induction of necrosis in transplantable solid tumors. The similarity of the histologic changes to those caused by administration of bacterial toxins

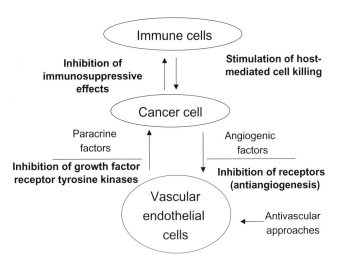

FIGURE 4   Relationships between tumor and host and their possible modulation in therapy. Factors secreted by vascular endothelial cells, together with other stromal components, contribute to the survival of tumor cells. Immune cells may contribute to increased rates of tumor cell death. The tumor cells secrete factors that support their own growth, the proliferation and remodeling of the vascular endothelium, and the inhibition of immune responses. All of these signals constitute potential targets for the development of new anticancer strategies.

suggested an effect on the tumor vasculature (Ludford, 1945). Subsequently, the synthetic drug flavone acetic acid, the antibiotic fostriecin, and the plant product homoharringtonine were also found to induce hemorrhagic necrosis of experimental tumors (Baguley *et al.*, 1989). Apart from colchicine, a variety of tubulin binders, including podophyllotoxin, vincristine, vinblastine, and combretastatin, were found to induce tumor necrosis (Baguley *et al.*, 1991; Hill *et al.*, 1993; Dark *et al.*, 1997). Flavone acetic acid and the structurally related 5,6-dimethylxanthenone-4-acetic acid appeared to act as a consequence of local production of TNF (Mace *et al.*, 1990; Zwi *et al.*, 1994), while the mitotic inhibitors appeared to change the shape of vascular endothelial cells (Dark *et al.*, 1997).

One particularly important class of tumor–host interactions concerns the vascular endothelial cells that provide the blood supply to tumors. Measurement of the proliferation rates of vascular endothelial cells in tumors showed them to divide more rapidly than in normal tissues (Hobson and Denekamp, 1984), leading to antivascular strategies for tumor management (Denekamp, 1990). At the same time, the factors responsible for tumor angiogenesis were being elucidated, and a basis for antiangiogenic drugs for cancer treatment was formulated (Folkman, 1985). This is discussed in Chapter 7.

B. Low-Molecular-Weight Modulators of Cytokine Effects

Research on cytokines led not only to clinical trials of individual cytokines but to the development of low-molecular-weight compounds that might modulate cytokine production. The anthelminthic drug levamisole was initially investigated as an immunostimulant (Amery *et al.*, 1977), has found clinical use in the treatment of colon and other tumors, and is currently thought to act by changing the balance of cytokine actions (Szeto *et al.*, 2000). Tilorone, a low-molecular-weight inducer of interferon (Zschiesche *et al.*, 1978), has been tested in phase II anticancer trials (Cummings *et al.*, 1981). Muramyl dipeptide was investigated as a low-molecular-weight inducer of TNF and appeared to act in concert with endotoxin to induce antitumor effects (Bloksma *et al.*, 1985). Thalidomide, infamous for its teratogenic effects in humans, was found to inhibit the synthesis of TNF (Sampaio *et al.*, 1991) and, more recently, has shown promising activity in the management of multiple myeloma (Singhal *et al.*, 1999). A complete understanding of how cytokine-modulating drugs act on tumor tissue requires further research.

5. Conclusions

In many ways, the scientific objectives of research into the drug-mediated treatment of cancer have not changed over the last few decades. We still search for selective poisons for cancer cells, we still wish to change, selectively, the regulation of growth of cancer cells, and we still wish to encourage the body's normal tissues to reject cancer tissue. While the incidence of radically new ideas in cancer treatment is relatively sparse, our understanding of the molecular makeup of the cancer cell has changed dramatically and the available technology is extraordinarily different. For instance, recent studies using microarray technology combined with the sequencing of the human genome provide the potential to investigate the activity of huge numbers of genes in response to anticancer agents (Scherf *et al.*, 2000). The challenge is to devise, from a deep understanding of the action of known anticancer drugs on human cancers, new strategies for cancer treatment.

References

Algire, G. H., Legallais, F. Y., and Park, H. D. (1947). Vascular reactions of normal and malignant tissue *in vivo*. II. The vascular reaction of normal and malignant tissues of mice to a bacterial polysaccharide from *Serratia marscens* (*Bacillus prodigiosus*) culture filtrates. *J. Natl. Cancer Inst.* **8**, 53–62.

Amery, W. K., Spreafico, F., Rojas, A. F., Denissen, E., and Chirigos, M. (1977). Adjuvant treatment with levamisole in cancer: a review of experimental and clinical data. *Cancer Treat. Rev.* **4**, 167–194.

Arcamone, F. (1985). Properties of antitumor anthracyclines and new developments in their application: Cain Memorial Award Lecture. *Cancer Res.* **45**, 5995–5999.

Arlin, Z. A. (1989). A special role for amsacrine in the treatment of acute leukemia. *Cancer. Inv.* **7**, 607–609.

Baguley, B. C., Calveley, S. B., Crowe, K. K., Fray, L. M., O'Rourke, S. A., and Smith, G. P. (1989). Comparison of the effects of flavone acetic acid, fostriecin, homoharringtonine and tumour necrosis factor alpha on Colon 38 tumors in mice. *Eur. J. Cancer Clin. Oncol.* **25**, 263–269.

Baguley, B. C., Holdaway, K. M., Thomsen, L. L., Zhuang, L., and Zwi, L. J. (1991). Inhibition of growth of colon 38 adenocarcinoma by vinblastine and colchicine—evidence for a vascular mechanism. *Eur. J. Cancer* **27**, 482–487.

Barry, M. A., Behnke, C. A., and Eastman, A. (1990). Activation of programmed cell death (apoptosis) by cisplatin, other anticancer drugs, toxins and hyperthermia. *Biochem. Pharmacol.* **40**, 2353–2362.

Been, M. D., and Champoux, J. J. (1980). Breakage of single-stranded DNA by rat liver nicking-closing enzyme with the formation of a DNA-enzyme complex. *Nucleic Acids Res.* **8**, 6129–6142.

Bertino, J. R. (1979). Nutrients, vitamins and minerals as therapy. *Cancer* **43**, 2137–2142.

Bissery, M.-C., Guénard, D., Guéritte-Voegelein, F., and Lavelle, F. (1991). Experimental antitumor activity of taxotere (RP 56976,NSC 628503) a taxol analogue. *Cancer Res.* **51**, 4845–4852.

Bloksma, N., Hofhuis, F. M., and Willers, J. M. (1985). Muramyl dipeptide analogues as potentiators of the antitumor action of endotoxin. *Cancer. Immunol. Immunother.* **19**, 205–210.

Carl, J. (1989). Drug-resistance patterns assessed from tumor marker analysis. *J. Natl. Cancer. Inst.* **81**, 1631–1639.

Carpenter, G., King, L., Jr., and Cohen, S. (1979). Rapid enhancement of protein phosphorylation in A-431 cell membrane preparations by epidermal growth factor. *J. Biol. Chem.* **254**, 4884–4891.

Carswell, E. A., Old, L. J., Kassel, R. L., Green, S., Fiore, N., and Williamson, B. (1975). An endotoxin-induced serum factor that causes necrosis of tumors. *Proc. Natl. Acad. Sci. USA* **25**, 3666–3670.

Crooke, S. T., and Bradner, W. T. (1976). Bleomycin, a review. *J. Med.* **7**, 333–428.

Cross, F., Roberts, J., and Weintraub, H. (1989). Simple and complex cell cycles. *Annu. Rev. Cell Biol.* **5**, 341–395.

Cummings, F. J., Gelman, R., Skeel, R. T., Kuperminc, M., Israel, L., Colsky, J., and Tormey, D. (1981). Phase II trials of Baker's antifol, bleomycin, CCNU, streptozotocin, tilorone, and 5-fluorodeoxyuridine plus arabinosyl cytosine in metastatic breast cancer. *Cancer* **48**, 681–685.

Curtis, S. W., Washburn, T., Sewall, C., Diaugustine, R., Lindzey, J., Couse, J. F., and Korach, K. S. (1996). Physiological coupling of growth factor and steroid receptor signaling pathways—estrogen receptor knockout mice lack estrogen-like response to epidermal growth factor. *Proc. Natl. Acad. Sci. USA* **93**, 12626–12630.

Dark, G. G., Hill, S. A., Prise, V. E., Tozer, G. M., Pettit, G. R., and Chaplin, D. J. (1997). Combretastatin A-4, an agent that displays potent and selective toxicity toward tumor vasculature. *Cancer Res.* **57**, 1829–1834.

Denekamp, J. (1990). Vascular attack as a therapeutic strategy for cancer. *Cancer Metastasis Rev.* **9**, 267–282.

Doolittle, R. F., Hunkapiller, M. W., Hood, L. E., Devare, S. G., Robbins K. C., Aaronson, S. A., and Antoniades, H. N. (1983). Simian sarcoma virus onc gene, v-sis, is derived from the gene (or genes) encoding a platelet-derived growth factor. *Science* **221**, 275–277.

Ellison, R. R., Holland, J. F., Weil, M., Jacquillat, C., Boiron, M., Bernard, J., Sawitsky, A., Rosner, F., Gussoff, B., Silver, R. T., Karanas, A., Cuttner, J., Spurr, C. L., Hayes, D. M., Blom, J., Leone, L. A., Haurani, F., Kyle, R., Hutchison, J. L., Forcier, R. J., and Moon, J. H. (1968). Arabinosyl cytosine: a useful agent in the treatment of acute leukemia in adults. *Blood* **32**, 507–523.

Evan, G., and Littlewood, T. (1998). A matter of life and cell death. *Science* **281**, 1317–1322.

Evans, T., Rosenthal, E. T., Youngblom, J., Distel, D., and Hunt, T. (1983). Cyclin: A protein specified by maternal mRNA in sea urchin eggs that is destroyed at each cleavage division. *Cell* **33**, 389–396.

Farber, S., Diamond, L. K., Mercer, D., Sylvester, R. F., and Wolff, J. A. (1948). Temporary remissions in acute leukemia in children produced by folic acid antagonist 4-amethophteroylglutamic acid (aminopterin). *N. Engl. J. Med.* **238**, 787–793.

Farber, S., D'Angio, G., Evans, A., and Mitus, A. (1960). Clinical studies of actinomycin D with special reference to Wilms' tumor in children. *Annu. NY. Acad. Sci.* **89**, 421–425.

Folkman, J. (1985). Tumor angiogenesis. *In* "Advances in Cancer Research" (G. Klein and S. Weinhouse, eds.), Vol. 43, pp. 175–203. Academic Press, New York.

Frank, R. T., Frank, M. L., Gustavosn, R. G., et al. (1925). Demonstration of the female sex hormone in the circulating blood. I. Preliminary report. *J. Am. Med. Assoc.* **85**, 510.

Gellert, M., Mizuuchi, K., O'Dea, M. H., and Nash, H. A. (1976). DNA gyrase: An enzyme that introduces superhelical turns into DNA. *Proc. Natl. Acad. Sci. USA* **73**, 3872–3876.

Glotzer, M., Murray, A. W., and Kirschner, M. W. (1991). Cyclin is degraded by the ubiquitin pathway. *Nature* **349**, 132–138.

Goldin, A., Venditti, J. M., Macdonald, J. S., Muggia, F. M., Henney, J. E., and DeVita, V. T., Jr. (1981). Current results of the screening program at the Division of Cancer Treatment, National Cancer Institute. *Eur. J. Cancer* **17**, 129–142.

Goldstein, S. (1990). Replicative senescence—the human fibroblast comes of age. *Science* **249**, 1129–1133.

Hayflick, L. (1965). The limited *in vitro* lifetime of human diploid cell strains. *Exp. Cell Res.* **37**, 614–636.

Hayflick, L., and Moorhead, P. S. (1961). The serial cultivation of human diploid cell strains. *Exp. Cell Res.* **25**, 585–621.

Heidelberger, C., Chaudhuari, N. K., and Danenberg, P. (1957). Fluorinated pyrimidines: A new class of tumor inhibitory compounds. *Nature* **179**, 1957.

Herwig, S., and Strauss, M. (1997). The retinoblastoma protein—a master regulator of cell cycle, differentiation and apoptosis. *Eur. J. Biochem.* **246,** 581–601.

Hill, S. A., Lonergan, S. J., Denekamp, J., and Chaplin, D. J. (1993). *Vinca* alkaloids—anti-vascular effects in a murine tumour. *Eur. J. Cancer* **29A,** 1320–1324.

Hitchings, G. H., and Elion, G. B. (1954). The chemistry and biochemistry of purine analogues. *Annu. NY. Acad. Sci.* **60,** 195–199.

Hobson, B., and Denekamp, J. (1984). Endothelial proliferation in tumours and normal tissues: continuous labelling studies. *Br. J. Cancer* **49,** 405–413.

Hsiang, Y. H., Hertzberg, R., Hecht, S., and Liu, L. F. (1985). Camptothecin induces protein-linked DNA breaks via mammalian DNA topoisomerase I. *J. Biol. Chem.* **260,** 14873–14878.

Issell, B. F., and Crooke, S. T. (1979). Etoposide (VP-16-213). *Cancer Treat. Rev.* **6,** 107–124.

James, R., and Bradshaw, R. A. (1984). Polypeptide growth factors. *Annu. Rev. Biochem.* **53,** 259–292.

Johnson, I. S., Armstrong, J. G., and Gorman, M. (1963). The *Vinca* alkaloids: A new class of oncolytic agents. *Cancer Res.* **23,** 1390–1427.

Juin, P., Hueber, A. O., Littlewood, T., and Evan, G. (1999). c-Myc-induced sensitization to apoptosis is mediated through cytochrome c release. *Genes Dev.* **13,** 1367–1381.

Karnofsky, D. A., Abelson, W. H., Craver, L. F., and Burchenal, J. H. (1948). The use of nitrogen mustards in the palliative treatment of carcinoma. *Cancer* **1,** 634–656.

Kerr, J. F., Wyllie, A. H., and Currie, A. R. (1972). Apoptosis: A basic biological phenomenon with wide ranging implications in tissue kinetics. *Br. J. Cancer* **26,** 239–257.

Kim, N. W., Piatyszek, M. A., Prowse, K. R., Harley, C. B., West, M. D., Ho, P. L., Coviello, G. M., Wright, W. E., Weinrich, S. L., and Shay, J. W. (1994). Specific association of human telomerase activity with immortal cells and cancer. *Science* **266,** 2011–2015.

King, K. L., and Cidlowski, J. A. (1998). Cell cycle regulation and apoptosis. *Annu. Rev. Physiol.* **60,** 601–617.

King, R. W., Deshaies, R. J., Peters, J. M., and Kirschner, M. W. (1996). How proteolysis drives the cell cycle. *Science* **274,** 1652–1659.

Kohn, K. W. (1996). Beyond DNA cross-linking—history and prospects of DNA-targeted cancer treatment—Fifteenth Bruce F. Cain Memorial Award Lecture. *Cancer Res.* **56,** 5533–5546.

Kohn, K. W., Spears, C. L., and Doty, P. (1966). Inter-strand crosslinking of DNA by nitrogen mustard. *J. Mol. Biol.* **19,** 266–288.

Lingner, J., Cooper, J. P., and Cech, T. R. (1995). Telomerase and DNA end replication: No longer a lagging strand problem. *Science* **269,** 1533–1534.

Ludford, R. J. (1945). Colchicine in the experimental chemotherapy of cancer. *J. Natl. Cancer Inst.* **6,** 411–441.

Mace, K. F., Hornung, R. L., Wiltrout, R. H., and Young, H. A. (1990). Correlation between *in vivo* induction of cytokine gene expression by flavone acetic acid and strict dose dependency and therapeutic efficacy against murine renal cancer. *Cancer Res.* **50,** 1742–1747.

Mathé, G., Weiner, R., Pouillart, P., Schwarzenberg, L., Jasmin, C., Schneider, M., Hayat, M., de Vassal, F., and Rosenfeld, C. (1973). BCG in cancer immunotherapy: experimental and clinical trials of its use in treatment of leukemia minimal and or residual disease. *J. Natl. Cancer Inst. Monogr.* **39,** 165–175.

McKnight, G. S., Pennequin, P., and Schimke, R. T. (1975). Induction of ovalbumin mRNA sequences by estrogen and progesterone in chick oviduct as measured by hybridization to complementary DNA. *J. Biol. Chem.* **250,** 8105–8110.

Meredith, J. E., Jr., Fazeli, B., and Schwartz, M. A. (1993). The extracellular matrix as a cell survival factor. *Mol. Biol. Cell.* **4,** 953–961.

Metcalf, D. (1971). Humoral regulators in the development and progression of leukemia. *In* "Advances in Cancer Research" (G. Klein, S. Weinhouse, and A. Haddow, Eds.), Vol. 14, pp. 181–230. Academic Press, New York.

Meyn, M. S. (1995). Ataxia-telangiectasia and cellular responses to DNA damage. *Cancer Res.* **55,** 5991–6001.

Miller, K. G., Liu, L. F., and Englund, P. T. (1981). A homogeneous type II DNA topoisomerase from HeLa cell nuclei. *J. Biol. Chem.* **256,** 9334–9339.

Morin, G. B. (1989). The human telomere terminal transferase enzyme is a ribonucleoprotein that synthesizes TTAGGG repeats. *Cell* **59,** 521–529.

Müller, W., and Crothers, D. (1968). Studies on the binding of actinomycin D and related compounds to DNA. *J. Mol. Biol.* **35,** 251–290.

Neidle, S., and Kelland, L. R. (1999). Commentary: Telomerase as an anti-cancer target: current status and future prospects. *Anticancer Drug Des.* **14,** 341–347.

Nelson, E. M., Tewey, K. M., and Liu, L. F. (1984). Mechanism of antitumor drug action: Poisoning of mammalian topoisomerase II on DNA by $4'$-(9-acridinylamino)-methanesulfon-*m*-anisidide. *Proc. Natl. Acad. Sci. USA* **81,** 1361–1364.

Pardee, A. B. (1974). A restriction point for control of normal animal cell proliferation. *Proc. Natl. Acad. Sci. USA* **71,** 1286–1290.

Pardoll, D. M. (1993). Cancer vaccines. *Trends Pharmacol. Sci.* **14,** 202–208.

Perry, P. J., and Jenkins Thomas, T. C. (1999). Recent advances in the development of telomerase inhibitors for the treatment of cancer. *Exp. Opin. Invest. Drugs* **8,** 1981–2008.

Pittillo, R. F., Schabel, F. M., Jr., Wilcox, W. S., and Skipper, H. E. (1965). Experimental evaluation of potential anticancer agents. XVI. Basic study of effects of certain anticancer agents on kinetic behavior of model bacterial cell populations. *Cancer. Chemother. Rep.* **47/1,** 1–26.

Plunkett, W., Huang, P., Searcy, C. E., and Gandhi, V. (1996). Gemcitabine: Preclinical pharmacology and mechanisms of action. *Semin. Oncol.* **23,** 3–15.

Pommier, Y. (1993). DNA topoisomerase-I and topoisomerase-II in cancer chemotherapy—update and perspectives. *Cancer Chemother. Pharmacol.* **32,** 103–108.

Pronk, G. J., and Bos, J. L. (1994). The role of p21(ras) in receptor tyrosine kinase signalling. *Biochim. Biophys. Acta Rev. Cancer* **1198,** 131–147.

Romanov, S. R., Kozakiewicz, B., Holst, C. B., Stampfer, M. R., Haupt, L. M., and Tisty, T. D. (2001). Normal human mannary epithelial cells spontaneously escape senescence and acquire genomic changes. *Nature* **409,** 633–637.

Rosenberg, B., Van Camp, L., and Krigas, T. (1965). Inhibition of cell division in *Escherichia coli* by electrolysis products from a platinum electrode. *Nature* **205,** 698.

Rous, P. (1983). Landmark article (JAMA 1911;56:198). Transmission of a malignant new growth by means of a cell-free filtrate. By Peyton Rous. *J. Am. Med. Assoc.* **250,** 1445–1449.

Rowinsky, E. K., and Donehower, R. C. (1991). The clinical pharmacology and use of antimicrotubule agents in cancer chemotherapeutics. *Pharmacol. Ther.* **52,** 35–84.

Rowinsky, E. K., Cazenave, L. A., and Donehower, R. C. (1990). Taxol: A novel investigational antimicrotubule agent. *J. Natl. Cancer. Inst.* **82,** 1247–1259.

Rygaard, J., and Povlsen, C. O. (1969). Heterotransplantation of a human malignant tumour to "nude" mice. *Acta. Path. Microbiol. Scand.* **77,** 758–760.

Sampaio, E. P., Sarno, E. N., Galilly, R., Cohn, Z. A., and Kaplan, G. (1991). Thalidomide selectively inhibits tumor necrosis factor-alpha production by stimulated human monocytes. *J. Exp. Med.* **173,** 699–703.

Scherf, U., Ross, D. T., Waltham, M., Smith, L. H., Lee, J. K., Tanabe, L., Kohn, K. W., Reinhold, W. C., Myers, T. G., Andrews, D. T., Scudiero, D. A., Eisen, M. B., Sausville, E. A., Pommier, Y., Botstein, D., Brown, P. O., and Weinstein, J. N. (2000). A gene expression database for the molecular pharmacology of cancer. *Nature Genet.* **24,** 236–244.

Schiff, P. B., Fant, J., and Horwitz, S. B. (1979). Promotion of microtubule assembly *in vitro* by taxol. *Nature* **277**, 665–667.

Singhal, S., Mehta, J., Desikan, R., Ayers, D., Roberson, P., Eddlemon, P., Munshi, N., Anaissie, E., Wilson, C., Dhodapkar, M., Zeldis, J., and Barlogie, B. (1999). Antitumour activity of thalidomide in refractory multiple myeloma. *N. Engl. J. Med.* **341**, 1565–1571.

Skipper, H. E. (1967). Criteria associated with destruction of leukemia and solid tumor cells in animals. *Cancer Res.* **27**, 2636–2645.

Smith, J. A., and Martin, L. (1973). Do cells cycle? *Proc. Natl. Acad. Sci. USA* **70**, 1263–1267.

Stahelin, H. F., and Von Wartburg, A. (1991). The chemical and biological route from podophyllotoxin glucoside to etoposide: Ninth Cain Memorial Lecture. *Cancer Res.* **51**, 5–15.

Stock, C. C. (1954). Experimental Cancer Chemotherapy. *In* "Advances in Cancer Research" (J. P. Greenstein and A. Haddow, Eds.), Vol. 2, pp. 426–492. Academic Press, New York.

Szeto, C., Gillespie, K. M., and Mathieson, P. W. (2000). Levamisole induces interleukin-18 and shifts type 1/type 2 cytokine balance. *Immunology* **100**, 217–224.

Tannock, I. (1978). Cell kinetics and chemotherapy: A critical review. *Cancer Treat. Rep.* **62**, 1117–1133.

Uppuluri, S., Knipling, L., Sackett, D. L., and Wolff, J. (1993). Localization of the colchicine-binding site of tubulin. *Proc. Natl. Acad. Sci. USA* **90**, 11598–11602.

Wani, M., Taylor, H. L., Wall, M. E., Coggan, P., and McPhail, A. T. (1971). Plant antitumor agents. VI. The isolation and structure of taxol a novel antileukemic and antitumor agent from *Taxus brevifolia*. *J. Am. Chem. Soc.* **93**, 2325–2327.

Ward, H. W. (1973). Anti-oestrogen therapy for breast cancer: A trial of tamoxifen at two dose levels. *Br. Med. J.* **1**, 13–14.

Watanabe, N., Niitsu, Y., Umeno, H., Kuriyama, H., Neda, H., Yamauchi, N., Maeda, M., and Urushizaki, I. (1988). Toxic effect of tumor necrosis factor on tumor vasculature in mice. *Cancer Res.* **48**, 2179–2183.

Waterfield, M. D., Scrace, G. T., Whittle, N., Stroobant, P., Johnsson, A., Wasteson, A., Westermark, B., Heldin, C. H., Huang, J. S., and Deuel, T. F. (1983). Platelet-derived growth factor is structurally related to the putative transforming protein p28sis of simian sarcoma virus. *Nature* **304**, 35–39.

Whittington, R. M., and Close, H. P. (1970). Clinical experience with mitomycin C (NSC-26980). *Cancer. Chemother. Rep.* **54**, 195–198.

Wieman, B., and Starnes, C. (1994). Coley's toxins, tumor necrosis factor and cancer research: A historical perspective. *Pharmacol. Ther.* **64**, 529–564.

Wilson, G. D., McNally, N. J., Dische, S., Saunders, M. I., Des Rochers, C., Lewis, A. A., and Bennett, M. H. (1988). Measurement of cell kinetics in human tumours *in vivo* using bromodeoxyuridine incorporation and flow cytometry. *Br. J. Cancer* **58**, 423–431.

Wilson, W. R., Baguley, B. C., Wakelin, L. P. G., and Waring, M. J. (1981). Interaction of the antitumour drug m-AMSA (4′-(9-acridinylamino) methanesulphon-m-anisidide) and related acridines with nucleic acids. *Mol. Pharmacol.* **20**, 404–414.

Wyllie, A. H. (1993). Apoptosis. *Br. J. Cancer* **67**, 205–208.

Zschiesche, W., Fahlbusch, B., Schumann, I., and Tonew, E. (1978). Induction of cytokines by tilorone hydrochloride. *Agents Actions* **8**, 515–522.

Zwelling, L. A., Michaels, S., Erickson, L. C., Ungerleider, R. S., Nichols, M., and Kohn, K. W. (1981). Protein-associated DNA strand breaks in L1210 cells treated with the DNA intercalating agents 4′-(9-acridinylamino)methanesulfon-m-anisidide and adriamycin. *Biochemistry* **20**, 6553–6563.

Zwi, L. J., Baguley, B. C., Gavin, J. B., and Wilson, W. R. (1994). Correlation between immune and vascular activities of xanthenone acetic acid antitumor agents. *Oncol. Res.* **6**, 79–85.

CHAPTER 2

NOVEL TARGETS IN THE CELL CYCLE AND CELL CYCLE CHECKPOINTS

Yves Pommier
Qiang Yu
Kurt W. Kohn

Laboratory of Molecular Pharmacology

Center for Cancer Research

National Institutes of Health

Bethesda, Maryland

Summary

Our knowledge of the functional relationship between the molecules that constitute the cell cycle and checkpoint pathways is expanding rapidly, thus providing us with new opportunities to further our understanding of the mechanisms of action of anticancer agents. This knowledge will undoubtedly lead to the development of novel strategies for the management of cancers based on the specific alterations in any given tumor. This chapter will outline the current knowledge in cell cycle and checkpoint control, discuss the rationale for targeting these pathways, and review the pharmacology of the agents that are currently known to act on the cell cycle control and checkpoint pathways.

1. Introduction

In the past decade, important milestones have been identified in the molecular pathways that control cell cycle progression. Knowledge of the functional relationships between the molecules that constitute the cell cycle and checkpoint pathways is expanding rapidly, providing us with a framework for understanding the potential effects of therapeutic intervention. New avenues for tumor-specific therapeutic intervention are now at close reach. The molecular characterization of tumors should identify the specific defects that drive cell cycle progression in particular cancers and provide us with a rationale for the type of treatment that would be most appropriate for a particular patient. New therapeutic approaches can now be validated genetically (e.g., gene knockout, antisense strategy, gene transfer) prior to a search for (a screening for) small-molecule inhibitors and for validating the activity of such inhibitors against a biochemical target in a given pathway. We will outline the molecular pathways that drive cell cycle progression and regulate the cell cycle checkpoints. We will next address the rationale for developing therapeutics that interfere with cell cycle progression and cell cycle checkpoint. Finally, we will review the various therapeutic approaches that are being developed for cancer treatment. This chapter will focus on the potential therapeutic aspects of the regulation of the G$_1$/S and G$_2$/M transition.

2. Molecular Regulation of Cell Cycle Progression

Cellular proliferation and division requires an orderly progression through the cell cycle, primarily driven by protein complexes composed of cyclins and cyclin-dependent kinases (Cdks) (Fig. 1). Initiation of the cell cycle takes place when cells pass the "restriction point," as defined by Arthur Pardee 30 years ago (Pardee, 1974), after which cells are committed to complete their cell cycle progression. Progression through the G$_1$-S transition requires the activity of at least two different types of kinases, cyclin D-Cdk4/6 and cyclin E/A-Cdk2 (Figs. 1 and 2). (For Fig. 2, see color insert.) At the G$_1$-S transition, Cdk4/6 and Cdk2 govern the entry into S phase. Cdk2 continues to be active through S phase, with its decline in activity signaling exit from S phase. Lastly, Cdk1 (Cdc2) becomes active in G$_2$ and its activity persists through mitosis (Figs. 1 and 3). (For Fig. 3, see color insert.)

The activity of the cyclin-Cdk kinases is regulated by two families of cyclin-dependent kinase inhibitors (CKI): Cip/Kip

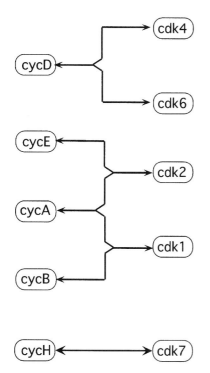

FIGURE 1   The binary association capabilities between the major cyclins and cdk's (cyclin-dependent kinases) involved in the mammalian G$_1$-S and G$_2$-M cell cycle transitions. (Modified from Kohn, 1999.)

and INK4. The members of the Cip/Kip family—p21^{Cip1}, p27^{Kip1}, and p57^{kip2}—can associate with and inactivate cyclin E/A-Cdk2 and cyclin B-Cdk1 complexes (Fig. 1). Binding of p27^{KIP} to cyclin E-Cdk2 prevents cells from entering into S phase, and binding of p27^{KIP} to cyclin A-Cdk2 prevents passage through S phase. p21^{Cip1} has a broader specificity. It can bind and inhibit both cyclin E/A-Cdk2 and cyclin B-Cdk1. In contrast, association of Cip/Kip family with cyclin D-Cdk4 or cyclin D-Cdk6 complexes appears to have a stimulatory effect (Blain *et al.*, 1997; Cheng *et al.*, 1999; LaBaer *et al.*, 1997; Soos *et al.*, 1996). Binding of Cip/Kip proteins to cyclin D-Cdk4/6 kinases can also prevent their interaction with cyclin E/A-Cdk2, thus facilitating the role of these kinases in completing the G$_1$ phase of the cell cycle and initiating DNA synthesis (Sherr and Roberts, 1999). The members of the INK4 family—p16^{INK4a}, p15^{INK4b}, p18^{INK4c} and p19^{INK4d}—specially target the Cdk4 and Cdk6 kinases, inhibiting their catalytic activity by preventing their binding to their regulatory cyclin D subunits (Sherr and Roberts, 1999) (Fig. 2).

The retinoblastoma tumor suppressor protein (pRb) is the primary substrate for cyclin-D-dependent kinases. pRb plays a critical role in regulating G$_1$ progression and is a key component of the molecular network controlling the restriction point. pRb can bind and suppress the transcriptional activity of various members of the E2F family (Chen *et al.*, 1996; Flemington *et al.*, 1993; Qin *et al.*, 1995). Cyclin-D-dependent Cdk's phosphorylate pRb in late G1, which disrupts the association of pRb, and E2F activation allows the coordinated expression of many genes that encode proteins necessary for S-phase entry and progression (Kato *et al.*, 1993) (Fig. 2). Among the E2F-regulated genes are cyclins E and A, whose association with Cdk2 is required for cells to make a transition from G$_1$ into S phase (Girard *et al.*, 1991; Pagano and Draetta, 1991).

The capacity of E2F to induce cyclin E, which in turn regulates Cdk2 to enforce pRb phosphorylation at additional sites, creates a positive-feedback loop for the accumulation of active E2F that helps contribute to the irreversibility of the G$_1$/S transition (Sherr, 1996; Taya, 1997; Weinberg, 1995). Cyclin-A- and B-dependent Cdk's activated later in the cell cycle maintain pRb in an hyperphosphorylated form until cells exit mitosis when pRb is returned to a hypophosphorylated state in the next G$_1$ phase (Ludlow *et al.*, 1993) (Fig. 2). Overexpression INK4 proteins arrest the cell cycle in G$_1$, which is consistent with the notion that INK4 proteins can antagonize the assembly of cyclin-D-dependent kinases by binding to Cdk4 or 6, thereby maintaining pRb in a growth-suppressive, hypophosphorylated state.

It is widely accepted that the onset of mitosis is driven by cyclin-B-dependent kinase Cdk1 (Cdc2) activation (Fig. 3). Cdk1 activation requires binding to its positive regulatory subunit, cyclin B. The kinase activity of Cdk1 is also regulated by phosphorylation. Phosphorylation on threonine 161 activates Cdk1, whereas phosphorylation on tyrosine 15 and threonine 14 by the Cdk1 inhibitory kinases Myt1 and Mik1 inhibits its activity. Cdc25C activates Cdk1 by removing the inhibitory phosphorylations of Cdk1 (Fig. 3). The activity of Cdc25C itself can be enhanced by Cdk1/cyclin B1-mediated phosphorylation (Hoffmann *et al.*, 1993; Izumi and Maller, 1993). Therefore, activation of Cdk1/cyclin B has been proposed to result in an autocatalytic feedback loop to ensure rapid activation of these complexes at the G_2-M transition (Hoffmann *et al.*, 1993).

3. Molecular Regulation of the Cell Cycle Checkpoints

Cell cycle checkpoints are mechanisms that monitor cell regulatory pathways and DNA structure before the cells enter the next phase of the cell cycle. Their activation in response to DNA damage either leads to cell cycle arrest, so as to allow repair of DNA damage, or leads to cell death by apoptosis or terminal growth arrest. In recent years, many genes involved in the regulation of DNA damage responses have been identified and related to the DNA damage checkpoint pathways (Figs. 2 and 3).

A. PI3K-Related Kinases: Key DNA Damage Signal Transducers

The mammalian DNA damage response pathway consists of several families of conserved protein kinases. Two members of the phosphoinositol kinase (PIK) family, Ataxia Telangiectasia Mutated (ATM) and ATR, share a COOH-terminal kinase domain bearing significant sequence homology to the catalytic domain of mammalian and yeast PIK family and are central to this signal transduction cascade (Fig. 3). ATM can bind directly to free DNA ends (Smith *et al.*, 1999) and act as a DNA damage sensor that signals to cell cycle checkpoint control. The ATM gene is mutated in the familial neural degeneration and cancer predisposition syndrome ataxia telangiectasia (AT) (Savitsky *et al.*, 1995). Cells derived from AT patients are defective for DNA damage checkpoints at G_1, S, and G_2 and are very sensitive to agents that cause DNA double-strand breaks, such as γ irradiation ((Morgan and Kastan, 1997; Morgan *et al.*, 1997; Rotman and Shiloh, 1998). A second mammalian PIK, ATR, carries out checkpoint-related functions that partially overlap with those performed by ATM (Cliby *et al.*, 1998; Wright *et al.*, 1998). The central roles of ATM and ATR in DNA damage response pathways have been demonstrated by their ability to activate p53 and other checkpoint kinases as discussed below.

B. Role of p53 and p21 in G_1-S Checkpoint Control

Of the various mammalian checkpoints, the G_1 checkpoint is now relatively well understood. Arrest in the G_1 phase of the cell cycle in mammalian cells exposed to DNA damage is mediated by the p53 gene product (Kastan *et al.*, 1991; Levine, 1997). The dependence of G_1 checkpoint on p53 is demonstrated by the observation that cells with wild-type p53 display a dose-dependent G_1 arrest in response to γ irradiation. However, cells lacking p53 function enter S phase due to a defective G_1 arrest. The p53 gene is a tumor suppressor gene most frequently mutated in human cancers (Cox and Lane, 1995). Loss of G_1-S checkpoint function has become a hallmark of human cancers with p53 mutations. p53 is a short-lived protein present at very low levels in the nuclei of normal cells. A variety of cellular insults, including DNA damage, hypoxia, and aberrant oncogenic signaling, elevate the levels of p53 due to enhanced stabilization. Stabilization of p53 in cells exposed to ionizing radiation (IR) or ultraviolet (UV) light is due to dissociation from Mdm2 (Shieh *et al.*, 1997), a protein that targets p53 for degradation through the ubiquitin pathway (Haupt *et al.*, 1997; Kubbutat *et al.*, 1997; Lane and Hall, 1997). p53 is a sequence-specific transcription factor that induces expression of several cell-cycle- and cell-death-related genes, including p21, Bax, and MDM2. G_1-S arrest results, at least in part, from p53-mediated p21 transactivation (Harper *et al.*, 1993). p21, also known as Cip1/Waf1, binds G_1-specific cyclin-CDK complex and acts as a CDK inhibitor, thus preventing cell cycle transition from G_1 to S phase (Deng *et al.*, 1995; Waldman *et al.*, 1995).

The mechanism that governs the p53 activation in response to DNA damage has been elucidated. Cells lacking ATM show reduced and delayed p53 activation in response to DNA damage, implicating the role of ATM in the regulation of p53 (Morgan and Kastan, 1997). Recently, it has been shown that ATM and ATR can phosphorylate p53 on Ser15 *in vivo* (Khanna *et al.*, 1998; Tibbetts *et al.*, 1999). They also contribute to the phosphorylation of p53 on Ser20 through activation of the checkpoint kinases Chk1 and Chk2 (Chehab *et al.*, 2000; Shieh *et al.*, 2000) (see below). Phosphorylation on Ser20 has been reported to decrease p53 binding to MDM2 and thereby contribute to the p53 stabilization (Chehab *et al.*, 1999; Unger *et al.*, 1999). Thus, ATM/ATR, p53, and p21 are three important genes that regulate the G_1-S checkpoint.

C. Role of Cdc25C in G_2-M Checkpoint Control

Cdc25 is one of the best characterized regulatory components of the eukaryotic cell cycle machinery. There are three human Cdc25 homologues: Cdc25A, B, and C. The three phosphatases share approximately 50% homology at the amino acid sequence level (Nilsson and Hoffmann, 2000). It appears that the phosphatases function differently in the cell cycle regulation. Cdc25A activity is required for S-phase entry, while Cdc25B and C activation is necessary for the regulation of entry into mitosis (Lammer *et al.*, 1998; Nilsson and Hoffmann, 2000). Cdc25C is best characterized for its function in G_2-M regulation by activation of Cdk1 (Fig. 3). In both human and yeast, inhibitory phosphorylation of Cdk1 is required for cell arrest in G_2 after DNA damage or DNA replication block (Blasina *et al.*, 1997; Rhind *et al.*, 1997). Although DNA-damage-induced activation of Wee1 kinase may be responsible for this inhibitory phosphorylation of Cdk1 (Den Haese *et al.*, 1995; O'Connell *et al.*, 1997; Rhind *et al.*, 1997), much evidence in both yeast and human cells points to the negative regulation of Cdc25C as a major event in G_2 checkpoint control.

It has been shown that Cdc25C is phosphorylated on Ser216 in asynchronously growing cells and throughout the G_1 and S phases of the cell cycle (Peng *et al.*, 1997). During mitosis, Ser216 becomes dephosphorylated and Cdc25C is hyperphosphorylated on NH_2-terminal serine and threonine residues (Peng *et al.*, 1997). It appears that the mitotic hyperphosphorylation of Cdc25C increases its intrinsic phosphatase activity (Lew and Kornbluth, 1996). In contrast, phosphorylation of Cdc25C on Ser216 throughout interphase negatively regulates Cdc25C. The negative effect of Ser216 phosphorylation is mediated by 14–3-3 binding, which sequesters Cdc25C in the cytoplasm and results in a decrease of Cdc25C access to Cdk1 (Peng *et al.*, 1997; Yang *et al.*, 1999). Thus, it has been proposed that DNA damage results in inactivation of Cdc25C by increased Ser216 phosphorylation. Two checkpoint kinases, Chk1 and Cds1, have been described to phosphorylate Cdc25C on Ser216 *in vitro* in response to genotoxic stress (Blasina *et al.*, 1999a; Brown *et al.*, 1999; Chen *et al.*, 1999a; Matsuoka *et al.*, 1998; Sanchez *et al.*, 1997), suggesting that Chk1 and Cds1 may regulate the DNA-damage-induced G_2 checkpoint by inactivation of Cdc25C to prevent mitotic entry (Fig. 3).

D. Checkpoint Effector Kinases Chk1 and Chk2

Studies in different species suggest that the two checkpoint kinases perform distinct roles in various checkpoint responses. In fission yeast, Cds1 is phosphorylated and activated when replication is inhibited by the DNA replication inhibitor hydroxyurea (HU) or when DNA is damaged in S phase (Brondello *et al.*, 1999; Lindsay *et al.*, 1998; Murakami and Nurse, 1999). However, Chk1 is normally only responsive to DNA damage but not to HU treatment (Walworth and Bernards, 1996). HU-induced Chk1 phosphorylation can only be detected when Cds1 is activated (58-59), indicating a cross-talk between the two checkpoint kinases.

However, human Chk1 and Cds1 (also called Chk2), appear to respond differently from their counterparts in fission yeast. In human cells, Chk2 is phosphorylated and activated upon exposure to a variety of signals, including ionizing and ultraviolet (UV) radiation, and hydroxyurea. Among them, the response to ionizing radiation is strongest (Brown *et al.*, 1999; Matsuoka *et al.*, 1998). By contrast, Chk1 phosphorylation appears to be most pronounced in cells treated with DNA-replication-interfering agents such as HU or UV, and, to a lesser extent, with ionizing radiation (Liu *et al.*, 2000). In addition, Chk1 activity is increased following UV irradiation (Mailand *et al.*, 2000) but displays no change following ionizing irradiation (Falck *et al.*, 2001; Kaneko *et al.*, 1999; Lukas *et al.*, 2001). It has been shown that Chk2 is regulated by ATM (Brown *et al.*, 1999; Matsuoka *et al.*, 1998), whereas Chk1 is regulated by ATR (Liu *et al.*, 2000; Zhao and Piwnica-Worms, 2001). These findings favor a model in which ATM-Chk2 and ATR-Chk1 represent two parallel pathways that respond to different types of DNA damage signals in mammalian cells. The ATM-Chk2 pathway primarily responds to DNA damage caused by ionizing radiation/double-strand DNA breaks, whereas the ATR-Chk1 pathway responds primarily to DNA-replication-blocking agents such as UV radiation and HU. In support of this model, a recent study showed that Chk1 is involved in the replication checkpoint through proteasome-dependent degradation of Cdc25A, whose activity is required for S-phase entry (Mailand *et al.*, 2000). However, both Chk1 and Chk2 pathways could overlap and cooperate with each other to ensure sufficient enforcement of checkpoints after DNA damage. When Chk2 is down-regulated by antisense inhibition, defective S and G_2 delays have been observed upon exposure, respectively, to the topoisomerase I inhibitor camptothecin that blocks DNA replication and to the topoisomerase II inhibitor etoposide (VP-16) that causes DNA double-strand breaks, suggesting that Chk2 is involved in both the DNA replication and damage checkpoints (Yu and Pommier, unpublished). Both Chk2-deficient mouse embryonic stem (ES) cells (Hirao *et al.*, 2000) and antisense Chk2-expressing human 293 cells (Yu and Pommier, unpublished) display normal onset of G_2 arrest but are defective in sustaining it, indicating that Chk2 is only required for maintaining the G_2 arrest. In contrast, Chk1 has been suggested to be required to initiate the G_2 arrest (Liu *et al.*, 2000). Therefore, human Chk1 and Chk2 appear to jointly enforce the G_2 checkpoint in response to DNA damage. It remains unclear whether Chk1 and Chk2 share the same substrate(s) *in vivo*. UCN-01 has been identified recently to inhibit Chk1 (Busby *et al.*, 2000; Graves *et al.*, 2000) (Fig. 3). Because UCN-01 inhibits Cdc25C phosphorylation *in vivo*, it has been suggested that Chk2 may not be the dominant kinase targeting Cdc25C (Busby *et al.*, 2000; Graves *et al.*, 2000). We recently found that UCN-01 inhibits Chk2 immunoprecipitated from human cancer cells (Yu and

Pommier, unpublished). Thus, it is likely that Chk2 may regulate checkpoint response through various substrate(s), including Cdc25C and p53. It would be interesting to develop anticancer drugs that target Chk2, since Chk2 down-regulation has been shown to enhance apoptotic response in p53-inactive human cells (Yu and Pommier, unpublished).

E. Role of p53 in G₂ Checkpoint Control

Contrary to the G_1 checkpoint, p53 did not appear to be required for G_2 arrest, since cells without p53 function are capable of DNA-damage-induced arrest in G_2. Recently, however, p53 has been implicated in the regulation of the G_2 checkpoint. By using gene targeting, it was shown that p53 and its effector gene p21 are essential to sustain DNA-damage-induced G_2 arrest (Bunz et al., 1998). Both p53- and p21-deficient cells display a normal initiation of G_2 arrest, but they prematurely escape the G_2 arrest (Bunz et al., 1998). Since p53 leads to accumulation of p21, it was generally thought that p53-mediated p21 induction contributes to the G_2 checkpoint by inactivation of Cdk1. However, given the poor inhibition of Cdk1/cyclin B1 by p21 (Harper et al., 1993, 1995), it does not appear to be a major event for the regulation of Cdk1/cyclin B1 activity. A more detailed mechanism has been described recently by Smits et al. showing that p21 blocks the CAK-mediated activating phosphorylation of Cdk1 on Thr161 (Smits et al., 2000), a different event from what has been well described on Tyr15 dephosphorylation by Cdc25C.

Another p53-responsive gene 14-3-3σ has been shown to be required for maintaining the DNA-damage-induced G_2 checkpoint. In the human colorectal cancer cell line, HCT116, expression of the 14-3-3σ gene is induced in a p53-dependent manner after DNA damage, and its overexpression leads to G_2 arrest by sequestering cyclin B1 and Cdk1 in the cytoplasm and preventing the cells from entering mitosis (Hermeking et al., 1997). Thus, cells lacking 14-3-3σ were unable to maintain G_2 arrest following DNA damage and underwent mitotic catastrophe as they entered mitosis (Chan et al., 1999).

Alternatively, p53 has been shown to transcriptionally down-regulate Cdk1 and cyclin B1 (perhaps indirectly) to modulate the G_2 checkpoint (Park et al., 2000; Passalaris et al., 1999). Treatment of p53 wild-type cells with the DNA damaging agent doxorubicin resulted in an arrest in G2, the maintenance of which correlated with down regulation of Cdk1 and cyclin B1 mRNA and protein (Park et al., 2000; Passalaris et al., 1999). Conversely, constitutive activation of Cdk1 kinase overrides p53-mediated G_2 arrest (Park et al., 2000). It appears that p53's role lies in the transcriptional repression of the cyclin B1 promoter (Innocente et al., 1999).

Taken together, current evidence indicated that Cdk1/cyclin B1 is regulated by multiple mechanisms, including p53-dependent and independent pathways (Fig. 3). However, deregulation of Cdk1 and cyclin B1 might not be the only

events that modulate the G_2 checkpoint. In contrast to p53 wild-type cells that abolish Cdk1-associated kinase activity when cells are arrested in G_2, cells lacking p53 function show a G_2 arrest despite high levels of cyclin B1 and Cdk1 kinase activity (Park et al., 2000; Passalaris et al., 1999). This observation suggests that there may exist a Cdk1/cyclin-B1-independent pathway(s) that maintains G_2 arrest in p53-deficient cells. Accordingly, it is possible that $p53^+$ and $p53^-$ cells use distinct pathways to regulate G_2 arrest. In cells with functional p53, p53-dependent regulation of Cdk1/cyclin B1 is a primary pathway that regulates G_2 arrest. However, in cells with defective p53 function, the p53-, Cdk1-independent pathway may become critical for G_2 arrest. Understanding of these mechanisms will better serve us in our search for novel therapeutic strategies to abrogate the G_2 checkpoint more efficiently and enhance cell killing by cancer therapeutic agents.

4. Rationale for Targeting Cyclin-Dependent Kinases and Cell Cycle Checkpoint Pathways

Uncontrolled cell proliferation and decreased apoptosis are basic dynamic mechanisms underlying cancer growth. In addition, genetic instability and defective checkpoints are key factors for carcinogenesis. Our understanding of the molecular elements that regulate these mechanisms has increased in the recent years. Cell cycle pathways and checkpoint controls have been found to be deregulated in human tumors and by oncogenic viruses. Genetic systems have also been used to demonstrate how the restoration of these pathways and/or interference with their molecular effectors can block cell proliferation. The fact that cyclin/Cdk's and checkpoint inhibitors, such as flavopiridol and UCN-01, demonstrate anticancer activity in animal models and in clinical trials is a demonstration that this strategy can work. Understanding how these agents achieve their selectivity for cancer cells should provide us with new approaches for cancer treatment.

1. Oncogenic viruses commonly activate cyclin-dependent kinases and inactivate the checkpoint pathways.
Tumor viruses commonly inactivate the pRb and p53 pathways to force cell division and block apoptosis. For instance, two genes (E6 and E7) are essential for replication of the human papillomaviruses (HPVs) that are associated with human cervical carcinomas. The E6 and E7 proteins bind and promote the degradation of p53 and pRb, respectively. The E1A and E1B gene products of adenoviruses inactivate pRb and p53, respectively. In the case of the papillomaviruses, p53 and pRb are inactivated by a single polypeptide, the SV40 T antigen.

Some tumor viruses can also activate the G_1 cyclins independently from p53. The herpesvirus associated with Kaposi's sarcoma (KSHV/HHV8) encodes a cyclin D2 homologue that forms a complex with Cdk6. This complex promotes the degradation of the CDK inhibitor, p27^{KIP1}, and thereby lifts the inhibition of cyclin D/Cdk complexes (Ills et al., 1999; Mann et al., 1999). The HPV E7 protein, in addition to inactivating pRb, also inactivates the other major CKIs, including p21$^{WAF1/CIP1}$ (Funk et al., 1997; Jones et al., 1997).

2. The $G_1 \rightarrow$ S transition pathways are commonly activated in human cancer.

There are numerous examples implicating enhanced/deregulated G_1-S cell cycle transition pathways in human cancer. The retinoblastoma gene protein, pRb, has been among the first tumor suppressor genes discovered. Inactivation and mutations of pRb that prevent the E2F binding and its inactivation by pRb predispose to cancers both in animal models and in humans. Cyclin-D-dependent kinases are activated directly or indirectly (through their negative regulators) in a large fraction of human cancers (Bartek et al., 1999; Bartkova et al., 1997; Donnellan and Chetty, 1999; Hall and Peters, 1996; Kaelin, 1997; Lavia and Jansen-Durr, 1999; Mansuri et al., 1997; Sellers and Kaelin, 1997). For instance, cyclin D1 is overexpressed in 70% of mantle cell lymphomas as a result of a translocation (t11:14) (Callanan et al., 1996). p27^{KIP1} is low in aggressive carcinomas (breast, colon, stomach, lung, and prostate) (Loda et al., 1997). Other genetic changes found in human cancers affect Cdk4, Cdk2, cyclin E, and the CKIs p15^{INK4B}, p16^{INK4A}, and p57^{KIP2} (Donnellan and Chetty, 1999). Up-regulation of the cyclin-D-dependent kinase pathways results in enhanced phosphorylation of pRb, which suppresses the negative regulatory effect of pRb on E2F and activates the E2F transcription factor (Fig. 2).

The proof of principle (validation) that inactivation of the G_1 Cdk's (Cdk4 and Cdk6) can effectively block cell proliferation has been demonstrated by overexpression of p16^{INK4A} in vitro and in vivo (McConnell et al., 1999; Nguyen et al., 1995; Schreiber et al., 1999; Serrano et al., 1993; Sumitomo et al., 1999; Wu et al., 1996). A 36-residue peptide (amino acid residues 84–103 of p16^{INK4A}) coupled with a peptide carrier has also been shown to be sufficient for inhibition of Cdk4 and of cell proliferation (Fahraeus et al., 1996). Because p16^{INK4A} selectively blocks Cdk4 and Cdk6, but not the other Cdk's (Serrano et al., 1993), it appears that selective targeting of the Cdk4 and Cdk6 kinases can selectively arrest cells that have functional pRb. Thus, assuming that pRb is the primary target for cyclin-D-dependent kinases, Cdk4 and Cdk6 inhibitors might be useful against cancers with normal pRb, and also possibly in patients with pRb deficiency for protecting normal tissues against the activity of cell-cycle-dependent anticancer agents.

Cyclin E is commonly amplified in human tumors. High cyclin E is correlated with low p27^{KIP1} levels and poor prognosis in young breast cancer patients (Donnellan and Chetty, 1999). A recent study indicated that inhibition of Cdk2 using

dominant negative forms of Cdk2 or oligonucleotides antisense to Cdk2 results in G_1 arrest and differentiation in some cells (Lee et al., 1999). However, because Cdk2 is associated with both cyclin E and the S-phase cyclin, cyclin A, it is questionable how selective Cdk2 inhibitors would be. It was recently observed that small peptides that block the activity of cyclin A and cyclin E were selectively toxic to transformed cells with pRb inactivation (Chen et al., 1999b). Because pRb-deficient cells have elevated E2F, which is negatively controlled by cyclin A/Cdk2, inhibition of Cdk2 would lead to high levels of E2F-1 and cell death by apoptosis.

To our knowledge there is no evidence that hyperactivation of the G2/M cyclin/Cdk's is a primary factor in human cancers and that the G2/M cyclin/Cdk's are differentially regulated in human cancers. Therefore, it is difficult to rationalize the development of cyclin B/Cdk1 inhibitors as anticancer agents. However, one interesting finding is that phosphorylation of survivin (Li et al., 1999), an inhibitor of apoptosis (IAP) by cyclin B/Cdk1, is necessary for binding of survivin to caspase 9 and inhibition of apoptosis. Thus, inhibition of Cdk1 might abrogate the antiapoptotic activity of survivin, which is selectively expressed in malignant tumors but not in adult tissues.

3. The cell cycle checkpoint pathways are commonly defective in human cancer.

A significant fraction of cancers are associated with cycle checkpoint deficiencies. The tumor suppressor gene p53 is defective (mutated or not expressed) in approximately 50% of human cancers, and patients with hereditary p53 mutations (Li–Fraumeni syndrome) have a high incidence of cancers (Lane, 1999). The sites of interaction of p53 can be related in two main functions: cell cycle checkpoint (including cell cycle arrest and DNA repair) and induction of apoptosis (Levine, 1997). Restoration of p53 activity has been validated for anticancer therapeutics by experiments showing that restoration of p53 activity in p53-negative tumors is effective both in experimental systems and in cancer patients (Ries et al., 2000).

Whether inhibition rather than restoration of checkpoint pathways is a valid approach for cancer chemotherapy is more debatable. It is plausible that the robustness of the cell cycle checkpoints relies on their redundancy. Since cancer cells are commonly defective in one or more checkpoint, it is plausible that abrogation of one checkpoint pathway might compromise cell survival. For instance, abrogation of the G2- or S-phase checkpoints by caffeine and UCN-01 selectively sensitizes p53-deficient cells to genotoxic agents (Powell et al., 1995; Yao et al., 1996). Furthermore, even in the absence of genotoxic stress (associated DNA-damaging treatment), it is conceivable that cell cycle checkpoint abrogation might be selectively toxic for cancer cells that exhibit genomic instability and spontaneous DNA lesions.

5. Agents and Strategies for Therapeutic Interference

A. Cdk Inhibitors

1. Small-Molecule Inhibitors of CDKs

A large number of Cdk inhibitors have been reported in the past 5 years by academic groups and the pharmaceutical industry. We refer the readers to recent and thorough reviews on this topic (Fry and Garrett, 2000; Meijer *et al.*, 1999), and we will only give an overview of the characteristics and structure of these inhibitors (Table 1). In spite of their diverse structures, these drugs generally bind to the ATP pocket in the Cdk catalytic site.

Not surprisingly, simple purine analogues were among the first reported cyclin B/Cdk1 inhibitors (Fig. 4). However, their IC_{50} values are relatively high (see Table 1) (Vesely *et al.*, 1994). For isopentenyladenine, olomucine, and roscovitine, crystal structures demonstrated that these drugs bind to the ATP pocket of Cdk2 (De Azevedo *et al.*, 1997; Noble *et al.*, 1999). Molecular modeling and screening of purine library and combinatorial chemistry led to more potent and

TABLE 1
Overview of Cdk Inhibitors

Name	*In vitro* potency selectivity	Preclinical and antitumor activity	Reference
6-Dimethylaminopurine	$IC_{50} = 120 \mu M$ for Cdk1		(Vesely *et al.*, 1994)
Isopentyladenine	$IC_{50} = 55 \mu M$ for Cdk1		(Vesely *et al.*, 1994)
Olomucine	$IC_{50} = 7 \mu M$ for Cdk1 More selective for Cdk1 than Cdk4 or Cdk6	G_1 arrest	(Abraham *et al.*, 1995; Alessi *et al.*, 1998; Buquet-Fagot *et al.*, 1997; Vesely *et al.*, 1994)
Roscovitine	$IC_{50} = 1 \mu M$ for Cdk1 and Cdk2	$GI_{50} = 16 \mu M$	(Alessi *et al.*, 1998; Meijer *et al.*, 1997)
CVT-313	$IC_{50} = 0.5 \mu M$ for Cdk2 Selective ($IC_{50} = 2 \mu M$ for Cdk1 and 200 μM for Cdk4)	G_1 and G_2 arrest	(Brooks *et al.*, 1997)
Purvanolols	Selective for Cdk1: $IC_{50} = 0.005 \mu M$ (0.07 μM for Cdk2)	$GI_{50} = 2 \mu M$ G_2 arrest and apoptosis > 10 μM	(Chang *et al.*, 1999; Gray *et al.*, 1998; Rosania *et al.*, 1999)
MDL-44	Selective for Cdk2 ($IC_{50} = 0.01 \mu M$) (0.25 μM Cdk4)	$IC_{50} = 0.5–1 \mu M$	(Dumont *et al.*, 1999a,b)
NU-2058	Weak: $IC_{50} = 6 \mu M$ for Cdk1; 16 μM for Cdk2		
Flavopiridol	Broad selectivity: $IC_{50} = 0.4 \mu M$ for Cdk1, Cdk2, Cdk4 and 7	G_1 and G_2 arrest; apoptosis	(Carlson *et al.*, 1999; De Azevedo *et al.*, 1996; Kaur *et al.*, 1992; Losiewicz *et al.*, 1994; Parker *et al.*, 1998; Sausville *et al.*, 1999; Senderowicz *et al.*, 1998; Stadler *et al.*, 2000)
2-Thio and 2-oxoflavopiridol	Selective for Cdk1 ($IC_{50} = 0.15 \mu M$) (7.5 μM for Cdk2; 23 μM for Cdk4)		
WO-09716447	$IC_{50} < 50 \mu M$ for Cdk4 (not reported for other Cdk's)		
PD-17851	Selective for Cdk4 ($IC_{50} = 0.04 \mu M$) (0.8 μM for Cdk2; 1.2 μM for Cdk1)	G_1 arrest in pRb wild-type cells	(Boschelli *et al.*, 1998; Nelson *et al.*, 1999)
AG-12275	Selective for Cdk4 ($IC_{50} = 0.003 \mu M$) (0.22 μM for Cdk2; 0.32 μM for Cdk1)	G_1 arrest in pRb wild-type cells	(Chong *et al.*, 1999; Lundgren *et al.*, 1999)
Kenpaullone	Broad selectivity: IC_{50}'s: 0.4 μM for Cdk1 0.7 for Cdk2; 8 for Cdk2; 0.9 for Cdk5	weak: $GI_{50} = 43 \mu M$ G_1 arrest	(Zaharevitz *et al.*, 1999)
Alsterpaullone	Selective for Cdk1 ($IC_{50} = 0.04 \mu M$) (0.7 μM for Cdk1 and Cdk2)	HCT116: $IC_{50} = 0.12 \mu M$ G_1 and G_2 arrest	(Kitagawa *et al.*, 1994; Yamamoto *et al.*, 1998)
Indirubin-5-sulfonic acid	Broad selectivity: 0.06 μM Cdk1, 0.035–0.15 μM for Cdk2, 0.15 Cdk/E, 0.3 Cdk4; 0.07 Cdk5	G_2 and G_1 arrest	(Hoessel *et al.*, 1999)

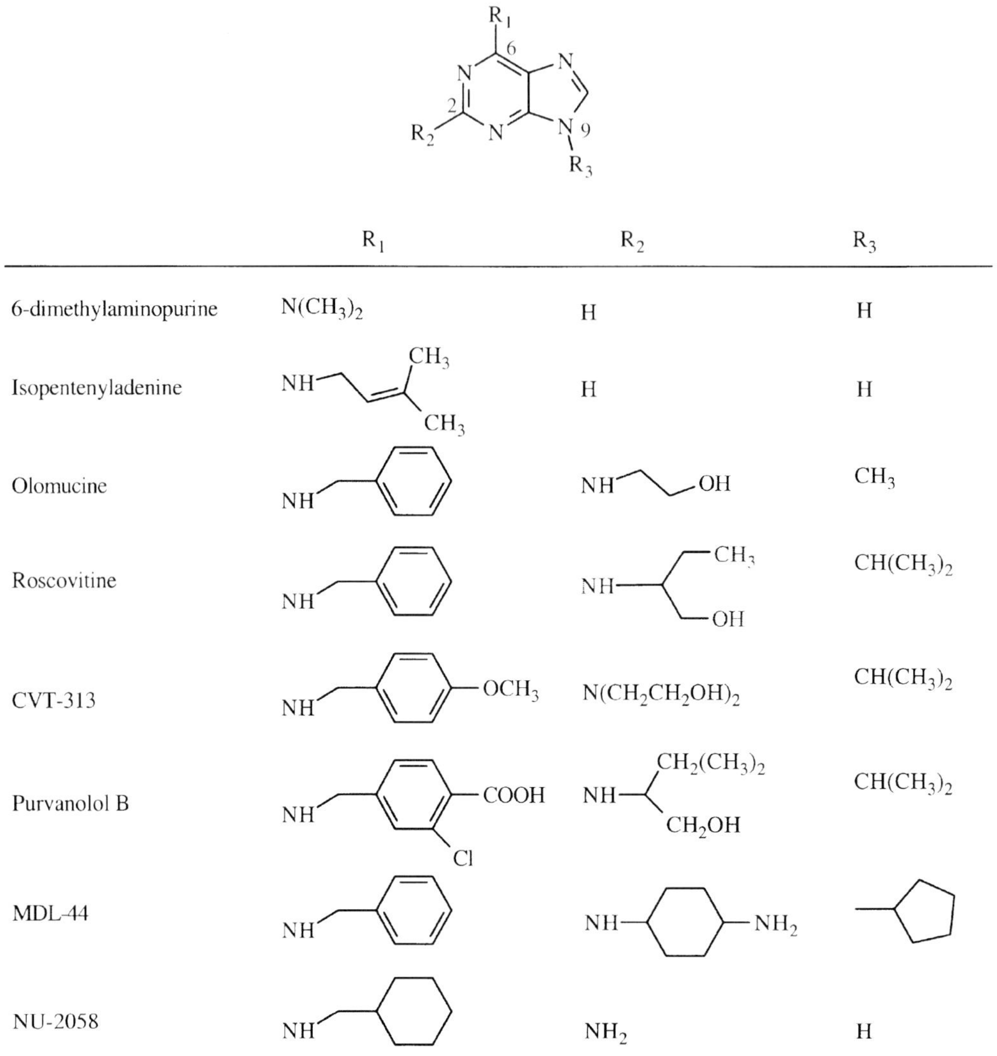

R_1, R_2, R_3 positions on purine ring (6, 2, 9 numbering)

	R_1	R_2	R_3
6-dimethylaminopurine	$N(CH_3)_2$	H	H
Isopentenyladenine	$NH-CH_2-CH=C(CH_3)CH_3$	H	H
Olomucine	$NH-CH_2-C_6H_5$ (benzyl)	$NH-CH_2CH_2-OH$	CH_3
Roscovitine	$NH-CH_2-C_6H_5$ (benzyl)	$NH-CH(CH_3)-CH_2OH$	$CH(CH_3)_2$
CVT-313	$NH-CH_2-C_6H_4-OCH_3$	$N(CH_2CH_2OH)_2$	$CH(CH_3)_2$
Purvanolol B	$NH-CH_2-C_6H_3(Cl)-COOH$	$NH-CH(CH_2(CH_3)_2)-CH_2OH$	$CH(CH_3)_2$
MDL-44	$NH-CH_2-C_6H_5$ (benzyl)	$NH-C_6H_{10}-NH_2$ (aminocyclohexyl)	cyclopentyl
NU-2058	$NH-CH_2-C_6H_{11}$ (cyclohexylmethyl)	NH_2	H

FIGURE 4 Structure of purine inhibitors of CDKs.

more specific inhibitors, such as CVT-313 and purvanolol which bear larger substitutions on the purine ring system and are most potent against Cdk1 (Brooks *et al.*, 1997; Gray *et al.*, 1998). The crystal structure of purvanolol bound to the ATP pocket of Cdk2 showed a binding similar to that of olomucine and roscovitine (Gray *et al.*, 1998). Another purine derivative, MDL-44, which is also selective for Cdk1, demonstrated activity in tumor models (Dumont *et al.*, 1999a,b).

The inhibitory activity of flavopiridol against cyclin B/Cdk1 was first reported in 1994 (Losiewicz *et al.*, 1994). Flavopiridol (Fig. 5) is a broad-spectrum Cdk inhibitor (IC_{50} approximately 100 nM for Cdk1, Cdk2, and Cdk4, and threefold higher for Cdk7 (CAK; see Table 1), causing G_1 and G_2 arrest (Carlson *et al.*, 1996; Kaur *et al.*, 1992) and apoptosis (Parker *et al.*, 1998) in cell culture. The deschloro derivative of flavopiridol has been crystallized with Cdk2 and found to bind to the ATP pocket of the enzyme (De Azevedo *et al.*,

1996). Flavopiridol arrests the cell cycle by at least three mechanisms: (1) direct inhibition of Cdk4, Cdk2, and Cdk1; (2) inactivation of these Cdk's by inhibition of Cdk7/cyclin H (CAK), which activates Cdk's by phosphorylation at threonine 160/161 (Worland *et al.*, 1993); and (3) decreased expression of cyclin D1 (Carlson *et al.*, 1999). Flavopiridol binding to DNA might contribute to the later effect (Bible *et al.*, 2000).

Flavopiridol exhibits antitumor activity in a preclinical model (Senderowicz and Sausville, 2000) and is synergistic with existing anticancer agents (Bible and Kaufmann, 1997). Flavopiridol is presently in phase II clinical trials as 72-hour continuous infusions. Plasma concentrations can reach 0.3–0.5 μM, which is in the concentration range that inhibits Cdk's *in vitro* (Table 1) (Senderowicz *et al.*, 1998; Senderowicz and Sausville, 2000; Stadler *et al.*, 2000). Derivatives have been reported by Bristol Myers Squibb and Mitotix

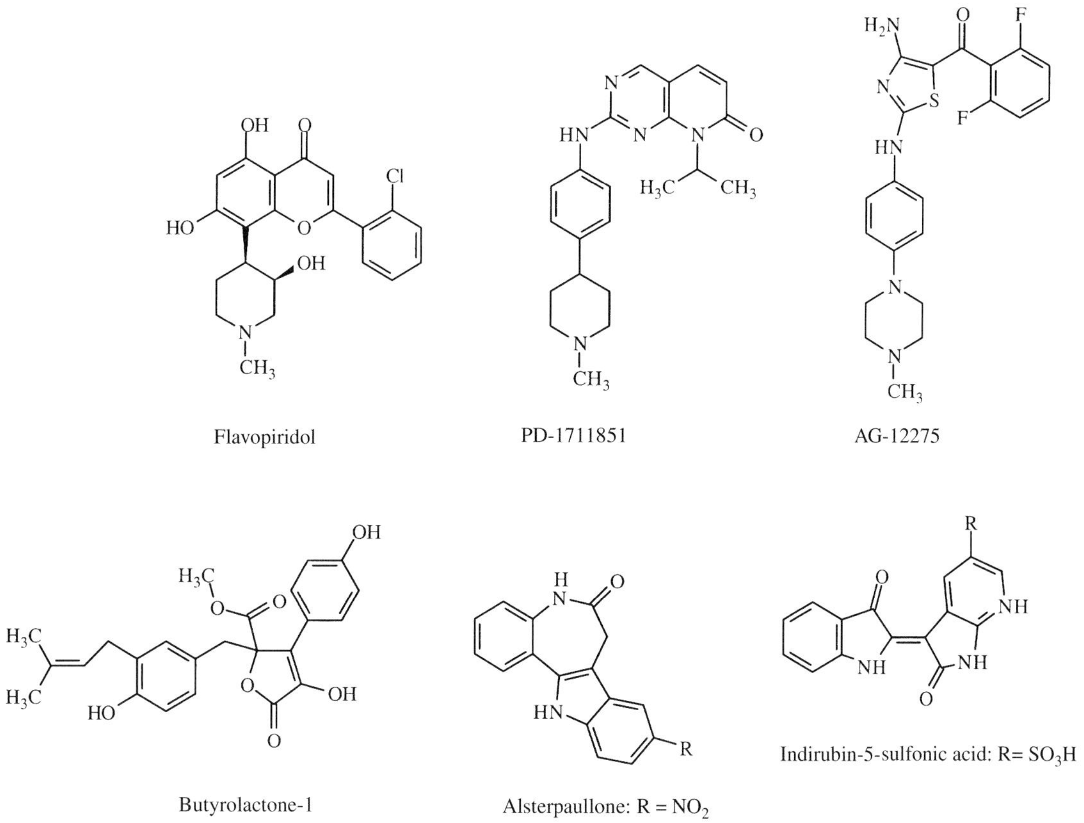

Flavopiridol   PD-1711851   AG-12275

Butyrolactone-1   Alsterpaullone: R = NO₂   Indirubin-5-sulfonic acid: R= SO₃H

FIGURE 5 Structure of CDK inhibitors.

(Table 1), which are more potent and more selective than flavopiridol (Griffin *et al.,* 1999; Mansuri *et al.,* 1997, 1998; Webster *et al.,* 1991). The antitumor activity of these later derivatives has not been reported.

Warner-Lambert recently disclosed a series of pyridopyrimidines that are competitive inhibitors of ATP in Cdk's (Boschelli *et al.,* 1998). PD-171851 (Fig. 5) is selective for Cdk4 with an IC$_{50}$ of 0.042 μM (Table 1). Consistently, PD-171851 arrests wild-type pRb cells in G$_1$ whereas pRb-defective cells continue to cycle.

Agouron disclosed 4-aminothiazole derivatives with excellent specificity toward Cdk4. AG-12275 (Fig. 5) binds to the Cdk's ATP pocket. It is approximately 100-fold more active on cyclin D3/Cdk4 than on cyclin A/Cdk2 or cyclin B/Cdk1, and arrests wild-type pRb cells in G$_1$ of the cell cycle (Lundgren *et al.,* 1999).

Kenpaullone was discovered in the NCI Anticancer Screen by COMPARE analysis using flavopiridol as a seed (Zaharevitz *et al.,* 1999). Kenpaullone is equally active against Cdk1, Cdk2, and Cdk5 but is much less effective against Cdk4 (Table 1). Molecular modeling suggests a mode of binding similar to that of olomucine and roscovitine, with room in the Cdk2 ATP binding pocket for further chemical substitutions, which should improve the drug potency and selectivity (Za-

harevitz *et al.,* 1999). One of the derivatives, alsterpaullone (Fig. 5), is markedly more potent both as a Cdk1 inhibitor (approximately 10-fold) and as a cytotoxic agent (IC$_{50}$ around 0.2 μM).

Recently, indirubin (Fig. 5), which has been used in the management of chronic myeloid leukemia in China, has been found, like flavopiridol, to selectively inhibit a broad range of cyclin/Cdk's (Hoessel *et al.,* 1999). One of its more potent derivatives, indirubin-5-sulfonic acid (Fig. 5 and Table 1), has been cocrystallized in the Cdk2 and found to bind to the ATP site in the enzyme. Treatment with indirubin-3'-monoxime results in G$_2$ arrest in various cell lines in culture and in G$_1$ arrest in Jurkat leukemia cells (Hoessel *et al.,* 1999). Whether Cdk's are the only targets for indirubin remains to be demonstrated since some of the derivatives have been reported to bind to DNA and affect microtubules (Hoessel *et al.,* 1999).

The specificity of the inhibitors described above varies among compounds. 6-Dimethylaminopurine, isopentenyladenine, staurosporine, and UCN-01 are relatively nonspecific protein kinase inhibitors that can affect other enzymes besides Cdk's. Olomucin, roscovitin, CVT-313, purvanolol, butyrolactone, and paullones are relatively selective for Cdk1 and Cdk2. By contrast, flavopiridol and indirubin have a broad range of specificity against different Cdk's. Other inhibitors have been reported at meetings and in patent applications (for review, see Fry and Garrett, 2000).

B. Checkpoint Kinase Inhibitors

As described above, the main checkpoint kinases include the PI3 kinases, ATM, ATR, and DNA-PK, and the checkpoint kinases, Chk1 and Chk2. Inhibitors have been identified for these kinases. However, their selectivity remains questionable.

1. UCN-01 and Other Indolocarbazoles

7-Hydroxystaurosporine (UCN-01, Fig. 6) is currently in phase II clinical trials. UCN-01 was originally isolated from the culture broth of *Streptomyces* sp. as a protein kinase C (PKC) inhibitor (for review, see Akinaga *et al.*, 2000). UCN-01 inhibits PKC more selectively than staurosporine or UCN-02, a stereoisomer of UCN-01 (Fig. 6). UCN-01 is most potent against the classical Ca^{2+}-dependent PKC isozymes (α, β, and γ) (IC_{50} approximately 30 nM) and does not inhibit the atypical PKC ξ. By contrast to other indolocarbazoles, such as rebecamycin and NB-506, UCN-01 and staurosporine do not bind to DNA and have no direct effect on DNA topoisomerase I.

UCN-01 is unique among anticancer drugs because, depending on the dose and the cell type used, it can have three different effects: cell cycle checkpoint abrogation, G_1 delay, and induction of apoptosis. The later two effects are generally observed at doses above 0.5 μM, where UCN-01 either blocks cell cycle progression from G_1 to S phase (Akinaga *et al.*, 1994; Seynaeve *et al.*, 1993) or induces apoptosis (Wang *et al.*, 1995) independently of p53 (Nieves-Neira and Pommier, 1999; Shao *et al.*, 1997b). Thus, UCN-01 differs from staurosporine, which induces G_1 delay at low concentrations (<0.01 μM) and G_2 delay with aneuploidy at higher concentrations (>0.03 μM) (Bruno *et al.*, 1992; Crissman *et al.*, 1991). The G_1 phase accumulation is apparently correlated with dephosphorylation of pRb and inhibition of Cdk2 by Cdk2 dephosphorylation and depletion of cyclin A as well as p21$^{WAF1/CIP1}$ activation (Akiyama *et al.*, 1997). The mechanisms by which UCN-01 (or staurosporine) induces apoptosis remain poorly understood.

At doses that have no significant effect on cell cycle progression (<0.3 μM) and can be achieved clinically (Fuse *et al.*, 1998; Senderowicz and Sausville, 2000), UCN-01 acts as a sensitizer for DNA-damaging agents and antimetabolite drugs, probably as a result of its inhibitory effects on the G_2- and S-phase checkpoints. Synergistic growth inhibition was observed in early studies in cell lines with mitomycin C, cisplatin, 5-fluorouracil, and methotrexate, and in mouse xenograft and syngenic models (Akinaga *et al.*, 1993, 2000). This synergism was later related to an abrogation of the G_2 delay/checkpoint (Bunch and Eastman, 1996; Wang *et al.*, 1996). Subsequent studies have shown that UCN-01 can also abrogate the S-phase accumulation induced by cisplatin or camptothecin (Bunch and Eastman, 1997; Shao *et al.*, 1997a). Remarkably, the potentiating effect of UCN-01 is greater for p53-deficient cells (Shao *et al.*, 1997a; Sugiyama *et al.*, 2000; Wang *et al.*, 1996). However, it should be noted that Hussain *et al.* (1997) found that the potentiation of cisplatin cytotoxicity by UCN-01 was not correlated with the p53 status of ovarian cancer cells. This raises the question of whether the expected selective potentiation of cisplatin cytotoxicity by UCN-01 is effectively greater and thereby provides a significantly enhanced therapeutic index in p53-defective tumor cells.

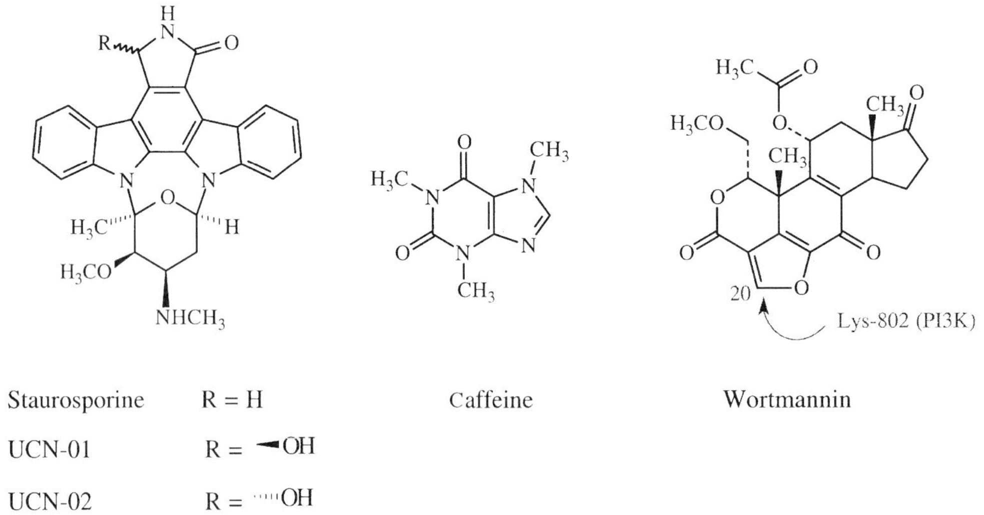

Staurosporine	R = H
UCN-01	R = ◂OH
UCN-02	R = ⁗OH

Caffeine

Wortmannin

Lys-802 (PI3K)

FIGURE 6 Structure of cell cycle checkpoint abrogators.

The molecular target(s) of UCN-01 for G_2- and S-phase abrogation have been identified recently. For G_2 checkpoint abrogation, the most plausible target of UCN-01 is Cdc25C, which becomes dephosphorylated on Ser216 in the presence of UCN-01 (Yu et al., 1998). This effect on Cdc25C is probably indirect and due to Chk1 inhibition by UCN-01. Chk1 inhibition has recently been demonstrated both with immunoprecipitated Chk1 (Busby et al., 2000; Sarkaria et al., 1999) and with recombinant Chk1 enzyme (Graves et al., 2000). Another mechanism by which UCN-01 might activate Cdk1 is inhibition of Wee1 (Yu et al., 1998), the kinase that inhibits Cdk1 activity by phosphorylating Tyr15 of Cdk1 (Fig. 3). More recently, we found that UCN-01 can also inhibit immunoprecipitated Chk2 kinase (Yu and Pommier, unpublished), which suggests that abrogation of the G_2- and S-phase checkpoints could be contributed by both Chk1 and Chk2 inhibition. Another effect of UCN-01 in relationship with S-phase checkpoint abrogation is the inhibition of camptothecin-induced RPA2 phosphorylation in cells pretreated with UCN-01 (Shao et al., 1999). Because the RPA2 kinase is DNA-dependent protein kinase (DNA-PK), and neither DNA-PK nor ATM is directly affected by UCN-01 (Sarkaria et al., 1999; Shao et al., 1999), these observations suggest that a UCN-01-sensitive kinase, such as Chk1 and Chk2, regulates DNA-PK. Recent observations also suggest that UCN-01 might potentiate the activity of cisplatin by inhibiting nucleotide excision repair via reduction of the interactions XPA/ERCC1(Jiang and Yang, 1999).

Phase I clinical trials showed that, in contrast to the preclinical animal studies, UCN-01 is tightly bound to α_1-acid glycoprotein and has very low distribution volumes and systemic clearance (Fuse et al., 1998; Sausville et al., 1998), and a very long half-life (approximately 30 days) (Senderowicz and Sausville, 2000). Phase II clinical trials are ongoing for UCN-01 in association with DNA-damaging agents and antimetabolites.

2. Caffeine

Caffeine (Fig. 6) was among the first cell cycle checkpoint abrogating drugs described. It served as a paradigm for agents that can sensitize cells to DNA damage by preventing cell cycle progression (Lau and Pardee, 1982; Schlegel and Pardee, 1986). Caffeine (at millimolar concentrations) has a broad range of activity on the cell cycle checkpoint controls. It abrogates the G_2 delay/checkpoint by inducing the removal of the inhibitory phosphorylation on cyclin B/Cdk1 and thereby activating cyclin B/Cdk1 (Yao et al., 1996). Caffeine overrides the G_1 checkpoints and attenuates p53 stabilization after irradiation (Kastan et al., 1991; Powell et al., 1995). Caffeine also overrides the replication delay (Dasso and Newport, 1990) and blocks checkpoint-dependent phosphorylation of Chk1 in *Xenopus* extracts (Kumagai et al., 1998) and fission yeast (Moser et al., 2000). Recently, several studies have indicated that these pleiotropic effects of caffeine could at least be in part related to direct inhibition of ATM (Blasina et al., 1999b; Sarkaria et al., 1999; Zhou et al., 2000), which can positively regulate the activity of Chk1 and Chk2 and the stabilization of p53 (see above). Caffeine is also active (at the same concentration: 1–10 mM) on ATR (Hall-Jackson et al., 1999; Sarkaria et al., 1999) and inhibits rad3, the fission yeast homologue of ATM and ATR (Moser et al., 2000).

3. Wortmannin

The fungal metabolite wortmannin (Fig. 6) is an irreversible inhibitor of the PI3K at low nanomolar concentrations (1–20 nM) (Arcaro and Wymann, 1993; Okada et al., 1994; Powis et al., 1994; Wymann et al., 1996). At higher concentrations (0.2–0.5 μM), wortmannin also inhibits DNA-PK and ATM (Hartley et al., 1995; Sarkaria et al., 1999) and the fission yeast homologue, rad3 (Moser et al., 2000), as well as mTOR (mammalian target of rapamycin) (Brunn et al., 1996). At submicromolar concentrations, wortmannin has no significant effect on PKC, cAMP- and cGMP-dependent protein kinases, mitogen-activated kinase, p70S6k, and the platelet-derived growth factor (PDGF) receptor tyrosine kinase (see references in Wymann et al., 1996). Experiments using radiolabeled wortmannin suggested that the C20 of wortmannin forms a covalent adduct on critical lysine residues of the phosphotransferase domains of PI3K (possibly Lys802) (Wymann et al., 1996) (Fig. 6). Wortmannin exhibits some antitumor activity in experimental systems (Schultz et al., 1995). However, the precise target(s) of the drug have not been identified (Lemke et al., 1999).

Treatment with wortmannin blocks the DNA-damage-induced p53 stabilization and results in radioresistant DNA synthesis (Boulton et al., 1996; Hosoi et al., 1998; Sarkaria et al., 1998) (consistent with inhibition of ATM; see above). Wortmannin is a highly effective sensitizer to ionizing radiation (Boulton et al., 1996, 2000; Price and Youmell 1996; Sarkaria et al., 1998), chlorambucil (Christodoulopoulos et al., 1998), as well as to the topoisomerase II inhibitor etoposide (VP-16) (Boulton et al., 2000). Because this radiosensitization is also observed in p53-deficient cells (Price and Youmell, 1996), it is plausible that wortmannin potentiates genotoxic lesions by mechanisms other than ATM inhibition and p53 destabilization. Other possible mechanisms of potentiation include DNA-PK inhibition (Boulton et al., 2000), which can result in inhibition of DNA double-strand break repair (Boulton et al., 1996), abrogation of the S-phase cell cycle checkpoints, and inhibition of RPA2 phosphorylation (Shao et al., 1999), and possibly radioresistant DNA synthesis (Boulton et al., 2000; Shao et al., 1999), as well as potentiation of apoptosis by PI3K inhibition.

The reactivity/instability of wortmannin precludes clinical use of the drug. However, other agents that selectively inhibit DNA-PK or ATM might be worth developing.

C. Other Sites for Intervention

1. Phosphatase Inhibitors (Cdc25 Phosphatase)

The dual-specificity protein phosphatase Cdc25 has recently emerged as a new target for drug development (for review, see Eckstein, 2000), because Cdc25 overexpression has been observed in a variety of cancers (Parsons, 1998) and because Cdc25C is a key substrate for checkpoint regulation by Chk1 and Chk2 kinases (see above). Cdc25A is also a transcriptional target of the proto-oncogene c-myc (Galaktionov et al., 1996). The crystal structure of its catalytic domain has recently been solved (Eckstein, 2000; Fauman et al., 1998). The Cdc25 family has been screened for inhibitors both in academia and the pharmaceutical industry.

2. Modulating E2F-1

Use of small molecule E2F-1 antagonists has been reported as a therapeutic approach (Chen et al., 1999b). Cdk 2 antagonists have also been shown to selectively kill cells with enhanced E2F-1 activity, suggesting that deregulation of E2F and inhibition of Cdk2 are synthetically lethal and provide a rationale for the development of Cdk2 antagonists as antineoplastic agents (Chen et al., 1999b).

Adenoviral vectors have been used to overexpress E2F-1 in order to activate apoptosis (Fueyo et al., 1998; Hunt et al., 1997) by p53-dependent (via p14^{INK4} which down-regulates MDM2 and therefore leads to increased stability of p53) and independent (via p73; Irwin et al., 2000; Lissy et al., 2000) pathways.

3. p53 Adenovirus Gene Transfer

The human group C adenovirus mutant dl1520 (Onyx-015) is an adenovirus that has been engineered to selectively replicate in and lyze p53-deficient cancer cells while sparing normal cells because it does not express the E1B 55-kDa gene (Heise et al., 1997). Although Onyx-015 and chemotherapy have demonstrated anti-tumoral activity in patients with recurrent head and neck cancer (Ganly et al., 2000), disease recurs rapidly with either therapy alone. Phase II clinical trials of a combination of intratumoral Onyx-015 injection with cisplatin and 5-fluorouracil in patients with recurrent squamous cell cancer of the head and neck recently demonstrated substantial objective responses, including a high proportion of complete responses. Tumor biopsies obtained after treatment showed tumor-selective viral replication and necrosis induction (Khuri et al., 2000). Onyx-015 acts synergistically with chemotherapeutic agents, such as cisplatin (Heise et al., 1997; Khuri et al., 2000; Osaki et al., 2000; Shimada et al., 2000). However, recent data indicate that Onyx-015 can replicate and kill cells with wild-type p53 very effectively, suggesting that this strategy is more complex than initially thought (Dix et al., 2000; Rogulski et al., 2000; Rothmann et al., 1998). Loss of p14^{ARF} has recently been shown to fa-

cilitate replication of Onyx-015, which suggests that Onyx-015 could be useful in tumors with lesions in the p53 pathway other than mutation of p53 (Ries et al., 2000).

4. Disrupting the p53–mdm2 Interaction

Mdm2 is the main cellular antagonist of p53, as evidence by the observations that mdm2 knockout mice embryo die early unless p53 is inactivated as well (Jones et al., 1995; Montes de Oca Luna et al., 1995). Thus, down-regulation of mdm2 and inhibition of the mdm2/p53 interaction have been proposed for the treatment of tumors with wild-type p53. In such cases, mdm2 inactivation should lead to p53 activation and cell death by apoptosis (or cell cycle arrest) (Levine, 1997). The human homologue of mdm2 is referred to either as hdm2 or mdm2. Hdm2 is also overexpressed in many different cancers, especially in soft-tissue tumors, such as sarcomas and osteosarcomas (Momand et al., 1998). In general, hdm2 amplification does not occur in tumors with p53 mutations (Momand et al., 1998).

Short peptides have been identified that bind to the mdm2 binding site on the N terminus of p53 and prevent the p53–mdm2 interaction without affecting p53 function (Bottger et al., 1997; Lane, 1999). Recently, Novartis reported an octamer synthetic peptide derived from p53 that inhibits p53–hdm2 interactions with high efficiency in vitro and kills tumor cells with hdm2 overexpression (Chene et al., 2000).

Inhibition of mdm2 expression by antisense oligodeoxynucleotides has been shown to activate p53 transcription, kill cells, and cause antitumor activity in xenograft models, alone and in synergy with doxorubicin and 10-hydroxycamptothecin (Moll and Zaika, 2000; Wang et al., 1999). Hybridon Inc. is advancing the commercial development of this approach, which is currently in the preclinical stage.

Inhibition of mdm2-dependent ubiquitination has been recently reported using an N-terminal p14^{ARF} peptide (Midgley et al., 2000). Thus, small peptides that are sufficient to block degradation of p53 could provide therapeutic agents capable of restoring p53-dependent cell death pathways in tumors that retain wild-type p53 expression.

6. Conclusions

It is increasingly clear that alterations of the cell cycle control and checkpoint pathways are generally present in human cancers and that such deficiencies can be identified in patient tumors. The dependence of tumors on activated cyclin-dependent kinases and the apparent deficiencies of tumor cells with respect to redundant pathways provide a rationale for the use of cyclin-dependent kinase inhibitors as anticancer agents. The key proteins in these pathways have been identified; these can be used to study the interactions of drugs at the molecular level and for the discovery of novel inhibitors. As discussed in this chapter, a variety of small-molecule inhibitors have already been discovered and some of them are in early clinical trials. Gene therapy has also been applied successfully for p53. An important challenge is to integrate the cell cycle and checkpoint pathways in a logical and comprehensive framework, to increase the selectivity of current therapies against specific targets, and to adapt these therapies to individual patients based on the molecular dissection of their tumors.

References

Abraham, R. T., Acquarone, M., Andersen, A., Asensi, A., Belle, R., Berger, F., Bergounioux, C., Brunn, G., Buquet-Fagot, C., Fagot, D., et al. (1995). Cellular effects of olomoucine, an inhibitor of cyclin-dependent kinases. *Biol. Cell.* **83,** 105–120.

Agami, R., and Bernards, R. (2000). Distinct initiation and maintenance mechanisms cooperate to induce G_1 cell cycle arrest in response to DNA damage. *Cell* **102,** 55–66.

Akinaga, S., Nomura, K., Gomi, K., and Okabe, M. (1993). Enhancement of antitumor activity of mitomycin C in vitro and in vivo by UCN-01, a selective inhibitor of protein kinase C. *Cancer Chemother. Pharmacol.* **32,** 183–189.

Akinaga, S., Nomura, K., Gomi, K., and Okabe, M. (1994). Effect of UCN-01, a selective inhibitor of protein kinase C, on the cell-cycle distribution of human epidermoid carcinoma, A431 cells. *Cancer Chemother. Pharmacol.* **33,** 273–280.

Akinaga, S., Sugiyama, K., and Akiyama, T. (2000). UCN-01 (7-hydroxy-staurosporine) and other indolocarbazole compounds: a new generation of anti-cancer agents for the new century? *Anticancer Drug. Des.* **15,** 43–52.

Akiyama, T., Yoshida, T., Tsujita, T., Shimizu, M., Mizukami, T., Okabe, M., and Akinaga, S. (1997). G1 phase accumulation induced by UCN-01 is associated with dephosphorylation of Rb and CDK2 proteins as well as induction of CDK inhibitor p21/Cip1/Sdi1 in p53-mutated human epidermoid carcinoma A431 cells. *Cancer Res.* **57,** 1495–1501.

Alessi, F., Quarta, S., Savio, M., Riva, F., Rossi, L., Stivala, L. A., Scovassi, A. I., Meijer, L., and Prosperi, E. (1998). The cyclin-dependent kinase inhibitors olomoucine and roscovitine arrest human fibroblasts in G1 phase by specific inhibition of CDK2 kinase activity. *Exp. Cell. Res.* **245,** 8–18.

Arcaro, A., and Wymann, M. P. (1993). Wortmannin is a potent phosphatidylinositol 3-kinase inhibitor: The role of phosphatidylinositol 3,4,5-trisphosphate in neutrophil responses. *Biochem. J.* **296,** 297–301.

Bartek, J., Lukas, J., and Bartkova, J. (1999). Perspective: defects in cell cycle control and cancer. *J. Pathol.* **187,** 95–99.

Bartkova, J., Lukas, J., and Bartek, J. (1997). Aberrations of the G1- and G1/S-regulating genes in human cancer. *Prog. Cell Cycle Res.* **3,** 211–220.

Bible, K. C., Bible, R. H., Jr., Kottke, T. J., Svingen, P. A., Xu, K., Pang, Y. P., Hajdu, E., and Kaufmann, S. H. (2000). Flavopiridol binds to duplex DNA. *Cancer Res.* **60,** 2419–2428.

Bible, K. C., and Kaufmann, S. H. (1997). Cytotoxic synergy between flavopiridol (NSC 649890, L86-8275) and various antineoplastic agents: The importance of sequence of administration. *Cancer Res.* **57,** 3375–3380.

Blain, S. W., Montalvo, E., and Massague, J. (1997). Differential interaction of the cyclin-dependent kinase (Cdk) inhibitor p27Kip1 with cyclin A-Cdk2 and cyclin D2-Cdk4. *J. Biol. Chem.* **272,** 25863–25872.

Blasina, A., de Weyer, I. V., Laus, M. C., Luyten, W. H., Parker, A. E., and McGowan, C. H. (1999a). A human homologue of the checkpoint kinase Cds1 directly inhibits Cdc25 phosphatase. *Curr. Biol.* **9,** 1–10.

Blasina, A., Paegle, E. S., and McGowan, C. H. (1997). The role of inhibitory phosphorylation of CDC2 following DNA replication block and radiation-induced damage in human cells. *Mol. Biol. Cell.* **8,** 1013–1023.

Blasina, A., Price, B. D., Turenne, G. A., and McGowan, C. H. (1999b). Caffeine inhibits the checkpoint kinase ATM. *Curr. Biol.* **9,** 1135–1138.

Boschelli, D. H., Dobrusin, E. M., Doherty, A. M., Fattacy, A., Fry, D. W., Baravian, M. R., Kallmeyer, S. T., and Wu, Z. (1998). Pyrido [2,3-D] pyrimidines and 4-aminopyrimidines as inhibitors of cellular proliferation. Warner-Lambert Co, WO-09833798.

Bottger, A., Bottger, V., Garcia-Echeverria, C., Chene, P., Hochkeppel, H. K., Sampson, W., Ang, K., Howard, S. F., Picksley, S. M., and Lane, D. P. (1997). Molecular characterization of the hdm2-p53 interaction. *J. Mol. Biol.* **269,** 744–756.

Boulton, S., Kyle, S., and Durkacz, B. W. (2000). Mechanisms of enhancement of cytotoxicity in etoposide and ionising radiation-treated cells by the protein kinase inhibitor wortmannin. *Eur. J. Cancer* **36,** 535–541.

Boulton, S., Kyle, S., Yalcintepe, L., and Durkacz, B. W. (1996). Wortmannin is a potent inhibitor of DNA double strand break but not single strand break repair in Chinese hamster ovary cells. *Carcinogenesis.* **17,** 2285–2290.

Brondello, J. M., Boddy, M. N., Furnari, B., and Russell, P. (1999). Basis for the checkpoint signal specificity that regulates Chk1 and Cds1 protein kinases. *Mol. Cell. Biol.* **19,** 4262–4269.

Brooks, E. E., Gray, N. S., Joly, A., Kerwar, S. S., Lum, R., Mackman, R. L., Norman, T. C., Rosete, J., Rowe, M., Schow, S. R., et al. (1997). CVT-313, a specific and potent inhibitor of CDK2 that prevents neointimal proliferation. *J. Biol. Chem.* **272,** 29207–29211.

Brown, A. L., Lee, C. H., Schwarz, J. K., Mitiku, N., Piwnica-Worms, H., and Chung, J. H. (1999). A human Cds1-related kinase that functions downstream of ATM protein in the cellular response to DNA damage. *Proc. Natl. Acad. Sci. USA* **96,** 3745–3750.

Brunn, G. J., Williams, J., Sabers, C., Wiederrecht, G., Lawrence, J. C., Jr., and Abraham, R. T. (1996). Direct inhibition of the signaling functions of the mammalian target of rapamycin by the phosphoinositide 3-kinase inhibitors, wortmannin and LY294002. *EMBO J.* **15,** 5256–5267.

Bruno, S., Ardelt, B., Skierski, J. S., Traganos, F., and Darzynkiewicz, Z. (1992). Different effects of staurosporine, an inhibitor of protein kinases, on the cell cycle and chromatin structure of normal and leukemic lymphocytes. *Cancer Res.* **51,** 470–473.

Bunch, R. T., and Eastman, A. (1996). Enhancement of cisplatin-induced cytotoxicity by 7-hydroxystaurosporine (UCN-01), a new G2-checkpoint inhibitor. *Clin. Cancer Res.* **2,** 791–797.

Bunch, R. T., and Eastman, A. (1997). 7-hydroxystaurosporine (UCN-01) causes redistribution of proliferating cell nuclear antigen and abrogates cisplatin-induced S-phase arrest in Chinese hamster ovary cells. *Cell Growth Diff.* **8,** 779–788.

Bunz, F., Dutriaux, A., Lengauer, C., Waldman, T., Zhou, S., Brown, J. P., Sedivy, J. M., Kinzler, K. W., and Vogelstein, B. (1998). Requirement for p53 and p21 to sustain G2 arrest after DNA damage. *Science* **282,** 1497–1501.

Buquet-Fagot, C., Lallemand, F., Montagne, M. N., and Mester, J. (1997). Effects of olomoucine, a selective inhibitor of cyclin-dependent kinases, on cell cycle progression in human cancer cell lines. *Anticancer Drugs.* **8,** 623–631.

Busby, E. C., Leistritz, D. F., Abraham, R. T., Karnitz, L. M., and Sarkaria, J. N. (2000). The radiosensitizing agent 7-hydroxystaurosporine (UCN-01) inhibits the DNA damage checkpoint kinase hChk1. *Cancer Res.* **60,** 2108–2112.

Callanan, M., Leroux, D., Magaud, J. P., and Rimokh, R. (1996). Implication of cyclin D1 in malignant lymphoma. *Crit. Rev. Oncog.* **7,** 191–203.

Carlson, B., Lahusen, T., Singh, S., Loaiza-Perez, A., Worland, P. J., Pestell, R., Albanese, C., Sausville, E. A., and Senderowicz, A. M. (1999). Downregulation of cyclin D1 by transcriptional repression in MCF-7 human breast carcinoma cells induced by flavopiridol. *Cancer Res.* **59**, 4634–4641.

Carlson, B. A., Dubay, M. M., Sausville, E. A., Brizuela, L., and Worland, P. J. (1996). Flavopiridol induces G1 arrest with inhibition of cyclin-dependent kinase (CDK) 2 and CDK4 in human breast carcinoma cells. *Cancer Res.* **56**, 2973–2978.

Chan, T. A., Hermeking, H., Lengauer, C., Kinzler, K. W., and Vogelstein, B. (1999). 14-3-3Sigma is required to prevent mitotic catastrophe after DNA damage. *Nature.* **401**, 616–620.

Chang, Y. T., Gray, N. S., Rosania, G. R., Sutherlin, D. P., Kwon, S., Norman, T. C., Sarohia, R., Leost, M., Meijer, L., and Schultz, P. G. (1999). Synthesis and application of functionally diverse 2,6,9-trisubstituted purine libraries as CDK inhibitors. *Chem. Biol.* **6**, 361–375.

Chehab, N. H., Malikzay, A., Appel, M., and Halazonetis, T. D. (2000). Chk2/hCds1 functions as a DNA damage checkpoint in G(1) by stabilizing p53. *Genes Dev.* **14**, 278–288.

Chehab, N. H., Malikzay, A., Stavridi, E. S., and Halazonetis, T. D. (1999). Phosphorylation of Ser-20 mediates stabilization of human p53 in response to DNA damage. *Proc. Natl. Acad. Sci. USA* **96**, 13777–13782.

Chen, L., Liu, T. H., and Walworth, N. C. (1999a). Association of Chk1 with 14-3-3 proteins is stimulated by DNA damage. *Genes Dev.* **13**, 675–685.

Chen, P. L., Riley, D. J., Chen-Kiang, S., and Lee, W. H. (1996). Retinoblastoma protein directly interacts with and activates the transcription factor NF-IL6. *Proc. Natl. Acad. Sci. USA* **93**, 465–469.

Chen, Y. N., Sharma, S. K., Ramsey, T. M., Jiang, L., Martin, M. S., Baker, K., Adams, P. D., Bair, K. W., and Kaelin, W. G., Jr. (1999b). Selective killing of transformed cells by cyclin/cyclin-dependent kinase 2 antagonists. *Proc. Natl. Acad. Sci. USA* **96**, 4325–4329.

Chene, P., Fuchs, J., Bohn, J., Garcia-Echeverria, C., Furet, P., and Fabbro, D. (2000). A small synthetic peptide, which inhibits the p53-hdm2 interaction, stimulates the p53 pathway in tumour cell lines. *J. Mol. Biol.* **299**, 245–253.

Cheng, M., Olivier, P., Diehl, J. A., Fero, M., Roussel, M. F., Roberts, J. M., and Sherr, C. J. (1999). The p21(Cip1) and p27(Kip1) CDK "inhibitors" are essential activators of cyclin D-dependent kinases in murine fibroblasts. *Embo. J.* **18**, 1571–1583.

Chong, W. K., Chu, S. S., Duvadie, R. R., Li, L., Xiao, W., and Yang, Y. (1999). 4-aminothiazole derivatives, their preparation and their use as inhibitors of cyclin-dependent kinases. Agouron Pharm Inc, WO-0992184.

Christodoulopoulos, G., Muller, C., Salles, B., Kazmi, R., and Panasci, L. (1998). Potentiation of chlorambucil cytotoxicity in B-cell chronic lymphocytic leukemia by inhibition of DNA-dependent protein kinase activity using wortmannin. *Cancer Res.* **58**, 1789–1792.

Cliby, W. A., Roberts, C. J., Cimprich, K. A., Stringer, C. M., Lamb, J. R., Schreiber, S. L., and Friend, S. H. (1998). Overexpression of a kinase-inactive ATR protein causes sensitivity to DNA-damaging agents and defects in cell cycle checkpoints. *EMBO J.* **17**, 159–169.

Cox, L. S., and Lane, D. P. (1995). Tumour suppressors, kinases and clamps: how p53 regulates the cell cycle in response to DNA damage. *Bioessays* **17**, 501–508.

Crissman, H. A., Gadbois, D. M., Tobey, R. A., and Bradbury, E. M. (1991). Transformed mammalian cells are deficient in kinase-mediated control of progression through the G_1 phase of the cell cycle. *Proc. Natl. Acad. Sci. USA* **88**, 7580–7584.

Dasso, M., and Newport, J. W. (1990). Completion of DNA replication is monitored by a feedback system that controls the initiation of mitosis in vitro: studies in Xenopus. *Cell* **61**, 811–823.

De Azevedo, W. F., Jr., Mueller-Dieckmann, H. J., Schulze-Gahmen, U., Worland, P. J., Sausville, E., and Kim, S. H. (1996). Structural basis for specificity and potency of a flavonoid inhibitor of human CDK2, a cell cycle kinase. *Proc. Natl. Acad. Sci. USA* **93**, 2735–2740.

Den Haese, G. J., Walworth, N., Carr, A. M., and Gould, K. L. (1995). The Wee1 protein kinase regulates T14 phosphorylation of fission yeast Cdc2. *Mol. Biol. Cell.* **6**, 371–385.

Deng, C., Zhang, P., Harper, J. W., Elledge, S. J., and Leder, P. (1995). Mice lacking p21CIP1/WAF1 undergo normal development, but are defective in G1 checkpoint control. *Cell* **82**, 675–684.

Dix, B. R., O'Carroll, S. J., Myers, C. J., Edwards, S. J., and Braithwaite, A. W. (2000). Efficient induction of cell death by adenoviruses requires binding of E1B55k and p53. *Cancer Res.* **60**, 2666–2672.

Donnellan, R., and Chetty, R. (1999). Cyclin E in human cancers. *FASEB J.* **13**, 773–780.

Dumont, J. A., Bitonti, A. J., Borcherding, D. R., Peet, N. P., Munson, H. R., and Shum, P. W. K. (1999a). 6,9-disubstituted 2-[trans-(4-aminocyclohexyl) amino] purines. Hoechst Marion Roussel Inc, WO-09943675.

Dumont, J. A., Borcherding, D., Loos, P. C., Shum, P. M. R., Tsay, J., Zhang, S., Peet, N. P., and Bitonti, A. J. (1999b). Novel adenine scaffold inhibitors of cyclin-dependent kinases. *Proc. Am. Assoc. Cancer Res.* **40**, 118.

Eckstein, J. W. (2000). Cdc25 as a potential target of anticancer agents. *Invest. New. Drugs* **18**, 149–156.

Fahraeus, R., Paramio, J. M., Ball, K. L., Lain, S., and Lane, D. P. (1996). Inhibition of pRb phosphorylation and cell-cycle progression by a 20-residue peptide derived from p16CDKN2/INK4A. *Curr. Biol.* **6**, 84–91.

Falck, J., Mailand, N., Syljuasen, R. G., Bartek, J., and Lukas, J. (2001). The ATM-Chk2-Cdc25A checkpoint pathway guards against radioresistant DNA synthesis. *Nature* **410(6830)**, 842–847.

Fauman, E. B., Cogswell, J. P., Lovejoy, B., Rocque, W. J., Holmes, W., Montana, V. G., Piwnica-Worms, H., Rink, M. J., and Saper, M. A. (1998). Crystal structure of the catalytic domain of the human cell cycle control phosphatase, Cdc25A. *Cell* **93**, 617–625.

Flemington, E. K., Speck, S. H., and Kaelin, W. G., Jr. (1993). E2F-1-mediated transactivation is inhibited by complex formation with the retinoblastoma susceptibility gene product. *Proc. Natl. Acad. Sci. USA* **90**, 6914–6918.

Fry, D. W., and Garrett, M. D. (2000). Inhibitors of cyclin-dependent kinases as therapeutic agents for the treatment of cancer. *Curr Opin Onc End Met Invest New Drugs* **2**, 40–59.

Fueyo, J., Gomez-Manzano, C., Yung, W. K., Liu, T. J., Alemany, R., McDonnell, T. J., Shi, X., Rao, J. S., Levin, V. A., and Kyritsis, A. P. (1998). Overexpression of E2F-1 in glioma triggers apoptosis and suppresses tumor growth in vitro and in vivo. *Nat. Med.* **4**, 685–690.

Funk, J. O., Waga, S., Harry, J. B., Espling, E., Stillman, B., and Galloway, D. A. (1997). Inhibition of CDK activity and PCNA-dependent DNA replication by p21 is blocked by interaction with the HPV-16 E7 oncoprotein. *Genes Dev.* **11**, 2090–2100.

Fuse, E., Tanii, H., Kurata, N., Kobayashi, H., Shimada, Y., Tamura, T., Sasaki, Y., Tanigawara, Y., Lush, R. D., Headlee, D., et al., (1998). Unpredicted clinical pharmacology of UCN-01 caused by specific binding to human alpha1-acid glycoprotein. *Cancer Res.* **58**, 3248–3253.

Galaktionov, K., Chen, X., and Beach, D. (1996). cdc25 cell-cycle phosphatase as a target of c-myc. *Nature* **382**, 511–517.

Ganly, I., Eckhardt, S. G., Rodriguez, G. I., Soutar, D. S., Otto, R., Robertson, A. G., Park, O., Gulley, M. L., Heise, C., Von Hoff, D. D., and Kaye, S. B. (2000). A phase I study of Onyx-015, an E1B attenuated adenovirus, administered intratumorally to patients with recurrent head and neck cancer. *Clin. Cancer Res.* **6**, 798–806.

Girard, F., Strausfeld, U., Fernandez, A., and Lamb, N. J. (1991). Cyclin A is required for the onset of DNA replication in mammalian fibroblasts. *Cell* **67**, 1169–1179.

Graves, P. R., Yu, L., Schwarz, J. K., Gales, J., Sausville, E. A., O'Connor, P. M., and Piwnica-Worms, H. (2000). The Chk1 protein kinase and the Cdc25C regulatory pathways are targets of the anticancer agent UCN-01. *J. Biol. Chem.* **275**, 5600–5605.

Gray, N. S., Wodicka, L., Thunnissen, A. M., Norman, T. C., Kwon, S., Espinoza, F. H., Morgan, D. O., Barnes, G., LeClerc, S., Meijer, L., et al.,

(1998). Exploiting chemical libraries, structure, and genomics in the search for kinase inhibitors. *Science* **281,** 533–538.

Griffin, R. J., Calvert, A. H., Curtin, N. J., Newell, D. R., Golding, B. T., Endicott, J. A., Nobel, M. E., Boyle, F. T., and Jewsbury, P. J. (1999). Cyclin dependent kinase inhibitors. Cancer Research Campaign, WO-09950251.

Hall, M., and Peters, G. (1996). Genetic alterations of cyclins, cyclin-dependent kinases, and Cdk inhibitors in human cancer. *Adv. Cancer Res.* **68,** 67–108.

Hall-Jackson, C. A., Cross, D. A., Morrice, N., and Smythe, C. (1999). ATR is a caffeine-sensitive, DNA-activated protein kinase with a substrate specificity distinct from DNA-PK. *Oncogene* **18,** 6707–6713.

Harper, J. W., Adami, G. R., Wei, N., Keyomarsi, K., and Elledge, S. J. (1993). The p21 Cdk-interacting protein Cip1 is a potent inhibitor of G_1 cyclin-dependent kinases. *Cell* **75,** 805–816.

Harper, J. W., Elledge, S. J., Keyomarsi, K., Dynlacht, B., Tsai, L. H., Zhang, P., Dobrowolski, S., Bai, C., Connell-Crowley, L., Swindell, E., et al. (1995). Inhibition of cyclin-dependent kinases by p21. *Mol. Biol. Cell* **6,** 387–400.

Hartley, K. O., Gell, D., Smith, G. C., Zhang, H., Divecha, N., Connelly, M., Admaon, A., Lees-Miller, S. P., Anderson, C. W., and Jackson, S. P. (1995). DNA-dependent protein kinase catalytic subunit: a relative of phosphatidylinositol 3-kinase and the ataxia telangiectasia gene product. *Cell* **82,** 849–856.

Haupt, Y., Maya, R., Kazaz, A., and Oren, M. (1997). Mdm2 promotes the rapid degradation of p53. *Nature* **387,** 296–299.

Heise, C., Sampson-Johannes, A., Williams, A., McCormick, F., Von Hoff, D. D., and Kirn, D. H. (1997). ONYX-015, an E1B gene-attenuated adenovirus, causes tumor-specific cytolysis and antitumoral efficacy that can be augmented by standard chemotherapeutic agents. *Nat. Med.* **3,** 639–645.

Hermeking, H., Lengauer, C., Polyak, K., He, T. C., Zhang, L., Thiagalingam, S., Kinzler, K. W., and Vogelstein, B. (1997). 14-3-3 sigma is a p53-regulated inhibitor of G2/M progression. *Mol. Cell.* **1,** 3–11.

Hirao, A., Kong, Y. Y., Matsuoka, S., Wakeham, A., Ruland, J., Yoshida, H., Liu, D., Elledge, S. J., and Mak, T. W. (2000). DNA damage-induced activation of p53 by the checkpoint kinase Chk2. *Science* **287,** 1824–1827.

Hoessel, R., Leclerc, S., Endicott, J. A., Nobel, M. E., Lawrie, A., Tunnah, P., Leost, M., Damiens, E., Marie, D., Marko, D., et al., (1999). Indirubin, the active constituent of a Chinese antileukaemia medicine, inhibits cyclin-dependent kinases. *Nat. Cell. Biol.* **1,** 60–67.

Hoffmann, I., Clarke, P. R., Marcote, M. J., Karsenti, E., and Draetta, G. (1993). Phosphorylation and activation of human cdc25-C by cdc2—cyclin B and its involvement in the self-amplification of MPF at mitosis. *EMBO J.* **12,** 53–63.

Hosoi, Y., Miyachi, H., Matsumoto, Y., Ikehata, H., Komura, J., Ishii, K., Zhao, H. J., Yoshida, M., Takai, Y., Yamada, S., et al. (1998). A phosphatidylinositol 3-kinase inhibitor wortmannin induces radioresistant DNA synthesis and sensitizes cells to bleomycin and ionizing radiation. *Int. J. Cancer* **78,** 642–647.

Hunt, K. K., Deng, J., Liu, T. J., Wilson-Heiner, M., Swisher, S. G., Clayman, G., and Hung, M. C. (1997). Adenovirus-mediated overexpression of the transcription factor E2F-1 induces apoptosis in human breast and ovarian carcinoma cell lines and does not require p53. *Cancer Res.* **57,** 4722–4726.

Husain, A., Yang, X. J., Rosales, N., Aghajamnian, C., Schwartz, G. K., and Spriggs, D. R. (1997). UCN-01 in ovary cancer cells: effective as a single agent and in combination with cis-diamminedichloroplatinum (II) independent of p53 status. *Clin. Cancer Res.* **3,** 2089.

Ills, M., Chew, Y. P., Fallis, L., Freddersdorf, S., Boshoff, C., Weiss, R. A., Lu, X., and Mittnacht, S. (1999). Degradation of p27(Klp) cdk inhibitor triggered by Kaposi's sarcoma virus cyclin-cdk6 complex. *EMBO J.* **1,** 644–653.

Innocente, S. A., Abrahamson, J. L., Cogswell, J. P., and Lee, J. M. (1999). p53 regulates a G_2 checkpoint through cyclin B1. *Proc. Natl. Acad. Sci. USA* **96,** 2147–2152.

Irwin, M., Marin, M. C., Phillips, A. C., Seelan, R. S., Smith, D. I., Liu, W., Flores, E. R., Tsai, K. Y., jacks, T., Vousden, K. H., and Kaelin, W. G. (2000). Role of the p53 homologue p73 in E2F-1 apoptosis. *Nature* **407,** 645–648.

Izumi, T., and Maller, J. L. (1993). Elimination of cdc2 phosphorylation sites in the cdc25 phosphatase blocks initiation of M-phase. *Mol. Biol. Cell.* **4,** 1337–1350.

Jiang, H., and Yang, L. Y. (1999). Cell cycle checkpoint abrogator UCN-01 inhibits DNA repair: association with attenuation of the interaction of XPA and ERCC1 nucleotide excision repair proteins. *Cancer Res.* **59,** 4529–4534.

Jones, D. L., Alani, R. M., and Munger, K. (1997). The human papillomavirus E7 oncoprotein can uncoupled cellular differentiation and proliferation in human keratinocytes by abrogating p21Clp1-mediated inhibition of cdk2. *Genes Dev.* **11,** 2101–2111.

Jones, S. N., Roe, A. E., Donehower, L. A., and Bradley, A. (1995). Rescue of embryonic lethality in Mdm2-deficient mice by absence of p53. *Nature* **378,** 206–208.

Kaelin, W. G., Jr. (1997). Alterations in G1-S cell-cycle control contributing to carcinogenesis. *Ann. NY. Acad. Sci.* **833,** 29–33.

Kaneko, Y. S., Watanabe, N., Morisaki, H., Akita, H., Fujimoto, A., Tominaga, K., Terasawa, M., Tachibana, A., Ikeda, K., Nakanishi, M., and Kaneko, Y. (1999). Cell-cycle-dependent and ATM-independent expression of human Chk1 kinase. *Oncogene* **18,** 3673–3681.

Kastan, M. B., Onyekwere, O., Sidransky, D., Vogelstein, B., and Craig, R. W. (1991). Participation of p53 protein in the cellular response to DNA damage. *Cancer Res.* **51,** 6304–6311.

Kato, J., Matsushime, H., Hiebert, S. W., Ewen, M. E., and Sherr, C. J. (1993). Direct binding of cyclin D to the retinoblastoma gene product (pRb) and pRb phosphorylation by the cyclin D-dependent kinase CDK4. *Genes Dev.* **7,** 331–342.

Kaur, G., Stetler-Stevenson, M., Sebers, S., Worland, P., Sedlacek, H., Myers, C., Czech, J., Naik, R., and Sausville, E. (1992). Growth inhibition with reversible cell cycle arrest of carcinoma cells by flavone L86-8275. *J. Natl. Cancer Inst.* **84,** 1736–1740.

Khanna, K. K., Keating, K. E., Kozlov, S., Scott, S., Gatei, M., Hobson, K., Taya, Y., Gabrielli, B., Chan, D., Lees-Miller, S. P., and Lavin, M. F. (1998). ATM associates with and phosphorylates p53: mapping the region of interaction. *Nat. Genet.* **20,** 398–400.

Khuri, F. R., Nemunaitis, J., Ganly, I., Arseneau, J., Tannock, I. F., Romel, L., Gore, M., Ironside, J., MacDougall, R. H., Heise, C., et al. (2000). A controlled trial of intratumoral ONYX-015, a selectively-replicating adenovirus, in combination with cisplatin and 5-fluorouracil in patients with recurrent head and neck cancer. *Nat. Med.* **6,** 879–885.

Kitagawa, M., Higashi, H., Takahashi, I. S., Okabe, T., Ogino, H., Taya, Y., Hishimura, S., and Okuyama, A. (1994). A cyclin-dependent kinase inhibitor, butyrolactone I, inhibits phosphorylation of RB protein and cell cycle progression. *Oncogene* **9,** 2549–2557.

Kohn, K. W. (1999). Molecular interaction map of the mammalian cell cycle control and DNA repair systems. *Mol. Biol. Cell.* **10,** 2703–2734.

Kubbutat, M. H., Jones, S. N., and Vousden, K. H. (1997). Regulation of p53 stability by Mdm2. *Nature* **387,** 299–303.

Kumagai, A., Guo, Z., Emami, K. H., Wang, S. X., and Dunphy, W. G. (1998). The Xenopus Chk1 protein kinase mediates a caffeine-sensitive pathway of checkpoint control in cell-free extracts. *J. Cell. Biol.* **142,** 1559–1569.

LaBaer, J., Garrett, M. D., Stevenson, L. F., Slingerland, J. M., Sandhu, C., Chou, H. S., Fattaey, A., and Harlow, E. (1997). New functional activities for the p21 family of CDK inhibitors. *Genes Dev.* **11,** 847–862.

Lammer, C., Wagerer, S., Saffrich, R., Mertens, D., Ansorge, W., and Hoffmann, I. (1998). The cdc25B phosphatase is essential for the G2/M phase transition in human cells. *J. Cell. Sci.* **111,** 2445–2453.

Lane, D. P. (1999). Exploiting the p53 pathway for cancer diagnosis and therapy. *Br. J. Cancer* **80**(Suppl 1), 1–5.

Lane, D. P., and Hall, P. A. (1997). MDM2—arbiter of p53's destruction. *Trends Biochem. Sci.* **22**, 372–374.

Lau, C. C., and Pardee, A. B. (1982). Mechanism by which caffeine potentiates lethality of nitrogen mustard. *Proc. Natl. Acad. Sci. USA* **79**, 2942–2946.

Lavia, P., and Jansen-Durr, P. (1999). E2F target genes and cell-cycle checkpoint control. *Bioessays* **21**, 221–230.

Lee, M., Simon, A. D., Stein, C. A., and Rabbani, L. E. (1999). Antisense strategies to inhibit restenosis. *Antisense Nucleic Acid Drug Dev.* **9**, 487–492.

Lemke, L. E., Paine-Murrieta, G. D., Taylor, C. W., and Powis, G. (1999). Wortmannin inhibits the growth of mammary tumors despite the existence of a novel wortmannin-insensitive phosphatidylinositol-3-kinase. *Cancer Chemother. Pharmacol.* **44**, 491–497.

Levine, A. J. (1997). p53, the cellular gatekeeper for growth and division. *Cell.* **88**, 323–331.

Lew, D. J., and Kornbluth, S. (1996). Regulatory roles of cyclin dependent kinase phosphorylation in cell cycle control. *Curr. Opin. Cell. Biol.* **8**, 795–804.

Li, F., Ackermann, E. J., Bennett, C. F., Rothermel, A. L., Plescia, J., Tognin, S., Villa, A., Marchisio, P. C., and Altieri, D. C. (1999). Pleiotropic cell-division defects and apoptosis induced by interference with survivin function. *Nat. Cell. Biol.* **1**, 461–466.

Lindsay, H. D., Griffiths, D. J., Edwards, R. J., Christensen, P. U., Murray, J. M., Osman, F., Walworth, N., and Carr, A. M. (1998). S-phase-specific activation of Cds1 kinase defines a subpathway of the checkpoint response in Schizosaccharomyces pombe. *Genes Dev.* **12**, 382–395.

Lissy, N. A., Davis, P. K., Irwin, M., Kealin, W. G., and Bowdy, S. F. (2000). A common E2F-1 and p73 pathway mediates cell death induced by TCR activation. *Nature* **407**, 642–644.

Liu, Q., Guntuku, S., Cui, X. S., Matsuoka, S., Cortez, D., Tamai, K., Luo, G., Carattini-Rivera, S., DeMayo, F., Bradley, A., et al., (2000). Chk1 is an essential kinase that is regulated by Atr and required for the G(2)/M DNA damage checkpoint. *Genes Dev.* **14**, 1448–1459.

Loda, M., Cukor, B., Tam, S. W., Lavin, P., Fiorentino, M., Draetta, G. F., Jessup, J. M., and Pagano, M. (1997). Increased proteasome-dependent degradation of the cyclin-dependent kinase inhibitor p27 in aggressive colorectal carcinomas. *Nat. Med.* **3**, 231–234.

Losiewicz, M. D., Carlson, B. A., Kaur, G., Sausville, E. A., and Worland, P. J. (1994). Potent inhibition of CDC2 kinase activity by the flavonoid L86-8275. *Biochem. Biophys. Res. Commun.* **201**, 589–595.

Ludlow, J. W., Glendening, C. L., Livingston, D. M., and DeCarprio, J. A. (1993). Specific enzymatic dephosphorylation of the retinoblastoma protein. *Mol. Cell. Biol.* **13**, 367–372.

Lukas, C., Bartkova, J., Latella, L., Falck, J., Mailand, N., Schroeder, T., Sehested, M., Lukas, J., and Bartek, J. (2001). DNA damage-activated kinase Chk2 is independent of proliferation or differentiation yet correlates with tissue biology. *Cancer Res.* **61(13)**, 4990–4993.

Lundgren, K., Price, S. M., Escobar, J., Huber, A., Chong, W., Li, L., Duvadie, R., Chu, S. S., Yang, Y., Nonomiya, J., et al., (1999). Diaminothiazoles: Potent, selective cyclin-dependent kinase inhibitors with antitumor efficacy. *Clin. Cancer Res.* **5**, 3755s.

Mailand, N., Falck, J., Lukas, C., Syljuasen, R. G., Welcker, M., Bartek, J., and Lukas, J. (2000). Rapid destruction of human Cdc25A in response to DNA damage. *Science* **288**, 1425–1429.

Mann, D. J., Chiled, E. S., Swanton, C., Laman, H., and Jones, N. (1999). Modulation of p27(Kip1) levels by the cyclin encoded by Kaposi's sarcoma-herpesvirus. *EMBO J.* **18**, 654–663.

Mansuri, M. M., Murthi, K. K., and Pal, K. (1997). Inhibitors of cyclin-dependent kinases. Mitotoxic Inc, WO-09716447.

Mansuri, M. M., Murthi, K. K., and Pal, K. (1998). Inhibitors of cyclin dependent kinases. Mitotix Inc, US-05733920.

Matsuoka, S., Huang, M., and Elledge, S. J. (1998). Linkage of ATM to cell cycle regulation by the Chk2 protein kinase. *Science* **282**, 1893–1897.

McConnell, B. B., Gregory, F. J., Stott, F. J., Hara, E., and Peters, G. (1999). Induced expression of p16(INK4a) inhibits both CDK4- and CDK2-associated kinase activity by reassortment of cyclin-CDK-inhibitor complexes. *Mol. Cell. Biol.* **19**, 1981–1989.

Meijer, L., Borgne, A., Mulner, O., Chong, J. P., Blow, J. J., Inagaki, N., Inagaki, M., Delcros, J. G., and Moulinoux, J. P. (1997). Biochemical and cellular effects of roscovitine, a potent and selective inhibitor of the cyclin-dependent kinases cdc2, cdk2 and cdk5. *Eur. J. Biochem.* **243**, 527–536.

Meijer, L., Leclerc, S., and Leost, M. (1999). Properties and potential-applications of chemical inhibitors of cyclin-dependent kinases. *Pharmacol. Ther.* **82**, 279–284.

Midgley, C. A., Desterro, J. M., Saville, M. K., Howard, S., Sparks, A., Hay, R. T., and Lane, D. P. (2000). An N-terminal p14ARF peptide blocks Mdm2-dependent ubiquitination in vitro and can activate p53 in vivo. *Oncogene* **19**, 2312–2323.

Moll, U. M., and Zaika, A. (2000). Disrupting the p53-mdm2 interaction as a potential therapeutic modality. *Drug Resistance Updates* **3**, 217–221.

Momand, J., Jung, D., Wilczynski, S., and Niland, J. (1998). The MDM2 gene amplification database. *Nucleic Acids Res.* **26**, 3453–3459.

Montes de Oca Luna, R., Wagner, D. S., and Lozano, G. (1995). Rescue of early embryonic lethality in mdm2-deficient mice by deletion of p53. *Nature* **378**, 203–206.

Morgan, S. E., and Kastan, M. B. (1997). p53 and ATM: Cell cycle, cell death, and cancer. *Adv. Cancer Res.* **71**, 1–25.

Morgan, S. E., Lovly, C., Pandita, T. K., Shiloh, Y., and Kastan, M. B. (1997). Fragments of ATM which have dominant-negative or complementing activity. *Mol. Cell. Biol.* **17**, 2020–2029.

Moser, B. A., Brondello, J. M., Baber-Furnari, B., and Russell, P. (2000). Mechanism of caffeine-induced checkpoint override in fission yeast. *Mol. Cell. Biol.* **20**, 4288–4294.

Murakami, H., and Nurse, P. (1999). Meiotic DNA replication checkpoint control in fission yeast. *Genes Dev.* **13**, 2581–2593.

Nelson, J. M., Boschelli, D., Dobrusin, E. M., Wu, Z., Fattaey, A., Garrett, M. D., Keller, P. R., Leopold, W. R., and Fry, D. W. (1999). Cell cycle and biological effects of PD 171851, a specific inhibitor of cyclin-dependent kinase 4 (CDK4). Keystone Symposia: The Molecular Basis of Cancer, 67.

Nguyen, X. J. D., Zhang, W. W. K. A. P., and Roth, J. A. (1995). Cell cycle arrest and inhibition of tumor cell proliferation by the p16INK4 gene mediated by an adenovirus vector. *Cancer Res.* **55**, 3250–3253.

Nieves-Neira, W., and Pommier, Y. (1999). Apoptotic response to camptothecin and 7-hydroxystaurosporine (UCN-01) in the eight human breast cancer cell lines of the NCI anticancer drug screen: multifactorial relationship with topoisomerase I, protein kinase C, bcl-2 and caspase pathways. *Int. J. Cancer* **82**, 396–404.

Nilsson, I., and Hoffmann, I. (2000). Cell cycle regulation by the Cdc25 phosphatase family. *Prog. Cell. Cycle Res.* **4**, 107–114.

Noble, M. E. and Endicott, J. A. (1999). Chemical inhibitors of cyclin-dependent kinases: Insights into design from X-ray crystallographic studies. *Pharmacol. Ther.* **82**, 269–278.

O'Connell, M. J., Raleigh, J. M., Verkade, H. M., and Nurse, P. (1997). Chk1 is a wee1 kinase in the G2 DNA damage checkpoint inhibiting cdc2 by Y15 phosphorylation. *EMBO J.* **16**, 545–554.

Okada, T., Kawano, Y., Sakakibara, T., Hazeki, O., and Ui, M. (1994). Essential role of phosphatidylinositol 3-kinase in insulin-induced glucose transport and antilipolysis in rat adipocytes. Studies with a selective inhibitor wortmannin. *J. Biol. Chem.* **269**, 3568–3573.

Osaki, S., Nakanishi, Y., Takayama, K., Pei, X. H., Ueno, H., and Hara, N. (2000). Alteration of drug chemosensitivity caused by the adenovirus-mediated transfer of the wild-type p53 gene in human lung cancer cells. *Cancer Gene. Ther.* **7**, 300–307.

Pagano, M., and Draetta, G. (1991). Cyclin A, cell cycle control and oncogenesis. *Prog. Growth Factor Res.* **3**, 267–277.

Pardee, A. B. (1974). A restriction point for control of normal animal cell proliferation. *Proc. Natl. Acad. Sci. USA* **71,** 1286–1290.

Park, M., Chae, H. D., Yun, J., Jung, M., Kim, Y. S., Kim, S. H., Han, M. H., and Shin, D. Y. (2000). Constitutive activation of cyclin B1-associated cdc2 kinase overrides p53-mediated G2-M arrest. *Cancer Res.* **60,** 542–545.

Parker, B. W., Kaur, G., Nieves-Neira, W., Taimi, M., Kohlhagen, G., Shimizu, T., Losiewicz, M. D., Pommier, Y., Sausville, E. A., and Senderowicz, A. M. (1998). Early induction of apoptosis in hematopoietic cell lines after exposure to flavopiridol. *Blood* **91,** 458–465.

Parsons, R. (1998). Phosphatases and tumorigenesis. *Curr. Opin. Oncol.* **10,** 88–91.

Passalaris, T. M., Benanti, J. A., Gewin, L., Kiyono, T., and Galloway, D. A. (1999). The G(2) checkpoint is maintained by redundant pathways. *Mol. Cell. Biol.* **19,** 5872–5881.

Peng, C. Y., Graves, P. R., Thoma, R. S., Wu, Z., Shaw, A. S., and Piwnica-Worms, H. (1997). Mitotic and G$_2$ checkpoint control: regulation of 14-3-3 protein binding by phosphorylation of Cdc25C on serine-216. *Science* **277,** 1501–1505.

Powell, S. N., De Frank, J. S., Connell, P., Eogan, M., Preffer, F., Dombkowski, D., Tang, W., and Friend, S. (1995). Differential sensitivity of p53(−) and p53(+) cells to caffeine-induced radiosensitization and override of G2 delay. *Cancer Res.* **55,** 1643–1648.

Powis, G., Bonjouklian, R., Berggren, M. M., Gallegos, A., Abraham, R., Ashendel, C., Zalkow, L., Matter, W. F., Dodge, J., Grindey, G., and Vlahos, C. J. (1994). Wortmannin, a potent and selective inhibitor of phosphatidylinositol-3-kinase. *Cancer Res.* **54,** 2419–2423.

Price, B. D., and Youmell, M. B. (1996). The phosphatidylinositol 3-kinase inhibitor wortmannin sensitizes murine fibroblasts and human tumor cells to radiation and blocks induction of p53 following DNA damage. *Cancer Res.* **56,** 246–250.

Qin, X. Q., Livingston, D. M., Ewen, M., Sellers, W. R., Arany, Z., and Kaelin, W. G., Jr. (1995). The transcription factor E2F-1 is a downstream target of RB action. *Mol. Cell. Biol.* **15,** 742–755.

Rhind, N., Furnari, B., and Russell, P. (1997). Cdc2 tyrosine phosphorylation is required for the DNA damage checkpoint in fission yeast. *Genes Dev.* **11,** 504–511.

Ries, S. J., Brandts, C. H., Chung, A. S., Biederer, C. H., Hann, B. C., Lipner, E. M., McCormick, F., and Michael Korn, W. (2000). Loss of p14ARF in tumor cells facilitates replication of the adenovirus mutant dl1520 (ONYX-015). *Nat. Med.* **6,** 1128–1133.

Rogulski, K. R., Freytag, S. O., Zhang, K., Gilbert, J. D., Paielli, D. L., Kim, J. H., Heise, C. C., and Kirn, D. H. (2000). In vivo antitumor activity of ONYX-015 is influenced by p53 status and is augmented by radiotherapy. *Cancer Res.* **60,** 1193–1196.

Rosania, G. R., Merlie, J., Jr., Gray, N., Chang, Y. T., Schultz, P. G., and Heald, R. (1999). A cyclin-dependent kinase inhibitor inducing cancer cell differentiation: biochemical identification using Xenopus egg extracts. *Proc. Natl. Acad. Sci. USA* **96,** 4797–4802.

Rothmann, T., Hengstermann, A., Whitaker, N. J., Scheffner, M., and zur Hausen, H. (1998). Replication of ONYX-015, a potential anticancer adenovirus, is independent of p53 status in tumor cells. *J. Virol.* **72,** 9470–9478.

Rotman, G., and Shiloh, Y. (1998). ATM: from gene to function. *Hum. Mol. Genet.* **7,** 1555–1563.

Sanchez, Y., Wong, C., Thoma, R. S., Richman, R., Wu, Z., Piwnica-Worms, H., and Elledge, S. J. (1997). Conservation of the Chk1 checkpoint pathway in mammals: Linkage of DNA damage to Cdk regulation through Cdc25. *Science* **277,** 1497–1501.

Sarkaria, J. N., Busby, E. C., Tibbetts, R. S., Roos, P., Taya, Y., Karnitz, L. M., and Abraham, R. T. (1999). Inhibition of ATM and ATR kinase activities by the radiosensitizing agent, caffeine. *Cancer Res.* **59,** 4375–4382.

Sarkaria, J. N., Tibbetts, R. S., Busby, E. C., Kennedy, A. P., Hill, D. E., and Abraham, R. T. (1998). Inhibition of phosphoinositide 3-kinase related kinases by the radiosensitizing agent wortmannin. *Cancer Res.* **58,** 4375–4382.

Sausville, E. A., Lush, R. D., Headlee, D., Smith, A. C., Figg, W. D., Arbuck, S. G., Senderowicz, A. M., Fuse, E., Tanii, H., Kuwabara, T., and Kobayashi, S. (1998). Clinical pharmacology of UCN-01: Initial observations and comparison to preclinical models. *Cancer Chemother. Pharmacol.* **42,** S54–S59.

Sausville, E. A., Zaharevitz, D., Gussio, R., Meijer, L., Louarn-Leost, M., Kunick, C., Schultz, R., Lahusen, T., Headlee, D., Stinson, S., et al. (1999). Cyclin-dependent kinases: Initial approaches to exploit a novel therapeutic target. *Pharmacol. Ther.* **82,** 285–292.

Savitsky, K., Bar-Shira, A., Gilad, S., Rotman, G., Ziv, Y., Vanagaite, L., Tagle, D. A., Smith, S., Uziel, T., Sfez, S., and et al., (1995). A single ataxia telangiectasia gene with a product similar to PI-3 kinase. *Science* **268,** 1749–1753.

Schlegel, R., and Pardee, A. B. (1986). Caffeine-induced uncoupling of mitosis from the completion of DNA replication in mammalian cells. *Science* **232,** 1264–1266.

Schreiber, M., Muller, W. J., Singh, G., and Graham, F. L. (1999). Comparison of the effectiveness of adenovirus vectors expressing cyclin kinase inhibitors p16INK4A, p18INK4C, p19INK4D, p21(WAF1/CIP1) and p27KIP1 in inducing cell cycle arrest, apoptosis and inhibition of tumorigenicity. *Oncogene* **18,** 1663–1676.

Schultz, R. M., Merriman, R. L., Andis, S. L., Bonjouklian, R., Grindey, G. B., Rutherford, P. G., Gallegos, A., Massey, K., and Powis, G. (1995). In vitro and in vivo antitumor activity of the phosphatidylinositol-3-kinase inhibitor, wortmannin. *Anticancer Res.* **15,** 1135–1139.

Sellers, W. R., and Kaelin, W. G., Jr. (1997). Role of the retinoblastoma protein in the pathogenesis of human cancer. *J. Clin. Oncol.* **15,** 3301–3312.

Senderowicz, A. M., Headlee, D., Stinson, S. F., Lush, R. M., Kalil, N., Villalba, L., Hill, K., Steinberg, S. M., Figg, W. D., Tompkins, A., et al. (1998). Phase I trial of continuous infusion flavopiridol, a novel cyclin-dependent kinase inhibitor, in patients with refractory neoplasms. *J. Clin. Oncol.* **16,** 2986–2999.

Senderowicz, A. M., and Sausville, E. A. (2000). Preclinical and clinical development of cyclin-dependent kinase modulators. *J. Natl. Cancer Inst.* **92,** 376–387.

Serrano, M., Hannon, G. J., and Beach, D. (1993). A new regulatory motif in cell-cycle control causing specific inhibition of cyclin D/CDK4. *Nature* **366,** 704–707.

Seynaeve, C. M., Stetler-Stevenson, M., Sebers, S., Kaur, G., Sausville, E. A., and Worland, P. J. (1993). Cell cycle arrest and growth inhibition by the protein kinase antagonist UCN-01 in human breast carcinoma cells. *Cancer Res.* **53,** 2081–2086.

Shao, R.-G., Cao, C.-X., Shimizu, T., O'Connor, P., Kohn, K. W., and Pommier, Y. (1997a). Abrogation of an S-phase checkpoint and potentiation of camptothecin cytotoxicity by 7-hydroxystaurosporine (UCN-01) in human cancer cell lines, possibly influenced by p53. *Cancer Res.* **57,** 4029–4035.

Shao, R.-G., Shimizu, T., and Pommier, Y. (1997b). 7-hydroxystaurosporine (UCN-01) induces apoptosis in human colon carcinoma and leukemia cells independently of p53. *Exp. Cell. Res.* **234,** 388–397.

Shao, R.-G., Cao, C.-X., Zhang, H., Kohn, K. W., Wold, M. S., and Pommier, Y. (1999). Replication-mediated DNA damage by camptothecin induces phosphorylation of RPA by DNA-dependent protein kinase and dissociates RPA:DNA-PK complexes. *EMBO J.* **18,** 1397–1406.

Sherr, C. J. (1996). Cancer cell cycles. *Science* **274,** 1672–1677.

Sherr, C. J., and Roberts, J. M. (1999). CDK inhibitors: positive and negative regulators of G1-phase progression. *Genes Dev.* **13,** 1501–1512.

Shieh, S. Y., Ahn, J., Tamai, K., Taya, Y., and Prives, C. (2000). The human homologs of checkpoint kinases Chk1 and Cds1 (Chk2) phosphorylate p53 at multiple DNA damage-inducible sites. *Genes Dev.* **14,** 289–300.

Shieh, S. Y., Ikeda, M., Taya, Y., and Prives, C. (1997). DNA damage-induced phosphorylation of p53 alleviates inhibition by MDM2. *Cell* **91**, 325–334.

Shimada, M., Kigawa, J., Kanamori, Y., Itamochi, H., Takahashi, M., Kamazawa, S., Sato, S., and Terakawa, N. (2000). Mechanism of the combination effect of wild-type TP53 gene transfection and cisplatin treatment for ovarian cancer xenografts. *Eur. J. Cancer* **36**, 1869–1875.

Smith, G. C., Cary, R. B., Lakin, N. D., Hann, B. C., Teo, S. H., Chen, D. J., and Jackson, S. P. (1999). Purification and DNA binding properties of the ataxia-telangiectasia gene product ATM. *Proc. Natl. Acad. Sci. USA* **96**, 11134–11139.

Smits, V. A., Klompmaker, R., Vallenius, T., Rijksen, G., Makela, T. P., and Medema, R. H. (2000). p21 inhibits thr161 phosphorylation of cdc2 to enforce the G_2 DNA damage checkpoint. *J. Biol. Chem.* **275**, 30638–30643.

Soos, T. J., Kiyokawa, H., Yan, J. S., Rubin, M. S., Giordano, A., DeBlasio, A., Bottega, S., Wong, B., Mendelsohn, J., and Koff, A. (1996). Formation of p27-CDK complexes during the human mitotic cell cycle. *Cell Growth Differ.* **7**, 135–146.

Stadler, W. M., Vogelzang, N. J., Amato, R., Sosman, J., Taber, D., Liebowitz, D., and Vokes, E. E. (2000). Flavopiridol, a novel cyclin-dependent kinase inhibitor, in metastatic renal cancer: a University of Chicago Phase II Consortium study. *J. Clin. Oncol.* **18**, 371–375.

Sugiyama, K., Shimizu, M., Akiyama, T., Tamaoki, T., Yamaguchi, K., Takahashi, R., Eastman, A., and Akinaga, S. (2000). UCN-01 selectively enhances mitomycin C cytotoxicity in p53 defective cells which is mediated through S and/or G(2) checkpoint abrogation. *Int. J. Cancer* **85**, 703–709.

Sumitomo, K., Shimizu, E., Shinohara, A., Yokota, J., and Sone, S. (1999). Activation of RB tumor suppressor protein and growth suppression of small cell lung carcinoma cells by reintroduction of p16INK4A gene. *Int. J. Oncol.* **14**, 1075–1080.

Taya, Y. (1997). RB kinases and RB-binding proteins: new points of view. *Trends Biochem. Sci.* **22**, 14–17.

Tibbetts, R. S., Brumbaugh, K. M., Williams, J. M., Sarkaria, J. N., Cliby, W. A., Shieh, S. Y., Taya, Y., Prives, C., and Abraham, R. T. (1999). A role for ATR in the DNA damage-induced phosphorylation of p53. *Genes Dev.* **13**, 152–157.

Unger, T., Juven-Gershon, T., Moallem, E., Berger, M., Vogt Sionov, R., Lozano, G., Oren, M., and Haupt, Y. (1999). Critical role for Ser20 of human p53 in the negative regulation of p53 by Mdm2. *EMBO J.* **18**, 1805–1814.

Vesely, J., Havlicek, L., Strnad, M., Blow, J. J., Donella-Deana, A., Pinna, L., Letham, D. S., Kato, J., Detivaud, L., Leclerc, S., et al. (1994). Inhibition of cyclin-dependent kinases by purine analogues. *Eur. J. Biochem.* **224**, 771–786.

Waldman, T., Kinzler, K. W., and Vogelstein, B. (1995). p21 is necessary for the p53-mediated G_1 arrest in human cancer cells. *Cancer Res.* **55**, 5187–5190.

Walworth, N. C., and Bernards, R. (1996). rad-dependent response of the chk1-encoded protein kinase at the DNA damage checkpoint. *Science* **271**, 353–356.

Wang, H., Zeng, X., Oliver, P., Le, L. P., Chen, J., Chen, L., Zhou, W., Agrawal, S., and Zhang, R. (1999). MDM2 oncogene as a target for cancer therapy: An antisense approach. *Int. J. Oncol.* **15**, 653–660.

Wang, Q., Fan, S., Eastman, A., Worland, P. J., Sausville, E. A., and O'Connor, P. M. (1996). UCN-01: A potent abrogator of G2 checkpoint function in cancer cells with disrupted p53. *J. Natl. Cancer Inst.* **88**, 956–961.

Wang, Q., Worland, P. J., Clark, J. L., Carlson, B. A., and Sausville, E. A. (1995). Apoptosis in 7-hydroxystaurosporine-treated T lymphoblasts correlates with activation of cyclin-dependent kinases 1 and 2. *Cell Growth Differ.* **6**, 927–936.

Webster, K. R., Mulheron, J. G., Qian, L., Wautlet, B. S., Chao, S. T., Stratton, L., Kelly, Y. F., Misra, R. N., Sack, J. S., Hunt, J. T., et al. (1991). Thio-flavopiridol, a selective inhibitor of CDK1. *Proc. Am. Assoc. Cancer Res.* **40**, 119.

Weinberg, R. A. (1995). The retinoblastoma protein and cell cycle control. *Cell* **81**, 323–330.

Worland, P. J., Kaur, G., Stetler-Stevenson, M., Sebers, S., Sartor, O., and Sausville, E. A. (1993). Alteration of the phosphorylation state of p34cdc2 kinase by the flavone L86-8275 in breast carcinoma cells. Correlation with decreased H1 kinase activity. *Biochem. Pharmacol.* **46**, 1831–1840.

Wright, J. A., Keegan, K. S., Herendeen, D. R., Bentley, N. J., Carr, A. M., Hoekstra, M. F., and Concannon, P. (1998). Protein kinase mutants of human ATR increase sensitivity to UV and ionizing radiation and abrogate cell cycle checkpoint control. *Proc. Natl. Acad. Sci. USA* **95**, 7445–7450.

Wu, Q., Possati, L., Montesi, M., Gualandi, F., Rimessi, P., Morelli, C., Trabanelli, C., and Barbanti-Brodano, G. (1996). Growth arrest and suppression of tumorigenicity of bladder-carcinoma cell lines induced by the P16/CDKN2 (p16INK4A, MTS1) gene and other loci on human chromosome 9. *Int. J. Cancer* **65**, 840–846.

Wymann, M. P., Bulgarelli-Leva, G., Zvelebil, M. J., Pirola, L., Vanhaesebroeck, B., Waterfield, M. D., and Panayotou, G. (1996). Wortmannin inactivates phosphoinositide 3-kinase by covalent modification of Lys-802, a residue involved in the phosphate transfer reaction. *Mol. Cell. Biol.* **16**, 1722–1733.

Yamamoto, H., Monden, T., Miyoshi, H., Izawa, H., Ikeda, K., Tsujie, M., Ohnishi, T., Sekimoto, M., Tomita, N., and Monden, M. (1998). Cdk2/cdc2 expression in colon carcinogenesis and effects of cdk2/cdc2 inhibitor in colon cancer cells. *Int. J. Oncol.* **13**, 233–239.

Yang, J., Winkler, K., Yoshida, M., and Kornbluth, S. (1999). Maintenance of G_2 arrest in the Xenopus oocyte: A role for 14-3-3- mediated inhibition of Cdc25 nuclear import. *EMBO J.* **18**, 2174–2183.

Yao, S. L., Akhtar, A. J., McKenna, K. A., Bedi, G. C., Sidransky, D., Mabry, M., Ravi, R., Collector, M. I., Jones, R. J., Sharkis, S. J., et al. (1996). Selective radiosensitization of p53-deficient cells by caffeine- mediated activation of p34cdc2 kinase. *Nat. Med.* **2**, 1140–1143.

Yu, L., Orlandi, L., Wang, P., Orr, M. S., Senderowicz, A. M., Sausville, E. A., Silvestrini, R., Watanabe, N., Piwnica-Worms, H., and O'Connor, P. M. (1998). UCN-01 abrogates G_2 arrest through a Cdc2-dependent pathway that is associated with inactivation of the Wee1Hu kinase and activation of the Cdc25C phosphatase. *J. Biol. Chem.* **273**, 33455–33464.

Zaharevitz, D. W., Gussio, R., Leost, M., Senderowicz, A. M., Lahusen, T., Kunick, C., Meijer, L., and Sausville, E. A. (1999). Discovery and initial characterization of the paullones, a novel class of small-molecule inhibitors of cyclin-dependent kinases. *Cancer Res.* **59**, 2566–2569.

Zhao, H. and Piwnica-Worms, H. (2001). Atr-mediated checkpoint pathways regulate phosphorylation and activation of human chk1. *Mol. Cell Biol.* **21(13)**, 4129–4139.

Zhou, B. B., Chaturvedi, P., Spring, K., Scott, S. P., Johanson, R. A., Mishra, R., Mattern, M. R., Winkler, J. D., and Khanna, K. K. (2000). Caffeine abolishes the mammalian G(2)/M DNA damage checkpoint by inhibiting ataxia-telangiectasia-mutated kinase activity. *J. Biol. Chem.* **275**, 10342–10348.

CHAPTER 3

GROWTH FACTOR AND SIGNAL TRANSDUCTION TARGETS FOR CANCER THERAPY

W. R. Leopold

Alex Bridges

Stuart Decker

David W. Fry

Alan Kraker

Judith Sebolt-Leopold

Pfizer Global Research and Development

Ann Arbor, Michigan

Summary

Dramatic advances in our understanding of the key mechanisms for misregulation of cell proliferation and survival in cancerous tissues have implicated a number of novel, as yet clinically unproven, targets as attractive foci of anticancer drug design strategies. Among the most intensely studied targets are those kinases associated with the aberrant signaling from growth factor receptors to the nucleus. Many of these signaling proteins have been demonstrated to have transforming activity, whereas others are thought to modulate the transforming potential of various oncogenes. Because of the breadth of the topic a comprehensive survey of all growth factor receptors and related signaling is not feasible. This chapter focuses on five major groups of targets that have been the object of particularly vigorous drug discovery research over the past decade. These include the erbB family of growth factor receptors, the ras/MAPK pathway components, src family kinases, the AKT family, and the nuclear hormone receptor family. Descriptions of physical structure, evidence of relevance as a potential target for therapeutic intervention, and, in some cases, discussion of prototype compounds in clinical development are provided.

1. Introduction

Over the past two decades it has become clear that one of the hallmarks of neoplastic transformation is the disregulation of signaling pathways that control cellular proliferation and survival. A large fraction of the identified oncogenes and tumor suppressor genes play key roles in these processes. Typically (in normal tissues) cell proliferation is initiated by the binding of extracellular growth factors (GFs) with growth-factor-specific receptors that reside either at the cell surface or in the cytoplasm. This interaction then triggers a signaling cascade mediated by the assembly of signaling complexes via specific protein–protein interactions and, in the case of cell surface GF receptors, the activation of multiple protein kinases. These processes are held tightly in check by counter-balancing signals in normal tissues but are activated by a variety of genetic defects in tumor cells that either lead to constitutive activation of growth-promoting proteins (oncogene activation) or the deletion of negative regulatory signals (suppressor gene loss). In the sections that follow, we have summarized data implicating disregulation of five major families of proteins currently thought to be important in the defective regulation of proliferation in human cancer (Fig. 1). Many of these families also play a role, either directly or indirectly, through the generation of paracrine signals in stro-

mal mechanisms that support tumor growth, such as angiogenesis and adhesion. This chapter is not meant to be comprehensive. A large number of other signaling systems exist that deserve attention as potential targets for therapeutic intervention in cancer, but because of space limitations we have chosen to focus on those that have received the most significant attention in recent years.

2. The erbB Family of Receptor Tyrosine Kinases (RTKs)

A. Structural Biology and Signal Transduction

The erbB receptor family comprises four distinct membrane glycoproteins consisting of epidermal growth factor (EGF) receptors erbB1, erbB2, erbB3, and erbB4 (also commonly referred to in the literature as HER1, HER2, HER3, and HER4). They are widely expressed in epithelial, mesenchymal, and neuronal tissues. These receptors are structurally similar and are composed of an extracellular ligand-

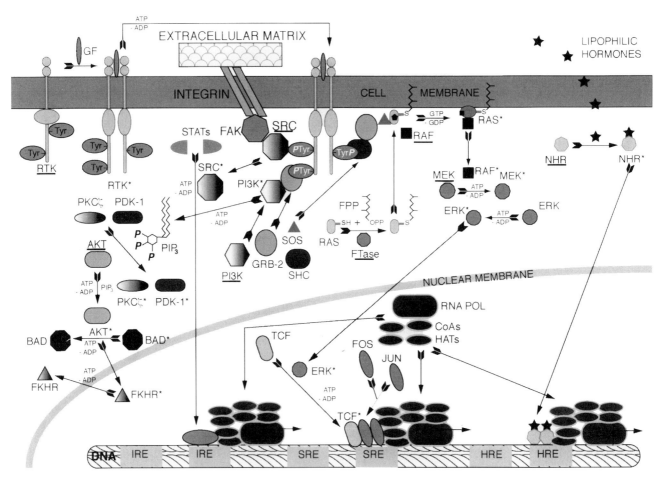

FIGURE 1 Signal transduction pathways covered in this chapter. Targets are underlined.

binding domain, a single transmembrane region, an intracellular domain possessing protein tyrosine kinase activity, and a C-terminal tail that contains specific tyrosine-containing sequences which, upon phosphorylation, become binding sites for src homology region 2 (SH2)–containing signaling proteins (Khazaie et al., 1993). The receptors also contain other phosphorylation sites that are believed to have a role in the regulation and function of the protein. Analogous structural and functional domains are present in all members of the receptor family. The overall amino acid sequence homology between this family of receptors is in the range of 50–60%; however, the similarity is not distributed evenly throughout the protein. The tyrosine kinase domains have the highest sequence homology at approximately 80%, whereas the C-terminal tails of the four receptors have little or no homology.

A complex system of different ligands and protein–protein interactions has evolved for this receptor family that produces a highly diverse network of signals associated with mitogenesis, differentiation, and cell survival. Several groups of ligands have been identified for this family of proteins, distinguished by their functional ability to bind and activate distinct sets of individual receptors (Riese and Stern, 1998; Daly, 1999; Hackel et al., 1999; Jones et al., 1999). The first group consists of EGF, transforming growth factor α (TGF-α), and amphiregulin, all of which bind exclusively to the EGF receptor (EGFr) (Stern et al., 1986; King et al., 1988; Stern and Kamps, 1988; Goldman et al., 1990; Wada et al., 1999; Johnson et al., 1993; Riese et al., 1996a, 1996b; Riese and Stern, 1998). Heparin-binding EGF and β-cellulin bind and activate both EGFr and erbB4 (Komurasaki et al., 1997; Riese et al., 1996a), whereas epiregulin appears to function as a broad-spectrum erbB receptor ligand binding all receptors except homodimers of erbB2 (Shelly et al., 1998). Another group of ligands consists of a large complex family of polypeptides called heregulins or neuregulins (also known as neu differentiation factors, glial growth factors, acetylcholine-receptor-inducing activity, or sensory- and motor-neuron-derived factor) and the neuregulin-2 proteins, also known as the cerebellum-derived growth factors (Hynes and Stern, 1994; Salomon et al., 1995; Fischbach and Rosen, 1997; Carraway, 1996; Meyer and Birchmeier, 1995; Marchionni et al., 1993; Chang et al., 1997; Carraway et al., 1997). These ligands appear to bind only erbB3 and erbB4 as individual receptors, but they can also bind the heterodimers erbB2/erbB3 and erbB2/erbB4 (Tzahar et al., 1996, 1997; Carraway and Cantley, 1994; Pinkas-Kramarski et al., 1996; Reese and Slamon, 1997; Burke et al., 1997; GrausPorta et al., 1997). Two recently identified members of this family were designated neuregulin-3 and neuregulin-4, both of which appear to bind only to erbB4 (Zhang et al., 1997; Harari et al., 1999). Thus far, no ligand has been identified that binds to erbB2 alone; however, this receptor is readily activated through transmodulation as a result of heterodimerization with the other receptors (Tzahar et al., 1996; Riese and Stern, 1998).

The ability of this receptor family to undergo homo- and heterodimerization both constitutively and in response to their different ligands (Riese and Stern, 1998) represents a unique property that provides enormous signaling diversity. All 10 possible dimeric complexes can exist, but there appears to be a graded hierarchy for the formation of heterodimers, and those containing erbB2 appear to be the most stable and preferred (Tzahar et al., 1996). For example, EGF, which binds only the EGFr, transmodulates erbB2 to a higher degree than erbB3 or erbB4, and heregulin-β, which binds to erbB3 and erbB4, induces interactions between these receptors more strongly with erbB2 than EGFr (Pinkas-Kramarski et al., 1996; Tzahar et al., 1996; Graus-Porta et al., 1997). Further signaling diversity within this family of receptors exists through differences in the amino acid sequences of their C-terminal domains. This area of the receptor contains key tyrosine residues which, when phosphorylated, represent a variety of consensus binding sites for SH2 domains that are present in various proteins involved in signal transmission (Pawson and Schlessinger, 1993; Schlessinger and Ullrich, 1992). These include Phosphatidyl inositol-3 (PI-3) kinase (Fiddes et al., 1995; Grasso et al., 1997; Ram and Ethier, 1996; Sepp-Lorenzino et al., 1996), Phospholipase C-γ (PLC-γ) (Fazioli et al., 1991; Jallal et al., 1992; Segatto et al., 1992), src (Lutrell et al., 1994; Muthuswamy et al., 1994), GRB2 (Fiddes et al., 1995; Janes et al., 1994), GRB7 (Stein et al., 1994; Fiddes et al., 1998), RAS-GAP (Sepp-Lorenzino et al., 1996), and shc (Fiddes et al., 1995; Sepp-Lorenzino et al., 1996). At least for erbB2, these phosphorylated binding sites have been shown to be essential for the transforming properties of the receptor (Ben-Levy et al., 1994; Dankort et al., 1997). Since the C-terminal tail represents an area where the least sequence homology exists between the four receptors, this represents a mechanism whereby different sets of signaling proteins can be recruited, depending on which receptors are activated and what binding sites are phosphorylated. Finally, each kinase can potentially exhibit additional selectivity through catalytic specificity (Songyang et al., 1995). This family of receptors, then, possesses the ability to provide enormous signaling diversity at four separate levels, including ligand selection, receptor homo- and heterodimerization, scaffolding sites for various signaling proteins at the C-terminal tails, and intrinsic substrate specificity for their kinase activities. Furthermore, diversity between different cells and tissue types can also exist, depending on expression levels and the preferred stoichiometry for interaction of these receptors and ligands. Stimulation of members of the erbB family can activate two major signal transduction pathways, ras/MAP kinase and PI-3 kinase/AKT (Fanger et al., 1997; Moghal and Sternberg, 1999; Reese and Slamon, 1997; Sepp-Lorenzino et al., 1996). Both of these pathways are involved in mitogenesis and cell survival.

B. Rationale for Inactivation of erbB Receptors as an Approach to Cancer Treatment

The rationale to pursue inhibitors of the erbB receptor kinase family as anticancer agents is based on more than a decade of clinical and preclinical evidence that implicates the EGF receptor and its family members, erbB2, erbB3 and erbB4, in the development, progression, and severity of a wide array of human cancers (Bacus et al., 1994; Depotter, 1994; Hynes and Stern, 1994; Davies and Chamberlin, 1996; Qian and Greene, 1997). In some cases, simple overexpression results in constitutive activation of the receptor (Janes et al., 1994). More recently, it has become clear that the four receptors within this family can intensify malignant transformation in a synergistic manner through their ability to form complex sets of homo- and heterodimers involving pairs of receptors in all permutations (Carraway and Cantley, 1994; Pinkas-Kramarski et al., 1996; Reese and Slamon, 1997; Burke et al., 1997; Graus-Porta et al., 1997; Tzahar et al., 1997). It has been shown that coexpression of the EGF receptor and erbB2 to levels where either receptor alone would have no effect were highly transforming when expressed simultaneously (Dougall et al., 1993; Qian et al., 1995; Muller et al., 1996). Members of this receptor family are overexpressed in a high percentage of tumor isolates from patients with breast, ovarian, and other cancers; and in many studies a correlation has been clearly established between high expression of EGFr or erbB2 and shorter survival times (Klijn et al., 1992; Rajkumar and Gullick, 1994; Bucci et al., 1997; Klijn et al., 1994; Toi et al., 1994; Bartlett et al., 1996; Scambia et al., 1995; Meden et al., 1995). These data, coupled with the fact that the tyrosine kinase activity is absolutely required for their mitogenic and transforming properties, provide a strong rationale to focus on these receptors as viable targets for cancer chemotherapy.

Thus far two approaches have been taken to attack this family of receptors on tumors. The first is antibodies directed to the extracellular domain that neutralize the receptor and/or prevent ligand from binding. Herceptin, which is directed specifically against erbB2, has been clinically approved for the treatment of patients with breast cancer whose tumors exhibit high expression of erbB2. Herceptin produces a significant number of responses in breast cancer patients whose disease in some cases is refractory to conventional therapies (Baselga et al., 2000; Cobleigh et al., 1998). Another successfully used antibody is IMC-C225, which binds specifically to the EGF receptor (erbB1) (Milas et al., 2000). This antibody, especially in combination with cytotoxic agents, has shown clinical responses in squamous cell carcinoma of the head and neck and colorectal cancer (Rubin et al., 2000; Bonner et al., 2000).

Perhaps the greatest effort toward targeting this receptor family has been through the development of specific inhibitors of their tyrosine kinase activities. Over the past 15 years a number of kinase inhibitors have been reported against the EGF receptor (Fry, 1994; Lawrence and Nui, 1998). Many of these earlier inhibitors suffered from a lack of potency and specificity, which compromised attempts to demonstrate an antitumor activity based solely on the proposed target. However, within the past 5 years, new structural classes of tyrosine kinase inhibitors, which exhibit enormous improvements in potency and specificity, have emerged against the EGF receptor as well as other members of this receptor family (Fry, 1999). The in vivo antitumor efficacy that was achieved with these more recently disclosed inhibitors paved the way for the clinical development. Three notable drugs that inhibit one or more members of the erbB family of tyrosine kinase are currently in clinical trials with very encouraging results thus far. These include Iressa (ZD-1839) (Baselga et al., 2000; Ferry et al., 2000), CP-358,774 (Karp et al., 1999; Siu et al., 1999), and CI-1033 (Fry, 2000; Sherwood et al., 1999; Vincent et al., 1999).

In summary, the preclinical and clinical results obtained thus far with agents that target the erbB family provide clinical confirmation of the attractiveness of these receptors as viable targets for cancer chemotherapy. However, the full potential for drugs that target this receptor family has yet to be realized. The ubiquitous nature of the erbB family in epithelial tissues provides an enormous potential for broad-spectrum antitumor activity. As oncologists optimize the clinical protocols for these unique drugs and explore combinations with conventional chemotherapy and radiation, there is a tremendous potential for drugs of this class to be part of a highly efficacious, broad-spectrum cancer therapy.

3. The Ras-Raf-MEK-ERK Signaling Pathway

Cell surface receptors for extracellular ligands initiate the transduction of proliferation signals to the cell nucleus (Fig. 1). As discussed in Section II for the erbB family, many of these GF receptors are tyrosine kinases, containing a cytoplasmic catalytic domain capable of auto- or transphosphorylation. Once phosphorylated, these receptors can serve as docking regions for proteins containing SH2 domains, such as Grb2, which plays a key role in the activation of Ras. Activated Ras then initiates a cascade of serine and threonine phosphorylations involving both Raf and MEK (MAP kinase kinase). This phosphorylation cascade leads to the activation of ERK (extracellular signal regulated kinase), which is a MAP kinase responsible for the activation of multiple transcription factors following its translocation to the cell nucleus. Of the many proteins that ultimately contribute to activation of the Ras pathway, including a number that are involved in protein–protein interactions, those receiving the most attention as targets for anticancer drug design are Ras, Raf, and MEK (Fig. 1).

A. Ras-Directed Approaches

The Ras family of G-proteins is diverse, composed of 21-kDa proteins that are critical to a broad array of cellular processes. Compared to other Ras family members, the *ras* proto-oncogenes (H-, K-, and N-) have received the most attention as anticancer drug targets. By virtue of its ability to bind guanine nucleotides, Ras acts as a molecular switch, which when GTP-bound transmits growth signals from the membrane to the nucleus. A single base activating mutation in one of the *ras* proto-oncogenes is sufficient to trigger neoplastic transformation. Colon and pancreatic tumors, which are notoriously refractory to conventional cancer treatment, exhibit an especially high incidence of activating *ras* mutations (roughly 50% and 90%, respectively). Across the broad spectrum of tumor types, approximately 30% of all human tumors possess an activating *ras* mutation. Still other tumors are characterized by high levels of activated Ras, driven by upstream stimulation of the pathway in the absence of Ras mutations (e.g. overexpression of erbB2). Pharmacologic interest has therefore focused on various approaches to interfering with the expression or function of Ras.

While the concept of repairing a single-base mutation by gene therapy is theoretically appealing, clinical application of such an approach is not imminent. However, investigators have made great strides in reducing expression of Ras at the translational level using antisense DNA to *ras*. ISIS 2503 is a phosphorothioate oligodeoxynucleotide that hybridizes to the translation initiation region of human H-ras mRNA (reviewed by Yuen and Sikic, 2000). While *in vivo* studies with ISIS 2503 have shown inhibition of growth in a variety of xenograft tumor models, phase 1 clinical testing of this agent failed to show objective responses (Gordon *et al.,* 1999; Dorr *et al.,* 1999).

The molecular target that has received the most attention for the design of anticancer agents to impair Ras function is farnesyltransferase (FTase). Ras must be anchored to the plasma membrane before it can initiate a cascade of signaling events that lead to cell proliferation. Ras has no transmembrane domain, but FTase posttranslationally modifies it by transfer of a farnesyl group, providing the requisite hydrophobicity for membrane attachment. All Ras proteins are prenylated by virtue of a common consensus sequence, referred to as the CAAX motif, located at their carboxy termini. The nature of the CAAX motif dictates its substrate specificity for various prenyltransferases. When CAAX is cysteine followed by two aliphatic amino acids and X is serine or methionine, the protein is a substrate for FTase. When leucine is present at the terminal position of the CAAX motif, the protein serves as a substrate for geranylgeranyltrans-ferase (GGTase). These prenylation enzymes also differ with respect to the size of their lipid substrate (15 vs 20 carbon for FTase and GGTase, respectively). Mutants lacking the CAAX motif cannot be prenylated, do not associate with the membrane, and consequently are not oncogenic (Kato *et al.,* 1992; Jackson *et al.,* 1990). Therefore, vigorous interest has been directed toward pharmacologic intervention of Ras prenylation as an approach to cancer treatment.

A number of farnesyltransferase inhibitors (FTIs) have been identified over the last 10 years possessing nanomolar activity *in vitro*. Historically, cellular screening of most FTIs has generally been carried out against H-ras-transformed cells. A caveat with this approach became apparent when it was discovered that FTIs are significantly less potent at blocking the membrane localization of k-Ras, which is encoded by the most prevalent *ras* oncogene in human tumors. This property is most likely due not only to the 10- to 30-fold higher affinity of K-ras for FTase compared with other Ras proteins, but also results from the ability of k-Ras to serve as a substrate for GGTase in the presence of an FTI (Reiss *et al.,* 1990, 1991; James *et al.,* 1996; Whyte *et al.,* 1997; Rowell *et al.,* 1997). Nonetheless, FTIs have demonstrated significant *in vivo* activity in a number of xenograft models, including tumors that are either wild type or mutated with respect to k-ras. In this regard, the data remind us that the true target under investigation here is FTase, not Ras. In support of this notion, prenylation of non-Ras proteins, such as Rho family members, is now thought to be important for the support of tumor cell growth (Sepp-Lorenzino *et al.,* 1995). RhoB, an endosomal protein that functions in receptor trafficking, is both farnesylated and geranylgeranylated (Zhang and Casey, 1996). Furthermore, it has been shown that geranylgeranylated RhoB suppresses human tumor cell proliferation by multiple mechanisms, promoting apoptosis in addition to inhibiting cell cycle progression (Du and Prendergast, 1999). The impact of these findings is significant since the clinical arena for prenylation inhibitors is conceivably larger and more diverse than originally anticipated.

Importantly, FTIs generally do not result in overt signs of clinical toxicity at efficacious dose levels in mouse models. This finding is consistent with the apparent lack of growth inhibitory activity of FTIs against nontransformed cells in culture (Kohl *et al.,* 1993; James *et al.,* 1993). These findings have positive implications for the potential of achieving high therapeutic indices in cancer patients treated with an FTI.

The reader is referred elsewhere for a review on current phase I trials being conducted with FTIs (Rowinsky, 1999). In several of these trials, achievement of biologically meaningful levels of drug can be assessed by measuring the extent to which a marker protein, e.g., prelamin A or HDJ-2, is farnesylated in clinical samples, e.g., buccal mucosal and peripheral blood mononuclear cells (Adjei *et al.,* 2000). Such translational assays will become increasingly important as clinical trials advance toward the phase II/phase III stage so as to correlate the degree of efficacy with the extent of target modulation. Early reports of partial responses in the clinic are encouraging. However, we will need to await the outcome of larger phase II clinical trials to gauge the potential activity of FTIs in a single-agent setting. It will likely prove particularly challenging to optimize FTI clinical trial design in the face of unresolved issues surrounding their cellular targets. Not only are multiple signaling protein prenylated, but also the extent to which these proteins contribute to the overall phenotype of a given tumor is likely to vary greatly.

B. Targeting Raf

Raf-1 is a serine/threonine protein kinase encoded by c-raf-1 that acts as a downstream effector of Ras in the mitogen-activated protein kinase (MAPK) pathway (Dunn et al., 1994; Stokoe et al., 1994). Mutated Raf-1 is constitutively active and has transforming potential in vitro (Stanton and Cooper, 1987). There is increasing evidence for a broad role for raf-1 in tumorigenesis, as evidenced by its ability to become activated by either protein kinase C α (PKCα) or the antiapoptotic protein Bcl-2 in a Ras-independent manner (Kolch et al., 1993; Wang et al., 1996). Importantly, raf mutations have been identified in a range of human tumors (Storm and Rapp, 1993). Raf is of course also activated in tumor cells containing enhanced GF signaling pathways and activating Ras mutations. Therefore, the collective evidence obtained to date suggests that Raf-1 may represent a viable anticancer drug target. However, the only Raf-directed approach for which early clinical data have been reported is that of a c-raf-1 antisense oligonucleotide (Stevenson et al., 1999; Yuen and Sikic, 2000). This agent was well tolerated, and suppression of target gene expression was observed in peripheral blood mononuclear cells (O'Dwyer et al., 1999). However, phase II data have not yet been published.

A Raf-1-interacting protein, RKIP, has also been recently reported (Yeung et al., 1999). This protein inhibits the phosphorylation and activation of MEK by Raf-1 and has also been shown to colocalize with Raf-1. However, until more is known regarding the mechanism by which RKIP disrupts the interaction between Raf-1 and MEK, its potential as a target for pharmacologic intervention in tumors remains unclear.

C. MEK Inhibitors Effectively Prevent Activation of MAPK

The MAPK pathway is considered essential for cellular growth. The family of MAPKs can be activated in response to a variety of extracellular stimuli (Lewis et al., 1998; Cobb and Goldsmith, 1995). ERK1 and ERK2, which were the first members of this family to be characterized, are activated by a cascade of phosphorylation events downstream from Ras (Fig.

1). After Ras interacts with and activates Raf1, it in turn phosphorylates and activates the dual-specificity kinases MEK1/MEK2 (MAP kinase kinase) on two distinct serine residues (Dent et al., 1992; Crews et al., 1992; Her et al., 1993). Activated MEK subsequently catalyzes the phosphorylation of ERK1 and ERK2 on both a tyrosine and a threonine residue (Anderson et al., 1990). No substrates for MEK have been identified other than ERK1 and ERK2 (Seger et al., 1992). Such tight selectivity coupled with the unique ability to phosphorylate both tyrosine and threonine residues points to this kinase playing a central role in integrating signals into the MAPK pathway. Furthermore, constitutive activation of MEK results in cellular transformation (Cowley et al., 1994; Mansour et al., 1994). Key studies have been carried out with the MEK inhibitor PD98059 showing that MEK inhibition not only impaired proliferation but also impacted a diverse array of cellular events, including differentiation, apoptosis, and angiogenesis (Dudley et al., 1995; Alessi et al., 1995; Pages et al., 1993; Pang et al., 1995; Finlay et al., 2000; Holmstrom et al., 1999; Elliceiri et al., 1998; Milanini et al., 1998). Based on these collective findings, MEK represents an attractive target for pharmacologic intervention in cancer.

An orally active small-molecule inhibitor of MEK has been reported providing in vivo validation for targeting MEK for anticancer drug design (Sebolt-Leopold et al., 1999). In this study, PD184352, which is a non-ATP-competitive, highly selective inhibitor of MEK, was found to significantly inhibit growth of colon carcinomas of both mouse and human origin. Importantly, efficacy was achieved with no signs of toxicity and was correlated with a reduction in the levels of activated MAPK in excised tumors. In addition to impairing tumor proliferation, PD184352 was found to block the disruption of cell–cell contact and motility required for invasion (Sebolt-Leopold et al., 1999). This finding is consistent with earlier reports indicating that hepatocyte growth factor (HGF) induces dispersion of epithelial cells by a Ras-dependent mechanism. The MEK/MAPK pathway is an essential mediator of HGF-induced cell scattering (Ridley et al., 1995; Herrera, 1998; Potempa and Ridley, 1998; Tanimura et al., 1998).

PD184352 (now called CI-1040) is presently entering phase I evaluation in cancer patients. As a mechanism-based therapy, the ultimate clinical utility of MEK inhibitors should be enhanced by the availability of a pharmacodynamic assay for monitoring inhibition of MAPK phosphorylation in ex vivo samples (Sebolt-Leopold et al., 1999). This assay not only allows for monitoring the degree of target suppression but has the potential to serve as a prognostic tool for identifying those patients most likely to derive benefit from treatment with a MEK inhibitor, as assessed by levels of activated MAPK in biopsied tumors. For example, overexpression of MAPK has been demonstrated in human breast cancer specimens and may be involved in both the onset and metastasis of this disease (Sivaraman et al., 1997).

The full scope of tumor types that rely on activation of MAPK for their proliferative and invasive phenotype remains to be determined. A study surveying more than 100 tumor cell lines and primary tumors of diverse origin for constitutive activation of the MAPK pathway suggests that the scope of tumors could be quite large (Hoshino *et al.*, 1999). In addition, it is conceivable that for those tumors that do not depend on the MAPK pathway to drive their proliferation, clinical benefit from MEK inhibition might still be derived by an antiangiogenic mechanism. Such speculation is based on the finding that sustained activation of MAPK in endothelial cells is a requirement for angiogenesis (Elliceiri *et al.*, 1998). Activated MAPK is not only important in angiogenic GF signaling, but it is also probably required for GF-induced secretion of angiogenic factors from tumors (Milanini *et al.*, 1998; Petit *et al.*, 1997).

While MEK has not been identified as an oncogene product, MEK is the focal point of many signal transduction mitogenic pathways mediated by proven oncogenes. The *ras* oncogene, which is mutated in a high proportion of tumors, as well as various oncogenic and angiogenic GF receptors that are frequently overexpressed in many cancers (e.g., erbB family of receptor tyrosine kinases), relies on activation of MEK and MAPK to produce proliferative signals. Thus, there exists compelling support for targeting the MEK/MAPK pathway in a mechanism-based approach to the development of new cancer therapies.

In summary, a number of interesting signaling antagonists targeting the Ras-MAPK pathway have been identified during the last decade. Pharmacologic hurdles have been overcome as we've witnessed their evolution into drug candidates exhibiting impressive efficacy in preclinical animal models. The more daunting task still confronts us as we begin to assess the full clinical utility of these various agents. It is important to remember that their full potential may not be appreciated until basic science leads us to the design of mechanistically driven combination regimens.

4. c-Src Kinase, Signal Transduction, Transformation, and Cancer

Another family of tyrosine kinases that may contain appropriate targets for therapeutic intervention in cancer is the nonreceptor, cytoplasmic c-Src kinase and other members of that kinase family. The amino acid sequence of this kinase family is composed of three major structural domains numbered from the C terminus. The first domain (<u>S</u>rc <u>H</u>omology 1, or SH1) encompasses the catalytic domain of the kinase while the SH2 domain (which contains tyrosine phosphorylation sites) and the SH3 domain (containing proline-rich regions) are likely involved in regulatory functions via intra- and intermolecular interactions (Thomas and Brugge, 1997;

Schwartzberg, 1998; Biscardi *et al.*, 1999b; Hubbard, 1999; Gonfloni *et al.*, 1999). Normal distribution of c-Src family kinases varies among tissue types, with the greatest abundance found in hematopoietic and neural tissue (Corey and Anderson, 1999).

A. c-Src and the Transformed Phenotype

The connection of c-Src kinase with cancer was initially supported by the observation that in cells derived from colon lesions ranging from premalignant adenomatous polyps through carcinoma *in situ* to metastatic adenocarcinoma, the specific activity of c-Src kinase was increased in comparison with that in normal colonic epithelium (Talamonti *et al.*, 1993; Iravani *et al.*, 1998). Other tumor types that have been found to express high levels of c-Src kinase include carcinomas of the breast (Verbeek *et al.*, 1996; Egan *et al.*, 1999), pancreas (Lutz *et al.*, 1998), and head and neck (van Oijen *et al.*, 1998).

Although apparently rare, src mutations have been described. In samples isolated from metastatic lesions, but not primary tumors, an activating mutation was identified in the C terminus of the protein that was found to be phenotypically transforming when transfected into normal cells. Transfection of this mutant src also caused an enhanced rate of metastasis in an experimental murine lung tumor metastasis assay (Irby *et al.*, 1999). A number of antisense approaches have also been used to implicate c-Src as an important facilitator of tumor cell proliferation *in vitro* and *in vivo*. c-Src antisense transfectants that expressed essentially no c-Src kinase activity did not form tumors in contrast to *c-src* sense transfected control cells (Staley *et al.*, 1997; Wiener, *et al.*, 1999).

B. c-Src Interactions with Proliferative and Survival Signaling Pathways

The mechanism by which c-Src influences tumor cell proliferation has been the subject of intense study. Although only limited evidence exists for the direct, single-agent, causative participation of overexpressed or overactive c-Src kinase in transforming events, many data support the participation of this kinase with other oncogenic signaling proteins and pathways (Fig. 1). EGF receptor (EGFr) family kinases, platelet-derived growth factor receptor (PDGFr) kinase, vascular endothelial growth factor receptor (VEGFr) kinase, and the proto-oncogenic tyrosine kinase receptor (Ret) have all been shown to interact with or require c-Src kinase activity for their signaling activity.

Transfection of ErbB2 into a human mammary epithelial cell line transformed those cells and resulted in increased specific activity of c-Src kinase. Clonogenicity of these transfected, transformed cells was markedly reduced by treatment with a c-Src kinase inhibitor, suggesting that the activity of c-Src kinase is an important contribution to maintenance of the transformed phenotype (Sheffield, 1998). Specific phosphorylation sites on EGFr have been shown to contribute to the association of c-Src kinase with EGFr upon EGF stimulation of the receptor with subsequent phosphorylations on EGFr likely catalyzed by c-Src. These phosphorylation events then resulted in recruitment of and further downstream signaling by other signaling molecules such as phosphatidylinositol 3-kinase (Sato *et al.*, 1995; Stover *et al.*, 1995). DNA synthesis in response to EGF stimulation may be dependent on c-Src kinase activity in at least some cells (Biscardi *et al.*, 1999a; Tice *et al.*, 1999; Roche *et al.*, 1995). c-Src has also been functionally associated with the PDGFr kinase by a number of investigators (Conway *et al.*, 1999; Gelderloos *et al.*, 1998). The implications of these interactions for tumor cell proliferation or angiogenesis are presently unclear since c-Src is not universally associated with PDGFr in all of its signaling functions (DeMali *et al.*, 1999; Klinghoffer *et al.*, 1999).

c-Src also appears to modulate the activity of the VEGF/VEGFr signaling pathway critical for tumor angiogenesis. Expression of VEGF has been found to correlate with c-Src kinase activity in colon tumor cells (Declan *et al.*, 1997). Furthermore, VEGF stimulation of Kaposi's sarcoma cells increased c-Src kinase activity, leading to increased cell proliferation that was blocked in the presence of an inhibitor of c-Src kinase (Munshi *et al.*, 2000). In an *in vivo* study, retroviral-mediated transfection of kinase-deleted c-Src prevented VEGF-stimulated vessel formation (Eliceiri *et al.*, 1999). Direct association of c-Src and the VEGF receptor Flk-1/KDR has also been noted (He *et al.*, 1999).

Another receptor tyrosine kinase that has been described that depends on c-Src kinase for its signaling activity to downstream effectors is Ret (Melillo *et al.*, 1999). The Ret receptor has been associated with multiple endocrine neoplasia syndromes. Ret stimulation induces c-Src activation, and a physical interaction between ret and c-Src via the c-Src SH2 domain has been demonstrated.

In addition to interactions of c-Src kinase with receptor tyrosine kinases, the association of c-Src has been made with the regulation of a transcriptional regulatory molecule involved in transformation. Members of the STAT (signal transducer and activator of transcription) family of molecules transduce mitogenic and cytokine-stimulated signals leading to cell proliferation (Bromberg *et al.*, 1999; Niu *et al.*, 1999). One of these STAT proteins, Stat3, has been shown to be activated by phosphorylation by c-Src kinase, an event that is required for its binding to DNA and thus its activity (Olayioye *et al.*, 1999; Cirri *et al.*, 1997; Schaefer *et al.*, 1999).

c-Src has also been shown to be associated with elements that regulate cellular adhesion and motility. Anchorage of cells to the extracellular matrix (ECM) is mediated through transmembrane receptors, called integrins, that are associated with cytoskeletal components. Intracellular structures called focal adhesions are sites of signal transduction from the ECM to the cell (Parsons and Parsons, 1997). Disruption of cell–cell and cell–ECM interactions is an important component of invasion and metastasis. Inhibition of c-Src appears to stabilize cell-to-cell contacts and reduce cell mobility in some models (Owens *et al.*, 2000; Felsenfeld *et al.*, 1999; Ishida *et al.*, 1999).

Although evidence for *src* as a human oncogene is lacking, the functional interaction of c-Src with a number of oncogene-based signal transduction pathways, its role in destabilizing cell–cell interactions, and the role of c-Src in STAT function suggest a number of opportunities for therapeutic intervention. The complex and ubiquitous biology of c-Src signaling also represents a significant challenge for those interested in the development of c-Src-based therapies.

5. Akt

The serine/threonine protein kinase known as Akt, PKB, or RAC-PK was discovered in 1991 by several groups. c-Akt is the cellular homologue of the v-Akt oncogene responsible for transformation by the AKT8 retrovirus originally isolated from a spontaneous murine thymoma (Bellacosa *et al.*, 1991; Staal, 1987). Concurrently, the protein was discovered by two groups searching for protein kinases (pKs) with kinase domains related to PKA and PKC. The kinase was termed PKB by Coffer and Woodgett (1991) and RAC-PK (for related to protein kinase A and C) by Jones *et al.* (1991). The kinase is no longer referred to as RAC-PK to avoid confusion with the Rho family GTPase Rac, but both Akt and PKB are still widely used. Three closely related isoforms of Akt have been described (Akt1, Akt2, and Akt3), which differ primarily at their carboxy termini. All isoforms contain an amino-terminal pleckstrin homology (PH) domain that binds phosphatidylinositol-3,4-bisphosphate [PI(3,4)P2] and phosphatidyinositol-3,4,5-trisphosphate [PI(3,4,5)P3] with high affinity (Franke *et al.*, 1997; Frech *et al.*, 1997; James *et al.*, 1996). These phosphoinositide second messengers are generated through activation of PI 3-kinases by growth factors, hormones, and G-protein agonists, and Akt has been shown to be one of the primary effectors in PI 3-kinase signaling. Interaction of the PH domain of Akt with PI(3,4)P2 or PI(3,4,5)P3 results in translocation of Akt to the plasma membrane, bringing Akt in proximity to upstream activating protein kinases (Andjelkovic *et al.*, 1997; Currie *et al.*, 1999; Klippel *et al.*, 1997; Meier *et al.*, 1997; Sable *et al.*, 1998; Zhang and Vik, 1997). Activation of Akt occurs through phosphorylation of residues Thr308 within the P loop of the kinase domain and Ser473 in a hydrophobic region near the carboxy terminus (Alessi *et al.*, 1996). The most well-characterized activator of Akt is 3-phosphoinositide-dependent protein kinase (PDK-1)

(Alessi *et al.,* 1997; Stokoe *et al.,* 1997), a serine/threonine kinase which also contains a PH domain and a kinase domain related to PKA and PKC. PDK-1 appears to be responsible for phosphorylation of Thr308 of Akt following PI 3-kinase activation. The identity of the Ser473 kinase remains uncertain, although data exist suggesting that under certain conditions PDK-1 may phosphorylate this site as well (Balendran *et al.,* 1999). Ser473 has also been reported to be an autophosphorylation site (Toker and Newton, 2000). In addition, Akt can be activated by agonists of the PKA pathway that increase intracellular calcium through phosphorylation of Thr308 by calcium/calmodulin-dependent kinase kinase (Sable *et al.,* 1997).

A. Akt as a Promoter of Cellular Survival

Akt is a critical mediator of cell survival. This was first shown for IGF-1-dependent survival of cultured cerebellar granule cells (Dudek *et al.,* 1997), and many subsequent studies have shown that activated Akt protects cells from apoptosis induced by ultraviolet radiation, ionizing radiation, GF withdrawal, detachment from ECM, and cell cycle irregularities (Blair *et al.,* 1999; Chen *et al.,* 1998; Crowder and Freeman, 1998; Dudek *et al.,* 1997; Eves *et al.,* 1998; Gerber *et al.,* 1998; Hausler *et al.,* 1998; Kauffmann Zeh *et al.,* 1997; Kennedy *et al.,* 1997; Khwaja *et al.,* 1997; Kulik *et al.,* 1997; Kulik and Weber, 1998; Philpott *et al.,* 1997; Rohn *et al.,* 1998; Songyang *et al.,* 1997; Xiong and Parsons, 1997). Dominant negative forms of Akt block the ability of GFs to promote survival (Dudek *et al.,* 1997; Kitamura *et al.,* 1998; van Weeren *et al.,* 1998). Identification of relevant substrates for Akt has been facilitated by the definition of a consensus sequence for phosphorylation by Akt (RXRXXS/T-F/L) (Datta *et al.,* 1999). There is evidence that Akt phosphorylates the proapoptotic protein BAD at Ser136 (Blume Jensen *et al.,* 1998; Datta *et al.,* 1997; del Peso *et al.,* 1997), resulting in sequestration of BAD by 14-3-3 proteins (Muslin *et al.,* 1996) and preventing the binding of BAD to BCL-X$_L$. It has been reported that caspase-9 activity is inhibited through phosphorylation by Akt, perhaps explaining observations that Akt can promote survival downstream of cytochrome *c.* Glycogen synthase kinase-3 (GSK-3) is another substrate for Akt, leading to inhibition of GSK-3 activity (Cross *et al.,* 1995; Hajduch *et al.,* 1998; Muslin *et al.,* 1996; Pap and Cooper, 1998; van Weeren *et al.,* 1998), accumulation of β-catenin, and activation of *myc* transcription (Franke *et al.,* 1997; Kikuchi, 2000).

Although phosphorylation of substrates such as BAD and caspase-9 indicates the importance of posttranslational modification in promoting survival, it is clear that GF-regulated gene expression affects the capacity of cells to undergo apoptosis. In this regard, members of the Forkhead family of transcription factors are substrates for Akt. Akt has been found to phosphorylate the human Forkhead family members FKHRL1 FKHR, and AFX (Biggs *et al.,* 1999; Brunet *et al.,* 1999; Kops *et al.,* 1999; Tang *et al.,* 1999). Phosphorylation by Akt regulates the subcellular localization of these proteins, preventing their translocation to the nucleus. Forkhead-dependent transcription appears necessary for induction of the apoptotic program in response to certain conditions. The *FasL* gene is one important proapoptotic gene up-regulated by Forkhead factors (Brunet *et al.,* 1999) and AFX transcriptionally activates the gene for the p27kip1 cell cycle inhibitor protein (Medema *et al.,* 2000). It has also been shown recently that Akt up-regulates Bcl-2 expression through the cAMP response element binding protein (Pugazhenthi *et al.,* 2000).

Several recent studies underscore the role of Akt in antiapoptotic signaling through NF-κB. Activated Ras has been shown to activate NF-κB (Downward, 1998; Kane *et al.,* 1999) through PI 3-kinase and Akt-dependent mechanisms, and this pathway is required for the survival-promoting effects of Ras. Akt has also been shown to positively regulate NF-κB activity in fibroblasts (Romashkova and Makarov, 1999), Jurkat cells (Kane *et al.,* 1999), and kidney cells (Ozes *et al.,* 1999). Akt-dependent activation of NF-κB appears to be mediated through effects on I κβ kinase, leading to degradation of the NF-κB inhibitor I-κB (Kane *et al.,* 1999).

B. Akt and Cancer

The initial discovery of Akt as a retroviral oncogene and the involvement of Akt in the promotion of cellular survival point to a more general role for Akt in oncogenesis. Tumor cells must evolve resistance to apoptosis triggered by a variety of conditions that would destroy normal cells. These include inappropriate activation of oncogenes, DNA damage, loss of attachment to substratum, hypoxia, and attack from the immune system, exposure to cytokines and Fas ligand, and others. Evidence suggests that increased signaling through Akt would give a clear survival advantage to tumor cells in the face of these challenges. Indeed, the Akt gene is amplified and Akt activity up-regulated in many tumor cell types. Akt1 is overexpressed in 20% of gastric adenocarinomas and in human breast cancer cells lines, particularly those overexpressing HER2 (Ahmad *et al.,* 1999; Cheng *et al.,* 1992, 1996; Liu *et al.,* 1999; Staal, 1987). In breast cancer cell lines Akt1 appears to be responsible for phosphorylation of BRCA1 (Altiok *et al.,* 1999), perhaps interfering with translocation of BRCA1 to the nucleus. Elevated Akt1 activity was also reported in about 5% of ovarian tumors and Akt2 has been shown to be amplified with high frequency in ovarian and pancreatic tumors (Cheng *et al.,* 1996; Ruggeri *et al.,* 1998; Yuan *et al.,* 2000). The kinase activity of Akt2 was activated in 36% of ovarian tumor specimens, with most of the tumors being high-grade stage III and IV (Yuan *et al.,* 2000).

Amplification of the Akt2 gene was found in 20% of pancreatic ductal adenomas (Ruggeri et al., 1998). Recently, Akt3 was found to be up-regulated in estrogen-receptor-deficient breast cancers and androgen-independent prostate cancer cell lines (Nakatani et al., 1999). The enzymatic activity of Akt3 was 20- to 60-fold higher in these cells relative to controls and correlated with increased levels of Akt3 mRNA and protein. Elevation of Akt activity has been shown to mediate resistance to tumor cells to chemotherapeutic agents such as paclitaxel (Page et al., 2000) and daunorubicin (Plo et al., 1999) and to contribute to resistance to hypoxic stress (Zhong et al., 2000).

Inactivating mutations in the PTEN/MMAC1 tumor suppressor gene also result in activation of Akt (Myers et al., 1998; Wu et al., 1998). The PTEN (phosphatase and tensin homologue deleted on chromosome 10) protein dephosphorylates the PI 3-kinase effector product PI(3,4,5)P3 at the 3′ position, thereby inactivating it. PTEN inactivation in tumor cells causes increased intracellular levels of PI(3,4,5)P3 and general enhancement of PI 3-kinase signaling. PTEN-deficient tumor cell lines and tumors derived from PTEN knockout mice display high basal levels of Akt activity and are resistant to numerous apoptotic-inducing stimuli (Stambolic et al., 1998; Suzuki et al., 1998). Ectopic expression of normal PTEN protein reduces Akt activity and restores sensitivity to apoptotic stimuli. Deletions at the PTEN locus of chromosome 10 have been found in glioblastoma multiforme and anaplastic astrocytomas as well as in prostate, endometrial, renal, small cell lung carcinoma, melanoma, and meningioma (Li et al., 1998; Steck et al., 1997, 1999). Homozygous inactivation of PTEN occurs in more than 30% of glioblastomas, more than 50% of melanomas and advanced prostate cancers, 30–50% of endometrial cancers, and about 10% of breast cancer lines (Guldberg et al., 1997; Rasheed et al., 1997; Risinger et al., 1997; Ruggeri et al., 1998; Suzuki et al., 1998; Tashiro et al., 1997; Wang et al., 1998). Mutation of PTEN appears to be one of the most common genetic defects in human cancer, occurring with a frequency approaching that of p53. Three rare autosomal dominant cancer syndromes are caused by germ line mutations in PTEN. These are Cowden disease (Liaw et al., 1997), Bannayan–Zonana syndrome (Marsh et al., 1997), and Lhermitte–Duclos disease (Liaw et al., 1997). Females carrying these mutations show a 30–50% incidence of breast cancer, with increased risk for glioblastomas, and thyroid cancer. A recent study also shows that germ line mutations in PTEN are more prevalent than thought previously, occurring in the general population at a rate of about 5% (De Vivo et al., 2000).

Within the past several years tumor-induced angiogenesis has become recognized as a potential target for innovative anticancer therapy. Numerous studies point to the importance of Akt in this process. Survival of endothelial cells is critical for angiogenesis, and key mediators of endothelial cell survival and proliferation, such as VEGF and angiopoietin-1 (Ang-1), promote survival through activation (Fujio and Walsh, 1999; Gerber et al., 1998; Papapetropoulos et al., 2000). In addition to its potential effects of Akt on BAD and caspase-9 in these cells, Akt has been shown to phosphorylate endothelial nitric oxide synthease leading to persistent activation of this enzyme (Dimmeler et al., 1999; Fulton et al., 1999). An extensive body of literature indicates an essential role for nitric oxide in neovascularization (Murohara et al., 1998; Papapetropoulos et al., 1997). Ang-1 treatment of endothelial cells has also been shown to enhance endothelial cell survival through up-regulation of the apoptosis inhibitor survivin (Papapetropoulos et al., 2000). Akt is activated by hypoxia and is responsible for hypoxic induction of VEGF (Mazure et al., 1997; Zhong et al., 2000) through stabilization of the transcriptional activator hypoxia-inducible factor-1α (Zundel et al., 2000). Taken together, these results suggest that inhibitors of Akt would negatively impact oncogenesis through effects on both the tumor cells and the tumor vasculature.

6. Nuclear Hormone Receptors as Targets for Cancer Therapy

Nuclear hormone receptors (NHRs) were first identified about 25 years ago as the high-affinity receptors for the steroid hormones, such as estrogen, testosterone, and cortisone (Yamamoto, 1985). Shortly afterward, other lipophilic hormones, such as thyroid hormone, vitamin D, and vitamin A (retinoic acid), were shown to bind to very similar NHRs, and it became apparent that there is an NHR superfamily, with several subfamilies (Evans, 1988). With the onset of cloning techniques aimed at the most highly conserved parts of the receptors, in excess of 150 members of this family have now been described (Beato et al., 1995; Giguere, 1999; Robertson et al., 1997). The NHRs appear to be among the most important controllers of organogenesis and cellular fate, and as such have very powerful effects on cellular proliferation and differentiation. With such properties it is not surprising that they have been implicated in several types of cancer, and that both positive and negative manipulation of NHR activity is being used in cancer therapy.

A. Structure of Nuclear Hormone Receptors

The NHRs are highly modular proteins in the 500- to 600-residue range, and are traditionally divided into several domains, which appear to fold independently of one another (Kumar and Thompson, 1999). The A/B domain is usually the most diverse, and may have an N-terminal activation domain (AF-1) plus domains involved in unique protein–protein interactions. The C domain is the most highly conserved and contains two zinc fingers, which make up the DNA binding domain (DBD). Rather than binding to a diverse array of DNA NHR response elements (NREs), most NHRs bind to hexanucleotide sequences that are AGGTCA or AGAACA or some minor variant thereof. The C domain also appears to contain a weak dimerization domain. The short D domain appears to contain a nuclear localization signal (NLS), a site for binding corepressor proteins, and acts as a hinge domain to the E domain. This domain, which appears to have the same overall gross structure regardless of sequence homology, contains a ligand binding domain (LBD), ligand-dependent dimerization domains, another NLS, and a ligand-dependent transcriptional activator function, AF-2. The C terminus contains a short F domain, which is not highly conserved. Isolated LBDs generally bind ligands with very similar affinity to the full length proteins. Several LBDs have been crystallized, some with agonists or antagonists bound, giving very valuable and consistent clues as to the molecular mechanisms of both the proteins and the drugs that interact with them (Brzozowski et al., 1997; Weatherman et al., 1999).

B. Mechanism of Action of the Nuclear Hormone Receptors

At present, it appears likely that many NHRs will be multifunctional devices with many modes of control and multiple utilities (perhaps along the lines of p53), but our understanding of these processes is very incomplete. Therefore, this chapter will contain a synopsis of the classically accepted and proven mode of action of NHRs, with the caveats that it is probably only a small facet of the real picture and that countermanding examples are already known for virtually everything described below.

Unliganded NHRs can exist as monomers in the cytosol, where they bind hydrophobic ligands, which have diffused into the cell through the plasma membrane (Beato, 1989) (Fig. 1). Once ligand is bound, the receptor adopts a new conformation exposing its NLS, which allows it access to the nucleus, where the NHR can bind to its NREs, which are almost always present in tandem (Beato et al., 1989). This arrangement leads to the NHRs binding to the NRE as dimers, and in fact the overall specificity of binding is determined largely by the distance between the two hexanucleotides (usually 1–5 base pairs) and by their orientation relative to one another (Kurokawa et al., 1993; Perlmann et al., 1993). Many NHRs bind as homodimers, including the classical steroid receptors, whereas others bind as heterodimers, e.g., VDR (vitamin D receptor), TR (thyroid receptor), RAR (retinoic acid receptor), and PPAR, (peroxisomal proliferator activated receptor), almost always with a member of the RXR (retinoid X receptor) family, which are receptors for 9-cis-retinoic acid. Once the appropriate agonist-bound dimeric complex is established on the DNA it adopts a conformation that exposes binding sites (the AF domains) for various coactivator proteins. There are already about 30 coactivator proteins known (Robyr et al., 2000), and they seem to have two important functions. The first is that they contain many protein–protein interaction surfaces, which have very important roles in recruiting TAF proteins to the transcriptional complex, stabilizing it as it is formed, leading eventually to recruitment of the TATA-binding protein, RNA polymerases, and gene transcription (Glass and Rosenfeld, 2000). The second function is that the coactivators either contain themselves or recruit the all-important histone acetyltransferases (HATs). These enzymes acetylate the ε-amino functionalities of lysines in histones (Hassig et al., 1998; Struhl, 1998). This causes the histones to lose their overall positive charge and destabilizes their interaction with the negatively charged phosphate backbone of DNA, leading to the disassembly of the nucleosomes, making the DNA accessible to the transcriptional machinery and thus allowing gene transcription to occur.

The most important exception to this picture is the fact that many NHRs can be found in the nucleus, bound to the NREs when unliganded (Fondell et al., 1993). There may well be cases where such binding is unproductive, simply having no effect on basal transcription from the downstream gene, but usually such unliganded NREs are bound to a second class of proteins, the corepressors. These compounds deny access to the coactivators and prevent the formation of transcriptional complexes. They also contain or recruit histone deacetylases, which unsurprisingly lead to reassembly of nucleosomes and complete silencing of the genes.

Some of the other variants that one sees on the classical model include NHRs that bind to DNA as monomers; NHRs that are constitutively activated when unliganded and are switched off by ligand binding; NHRs that are activated or deactivated by reversible posttranslational modification, usually phosphorylation, but possibly also HAT-mediated acetylation (Cenni and Picard, 1999); and splicing variants that may have lost the ability to bind to DNA or that may only be capable of binding either coactivators or corepressors.

C. Tissue-Selective Ligands

Additional levels of complexity have been introduced by the study of artificial ligands. Initially both agonists and antagonists were sought, especially those of estrogen, where agonists were expected to be fertility drugs or contraceptives, and antagonists were expected to have anticancer activity, especially in breast cancer. Although both pure agonists and pure antagonists were found, it became obvious that many compounds could act as agonists or antagonists, depending on the tissue being treated. For example, tamoxifen, which is used to treat patients with estrogen-dependent breast cancer, is clearly an estrogen antagonist in most such breast cancers but is an estrogen agonist in uterus, causing a hyperplasia that can be blocked by a pure antagonist (Dhingra, 1999). This has led to the concept of selective estrogen receptor modulators (SERMs), which postulates that the estrogen receptor (ER) can bind ligands that induce conformations different from the natural liganded or unliganded conformations, and that such unnatural conformations can behave differently in different settings. If one assumes that the unliganded ER binds both corepressors R_A and R_B but no coactivators, whereas the estrogen-bound ER binds no corepressors but binds two coactivators C_A and C_B, then in tissue A (which expresses only R_A and C_A) the liganded or unliganded ER should have the same effect as in tissue B (which expresses only R_B and C_B). If one had a ligand that induced an artificial conformation of the receptor which allowed for the unbinding of R_A but not R_B, and the recruitment of C_A but not C_B, such a compound would act as an estrogen agonist in tissue A but as an estrogen antagonist in tissue B. Although such a happenstance may seem unlikely, most aspects of this model have been demonstrated. For example, x-ray crystal structures of raloxifene and tamoxifen in the LBD of ERβ clearly show differences in protein conformation from the same receptor binding estradiol (Brzozowski *et al.*, 1997), and the major change in conformation comes in a helix known to be important in binding coactivators. Furthermore, association assays (CARLAs) show that some of the coactivators normally recruited to ER by estradiol are still associated with it, but others are no longer associated with the liganded receptor. The reality will probably turn out to be more complex than even this suggests, as different promotor elements in the same cell type may also affect coactivator recruitment, so that a ligand may act as an agonist on one response element and an antagonist on another in the same cell. Although such complexity has been best demonstrated for estrogen ligands, there is little reason to doubt that such mixed agonist and antagonist activity will be inducible at many of the NHRs.

D. Use of NHR Agonists and Antagonists in Cancer Therapy

Generally speaking, the manipulation of NHRs in cancer treatment is designed to reduce the proliferative rate of the tumor. Whether it is designed to increase or decrease transcription from NHR-controlled genes depends on the effects that such transcription has in the tissue from which the tumor is derived. The two extremes are probably best represented by the roles of retinoids in acute promyelocytic leukemia (APL) and estrogens in breast cancer. APL usually involves a chromosomal translocation, causing a chimeric RAR-PML protein to be produced. This acts as a dominant negative retinoic acid receptor, and prevents transcription of retinoic-acid-controlled genes, which would normally force terminal differentiation of proleukemic blasts, thus repressing their ability to proliferate (Ruthardt *et al.*, 1997). By contrast, in the breast epithelial tissue, from which most breast cancers arise, estrogen plays a strongly mitogenic role, and early breast tumors are often very responsive to hormone therapy, which involves compounds which are estrogen antagonists in breast tissue, such as tamoxifen (Grese and Dodge, 1998). Studies suggest that tamoxifen may also be used in a chemopreventative mode to reduce the occurrence of breast cancer (Radmacher and Simon, 2000).

E. Some Nuclear Hormone Receptors Targeted by Antagonists in Cancer Therapy

1. Estrogen Receptor

The relationship between estrogen and breast cancer may be one of the most intensely studied in all oncology. Correlations between breast cancer and early menarche, late menopause, high endogenous estrogen levels, and the taking of therapeutic estrogens have all been established, and all point to the conclusion that breast cancer risk increases with increasing estrogen exposure. The estrogen antagonist tamoxifen proved efficacious against about 50% of breast cancers, which express estrogen receptor (ER), and extensive studies have shown that tamoxifen therapy for 5 years produces a 5-year delay in cancer recurrence but that 10 years of treatment does not significantly extend that delay. About 50% of breast cancers at diagnosis do not express appreciable levels of ER, and these ER-negative tumors have a poorer prognosis than ER-positive tumors, with shorter times to relapse and shorter survival times. There are several possible causes of the rise of tamoxifen resistance. The most common cause is probably the repressed tumor selecting slowly for a slower growing but ER-negative fraction, although mutation may also allow the development of ER-negative status. Mechanisms of estrogen negativity are not well understood; however, it does appear in many cases that the ER is still present in low amounts, and that signaling through it may be both intense and ligand independent. One mechanism involves the oncogene erbB2 (see above), which activates a signaling pathway leading to a phosphorylated ER that binds to ER response elements, leading to ligand-independent transcription. Evidently the binding of tamoxifen is not sufficient to block the adoption of an active conformation by the phosphorylated ER, but more potent antagonists, such as ICI 182780 (Wakeling, 1993), the "pure antiestrogen," sometimes have a therapeutic effect in tamoxifen-resistant, "ER-negative" tumors. Another mechanism involves the induction of breast cancer antiestrogen resistance (BCAR) genes, which are adaptor-like proteins of currently unknown function. The BCAR-1 gene is widely expressed, but its overexpression is detected in ER-positive tamoxifen-resistant tumors, and its overexpression in MCF-7 cells makes them tamoxifen (and ICI 182780) resistant (Brinkman *et al.*, 2000).

2. Progesterone Receptor

Although not as important a breast mitogen as estrogen, progesterone appears to be a risk factor for breast cancer. In most hormone replacement therapies (HRTs) a progestin is given along with the estrogen to counteract estrogenic side effects in the uterus. Such combined HRT results in a significantly larger increase in breast cancer risk than does administration of a pure estrogen (Ross *et al.*, 2000). The antiprogestin RU-486—the "abortion pill"—was originally developed for breast cancer therapy, for which it has shown promise in clinical trials (Koide, 1998). However, the controversy surrounding it has impeded full evaluation of this indication.

3. Androgen Receptor

Testosterone is a known mitogen in the prostate, and prostate cancer is the most common cancer in aging men. Those surgically castrated before puberty never develop prostate cancer, and orchiectomy is one of the standard treatments for prostate cancer. Like breast cancer, a large percentage of prostate cancers are at diagnosis hormone refractory, expressing very little androgen receptor (AR). Antiandrogens, such as cyproterone (Barradell and Foulds, 1994) and bicalutamide (Casodex) (Kolvenbag *et al.*, 1998), can be used in hormone-positive prostate cancers and can appreciably slow progression of the disease in such cases. But once again by analogy with breast cancers, prostate cancers tend to become androgen negative and hormone refractory upon prolonged treatment. The presence of erbB2 in many prostate tumors raises the possibility that the same mechanisms are involved in many hormone resistance cases in both tumor types.

F. Some Nuclear Hormone Receptors Targeted by Agonists in Cancer Therapy

1. Retinoic Acid Receptors (RARs, RXRs)

As discussed above, in APL genetic translocations can lead to suppression of retinoid differentiative signaling in lymphoblasts in the granulocyte lineage, to an undifferentiated phenotype, which continues to proliferate. The PML-RARα fusion protein can still bind to retinoic acid receptor (RAR) response elements and can recruit corepressors to these sites, preventing gene transcription. Supraphysiologic concentrations of retinoic acid agonists can lead to the normal retinoid differentiative signaling and thus to amelioration or cure of the leukemia (Smith *et al.*, 1992). Although this is suggestive that the affinity of the receptor for agonists is reduced by the fusion and that this is being compensated for by increasing the concentration of the ligand, current evidence is not equivocal here, as, for example, RARα[-/-] KO mice develop granulocytes normally. Other genetic translocations

with RARα lead to fusion proteins that are insensitive to retinoid therapy (Slack and Gallagher, 1999), and loss of RARβ has been implicated in hepatocellular carcinoma and oral leukoplakia (Lotan, 1997). The latter disease can be successfully managed with retinoids. As retinoids are powerful differentiative agents, one might expect them to produce differentiation in cancers, where disregulated retinoid signaling is not directly implicated in carcinogenesis. Both breast and prostate tumor lines have been shown to be sensitive to retinoids. As the retinoid X receptors (RXRs) are obligate heterodimeric partners for a number of NHRs that have been targeted for cancer therapy, one might expect RXR ligands to have potential in this field also (Benoit *et al.*, 1999), and their use is certainly under intense preclinical scrutiny. Experimentally, retinoids also show cancer chemopreventative properties, due to activation of RARs/RXRs and probably to their antioxidant properties also. However, a large clinical trial involving vitamin A supplementation for smokers had to be abandoned when the lung cancer rate in the treated group was found to be greater than that of the control group—a finding that is currently unexplained. It may be due to the antioxidant effects of the vitamin suppressing apoptosis of newly transformed cells, which involves various reactive oxygen intermediates.

2. Peroxisome Proliferator Activated Receptor

There are three subfamilies of PPAR: PPARα, PPARβ/δ, and PPARγ. All of these receptors appear to be involved in regulation of lipid metabolism, and many of their natural ligands are lipids or lipid-like molecules (Gelman *et al.*, 1999). All of the receptor subtypes have been implicated in cancer—α for hepatocellular cancer mediated by peroxisomal proliferators (Corton *et al.*, 2000), β/δ because of possible ties to nonsteroidal anti-inflammatory drug mechanisms of action (He *et al.*, 1999), and γ due to its prodifferentiative effects. One of the effects of PPARγ stimulation is the differentiation of preadipocytes to adipocytes, and a thiazolinedione PPARγ agonist Rezulin (Pfizer) has been shown in a clinical trial to suppress liposarcoma, presumably by forcing the proliferating immature adipocytes that make up the tumor into terminal differentiation (Demetri *et al.*, 1999). Preclinical models suggest that the prodifferentiative effects may extend to other tissues, such as prostate (Kubota *et al.*, 1998) and breast (Mueller *et al.*, 1998). PPARγ activators are being investigated for both indications.

7. Implications for Drug Discovery and Development

The identification of these and other specific molecular targets for anticancer drug design and the delineation of the signaling pathways in which they act not only raises the possibility of qualitatively novel cancer therapies but also has important implications for the drug discovery and development processes themselves. Historically the cancer drug discovery process has consisted of an *in vitro* assay of cell death or enzyme function followed by either efficacy testing in syngeneic (or xenograft) models or, less frequently, pharmacokinetic profiling designed to estimate exposure relative to that assumed to be active from the *in vitro* studies. This paradigm placed a heavy emphasis on efficacy testing, which can consume large amounts of limited drug supplies, manpower, and vivarium space. In addition, these studies are time consuming, requiring a month to several months for a single experiment. Drug discovery is a largely iterative process, and once activity was confirmed, the usual result was many cycles of synthesis and testing to improve various attributes of the chemical series, often without an informed focus on the root causes of the perceived deficiencies.

Most of the targets described above directly modify specific substrates in ways that can be measured directly from tumor tissues. In other cases, target-specific effects several steps removed from a direct substrate can be informative because of our knowledge of the signaling pathways involved. Application of these pharmacodynamic readouts offers the potential of dramatically increasing the speed of drug evaluation in the preclinical drug discovery cycle. We have made extensive use of pharmacodynamic readouts of substrate modification by our signal transduction targets for the larger part of the past decade (Fry *et al.*, 1994, 1998; Sebolt-Leopold *et al.*, 1999). Our current drug candidate evaluation paradigm now typically consists of the following steps: (1) biochemical assay of enzyme activity and counterscreening for specificity against similar enzymes; (2) pharmacodynamic assessment of potency and duration of cellular effects in cell culture; (3) pharmacodynamic assessment of both potency and duration of effect in human tumor xenografts coupled with tolerance testing in small numbers of animals; and finally (4) efficacy testing on the very few compounds that are passed through to this point. Pharmacokinetic analysis usually accompanies the activities of step 3, but if a robust pharmacodynamic assay is available, compounds can often be successfully optimized in the absence of extensive pharmacokinetic data. The effort involved in step 3 usually generates a matrix of dose-response and time course of drug effect data in tumors from treated animals simultaneously with testing to grossly establish tolerated levels on repeated dosing. Reliable and informative data for *in vivo* assessment of potential therapeutic effect can be generated with three- to fourfold fewer animals. In addition, the pharmacodynamic/tolerance experiments take less than a week to complete, compared with an average of 8–12 weeks for efficacy experiments with active compounds in human tumor xenograft systems. Finally, the dose potency and duration of response data generated in the

pharmacodynamic assays can be used to optimize protocols for the efficacy testing, reducing animal waste and the need for repeated experiments because of missed dose ranges, etc. The power and speed of this approach is a clear advantage afforded to those who work with targets similar to those delineated above, and we now routinely optimize inhibitors of targets proven to generate *in vivo* efficacy on the basis of the pharmacodynamic assays.

It should be clear that a similar approach might be taken in clinical trials via pre- and posttreatment biopsy of tumors. A significant application of this data would be to set relevant dose levels for phase II clinical trials. The preclinical discovery of highly specific inhibitors of selected targets (Fry *et al.*, 1994, 1998; Sebolt-Leopold *et al.*, 1999) suggests the possibility of a concentration or dose threshold that delivers total suppression of the desired target. For targets that are thought to offer tumor-specific pharmacologic effects, it is not clear that phase II trials should be carried out at the traditionally sought maximum tolerated dose from phase I trials if suppression of the primary target can be demonstrated with a pharmacodynamic readout at lower and better tolerated dose levels.

The recent expansion of our understanding of the signaling pathways involved in the dysregulation of human tumors has led to the identification of a multitude of clinically unprecedented targets for anticancer drug discovery. In addition, new paradigms for the drug discovery process offer the promise of increased preclinical throughput and precision. Combined these developments portend a future filled with promise for the rapid development of qualitatively different therapies for cancer. These will likely offer opportunities not only for curative therapy in the acute setting but also for management of cancer as a chronic disease involving the use of very well-tolerated agents, and even the possibility of chemoprevention therapies for use in high-risk patients.

References

Adjei, A. A., Davis, J. N., Erlichman, C., Svingen, P. A., and Kaufmann, S. H. (2000). Comparison of potential markers of farnesyltransferase inhibition. *Clin. Cancer. Res.* **23**, 18–25.

Ahmad, S., Singh, N., and Glazer, R. I. (1999). Role of AKT1 in 17beta-estradiol- and insulin-like growth factor I (IGF-I)-dependent proliferation and prevention of apoptosis in MCF-7 breast carcinoma cells. *Biochem. Pharmacol.* **58**, 425–430.

Alessi, D. R., Andjelkovic, M., Caudwell, B., Cron, P., Morrice, N., Cohen, P., and Hemmings, B. A. (1996). Mechanism of activation of protein kinase B by insulin and IGF-1. *EMBO J.* **15**, 6541–6551.

Alessi, D. R., Cuenda, A., Cohen, P., Dudley, D. T., and Saltiel, A. R. (1995). PD 098059 is a specific inhibitor of the activation of mitogen-activated protein kinase kinase in vitro and in vivo. *J. Biol. Chem.* **270**, 27489–27494.

Alessi, D. R., Deak, M., Casamayor, A., Caudwell, F. B., Morrice, N., Norman, D. G., Gaffney, P., Reese, C. B., MacDougall, C. N., Harbison, D., Ashworth, A., and Bownes, M. (1997). 3-Phosphoinositide-dependent protein kinase-1 (PDK1): Structural and functional homology with the Drosophila DSTPK61 kinase. *Curr. Biol.* **7,** 776–789.

Altiok, S., Batt, D., Altiok, N., Papautsky, A., Downward, J., Roberts, T. M., and Avraham, H. (1999). Heregulin induces phosphorylation of BRCA1 through phosphatidylinositol 3-kinase/AKT in breast cancer cells. *J. Biol. Chem.* **274,** 32274–32278.

Anderson, N. G., Maller, J. L., Tonks, N. K., and Sturgill, T. W. (1990). Requirement for integration of signals from two distinct phosphorylation pathways for activation of MAP kinase. *Nature* **343,** 651–653.

Andjelkovic, M., Alessi, D. R., Meier, R., Fernandez, A., Lamb, N. J., Frech, M., Cron, P., Cohen, P., Lucocq, J. M., and Hemmings, B. A. (1997). Role of translocation in the activation and function of protein kinase B. *J. Biol. Chem.* **272,** 31515–31524.

Bacus, S. S., Zelnick, C. R., Plowman, G., and Yarden, Y. (1994). Expression of the erbB-2 family of growth factor receptors and their ligands in breast cancers—Implication for tumor biology and clinical behavior. *Am. J. Clin. Pathol.* **102,** S13-S24.

Balendran, A., Casamayor, A., Deak, M., Paterson, A., Gaffney, P., Currie, R., Downes, C. P., and Alessi, D. R. (1999). PDK1 acquires PDK2 activity in the presence of a synthetic peptide derived from the carboxyl terminus of PRK2. *Curr. Biol.* **9,** 393–404.

Barradell, L. B. and Faulds, D. (1994). Cyproterone. A review of its pharmacology and therapeutic efficacy in prostate cancer. *Drugs Aging* **5,** 59–80.

Bartlett, J. M., Langdon, S. P., Simpson, B. J., Stewart, M., Datsaros, D., Sismondi, P., Love, S., Scott, W. N., Williams, A. R., Lessells, A. M., Macleod, K. G., Smyth, J. F., and Miller, W. R. (1996). The prognostic value of epidermal growth factor receptor mRNA expression in primary ovarian cancer. *Br. J. Cancer* **73,** 301–306.

Baselga, J., Herbst, R., LoRusso, P., Rischin, D., Ranson, M., Plummer, R., Raymond, E., Maddox, A., Kaye, S. B., Kieback, D. G., Harris, A., and Ochs, J. (2000). Continuous administration of ZD 1839 (Iressa), a novel oral epidermal growth factor receptor tyrosine kinase inhibitor (EGFR-TKI), in patients with five selected tumor types: evidence of activity and good tolerability. *Proc. Am. Assoc. Clin. Oncol.* **19,** 177a.

Beato, M. (1989). Gene regulation by steroid hormones. *Cell.* **56,** 335–344.

Beato, M., Chalepakis, G., Schauer, M., and Slater, E. P. (1989). DNA regulatory elements for steroid hormones. *J. Steroid Biochem.* **32,** 737–748.

Beato, M., Herrlich, P., and Schutz, G. (1995). Steroid hormone receptors: Many actors in search of a plot. *Cell* **83,** 851–857.

Bellacosa, A., Testa, J. R., Staal, S. P., and Tsichlis, P. N. (1991). A retroviral oncogene, akt, encoding a serine-threonine kinase containing an SH2-like region. *Science* **354,** 274–277.

Ben-Levy, R., Paterson, H. F., Marshall, C. J., and Yarden, Y. (1994). A single autophosphorylation site confers oncogenicity to the neu/erbB-2 receptor and enables coupling to the MAP kinase pathway. *EMBO J.* **13,** 3302–3311.

Benoit, G., Altucci, L., Flexor, M., Ruchaud, S., Lillehaug, J., Raffelsberger, W., Gronemeyer, H., and Lanotte, M. (1999). RAR-independent RXR signaling induces t(15;17) leukemia cell maturation. *EMBO J.* **18,** 7011–7018.

Biggs, W. H., III, Meisenhelder, J., Hunter, T., Cavenee, W. K., and Arden, K. C. (1999). Protein kinase B/Akt-mediated phosphorylation promotes nuclear exclusion of the winged helix transcription factor FKHR1. *Proc. Natl. Acad. Sci. USA* **96,** 7421–7426.

Biscardi, J. S., Maa, M.-C., Tice, D. A., Cox, M. E., Leu, T.-H., and Parsons, S. J. (1999a). c-Src mediated phosphorylation of the epidermal growth factor receptor on Tyr[845] and Tyr[1101] is associated with modulation of receptor function. *J. Biol. Chem.* **274,** 8335–8343.

Biscardi, J. S., Tice, D. A., and Parsons, S. J. (1999b). c-Src, receptor tyrosine kinases, and human cancer. *Adv. Cancer. Res.* **76,** 61–119.

Blair, L. A., Bence Hanulec, K. K., Mehta, S., Franke, T., Kaplan, D., and Marshall, J. (1999). Akt-dependent potentiation of L channels by insulin-like growth factor-1 is required for neuronal survival. *J. Neurosci.* **19,** 1940–1951.

Blume Jensen, J. P., Janknecht, R., and Hunter, T. (1998). The kit receptor promotes cell survival via activation of PI 3-kinase and subsequent Akt-mediated phosphorylation of Bad on Ser136. *Curr. Biol.* **8,** 779–782.

Bonner, J. A., Ezekiel, M. P., Robert, F., Meredith, R. F., Spencer, S. A., and Waksal, H. W. (2000). Continued response following treatment with IMC-C225, an EGFr MoAb, combined with RT I advanced head and neck malignancies. *Proc. Am. Assoc. Clin. Oncol.* **19,** 4a.

Brinkman, A., van der Flier, S., Kok, E. M., and Dorssers, L. C. J. (2000). BCAR1, a human homologue of the adapter protein p130Cas, and anti-estrogen resistance in breast cancer cells. *J. Natl. Cancer. Inst.* **92,** 112–120.

Bromberg, J. F., Wrzeszczynska, M. H., Devgan, G., Zhao, Y. X., Pestell, R. G., Albanese, C., and Darnell, J. (1999). Stat3 as an oncogene. *Cell.* **98,** 295–303.

Brunet, A., Bonni, A., Zigmond, M. J., Lin, M. Z., Juo, P., Hu, L. S., Anderson, M. J., Arden, K. C., Blenis, J., and Greenberg, M. E. (1999). Akt promotes cell survival by phosphorylating and inhibiting a Forkhead transcription factor. *Cell* **96,** 857–868.

Brzozowski, A. M., Pike, A. C. W., Dauter, Z., Bonn, T., Engstrom, O., Ohman, L., Greene, G. I., Gustafsson, J-A., and Carlquist, M. (1997). Molecular basis of agonism and antagonism in the estrogen receptor. *Nature* **389,** 753–758.

Bucci, B., D'Agnano, I., Botti, C., Mottolese, M., Carico, E., Zupi, G., and Vecchione, A. (1997). EGF-R expression in ductal breast cancer: Proliferation and prognostic implications. *Anticancer Res.* **17,** 769–774.

Burke, C. L., Lemmon, M. A., Coren, B. A., Engelman, D. M., and Stern, D. F. (1997). Dimerization of the p185(neu) transmembrane domain is necessary but not sufficient for transformation. *Oncogene* **14,** 687–696.

Carraway, K. L., and Cantley, L. C. (1994). A neu acquaintance for ErbB3 and ErbB4: A role for receptor heterodimerization in growth signaling. *Cell* **78,** 5.

Carraway, K. L. III. (1996). Involvement of the neuregulins and their receptors in cardiac and neural development. *Bioessays* **18,** 263–266.

Carraway, K. L., Weber, J. L., Unger, M. J., Ledesma, J., Yu, N., Gassmann, M., and Lai, C. (1997). Neuregulin-2, a new ligand of ErbB3/ErbB4-receptor tyrosine kinases. *Nature* **387,** 512–516.

Cenni, B. and Picard, D. (1999). Ligand-independent activation of steroid receptors: New roles for old players. *Trends Endo. Metab.* **10,** 41–46.

Chang, H., Riese, D. J., Gilbert, W., Stern, D. F., and McMahan, U. J. (1997). Ligands for ErbB-family receptors encoded by a newly characterized neuregulin-like gene. *Nature* **387,** 509–512.

Chen, R. H., Su, Y. H., Chuang, R. L., and Chang, T. Y. (1998). Suppression of transforming growth factor-beta-induced apoptosis through a phosphatidylinositol 3-kinase/Akt-dependent pathway. *Oncogene* **17,** 1959–1968.

Cheng, J. Q., Godwin, A. K., Bellacosa, A., Taguchi, T., Franke, T. F., Hamilton, T. C., Tsichlis, P. N., and Testa, J. R. (1992). AKT2, a putative oncogene encoding a member of a subfamily of protein-serine/threonine kinases, is amplified in human ovarian carcinomas. *Proc. Natl. Acad. Sci. USA* **89,** 9267–9271.

Cheng, J. Q., Ruggeri, B., Klein, W. M., Sonoda, G., Altomare, D. A., Watson, D. K., and Testa, J. R. (1996). Amplification of AKT2 in human pancreatic cells and inhibition of AKT2 expression and tumorigenicity by antisense RNA. *Proc. Natl. Acad. Sci. USA.* **93,** 3636–3641.

Cirri, P., Chiarugi, P., Marra, F., Raugei, G., Camici, G., Manao, G., and Ramponi, G. (1997). C-Src activates both STAT1 and STAT3 in PDGF-stimulated NIH3T3 cells. *Biochem. Biophys. Res. Commun.* **239,** 493–497.

Cobb, M. H., and Goldsmith, E. J. (1995). How MAP kinases are regulated. *J. Biol. Chem.* **270,** 14843–14846.

Cobleigh, M. A., Vogel, C. L., Tripathy, D., Robert, N. J., Scholl, R. S., Fehrenbacher, L., Paton, V., Shak, S., Lieberman, G., and Slamon, D.

(1998). Efficacy and safety of Herceptin (humanized anti-HER2 antibody) as a single agent in 222 women with HER2 overexpression who relapsed following chemotherapy for metastatic breast cancer. *Proc. Am. Soc. Clin. Oncol.* **17,** 97a.

Coffer, P. J., and Woodgett, J. R. (1991). Molecular-cloning and characterization of a novel putative protein-serine kinase related to the cAMP-dependent and protein kinase C families. *Eur. J. Biochem.* **201,** 475–481.

Conway, A. M., Rakhit, S., Pyne, S., and Pyne, N. J. (1999). Platelet-derived-growth-factor stimulation of the p42/p44 mitogen-activated protein kinase pathway in airway smooth muscle: role of pertussis-toxin-sensitive G-proteins, C-Src tyrosine kinases and phosphoinositide 3-kinase. *Biochem. J.* **337,** 171–177.

Corey, S. J., and Anderson, S. M. (1999). Src-related protein tyrosine kinases in hematopoiesis. *Blood* **93,** 1–14.

Corton, J. C., Lapinskas, P. J., and Gonzalez, F. J. (2000). Central role of PPARalpha in the mechanism of hepatocarcinogenic peroxisome proliferators. *Mutat. Res.* **448,** 139–151.

Cowley, S., Paterson, H., Kemp, P., and Marshall, C. J. (1994). Activation of MAP kinase kinase is necessary and sufficient for PC12 differentiation and for transformation of NIH3T3 cells. *Cell* **77,** 841–852.

Crews, C. M., Alessandrini, A., and Erickson, R. L. (1992). The primary structure of MEK, a protein kinase that phosphorylates the ERK gene product. *Science* **258,** 478–480.

Cross, D. A., Alessi, D. R., Cohen, P., Andjelkovich, M., and Hemmings, B. A. (1995). Inhibition of glycogen synthase kinase-3 by insulin mediated by protein kinase B. *Nature* **378,** 785–789.

Crowder, R. J., and Freeman, R. S. (1998). Phosphatidylinositol 3-kinase and Akt protein kinase are necessary and sufficient for the survival of nerve growth factor-dependent sympathetic neurons. *J. Neurosci.* **18,** 2933–2943.

Currie, R. A., Walker, K. S., Gray, A., Deak, M., Casamayor, A., Downes, C. P., Cohen, P., Alessi, D. R., and Lucocq, J. (1999). Role of phosphatidylinositol 3,4,5-trisphosphate in regulating the activity and localization of 3-phosphoinositide-dependent protein kinase-1. *Biochem. J.* **337,** 575–583.

Daly, R. J. (1999). Take your partners, please—Signal diversification by the erbB family of receptor tyrosine kinases. *Growth Factors* **16,** 255–263.

Dankort, D. L., Wang, Z., Blackmore, V., Moran, M. F., and Muller, W. J. (1997). Distinct tyrosine autophosphorylation sites negatively and positively modulate neu-mediated transformation. *Mol. Cell. Biol.* **17,** 5410–5425.

Datta, S. R., Brunet, A., and Greenberg, M. E. (1999). Cellular survival: A play in three Akts. *Genes Dev.* **13,** 2905–2927.

Datta, S. R., Dudek, H., Tao, X., Masters, S., Fu, H., Gotoh, Y., and Greenberg, M. E. (1997). Akt phosphorylation of BAD couples survival signals to the cell-intrinsic death machinery. *Cell* **91,** 231–241.

Daum, G., Eisenmann-Tappe, I., Fries, H. W., Troppmair, J., and Rapp, U. R. (1994). The ins and outs of Raf kinases. *Trends Biochem. Sci.* **19,** 474–480.

Davies, D. E. and Chamberlin, S. G. (1996). Targeting the epidermal growth factor receptor for therapy of carcinomas. *Biochem. Pharmacol.* **51,** 1101–1110.

De Vivo, I., Gertig, D. M., Nagase, S., Hankinson, S. E., O'Brien, R., Speizer, F. E., Parsons, R., and Hunter, D. J. (2000). Novel germline mutations in the PTEN tumour suppressor gene found in women with multiple cancers. *J. Med. Genet.* **37,** 336–341.

Declan, F. R. Y., Ellis, L. M., Parikh, N. U., Liu, W., Staley, C. A., and Gallick, G. E. (1997). Regulation of vascular endothelial growth factor expression in human colon carcinoma cells by activity of src kinase. *Surgery* **122,** 501–507.

del Peso, L., Gonzalez Garcia, M., Page, C., Herrera, R., and Nunez, G. (1997). Interleukin-3-induced phosphorylation of BAD through the protein kinase Akt. *Science* **278,** 687–689.

DeMali, K. A., Godwin, S. L., Soltoff, S. P., and Kazlauskas, A. (1999). Multiple roles for Src in a PDGF-stimulated cell. *Exp. Cell Res.* **253,** 271–279.

Demetri, G. D., Fletcher, C. D. M., Mueller, E., Sarraf, P., Naujoks, R., Campbell, N., Spiegelman, B. M., and Singer, S. (1999). Induction of solid tumor differentiation by the peroxisome proliferator-activated receptor-gamma ligand troglitazone in patients with liposarcoma. *Proc. Natl. Acad. Sci. USA* **96,** 3951–3956.

Dent, P., Haser, W., Haystead, T. A., Vincent, L. A., Roberts, T. M., and Sturgill, T. W. (1992). Activation of mitogen-activated protein kinase kinase by v-Raf in NIH 3T3 cells and in vitro. *Science* **257,** 1404–1407.

Depotter, C. R. (1994). The neu-*Oncogene:* More than a prognostic indicator? *Human Pathol.* **25,** 1264–1268.

Dhingra, K. (1999). Antiestrogens—taxmoxifen, SERMs and beyond. *Invest. New Drugs* **17,** 285–311.

Dimmeler, S., Fleming, I., Fisslthaler, B., Hermann, C., Busse, R., and Zeiher, A. M. (1999). Activation of nitric oxide synthase in endothelial cells by Akt-dependent phosphorylation. *Nature* **399,** 601–605.

Dorr, A., Burce, J., Monia, B., Johnston, J., Geary, R., Kwoh, T. J., Holmlund, J. T., and Nemunaitis, J. (1999). Phase I and pharmacokinetic trial of ISIS 2503, a 20-mer antisense oligonucleotide against H-ras, by 14-day continuous infusion in patients with advanced cancer. *Proc. Am. Soc. Clin. Oncol.* **18,** 157a.

Dougall, W. C., Qian, X., and Greene, M. I. (1993). Interaction of the neu/p185 and EGF receptor tyrosine kinases: Implications for cellular transformation and tumor therapy. *J. Cell. Biochem.* **53,** 61–73.

Downward, J. (1998). Ras signaling and apoptosis. *Curr. Opin. Genet. Dev.* **8,** 49–54.

Du, W., and Prendergast, G. C. (1999). Geranylgeranylated RhoB mediates suppression of human tumor cell growth by farnesyltransferase inhibitors. *Cancer Res.* **59,** 5492–5496.

Dudek, H., Datta, S. R., Franke, T. F., Birnbaum, M. J., Yao, R., Cooper, G. M., Segal, R. A., Kaplan, D. R., and Greenberg, M. E. (1997). Regulation of neuronal survival by the serine-threonine protein kinase Akt. *Science* **275,** 661–665.

Dudley, D. T., Pang, L., Decker, S. J., Bridges, A. J., and Saltiel, A. R. (1995). A synthetic inhibitor of the mitogen-activated protein kinase cascade. *Proc. Natl. Acad. Sci. USA* **92,** 7686–7689.

Egan, C., Pang, A., Durda, D., Cheng, H.-C., Wang, J. H., and Fujita, D. J. (1999). Activation of src in human breast tumor cell lines: elevated levels of phosphotyrosine phosphatase activity that preferentially recognizes the src carboxy terminal negative regulatory tyrosine 530. *Oncogene* **18,** 1227–1237.

Eliceiri, B. P., Paul, R., Schwarzberg, P. L., Hood, J. D., Leng, J., and Cheresh, D. L. (1999). Selective requirement for Src kinases during VEGF-induced angiogenesis and vascular permeability. *Mol. Cell* **4,** 915–924.

Eliceiri, B. P., Klemke, R., Stromblad, S., and Cheresh, D. A. (1998). Integrin alphavbeta3 requirement for sustained mitogen-activated protein kinase activity during angiogenesis. *J. Cell Biol.* **140,** 1255–1263.

Evans, R. M. (1988). The steroid and thyroid hormone receptor superfamily. *Science* **240,** 889–895.

Eves, E. M., Xiong, W., Bellacosa, A., Kennedy, S. G., Tsichlis, P. N., Rosner, M. R., and Hay, N. (1998). Akt, a target of phosphatidylinositol 3-kinase, inhibits apoptosis in a differentiating neuronal cell line. *Mol. Cell Biol.* **18,** 2143–2152.

Fanger, G. R., Johnson, N. L., and Johnson, G. L. (1997). MEK kinases are regulated by EGF and selectively interact with rac/cdc42. *EMBO J.* **16,** 4961–4972.

Fazioli, F., Kim, U.-H., Rhee, S. G., Molloy, C. J., Segatto, O., and DiFiore, P. P. (1991). The erbB-2 mitogenic signaling pathway: tyrosine phosphorylation of phopholipase C-γ and GTPase-activating protein does not correlate with erbB-2 mitogenic potency. *Mol. Cell. Biol.* **11,** 2040–2048.

Felsenfeld, D. P., Schwartzberg, P. L., Venegas, A., Tse, R., and Sheetz, M. P. (1999). Selective regulation of integrin-cytoskelton interactions by the tyrosine kinase Src. *Nature Cell Biol.* **1,** 200–206.

Ferry, D., Hammond, L., Ranson, M., Kris, M., Miller, V., Murray, P., Tullo, A., Feyereislova, A., Averbuch, S., and Rowinsky, E. (2000). Intermittent oral Zd1839 (Iressa), A novel epidermal growth factore receptor tyrosine kinase inhibitor (Egfr-Tki), shows evidence of good tolerability and activity: Final results from a phase I study. *Proc. Am. Assoc. Clin. Oncol.* **19,** 3a.

Fiddes, R. J., Campbell, D. H., Janes, P. W., Sivertsen, S. P., Sasaki, H., Wallasch, C., and Daly, R. J. (1998). Analysis of Grb7 recruitment by heregulin-activated erbB receptors reveals a novel target selectivity for erbB3. *J. Biol. Chem.* **273,** 7717–7724.

Fiddes, R. J., Janes, P. W., Sanderson, G. M., Sivertsen, S. P., Sutherland, R. L., and Daly, R. J. (1995). Heregulin (HRG)-induced mitogenic signaling and cytotoxic activity of a HRG/PE40 ligand toxin in human breast cancer cells. *Cell Growth Different.* **6,** 1567–1577.

Finlay, D., Healy, V., Furlong, F., O'Connell, F. C., Keon, N. K., and Martin, F. (2000). MAP kinase pathway signaling is essential for extracellular matrix determined epithelial cell survival. *Cell Death Differ.* **7,** 303–313.

Fischbach, G. D., and Rosen, K. M. (1997). ARIA: A neuromuscular junction neuregulin. *Ann. Rev. Neurosci.* **20,** 429–458.

Fondell, J. D., Roy, A. L., and Roeder, R. G. (1993). Unliganded thyroid hormone receptor inhibits formation of a functional preiniation complex: implications for active repression. *Genes Dev.* **7,** 1400–1410.

Franke, T. F., Kaplan, D. R., Cantley, L. C., and Toker, A. (1997). Direct regulation of the Akt proto-oncogene product by phosphatidylinositol-3,4-bisphosphate. *Science* **275,** 665–668.

Frech, M., Andjelkovic, M., Ingley, E., Reddy, K. K., Falck, J. R., and Hemmings, B. A. (1997). High affinity binding of inositol phosphates and phosphoinositides to the pleckstrin homology domain of RAC/protein kinase B and their influence on kinase activity. *J. Biol. Chem.* **272,** 8474–8481.

Fry, D. W. (1994). Protein tyrosine kinases as therapeutic targets in cancer chemotherapy and recent advances in the development of new inhibitors. *Exp. Opin. Invest. Drugs* **3,** 577–595.

Fry, D. W. (1999). Inhibition of the epidermal growth factor receptor family of tyrosine kinases as an approach to cancer chemotherapy: Progression from reversible to irreversible inhibitors. *Pharm. Ther.* **82,** 207–218.

Fry, D. W. (2000). Site-directed irreversible inhibitors of the erbB family of receptor tyrosine kinases as novel chemotherapeutic agents for cancer. *Anticancer. Drug. Design.* **15,** 3–16.

Fry, D. W., Bridges, A. J., Denny, W. A., Doherty, A., Greis, K., Hicks, J. L., Hook, K. E., Keller, P. R., Leopold, W. R., Loo, J., McNamara, D. J., Nelson, J. M., Sherwood, V., Smaill, J. B., Trumpp-Kallmeyer, S., and Dobrusin, E. M. (1998). Specific, irreversible inactivation of the epidermal growth factor receptor and erbB2, by a new class of tyrosine kinase inhibitor. *Proc. Natl. Acad. Sci. USA* **95,** 12022–12027.

Fry, D. W., Kraker, A. J., McMichael, A., Ambroso, L. A., Nelson, J. M., Connors, R., Leopold, W. R., and Bridges, A. J. (1994). A specific inhibitor of the epidermal growth factor receptor tyrosine kinase. *Science* **265,** 1093–1095.

Fujio, Y., and Walsh, K. (1999). Akt mediates cytoprotection of endothelial cells by vascular endothelial growth factor in an anchorage-dependent manner. *J. Biol. Chem.* **274,** 16349–16354.

Fulton, D., Gratton, J. P., McCabe, T. J., Fontana, J., Fujio, Y., Walsh, K., Franke, T. F., Papapetropoulos, A., and Sessa, W. C. (1999). Regulation of endothelium-derived nitric oxide production by the protein kinase Akt. *Nature* **399,** 597–601.

Gelderloos, J. A., Rosenkranz, S., Bazenet, C., and Kazlauskas, A. (1998). A role for src in signal relay by the platelet-derived growth factor α receptor. *J. Biol. Chem.* **273,** 5908–5915.

Gelman, L., Fruchart, J. C., and Auwerx, J. (1999). An update on the mechanisms of action of the peroxisome proliferator-activated receptors (PPARs) and their roles in inflammation and cancer. *Cell. Mol. Life Sci.* **55,** 932–943.

Gerber, H. P., McMurtrey, A., Kowalski, J., Yan, M., Keyt, B. A., Dixit, V., and Ferrara, N. (1998). Vascular endothelial growth factor regulates endothelial cell survival through the phosphatidylinositol 3′-kinase/Akt signal transduction pathway. Requirement for Flk-1/KDR activation. *J. Biol. Chem.* **273,** 30336–30343.

Giguere, V. (1999). Orphan nuclear receptors: From gene to function. *Endocrine Rev.* **20,** 689–725.

Glass, C. K., and Rosenfeld, M. G. (2000). The coregulator exchange in transcriptional functions of nuclear receptors. *Genes Dev.* **14,** 121–141.

Goldman, R., Ben Levy, R., Peles, E., and Yarden, Y. (1990). Heterodimerization of the erbB1 and erbB2 receptors in human breast carcinoma cells: A mechanism for receptor transregulation. *Biochemistry.* **29,** 11024–11028.

Gonfloni, S., Frischknecht, Way, M., and Superti-Furga, G. (1999). Leucine 255 of Src couples intramolecular interactions to inhibition of catalysis. *Nature Struct. Biol.* **6,** 760–764.

Gordon, M. S., Sandler, A. B., Holmlund, J. T., Dorr, A., Battiato, L., Fife, K., Geary, R., Kwoh, T. J., and Sledge, G. W. (1999). A phase I trial of ISIS 2503, an antisense inhibitor of H-ras, administered by a 24-hour weekly infusion to patients with advanced cancer. *Proc. Am. Soc. Clin. Oncol.* **18,** 157a.

Grasso, A. W., Wen, D., Miller, C. M., Rhim, J. S., Pretlow, T. G., and Kung, H.-J. (1997). ErbB kinases and NDF signaling in human prostate cancer cells. *Oncogene* **15,** 2705–2716.

GrausPorta, D., Beerli, R. R., Daly, J. M., and Hynes, N. E. (1997). ErbB-2, the preferred heterodimerization partner of all ErbB receptors, is a mediator of lateral signaling. *EMBO J.* **16,** 1647–1655.

Grese, T. A., and Dodge, J. A. (1998). Selective estrogen receptor modulators (SERMs). *Curr. Pharm. Des.* **4,** 71–92.

Guldberg, P., thor Straten, P., Birck, A., Ahrenkiel, V., Kirkin, A. F., and Zeuthen, J. (1997). Disruption of the MMAC1/PTEN gene by deletion or mutation is a frequent event in malignant melanoma. *Cancer Res.* **57,** 3660–3663.

Hackel, P. O., Zwick, E., Prenzel, N., and Ullrich, A. (1999). Epidermal growth factor receptors: critical mediators of multiple receptor pathways. *Curr. Opin. Cell Biol.* **11,** 184–189.

Hajduch, E., Alessi, D. R., Hemmings, B. A., and Hundal, H. S. (1998). Constitutive activation of protein kinase B alpha by membrane targeting promotes glucose and system A amino acid transport, protein synthesis, and inactivation of glycogen synthease kinase 3 in L6 muscle cells. *Diabetes* **47,** 1006–1013.

Harari, D., Tzahar, E., Romano, J., Shelly, M., Pierce, J. H., Andrews, G. C., and Yarden, Y. (1999). Neuregulin-4: a novel growth factor that acts through the erbB-4 receptor tyrosine kinase. *Oncogene* **18,** 2681–2689.

Hassig, C. A., and Schreiber, S. L., (1998). Nuclear histone acetylases and deacetylases and transcriptional regulation: HATs off to the HDACs. *Curr. Opin. Chem. Biol.* **1,** 300–308.

Hausler, P., Papoff, G., Eramo, A., Reif, K., Cantrell, D. A., and Ruberti, G. (1998). Protection of CD95-mediated apoptosis by activation of phosphatidylinositide 3-kinase and protein kinase B. *Eur. J. Immunol.* **28,** 57–69.

He, H., Venema, V. J., Gu, X., Venema, R. C., Marrero, M. B., and Caldwell, R. B. (1999). Vascular endothelial growth factor signals endothelial cell production of nitric oxide and prostacyclin through Flk-1/KDR activation of c-Src. *J. Biol. Chem.* **274,** 25130–25135.

He, T. C., Chan, T. A., Vogelstein, B., and Kinzler, K. W. (1999). PPAR delta is an APC-regulated target of nonsteroidal anti-inflammatory drugs. *Cell* **99,** 335–345.

Her, J. H., Lakhani, S., Zu, K., Vila, J., Dent, P., Sturgill, T. W., and Weber, M. J. (1993). Dual phosphorylation and autophosphorylation in mitogen-activated protein (MAP) kinase activation. *Biochem. J.* **296,** 25–31.

Herrera, R. (1998). Modulation of hepatocyte growth factor-induced scattering of HT29 colon carcinoma cells. Involvement of the MAPK pathway. *J. Cell Sci.* **111**, 1039–1049.

Holmstrom, T. H., Tran, S. E., Johnson, V. L., Ahn, N. G., Chow, S. C., and Eriksson, J. E. (1999). Inhibition of mitogen-activated kinase signaling sensitizes HeLa cells to Fas apoptosis. *Mol. Cell. Biol.* **19**, 5991–6002.

Hoshino, R., Chatani, Y., Yamori, T., Tsuruo, T., Oka, H., Yoshida, O., Shimada, Y., Ari-i, S., Wada, H., Fujimoto, J., and Kohno, M. (1999). Constitutive activation of the 41-/43-kDa mitogen-activated protein (MAP) kinases in human tumors. *Oncogene* **18**, 813–822.

Hubbard, S. R. (1999). Src autoinhibition: Let us count the ways. *Nat. Struct. Biol.* **6**, 711–714.

Hynes, N. E., and Stern, D. F. (1994). The biology of erbB-2/neu/HER-2 and its role in cancer. *Biochim. Biophys. Acta* **1198**, 165–184.

Iravani, S., Mao, W., Fu, L., Karl, R., Yeatman, T., Jove, R., and Coppola, D. (1998). Elevated c-src protein expression is an early event in colonic neoplasia. *Lab. Invest.* **78**, 365–371.

Irby, R. B., Mao, W., Coppola, D., Kang, J., Loubeau, J. M., Trudeau, W., Karl, R., Fujita, D. J., Jove, R., and Yeatman, T. J. (1999). Activating SRC mutation in a subset of advanced human colon cancers. *Nat. Gene.* **21**, 187–190.

Ishida, T., Ishida, M., Suero, J., Takahashi, M., and Berk, B. C. (1999). Agonist-stimulated cytoskeletal reorganization and signal transduction at focal adhesions in vascular smooth muscle cells requires c-Src. *J. Clin. Invest.* **103**, 789–797.

Jackson, J. H., Cochrane, C. G., Bourne, J. R., Solski, P. A., Buss, J. E., and Der, C. J. (1990). Farnesyl modification of Kirsten-ras exon 4B protein is essential for transformation. *Proc. Natl. Acad. Sci. USA* **87**, 3042–3046.

Jallal, B., Schlessinger, J., and Ullrich, A. (1992). Tyrosine phosphatase inhibition permits analysis of signal transduction complexes in p185HER2/neu-overexpressing human tumor cells. *J. Biol. Chem.* **267**, 4357–4363.

James, G., Goldstein, J. L., and Brown, M. S. (1996). Resistance of K-RasBV12 proteins to farnesyltransferase inhibitors in Rat1 cells. *Proc. Natl. Acad. Sci. USA* **93**, 4454–4458.

James, G. L., Goldstein, J. L., Brown, M. S., Rawson, T. E. Somers, T. C., McDowell, R. S., Crowley, C. W., Lucas, B. I., Levinson, A. D., and Marsters, Jr., J. C. (1993). Benzodiazepine peptidomimetics: potent inhibitors of ras farnesylation in animal cells. *Science* **260**, 1937–1942.

James, S. R., Downes, C. P., Gigg, R., Grove, S. J., Holmes, A. B., and Alessi, D. R. (1996). Specific binding of the Akt-1 protein kinase to phosphatidylinositol 3,4,5-triphosphate without subsequent activation. *Biochem. J.* **315**, 709–713.

Janes, P. W., Daly, R. J., deFazio, A., and Sutherland, R. L., (1994). Activation of the ras signaling pathway in human breast cancer cells overexpressing erbB-2. *Oncogene* **9**, 3601–3608.

Johnson, G. R., Kannan, B., Shoyab, M., and Stromberg, K. (1993). Amphiregulin induces tyrosine phosphorylation of the epidermal growth factor receptor and p185erbB2. *J. Biol. Chem.* **268**, 2924–2931.

Jones, J. T., Akita, R. W., and Sliwkowski, M. X. (1999). Binding specificities and affinities of EGF domains for ErbB receptors. *FEBS Lett.* **447**, 227–231.

Kane, L. P., Shapiro, V. S., Stokoe, D., and Weiss, A. (1999). Induction of NF-kappaB by the Akt/PKB kinase. *Curr. Biol.* **9**, 601–604.

Karp, D. D., Silberman, S. L., and Csudae, R., Wirth, F., Gaynes, L., Posner, M., Bubley, G., Koon, H., Bergman, M., Huang, M., and Schnipper, L. E. (1999). Phase I dose escalation study of epidermal growth factor receptor (EGFR) tyrosine kinase (TK) inhibitor CP-358,774 in patients with advanced solid tumors. *Proc. Am. Soc. Clin. Oncol.* **18**, 388a.

Kato, K., Cox, A. D., Kisaka, M. M., Graham, S. M., Buss, J. E., and Der, C. J. (1992). Isoprenoid addition to ras protein is the critical modification for its membrane association and transforming activity. *Proc. Natl. Acad. Sci. USA* **89**, 6403–6407.

Kauffmann Zeh, A., Rodriguez Viciana, P., Ulrich, E., Gilbert, C., Coffer, P., Downward, J., and Evan, G. (1997). Suppression of c-Myc-induced apoptosis by Ras signaling through PI(3)K and PKB. *Nature* **385**, 544–548.

Kennedy, S. G., Wagner, A. J., Conzen, S. D., Jordan, J., Bellacosa, A., Tsichlis, P. N., and Hay, N. (1997). The PI 3-kinase/Akt signaling pathway delivers an anti-apoptotic signal. *Genes Dev.* **11**, 701–713.

Khazaie, K., Schirrmacher, V., and Lichtner, R. B. (1993). EGF receptor in neoplasia and metastasis. *Cancer Metab. Rev.* **12**, 255–274.

Khwaja, A., Rodriguez Viciana, P., Wennstrom, S., Warne, P. H., and Downward, J. (1997). Matrix adhesion and Ras transformation both activate a phosphoinositide 3-OH kinase and protein kinase B/Akt cellular survival pathway. *EMBO J.* **16**, 2783–2793.

Kikuchi, A. (2000). Regulation of beta-catenin signaling in the Wnt pathway. *Biochem. Biophys. Res. Commun.* **268**, 243–248.

King, C. R., Borrello, I., Bellot, G., Comoglio, P., and Schlessinger, J. (1988). EGF binding to its receptor triggers a rapid tyrosine phosphorylation of the erbB-2 protein in the mammary tumor cell line SK-BR-3. *EMBO J.* **7**, 1647–1651.

Kitamura, T., Ogawa, W., Sakaue, H., Hino, Y., Kuroda, S., Takata, M., Matsumoto, M., Maeda, T., Konishi, H., Kikkawa, U., and Kasuga, M. (1998). Requirement for activation of the serine-threonine kinase Akt (protein kinase B) in insulin stimulation of protein synthesis but not of glucose transport. *Mol. Cell Biol.* **18**, 3708–3717.

Klijn, J. G., Look, M. P., Portengen, H., Alexieva-Figusch, J., van Putten, W. L., and Foekens, J. A. (1994). The prognostic value of epidermal growth factor receptor (EGF-R) in primary breast cancer: results of a 10 year follow-up study. *Breast Cancer Res. Treat.* **29**, 73–83.

Klijn, J. G. M., Berns, P. M. J. J., Schmitz, P. I. M., and Foekens, J. A. (1992). The clinical significance of epidermal growth factor receptor (EGF-R) in human breast cancer—A review on 5232 patients. *Endocrine Rev.* **13**, 3–17.

Klinghoffer, R. A., Sachsenmaier, C., Cooper, J. A., and Soriano, P. (1999). Src family kinases are required for integrin but not PDGFR signal transduction. *EMBO J.* **18**, 2459–2471.

Klippel, A., Kavanaugh, W. M., Pot, D., and Williams, L. T. (1997). A specific product of phosphatidylinositol 3-kinase directly activates the protein kinase Akt through its pleckstrin homology domain. *Mol. Cell Biol.* **17**, 338–344.

Kohl, N. E., Mosser, S. D., deSolms, S. J., Giuliani, E. A., Pompliano, D. L., Graham, S. L., Smith, R. L., Scolnick, E. M., Oliff, A., and Gibbs, J. B. (1993). Selective inhibition of ras-dependent transformation by a farnesyltransferase inhibitor. *Science* **260**, 1934–1937.

Koide, S. S. (1998). Mifepristone. Auxiliary therapeutic use in cancer and related disorders. *J. Reprod. Med.* **43**, 551–560.

Kolch, W., Heidecker, G., Kochs, G., Hummel, R., Vahidi, H., Mischak, H., Finkenzeller, G., Marme, D., and Rapp, U. R. (1993). Protein kinase C alpha activates RAF-1 by direct phosphorylation. *Nature* **364**, 249–252.

Kolvenbag, G. J., Blackledge, G. R., and Gotting-Smith, K. (1998). Bicalutamide (Casodex) in the treatment of prostate cancer: history of clinical development. *Prostate* **34**, 61–72.

Komurasaki, T., Toyoda, H., Uchida, D., and Morimoto, S. (1997). Epiregulin binds to epidermal growth factor receptor and erbB-4 and induces tyrosine phosphorylation of epidermal growth factor receptor, erbB-2, erbB-3 and erbB-4. *Oncogene* **15**, 2841–2848.

Kops, G. J., de Ruiter, N. D., De Vries Smits, A. M., Powell, D. R., Bos, J. L., and Burgering, B. M. (1999). Direct control of the Forkhead transcription factor AFX by protein kinase B. *Nature* **398**, 630–634.

Kubota, T., Koshizuka, K., Williamson, E. A., Asou, H., Said, J. W., Holden, S., Miyoshi, I., and Koeffler, H. P. (1998). Ligand for peroxisome proliferator-activated receptor gamma (troglitazone) has potent antitumor effect against human prostate cancer both *in vitro* and *in vivo*. *Cancer Res.* **58**, 3344–3352.

Kulik, G., and Weber, M. J. (1998). Akt-dependent and -independent survival signaling pathways utilized by insulin-like growth factor I. *Mol. Cell Biol.* **18,** 6711–6718.

Kulik, G., Klippel, A., and Weber, M. J. (1997). Antiapoptotic signalling by the insulin-like growth factor I receptor, phosphatidylinositol 3-kinase, and Akt. *Mol. Cell Biol.* **17,** 1595–1606.

Kumar, R., and Thompson, E. B. (1999). The structure of the nuclear hormone receptors. *Steroids* **64,** 310–319.

Kurokawa, R., Yu, V. C., Naar, A., Kyakumoto, S., Han, Z., Silverman, S., Rosenfeld, M. G., and Glass, C. K. (1993). Differential orientations of the DNA-binding domain and carboxy terminal dimerization interface regulate binding site selection by nuclear hormone heterodimers. *Genes Dev.* **7,** 1423–1435.

Lawrence, D. S., and Niu, J. K. (1998). Protein kinase inhibitors: The tyrosine-specific protein kinases. *Pharm. Ther.* **77,** 81–114.

Lewis, T. S., Shapiro, P. S., and Ahn, N. G. (1998). Signal transduction through MAP kinase cascades. *Adv. Cancer Res.* **74,** 49–139.

Li, J., Simpson, L., Takahashi, M., Miliaresis, C., Myers, M. P., Tonks, N., and Parsons, R. (1998). The PTEN/MMAC1 tumor suppressor induces cell death that is rescued by the AKT/protein kinase B oncogene. *Cancer Res.* **58,** 5667–5672.

Liaw, D., Marsh, D. J., Li, J., Dahia, P. L., Wang, S. I., Zheng, Z., Bose, S., Call, K. M., Tsou, H. C., Peacocke, M., Eng, C., and Parsons, R. (1997). Germline mutations of the PTEN gene in Cowden disease, an inherited breast and thyroid cancer syndrome. *Nat. Genet.* **16,** 64–67.

Liu, W., Li, J., and Roth, R. A. (1999). Heregulin regulation of Akt/protein kinase B in breast cancer cells. *Biochem. Biophys. Res. Commun.* **261,** 897–903.

Lotan, R. (1997). Retinoids and chemoprevention of aerodigestive tract cancers. *Cancer Metastasis Rev.* **16,** 349–356.

Lutrell, d. K., Lee, A., Lansing, T. J., Crosby, R. M., Jung, K. D., Willard, M., Rodriguez, M., Berman, J., and Gilmer, T. M. (1994). Involvement of pp60c-src with two major signaling pathways in human breast cancer. *Proc. Natl. Acad. Sci.* **19,** 83–97.

Lutz, M. P., Silke Eβer, I. B., Flossmann-Kast, B. B. M., Vogelmann, R., Lührs, H., Friess, H., Büchler, M. W., and Adler, G. (1998). Overexpression and activation of the tyrosine kinase src in human pancreatic carcinoma. *Biochem. Biophys. Res. Commun.* **243,** 503–508.

Mansour, S. J., Matten, W. T., Hermann, A. S., Candia, J. M., Rong, S., Fukasawa, K., Vande Woude, G. F., and Ahn, N. G. (1994). Transformation of mammalian cells by constitutively active MAP kinase kinase. *Science* **265,** 966–970.

Marchionni, M. A., Goodearl, A. D. J., Chen, M. S., Berminghan-McDonogh, O., Kirk, C., Hendricks, M., Danehy, F., Misumi, D., Sudhalter, J., Kobayashi, K., Wroblewski, D., Lynch, C., Baldassare, M., Hiles, I., Davis, J. B., Hsuan, J. J., Totty, N. F., Otsu, M., McBurney, R. N., Waterfield, M. D., Stroobant, P., and Gwynne, D. (1993). Glial growth factors are alternatively spliced erbB2 ligands expressed in the nervous system. *Nature* **362,** 312–318.

Marsh, D. J., Dahia, P. L., Zheng, Z., Liaw, D., Parsons, R., Gorlin, R. J., and Eng, C. (1997). Germline mutations in PTEN are present in Bannayan-Zonana syndrome. *Nat. Genet.* **16,** 333–334.

Mazure, N. M., Chen, E. Y., Laderoute, K. R., and Giaccia, A. J. (1997). Induction of vascular endothelial growth factor by hypoxia is modulated by a phosphatidylinositol 3-kinase/Akt signaling pathway in Ha-ras-transformed cells through a hypoxia inducible factor-1 transcriptional element. *Blood* **90,** 3322–3331.

Medema, R. H., Kops, G. J., Bos, J. L., and Burgering, B. M. (2000). AFX-like Forkhead transcription factors mediate cell-cycle regulation by Ras and PKB through p27kip1. *Nature.* **404,** 782–787.

Meden, H., Marx, D., Raab, T., Schauer, K. M., and Kuhn, W. (1995). EGF-R and overexpression of the Oncogene c-erbB-2 in ovarian cancer: immunohistochemical findings and prognostic value. *J. Obstet. Gynecol.* **21,** 167–178.

Meier, R., Alessi, D. R., Cron, P., Andjelkovic, M., and Hemmings, B. A. (1997). Mitogenic activation, phosphorylation, and nuclear translocation of protein kinase B-beta. *J. Biol. Chem.* **272,** 30491–30497.

Melillo, R. M., Barone, M. V., Lupoli, G., Cirafici, A. M., Carlomagno, F., Visconti, R., Matoskova, B., DiFiore, P. P., Vecchio, G., Fusco, A., and Santoro, M. (1999). Ret-mediated mitogenesis requires Src kinase activity. *Cancer Res.* **59,** 1120–1126.

Meyer, D., and Birchmeier, C. (1995). Multiple essential functions of neuregulin in development. *Nature* **378,** 386–398.

Milanini, J., Vinals, F., Pouyssegur, J., and Pages, G. (1998). p42/p44 MAP kinase module plays a key role in the transcriptional regulation of the vascular endothelial growth factor gene in fibroblasts. *J. Biol. Chem.* **273,** 18165–18172.

Milas, L., Mason, K., Hunter, N., Petersen, S., Yamakawa, M., Ang, K., Mendelsohn, J., and Fan, Z. (2000). In vivo enhancement of tumor radioresponse by C225 antiepidermal growth factor receptor antibody. *Clin. Cancer. Res.* **6,** 701–708.

Moghal, N., and Sternberg, P. W. (1999). Multiple positive and negative regulators of signaling by the EGF-receptor. *Curr. Opin. Cell Biol.* **11,** 190–196.

Mueller, E., Sarraf, P., Tontonoz, P., Evans, R. M., Martin, K. J., Zhang, M., Fletcher, C., Singer, S., and Spiegelman, B. M. (1998). Terminal differentiation of human breast cancer through PPAR gamma. *Mol. Cell* **1,** 465–470.

Muller, W. J., Arteaga, C. L., Muthuswamy, S. K., Siegel, P. M., Webster, M. A., Cardiff, R. D., Meise, K. S., Li, F., Halter, S. A., and Coffey, R. J. (1996). Synergistic interaction of the neu proto-Oncogene product and transforming growth factor alpha in the mammary epithelium of transgenic mice. *Mol. Cell. Biol.* **16,** 5726–5736.

Munshi, N., Groopman, J. E., Gill, P. S., and Ganju, R. K. (2000). C-Src mediates mitogenic signals and associates with cytoskeletal proteins upon vascular endothelial growth factor stimulation in Kaposi's sarcoma cells. *J. Immunol.* **164,** 1169–1174.

Murohara, T., Asahara, T., Silver, M., Bauters, C., Masuda, H., Kalka, C., Kearney, M., Chen, D., Symes, J. F., Fishman, M. C., Huang, P. L., and Isner, J. M., (1998). Nitric oxide synthase modulates angiogenesis in response to tissue ischemia. *J. Clin. Invest.* **101,** 2567–2578.

Muslin, A. J., Tanner, J. W., Allen, P. M., and Shaw, A. S. (1996). Interaction of 14-3-3 with signaling proteins is mediated by the recognition of phosphoserine. *Cell* **84,** 889–897.

Muthuswamy, S. K., Siegel, P. S., Dankort, D. L., Webster, M. A., and Muller, W. J. (1994). Mammary tumors expressing the new proto-oncogene possess elevated c-src tyrosine kinase activity. *Mol. Cell. Biol.* **14,** 735–743.

Myers, M. P., Pass, I., Batty, I. H., Van der Kaay, J., Stolarov, J. P., Hemmings, B. A., Wigler, M. H., Downes, C. P., and Tonks, N. K. (1998). The lipid phosphatase activity of PTEN is critical for its tumor suppressor function. *Proc. Natl. Acad. Sci. USA* **95,** 13513–13518.

Nakatani, K., Thompson, D. A., Barthel, A., Sakaue, H., Liu, W., Weigel, R. J., and Roth, R. A. (1999). Up-regulation of Akt3 in estrogen receptor-deficient breast cancers and androgen-independent prostate cancer lines. *J. Biol. Chem.* **274,** 21528–21532.

Niu, G., Heller, R., Catlett-Falcone, R., Coppola, D., Jaroszeski, M., Dalton, W., Jove, R., and Yu, H. (1999). Gene therapy with dominant-negative Stat3 suppresses growth of the murine melanoma B16 tumor in vivo. *Cancer Res.* **59,** 5059–5063.

O'Dwyer, P. J., Stevenson, J. P., Gallagher, M., Cassella, A., Vasilevskaya, I., Monia, B. P., Holmlund, J., Dorr, F. A., and Yao, K. S. (1999). c-Raf-1 depletion and tumor responses in patients treated with the c-raf-1 antisense oligodeoxynucleotide ISIS 5132 (CGP 69846A). *Clin. Cancer Res.* **5,** 3977–3982.

Olayioye, M. A., Beuvink, I., Horsch, K., Daly, J. M., and Hynes, N. E. (1999). ErbB receptor-induced activation of Stat transcription factors is mediated by src tyrosine kinases. *J. Biol. Chem.* **274,** 17209–17218.

Owens, D. W., McLean, G. W., Wyke, A. W., Paraskeva, C., Parkinson, E. K., Frame, M. C., and Brunton, V. G. (2000). The catalytic activity of the Src family kinases is required to disrupt cadhedrin-dependent cell-cell contacts. *Mol. Biol. Cell* **11**, 51–64.

Ozes, O. N., Mayo, L. D., Gustin, J. A., Pfeffer, S. R., Pfeffer, L. M., and Donner, D. B. (1999). NF-kappaB activation by tumour necrosis factor requires the Akt serine-threonine kinase. *Nature* **401**, 82–85.

Page, C., Lin, H. J., Jin, Y., Castle, V. P., Nunez, G., Huang, M., and Lin, J. (2000). Overexpression of Akt/AKT can modulate chemotherapy-induced apoptosis. *Anticancer Res.* **20**, 407–416.

Pages, G., Lenormand, P., L'Allemain, G., Chambard, J. C., Meloche, S., and Pouyssegur, J. (1993). Mitogen-activated protein kinases p42mapk and p44mapk are required for fibroblast proliferation. *Proc. Natl. Acad. Sci. USA* **90**, 8319–8323.

Pang, L., Sawada, T., Decker, S. J., and Saltiel, A. R. (1995). Inhibition of MAP kinase kinase blocks the differentiation of PC-12 cells induced by nerve growth factor. *J. Biol. Chem.* **270**, 13585–13588.

Pap, M., and Cooper, G. M. (1998). Role of glycogen synthase kinase-3 in the phosphatidylinositol 3-Kinase/Akt cell survival pathway. *J. Biol. Chem.* **273**, 19929–19932.

Papapetropoulos, A., Fulton, D., Mahboubi, K., Kalb, R. G., O'Connor, D. S., Li, F., Altieri, D. C., and Sessa, W. C. (2000). Angiopoietin-1 inhibits endothelial cell apoptosis via the Akt/survivin pathway. *J. Biol. Chem.* **275**, 9102–9105.

Papapetropoulos, A., Garcia-Cardena, G., Madri, J. A., and Sessa, W. C. (1997). Nitric oxide production contributes to the angiogenic properties of vascular endothelial growth factor in human endothelial cells. *J. Clin. Invest.* **100**, 3131–3139.

Parsons, J. T., and Parsons, S. J. (1997). Src family protein tyrosine kinases: Cooperating with growth factor and adhesion signaling proteins. *Curr. Opin. Cell Biol.* **9**, 187–192.

Pawson, T., and Schlessinger, J. (1993). SH2 and SH3 domains. *Curr. Biol.* **3**, 434–442.

Perlmann, T., Rangarajan, P. N., Umesono, K., and Evans, R. M. (1993). Determinants for selective RAR and TR recognition of direct repeat HREs. *Genes Dev.* **7**, 1411–1422.

Petit, A. M., Rak, J., Hung, M. C., Rockwell, P., Goldstein, N., Fendly, B., and Kerbel, R. S. (1997). Neutralizing antibodies against epidermal growth factor and ErbB-2/neu receptor tyrosine kinases down-regulate vascular endothelial growth factor production by tumor cells in vitro and in vivo: Angiogenic implications for signal transduction therapy of solid tumors. *Am. J. Pathol.* **151**, 1523–1530.

Philpott, K. L., McCarthy, M. J., Klippel, A., and Rubin, L. L. (1997). Activated phosphatidylinositol 3-kinase and Akt kinase promote survival of superior cervical neurons. *J. Cell Biol.* **139**, 809–815.

Pinkas-Kramarski, R., Soussan, L., Waterman, H., Levkowitz, G., Alroy, I., Klapper, L., Lavi, S., Seger, R., Ratzkin, B. J., Sela, M., and Yarden, Y. (1996). Diversification of Neu differentiation factor and epidermal growth factor signaling by combinatorial receptor interactions. *EMBO J.* **15**, 2452–2467.

Plo, I., Bettaieb, A., Payrastre, B., Mansat De Mas, V., Bordier, C., Rousse, A., Kowalski Chauvel, A., Laurent, G., and Lautier, D. (1999). The phosphoinositide 3-kinase/Akt pathway is activated by daunorubicin in human acute myeloid leukemia cell lines. *FEBS Lett.* **452**, 150–154.

Potempa, S., and Ridley, A. J. (1998). Activation of both MAP kinase and phosphatidylinositide 3-kinase by Ras is required for hepatocyte growth factor/scatter factor-induced adherens junction disassembly. *Mol. Biol. Cell* **9**, 2185–2200.

Pugazhenthi, S., Nesterova, A., Sable, C., Heidenreich, K. A., Boxer, L. M., Heasley, L. E., and Reusch, J. E. (2000). Akt/protein kinase B up-regulates Bcl-2 expression through cAMP-response element-binding protein. *J. Biol. Chem.* **275**, 10761–10766.

Qian, X., and Greene, M. I. (1997). Her2/neu: A receptor tyrosine kinase with developmental and oncogenic activity. *Encyclopedia Cancer* **2**, 835–856.

Qian, X. L., Dougall, W. C., Fei, Z. Z., and Greene, M. I. (1995). Intermolecular association and trans-phosphorylation of different neu-kinase forms permit SH2-dependent signaling and oncogenic transformation. *Oncogene* **10**, 211–219.

Radmacher, M. D., and Simon, R. (2000). Estimation of tamoxifen's efficacy for preventing the formation and growth of breast tumors. *J. Natl. Cancer Inst.* **92**, 48–53.

Rajkumar, T., and Gullick, W. J. (1994). The type I growth factor receptors in human breast cancer breast. *Cancer Res. Treat.* **29**, 3–9.

Ram, T. G., and Ethier, S. P. (1996). Phosphatidylinositol 3-kinase recruitment by p185erbB-2 and erbB-3 is potently induced by neu differentiation factor/heregulin during mitogenesis and is constitutively elevated in growth factor-independent breast carcinoma cells with c-erbB-2 gene amplification. *Cell Growth Different.* **7**, 551–561.

Rasheed, B. K., Stenzel, T. T., McLendon, R. E., Parsons, R., Friedman, A. H., Friedman, H. S., Bigner, D. D., and Bigner, S. H. (1997). PTEN gene mutations are seen in high-grade but not in low-grade gliomas. *Cancer Res.* **57**, 4187–4190.

Reese, D. M., and Slamon, D. J. (1997). HER-2/neu signal transduction in human breast and ovarian cancer. *Stem Cells* **15**, 1–8.

Reiss, Y., Goldstein, J. L., Seabra, M. C., Casey, P. J., and Brown, M. S. (1990). Inhibition of purified p21 ras farnesyl:protein transferase by Cys-AAX tetrapeptides. *Cell.* **62**, 81–88.

Reiss, Y., Stradley, S. J., Gierasch, L. M., Brown, M. S., and Goldstein, J. L. (1991). Sequence requirement for peptide recognition by rat brain p21 ras protein farnesyltransferase. *Proc. Natl. Acad. Sci. USA* **88**, 732–736.

Ridley, A. J., Comoglio, P. M., and Hall, A. (1995). Regulation of scatter factor/hepatocyte growth factor responses by Ras, Rac and Rho in MDCK cells. *Mol. Cell Biol.* **15**, 1110–1122.

Riese, D. J., and Stern, D. F. (1998). Specificity within the EGF family/erbB receptor family signaling network. *Bioessays* **20**, 41–48.

Riese, D. J., II, Bermingham, Y., van Raaij, T. M., Buckely, S., Plowman, G. D., and Stern, D. F. (1996a). Betacellulin activates the epidermal growth factor receptor and erbB4, and induces cellular response patterns distinct from those stimulated by epidermal growth factor or neuregulin-β. *Oncogene* **12**, 345–353.

Riese, D. J., II, Kim, E. D., Elinius, K., Buckely, S., Klagsgrun, M., Plowman, G. D., and Stern, D. F. (1996b). The epidermal growth factor receptor couples transforming growth factor-α, heparin-binding epidermal growth factor-like factor, and amphiregulin to neu, erbB3, and erbB4. *J. Biol. Chem.* **271**, 20047–20052.

Risinger, J. I., Hayes, A. K., Berchuck, A., and Barrett, J. C. (1997). PTEN/MMAC1 mutations in endometrial cancers. *Cancer Res.* **57**, 4736–4738.

Robertson, D. W., Willy, P. J., Heyman, R. A., and Mangelsdorf, D. J. (1997). Nuclear orphan receptors: Scientific progress and therapeutic opportunities. *In* "Annual Reports in Medicinal Chemistry" (J. A. Bristol, ed.), Vol. 32, pp. 251–260. Academic Press, San Diego.

Robyr, D., Wolffe, A. P., and Wahli, W. (2000). Nuclear hormone receptor coregulators in action: diversity for shared tasks. *Mol. Endocrinol.* **14**, 329–347.

Roche, S., Koegl, M., Barone, M. V., Roussel, M. F., and Courtneidge, S. A. (1995). DNA synthesis induced by some but not all growth factors requires src family protein tyrosine kinases. *Mol. Cell Biol.* **15**, 1102–1109.

Rohn, J. L., Hueber, A. O., McCarthy, N. J., Lyon, D., Navarro, P., Burgering, B. M., and Evan, G. I. (1998). The opposing roles of the Akt and c-Myc signalling pathways in survival from CD95-mediated apoptosis. *Oncogene* **17**, 2811–2818.

Romashkova, J. A., and Makarov, S. S. (1999). NF-kappaB is a target of AKT in anti-apoptotic PDGF signaling. *Nature* **401**, 86–90.

Ross, R. K., Paganini-Hill, A., Wan, P. C., and Pike, M. C. (2000). Effect of hormone replacement therapy on breast cancer risk: Estrogen versus estrogen plus progestin. *J. Natl. Cancer Inst.* **92,** 328–332.

Rowell, C. A., Kowalczyk, J. J., Lewis, M. D., and Garcia, A. M. (1997). Direct demonstration of geranylgeranylation and farnesylation of Ki-Ras in vivo. *J. Biol. Chem.* **272,** 14093–14097.

Rowinsky, E. K., Windle, J. J., and Von Hoff, D. D. (1999). Ras protein farnesyltransferase: a strategic target for anticancer therapeutic development. *J. Clin. Oncol.* **17,** 3631–3652.

Rubin, M. S., Shin, D. M., Pasmantier, M., Falcey, J. W., Paulter, V. J., Fetzer, K. M., Waksal, H. W., Mendelsohn, J., and Hong, W. K. (2000). Monoclonal antibody (MoAb) IMC-C225, an anti-epidermal growth factor receptor (EGFr), for patients (Pts) with EGFr-positive tumors refractory to or in relapse from previous therapeutic regimens. *Proc. Am. Assoc. Clin. Oncol.* **19,** 474a.

Ruggeri, B. A., Huang, L., Wood, M., Cheng, J. Q., and Testa, J. R. (1998). Amplification and overexpression of the AKT2 oncogene in a subset of human pancreatic ductal adenocarcinomas. *Mol. Carcinog.* **21,** 81–86.

Ruthardt, M., Testa, U., Nervi, C., Ferrucci, P. F., Grignani, F., Puccetti, E., Grignani, F., Pesche, C., and Pelicci, P. G. (1997). Opposite effects of the acute promyelocytic leukemia PML-retinoic acid receptor alpha (RARalpha) and PLZF-RAR alpha fusion proteins on retinois acid signalling. *Mol. Cell. Biol.* **17,** 4859–4869.

Sable, C. L., Filippa, N., Filloux, C., Hemmings, B. A., and Van Obberghen, E. (1998). Involvement of the pleckstrin homology domain in the insulin-stimulated activation of protein kinase B. *J. Biol. Chem.* **273,** 29600–29606.

Sable, C. L., Filippa, N., Hemmings, B., and Van Obberghen, E. (1997). cAMP stimulates protein kinase B in a Wortmannin-insensitive manner. *FEBS Lett* **409,** 253–257.

Salomon, D. S., Brandt, R., Ciardiello, F., and Normanno, N. (1995). Epidermal growth factor-related peptides and their receptors in human malignancies. *Crit. Rev. Oncol. Hematol.* **19,** 183–232.

Sato, K. I., Sato, A., Aoto, M., and Fukami, Y. (1995). Site-specific association of c-src with epidermal growth factor receptor in A431 cells. *Biochem. Biophys. Res. Commun.* **210,** 844–851.

Scambia, G., Benedetti-Panici, P., Ferrandina, G., Distefano, M., Salerno, G., Romanini, M. E., Fagotti, A., and Mancuso, S. (1995). Epidermal growth factor, estrogen and progesterone receptor expression in primary ovarian cancer: correlation with clinical outcome and response to chemotherapy. *Br. J. Cancer* **72,** 361–366.

Schaefer, L. K., Wang, S. G., and Schaefer, T. S. (1999). C-Src activates the DNA binding and transcriptional activity of Stat3 molecules: serine 727 is not required for transcriptional activation under certain circumstances. *Biochem. Biophys. Res. Commun.* **266,** 481–487.

Schlessinger, J., and Ullrich, A. (1992). Growth factor signaling by receptor tyrosine kinases. *Neuron* **9,** 383–391.

Schwartzberg, P. L. (1998). The many faces of Src: multiple functions of a prototypical tyrosine kinase. *Oncogene* **17,** 1463–1468.

Sebolt-Leopold, J. S., Dudley, D. T., Herrera, R., Van Becelaere, K., Wiland, A., Gowan, R. C., Tecle, H., Barrett, S. D., Bridges, A., Przybranowski, S., Leopold, W. R., and Saltiel, A. R. (1999). Blockade of the MAP kinase pathway suppresses growth of colon tumors in vivo. *Nat. Med.* **5,** 810–816.

Segatto, O., Lonardo, F., Helin, K., Wexler, D., Fazioli, F., Rhee, S. G., and Di Fiore, P. P. (1992). erbB-2 autophosphorylation is required for mitogenic action and high-affinity substrate coupling. *Oncogene* **7,** 1339–1346.

Seger, R., Ahn, N. G., Posada, J., Munar, E. S., Jensen, A. M., Cooper, J. A., Cobb, M. H., and Krebs, E. G. (1992). Purification and characterization of mitogen-activated protein kinase activated epidermal growth factor-stimulated A431 cells. *J. Biol. Chem.* **267,** 14373–14381.

Sepp-Lorenzino, L., Eberhard, I., Ma, Z., Cho, C., Serve, H., Liu, F., Rosen, N., and Lupu, R. (1996). Signal transduction pathways induced by heregulin in MDA-MB-453 breast cancer cells. *Oncogene* **12,** 1679–1687.

Sepp-Lorenzino, L., Ma, Z., Rands, E., Kohl, N. E., Gibbs, J. B., Oliff, A., and Rosen, N. (1995). A peptidomimetic inhibitor of farnesyl:protein transferase blocks the anchorage-dependent and -independent growth of human tumour cell lines. *Cancer Res.* **55,** 5302–5309.

Sheffield, L. G. (1998). C-src activation by erbB2 leads to attachment-independent growth of human breast epithelial cells. *Biochem. Biophys. Res. Commun.* **250,** 27–31.

Shelly, M., Pinkas-Kramarski, R., Guarino, B. C., Waterman, H., Wang, L.-M., Lyass, L., Alimandi, M., Kuo, A., Bacus, S. S., Pierce, J. H., Andrews, G. c., and Yarden, Y. (1998). Epiregulin is a potent pan-erbB ligand that preferentially activates heterodimeric receptor complexes. *J. Biol. Chem.* **17,** 10496–10505.

Sherwood, V., Bridges, A. J., Denny, W. A., Rewcastle, G. W., and Smaill, J. B., and Fry, D. W. (1999). Selective inhibition of heregulin-dependent tyrosine phosphorylation and cellular signaling through erbB2, erbB3 and erbB4 by PD 158780 and a new irreversible inhibitor, PD 183805. *Proc. Am. Assoc. Cancer Res.* **40,** 723.

Siu, L. L., Hidalgo, M., Nemunaitis, J., Rizzo, J., Moczygemba, J., Eckhardt, S. G., Tolcher, A., Smith, L., Hammond, L., Blackburn, A., Tensfeldt, T., Silberman, S., Von Hoff, D. D., and Rowinsky, E. K. (1999). Dose and schedule-duration escalation of the epidermal growth factor receptor (EGFR) tyrosine kinase (TK) inhibitor CP-358,774: A phase I and pharmacokinetic (PK) study. *Proc. Am. Soc. Clin. Oncol.* **18,** 388a.

Sivaraman, V. S., Wang, H., Nuovo, G. J., and Malbon, C. C. (1997). Hyperexpression of mitogen-activated protein kinase in human breast cancer. *J. Clin. Invest.* **99,** 1478–1483.

Slack, J. L., and Gallagher, R. E. (1999). The molecular biology of acute promyelocytic leukemia. *Cancer Treat. Res.* **99,** 75–124.

Smith, M. A., Parkinson, D. R., Cheson, B. D., and Friedman, M. A. (1992). Retinoids in cancer therapy. *J. Clin. Oncol.* **10,** 839–864.

Songyang, Z., Baltimore, D., Cantley, L. C., Kaplan, D. R., and Franke, T. F. (1997). Interleukin 3-dependent survival by the Akt protein kinase. *Proc. Natl. Acad. Sci. USA* **94,** 11345–11350.

Songyang, Z., Carraway III, K. L., Eck, M. J., Harrison, S. C., Feldman, R. A., Mohammadi, M., Schlessinger, J., Hubbard, S. R., Smith, D. P., Eng, C., Lorenzo, M. J., Ponder, B. A. J., Mayer, B. J., and Cantley, L. C. (1995). Catalytic specificity of protein-tyrosine kinases is critical for selective signalling. *Nature* **373,** 536–539.

Staal, S. P. (1987). Molecular cloning of the akt oncogene and its human homologues AKT1 and AKT2: amplification of AKT1 in a primary human gastric adenocarcinoma. *Proc. Natl. Acad. Sci. USA* **84,** 5034–5037.

Staley, C. A., Parikh, N. U., and Gallick, G. E. (1997). Decreased tumorigenicity of human colon adenocarcinoma cell line by an antisense expression vector specific for c-src. *Cell Growth Different.* **8,** 269–274.

Stambolic, V., Suzuki, A., de la Pompa, J. L., Brothers, G. M., Mirtsos, C., Sasaki, T., Ruland, J., Penninger, J. M., Siderovski, D. P., and Mak, T. W. (1998). Negative regulation of PKB/Akt-dependent cell survival by the tumor suppressor PTEN. *Cell* **95,** 29–39.

Stanton, V. P. Jr., and Cooper, G. M. (1987). Activation of human raf transforming genes by deletion of normal amino-terminal coding sequences. *Mol. Cell. Biol.* **7,** 1171–1179.

Steck, P. A., Lin, H., Langford, L. A., Jasser, S. A., Koul, D., Yung, W. K., and Pershouse, M. A. (1999). Functional and molecular analyses of 10q deletions of human gliomas. *Genes Chromosomes Cancer* **24,** 135–143.

Steck, P. A., Pershouse, M. A., Jasser, S. A., Yung, W. K., Lin, H., Ligon, A. H., Langford, L. A., Baumgard, M. L., Hattier, T., Davis, T., Frye, C., Hu, R., Swedlund, B., Teng, D. H., and Tavtigian, S. V. (1997). Identification of a candidate tumour suppressor gene, MMAC1, at chromosome 10q23.3 that is mutated in multiple advanced cancers. *Nat. Genet.* **15,** 356–362.

Stein, D., Wu, J., Fuqua, S. A., Roonprapunt, C., Yajnik, V., D'Eustachio, P., Moskow, J. J., Buchberg, A. M., Osborne, C. K., and Margolis, B. (1994). The SH2 domain protein GRB7 is co-amplified, overexpressed and in a tight complex with HER2 in breast cancer. *EMBO J.* **13,** 1331–1340.

Stern, D. F., Heffernan, P. A., and Weinberg, R. A. (1986). P185, a product of the neu proto-*Oncogene,* is a receptor-like protein associated with tyrosine kinase activity. *Mol. Cell. Biol.* **6,** 1729–1740.

Stern, D. F., and Kamps, M. P. (1988). EGF-stimulated tyrosine phosphorylation of p185^{neu}. A potential model for receptor interactions. *EMBO J.* **7,** 995–1001.

Stevenson, J. P., Yao, K.-S., Gallagher, M., Friedland, D., Mitchell, E. P., Cassella, A., Monia, B., Kwoh, T. J., Yu, R., Holmlund, J., Dorr, F. A., and O'Dwyer, P. J. (1999). Phase I clinical/pharmacokinetic and pharmacodynamic trial of the c-raf-1 antisense oligonucleotide ISIS 5132 (CGP 69846A). *J. Clin. Oncol.* **17,** 2227–2236.

Stokoe, D., Macdonald, S. G., Cadwallader, K., Symons, M., and Hancock, J. F. (1994). Activation of Raf as a result of recruitment to the plasma membrane. *Science* **264,** 1463–1467.

Stokoe, D., Stephens, L. R., Copeland, T., Gaffney, P. R., Reese, C. B., Painter, G. F., Holmes, A. B., McCormick, F., and Hawkins, P. T. (1997). Dual role of phosphatidylinositol-3,4,5-trisphosphate in the activation of protein kinase B. *Science* **277,** 567–570.

Storm, S. M., and Rapp, U. R. (1993). Oncogene activation: c-raf-1 gene mutations in experimental and naturally occurring tumors. *Toxicol. Lett.* **67,** 201–210.

Stover, D. R., Becker, M., Liebetanz, J., and Lydon, N. B. (1995). Src phosphorylation of the epidermal growth factor receptor at novel sites mediates receptor interaction with src and p85 alpha. *J. Biol. Chem.* **270,** 15591–15597.

Struhl, K. (1998). Histone acetylation and transcriptional regulatory mechanisms. *Genes Dev.* **12,** 599–606.

Suzuki, H., Freije, D., Nusskern, D. R., Okami, K., Cairns, P., Sidransky, D., Isaacs, W. B., and Bova, G. S. (1998). Interfocal heterogeneity of PTEN/MMAC1 gene alterations in multiple metastatic prostate cancer tissues. *Cancer Res.* **58,** 204–209.

Talamonti, M. S., Roh, M. S., Curley, S. A., and Gallick, G. E. (1993). Increase in level and activity of pp60^{c-src} in progressive stages of human colorectal carcinoma. *J. Clin. Invest.* **91,** 53–60.

Tang, E. D., Nunez, G., Barr, F. G., and Guan, K. L. (1999). Negative regulation of the forkhead transcription factor FKHR by Akt. *J. Biol. Chem.* **274,** 16741–16746.

Tanimura, S., Chatani, Y., Hoshino, R., Sato, M., Watanabe, S., Kataoka, T., Nakamura, T., and Kohno, M. (1998). Activation of the 41/43 kDa mitogen-activated protein kinase signaling pathway is required for hepatocyte growth factor-induced cell scattering. *Oncogene* **17,** 57–65.

Tashiro, H., Blazes, M. S., Wu, R., Cho, K. R., Bose, S., Wang, S. I., Li, J., Parsons, R., and Ellenson, L. H. (1997). Mutations in PTEN are frequent in endometrial carcinoma but rare in other common gynecological malignancies. *Cancer Res.* **57,** 3935–3940.

Thomas, S. M., and Brugge, J. S. (1997). Cellular functions regulated by src family kinases. *Ann. Rev. Cell Dev. Biol.* **13,** 513–609.

Tice, D. A., Biscardi, J. S., Nickles, A. L., and Parsons, S. J. (1999). Mechanism of biological synergy between cellular src and epidermal growth factor receptor. *Proc. Natl. Acad. Sci. USA* **96,** 1415–1420.

Toi, M., Tominaga, T., Osaki, A., and Toge, T. (1994). Role of epidermal growth factor receptor expression in primary breast cancer: Results of a biochemical study and an immunocytochemical study. *Breast Cancer Res.* **29,** 51–58.

Toker, A., and Newton, A. C. (2000). Akt/protein kinase B is regulated by autophosphorylation at the hypothetical PDK-2 site. *J. Biol. Chem.* **275,** 8271–8274.

Tzahar, E., PinkasKramarski, R., Moyer, J. D., Kapper, L. N., Alroy, I., Lev-

kowitz, G., Shelly, M., Henis, S., Eisenstein, M., Ratzkin, B. J., Sela, M., Andrews, G. C., and Yarden, Y. (1997). Bivalence of EGF-like ligands drives the ErbB signaling network. *EMBO J.* **16,** 4938–4950.

Tzahar, E., Waterman, H., Chen, X. M., Levkowitz, G., Karunagaran, D., Lavi, S., Ratzkin, B. J., and Yarden, Y. (1996). A hierarchical network of interreceptor interactions determines signal transduction by neu differentiation factor/neuregulin and epidermal growth factor. *Mol. Cell. Biol.* **16,** 5276–5287.

van Oijen, M. G. C. T., Rijksen, G., ten Broek, F. W., and Slootweg, P. J. (1998). Overexpression of c-src in areas of hyperproliferation in head and neck cancer, premalignant lesions and benign mucosal disorders. *J. Oral Pathol. Med.* **27,** 147–152.

van Weeren, P. C., de Bruyn, K. M., de Vries Smits, A. M., van Lint, J., and Burgering, B. M. (1998). Essential role for protein kinase B (PKB) in insulin-induced glycogen synthase kinase 3 inactivation. Characterization of dominant-negative mutant of PKB. *J. Biol. Chem.* **273,** 13150–13156.

Verbeek, B. S., Vroom, T. M., Adriaansen-Slot, S. S., Ottenhoff-Kalff, A. E., Geertzema, J. G. N., Hennipman, A., and Rijksen, G. (1996). c-Src protein expression is increased in human breast cancer. An immunohistochemical and biochemical analysis. *J. Pathol.* **180,** 383–388.

Vincent, P. W., Patmore, S. J., Atkinson, B. E., Bridges, A. J., Kirkish, L. S., Dudeck, R. C., Leopold, W. R., Zhou, H., and Elliott, W. L. (1999). Optimal in vivo treatment schedule for the novel EGF receptor family tyrosine kinase inhibitor, PD 183805, correlates with the inhibition of receptor tyrosine phosphorylation. *Proc. Am. Assoc. Cancer Res.* **39,** 117.

Wada, T., Qian, X., and Green, M. I. (1999). Intermolecular association of the p185neu protein and EGF receptor modulates EGF receptor function. *Cell* **61,** 1339–1347.

Wakeling, A. E. (1993). The future of new pure antiestrogens in clinical breast cancer. *Breast Cancer Res. Treat.* **25,** 1–9.

Wang, H-G., Rapp, U. R., and Reed, J. C. (1996). Bcl-2 targets the protein kinase Raf-1 to mitochondria. *Cell* **87,** 629–638.

Wang, S. I., Parsons, R., and Ittmann, M. (1998). Homozygous deletion of the PTEN tumor suppressor gene in a subset of prostate adenocarcinomas. *Clin. Cancer Res.* **4,** 811–815.

Weatherman, R. V., Fletterick, R. J., and Scanlan, T. S. (1999). Nuclear-receptor ligands and ligand-binding domains. *Ann. Rev. Biochem.* **68,** 559–581.

Whyte, D. B., Kirschmeier, P., Hockenberry, T. N., Nunez-Oliva, I., James, L., Catino, J. J., Bishop, W. R., and Pai, J. K. (1997). K- and N-Ras are geranylgeranylated in cells treated with farnesyl protein transferase inhibitors. *J. Biol. Chem.* **272,** 14459–14464.

Wiener, J. R., Nakano, K., Kruzelock, R. P., Bucana, C. D., Bast, R. C., and Gallick, G. E. (1999). Decreased Src tyrosine kinase activity inhibits malignant human ovarian cancer tumor growth in a nude mouse model. *Clin. Cancer Res.* **5,** 2164–2170.

Wu, X., Senechal, K., Neshat, M. S., Whang, Y. E., and Sawyers, C. L. (1998). The PTEN/MMAC1 tumor suppressor phosphatase functions as a negative regulator of the phosphoinositide 3-kinase/Akt pathway. *Proc. Natl. Acad. Sci. USA* **95,** 15587–15591.

Xiong, W., and Parsons, J. T. (1997). Induction of apoptosis after expression of PYK2, a tyrosine kinase structurally related to focal adhesion kinase. *J. Cell Biol.* **139,** 529–539.

Yamamoto, K. (1985). Steroid receptor regulated transcription of specific genes and gene networks. *Annu. Rev. Genet.* **19,** 209–252.

Yeung, K., Setiz, T., Li, S., Janosch, P., McFerran, B., Kaiser, C., Fee, F., Katsanakis, K. D., Rose, D. W., Mischak, H., Sedivy, J. M., and Kolch, W. (1999). Suppression of Raf-1 kinase activity and MAP kinase signalling by RKIP. *Nature* **401,** 173–177.

Yuan, Z. Q., Sun, M., Feldman, R. I., Wang, G., Ma, X., Jiang, C., Coppola,

D., Nicosia, S. V., and Cheng, J. Q. (2000). Frequent activation of AKT2 and induction of apoptosis by inhibition of phosphoinositide-3-OH kinase/Akt pathway in human ovarian cancer. *Oncogene* **19,** 2324–2330.

Yuen, A. R., and Sikic, B. I. (2000). Clinical studies of antisense therapy in cancer. *Front. Biosci.* **5,** 588–593.

Zhang, D., Sliwkowski, M. X., Mark, M., Frantz, G., Akita, R., Sun, Y., Hillan, K., Crowley, C., Brush, J., and Godowski, P. J. (1997). Neuregulin-3 (NRG3): A novel neural tissue-enriched protein that binds and activates erbB4. *Proc. Natl. Acad. Sci.* **94,** 9562–9567.

Zhang, F. L., and Casey, P. J. (1996). Protein prenylation: Molecular mechanisms and functional consequences. *Annu. Rev. Biochem.* **65,** 241–269.

Zhang, X., and Vik, T. A. (1997). Growth factor stimulation of hematopoi-etic cells leads to membrane translocation of AKT1 protein kinase. *Leuk. Res.* **21,** 849–856.

Zhong, H., Chiles, K., Feldser, D., Laughner, E., Hanrahan, C., Georgescu, M. M., Simons, J. W., and Semenza, G. L. (2000). Modulation of hypoxia-inducible factor 1 alpha expression by the epidermal growth factor/phosphatidylinositol 3-kinase/PTEN/AKT/FRAP pathway in human prostate cancer cells: implications for tumor angiogenesis and therapeutics. *Cancer Res.* **60,** 1541–1545.

Zundel, W., Schindler, C., Haas Kogan, D., Koong, A., Kaper, F., Chen, E., Gottschalk, A. R., Ryan, H. E., Johnson, R. S., Jefferson, A. B., Stokoe, D., and Giaccia, A. J. (2000). Loss of PTEN facilitates HIF-1-mediated gene expression. *Genes Dev.* **14,** 391–396.

CHAPTER 4

CELL DEATH PATHWAYS AS TARGETS FOR ANTICANCER DRUGS

Eric Solary*,†
Nathalie Droin*
Olivier Sordet*
Cédric Rebe*
Rodolphe Filomenko*
Anne Wotawa*
Stephanie Plenchette*
Patrick Ducoroy*

*INSERM 517, Dijon, France;
and †Hematology Unit, CHU Le Bocage, Dijon, France

Summary

Biochemical and molecular analyses have indicated that currently used anticancer drugs simultaneously activate several pathways that either positively or negatively regulate cell death induction. The main pathway from specific damage induced by these drugs to apoptosis involves activation of caspases in the cytosol by proapoptotic molecules, such as cytochrome c, released from the mitochondria under the control of the Bcl-2 family of proteins. Anticancer drugs modulate this pathway by modifying the expression of Bcl-2 proteins (e.g., through $p53$-dependent gene transcription), their activity (e.g., by phosphorylating Bcl-2), and their subcellular localization (e.g., by inducing the translocation of specific BH3-only proapoptotic proteins). Anticancer drugs can also up-regulate the expression of death receptors, such as Fas (APO-1/CD95) and TRAIL receptors, and sensitize tumor cells to their cognate ligands. The Fas–FasL interaction could amplify early steps of drug-induced apoptosis while up-regulation of TRAIL receptors offers the opportunity for a synergistic administration of an anticancer drug and TRAIL. In addition, anticancer drugs activate in tumor cells several lipid-dependent signal transduction pathways that either increase or decrease their ability to die by apoptosis. Additional protective pathways activated by chemotherapeutic agents involve the NF-κB transcription factor, heat-shock proteins such as Hsp27, and cell cycle regulatory molecules. In this chapter we discuss how modulation of the balance between noxious and protective signals that modulate cell death pathways could improve the efficacy of currently used anticancer agents or suggest new therapeutic targets.

55

1. Introduction

Biochemical and molecular pharmacology studies have identified the cellular target of currently used anticancer agents, e.g., topoisomerase inhibitors, alkylating agents, and X-irradiation damage DNA. Spindle poisons inhibit the functions of microtubules, and antimetabolites inhibit DNA synthesis by disrupting nucleotide pools. These studies also identified several mechanisms that can limit anticancer drug efficacy by decreasing drug interaction with its specific intracellular target, e.g., decreased accumulation of the drug in the tumor cell as a consequence of an increased energy-dependent efflux (so-called multidrug resistance), altered cellular metabolism of the chemotherapeutic agent, or mutation of its main intracellular target. Based on these studies, various strategies have been proposed to improve the clinical usefulness of anticancer drugs, such as addition of leucovorin to 5-fluorouracil treatment (Erlichman *et al.,* 1988) or inhibition of P-glycoprotein-mediated efflux with a noncytotoxic "multidrug resistance reversing agent" (Solary *et al.,* 1996). During the past 10 years, our knowledge of the signaling pathways that regulate cell death has risen dramatically. Virtually all anticancer drugs can kill tumor cells by inducing apoptosis. In addition, apoptotic blast cells can be detected in the peripheral blood from patients who receive chemotherapeutic drugs for treatment of acute leukemia (Yang *et al.,* 1994). Thus, apoptosis may be a clinically relevant mode of tumor cell death triggered by anticancer agents, and the ability of tumor cells to die by apoptosis in response to specific damage induced by an anticancer drug may be an additional determinant of their sensitivity to this drug. This chapter will discuss the different pathways that positively and negatively regulate the cell death process in response to anticancer-drug-induced damage. Targeting of these noxious or protective signals could provide new strategies to improve the efficacy of current chemotherapeutic regimens.

2. Two Main Pathways for Drug-Induced Apoptosis

Apoptosis is a physiologic process that engages a well-ordered signaling cascade, eventually leading to cell demise and dead-cell clearance by neighboring phagocytes. In many tumor cells, the main signaling pathway leading from drug-induced damage to cell death involves the mitochondrial release of proapoptotic molecules under the control of the Bcl-2 family of proteins. Death receptors of the tumor necrosis factor (TNF) receptor superfamily, mainly Fas (APO-1/CD95), may play a role in linking drug-induced damage to the apoptotic machinery and modulating drug response (Fig. 1).

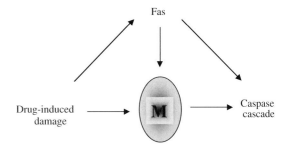

FIGURE 1 Two main pathways involved in drug-induced cell death. In most tumor cells, the main signaling pathway leading from drug-induced damage to cell death involves the mitochondrial release of molecules that activate the caspase cascade. Death receptors such as Fas (APO-1/CD95) may also play a role in linking drug-induced damage to the apoptotic machinery.

A. The Mitochondrial Pathway

Like many other apoptotic stimuli, chemotherapeutic agents can induce mitochondrial membrane permeabilization. This permeabilization concerns the inner membrane and induces a dissipation of the proton gradient that results from the respiration driven, electron transport chain mediated pumping of these protons and is responsible for the mitochondrial transmembrane potential $\Delta\psi_m$. Permeabilization also concerns the outer membrane of the mitochondria, which induces the leakage of soluble proteins normally confined to the intermembrane space of these organelles (Kluck *et al.,* 1997).

Various alternative mechanisms have been proposed to account for mitochondrial membrane permeabilization (for review, see Kroemer and Reed, 2000). One of the proposed models involves autonomous pore formation in the external mitochondrial membrane by proapoptotic proteins of the Bcl-2 family such as Bax, which requires Bax oligomerization and may be enhanced by the truncated protein Bid (a BH3-domain-only protein of the Bcl-2 family that will be further described in Section 2.A) and antagonized by Bcl-2 (Antonsson *et al.,* 1997; Schlesinger *et al.,* 1997; Eskes *et al.,* 2000). Another model suggests that inner membrane permeabilization occurs first as a consequence of pore formation by the adenine nucleotide translocator (ANT), an ATP/ADP-specific antiporter that, in response to apoptotic stimuli, would become a nonspecific pore. Then the rapid loss of the mitochondrial transmembrane potential $\Delta\psi_m$ could induce osmotic matrix swelling and consequent outer-membrane rupture (Zamzami *et al.,* 1995; Marzo *et al.,* 1998; Crompton, 1999). The third model involves the voltage-dependent anion channel (VDAC), the most abundant protein in the outer membrane of the mitochondria. In normal conditions, this channel is permeable to solutes up to 5000 Da. Interaction with Bax could render the channel permeant to higher molecular weight molecules, such as cytochrome *c* (Shimizu *et al.,* 1999). A fourth hypothesis is that both VDAC and ANT are involved in mitochondrial permeabilization by forming a multimolecular complex known as the permeability transition pore, under the control of Bcl-2 and related anti-apoptotic proteins. Alteration of this complex may affect both inner and outer membranes of the mitochondria (Kroemer and Reed, 2000). Actually, the exact mechanism may depend on the cell type due to the tissue-specific expression of some components of the permeability transition pore.

Among the molecules released from the intermembrane space of the mitochondria is 14.5-kDa heme-binding holocytochrome c, which upon entry in the cytosol induces oligomerization of APAF-1 (apoptotic protease activating factor 1) and exposes its caspase recruitment domain (ARD) in the presence of ATP (Li et al., 1997; Hu et al., 1999). In turn, oligomerized APAF-1 binds to cytosolic procaspase-9 in a so-called apoptosome complex and induces juxtaposition of two procaspase-9 molecules, resulting in autoactivation and release of mature caspase-9 (Fig. 2). This latter enzyme then activates additional caspase-9 molecules, as well as caspase-3 and caspase-7, which in turn activate a downstream caspase cascade (Slee et al., 1999). Mitochondrial caspases and certain heat-shock proteins (Hsp's), such as Hsp60 and Hsp10, that are also released from the mitochondrial intermembrane space may facilitate initiation of these catabolic reactions (Samali et al., 1999a; Xanthoudakis et al., 1999).

In some cells, cytochrome c release could inhibit the respiratory chain in the mitochondria, resulting in ATP depletion that precludes procaspase-9 recruitment by APAF-1. This situation prevents caspase-dependent features of apoptosis such as oligonucleosomal DNA fragmentation and advanced chromatin condensation. The death phenotype observed in such a situation could involve the 57-kDa flavoprotein apoptosis inducing factor (AIF), which translocates from the mitochondria to the nucleus and triggers ATP- and caspase-independent nuclear changes (Susin et al., 1999b) (Fig. 2). Inhibition of the respiratory chain also enhances generation of radical oxygen species that contribute to cell damage. Changes in mitochondrial function may also be responsible for cytoplasmic acidification that was reported as an early event during apoptosis (Kroemer and Reed, 2000).

B. The Death-Receptor-Dependent Pathway

At least in some cell types, cytotoxic-drug-induced apoptosis also involves the death receptor Fas (also known as APO-1 or CD95), a 45-kDa, type I membrane, death receptor protein that belongs to the TNF receptor superfamily. Its natural ligand, Fas ligand (FasL, APO-1L, CD95L), exists mainly as a 40-kDa membrane-bound protein (Pinkoski and Green, 1999). The apoptotic cell death pathway triggered by FasL is believed to proceed as follows: FasL binds to and induces clustering of Fas, the intracellular part of which contains a characteristic 85-amino-acid region known as the death domain (DD). A complex known as the death-initiating signaling complex (DISC) is formed that involves an adaptor protein named FADD (for Fas-associated death domain) (Chinnaiyan et al., 1995) and procaspase-8 (Medema et al., 1997). FADD binds to the cytoplasmic region of Fas through homophilic interactions of their respective DD and to the N-terminal domain of procaspase-8 through a second interacting region called the death effector domain (DED). Oligomerization of procaspase-8 in the DISC results in autoactivation with release in the cytosol of fully active caspase-8. This process may involve additional proteins, such as FLASH, though the role of this latter protein in Fas signaling remains controversial (Imai et al., 1999). Depending on the level of DISC formed in each cell type, caspase-8 can either directly activate the effector caspases (type I cells) or cleave the carboxy-terminal part of a BH3 domain-only proapoptotic member of the Bcl-2 family designated Bid (type II cells) (Li et al., 1998b; Luo et al., 1998; Scaffidi et al., 1999). In turn, translocation of the truncated Bid to the mitochondria activates, in combination with Bax, the previously described mitochondrial pathway to cell death (Fig. 3). The Fas–FasL system plays an important role in the normal development of T lymphocytes and self-destruction of activated T cells. Fas–FasL interaction is also one of the mechanisms by which cytotoxic immune cells can kill Fas-expressing target cells (Pinkoski and Green, 1999).

Ionizing radiation (Ogawa et al. 1997; Albanese and Dainiak, 2000) and various anticancer drugs (Friesen et al., 1996; Fulda et al., 2000) were shown to cause up-regulation of FasL. In some cell types, this up-regulation could depend on the presence of a functional wild-type p53 gene (Muller et al., 1998). Then interaction of FasL with Fas at the surface of tumor cells could define an autocrine/paracrine pathway similar to that observed in activation-induced cell death of T lymphocytes. However, the role of the FasL–Fas system in drug-induced apoptosis has been challenged by several studies in which the cell death process was not influenced by antagonistic antibodies or molecules that prevent FasL interaction with Fas. In addition, apoptosis induced by chemotherapeutic drugs is not altered in embryonic fibroblasts from FADD (Yeh et al., 1998) and

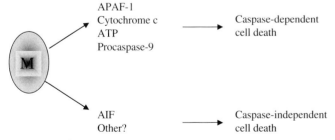

FIGURE 2 Caspase-dependent and independent cell death pathways. While caspases play a role in most apoptotic pathways, e.g., through the mitochondrial release of cytochrome c and the formation of the apoptosome (APAF-1/cytochrome c/ATP/procaspase-9), a caspase-independent pathway has been identified that could involved the flavoprotein apoptosis-inducing factor.

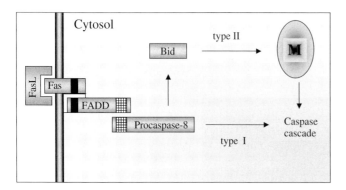

FIGURE 3 Two pathways for Fas-mediated cell death. FasL interaction with Fas induces its trimerization (not shown) and the recruitment of the adaptor molecule FADD through death domain interactions *(black boxes)*. In turn, FADD recruits procaspase-8. Depending on the cell content in active caspase-8, this enzyme either directly activates the downstream caspases (type I cells) or cleaves Bid (type II cells). Truncated Bid, in combination with Bax (not shown), activates the mitochondrial pathway to cell death.

caspase-8 (Varfolomeev *et al.,* 1998) knockout (KO) mice. A first hypothesis that could account for these observations is that DISC formation could be dispensable for drug-induced cell death, depending on the cell type. Another possibility is that anticancer drugs, like UV radiation and other compounds, could induce Fas clustering at the surface of tumor cells in the absence of FasL (Micheau *et al.,* 1999b). Whatever the exact mechanism, Fas alone or the FasL–Fas interaction may be involved in the initiation phase of apoptosis triggered by anticancer drugs while requirement for this system may be bypassed at later stages, when alterations of the mitochondria occur as a direct consequence of specific damage induced by the drug (Fulda *et al.,* 2000).

Fas gene mutations that characterize some congenital autoimmune lymphoproliferative syndromes (ALPSs) and inhibit Fas-mediated apoptosis by a dominant-negative mechanism (Rieux-Laucat *et al.,* 1999) have now been identified in several malignancies (Landowski *et al.,* 1997; Beltinger *et al.,* 1998; Tamiya *et al.,* 1998). These mutations of Fas could account for some chemoresistance, e.g., in acute T-cell leukemias. Caspase-10 mutations, which account for some congenital ALPSs without Fas mutation (Wang *et al.,* 1999b), have not been so far identified in human lymphoid tumors, but caspase-8 was recently shown to be inactivated or deleted in neuroblastoma cells (Teitz *et al.,* 2000), thus rendering these cells more resistant to chemotherapeutic drugs.

3. Modulation of Drug-Induced Cell Death by Bcl-2 and Related Proteins

A. The *Bcl-2* Gene Family

The *Bcl-2* (B-cell leukemia/lymphoma 2) gene was identified at the chromosomal breakpoint of the t(14;18)(q32;q21) that characterizes follicular B-cell lymphomas (Bakhshi *et al.,* 1985; Cleary *et al.,* 1986). Overexpressed Bcl-2 protein antagonizes apoptosis induced by a number of different stimuli, including anticancer drugs (for review, see Zamzami *et al.,* 1998; Gross *et al.,* 1999). Overexpression of *bcl-2* in various human tumors contributes to cell accumulation and, in combination with abnormal expression of other oncogenes such as *c-myc,* to malignant transformation (Strasser *et al.,* 1990; McDonnell *et al.,* 1989; 1991).

A number of *bcl-2*-related genes have been identified that either prevent cell death and function as potential oncogenes (Bcl-2, Bcl-X$_L$, Mcl-1, A1/ Bfl-1, Bcl-W), or encourage cell demise and behave as tumor suppressor genes (Bax, Bak, Bok, Bcl-X$_S$, Bad, Bim, Bid, Bik, Hrk) (Zamzami *et al.,* 1998; Gross *et al.,* 1999). For example, missense mutations in Bax, which were recently identified in primary human tumors, could contribute to disease progression and drug resistance (Meijerink *et al.,* 1998). In addition, the genome of several pathogenic viruses, such as Epstein–Barr virus and Kaposi's sarcoma virus (Henderson *et al.,* 1993; Sarid *et al.,* 1997; Cheng *et al.,* 1997a), encodes Bcl-2 analogues.

Structural analysis of Bcl-2 and related proteins led to the distinction of three subfamilies. Antiapoptotic Bcl-2 proteins possess up to four conserved Bcl-2-homology (BH) domains designated BH1 to BH4. Proapoptotic Bcl-2-related proteins can be divided in those with at least three BH domains, such as Bax, Bak and Bok/mtd, and more distantly related proteins that share only the BH3 domain with Bcl-2, such as Bid, Bim, or Bad (also designated BH3-only proteins). In addition, many of these proteins contain a carboxy-terminal transmembrane domain that targets them to cellular membranes, e.g., the mitochondrial outer membrane (Gross *et al.,* 1999) (Table 1).

In the absence of death signal, many proapoptotic members of the Bcl-2 family actually localize to cytosol or cytoskeleton. Following a death signal, these proteins undergo a conformational change that enables them to target and integrate into membranes, especially the mitochondrial outer membrane. Then interactions between antiapoptotic and proapoptotic members of the Bcl-2 family modulate cytochrome *c* redistribution from the mitochondria. However, some proapoptotic proteins such as Bax or Bak have autonomous death-inducing activity, apart from their ability to bind Bcl-2 or other antiapoptotic members of the family (Inohara *et al.,* 1997; Simonian *et al.,* 1997; Zha and Reed, 1997).

B. Bcl-2 Proteins Modulate Cell Death

1. Mechanisms of Action of Bcl-2 Proteins

The Bcl-2 family of proteins modulates cell death in part by affecting the mitochondrial compartmentalization of cytochrome *c* and several other proteins. Expression of Bcl-2 protein also stabilizes the mitochondrial transmembrane potential by regulating the proton flux, inhibits generation of

TABLE 1
Antiapoptotic and Proapoptotic Molecules That Modulate
Cytotoxic-Agent-Induced Apoptosis

	Antiapoptotic	Proapoptotic
Bcl-2-family of proteins	Bcl-2, Bcl-X$_L$, Mcl-1	Bax, Bak, Bcl-X$_S$, Bim, Bid, Bad Caspase-cleaved Bcl-2 Phosphorylated Bcl-2
Caspases	Caspase isoforms (2S, 9b) Nitrosylated caspase-3 Phosphorylated caspase-9	Initiator caspases (2L, 8, 9, 10) Effector caspases (3, 6, 7)
Other modulators	IAPs (inhibitors of apoptosis) FLIP (FLICE inhibitory protein) NF-κB (nuclear factor–kappa B	Death receptors
Heat-shock proteins	Hsp27, Hsp70	Hsp60, Hsp90
Cell cycle	p21$^{CIP1/WAF1}$, p27^{Kip1}	p53, (p73?)
Lipid signals	Ceramide	Diacylglycerol
Kinases	Phosphatidylinositol 3′-kinase (PI-3K) Protein kinase C (PKC) Mitogen activated protein kinase (MAPK)	c-Jun N-terminal kinase (JNK)

radical oxygen species, and prevents cytoplasmic acidification. Thus, Bcl-2 proteins can be envisioned as general regulators of mitochondrial physiology. More specifically, their structural similarities with pore-forming domains of certain bacterial toxins have suggested that some of these proteins may form channels in the outer mitochondrial membrane (Schendel et al., 1998).

Indirect mechanisms of action have also been proposed to account for Bcl-2 antiapoptotic activity. Bcl-2 interacts with a series of proteins involved in cell cycle regulation and gene transcription. For example, Bcl-2 binds to and sequesters calcineurin, a calcium-dependent phosphatase. As a consequence, the nuclear factor of activated T lymphocytes (NFAT) is not dephosphorylated in response to cytotoxic drugs, and then does not move to the nucleus to activate the transcription of FasL and trigger apoptosis through a FasL–Fas interaction (Shibasaki et al., 1997). Lastly, at least in some cell types, the antiapoptotic protein Bcl-2 can become a proapoptotic factor when cleaved by caspases during the apoptotic process (Cheng et al., 1997b).

2. Translocation of Proapoptotic Bcl-2 Proteins

In healthy cells, the proapoptotic proteins are maintained by various mechanisms in a latent form in the cytoplasm until unleashed by apoptotic signals. For example, in viable cells, the proapoptotic molecule Bax is monomeric and found either in the cytosol or loosely attached to membranes. Fol-

lowing a death stimulus, Bax dimerizes, translocates to the mitochondria, inserts into outer mitochondria membranes, and alters the exposure of its amino-terminal domain. Bak demonstrates similar conformational changes in response to some apoptotic stimuli (Gross et al., 1999), suggesting that the amino-terminal part of Bax and Bak acts as an inhibitory domain.

The BH3-only protein 22-kDa protein known as Bid is cleaved by caspase-8 in some cells exposed to Fas agonists or TNF-α (Nagata, 1999). The 15-kDa truncated carboxy-terminal part of Bid then translocates to the mitochondria and, in cooperation with Bax (Desagher et al., 1999), releases cytochrome c. Another BH3-only protein is Bad, which is inactivated by survival-promoting factors such as interleukin-3 (IL-3) through several phosphorylation pathways (Downward, 1999). Dephosphorylation of Bad upon growth factor deprivation induces its translocation from a cytosolic 14-3-3 protein to the mitochondria (Wang et al., 1999a).

A third BH3-only protein, Bim, could play an important role in microtubule-agent-induced apoptosis (Puthalakath et al., 1999). Bim is expressed in many hematopoietic cell types. Studies on Bim$^{-/-}$ mice have shown that the protein might have a role in regulating blood leukocyte number including B and T lymphocytes, monocytes, and granulocytes and in platelet shedding from megakaryocytes. Bim is normally sequestered to the microtubule dynein motor complex by interaction with dynein light chain LC8. Apoptotic stimuli provoke release of Bim and LC8, allowing Bim to associate with Bcl-2-like proteins (Bouillet et al., 1999). When treated with taxol, purified Bim$^{-/-}$ pre-T cells demonstrated extended survival. These cells were also more resistant to dexamethasone and ionizing radiation than wild-type cells but demonstrated similar sensitivity to etoposide (Bouillet et al., 1999). Bim is essential for responses to certain apoptotic stimuli that can be antagonized by Bcl-2 but is largely dispensable for others. It thus appears that different BH3-only proteins are required to execute particular death responses in individual cell types (Fig. 4).

3. Bcl-2 Phosphorylation

Bcl-2 activity can also be regulated by phosphorylation at serine residues 70 and 87 that is associated with loss of its antiapoptotic function (Haldar et al., 1995; Chang et al., 1997; Basu and Holder, 1998a; Deng et al., 1998; Poommipanit et al., 1999). Bcl-2 phosphorylation is specifically induced by anticancer drugs that interact with monomeric tubulin and affect microtubule polymerization, such as the Vinca alkaloids, and those that interact with polymerized tubulin and prevent depolymerization, such as the taxanes. This effect is not seen with DNA-damaging agents. Bcl-2 phosphorylation has been shown to prevent the protein from forming heterodimers with Bax. Several signal transduction pathways could be involved in antimicrotubule-agent-mediated Bcl-2 phosphorylation (Srivastava et al., 1998; Basu et al., 2000).

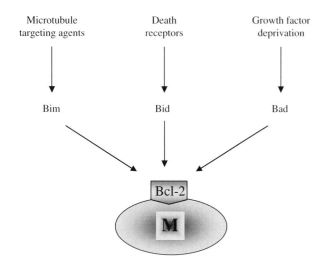

FIGURE 4 Recruitment of BH3-only proteins. Different BH3-domain only proteins (proapoptotic molecules of the Bcl-2 family) are required to execute specific death responses to specific stimuli and in specific cell types. In response to a given stimulus, these proteins migrate from the cytosol to the mitochondria where they interact with and neutralize the antiapoptotic proteins of the Bcl-2 family, e.g., Bcl-2 itself.

One of these pathways involves Raf-1, a ubiquitously expressed serine/threonine kinase that is activated in cells treated with paclitaxel and whose expression is decreased in cell lines resistant to this drug. Raf-1-mediated phosphorylation of Bcl-2 could involve induction of the cyclin-dependent kinase inhibitor p21$^{WAF1/CIP1}$, either as a consequence of p53 induction or not (Basu et al., 2000). Another kinase that was suggested to be involved in Bcl-2 phosphorylation is protein kinase A (PKA), which is activated in response to microtubule damage (Srivastava et al., 1998). The role of p34^{cdc2} kinase and the mitogen-activated protein kinases (MAPKs) that include extracellular signal-regulated protein kinases (ERKs), c-Jun N-terminal kinase/stress-activated protein kinases (JNK/SAPKs) and p38, in modulating Bcl-2 phosphorylation is still unclear and could depend on the cell type and the cytotoxic agent (Wang et al., 1999c). For example, a transient and early activation of JNK/SAPK rather than Raf-1 phosphorylation might account for Bcl-2 phosphorylation in K562 myelogenous leukemic cells exposed to 2-methoxyestradiol, which inhibits microtubule dynamics (Attala et al., 1998; Wang et al., 1999c). Whatever the pathway, phosphorylation/dephosphorylation of Bcl-2 appears as a molecular determinant of cell survival or death in response to microtubule-damaging anticancer drugs.

4. Transcriptional Regulation of Bcl-2-Related Proteins

A last mechanism that modulates the expression and activity of Bcl-2 proteins is their transcriptional regulation. The transcription factor p53 was demonstrated to bind to typical recog-

nition elements located in the *bax* gene promoter while down-regulating *bcl-2* gene expression (Miyashita et al., 1994; Selvakumaran et al., 1994; Miyashita and Reed, 1995; Basu and Haldar, 1998b). A transcriptional regulation of the BH3-only protein Hrk has also been demonstrated (Inohara et al., 1997). The ability of DNA-damaging agents to up-regulate *bax* gene was proposed to explain why some tumors with high levels of Bcl-2 protein could initially respond to these agents.

Thus, proapoptotic members of the Bcl-2 family behave as sentinels for cellular damage. To avoid toxicity in healthy cells, these sentinels are either transcriptionally silent or sequestered in various parts of the cells. Each of them monitors specific damage, e.g., Bim is on the lookout for microtubule disruption, Bax and Bad for metabolic stress, and Bid for limited caspase-8 activation. Whether specific alteration of the pathway could account for specific resistance to a given anticancer agent is still undetermined.

C. Bcl-2 Proteins as Targets for Cancer Therapy

Various mechanisms can account for abnormal expression of Bcl-2 proteins in malignant cells, including chromosomal translocation that structurally alters *bcl-2* or a related gene, single-nucleotide substitutions or frameshift mutations that inactivate Bax, retrovirus insertion that activates Bcl-X$_L$, and abnormal transcriptional or posttranscriptional regulation of the protein. Imbalance in the ratios of anti- and proapoptotic Bcl-2 family members can render the cells more resistant to a variety of apoptotic stimuli, including chemotherapeutic agents, radiation, and more recent anticancer therapies. This defines a new multidrug resistance phenotype in which translation of drug-induced damage in a death signal is altered (Miyashita and Reed, 1993; Schmitt et al., 1998).

The prognostic value of Bcl-2 and Bcl-2-related protein expression remains a controversial issue due to the complexity of dealing with a large multigene family and the potential alteration of their expression or sequence. A number of studies have correlated Bcl-2 increased expression and Bax reduced levels to poor clinical outcome in various malignancies (Reed, 1999; Kornblau et al., 1999). An increase in Mcl-1 expression was also associated with the relapse of acute leukemias (Kaufmann et al., 1998). However, the results of these clinical correlative studies are not uniform. High Bcl-2 expression has been sometimes associated with a better outcome, and increased expression of Bax was associated with unfavorable prognosis in several types of tumors (Meijerink et al., 1998; Hogarth and Hall, 1999). In addition, although overexpression of Bcl-2 prevents apoptosis and its cytoprotective effect extends to some types of necrosis, some cells could die through another death mechanism (Houghton, 1999; Vander Heiden and Thompson, 1999).

Although the interpretation of correlative clinical studies remains difficult, antisense strategies using oligonucleotides and hammerhead ribozymes to inhibit Bcl-2 expression have demonstrated some efficacy *in vitro* (Kitada *et al.,* 1994) and *in vivo* (Jansen *et al.,* 1998). Bcl-2 antisense oligonucleotides have also been tested in a phase I study of patients with relapsed and refractory lymphomas, yielding promising results (Webb *et al.,* 1997). The use of small peptides that bind to antiapoptotic proteins of the Bcl-2 family and mimic the effects of proapoptotic members of this family is currently investigated (Muchmore *et al.,* 1996; Sattler *et al.,* 1997). Another approach is tumor-selective expression of Bax, e.g., through adenoviral gene transfer, which demonstrated highly selective toxicity on tumor cells both in *in vitro* clonogenic assays and in animal models (Reed, 1997; Tai *et al.,* 1999).

4. The Central Role of Caspases in Drug-Induced Apoptosis

A. The Caspase Family

The core apoptotic machinery involves a family of mammalian cysteine aspartic proteases referred to as caspases (Budihardjo *et al.,* 1999; Kumar, 1999). Fourteen caspases have been identified in mammalian cells, of which 11 enzymes are known in humans. These enzymes are synthesized as inactive proenzymes that must be cleaved at conserved aspartate residues to generate the active tetrameric enzyme (Nicholson, 1999) containing two large and two small subunits (Walker *et al.,* 1994; Rotonda *et al.,* 1996) (Fig. 5A). Caspases cleave their substrates at aspartate residues and function as a proteolytic cascade. To some extent, this cascade involves initiator caspases characterized by a long prodomain (caspase-2, 3, 6, 7, 8, 9, 10) upstream of effector enzymes with a short prodomain (caspase-3, 6, and 7) (Fig. 5B). Other enzymes (caspase-1, 4, 5, 11, 12, and 14) are mainly involved in cytokine maturation and inflammation. Activation of initiator caspases usually involves the recruitment of multiple homologous enzymes to an adaptor molecule, such as APAF-1, FADD, or RAIDD (Chinnaiyan *et al.,* 1995; Zou *et al.,* 1997; Duan and Dixit, 1997; Ahmad *et al.,* 1997). Then the proteolytic cascade propagates the death signal and effector enzymes cleave a series of key cellular protein substrates (Slee *et al.,* 1999). However, some caspases with a short prodomain, such as caspase-3, could be involved in a feedback amplification loop by activating certain caspases with a long prodomain. In most cases, cleavage of intracellular proteins contributes to the death process. However, we have shown that caspase-mediated cleavage of the CDKK inhibitor p27^{Kip1} could negatively regulate the feedback amplification loop involved in apoptosis (Eymin *et al.,* 1999a, 1999b) (Fig. 6).

All anticancer agents can induce apoptosis and activate caspases in tumor cells. For example, in U937 human leukemic cells, caspase-3 and caspase-6 play a central role in apoptosis triggered by topoisomerase inhibitors while the various isoforms of caspase-2 modulate their activity (Dubrez *et al.,* 1996; 1998; Droin *et al.,* 1998; Sordet *et al.,* 1999; Droin *et al.,* 2000; Droin *et al.* 2001a,b). In addition, data in caspase-9 (Kuida *et al.,* 1998; Hakem *et al.,* 1998) and APAF-1 (Cecconi *et al.,* 1998; Yoshida *et al.,* 1998) KO mice have suggested that the generation of a caspase-9-containing apoptosome complex was crucial for drug-induced apoptosis. Caspase-3 is required for some typical hallmarks of apoptosis, such as DNA fragmentation and membrane blebbing (Sakahira *et al.,* 1998; Sahara *et al.,* 1999). Inactivation of specific caspase genes such as caspase-3 or caspase-8 has now been documented in cell lines or specific tumors. Whether such change in caspase gene expression only modulates the phenotype of death induced by chemotherapeutic drugs or

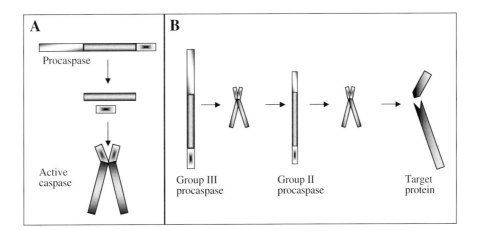

FIGURE 5 The caspase cascade. (**A**) Caspases are synthesized as inactive proenzymes that must be cleaved at conserved aspartate residues to generate the active tetrameric enzyme containing two large and two small subunits. (**B**) To some extent, caspases function as a proteolytic cascade involving initiator caspases characterized by a long prodomain upstream of effector enzymes with a short prodomain.

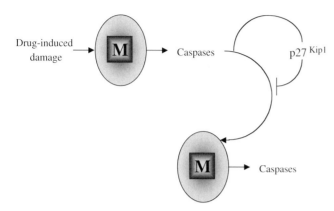

FIGURE 6 Caspase-mediated cleavage of p27[Kip1]. While caspase-mediated cleavage of most cellular proteins actively contributes to the death process, cleavage of the cyclin-dependent kinase inhibitor generates an N-terminal fragment that negatively interacts with an amplification loop leading to apoptosis.

induces some resistance to these drugs is still a matter of controversy. The caspases involved in the cell death process could vary, depending of the cell type and the apoptotic stimulus. The reason for the cells' using different caspases for undergoing cell death, depending on the cell context, is not clear, but several observations provide possible explanations.

B. Caspase Cellular Compartmentalization

While caspases are localized in the cytosol, a fraction of these enzymes are also localized in specific organelles. For example, in several tissues, procaspase-3 is present in the intermembrane space of the mitochondria, in a complex with Hsp60 and Hsp10 (Samali et al., 1999a; Xanthoudakis et al., 1999). Upon activation of the death process, procaspase-3 is activated and dissociated from the Hsp complex. A substantial proportion of cellular procaspases 2 and 9 is also found in the mitochondria (Susin et al., 1999a). Death signals can induce the translocation of mitochondrial caspase-2 and caspase-9 to the nucleus (Krajewski et al., 1999) or the translocation of active caspase-7 to mitochondria and microsomes (Chandler et al., 1998). Lastly, several caspases were shown to translocate to the nucleus in response to death stimuli (Kumar, 1999; Martins et al., 1997). The role of caspase compartmentalization in regulating cell response to anticancer drugs and other apoptotic stimuli remains poorly understood, though it was proposed that it might restrain caspase activation and separate these enzymes from their substrate in living cells.

C. Transcriptional Regulation of Caspases

Cytotoxic drugs up-regulate the transcription of several molecules involved in cell death pathways, including Fas, FADD, and caspases, before undergoing cell death (Droin et al., 1998; Micheau et al., 1997; 1999b). Although the reg-

ulation of *CASP* gene transcription remains poorly known (Kumar et al., 1997) and the role of this upregulation is unclear, accumulation of these proteolytic enzymes in tumor cells might sensitize them to apoptotic stimuli. Up-regulation of death receptors and downstream caspases in cells exposed to anticancer drugs suggests new therapeutic strategies combining the drugs with death receptors agonists (see Section 5.A) or lymphokine-activated immune cells.

In addition, several *CASP* genes, including *CASP-1, CASP-2, CASP-6, CASP-8, CASP-9,* and *CASP-10,* generate one or several alternative spliced isoforms whose function is mostly unknown. However, the short isoforms of procaspase-2 (Wang et al., 1994) and procaspase-9 (Srinivasula et al., 1999) prevent rather than facilitate apoptotic cell death (Table 1). Procaspase-9b, the short isoform of procaspase-9, was shown to antagonize activation of the long isoform of procaspase-9 by interfering with its recruitment in the apoptosome (Srinivasula et al., 1999; Seol and Billiar, 1999). The prodomain of caspases, generated either by cleavage/activation of the proenzyme or as a specific mRNA isoform (Droin et al., 2000), could also function as an endogenous modulator of the caspase cascade.

D. Posttranslational Modifications of Caspases

Procaspase-9 can be phosphorylated by the protein kinase B (also known as Akt) in response to growth factors such as IL-3 (Cardone et al., 1998). This phosphorylation prevents procaspase-9 activation at the level of the apoptosome. Simultaneously, Akt could be involved in the phosphorylation of the BH3-only protein Bad. In turn, Bad interacts with a 14-3-3 protein in the cytosol, which prevents the proapoptotic protein from neutralizing Bcl-2 on the mitochondrial membrane. Another described posttranslational modification of caspases is the S-nitrosylation of the active-site cysteine of procaspase-3 that inhibits recombinant enzyme activity in cell-free systems (Dimmeler et al., 1997). This reversible nitrosylation was demonstrated to occur in the absence of nitric oxide donor in human B and T cells while the signal transduction pathway activated by Fas ligation induced both the denitrosylation of the active site and procaspase-3 cleavage in its active fragments (Mannick et al., 1999).

E. Endogenous Modulators of Caspases

1. IAP Family Proteins

Several endogenous proteins directly or indirectly interfere with caspase activation. Inhibitors of apoptosis proteins (IAPs) are highly conserved proteins (Deveraux et al., 1999) that are structurally characterized by at least one BIR (for baculoviral inhibitor of apoptosis repeat) domain. This domain has been identified so far in five human proteins (NAIP, cIPA1, cIAP2, XIAP, and survivin) (Fig. 7 and Table 1). One

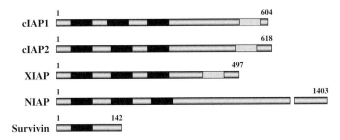

FIGURE 7 IAP family of proteins. IAPs are endogenous inhibitors of caspase activation that contain at least one BIR domain *(black box)* that is responsible for caspase inhibition. Some IAPs also contain a C-terminal ring domain *(white box)* whose role is still controversial.

of these proteins, survivin, shows strong up-regulation in a number of human tumors, e.g., in high-grade lymphomas. This small IAP with a single BIR domain, which is highly expressed in embryonic tissues but cannot be detected in normal adult differentiated tissues, correlates with survival in several human tumors (Ambrosini *et al.,* 1997). The majority of IAPs inhibit selective members of the caspase family, either directly or indirectly. The caspases inhibited by IAPs are mostly those that operate in the distal portion of the proteolytic cascade. IAPs also demonstrated caspase-independent inhibitory mechanisms such as those mediated by activation of the transcriptional factor NF-κB (Deveraux *et al.,* 1999). These proteins were demonstrated to block apoptosis induced by a variety of anticancer drugs (etoposide, cisplatin, taxol, actinomycin D, doxorubicin) and ionizing radiation (Ambrosini *et al.,* 1997, 1998; Tamm *et al.,* 1998). Interestingly, survivin associates with mitotic spindles and demonstrates cell-cycle-specific expression in G_2/M, which is mediated by G_1 transcriptional repressor elements in the survivin promoter (Li *et al.,* 1998a; Kobayashi *et al.,* 1999). In malignant cells, however, the protein is expressed in a cell-cycle-independent manner. Survivin specifically protects against taxol while demonstrating limited inhibitory effect against vincristine. Conversely, plasmids encoding antisense *survivin* cDNA were claimed to sensitize tumor cells to anticancer-drug-induced apoptosis (Li *et al.,* 1999). Thus, survivin is an exciting tumor marker that could also modulate cell response to anticancer drugs. Compounds that block IAP binding to caspases have also been proposed as a strategy for killing tumor cells by releasing caspases. Analysis of cell death proteins in *Drosophilia melanogaster* has identified such proteins in which a common 14-amino-acid domain binds IAPs and induces cell death (Vucic *et al.,* 1997; 1998).

2. DED-Containing Inhibitors of Death Receptors

Another protein that negatively interferes with caspase activation is the cellular FLICE inhibitory protein (c-FLIP, also called Casper/I-FLICE/FLAME-1/CASH/CLARP/MRIT/Usurpin), an inactive homologue of caspase-8 and caspase-

10 that contains a DED but lacks a catalytic active site and the residues that form the substrate-binding pocket. Thus, c-FLIP may act as a competitive inhibitor by preventing the binding of these caspases to the cytosolic domain of death receptors (Tschopp *et al.,* 1998) (Table 1). Several other DED-containing inhibitors of death signaling have been identified in viruses. c-FLIP plays a role in the resistance of resting T cells to Fas-induced cell death. Elevated expression of c-FLIP has been associated with Fas resistance and in the progression and immune escape of some human tumors *in vivo* (Tschopp *et al.,* 1998).

3. Heat Shock Proteins

The highly conserved proteins known as Hsp's (Jaattela, 1999) include proteins that are either constitutively expressed in mammalian cells, such as Hsp90, Hsc70, and Hsp60, or induced/activated in response to stressful stimuli, such as Hsp70 and Hsp27 (Table 1). The constitutively expressed Hsp's behave as chaperones for other cellular proteins, e.g., to maintain these proteins in an active conformation, to prevent premature folding of nascent polypeptides, or to facilitate their intracellular translocation. Like the Bcl-2 family of proteins, Hsp's include antiapoptotic and proapoptotic proteins whose expression level could determine the cell fate in response to death stimuli. As described in Sections 2.A and 4.B, Hsp60 and Hsp10 form complexes with procaspase-3 in the mitochondrial fraction of various cell types (Samali *et al.,* 1999a, 1999b; Xanthoudatis *et al.,* 1999) and could accelerate the activation of procaspases when released in combination with cytochrome *c* from the mitochondrial intermembrane space (Samali *et al.,* 1999a; Xanthoudatis *et al.,* 1999). Overexpression of Hsp90 has also been shown to increase the rate of apoptosis in U937 myelogenous leukemic cells exposed to TNF-α or cycloheximide (Galea-Lauri *et al.,* 1996).

In contrast, overexpression of Hsp70 protects the cells from apoptosis, both upstream and downstream of the effector caspase activation (Gabai *et al.,* 1997; Jaattela *et al.,* 1998). It was proposed that Hsp70 could protect the cells from energy deprivation and/or ATP depletion associated with cell death. Hsp70 could also interfere with the signal transduction pathway leading to activation of JNK in response to stress (Mosser *et al.,* 1997; Stuart *et al.,* 1998; Buzzard *et al.,* 1998). Lastly, Hsp70 was reported to chaperone altered protein products generated upon caspase activation (Jaattela *et al.,* 1998) (Fig. 8). According to this latter observation, Hsp70 could rescue cells in a later phase of the apoptosis signaling cascade than any other known survival-enhancing protein or drug.

Another Hsp involved in cell death regulation is Hsp27, a small Hsp that is constitutively expressed in many cell types and tissues, at specific stages of development and differentiation. When overexpressed in tumor cells, e.g., as a response to stress or when epithelial tumor cells are grown at conflu-

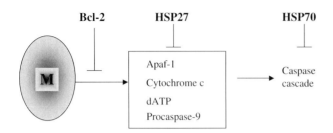

FIGURE 8 Heat-shock proteins. While Bcl-2 prevents cytochrome c release from the mitochondria, HSP27 does not. This latter protein prevents the activation of procaspase-9 in the apoptosome. HSP70 was proposed to negatively interfere with cell death pathways at various levels, including the chaperoning of peptides generated upon caspase activation.

ence, this protein increases malignant cell tumorigenicity (Garrido *et al.*, 1998). It also protects these cells against apoptotic cell death triggered by various stimuli, including hyperthermia, oxidative stress, staurosporine, FasL, and cytotoxic drugs (Mehlen *et al.*, 1996a,b; Garrido *et al.*, 1997). These stimuli often induce Hsp27 (and Hsp70) overexpression, providing an example of a protective signal being triggered by an apoptotic stimulus while simultaneously activating a death pathway. Among the mechanisms that could account for Hsp27 antiapoptotic activity, the protein was suggested to increase the antioxidant defense of cells by increasing glutathione cell content (Mehlen *et al.*, 1996a) and neutralizing the toxic effects of oxidized proteins by its chaperone-like activity (Lavoie *et al.*, 1995). Hsp27 also binds to activated protein kinase B/Akt, a protein that generates a survival signal in response to growth factor stimulation; however, the effect of this binding on the protective activity of Akt remain unclear (Konishi *et al.*, 1997). In addition, we have recently demonstrated that Hsp27, like Bcl-2, could prevent the activation of procaspase-9 and procaspase-3 in U937 human leukemic cells exposed to anticancer drugs (Garrido *et al.*, 1999). However, in contrast to Bcl-2, Hsp27 does not prevent the release of cytochrome c from the mitochondria into the cytosol. Hypothetically, this could occur through Hsp binding to APAF-1, cytochrome c, or procaspase-9 (Fig. 8).

Based on the role of Hsp27 and Hsp70 in the negative regulation of drug-induced cell death, their abundant expression in many human tumors, and their role in tumorigenesis, specific pharmaceutical compounds binding to the active site of the protein or specific antisense oligonucleotides inhibiting their expression might enhance anticancer drug activity (Jaattela *et al.*, 1998). Another potential target for modulating Hsp70 expression in tumor cells is the Ku autoantigen, whose negative influence on anticancer-drug-induced apoptosis could be mediated by Hsp's (Kim *et al.*, 1999). Conversely, pharmacologic stimuli or cytokines that induce Hsp expression could be proposed to protect normal tissues from stressful stimuli.

5. Synergy between Death Receptors and Cytotoxic Drugs

A. Up-regulation of Fas by Anticancer Drugs

Tumor cells have developed multiple mechanisms to resist Fas-mediated cell death, including reduction or loss of Fas from the leukemic cell surface (Martinez-Lorenzo *et al.*, 1998), mutation of the cytoplasmic domain of Fas (Landowski *et al.*, 1997; Beltinger *et al.*, 1998; Tamiya *et al.*, 1998; Maeda *et al.*, 1999), secretion of the soluble form of Fas, overexpression of antiapoptotic proteins of the Bcl-2 family (von Reyher *et al.*, 1998), and overexpression of the previously described inhibitor c-FLIP (Tschopp *et al.*, 1998; Algeciras-Schimnich *et al.*, 1999). Interestingly, some tumor cells that are resistant to Fas-mediated signaling can be sensitized by treatment with cycloheximide, actinomycin D, or interferon-γ (Micheau *et al.*, 1997). We and others have shown that cytotoxic drugs and ionizing radiation could up-regulate the expression of the receptor Fas at the surface of tumor cells, thereby increasing tumor cell response to Fas-mediated apoptotic signals (Sheard *et al.*, 1999; Posovsky *et al.*, 1999). Thus, drug-resistant tumor cell lines that are cross-resistant to Fas triggering become highly sensitive to Fas-induced apoptosis upon exposure to anticancer drugs (Morimoto *et al.*, 1993). Resistance to Fas-mediated cell death decreases tumor cell susceptibility to lymphokine-activated killer cells (Knight *et al.*, 1993; Lee *et al.*, 1996) that could be restored by drug-induced sensitization to Fas agonists (Micheau *et al.*, 1997). This observation has suggested that combining FasL with anticancer drug treatment might be an efficient strategy to trigger apoptosis of tumor cells, which is true in cultured cells. Unfortunately, intravenous infusion of agonistic anti-Fas antibody induces the rapid killing of animals due to lethal liver damage. This damage is caused by induction of Fas-dependent apoptosis in hepatocytes that express high levels of Fas (Kondo *et al.*, 1997). Since TNF-α also induces severe toxic side effects when administered systemically, the benefit of combining cytokines of the TNF superfamily to systemic anticancer therapy appeared limited until the identification of TRAIL.

B. Synergy between TRAIL and Anticancer Drugs

The FasL and TNF homologue designated TNF-related apoptosis inducing ligand (TRAIL) (Wiley *et al.*, 1995), also known as Apo-2 ligand (Pitti *et al.*, 1996), is a transmembrane protein that also exists as a soluble molecule (Bodmer *et al.*, 2000). Interestingly, a wide range of normal tissues express TRAIL mRNA while being resistant to TRAIL-induced cell death, but transformed cells are sensitive to the cytokine. In addition, intravenous infusion of a soluble trimerized form of recombinant TRAIL did not induce any significant side effects in mice and monkeys (Walczack *et al.,* 1999; Ashkenazi *et al.,* 1999b). Thus, soluble TRAIL may have potential utility in systemic therapy for malignant tumors.

The differential sensitivity of normal and tumor cells to TRAIL is still unexplained. Receptors for TRAIL include two type I transmembrane proteins, with a death domain similar to that of Fas and TNF-R1 in their cytoplasmic carboxy-terminal portion. In addition to these receptors, designated TRAIL-R1 (or DR4) and TRAIL-R2 (or DR5), two other receptors, known as TRAIL-R3 (or DcR1/ TRID) and TRAIL-R4 (or DcR2), bind TRAIL. They bind with an affinity comparable to that of TRAIL-R1 and TRAIL-R2 but differ in their cytoplasmic domain and do not mediate apoptosis upon ligation (Pan *et al.,* 1997; Griffith and Lynch, 1998; Ashkenazi and Dixit, 1999). TRAIL-R3 is devoid of any transmembrane or cytoplasmic domain and is glycosylphosphosphatidylinositol-linked to the cell surface whereas TRAIL-R4 contains only a partial death domain (Fig. 9). Thus, TRAIL-R3 and TRAIL-R4 could act as decoy receptors that determine whether a cell is resistant or sensitive to TRAIL (Chan *et al.,* 1999). An alternative hypothesis for the differential sensitivity of normal and tumor cells to TRAIL involves the differential expression of c-FLIP (see Section 4.E.2).

The selective response of tumor cells to TRAIL, its safety when administered to animals (Walczack *et al.,* 1999; Ashkenazi *et al.,* 1999), and its efficacy in suppressing tumor growth suggested that TRAIL-based tumor therapy might be an efficient anticancer strategy. In addition, subtoxic concentrations of chemotherapeutic drugs were shown to increase or restore the response to TRAIL in cell lines that were resistant to the cytokine (Mizutani *et al.,* 1999; Gibson *et al.,* 2000). Thus, combination of an anticancer drug with TRAIL may rein-

force TRAIL-based therapy. Interestingly, the synergy of TRAIL with anticancer drugs such as etoposide was observed in cell lines selected for their resistance to cytotoxic drugs and Fas-mediated apoptosis (Bonavida *et al.,* 1999). The mechanisms proposed to account for the anticancer drug/TRAIL synergy include the p53-dependent or independent transcriptional induction of TRAIL-R1 and R2, the decreased expression of intracellular inhibitors of TRAIL-induced apoptosis such as c-FLIP (Tschopp *et al.,* 1998), and the up-regulation of proapoptotic molecules such as FADD and procaspases (Lacour *et al.,* 2001). The precise mechanism could depend on the tumor cell type, the cytotoxic drug, and the concentration used to sensitize tumor cells to TRAIL-induced cell death. Whatever this molecular mechanism, preliminary studies testing the combination of TRAIL to 5-fluorouracil or camptothecin *in vivo* have confirmed the great potential interest of this strategy in the management of human tumors (Ashkenazi *et al.,* 1999). However, the toxicity of TRAIL toward human hepatocytes in culture suggests that caution is still required before there can be further testing of TRAIL for the treatment of humans (Jo *et al.,* 2000).

C. The Cell Cycle Checkpoints

Progression through a series of phases that allow cells to accurately duplicate themselves is regulated by protein complexes consisting of cyclins and cyclin-dependent protein kinases (CDKs). To prevent the replication of damaged DNA during S phase or its segregation during mitosis, DNA integrity is monitored by signal transduction pathways whose effectors can inhibit cell cycle progression by interacting with cyclin–CDK complexes, e.g., to facilitate DNA repair. These checkpoints exist at the G_1 stage, before DNA replication (G_1 checkpoint), or at the G_2 stage, just before mitosis (G_2 checkpoint).

These G_1 DNA damage checkpoints implicate at least two kinases: the DNA dependent protein kinase (DNA-PK) (Woo *et al.,* 1998) and the ataxia-telangiectasia mutated protein kinase (ATM-PK) (Yuan *et al.,* 1999) (Fig. 10). Both kinases phosphorylate the tumor suppressor p53. ATM phosphorylates a network of other proteins involved in cell cycle arrest and/or DNA repair, such as NBS1, a protein mutated in the Nijmegen breakage syndrome; BRCA1, a protein whose mutation plays a role in familial breast and ovarian cancers; and the nonreceptor tyrosine kinase c-Abl (Wang, 2000). DNA-PK and ATM-PK phosphorylate p53, which stabilizes the protein or disrupts its interaction with MDM2 (a protein that regulates p53) and activates p53-dependent transcription (Yuan *et al.,* 1999). One of the targets of p53 transcriptional activity is a 21-kDa inhibitor of CDKs known as $p21^{Cip1/Waf1}$ that mediates cell cycle arrest in G_1 phase through dephosphorylation of the retinoblastoma protein (Rb). This effect could be enforced by c-Abl-mediated activation of p73, the

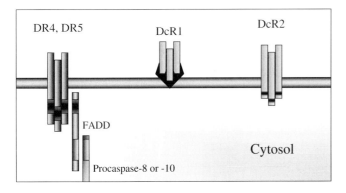

FIGURE 9 TRAIL receptors. A series of TRAIL receptors have been described including complete death receptors DR4 and DR5 that, upon ligation of TRAIL, recruit FADD and procaspase-8 or procaspase-10 and trigger a cell death signal. DcR1 is devoid of any transmembrane or cytoplasmic domain and is glycosylphosphosphatidylinositol linked to the cell surface, whereas DcR2 contains only a partial death domain. Thus, DcR1 and DcR2 were suggested to act as decoy receptors that determine whether a cell is resistant or sensitive to TRAIL.

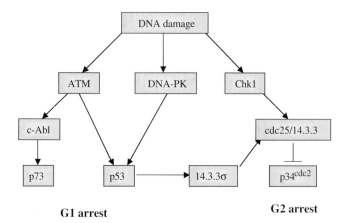

G1 arrest   **G2 arrest**

FIGURE 10 DNA damage checkpoints. DNA damage activates both the DNA protein kinase that phosphorylates p53 and the ataxia-telangiectasia-mutated (ATM) protein that activates the nonreceptor tyrosine kinase c-Abl and p73 or p53. The p73 and the p53 proteins can induce cell cycle arrest in the G_1 phase. p53 can also trigger apoptosis. p53-independent interaction of one of the seven human members of the 14-3-3 family of proteins with cdc25C is required for initiating the G_2 DNA damage checkpoint. p53 could sustain the DNA damage G_2 checkpoint by interacting with the 14-3-3σ protein.

product of one of the two recently discovered p53-related genes (Agami *et al.,* 1999; Gong *et al.,* 1999; White and Prives, 1999). Cell cycle arrest in late G_1 is supposed to allow for repair of damaged DNA prior to DNA replication (Lowe *et al.,* 1993, 1994). p53 contributes to DNA damage repair by up-regulating the newly described p53R2 gene that encodes a subunit of the ribonucleotide reductase (Tanaka *et al.,* 2000). p53 transcriptional activity can also trigger apoptosis, e.g., through down-regulation of *bcl-2* and *NF-κB,* and upregulation of *bax,* to selectively eliminate severely damaged cells.

In the absence of p53, cell cycle arrest in response to DNA damage occurs in G_2. This G_2 DNA damage pathway is initiated by phosphorylation of a kinase known as Chk1. In turn, this kinase phosphorylates the phosphatase Cdc25 on serine 216. This phosphorylation induces interaction of Cdc25 with one of the seven human members of the 14-3-3 family of proteins. The highly conserved 14-3-3 proteins are phosphoserine-binding proteins. Binding of phosphorylated Cdc25 to one of these proteins prevents Cdc25 from accumulating in the nucleus and activating p34^{cdc2} by dephosphorylation. p34^{cdc2} is maintained in an inactive state by phosphorylation on tyrosine 15 by the nuclear kinase Wee1 and/or on threonine 14 and tyrosine 15 by the cytoplasmic kinase Myt1. p53 was shown recently to play some role in G_2 DNA damage checkpoint (Waterman *et al.,* 1998) (Fig. 10). While p53-independent interaction of a 14-3-3 protein with cdc25C is required for initiating the G_2 DNA damage checkpoint, p53 contributes to sustaining this checkpoint by inducing expression of the 14-3-3σ protein (Chan *et al.,* 1999).

The consequence of 14-3-3σ expression is the nuclear export of p34^{cdc2}/cyclin B1 complexes to prevent the G_2 checkpoint bypass. Despite this role of p53, cancer cells that lack p53 still arrest in G_2 in response to DNA damage, and this G_2 checkpoint can be altered by agents, such as methylxanthines and 7-hydroxystaurosporine (UCN01), that selectively potentiate the cytotoxic effects of DNA-damaging agents (Sugiyama *et al.,* 2000). Molecules designed to more specifically inhibit the components of the pathway, such as Chk1, 14-3-3/cdc25C, and 14-3-3σ/p53, might be tested as potential enhancers of the antitumor activity of DNA-damaging agents by inducing apoptosis or mitotic catastrophe.

D. Checkpoint Status and Cell Sensitivity to Chemotherapeutic Agents

Although checkpoint status, e.g., p53 expression, influences the decision of whether a cell undergoes apoptosis after a genotoxic insult and the rate at which the cell dies, the question remains as to whether and how the checkpoint status affects the overall sensitivity of cells to anticancer drugs inducing genotoxic damage. Studies performed in dominant oncogene-transformed fibroblasts from embryos of *p53* wild-type and *p53* KO mice have suggested a role of *p53* mutations in resistance to apoptosis induced by radiation and anticancer drugs (Lowe *et al.,* 1993, 1994). This observation was enforced by the highly significant association of *p53* mutation with drug resistance in a series of 60 cell lines used for screening anticancer agents by the use of a short-term cytotoxic assay (Weinstein *et al.,* 1997). However, this hypothesis was challenged when *in vitro* cell killing was measured with long-term colony-forming assays rather than short-term assays measuring growth inhibition, functional changes such as trypan blue or propidium iodide uptake, or apoptosis. It was proposed that, in many leukemia and lymphoma cell lines that are highly sensitive to chemotherapeutic agents and radiation and die rapidly through apoptosis in response to drug-induced DNA damage, mutation of *p53* could behave as a true resistance factor to some specific genotoxic insults. In other cells, short-term assays can be misleading and apoptosis does not necessarily predict overall sensitivity to DNA-damaging agents.

One of the reasons for which no clear correlation can be established between *p53* status and cell sensitivity to DNA-damaging agents could be the role of wild-type p53 protein in nucleotide excision repair, e.g., by activating the recently described p53 target gene p53R2, which plays a crucial role in supplying deoxyribonucleotides for DNA repair (Tanaka *et al.,* 2000). Due to this function, inactivation of p53 protein could enhance cell sensitivity rather than cell resistance to chemotherapeutic drugs that activate a p53-dependent repair mechanism.

The best way for identifying efficient therapeutic compounds according to the integrity of cell cycle checkpoints has been further challenged in a recent study testing the influence of p21$^{WAF1/CIP1}$ mutation on tumor cell response to DNA-damaging agents. p21 is transcriptionally activated by p53 and is responsible for the p53-dependent G_1 checkpoint. Normal cells or cancer cells with an intact p21 enter a stable arrest following DNA damage by radiation or anticancer drugs. Mutation of p21 sensitizes tumor cells to DNA-damaging agent-induced apoptosis, as a consequence of uncoupling between mitosis and S phase. A standard clonogenic assay failed to detect any influence of p21 mutations on cell response to DNA-damaging agents, suggesting that although p21 mutation could sensitize the cell to drug-induced apoptosis, cells with a wild-type p21 will die with the same efficacy, although through a slower process. Actually, xenografts established from tumor cells with altered p21 checkpoint were dramatically more sensitive to radiation than those obtained with wild-type p21, otherwise isogenic cell lines (Waldman *et al.*, 1997). Thus, the *in vitro* clonogenic assay did not predict the dramatically different sensitivities found *in vivo*, probably because this assay did not distinguish cell cycle arrest from cell death. Thus, in this situation, apoptosis induction is more predictive of the *in vivo* response than long-term *in vitro* clonogenic assays.

Interestingly, a promising application of understanding the role of p53 in DNA-damage-induced apoptosis could be the protection of healthy tissues. In *p53*-deficient mice, these healthy tissues were shown to suffer less damage from γ-irradiation than the healthy tissues from normal mice. A new pharmacologic compound, pifithrin-α, was shown to protect vulnerable tissues by temporarily and reversibly blocking p53. A single injection of pifithrin-α rescued normal mice from a near-lethal radiation exposure without changing the response of p53-deficient tumor xenografts, providing a potential way to give patients optimal doses of chemotherapy, at least when bearing a p53-deficient tumor (Brown and Wouters, 1999; Komarov *et al.*, 1999).

E. Lipid-Dependent Signaling Pathways

In addition to specific damage induced in target cells, e.g., DNA damage, anticancer agents simultaneously activate several lipid-dependent signaling pathways that can either stimulate or prevent the activation of the cell death machinery in response to this damage. One of the most studied of these signaling pathways that could modulate cell sensitivity to chemotherapeutic drugs and ionizing radiation is the sphingomyelin-ceramide pathway, a pathway that is activated within a few minutes after drug interaction with the target cell (Tepper *et al.*, 1995; Hannun, 1996; Jarvis *et al.*, 1996; Liu *et al.*, 1999) (Fig. 11).

Sphingomyelin was initially considered as a structural element in eukaryotic cell membranes. Then, hydrolysis of sphingomyelin leading to ceramide generation was identified to occur in response to a large number of natural and pharmacologic effectors and to play a role in cell sensitivity to apoptosis induction by these effectors. Several chemotherapeutic drugs were shown to activate a sphingomyelinase in

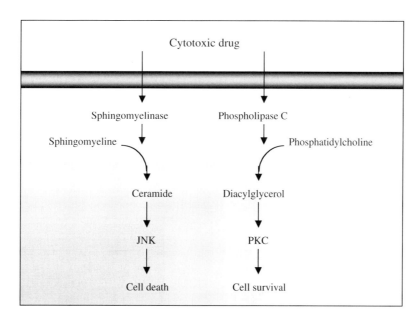

FIGURE 11 Lipid-dependent signaling pathways. Anticancer drugs can activate a sphingomyelinase that generates ceramide, activates the JNK1/SAPK pathway, and facilitates cell death by apoptosis. Simultaneously, drug-induced activation of a phospholipase C generates diacylglycerol that activates protein kinase C. This kinase inhibits the ceramide pathway both upstream and downstream of ceramide generation. The reality is more complex since ceramide itself can activate both pro- (e.g., JNK1/SAPK) and anti- (e.g., PKC·ξ) apoptotic pathways. Cross-talk between these pathways contributes to determining the fate of the cell.

leukemic cells, including daunorubicin, mitoxantrone, etoposide, vincristine, dexamethasone, ara-C, and cisplatin (Strum et al., 1994; Jaffrezou et al., 1996; Bettaieb et al., 1999). In addition, hydrolysis of sphingomyelin was identified in cells exposed to ionizing radiation, FasL and TNF-α (Quintans et al., 1994; Tepper et al., 1995; Bettaieb et al., 1996). The pool of sphingomyelin and the nature of the sphingomyelinase involved in ceramide generation remain controversial and could vary, depending on the cell type and the death stimulus. Ceramide generated in response to apoptotic stimuli activates several intracellular targets in which the JNK/SAPK cascade may play an essential role in ceramide-mediated cell death (Verheij et al., 1996) (Fig. 11).

PKC activators, including phorbol esters and diacylglycerol, can negatively interfere with the sphingomyelin-ceramide pathway both upstream of ceramide generation by preventing sphingomyelinase activity and downstream of ceramide by inhibiting its ability to induce apoptosis (Grant and Jarvis, 1996; Mansat et al., 1997) (see Section 5.F.1). Interestingly, most anticancer drugs as well as cytokines such as TNF-α are capable of activating the production of diacylglycerol in parallel with activating ceramide generation (Fig. 11 and Table 1). Thus, the cytotoxic activity of an anticancer agent may be modulated by the balance between the noxious pathway mediated by ceramide and the protective pathway mediated by diacylglycerol (Jaffrezou et al., 1998). This observation opens perspectives of pharmacologic manipulations aimed at increasing the lethal pathways while inhibiting the protective signals. For example, neutralization of oncogenes, such as c-Abl, that may contribute to accelerate diacylglycerol turnover could sensitize the cells to drug-induced cell death.

F. Modulation of Apoptosis by Kinases

1. Protein Kinase C

As indicated in Section 5.E, several PKCs are targets for diacylglycerol. PKCs compose a family of lipid-regulated serine/threonine kinases containing at least 12 mammalian isoforms in which three subfamilies have been identified. These include classical PKCs that respond to Ca^{2+} and diacylglycerol or phosphatidylserine, novel PKCs that respond to diacylglycerol but are insensitive to Ca^{2+}, and atypical PKCs that do not respond to diacylglycerol or to Ca^{2+} but can be activated by the phosphatidylinositol 3-kinase (PI-3K) (Grant and Jarvis, 1996).

PKC activators were shown to prevent apoptosis induced by various stimuli. The mechanisms involved in this negative effect include inhibition of ceramide generation and ceramide-mediated activation of the JNK/SAPK pathway (Mansat et al., 1997); phosphorylation of kinases such as Raf-1, which is involved in Bcl-2 phosphorylation (Basu et al., 2000); and activation of the Na^+/H^+ antiporter to prevent intracellular pH acidification (Grant and Jarvis, 1996). Down-regulation

of PKCs by long-term exposure to the macrocyclic lactone bryostatin-1 increases tumor cell sensitivity to apoptosis induced by cytarabine, cisplatin, vincristine, and melphalan. Another PKC inhibitor, safingol, sensitizes tumor cells to apoptosis induced by mitomycin C. Thus, interruption of the PKC pathway may enhance the cytotoxic activity of various antineoplastic drugs by increasing their ability to trigger tumor cell apoptosis (Grant and Jarvis, 1996).

The atypical isoform ξ of PKCs is a critical mediator in mitogenic signal transduction by activating the MAPK pathway (Moscat and Diaz-Meco, 1996; Takeda et al., 1999). This isoform was also shown to specifically interact with the product of par-4, a gene that is induced during apoptosis (Diaz-Meco et al., 1996), and to activate the antiapoptotic transcription factor NF-κB (see Section 6). Atypical isoforms of PKCs also protect cells from drug-induced apoptosis, suggesting that these isoforms are potential targets for anticancer drug activity modulation.

2. Phosphatidylinositol 3-Kinase

PI-3Ks are a family of enzymes that catalyze the phosphorylation of inositol lipids at the D3 position of the inositol ring, generating new intracellular second messengers. These PI-3Ks play an important role among other kinases involved in signal transduction pathways. Some of the lipid products of PI-3K interact with downstream effectors, such as the serine/threonine kinase known as protein kinase B or Akt (PKB/Akt). For example, survival factors such as hematopoietic growth factors (e.g., IL-3) engage a survival-signaling pathway that involves the activation of PI-3K, the production of 3′-phosphoinositides, the activation and recruitment of phospholipid-dependent kinases, and the phosphorylation of PKB/Akt on serine 473 and threonine 308. Activated PKB/Akt then inhibits apoptosis by phosphorylating Bad (Downward, 1999; Schurmann, 2000), procaspase-9 (Cardone et al., 1998; Azuma et al., 2000), and other proteins as well, increasing NF-κB activity (Nidai Ozes et al., 1999; Romashkova and Makarov, 1999), decreasing FasL transcription, and modulating the production of nitric oxide (Khwaja, 1999). The PTEN phosphatase dephosphorylates phosphoinositides, and dependence on this pathway is abrogated in tumor cells in which the PTEN activity is lost (as is observed in about 50% of prostate tumors). Inhibitors of PI-3K can induce apoptosis of tumor cells in which this pathway is constitutively activated as a consequence of Ras oncogene or PTEN phosphatase mutations. In addition, the PI-3K pathway is one of the antiapoptotic signaling pathways that can be activated by anticancer drugs, such as the anthracyclines. Inhibition of PI-3K by wortmannin and LY294002 accelerates daunorubicin-induced apoptosis in U937 cells (Plo et al., 1999). Thus, control of PI-3K activity is an attractive target for modulating the cytotoxicity of chemotherapeutic drugs in cancer cells.

3. Mitogen-Activated Protein Kinases

The mitogen-activated protein kinases (MAPKs) are a group of conserved signaling molecules that include three major subfamilies, including ERKs, JNK/SAPKs, and p38-MAPKs. These kinases are activated by phosphorylation and their major targets are transcription factors that regulate gene expression. ERK and JNK/p38-MAPK have opposite functions in regulating apoptosis and define one of the dynamic balances that determines cell fate in response to apoptosis inducers (Xia et al., 1995). Activation of the JNK pathway is observed in apoptosis and is triggered by a variety of stimuli, including anticancer drugs, while interference with the JNK pathway can suppress drug-induced apoptosis (Chen and Tan, 2000). JNK activation can involve various sensors of oxidative stress or ATM-mediated activation of the c-Abl tyrosine kinase in response to DNA damage. Downstream targets of JNK include transcription factors such as c-Jun (which enhances FasL expression), p53 (whose influence on apoptosis has been previously discussed), and c-Myc. In addition, JNK may be a mediator of Bcl-2 phosphorylation in response to paclitaxel treatment (Wang et al., 1999c).

4. Other Kinases

Several other signaling pathways can be activated directly or indirectly by cytotoxic agents. Protein tyrosine kinase inhibitors are potent inducers of apoptosis. Compounds such as quercetin, genistein, and tyrphostins could potentiate the lethal effect of cytarabine and taxol by facilitating apoptosis.

6. The Rel/NF-κB/IκB Proteins

NF-κB was first identified as a B-cell-specific nuclear protein that activates immunoglobulin kappa light chain gene transcription during B-cell maturation (Sen and Baltimore, 1986). This sequence-specific transcription factor is now known to be ubiquitously expressed and involved in the generation of a number of gene products that play a role in immune and inflammatory reactions, cell cycle control, oncogenesis, or viral replication (Lee and Burckart, 1998). In many cell types, NF-κB is in the cytoplasm as an inactive complex when associated with the molecule IκB. Serine phosphorylation of this inhibitor by an IκB kinase (IKK) triggers IκB proteolytic degradation through the ubiquitin/proteasome pathway for NF-κB to be activated and translocated in the nucleus. The nuclear NF-κB then binds to specific κB DNA motifs and modulates the transcription of target genes.

The NF-κB/Rel mammalian family of proteins includes five members classified into two groups. Group I proteins, which include NF-κB1/p50 and NF-κB2/p52, are produced as p105 and p100 precursor proteins, respectively, whereas group II proteins, including RelA/p65, RelB, and c-Rel, do not require proteolysis of a precursor. The transcription factor is a homo- or heterodimeric combination of NF-κB/Rel proteins. The I-κB family includes IκB-γ and IκB-δ produced by p105 and p100 proteolysis, the extensively studied IκB-α, and the less well known IκB-β, IκB-ε, and Bcl-3 (Thanos and Maniatis, 1995). Amplification and rearrangements of Rel/NF-κB/I-κB gene family members have been identified in various malignancies (Luque and Gelinas, 1997; Furman et al., 2000; Kordes et al., 2000).

The role of NF-κB in modulating apoptotic pathways was suggested by the massive apoptosis of liver cells observed in embryonic NF-κB KO mice (Beg et al., 1995). Various strategies then demonstrated that turning off NF-κB could sensitize tumor cells to death induced by TNF-α and anticancer drugs (Beg and Baltimore, 1996; Wang et al., 1996). NF-κB up-regulates several survival factors in lymphoid cells, including the expression of some IAPs (Chu et al., 1997; Stehlick et al., 1998), which in turn activate NF-κB in a positive-feedback loop (LaCasse et al., 1998). For example, it was proposed that following infection with the Epstein–Barr virus, the host cell surface late antigen LMP1 acts as a constitutively active receptor molecule triggering NF-κB activation, which could explain the high level of c-IAP1 in Reed-Sternberg cells that characterize Hodgkin's disease (Bargou et al., 1986; Messineo et al., 1998). NF-κB was recently shown also to play an essential role in p53-induced apoptosis (Ryan et al., 2000) and to directly transactivate the cytotoxic ligand FasL in response to anticancer drugs or radiation (Khwaja, 1999; Kuhnel et al., 2000). Thus, the transcription factor NF-κB could either protect from or contribute to apoptosis.

Inhibition of NF-κB activation has been proposed as a potential therapeutic strategy in the treatment of immune and inflammatory diseases. The role of NF-κB in modulating tumor cell sensitivity to cytotoxic drugs and the alteration of this pathway in various malignancies (Rayet and Gelinas, 1999) suggest that this strategy could also apply to cancer therapy. Several classes of drugs have been identified as NF-κB inhibitors, including corticosteroids, immunosuppressants, nonsteroidal anti-inflammatory drugs, gold-containing compounds, antioxidants, and the fungal metabolite gliotoxin (Lee and Burckart, 1998). These drugs either induce up-regulation of I-κB-α or prevent its degradation, or directly inhibit NF-κB or prevent its nuclear translocation. Their efficacy is precluded by their lack of specificity, their weak inhibitory effect, and their unrelated pharmacologic effects. In the future, testing agents that target specific components of NF-κB activation pathway more specifically, such as synthetic peptide aldehyde inhibitors of proteasome that prevent I-κB proteolysis, may indicate whether this pathway could be a good target for modulating anticancer drug activity, e.g., by preventing p53-mediated apoptosis of normal cells exposed to DNA-damaging agents while increasing their efficacy toward p53-null or defective tumor cells.

7. Conclusion

Classical pharmacology has provided critical insights regarding drug–target interaction, cell cycle kinetics, or DNA damage/repair systems. In response to specific damage, tumor cells activate a death program. Apoptosis is not the only mode of cell death triggered by anticancer drugs. Nevertheless, better understanding of apoptotic pathways and their modulation by various negative and positive signals simultaneously activated by anticancer agents may prove particularly valuable in cancer therapy. Proteins involved in cell death regulation could be used as new targets for anticancer drugs, and simultaneous signals may be manipulated to increase the efficacy of classical anticancer drugs and radiation. For example, a monoclonal antibody targeting the ErbB-1 receptor showed promise across a spectrum of epithelial tumors by enhancing their radiosensitivity, possibly as a consequence of radiation-induced apoptosis promotion (Harari and Huang, 2000). Continuous administration of low doses of chemotherapeutic drugs may also sensitize the tumor endothelium to antiangiogenic therapy that induces endothelial cell apoptosis and increase tumor cell sensitivity to death receptor agonists such as TRAIL. Thus, analysis of the molecular mechanisms of cell death has dramatically increased the field of anticancer drug pharmacology and suggested new strategies for tumor cell sensitization or normal cell protection, some of which might be tested in clinics in the near future.

References

Agami, R., Blandino, G., Oren, M., and Shaul, Y. (1999) Interaction of c-Abl and p73 alpha and their collaboration to induce apoptosis. *Nature* **399**, 809–813.

Ahmad, M., Srinivasula, S. M., and Wang, L. (1997). CRADD, a novel human apoptotic adaptor molecule for caspase-2, and FasL/tumor necrosis factor receptor-interacting protein RIP. *Cancer Res.* **57**, 615–619.

Albanese, J., and Dainiak, N.(2000). Ionizing radiation alters Fas antigen ligand at the cell surface and on exfoliated plasma membrane-derived vesicles: implications for apoptosis and intercellular signaling. *Radiat. Res.* **153**, 49–61.

Algeciras-Schimnich, A., Griffith, T. S., Lynch, D. H., and Paya, C. V. (1999). Cell cycle-dependent regulation of FLIP levels and susceptibility to Fas-mediated apoptosis. *J. Immunol.* **162**, 5205–5211.

Ambrosini, G., Adida, C., and Altieri, D. C. (1997). A novel anti-apoptosis gene, survivin, expressed in cancer and lymphoma. *Nat. Med.* **3**, 917–921.

Ambrosini, G., Adida, C., Sirugo, G., and Altieri, D. C. (1998). Induction of apoptosis and inhibition of cell proliferation by survivin gene targeting. *J. Biol. Chem.* **273**, 11177–11182.

Antonsson, B., Conti, F., Ciavatta, A., Montessuit, S., Lewis, S., Martinou, I., Bernasconi, L., Bernard, A., Mermod, J. J., Mazzei, G., Maundrell, K., Gambale, F., Sadoul, R., and Martinou, J. C. (1997). Inhibition of Bax channel-forming activity by Bcl-2. *Science* **277**, 370–372.

Ashkenazi, A., and Dixit, V. M. (1999). Apoptosis control by death and decoy receptors. *Curr. Opin. Cell Biol.* **11**, 255–260.

Ashkenazi, A., Pai, R. C., Fong, S., Leung, S., Lawrence, D. A., Marsters, S. A., Blackie, C., Chang, L., McMurtrey, A. E., Hebert, A., DeForge, L.,

Koumenis, I. L., Lewis, D., Harris, L., Bussiere, J., Koeppen, H., Shahrokh, Z., and Schwall, R. H. (1999). Safety and antitumor activity of recombinant soluble Apo2 ligand. *J. Clin. Invest.* **104**, 155–162.

Attala, H., Westberg, J. A., Andersson, L. C., Adlercreutz, H., and Makela, T. P. (1998). 2-Methyoxyestradiol-induced phosphorylation of bcl-2: Uncoupling from JNK/SAPK activation. *Biochem. Biophys. Res. Commun.* **247**, 616–621.

Azuma, T., Koths, K., Flanagan, L., and Kwiatkowski, D. (2000). Gelsolin in complex with phosphatidylinositol 4,5-bisphosphate inhibits caspase-3 and -9 to retard apoptotic progression. *J. Biol. Chem.* **275**, 3761–3766.

Bakhshi, A., Jensen, J. P., Goldman, P., Wright, J. J., McBride, O. W., Epstein, A. L., and Korsmeyer, S. J. (1985). Cloning the chromosomal breakpoint of t(14;18) human lymphomas: clustering around JH on chromosome 14 and near a transcriptional unit on 18. *Cell* **41**, 899–906.

Bargou, R. C., Emmerich, F., Krappmann, D., Bommert, K., Mapara, M. Y., Arnold, W., Royer, H. D., Grinstein, E., Greiner, A., Scheidereit, C., and Dorken, B. (1997). Constitutive nuclear factor-κ B-RelA activation is required for proliferation and survival of Hodgkin's disease tumor cells. *J. Clin. Invest.* **100**, 2961–2969.

Basu, A., and Haldar, S. (1998a). Microtubule-damaging drugs triggered bcl2 phosphorylation-requirement of phosphorylation on both serine-70 and serine-87 residues of bcl2 protein. *Int. J. Oncol.* **13**, 659–664.

Basu, A., and Haldar, S. (1998b). The relationship between Bcl-2, Bax and p53: consequences for cell cycle progression and cell death. *Mol. Human Reprod.* **4**, 1099–1109.

Basu, A., You, S. A., and Haldar, S. (2000). Regulation of Bcl2 phosphorylation by stress response kinase pathway. *Int. J. Oncol.* **16**, 497–500.

Beg, A., Sha, W., Bronson, R., Ghosh, S., and Baltimore, D. (1995). Embryonic lethality and liver degeneration in mice lacking the RelA component of NF-κB. *Nature* **376**, 167–170.

Beg, A. A., and Baltimore, D. (1996). An essential role for NF-κB in preventing TNF-α-induced apoptosis by NF-κB. *Science* **274**, 787–789.

Beltinger, C., Kurz, E., Bohler, T., Schrappe, M., Ludwig, W. D., and Debatin, K. M. (1998). CD95 (APO-1/Fas) mutations in childhood T-lineage acute lymphoblastic leukemia. *Blood* **91**, 3943–3951.

Bettaieb, A., Plo, I., Mansat-De Mas, V., Quillet-Mary, A., Levade, T., Laurent, G., and Jaffrezou, J. P. (1999). Daunorubicin- and mitoxantrone-triggered phosphatidylcholine hydrolysis: implication in drug-induced ceramide generation and apoptosis. *Mol. Pharmacol.* **55**, 118–125.

Bettaieb, A., Record, M., Come, M. G., Bras, A. C., Chap, H., Laurent, G., and Jaffrezou, J. P. (1996). Opposite effects of tumor necrosis factor alpha on the sphingomyelin-ceramide pathway in two myeloid leukemia cell lines: role of transverse sphingomyelin distribution in the plasma membrane. *Blood* **88**, 1465–1472.

Bodmer, J. L., Holler, N., Reynard, S., Vinciguerra, P., Schneider, P., Juo, P., Blenis, J., and Tschopp, J. (2000). TRAIL receptor-2 signals apoptosis through FADD and caspase-8. *Nat. Cell Biol.* **2**, 241–243.

Bonavida, B., Ng, C. P., Jazirehi, A., Schiller, G., and Mizutani, Y. (1999). Selectivity of TRAIL-mediated apoptosis of cancer cells and synergy with drugs: the trail to non-toxic cancer therapeutics. *Int. J. Oncol.* **15**, 793–802.

Bouillet, P., Metcalf, D., Huang, D. C., Tarlinton, D. M., Kay, T. W., Kontgen, F., Adams, J. M., and Strasser, A. (1999). Proapoptotic Bcl-2 relative Bim required for certain apoptotic responses, leukocyte homeostasis, and to preclude autoimmunity. *Science* **286**, 1735–1738.

Brown, J. M., and Wouters, B. G. (1999). Apoptosis, p53 and tumor cell sensitivity to anticancer agents. *Cancer Res* 1999; 59: 1391–1399.

Budihardjo, I., Oliver, H., Lutter, M., Luo, X., and Wang, X. (1999). Biochemical pathways of caspase activation during apoptosis. *Annu. Rev. Cell. Dev. Biol.* **15**, 269–290.

Buzzard, K. A., Giaccia, A. J., Killender, M., and Anderson, R. L. (1998). Heat shock protein 72 modulates pathways of stress-induced apoptosis. *J. Biol. Chem.* **273**, 17147–17153.

Cardone, M. H., Roy, N., Stennicke, H. R., Salvesen, G. S., Franke, T. F., Stanbridge, E., Frisch, S., and Reed, J. C. (1998). Regulation of cell death protease caspase-9 by phosphorylation. *Science* **282**, 1318–1321.

Cecconi, F., Alvarez-Bolado, G., Meyer, B. I., Roth, K. A., and Gruss, P. (1998). Apaf1 (CED-4 homolog) regulates programmed cell death in mammalian development. *Cell* **94**, 727–737.

Chan, T. A., Hermeking, H., Lengauer, C., Kinzler, K. W., and Vogelstein, B. (1999). 14-3-3· is required to prevent mitotic catastrophe after DNA damage. *Nature* **401**, 616–620.

Chandler, J. M., Cohen, G. M., and MacFarlane, M. (1998). Different subcellular distribution of caspase-3 and caspase-7 following Fas-induced apoptosis in mouse liver. *J. Biol. Chem.* **273**, 10815–10818.

Chang, B. S., Minn, A. J., Muchmore, S. W., Fesik, S. W., and Thompson, C. B. (1997). Identification of a novel regulatory domain in Bcl-X(L) and Bcl-2. *EMBO J.* **16**, 968–977.

Chen, Y-R., and Tan, T-H. (2000). The c-Jun N-terminal kinase pathway and apoptotic signal. *Int. J. Oncol.* **16**, 651–662.

Cheng, E.H-Y, Nicholas, J., Bellows, D. S., Hayward, G. S., Guo, H., and Hardwick, J. M. (1997a). A Bcl-2 homolog encoded by Kaposi sarcoma-associated virus, human herpes virus 8, inhibits apoptosis but does not heterodimerize with Bax or Bak. *Proc. Natl. Acad. Sci. USA* **94**, 690–694.

Cheng, E.H-Y, Kirsch, D. G., Clem, R. J., Ravi, R., Kastan, M. B., Bedi, A., Ueno, K., and Hardwick, J. M. (1997b). Conversion of Bcl-2 to a Bax-like death effector by caspases. *Science* **278**, 1966–1968.

Chinnaiyan, A. M., O'Rourke, K., Tewari, M., and Dixit, V. M. (1995). FADD, a novel death domain-containing protein, interacts with the death domain of Fas and initiates apoptosis. *Cell* **81**, 505–512.

Chu, Z. L., McKinsey, T. A., Liu, L., Gentry, J. J., Malim, M. H., and Ballard, D. W. (1997). Suppression of tumor necrosis factor-induced cell death by inhibitor of apoptosis c-iap2 is under NF-κB control. *Proc. Natl. Acad. Sci.USA* 1997; **94**, 10057–10062.

Cleary, M. L., Smith, S. D., and Sklar, J. (1986). Cloning and structural analysis of cDNAs for bcl-2 and a hybrid bcl-2/immunoglobulin transcript resulting from the t(14;18) translocation. *Cell* **47**, 19–28.

Crompton, M. (1999). The mitochondrial permeability transition pore and its role in cell death. *Biochem J* **341**, 233–249.

Deng, X., Ito, T., Carr, B., Mumby, M., and May, W. S. Jr. (1998). Reversible phosphorylation of Bcl2 following interleukin 3 or bryostatin 1 is mediated by direct interaction with protein phosphatase 2A. *J Biol Chem* **273**, 34157–34163.

Desagher, S., Osen-Sand, A., Nichols, A., Eskes, R., Montessuit, S., Lauper, S., Maundrell, K., Antonsson, B., and Martinou, J. C. (1999). Bid-induced conformational change of Bax is responsible for mitochondrial cytochrome c release during apoptosis. *J. Cell. Biol.* **144**, 891–901.

Deveraux, Q. L., Stennicke, H. R., Salvesen, G. S., and Reed J. C. (1999). Endogenous inhibitors of caspases. *J. Clin. Immunol.* **19**, 388–398.

Diaz-Meco, M. T., Municio, M. M., Frutos, S., Sanchez, P., Lozano, J., Sanz, L., and Moscat, J. (1996) The product of par-4, a gene induced during apoptosis, interacts selectively with the atypical isoforms of protein kinase C. *Cell* **86**, 777–786.

Dimmeler, S., Haendeler, J., Nehls, M., and Zeiher, A. M. (1997). Suppression of apoptosis by nitric oxide via inhibition of interleukin-1beta-converting enzyme (ICE)-like and cysteine protease protein (CPP)-32-like proteases. *J. Exp. Med.* **185**, 601–607.

Downward, J. (1999). How BAD phosphorylation is good for survival. *Nat. Cell Biol.* **1**, E33–E35.

Droin, N., Beauchemin, M., Solary, E., and Bertrand, R. (2000). Identification of a caspase-2 isoform that behaves as an endogenous inhibitor of the caspase cascade. *Cancer Res.* **60**, 7039–7047.

Droin, N., Bichat, F., Rebe, C., Wotawa, A., Sordet, O., Hammann, A., Bertrand, R., and Solary, E. (2001). Involvement of caspase-2 long isoform in Fas-mediated cell death of human leukemic cells. *Blood* **97**, 1835–1844.

Droin, N., Dubrez, L., Eymin, B., Renvoizé, C., Bréard, J., Dimanche-Boitrel, M. T., and Solary, E. (1998). Upregulation of CASP genes in human tumor cells undergoing etoposide-induced apoptosis. *Oncogene* **16**, 2885–2894.

Droin, N., Rebe, C., Bichat, F., Hammann, A., Bertrand, R., and Solary, E. (2001). Modulation of apoptosis by procaspase-2 short isoform: selective inhibition of chromatin condensation, apoptotic body formation and phosphatidylserine externalization. *Oncogene* **20**, 260–269.

Duan, H., and Dixit, V. M. (1997). RAIDD is a new "death" adaptor molecule. *Nature* **385**, 86–89.

Dubrez, L., Savoy, I., Hamman, A., and Solary, F. (1996). Pivotal role of a DEVD-sensitive step in etoposide-induced and Fas-mediated apoptotic pathways. *EMBO J.* **15**, 5504–5512.

Dubrez, L., Eymin, B., Sordet, O., Droin, N., Turhan, A. G., and Solary, E. (1998). BCR-ABL delays apoptosis upstream of procaspase-3 activation. *Blood* **91**, 2415–2422.

Erlichman, C., Fine, S., Wong, A., and Elhakim, T. A. (1988) A randomized trial of fluorouracil and folinic acid in patients with metastatic colon carcinoma. *J. Clin. Oncol.* **10**, 210–219.

Eskes, R., Desagher, S., Antonsson, B., and Martinou, J. C. (2000). Bid induces the oligomerization and insertion of Bax into the outer mitochondrial membrane. *Mol. Cell. Biol.* **20**, 929–935.

Eymin, B., Haugg, M., Droin, N., Sordet, O., Dimanche-Boitrel, M. T., and Solary, E. (1999a). p27^{Kip1} induces drug resistance by preventing apoptosis upstream of cytochrome c release from mitochondria and procaspase-3 activation. *Oncogene* **18**, 1411–1418

Eymin, B., Sordet, O., Droin, N., Munsch, B., Haugg, M., Van de Craen, M., Vandenabeele, P., and Solary, E. (1999b). Caspase-induced proteolysis of the cyclin-dependent kinase inhibitor p27^{Kip1} mediates its anti-apoptotic activity. *Oncogene* **18**, 4839–4847.

Friesen, C., Herr, I., Krammer, P. H., and Debatin, K. M. (1996). Involvement of the CD95 (APO-1/FAS) receptor/ligand system in drug-induced apoptosis in leukemia cells. *Nat. Med.* **2**, 574–577.

Fulda, S., Strauss, G., Meyer, E., and Debatin, K. M. (2000). Functional CD95 ligand and CD95 death-inducing signaling complex in activation-induced cell death and doxorubicin-induced apoptosis in leukemic T cells. *Blood* **95**, 301–308.

Furman, R. R., Asgary, Z., Mascarenhas, J. O., Liou, H. C., and Schattner, E. J. (2000). Modulation of NF-kappa B activity and apoptosis in chronic lymphocytic leukemia B cells. *J. Immunol.* **164**, 2200–2206.

Gabai, V. L., Meriin, A. B., Mosser, D. D., Caron, A. W., Rits, S., Shifrin, V. I., and Sherman, M. Y. (1997). Hsp70 prevents activation of stress kinases. A novel pathway of cellular thermotolerance. *J. Biol. Chem.* **272**, 18033–18037.

Galea-Lauri, J., Richardson, A. J., Latchman, D. S., and Katz, D. R. (1996). Increased heat shock protein 90 (hsp90) expression leads to increased apoptosis in the monoblastoid cell line U937 following induction with TNF-alpha and cycloheximide: a possible role in immunopathology. *J. Immunol.* **157**, 4109–4118.

Garrido, C., Ottavi, P., Fromentin, A., Hammann, A., Arrigo, A. P., Chauffert, B., and Mehlen, P. (1997). HSP27 as a mediator of confluence-dependent resistance to cell death induced by anticancer drugs. *Cancer Res.* **57**, 2661–2667.

Garrido, C., Fromentin, A., Bonnotte, B., Favre, N., Moutet, M., Arrigo, A. P., Mehlen, P., and Solary, E. (1998). Heat shock protein 27 enhances the tumorigenicity of immunogenic rat colon carcinoma cell clones. *Cancer Res.* **58**, 5495–5499.

Garrido, C., Bruey, J. M., Fromentin, A., Hammann, A., Arrigo, A. P., and Solary, E. (1999). HSP27 inhibits cytochrome c-dependent activation of procaspase-9. *FASEB J.* **13**, 2061–2070.

Gibson, S. B., Oyer, R., Spalding, A. C., Anderson, S. M., and Johnson, G. L. (2000). Increased expression of death receptors 4 and 5 synergizes the apoptosis response to combined treatment with etoposide and TRAIL. *Mol. Cell. Biol.* **20**, 205–212.

Gong, J. G., Costanzo, A., Yang, H. Q., Melino, G., Kaelin, W. G. Jr, Levrero, M., and Wang, J. Y. (1999). The tyrosine kinase c-Abl regulates p73 in apoptotic response to cisplatin-induced DNA damage. *Nature* **399**, 806–809.

Grant, S., and Jarvis, W. D. (1996). Modulation of drug-induced by interruption of the protein kinase C signal transduction pathway: a new therapeutic strategy. *Clin. Cancer Res.* **2**, 1915–1920.

Griffith, T. S., and Lynch, D. H. (1998). TRAIL: A molecule with multiple receptors and control mechanisms. *Curr .Op. Immunol.* **10**, 559–563

Gross, A., McDonnell, J. M., and Korsmeyer, S. J. (1999). BCL-2 family members and the mitochondria in apoptosis. *Genes Dev.* **13**, 1899–1911.

Hakem, R., Hakem, A., Duncan, G. S., Henderson, J. T., Woo, M., Soengas, M. S., Elia, A., de la Pompa, J. L., Kagi, D., Khoo, W., Potter, J., Yoshida, R., Kaufman, S. A., Lowe, S. W., Penninger, J. M., and Mak T. W. (1998). Differential requirement for caspase-9 in apoptotic pathways in vivo. *Cell* **94**, 339–352.

Haldar, S., Jena, N., and Croce, C. M. (1995). Inactivation of Bcl-2 by phosphorylation. *Proc. Natl. Acad. Sci. USA* **92**, 4507–4511.

Hannun, Y. A. (1996). Functions of ceramide in coordinating cellular responses to stress. *Science* **274**, 1855–1859.

Harari, P. M., and Huang, S. M. (2000) Modulation of molecular targets to enhance radiation. *Clin. Cancer Res.* **6**, 323–325.

Henderson, S., Huen, D., Rowe, M., Dawson, C., and Johnson, G. (1993) Epstein-Barr virus-coded BHRF1 protein, a viral homologue of Bcl-2, protects human B cells from programmed cell death. *Proc. Natl. Acad. Sci. USA* **90**, 8479–8483.

Hogarth, L. A., and Hall, A. G. (1999). Increased BAX expression is associated with an increased risk of relapse in childhood acute lymphocytic leukemia. *Blood* **93**, 2671–2678.

Houghton, J. A. (1999). Apoptosis and drug response. *Curr. Opin. Oncol.* **11**, 475–481.

Hu, Y., Benedict, M. A., Ding, L., and Nunez, G. (1999). Role of cytochrome c and dATP/ATP hydrolysis in Apaf-1-mediated caspase-9 activation and apoptosis. *EMBO J.* **18**, 3586–3595.

Imai, Y., Kimura, T., Murakami, A., Yajima, N., Sakamaki, K., and Yonehara, S. (1999). The CED-4-homologous protein FLASH is involved in Fas-mediated activation of caspase-8 during apoptosis. *Nature,* **398**, 777–785.

Inohara, N., Ding, L., Chen, S., and Nunez, G. (1997). Harakiri, a novel regulator of cell death, encodes a protein that activates apoptosis and interacts selectively with survival-promoting proteins Bcl-2 and Bcl-X(L). *EMBO J.* **16**, 1686–1694.

Jaattela, M., Wissing, D., Kokholm, K., Kallunki, T., and Egeblad, M. (1998). Hsp70 exerts its anti-apoptotic function downstream of caspase-3-like proteases. *EMBO J.* **17**, 6124–6134.

Jaattela, M. (1999). Heat shock proteins as cellular lifeguards. *Ann. Med.* **31**, 261–271.

Jaffrézou, J. P., Levade, T., Bettaieb, A., Andrieu, N., Bezombes, C., Maestre, N., Vermeersch, S., Rousse, A., and Laurent, G. (1996). Daunorubicin-induced apoptosis: triggering of ceramide generation through sphingomyelin hydrolysis. *EMBO J.* **15**, 2417–2424.

Jaffrézou, J. P., Bettaieb, A., Levade, T., and Laurent, G. (1998). Antitumor-agent-induced apoptosis in myeloid leukemia cells: a controlled suicide. *Leuk. Lymph.* **29**, 453–463.

Jansen, B., Schlagbauer-Wald, H., Brown, B. D., Bryan, R. N., Van Elsas, A., Müller, M., Wolff, K., Eichler, H-G., and Pehamberger, H. (1998). Bcl-2 antisense therapy chemosensitizes human melanoma in SCID mice. *Nat. Med.* **4**, 232–234.

Jarvis, W. D., Grant, S., and Kolesnick, R. N. (1996). Ceramide and the induction of apoptosis. Clin. *Cancer Res.* **2**, 1–6.

Jo, M., Kim, T. H., Seol, D. W., Esplen, J. E., Dorko, K., Billiar, T. R., and Strom, S. C. (2000). Apoptosis induced in normal human hepatocytes by tumor necrosis factor-related apoptosis inducing ligand. *Nature Med.* **6**, 564–567.

Kaufmann, S. H., Karp, J. E., Svingen, P. A., Krajewski, S., Burke, P. J.,

Gore, S. D., and Reed, J. C. (1998). Elevated expression of the apoptotic regulator Mcl-1 at the time of leukemic relapse. *Blood* **91**, 991–1000.

Khwaja, A. (1999). Akt is more than just a Bad kinase. *Nature* **401**, 33–34.

Kim, S. H., Kim, D., Han, J. S., Jeong, C. S., Chung, B. S., Kang, C. D., and Li, G. C. (1999). Ku autoantigen affects the susceptibility to anticancer drugs. *Cancer Res.* **59**, 4012–4017.

Kitada, S., Takayama, S., De Riel, K., Tanaka, S., and Reed, J. C. (1994). Reversal of chemoresistance of lymphoma cells by antisense-mediated reduction of bcl-2-gene expression. *Antisense Res. Dev.* **4**, 71–79.

Kluck, R. M., Bossy-Wetzel, E., Gree, D. R., and Newmeyer, D. D. (1997) The release of cytochrome c from mitochondria: a role for Bcl-2 regulation of apoptosis. *Science* **275**, 1132–1136.

Knight, C. R. L., Rees, R. C., Platts, A., Johnson, T., and Griffin, M. (1993). Interleukin-2-activated human effector lymphocytes mediate cytotoxicity by inducing apoptosis in human leukaemia and solid tumour target cells. *J. Immunol.* **79**, 535–541.

Kobayashi, K., Hatano, M., Otaki, M., Ogasawara, T., and Tokuhisa, T. (1999). Expression of a murine homologue of the inhibitor of apoptosis protein is related to cell proliferation. *Proc. Natl. Acad. Sci. USA* **96**, 1457–1462.

Komarov, P. G., Komarova, E. A., Kondratov, R. V., Christov-Tselkov, K., Coon, J. S., Chernov, M. V., and Gudkov, A. V. (1999). A chemical inhibitor of p53 that protects mice from the side effects of cancer therapy. *Science* **285**, 1733–1737.

Kondo, T., Suda, T., Fukuyama, H., Adachi, M., and Nagata, S. (1997). Essential roles of the Fas ligand in the development of hepatitis. *Nat. Med.* **3**, 409–413.

Konishi, H., Matsuzaki, H., Tanaka, M., Takemura, Y., Kuroda, S., Ono, Y., and Kikkawa, U. (1997). Activation of protein kinase B (Akt/RAC-protein kinase) by cellular stress and its association with heat shock protein Hsp27. *FEBS Lett.* **410**, 493–498.

Kordes, U., Krappmann, D., Heissmeyer, V., Ludwig, W. D., and Scheidereit, C. (2000). Transcription factor NF-kappaB is constitutively activated in acute lymphoblastic leukemia cells. *Leukemia* **14**, 399–402.

Kornblau, S. M., Thall, P. F., Estrov, Z., Walterscheid, M., Patel, S., Theriault, A., Keating, M. J., Kantarjian, H., Estey, E., and Andreeff, M. (1999). The prognostic impact of BCL2 protein expression in acute myelogenous leukemia varies with cytogenetics. *Clin. Cancer Res.* 1999; **5:** 1758–1766.

Krajewski, S., Krajewska, M., Ellerby, L. M., Welsh, K., Xie, Z., Deveraux, Q. L., Salvesen, G. S., Bredesen, D. E., Rosenthal, R. E., Fiskum, G., and Reed, J. C. (1999). Release of caspase-9 from mitochondria during neuronal apoptosis and cerebral ischemia. *Proc. Natl. Acad. Sci. USA* **96**, 5752–5757.

Kroemer, G., and Reed, J. C. (2000). Mitochondrial control of cell death. *Nat. Med* **6**, 513–519.

Kuhnel, F., Zender, L., Paul, Y., Tietze, M. K., Trautwein, C., Manns, M., and Kubicka, S. (2000). NKkappaB mediated apoptosis through transcriptional activation of Fas (CD95) in adenoviral hepatitis. *J. Biol. Chem.* **275**, 6421–6427.

Kuida, K., Haydar, T. F., Kuan, C. Y., Gu, Y., Taya, C., Karasuyama, H., Su, M. S., Rakic, P., and Flavell, R. A. (1998). Reduced apoptosis and cytochrome c-mediated caspase activation in mice lacking caspase-9. *Cell* **94**, 325–337.

Kumar, A., Commane, M., Flickinger, T. W., Horvath, C. M., and Stark, G. R. (1997). Defective TNFα-induced apoptosis in STAT1-null cells due to low constitutive levels of caspases. *Science* **278**, 1630–1632.

Kumar, S. (1999). Mechanisms mediating caspase activation in cell death. *Cell Death Differ.* **6**, 1060–1066.

LaCasse, E. C., Baird, S., Korneluk, R. G., and MacKenzie, A. E. (1998). The inhibitors of apoptosis (IAPs) and their emerging role in cancer. *Oncogene* **17**, 3247–3259.

Lacour, S., Hammann, A., Wotawa, A., Corcos, L., Solary, E., and Dimanche-

Boitrel, M. T. (2001). Anticancer agents sensitize tumor cells to tumor necrosis factor-related apoptosis-inducing ligand-mediated caspase-8 activation and apoptosis. *Cancer Res.* **61,** 1645–1651.

Landowski, T. H., Qu, N., Buyuksal, I., Painter, J. S., and Dalton, W. S. (1997). Mutations in the Fas antigen in patients with multiple myeloma. *Blood* **90,** 4266–4270.

Lavoie, J. N., Lambert, H., Hickey, E., Weber, L. A., and Landry, J. (1995). Modulation of cellular thermoresistance and actin filament stability accompanies phosphorylation-induced changes in the oligomeric structure of heat shock protein 27. *Mol. Cell. Biol.* **15,** 505–516.

Lee, K. L., Spielmann, J., Zhao, D. J., Olsen, K. J., and Podack, E. R. (1996). Perforin, Fas ligand, and tumor necrosis factor are the major cytotoxic molecules used by lymphokine-activated killer cells. *J. Immunol.* **157,** 1919–1925.

Lee, J-I., and, Burckart, G. J. (1998). Nuclear factor kappa B: important transcription factor and therapeutic target. *Clin. Pharmacol.* **38,** 981–993.

Li, P., Nijhawan, D., Budihardjo, I., Srinivasula, S. M., Ahmad, M., Alnemri, E. S., and Wang, X. (1997). Cytochrome c and dATP-dependent formation of Apaf-1/caspase-9 complex initiates an apoptotic protease cascade. *Cell* **91,** 479–489.

Li, F., Ambrosini, G., Chu, E. Y., Plescia, J., Tognin, S., Marchisio, P.C., and Altieri, D.C. (1998a). Control of apoptosis and mitotic spindle checkpoint by survivin. *Nature* **396,** 580–584.

Li, H., Zhu, H., Xu, C. J., and Yuan, J. (1998b). Cleavage of Bid by caspase 8 mediates the mitochondrial damage in the Fas pathway of apoptosis. *Cell* **94,** 491–501.

Li, F., Ackermann, E. J., Bennett, C. F., Rothermel, A. L., Plescia, J., Tognin, S., Villa, A., Marchisio, P. C., and Altieri, D. C. (1999). Pleiotropic cell-division defects and apoptosis induced by interference with survivin function. *Nat. Cell Biol.* **1,** 461–466.

Liu, G., Kleine, L., and Hebert, R. L. (1999). Advances in the signal transduction of ceramide and related sphingolipids. *Crit. Rev. Clin. Lab. Sci.* **36,** 511–573.

Lowe, S. W., Ruley, H. E., Jacks, T., and Housman, D. E. (1993). p53-dependent apoptosis modulates the cytotoxicity of anticancer agents. *Cell* **74,** 957–967.

Lowe, S. W., Bodis, S., McClatchey, A., Remington, L., Ruley, H. E., Fisher, D. E., Housman, D. E., and Jacks, T. (1994). p53 status and the efficacy of cancer therapy in vivo. *Science* **266,** 807–810.

Luo, X., Budihardjo, I., Zou, H., Slaughter, C., and Wang, X. (1998). Bid, a Bcl2 interacting protein, mediates cytochrome c release from mitochondria in response to activation of cell surface death receptors. *Cell* **94,** 481–490.

Luque, I., and Gelinas, C. (1997) Rel/NF-κB and I-κB factors in oncogenesis. *Semin. Cancer Biol.* **8,** 103–111.

Maeda, T., Yamada, Y., Moriuchi, R., Sugahara, K., Tsuruda, K., Joh, T., Atogami, S., Tsukasaki, K., Tomonaga, M., and Kamihira, S. (1999) Fas gene mutation in the progression of adult T cell leukemia. *J. Exp. Med.* **189,** 1063–1071.

Mannick, J. B., Hausladen, A., Liu, L., Hess, D. T., Zeng, M., Miao, Q. X., Kane, L. S., Gow, A. J., and Stamler, J. S. (1999). Fas-induced caspase denitrosylation. *Science* **284,** 651–654.

Mansat, V., Laurent, G., Bettaieb, A., Levade, T., and Jaffrézou, J. P. (1997). The protein kinase C activators phorbol esters and phosphatidylserines inhibit neutral sphingomyelinase activation, ceramide and apoptosis triggered by daunorubicin. *Cancer Res.* **57,** 5300–5304.

Martinez-Lorenzo, M. J., Gamen, S., Etxeberria, J., Lasierra, P., Larrad, L., Pineiro, A., Anel, A., Naval, J., and Alava, M. A. (1998). Resistance to apoptosis correlates with a highly proliferative phenotype and loss of Fas and CPP32 (caspase-3) expression in human leukemia cells. *Int. J. Cancer* **75,** 473–481.

Martins, L. M., Mesner, P. W., Kottke, T. J., Basi, G. S., Sinha, S., Tung, J. S., Svingen, P. A., Madden, B. J., Takahashi, A., McCormick, D. J.,

Earnshaw, W. C., and Kaufmann, S. H. (1997). Comparison of caspase activation and subcellular localization in HL-60 and K562 cells undergoing etoposide-induced apoptosis. *Blood* **90,** 4283–4296.

Marzo, I., Brenner, C., Zamzami, N., Jurgensmeier, J. M., Susin, S. A., Vieira, H. L., Prevost, M. C., Xie, Z., Matsuyama, S., Reed, J. C., and Kroemer, G. (1998). Bax and adenine nucleotide translocator cooperate in the mitochondrial control of apoptosis. *Science* **281,** 2027–2031.

McDonnell, T. J., Deane, N., Platt, F. M., Nunez, G., Jaeger, U., McKearn, J. P., and Korsmeyer, S. J. (1989). bcl-2-immunoglobulin transgenic mice demonstrate extended B cell survival and follicular lymphoproliferation. *Cell* **57,** 79–88.

McDonnell, T. J., and Korsmeyer, S. J. (1991). Progression from lymphoid hyperplasia to high-grade malignant lymphoma in mice transgenic for the t(14; 18). *Nature* **349,** 254–256.

Medema, J. P., Scaffidi, C., Kischkel, F. C., Shevchenkon, A., Mann, M., Krammer, P. H., and Peter, M. E. (1997). FLICE is activated by association with the CD95 death-inducing signaling complex (DISC). *EMBO J.* **16,** 2794–2804.

Mehlen, P., Kretz-Remy, C., Preville, X., and Arrigo, A. P. (1996a). Human hsp27, Drosophila hsp27 and human alphaB-crystallin expression-mediated increase in glutathione is essential for the protective activity of these proteins against TNFalpha-induced cell death. *EMBO J.* **15,** 2695–2706.

Mehlen, P., Schulze-Osthoff, K., and Arrigo, A. P. (1996b). Small stress proteins as novel regulators of apoptosis. Heat shock protein 27 blocks Fas/APO-1- and staurosporine-induced cell death. *J. Biol. Chem.* **271,** 16510–16514.

Meijerink, J. P., Mensink E. J., Wang K., Sedlak T. W., Sloetjes A. W., de Witte T., Waksman G., and Korsmeyer S. J. (1998). Hematopoietic malignancies demonstrate loss-of-function mutations of BAX. *Blood* **91,** 2991–2997.

Messineo, C., Jamerson, M. H., Hunter, E., Braziel, R., Bagg, A., Irving, S. G., and Cossman, J. (1998). Gene expression by single Reed-Sternberg cells: pathways of apoptosis and activation. *Blood* **91,** 2443–2451.

Micheau, O., Solary, E., Hammann, A., Martin, F., and Dimanche-Boitrel, M. T. (1997). Sensitization of cancer cells treated with cytotoxic drugs to fas-mediated cytotoxicity. *J. Natl. Cancer Inst.* **89,** 783–789.

Micheau, O., Hammann, A., Solary, E., and Dimanche-Boitrel, M. T. (1999a). STAT-1-independent upregulation of FADD and procaspase-3 and -8 in cancer cells treated with cytotoxic drugs. *Biochem. Biophys. Res. Commun.* **256,** 603–607.

Micheau, O., Solary, E., Hammann, A., and Dimanche-Boitrel, M. T. (1999b) Fas ligand-independent, FADD-mediated activation of the Fas death pathway by anticancer drugs. *J. Biol. Chem.* **274,** 7987–7992.

Miyashita, T., and Reed, J. C. (1993). Bcl-2 oncoproteins blocks chemotherapy-induced apoptosis in a human leukemia cell line. *Blood* **81,** 151–157.

Miyashita, T., Harigal, M., Hanada, M., and Reed, J. C. (1994) Identification of a p53-dependent negative responsive element in the bcl-2 gene. *Cancer Res.* **54,** 3131–3135.

Miyashita, T., and Reed, J. C. (1995) Tumor suppressor p53 is a direct transcriptional activator of the human bax gene. *Cell* **80,** 293–299.

Mizutani, Y., Yoshida, O., Miki, T., and Bonavida, B. (1999). Synergistic cytotoxicity and apoptosis by Apo-2 ligand and adriamycin against bladder cancer cells. *Clin. Cancer Res.* **5,** 2605–2612.

Morimoto, H., Yonehara, S., Bonavida, B. (1993). Overcoming tumor necrosis factor and drug resistance of human tumor cell lines by combination treatment with anti-Fas antibody and drugs or toxins. *Cancer Res.* **53,** 2591–2596.

Moscat, J., Diaz-Meco, M. T. (1996). Zeta protein kinase C: a new target for antiproliferative interactions. *Anticancer Drugs* **7,** 143–148.

Mosser, D. D., Caron, A. W., Bourget, L., Denis-Larose, C., Massie, B. (1997). Role of the human heat shock protein hsp70 in protection against stress-induced apoptosis. *Mol. Cell. Biol.* **17,** 5317–5327.

Muller, M., Wilder, S., Bannasch, D., Israeli, D., Lehlbach, K., Li-Weber, M., Friedman, S. L., Galle, P. R., Stremmel, W., Oren, M., and Krammer, P. H. (1998). p53 activates the CD95 (APO-1/Fas) gene in response to DNA damage by anticancer drugs. *J. Exp. Med.* **188,** 2033–2045.

Muchmore, S. W., Sattler, M., Liang, H., Meadows, R. P., Nettesheim, D., Chang, B. S., Thompson, C. B., Wong, S. L., and Ng, S. H. (1996). X-ray and NMR structure of human Bcl-XL, an inhibitor of programmed cell death. *Nature* **381,** 335–341.

Nagata, S. (1999). Biddable death. *Nat. Cell Biol.* **1,** E143–E145.

Nicholson, D. W. (1999). Caspase structure, proteolytic substrates, and function during apoptotic cell death. *Cell Death Differ.* **6,** 1028–1042.

Nidai Ozes, O., Mayo, L. D., Gustin, J. A., Pfeffer, S. R., Pfeffer, L. M., and Bonner, D. B. (1999). NF-κB activation by tumour necrosis factor requires the Akt serine-threonine kinase. *Nature* **401,** 82–85.

Ogawa, Y., Nishioka, A., Hamada, N., Terashima, M., Inomata, T., Yoshida, S., Seguchi, H., and Kishimoto, S. (1997). Expression of Fas (CD95/APO-1) antigen induced by radiation therapy for diffuse B-cell lymphoma: immunohistochemical study. *Clin. Cancer Res.* **3,** 2211–2216.

Pan, G., O'Rourke, K., Chinnaiyan, A. M., Gentz, R., Ebner, R., Ni, J., and Dixit, V. M. (1997). The receptor for the cytotoxic ligand TRAIL. *Science* **276,** 111–113.

Pinkoski, M. J., and Green, D. R. (1999). Fas ligand, death gene. *Cell Death Differ.* **6,** 1174–1181.

Pitti, R. M., Marters, S. A., Ruppert, T. S., Donahue, C. J., Moore, A., and Ashkenazi, A. (1996). Induction of apoptosis by Apo-2 ligand, a new member of the tumor necrosis factor family. *J. Biol. Chem.* **271,** 12687–12690.

Plo, I., Bettaieb, A., Payrastre, B., Mansat-De Mas, V., Bordier, C., Rousse, A., Kowalski-Chauvel, A., Laurent, G., and Lautier, D. (1999). The phosphoinositide 3-kinase/Akt pathway is activated by daunorubicin in human acute myeloid leukemia cell lines. *FEBS Lett.* **452,** 150–154.

Poommipanit, P. B., Chen, B., and Oltvai, Z. N. (1999). Interleukin-3 induces the phosphorylation of a distinct fraction of bcl-2. *J. Biol. Chem.* **274,** 1033–1039.

Posovsky, C., Friesen, C., Herr, I., and Debatin, K. M. (1999). Chemotherapeutic drugs sensitize pre-B ALL cells for CD95- and cytotoxic T-lymphocyte-mediated apoptosis. *Leukemia* **13,** 400–409.

Puthalakath, H., Huang, D. C., O'Reilly, L. A., King, S. M., and Strasser, A. (1999). The proapoptotic activity of the Bcl-2 family member Bim is regulated by interaction with the dynein motor complex. *Mol. Cell* **3,** 287–296.

Quintans, J., Kilkus, J., McShan, C. L., Gottschalk, A. R., and Dawson, G. (1994). Ceramide mediates the apoptotic response of WEHI 231 cells to anti-immunoglobulin, corticosteroids and irradiation. *Biochem. Biophys. Res. Commun.* **202,** 710–714.

Rayet, B., and Gelinas, C. (1999). Aberrant rel/NF-kB genes and activity in human cancer. *Oncogene* **18,** 6938–6947.

Reed, J. C. (1997). Promise and problems of Bcl-2 antisense therapy. *J. Natl. Cancer Inst.* **89,** 988–990.

Reed, J. C. (1999). Bcl-2 family proteins: relative importance as determinants of chemoresistance in cancer. *In* "Apoptosis and Cancer Chemotherapy" (J.A. Hickman and C. Dive, eds.), pp. 99–116, Humana Press, Totowa, NJ.

Rieux-Laucat, F., Blachere, S., Danielan, S., de Villartay, J.P., Oleastro, M., Solary, E., Badre Meunier, B., Arkwright, P., Pondaré, C., Bernaudin, F., Chapel, H., Nielsen, S., Berah, M., Fisher, A., and Le Deist, F. (1999). Lymphoproliferative syndrome with autoimmunity : a possible genetic basis for dominant expression of the clinical manifestations. *Blood* **94,** 1192–1199.

Romashkova, J. A., and Makarov, S. S. (1999) NK-κB is a target of Akt in anti-apoptotic PDGF signalling. *Nature* **401,** 86–90.

Rotonda, J., Nicholson, D. W., Fazil, K. M., Gallant, M., Gareau, Y., Labelle, M., Peterson, E. P., Rasper, D. M., Ruel, R., Vaillancourt, J. P., Thorn-

berry, N. A., and Becker, J. W. (1996). The three-dimensional structure of apopain/CPP32, a key mediator of apoptosis. *Nat. Struct. Biol.* **3,** 619–625.

Ryan, K. M., Ernst, M. K., Rice, N. R., and Vousden, K. H. (2000). Role of NF-kappaB in p53-mediated programmed cell death. *Nature* **404,** 892–897.

Sahara, S., Aoto, M., Eguchi, Y., Imamoto, N., Yoneda, Y., and Tsujimoto, Y. (1999). Acinus is a caspase-3-activated protein required for apoptotic chromatin condensation. *Nature* **401,** 168–173.

Sakahira, H., Enari, M., and Nagata, S. (1998). Cleavage of CAD inhibitor in CAD activation and DNA degradation during apoptosis. *Nature* **391,** 96–99.

Samali, A., Cai J., Zhivotovsky, B., Jones, D. P., and Orrenius, S. (1999a). Presence of a preapoptotic complex of pro-caspase-3, Hsp60 and Hsp10 in the mitochondrial fraction of Jurkat cells. *EMBO J.* **18,** 2040–2048.

Samali, A., Holmberg, C. I., Sistonen, L., and Orrenius, S. (1999b). Thermotolerance and cell death are distinct cellular responses to stress: dependence on heat shock proteins. *FEBS Lett.* **461,** 306–310.

Sarid, R., Sato, T., Bohenzky, R. A., Russo, J. J., and Chang, Y. (1997). Kaposi's sarcoma-associated herpesvirus encodes a functional Bcl-2 homolog. *Nat. Med.* **3,** 293–298.

Sattler, M., Liang, H., Nettesheim, D., Meadows, R. P., Harlan, J. B., Yoon, H. S., Shuker, S. B., Chang, B. S., Minn, A. J., and Thompson, C. B. (1997). Structure of Bcl-XL-Bak peptide complex: recognition between regulators of apoptosis. *Science* **275,** 983–986.

Scaffidi, C., Schmitz, I., Zha, J., Korsmeyer, S. J., Krammer, P. H., and Peter, M. E. (1999). Differential modulation of apoptosis sensitivity in CD95 type I and type II cells. *J. Biol. Chem.* **274,** 22532–22538.

Schendel, S. L., Montal, M., and Reed, J. C. (1998). Bcl-2 family proteins as ion-channels. *Cell Death Differ.* **5,** 372–380.

Schlesinger, P. H., Gross, A., Yin, X. M., Yamamoto, K., Saito, M., Waksman, G., and Korsmeyer, S. J. (1997). Comparison of the ion channel characteristics of proapoptotic BAX and antiapoptic BCL-2. *Proc. Natl. Acad. Sci. USA* **94,** 11357–11362.

Schmitt, E., Cimoli, G., Steyaert, A., and Bertrand, R. (1998). Bcl-xL modulates apoptosis induced by anticancer drugs and delays DEVDase and DNA fragmentation-promoting activities. *Exp. Cell Res.* **240,** 107–121.

Schurmann, A., Mooney, A. F., Sanders, L. C., Sells, M. A., Wang, H. G., Reed, J. C., and Bokoch, G. M. (2000). p21-activated kinase 1 phosphorylates the death agonist Bad and protects cells from apoptosis. *Mol. Cell. Biol.* **20,** 453–461.

Selvakumaran, M., Lin, H. K., Miyashita, T., Wang, H. G., Krajewski, S., Reed, J. C., Hoffman, B., and Liebermann, D. (1994). Immediate early up-regulation of bax expression by p53 but not TGF beta 1: a paradigm for distinct apoptotic pathways. *Oncogene* **9,** 1791–1798.

Seol, D. W., and Billiar, T. R. (1999). A caspase-9 variant missing the catalytic site is an endogenous inhibitor of apoptosis. *J. Biol. Chem.* **274,** 2072–2076.

Sen, R., and Baltimore, D. (1986). Multiple nuclear factors interact with the immunoglobulin enhancer sequence. *Cell* **46,** 705–716

Sheard, M. A., Krammer P. H., Zaloudik J. (1999). Fractionated gamma-irradiation renders tumour cells more responsive to apoptotic signals through CD95. *Br. J. Cancer* **80,** 1689–1696.

Shibasaki, F., Kondo E., Akagi T., and McKeon F. (1997). Suppression of signalling through transcription factor NF-AT by interactions between calcineurin and Bcl-2. *Nature* **386,** 728–731.

Shimizu, S., Narita, M., and Tsujimoto, Y. (1999). Bcl-2 family proteins regulate the release of apoptogenic cytochrome c by the mitochondrial channel VDAC. *Nature* **399,** 483–487.

Simonian, P. L., Grillot, D. A., and Nunez, G. (1997). Bak can accelerate chemotherapy-induced cell death independently of its heterodimerization with Bcl-XL and Bcl-2. *Oncogene* **15,** 1871–1875.

Slee, E. A., Harte, M. T., Kluck, R. M., Wolf, B. B., Casiano, C. A., Newmeyer,

D. D., Wang, H. G., Reed, J. C., Nicholson, D. W., Alnemri, E. S., Green, D. R., and Martin, S. J. (1999). Ordering the cytochrome c-initiated caspase cascade: hierarchical activation of caspases-2, -3, -6, -7, -8, and -10 in a caspase-9-dependent manner. *J. Cell Biol.* **144,** 281–292.

Solary, E., Witz, F., Caillot, D., Moreau, P., Desablens, B., Cahn, J. Y., Sadoun, A., Berthou, C, Maloisel, F., Guyotat, D., Casassus, P., Ifrah, N., Lamy, T., Audhuy, B., Colombat, P., and Harousseau, J. L. (1996). Combination of quinine as a potential reversing agent with mitoxantrone and cytarabine for the treatment of acute leukemias: a randomised multicentric study. *Blood* **88,** 1198–1205.

Sordet, O., Bettaieb, A., Bruey, J. M., Eymin, B., Droin, N., Ivarsson, M., Garrido, C., and Solary, E. (1999). Selective inhibition of apoptosis by TPA-induced differentiation of U937 leukemic cells. *Cell Death Differ.* **6,** 351–361.

Srinivasula, S. M., Ahmad, M., Guo, Y., Zhan, Y., Lazebnik, Y., Fernandes-Alnemri, T., and Alnemri, E. S. (1999). Identification of an endogenous dominant-negative short isoform of caspase-9 that can regulate apoptosis. *Cancer Res.* **59,** 999–1002.

Srivastava, R. K., Srivastava, A. R., Korsmeyer, S. J., Nesterova, M., Cho-Chung, Y. S., and Longo, D. L. (1998). Involvement of microtubules in the regulation of Bcl2 phosphorylation and apoptosis through cyclic AMP-dependent protein kinase. *Mol. Cell. Biol.* **18,** 3509–3517.

Stehlik, C., de Martin, R., Kumabashiri, I., Schmid, J. A., Binder, B. R., and Lipp, J. (1998). Nuclear Factor (NF)-κB-regulated X-chromosome-linked iap gene expression protects endothelial cells from tumor necrosis factor-a-induced apoptosis. *J. Exp. Med.* **188,** 211–216.

Strasser, A., Harris, A. W., Bath, M. L., and Cory, S. (1990). Novel primitive lymphoid tumours induced in transgenic mice by cooperation between myc and bcl-2. *Nature* **348,** 331–333.

Strum, J. C., Small, G. W., Pauig, S. B., and Daniel, L. W. (1994). 1-beta-D-Arabinofuranosylcytosine stimulates ceramide and diglyceride formation in HL-60 cells. *J. Biol. Chem.* **269,** 15493–15497.

Stuart, J. K., Myszka, D. G., Joss, L., Mitchell, R. S., McDonald, S. M., Xie, Z., Takayama, S., Reed, J. C., and Ely K. R. (1998). Characterization of interactions between the anti-apoptotic protein BAG-1 and Hsc70 molecular chaperones. *J. Biol. Chem.* **273,** 22506–22514.

Sugiyama, K., Shimizu, M., Akiyama, T., Tamaoki, T., Yamaguchi, K., Takahashi, R., Eastman, A., and Akinaga, S. (2000). UCN-01 selectively enhances mitomycin C cytotoxicity in p53 defective cells which is mediated through S and/or G(2) checkpoint abrogation. *Int. J. Cancer* **85,** 703–709.

Susin, S. A., Lorenzo, H. K., Zamzami, N., Marzo, I., Brenner, C., Larochette, N., Prevost, M. C., Alzari, P. M., and Kroemer, G. (1999a). Mitochondrial release of caspase-2 and -9 during the apoptotic process. *J. Exp. Med.* **189,** 381–394.

Susin, S. A., Lorenzo, H. K., Zamzami, N., Marzo, I., Snow, B. E., Brothers, G. M., Mangion, J., Jacotot, E., Costantini, P., Loeffler, M., Larochette, N., Goodlett, D. R., Aebersold, R., Siderovski, D. P., Penninger, J. M., and Kroemer, G. (1999b). Molecular characterization of mitochondrial apoptosis-inducing factor. *Nature* **397,** 441–446.

Tai, Y. T., Strobel, T., Kufe, D., and Cannistra, S. A. (1999). In vivo cytotoxicity of ovarian cancer cells through tumor-selective expression of the BAX gene. *Cancer Res.* **59,** 2121–2126.

Takeda, H., Matozaki, T., Takada, T., Noguchi, T., Yamao, T., Tsuda, M., Ochi, F., Fukunaga, K., Inagaki, K., and Kasuga, M. (1999). PI 3-kinase γ and protein kinase ξ mediate RAS-independent activation of MAP kinase by a Gi protein-coupled receptor. *EMBO J.* **18,** 386–395.

Tamiya, S., Etoh, K., Suzushima, H., Takatsuki K., and Matsuoka, M. (1998). Mutation of CD95 (Fas/Apo-1) gene in adult T-cell leukemia cells. *Blood* **91,** 3935–3942.

Tamm, I., Wang, Y., Sausville, E., Scudiero, D. A., Vigna, N., Oltersdorf, T., and Reed, J. C. (1998). IAP-family protein survivin inhibits caspase activity and apoptosis induced by Fas (CD95), Bax, caspases, and anticancer drugs. *Cancer Res.* **58,** 5315–5320.

Tanaka, H., Arakawa, H., Yamaguchi, T., Shiraishi, K., Fukuda, S., Matsui, K., Takei, Y., and Nakamura Y. (2000). A ribonucleotide reductase gene involved in a p53-dependent cell-cycle checkpoint for DNA damage. *Nature* **404,** 42–49.

Teitz, T., Wei, T., Valentine, M. B., Vanin, E. F., Grenet, J., Valentine, V. A., Behm, F. G, Look, A. T., Lahti, J. M., and Kidd, V. J. (2000). Caspase 8 is deleted or silenced preferentially in childhood neuroblastomas with amplification of MYCN. *Nature Med.* **6,** 529–535.

Tepper, C. G., Jayadev, S., Liu, B., Bielawska, A., Wolff, R., Yonehara, S., Hannun, Y. A., and Seldin, M. F. (1995). Role of ceramide as an endogenous mediator of Fas-induced cytotoxicity. *Proc. Natl. Acad. Sci. USA* **92,** 8443–8447.

Thanos, D., and Maniatis, T. (1995) NF-κB: a lesson in family values. *Cell* **80,** 529–532.

Torii, S., Egan, D. A., Evans, R. A., and Reed, J. C. (1999). Human Daxx regulates Fas-induced apoptosis from nuclear PML oncogenic domains (PODs). *EMBO J.* **18,** 6037–6049.

Tschopp, J., Irmler, M., and Thome, M. (1998). Inhibition of Fas death signals by FLIPs. *Current. Op. Immunol.* **10,** 552–558.

Vander Heiden, M. G., and Thompson, C. B. (1999). Bcl-2 proteins: regulators of apoptosis or of mitochondrial homeostasis? *Nat. Cell Biol.* **1,** E209–E216.

Varfolomeev, E. E., Schuchmann, M., Luria, V., Chiannilkulchai, N., Beckmann, J. S., Mett, I. L., Rebrikov, D., Brodianski, V. M., Kemper, O. C., Kollet, O., Lapidot, T., Soffer, D., Sobe, T., Avraham, K. B., Goncharov, T., Holtmann, H., Lonai, P., and Wallach, D. (1998). Targeted disruption of the mouse Caspase 8 gene ablates cell death induction by the TNF receptors, Fas/Apo1, and DR3 and is lethal prenatally. *Immunity* **9,** 267–276.

Verheij, M., Bose, R., Lin, X. H., Yao, B., Jarvis, W. D., Grant, S., Birrer, M. J., Szabo, E., Zon, L. I., Kyriakis, J. M., Haimovitz-Friedman, A., Fuks, Z., and Kolesnick, R. N. (1996). Requirement for ceramide-initiated SAPK/JNK signalling in stress-induced apoptosis. *Nature* **380,** 75–79.

von Reyher, U., Strater, J., Kittstein, W., Gschwendt, M., Krammer, P. H., and Moller, P. (1998). Colon carcinoma cells use different mechanisms to escape CD95-mediated apoptosis. *Cancer Res* **58,** 526–534.

Vucic, D., Kaiser, W. J., Harvey, A. J., and Miller, L. K. (1997) Inhibition of reaper-induced apoptosis by interaction with inhibitor of apoptosis proteins (IAPs). *Proc. Natl. Acad. Sci.USA* **94,** 10183–10188.

Vucic, D., Kaiser, W. J., and Miller, L. K. (1998) Inhibitor of apoptosis proteins physically interact with and block apoptosis induced by Drosophilia proteins HID and GRIM. *Mol. Cell Biol.* **18,** 3300–3309.

Walczak, H., Miller, R. E., Ariail, K., Gliniak, B., Griffith, T. S., Kubin, M., Chin, W., Jones, J, Woodward, A., Le, T., Smith, C., Smolak, P., Goodwin, R. G., Rauch, C. T., Schuh, J. C., and Lynch, D. H. (1999). Tumoricidal activity of tumor necrosis factor-related apoptosis-inducing ligand in vivo. *Nat. Med.* **5,** 157–163.

Waldman, T., Zhang, Y., Dillehay, L., Yu, J., Kinzler, K., Vogelstein, B., and Williams, J. (1997). Cell-cycle arrest versus cell death in cancer therapy. *Nat. Med.* **3,** 1034–1036.

Walker, N. P., Talanian, R. V., Brady, K. D., Dang, L. C., Bump, N. J., Ferenz, C. R., Franklin, S., Ghayur, T., Hackett, M. C., Hammill, L. D., Herzog, L., Hugunin, M., Houy, W., Mankovich, J. A., McGuiness, L., Orlewicz, E., Paskind, M., Pratt, C. A., Reis, P., Summani A., Terranova, M., Welch, J. P., Xiong L., Möller, A., Tracey, D. E., Kamen, R., and Wong, W. W. (1994). Crystal structure of the cysteine protease interleukin-1 beta-converting enzyme: a (p20/p10)$_2$ homodimer. *Cell* **78,** 343–352.

Wang, C. Y., Mayo M. W., and Baldwin A. S. Jr. (1996). TNF- and cancer therapy-induced apoptosis: potentiation by inhibition of NF-κB. *Science* **274,** 784–787.

Wang, H. G., Pathan, N., Ethell, I. M., Krajewski, S., Yamaguchi, Y.,

Shibasaki, F., McKeon, F., Bobo, T., Franke, T. F., and Reed, J. C. (1999a). Ca^{2+}-induced apoptosis through calcineurin dephosphorylation of BAD. *Science* **284**, 339–343.

Wang, J., Zheng, L., Lobito, A., Chan, F. K., Dale, J., Sneller, M., Yao, X., Puck, J. M., Straus, S. E., and Lenardo, M. J. (1999b). Inherited human Caspase 10 mutations underlie defective lymphocyte and dendritic cell apoptosis in autoimmune lymphoproliferative syndrome type II. *Cell* **98**, 47–58.

Wang, J. Y. J. (2000). New link in a web of human genes. *Nature* **405**, 404–405.

Wang, L., Miura, M., Bergeron, L., Zhu, H., and Yuan, J. (1994). Ich-1, an Ice/ced-3-related gene, encodes both positive and negative regulators of programmed cell death. *Cell* **78**, 739–750.

Wang, L. G., Liu, X. M., Kreis, W., and Budman, D. R. (1999c). The effect of antimicrotubule agents on signal transduction pathways of apoptosis. *Cancer Chemother. Pharmacol.* **44**, 355–361.

Waterman, M. J, Stavridi, E. S., Waterman, J. L., and Halazonetis, T. D. (1998). ATM-dependent activation of p53 involves dephosphorylation and association with 14-3-3 proteins. *Nat. Genet.* **19**, 175–178.

Webb, A., Cinnuingham, D., Cotter, F., Clarke, P. A., di Stefano, F., Ross, P., Corbo, M., and Dziewanowska, Z. (1997). Bcl-2 antisense therapy in patients with non-Hodgkin lymphoma. *Lancet* **349**, 1137–1141.

Weinstein, J. N., Myers, T. G., O'Connor, P. M., Friend, S. H., Fornace, A. J. Jr, Kohn, K. W., Fojo, T., Bates, S. E., Rubinstein, L. V., Anderson, N. L., Buolamwini, J. K., van Osdol, W. W., Monks, A. P., Scudiero, D. A., Sausville, E. A., Zaharevitz, D. W., Bunow B., Viswanadhan, V. N., Johnson, G. S., Wittes, R. E., and Paull, K. D. (1997). An information-intesive approach to the molecular pharmacology of cancer. *Science* **275**, 343–349.

White, E., and Prives, C. (1999). DNA damage enables p73. *Nature* **399**, 734–535.

Wiley, S. R., Schooley, K., Smolak, P. J., Din, W. S., Huang, C. P., Nicholl, J. K., Sutherland, G. R., Smith, T. D., Rauch, C., Smith, C. A., and Goodwin, R. G. (1995). Identification and characterization of a new member of the TNF family that induces apoptosis. *Immunity* **3**, 673–682.

Woo, R. A., McLure, K. G., Lees-Miller, S. P., Rancourt, D. E., and Lee, P. M. K. (1998). DNA-dependent kinase acts upstream of p53 in response to DNA damage. *Nature* **394**, 700–704.

Xanthoudakis, S., Roy, S., Rasper, D., Hennessay, T., Aubin, Y., Cassady, R., Tawa, P., Ruel, R., Rosen, A., and Nicholson, D. W. (1999). Hsp60 accelerates the maturation of pro-caspase-3 by upstream activator proteases during apoptosis. *EMBO J* **18**, 2049–2056.

Xia, Z., Dickens, M., Raingeaud, J., Davis, R. J., and Greenberg, M. E. (1995). Opposing effects of ERK and JNK-p38 MAP kinases on apoptosis. *Science* **270**, 1326–1331.

Yang, J., Liu, X. S., Bhalla, K., Kim, C. N., Ibrado, A. M., Cai, J. Y., Peng, T. I., Jones, D. P., and Wang, X. D. (1997). Prevention of apoptosis by Bcl-2. Release of cytochrome C from mitochondria blocked. *Science* **275**, 1129–1132.

Yang, S., Wang, C., Minden, M. D., and McCulloch, E. A. (1994). Fluorescence labeling of nicks in DNA from leukemic blast cells as a measure of damage following cytosine arabinoside: application to the study of drug sensitivity. *Leukemia* **8**, 2052–2059.

Yeh, W. C., Pompa, J. L., McCurrach, M. E., Shu, H. B., Elia, A. J., Shahinian, A., Ng, M., Wakeham, A., Khoo, W., Mitchell, K., El-Deiry, W. S., Lowe, S. W., Goeddel, D. V., and Mak, T. W. (1998). FADD: essential for embryo development and signaling from some, but not all, inducers of apoptosis. *Science* **279**, 1954–1958.

Yoshida, H., Kong, Y. Y., Yoshida, R., Elia, A. J., Hakem, A., Hakem, R., Penninger, J. M., and Mak, T. W. (1998). Apaf1 is required for mitochondrial pathways of apoptosis and brain development. *Cell* **94**, 739–750.

Yuan, Z. M., Shioya, H., Ishiko, T., Sun, X., Gu, J., Huang, Y. Y., Lu, H., Kharbanda, S., Weichselbaum, R., and Kufe, D. (1999). p73 is regulated by tyrosine kinase c-Abl in the apoptotic response to DNA damage. *Nature* **399**, 814–817.

Zamzami, N., Marchetti, P., Castedo, M., Zanin, C., Vayssiere, J. L., Petit, P. X., and Kroemer, G. (1995). Reduction in mitochondrial potential constitutes an early irreversible step of programmed lymphocyte death in vivo. *J. Exp. Med.* **181**, 1661–1672.

Zamzami, N., Brenner, C., Marzo, I., Susin, S. A., and Kroemer, G. (1998). Subcellular and submitochondrial mode of action of Bcl-2-like oncoproteins. *Oncogene*, **16**, 2265–2282.

Zha, H., and Reed, J. C. (1997) Heterodimerization-independent functions of cell death regulatory proteins Bax and Bcl-2 in yeast and mammalian cells. *J. Biol. Chem.* **272**, 31482–31488.

Zhang, X. D., Franco, A., Myers, K., Gray, C., Nguyen, T., and Hersey, P. (1999). Relation of TNF-related apoptosis-inducing ligand (TRAIL) receptor and FLICE-inhibitory protein expression to TRAIL-induced apoptosis of melanoma. *Cancer Res.* **59**, 2747–2753.

Zou, H., Henzel, W. J., Liu, X., Lutschg, A., and Wang, X. (1997). Apaf-1, a human protein homologous to *C. elegans* CED-4, participates in cytochrome c-dependent activation of caspase-3. *Cell* **90**, 405–413.

CHAPTER 5

DRUG RESISTANCE PATHWAYS AS TARGETS

Akihiro Tomida*

Takashi Tsuruo*,†

*Institute of Molecular and Cellular Biosciences, University of Tokyo, Tokyo, Japan;

and †Cancer Chemotherapy Center, Japanese Foundation for Cancer Research, Tokyo, Japan

Summary

Resistance to chemotherapeutic drugs is a principal problem in the treatment of cancer. Drug resistance may already exist before the initiation of therapy or may be acquired after successful initial therapy. Cancer cells in culture can become resistant to virtually all of the cytotoxic drugs currently in use for chemotherapy. There has been much effort to understand the mechanisms of drug resistance of cancer cells. Multidrug resistance due to overexpression of P-glycoprotein has been extensively investigated. Several inhibitors for P-glycoprotein-mediated drug transport have been developed, and clinical trials have shown promise for their use in hematologic malignancies. Thus, an understanding of drug resistance pathways can provide targets to overcoming drug resistance in humans. In this chapter, we discuss several drug resistance pathways, including drug transporters, cellular stress response, and DNA repair, as potential therapeutic targets.

1. Introduction

Cancer chemotherapy has gradually improved with the discovery of various antitumor drugs and has profound, positive results when applied to many hematologic malignancies and to a few solid tumors, especially germ cell and some childhood malignancies. Successful treatment of patients with certain malignancies suggests a high potential of current chemotherapeutic agents. However, the effectiveness of chemotherapy has been often limited by drug resistance of tumors and by the side effects on normal tissues and cells. In fact, many tumors are intrinsically resistant to many of the most potent cytotoxic agents used in cancer therapy. Other tumors, initially sensitive, recur and are resistant not only to the initial therapeutic agents but to other drugs that were not used for the treatment. Because of the serious problem of clinical drug resistance, much effort has been expended to advance our understanding of the mechanisms of drug resistance of cancer cells.

Drug resistance, intrinsic or acquired, can be attributed to mutational (genetic) or nonmutational (epigenetic) processes in cancer cells. These processes frequently lead to the same biochemical mechanisms of drug resistance. Cancer cells become resistant to anticancer drugs by a wide variety of biochemical mechanisms (Harrison, 1995). These include (1) decreased intracellular drug accumulation by decreased inward transport or by increased drug efflux; (2) increased drug inactivation or detoxification; (3) decreased conversion of drug to an active form; (4) altered quantity or activity of target proteins; (5) increased DNA repair capacity; and (6) decreased susceptibility of apoptotic response. Although drug resistance is a problem, these biochemical changes can be exploited for selective killing of the resistant tumor cells and ultimately for developing novel strategies and therapeutics to overcome the problem of drug resistance in the clinic. In this chapter, we discuss the drug resistance pathways, including drug transport, cellular stress response, and DNA repair, as targets for the development of new anticancer drugs.

2. Targeting Drug Transport

A. The Multidrug Transporter P-glycoprotein

1. P-glycoprotein in Multidrug Resistance

Resistance to a broad spectrum of chemotherapeutic agents in cancer cell lines and human tumors has been called multidrug resistance (MDR) (reviewed in Ling, 1997). *In vitro* selection of tumor cells for resistance to lipophilic cytotoxic agents often results in development of cross-resistance to different types of cytotoxic drugs. The MDR phenotype is associated with an increased drug efflux from the cell, which is mediated by an energy-dependent mechanism. Studies on the MDR phenotype have led to discovery of ATP-binding cassette (ABC) transporters, such as P-glycoprotein (P-gp) and multidrug-resistance-associated protein (MRP). Much progress has been made in developing strategies to overcome the transporter-mediated MDR, especially for P-gp.

P-gp, encoded by the *MDR-1* gene, is the first identified mammalian multidrug transporter that pumps various cytotoxic drugs out of the cell (reviewed in Ambudkar *et al.*, 1999). Overexpression of P-gp causes cancer cells to become resistant to a great variety of structurally and functionally dissimilar antitumor drugs, including vinblastine, vincristine, doxorubicin, daunorubicin, etoposide, teniposide, paclitaxel, and many others. Transfection of *MDR-1* cDNA confers MDR on sensitive cells (Shen *et al.*, 1986; Gros *et al.*, 1986; Ueda *et al.*, 1987). P-gp has been shown to bind anticancer drugs and to be an ATPase localized at the plasma membrane of resistant cancer cells. Although many aspects of P-gp structure and function have been clarified over the past two decades (Ambudkar *et al.*, 1999), it is still unclear precisely how P-gp recognizes and transports a wide variety of drugs. Furthermore, its role in preventing apoptosis induction in cells (Johnstone *et al.*, 2000) suggests that P-gp has a multifunctional property in addition to acting as a drug transporter. However, P-gp has an important feature for the molecular target: binding and transport of a particular drug substrate by P-gp can be inhibited by another drug substrate and by agents that reverse MDR in cancer cells.

The expression of P-gp has been elevated in intrinsically drug-resistant cancers of the colon, kidney, and adrenal as well as in some tumors that acquired drug resistance after chemotherapy (Ling, 1997; Ambudkar *et al.*, 1999). The expression of *MDR-1* mRNA in tumors correlates well with certain clinical drug resistance. Although gene amplification is often observed in highly drug-resistant cell lines selected *in vitro,* it has never been seen in clinical samples. Therefore, transcriptional up-regulation of *MDR-1* mRNA and/or chromosomal abnormalities (e.g., DNA methylation) near the *MDR-1* locus may be involved in the elevated expression of P-gp in clinically resistant tumors (reviewed in Kantharidis *et al.,* 2000). In support of this, *MDR-1* promoter activity is up-regulated by various stimuli, such as anticancer drugs, DNA-damaging agents, heat shock, serum starvation, and ultraviolet irradiation. Recently, transient activation of *MDR-1* gene expression was observed in human metastatic sarcoma after *in vivo* exposure to doxorubicin (Abolhoda *et al.*, 1999). The expression of *MDR-1* can also be up-regulated as a consequence of tumor progression, such as mutation of the tumor suppressor gene *p53* and activation of the oncogene *ras* (Kantharidis *et al.,* 2000). Furthermore, a transcription factor YB-1 can positively regulate the *MDR-1* promoter containing a Y box (Kantharidis *et al.,* 2000), and nuclear expression of YB-1 correlates with *MDR-1* expression in breast cancer and osteosarcoma (Bargou *et al.,* 1997; Oda *et al.,* 1998).

P-gp is also expressed in such normal tissues as adrenal, gravid uterus, kidney, liver, colon, and capillary endothelium in brain (reviewed in Schinkel, 1997; Silverman, 1999). P-gp expressed in normal tissue could have physiologic functions specific to those tissues. For example, P-gp expressed in brain capillary endothelium could be functionally involved in the blood–brain barrier. P-gp in the adrenal gland could be responsible for secretion of steroid hormones. P-gp in luminal surface of colon, brush border of proximal tubules in kidney, and biliary canalicular surface of hepatocytes could contribute to excretion of natural toxic substances into the lumen of gastrointestinal tract, urine, and bile, respectively. At least in mice, P-gp does not appear essential for basic physiologic functions because simultaneous genetic knockout of *mdr1a* and *mdr1b* resulted in healthy mice (Schinkel, 1998). However, the mice exhibited increased sensitivity to cytotoxic drugs with decreased blood–brain barrier function and increased intestinal absorption of drugs. These observations support the notion that P-gp in normal tissues plays an important role in preventing uptake of xenobiotics. When targeting P-gp in resistant tumors, we must be concerned about the normal functions of P-gp.

2. Pharmacologic Inhibition of P-glycoprotein

Because P-gp appears to be involved in both acquired and intrinsic MDR in human cancers, the selective killing of tumor cells expressing P-gp could be very important for cancer therapy. In 1981, we reported that the calcium channel blocker verapamil inhibited active drug efflux and restored drug sensitivity in MDR cells (Tsuruo *et al.*, 1981). Various compounds, including calcium channel blockers and calmodulin inhibitors, have been shown to enhance the cytotoxic activity of various antitumor agents (reviewed in Tsuruo, 1988; Ford *et al.*, 1996;

Robert, 1999). All of these agents antagonize MDR by increasing the drug accumulation in MDR cells, whereas they show little or no effect on drug-sensitive cells. Most of the reversing agents, such as verapamil, cyclosporin A, diltiazem, and FK-506, are substrates for P-gp-mediated transport and competitively inhibit the transport of antitumor drugs by P-gp. Some chemosensitizers, such as progesterone and nitredipine, have been thought to act as nonsubstrate inhibitors of P-gp.

In clinical trials, the first-generation modulators, such as verapamil and cyclosporin A, showed various adverse effects mediated by their original pharmacologic activities. Recently, promising MDR-reversing agents, which lack the original or other pharmacologic activities, have been developed. For example, PSC-833, a nonimmunosuppressive analogue of cyclosporine, was superior to cyclosporin A in overcoming of MDR *in vitro*—10-fold more effective—and *in vivo* (reviewed in Atadja *et al.*, 1998). Moreover, PSC-833 surpassed cyclosporin A and verapamil in prolonging life in P388/VCR-bearing mice when chemosensitizers were administered orally along with vincristine and doxorubicin administered intraperitoneally or intravenously. PSC-833 is currently in clinical trials (for example, see Advani *et al.*, 1999; Lee *et al.*, 1999; Fracasso *et al.*, 2000; Tidefelt *et al.*, 2000). The clinical trial findings are promising in acute myeloid leukemia (Advani *et al.*, 1999). MS-209, a quinoline derivative, is also a potent MDR-reversing agent (Nakanishi and Tsuruo, 1996). It is undergoing clinical trials because of its efficient oral bioavailability and potentiating effects.

It is important to note that any P-gp inhibitor has the potential to have deleterious effects on normal cells. In fact, clinical trials with the first-generation modulators or PSC-833 revealed alterations in anticancer drug pharmacokinetics with an increase in the area under the urine and/or a decrease in anticancer drugs clearance (Sikic *et al.*, 1997). To improve combined chemotherapy, we must consider the pharmacokinetic features of the MDR-reversing agents and the anticancer drugs when given together. Interestingly, some new-generation P-gp inhibitors lack significant pharmacokinetic interaction with doxorubicin (GF120918), with doxorubicin or paclitaxel (OC144-093), or plasma levels of doxorubicin, etoposide, and paclitaxel (LY335979) (Hyafil *et al.*, 1993; Starling *et al.*, 1997; Newman *et al.*, 2000). In addition, the new-generation P-gp inhibitors, if not all, exhibit nanomolar potency, low nonspecific cytotoxicity, high P-gp specificity with direct interaction, relatively long duration of action with reversibility, and good oral bioavailability. These properties with the lack of pharmacokinetic interaction would be important for the development of new P-gp inhibitors.

3. Monoclonal Antibodies against P-glycoprotein

A number of monoclonal antibodies (MAb's) against P-gp have been established. They are useful for basic research and for diagnosis (reviewed in Okochi *et al.*, 1997; Ramachan-

dran and Melnick, 1999). MAb's that recognize the extracellular epitope of P-gp can be used for targeting P-gp. Our research group has developed immunotherapeutic approaches for overcoming MDR using anti-P-gp MAb's MRK-16 and MRK-17 (Hamada and Tsuruo, 1986). We have evaluated the effect of MRK-16 and MRK-17 on the growth of human MDR ovarian cancer cells, 2780AD, in nude mice and found that these MAb's by themselves inhibited growth of MDR tumors (Tsuruo *et al.*, 1989). The benefit of MRK-16 use *in vivo* has also been verified in a xenograft of MDR human colon cancer, HT29mdr1 (Pearson *et al.*, 1991). In addition to its immunotherapeutic effects, MRK-16 inhibits the transport of antitumor drugs by P-gp and enhances the sensitivity of MDR cells to the drugs (Hamada and Tsuruo, 1986). The combination of antitumor drugs and MRK-16 was also examined in nude mice bearing MDR tumors and was shown to overcome MDR *in vivo* (Pearson *et al.*, 1991). The inhibition of drug transport by MAb's was also observed with other anti-P-gp MAb's, such as UIC2 (Mechetner and Roninson, 1992), 4E3 (Arceci *et al.*, 1993), and a series of HYB antibodies (Rittmann-Grauer *et al.*, 1992). Reversal of MDR by HYB-241 was demonstrated in the human MDR tumor xenograft model (Rittmann-Grauer *et al.*, 1992). Thus, anti-P-gp MAb's can inhibit the transport of antitumor drugs by P-gp, which when combined with drugs would contribute to additional therapeutic effects.

The combination of anti-P-gp MAb with chemosensitizers may also be useful in reversing P-gp-mediated MDR. The combination of MRK-16 with cyclosporin A or PSC-833 synergistically reversed doxorubicin resistance in K562/ADM cells (Naito *et al.*, 1993). This same MDR-reversing effect was also obtained in 2780AD, intrinsically MDR HCT-15 and its doxorubicin-resistant HCT-15/ADM2-2 cells (Naito *et al.*, 1996; Watanabe *et al.*, 1997). The antitumor activity of combination therapy with MRK-16 (low doses, at which the MAb by itself did not show tumor growth inhibition), cyclosporine derivatives (either cyclosporin A or PSC-833), and doxorubicin was examined in athymic mice bearing HCT-15/ADM2-2 xenografts (Watanabe *et al.*, 1997). The ternary combinations significantly inhibited tumor growth, including some cures, while MRK-16 combined with doxorubicin but without cyclosporine derivatives resulted in moderate inhibition. The mechanistic analysis showed that MRK-16 increased the accumulation of cyclosporin A in MDR cells. On the other hand, MRK-16 did not affect intracellular accumulation of PSC-833 in MDR cells. Instead, PSC-833 increased MRK-16 binding to P-gp. Cyclosporin A also increased MRK-16 binding to P-gp. These interactions between MRK-16 and cyclosporine derivatives could explain the synergistic MDR reversal activity.

4. Other Approaches

MDR-reversing agents can inhibit the emergence of P-gp-mediated drug resistance (Sikic *et al.*, 1997). In *in vitro* experiments with a human sarcoma cell line, doxorubicin predominantly selected the MDR mutants expressing P-gp. PSC-833 reduced the mutation rate for resistance to doxorubicin and suppressed activation of *MDR-1* gene and the appearance of MDR mutants (Beketic-Oreskovic *et al.,* 1995). These observations have a clinical implication that treatment of drug-sensitive P-gp-negative cancers with effective MDR-reversing agents might suppress the emergence of resistant subclones that express P-gp.

Antisense oligodeoxynucleotides (ODNs) and ribozymes have attracted considerable interest as a tool to inhibit gene expression. Several studies have demonstrated that these agents can be used to inhibit *MDR-1* gene expression and to reverse MDR in cultured cells (Byrne *et al.,* 1998). Recently, Cucco and Calabretta (1996) reported antisense ODN-mediated reversal of MDR *in vivo.* They used an 18-mer *MDR-1* antisense phosphorothioate ODN in combination with vincristine. *In vitro* treatment with the antisense ODNs restored vincristine sensitivity of MDR human leukemia HL-60 (HL-60/Vinc) cells. The *in vitro* reversion of MDR correlated with inhibition of P-gp expression in HL-60/Vinc cells exposed to the *MDR-1* antisense ODNs. Combination therapy with *MDR-1* antisense ODNs and vincristine resulted in significant prolonged survival in mice. Treatment with *MDR-1* antisense ODNs or vincristine alone had no effect on survival. These results suggest that the use of *MDR-1* antisense ODNs in combination with standard antineoplastic drugs may be useful in reversing MDR *in vivo.*

The maturation process of P-gp can be a target for overcoming MDR. Recently, Loo and Clark (2000) showed that P-gp maturation can be blocked by disulfiram, a drug used to treat persons with alcoholism. Disulfiram at 100 nM increased sensitivity of P-gp-transfected HEK293 cells to vinblastine and colchicine. Treatment of the P-gp-transfected cells with disulfiram as low as 50 nM blocked maturation of recombinant P-gp. Although disulfiram also inhibited P-gp activity (assessed by verapamil-stimulated ATPase activity), these data raised the possibility that it could be used as an antichaperone to prevent P-gp maturation and transport to the cell surface. Because cyclosporin A and modulators of P-gp can act as a chemical chaperone by stabilizing newly synthesized P-gp for transport to the cell surface (Loo and Clarke, 1997), targeting P-gp maturation may provide a novel strategy to control MDR tumors.

Liposomal carriers have been demonstrated to provide tumor-specific delivery of antitumor agents as well as to circumvent many associated toxicities by altering the pharmacodistribution properties of encapsulated drugs (Krishna and Mayer, 1999). As described above, some modulators of P-gp alter anticancer drug pharmacokinetics and significantly reduce the elimination of many anticancer drugs from circulation, creating the need to reduce the dosages of the anticancer agents. These adverse interactions may be avoided by optimizing drug delivery using liposomal carriers. For example, Krishna and Mayer (1997) showed that, in BDF1 mice, liposomal doxorubicin exhibited comparable plasma elimination and tissue distribution properties in the presence and absence of MDR modulator PSC-833, whereas free doxorubicin displayed reduced plasma elimination rates and altered tissue distribution in the presence of PSC-833.

It may be possible to use gene therapy to augment hematopoietic cell function by expressing drug resistance genes, including the *MDR-1* gene, to reduce toxic side effects of cancer chemotherapy (Koc *et al.,* 1996; Sugimoto *et al.,* 1998). Although the *MDR-1* gene is expressed in various normal tissues, as above, it is not widely expressed in bone marrow cells. Lack of protection by the drug transporter may be one of the reasons for severe bone marrow cell suppression by many chemotherapeutic agents. Therefore, successful introduction of the *MDR-1* gene would allow the hematopoietic cells to survive escalated doses of chemotherapy. For this purpose, retrovirus-mediated gene transfer can be used because of the potential for stable vector integration and expression (Sugimoto *et al.,* 1998). Although clinical application of this therapy has been limited by low gene transfer into long-term repopulating cells (Hanania *et al.,* 1996; Hesdorffer *et al.,* 1998), a recent study reported a substantial advance in the use of retroviral vectors to transduce human hematopoietic progenitor cells (Abonour *et al.,* 2000). This therapeutic approach is interesting because it would be applicable to a wide range of currently resistant solid tumors.

B. Other Drug Transporters

Resistance to multiple drugs associated with reduced drug accumulation in human tumor cells can be conferred by the 190-kDa multidrug resistance protein MRP1 (reviewed in Hipfner *et al.,* 1999). The *MRP1* cDNA was cloned from an MDR small cell lung cancer cell line, H69AR (Cole *et al.,* 1992). Transfection of the *MRP1* cDNA confers MDR (Zaman *et al.,* 1994; Grant *et al.,* 1994; Kruh *et al.,* 1994; Zaman *et al.,* 1995). The MRP1-transfected cells, like P-gp-transfected cells, have become resistant to vincristine, doxorubicin, daunorubicin, and etoposide with reduced drug accumulation. Unlike P-gp-transfected cells, the *MRP1*-transfected cells showed no or marginal resistance to colchicine and paclitaxel. Besides the antitumor drugs, *MRP1* transfection confers resistance to certain antimonial and arsenical oxyanions. Thus, the drug resistance pattern by P-gp and MRP1 are similar but not identical. MRP1 can actually function as an ATP-dependent drug transporter (Hipfner *et al.,* 1999). Using inside-out membrane vesicles from cells overexpressing MRP1, an ATP-dependent transport was shown for vincristine and daunorubicin in the presence of reduced glutathione. In contrast, an anionic drug, methotrexate, can be transported in its native form. The *MRP1* gene has been expressed in various tumor types, and MRP1 expression has been associated with drug resistance in or prognosis of breast cancer, neuroblastomas, retinoblastomas, and lung cancers (Hipfner *et al.*, 1999).

In addition to *MRP1*, five human *MRP* subfamily members have been identified, including MRP2 (cMOAT), MRP3 (MOAT-D), MRP4 (MOAT-B), MRP5 (MOAT-C), and MRP6 (MOAT-E) (reviewed in Konig *et al.*, 1999). The genes encoding *MRP1-6* are on different chromosomes, and the mRNAs are expressed in a variety of normal tissues. MRP1 and other subfamily members can transport organic anions or conjugates of lipophilic substances with glutathione, glucuronate, or sulfate. Among them, MRP2, MRP3, and MRP5 have the capacity to confer resistance to chemotherapeutic agents. Transfection studies with *MRP2* cDNA have shown that it can confer resistance to a variety of chemotherapeutic agents, including vinblastine, vincristine, methotrexate, camptothecin derivatives, etoposide, doxorubicin, and cisplatin (Sugiyama *et al.*, 1998; Cui *et al.*, 1999; Hooijberg *et al.*, 1999). Conversely, stable transfectants of antisense *MRP2* cDNA in hepatic cancer cell lines exhibited an increased sensitivity to cisplatin, vincristine, and camptothecins (Koike *et al.*, 1997). Recently, mRNA expression of *MRP2* was shown to be associated with resistance to cisplatin in colorectal cancer (Hinoshita *et al.*, 2000). Transfection of *MRP3* cDNA also conferred drug resistance against etoposide and methotrexate (Kool *et al.*, 1999), and *MRP5* cDNA transfection conferred resistance against the thiopurine anticancer drugs 6-mercaptopurine and thioguanine (Wijnholds *et al.*, 2000). Thus, MRPs appear to confer distinct (but overlapping) drug resistance patterns.

MXR1, also known as BCRP or ABCP, is a recently discovered ABC half-transporter (Doyle *et al.*, 1998; Miyake *et al.*, 1999; Allikmets *et al.*, 1998), and overexpression of MXR1/BCRP/ABCP is often found in cell lines resistant to mitoxantrone or topotecan (Ross *et al.*, 1999; Maliepaard *et al.*, 1999; Scheffer *et al.*, 2000). In the resistant cell lines, decreased drug accumulation has been observed with enhanced, energy-dependent efflux of the drugs. The resistance pattern was different from that generally observed in the cases of P-gp or MRP1 overexpression. Transfection of *MXR1/BCRP/ABCP* cDNA into drug-sensitive MCF-7 cells conferred resistance to mitoxantrone, doxorubicin, daunorubicin, and topotecan but not to paclitaxel, vincristine, and cisplatin (Doyle *et al.*, 1998; Rabindran *et al.*, 2000). In addition, lower intracellular accumulation and retention of daunorubicin and an ATP-dependent enhancement of the efflux of rhodamine 123 were observed in the transfected cells (Doyle *et al.*, 1998). Recently, a wide range of MXR1/BCRP/ABCP mRNA expression was found among blast cell samples obtained from AML patients (Ross *et al.*, 2000). Thus, MXR1/BCRP/ABCP, similar to P-gp and MRPs, seems to play a role in the development of clinical drug resistance.

Similar approaches against P-gp-mediated MDR, as described above, could aid in overcoming drug resistance mediated by other ABC transporters. Pharmacologic inhibition of the ABC transporters may be a realistic approach to resensitizing cells to the action of antitumor agents. In fact, a number of compounds have been reported as inhibitors of MRPs and MXR1/BCRP/ABCP (Konig *et al.*, 1999; Rabindran *et al.*, 2000). Such agents would also be valuable tools in understanding the interaction of small molecules with ABC transporters. Interestingly, some P-gp inhibitors currently in development have the potency to inhibit other drug transporters and to increase drug sensitivity in non-P-gp MDR cells. For example, MS-209 can increase drug sensitivity of MRP1-overexpressing tumor cells (Nakamura *et al.*, 1999), and GF120918 can reverse increased efflux of mitoxantrone in MXR1/BCRP/ABCP-overexpressing cells (Allen *et al.*, 1999). These compounds may be attractive as a dual inhibitor of P-gp and MRP1 or MXR1/BCRP/ABCP because coexpression of drug transporters in the same cells can occur (Brock *et al.*, 1995). Although the *in vitro* studies with MDR cancer cells have revealed the involvement of multiple ABC transporters as well as LRP (Izquierdo *et al.*, 1996; Kitazono *et al.*, 1999) and have led to the discovery of several inhibitors, the clinical relevance of each transporter has not been determined fully. Future studies will be necessary to clarify which ABC transporters are important to or responsible for clinical resistance, ultimately, in each patient.

3. Targeting Cellular Stress Responses

The mechanisms of drug resistance have been intensively studied in established drug-resistant cell lines. In addition to relatively stable resistance, transient or inducible drug resistance can be associated with clinical drug resistance. Recent studies have revealed drug resistance that was induced transiently by the exposure of cancer cells to antitumor agents. Tumor cells can also exhibit drug resistance in microenvironmental conditions, such as hypoxia and glucose starvation. Such inducible drug resistance may also provide important targets for improving cancer chemotherapy.

A. NF-κB Pathway

The transcriptional factor NF-κB/Rel family regulates expression of genes involved in diverse biological processes, such as inflammation and immune responses, cell growth, and apoptosis (Ghosh *et al.*, 1998; Mercurio and Manning, 1999). This family is composed of several structurally related proteins, including p50, p52, RelA (p65), RelB, and c-Rel. They can form homo- and heterodimers that bind to DNA regulatory sites and generally activate specific target gene expression. In mammals, the most common NF-κB/Rel dimer contains p50-RelA (p65) and is specifically called NF-κB. NF-κB is normally retained in the cytoplasm in an inactive form through association with members of the IκB family proteins, most notably IκBα. Dissociation from IκBα is essential for NF-κB to enter the nucleus and to activate gene expression. Several signaling cascades for NF-κB activation converge at an IκB kinase (IKK) complex, responsible for phosphorylation of IκBα at serines 32 and 36 (Karin, 1999; Israel, 2000). Once phosphorylated, IκBα is ubiquitinated and degraded through the ubiquitin-proteasome proteolytic mechanism (Karin and Delhase, 2000). The sequential events can be induced by multiple extracellular stimuli, typically by tumor necrosis factor α (TNF-α). NF-κB activation can also be achieved through distinct regulatory pathways, such as calpain-dependent degradation of IκBα and tyrosine-phosphorylation-induced dissociation of IκBα from NF-κB, depending on the stimuli (Mercurio and Manning, 1999).

Several studies have shown that NF-κB is activated by treatments of cancer cells with antitumor agents, including ionizing radiation, topoisomerase (topo) I and II inhibitors, antimetabolites, taxanes, and *Vinca* alkaloids (reviewed in Pahl, 1999). Although the mechanisms of drug-induced NF-κB activation are not well understood, a recent study showed that the topo I inhibitors camptothecin and topotecan induce NF-κB activation by a mechanism that is dependent on the drug-induced DNA damage followed by the IKK-dependent cytoplasmic signaling events (Huang *et al.*, 2000). Thus, antitumor agents can activate NF-κB through phosphorylation and subsequent degradation of IκBα in the cytoplasm. In supporting this notion, mutant forms of IκBα, called super-repressors, which are resistant to the signal-induced phosphorylation and degradation (typically by mutations at serines 32 and 36), inhibit NF-κB activation induced by various chemotherapeutic agents (Wang *et al.*, 1999; Cusack *et al.*, 2000; Huang *et al.*, 2000).

It is important to note that inhibition of NF-κB, using the IκBα superrepressor, has been shown to sensitize tumor cells to apoptosis induced by ionizing radiation, TNF-α, and chemotherapeutic agents, including daunorubicin and camptothecins (Wang *et al.*, 1996,1999; Cusack *et al.*, 2000; Huang *et al.*, 2000). Notably, adenovirus-mediated transfer of the superrepressor IκBα enhanced the antitumor activity of CPT-11 against human fibrosarcoma HT1080 and colorectal cancer LoVo xenografts (Wang *et al.*, 1999; Cusack *et al.*, 2000). Furthermore, CPT-11 actually induced NF-κB activation in the LoVo tumors, and the adenoviral delivery of IκBα into the tumors inhibited the drug-induced NF-κB activation (Cusack *et al.*, 2000). These studies, together with identification of antiapoptotic *bcl-2* homologues and inhibitors of apoptosis (IAPs) as NF-κB target genes (Pahl, 1999), demonstrate that the activation of NF-κB may play a protective role against drug-induced apoptosis (Fig. 1). Thus, NF-κB activation in response to chemotherapy can be an important mechanism of inducible chemoresistance, and the NF-κB pathways may provide potential targets for improving chemotherapy's effectiveness (Waddick and Uckun, 1999; Mayo and Baldwin, 2000).

However, the NF-κB story is not as simple as it seems. There are controversial reports showing that NF-κB inhibition fails to sensitize cancer cells to apoptosis induced by

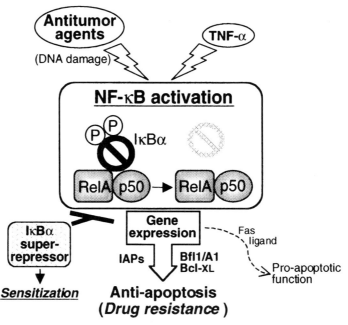

FIGURE 1   Schematic representation of inducible resistance mediated by NF-κB activation.

TNF-α or cytotoxic drugs (Cai *et al.,* 1997; Bentires-Alj *et al.,* 1999; Cusack *et al.,* 1999). In addition, NF-κB can exert not only antiapoptotic but also proapoptotic effects in different cell types (Barkett and Gilmore, 1999). For example, the physiologic apoptosis inducer Fas ligand has recently been shown to contain NF-κB consensus sequences in its promoter region (Kasibhatla *et al.,* 1999) and to be up-regulated in response to DNA damage (Mo and Beck, 1999). More recently, it was shown that the tumor suppressor p53 can induce activation of NF-κB and that inhibition or loss of NF-κB activity specifically abrogates the p53-mediated apoptotic response, without impinging on the ability to activate expression of target genes, such as p21$^{WAF1/CIP1}$, or to induce cell cycle arrest (Ryan *et al.,* 2000). The same study also showed that p53 uses a different signaling pathway to activate NF-κB than TNF-α does (Ryan *et al.,* 2000). These controversial observations might be due to complex features of NF-κB both in its regulation and in its function. In fact, to date, it has been described that NF-κB is activated by more than 150 different stimuli and that, in turn, active NF-κB participates in the control of transcription of more than 150 target genes (Pahl, 1999). Further understanding of mechanisms of NF-κB pathways, as well as development of specific inhibitors for the pathways (Epinat and Gilmore, 1999), may help to improve current chemotherapy by identifying targets to circumvent the NF-κB-mediated inducible drug resistance.

B. Microenvironment-Induced Drug Resistance Pathways

1. Unique Physiology of Solid Tumors

Solid tumors generally have regions of low oxygen (hypoxia) (reviewed in Brown and Giaccia, 1998; Rofstad, 2000). Tissue oxygen electrode measurements taken in cancer patients showed a median range of oxygen partial pressure of 10–30 mm Hg in tumors, with a significant proportion of readings below 2.5 mm Hg. Readings in normal tissues ranged from 24 to 66 mm Hg. Tumor hypoxia occurs in well-differentiated, slowly growing, nonmetastatic tumors, as well as in rapidly growing, anaplastic, aggressive malignancies. Hypoxic areas of solid tumors typically have low pH and low levels of glucose and other nutrients. The microenvironment is primarily based on inadequate vascularization in solid tumors.

The microenvironment itself has been thought to be a major mechanism of drug resistance because it reduces drug accessibility to tumor cells and reduces the oxygen radicals generated by antitumor drugs (Brown and Giaccia, 1998). The drug resistance can also be associated with decrease in the fraction of proliferating cells or the rate of cell proliferation as a function of distance from the blood vessels. Such situations can be reproduced *in vitro* by growing cells as multicelluar spheroids (Sutherland, 1988; Hamilton, 1998). In-

terestingly, it has been shown that resistance to alkylating agents can be acquired in a multicellular, spheroid-dependent manner (St. Croix *et al.,* 1998; Green *et al.,* 1999). In the tumor microenvironment, cell–cell contact may provide another mechanism of drug resistance, as suggested by the fact that confluent cancer cells in culture are more resistant to anticancer drugs than nonconfluent cells (Garrido *et al.,* 1997). Adhesion of cancer cells to extracellular matrix can also confer drug resistance through protection of cells from drug-induced apoptosis (Sethi *et al.,* 1999). In addition, the microenvironmental stress conditions, such as hypoxia and glucose deprivation, may produce selective pressure on tumor cells that have decreased apoptotic potential through genetic alterations (Shim *et al.,* 1998; Graeber *et al.,* 1996), thereby leading to apoptosis resistance induced by antitumor drugs that have different mechanisms of action. What is also important is that the stress conditions also induce drug resistance without such genetic alterations in tumor cells (Tomida and Tsuruo, 1999).

As illustrated in Fig. 2, there are several approaches to circumvent the microenvironment-associated drug resistance (Brown and Giaccia, 1998), such as (1) hypoxia-selective cytotoxins, which are activated by hypoxia; (2) liposomal drug delivery, which exploits leakiness of tumor vessels; (3) antiangiogenetic agents, which target the dependency of tumor growth on new blood vessel formation; and (4) gene therapy, activated either by hypoxia or by necrotic regions of tumors. These approaches are interesting, and some of them, such as the hypoxia-selective cytotoxin tirapazamine (Brown and Giaccia, 1998) and antiangiogenetic agents (Boehm *et al.,* 1997; Kerbel, 2000), show great promise. In addition, it can be useful to modulate the drug sensitivity of cancer cells under stress conditions. In the following two sections, we discuss the mechanisms of stress-mediated resistance and the potential targets for its reversal.

2. Stress-Inducible Drug Resistance

Cellular responses to microenvironmental stresses, such as hypoxia and glucose deprivation, can induce cellular drug resistance. The pathophysiologic stress conditions, in culture, commonly cause the glucose-regulated response of cancer cells, which is characterized by induction of endoplasmic reticulum (ER)–resident stress proteins, GRP78 and GRP94 (Lee, 1992). This stress response in cancer cells is also induced by various chemical stressors, such as calcium ionophore A23187, 2-deoxyglucose, and glucosamine, which disturb the ER functions (Lee, 1992). The stress response can be mediated, at least in part, by the unfolded protein response or ER stress response pathway that is induced following the accumulation of unfolded proteins in the ER (Kaufman, 1999). Activation of this pathway results in up-regulation of genes that encode ER-resident enzymes involved in protein folding. In fact, GRP78 and GRP94 are molecular chaper-

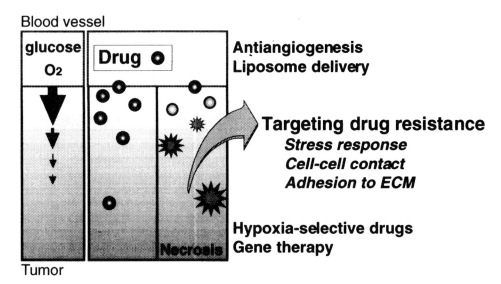

FIGURE 2 Strategies to circumvent microenvironment-associated drug resistance.

ones that play an important role in protein folding in the ER (Gething and Sambrook, 1992). It is important to recall that the induction of GRPs is observed during murine tumor growth (Shen *et al.*, 1987; Cai *et al.*, 1993).

A possible link between glucose-regulated stress response and drug resistance was first reported by Shen *et al.* (1987). They showed that GRP-inducing conditions, such as glucose deprivation and hypoxia, caused significant resistance induction to doxorubicin in Chinese hamster ovary (CHO) cells. Removal of GRP-inducing conditions resulted in the rapid disappearance of this resistance in a manner that correlated with the repression of the GRPs. Subsequently, the stressed CHO cells were shown to become resistant to etoposide as well as to doxorubicin (Hughes *et al.*, 1989), both of which are antitumor topo II poisons. After these reports, the deficiency of poly(ADP-ribose) synthesis was also reported to induce the expression of GRP78 and the development of etoposide resistance in Chinese hamster V79 cells (Chatterjee *et al.*, 1995). Furthermore, we showed that etoposide resistance was induced in human cancer cell lines under stress conditions (Yun *et al.*, 1995). Thus, a glucose-regulated stress response is associated with development of cellular resistance to topo II poisons. Topo II poisons stabilize the cleavable complex, an intermediate product of the topo-IIα-catalyzed reaction (Rubin *et al.*, 1996). Accumulation of the cleavable complexes is thought to lead to eventual cell death, and a decrease in the number of cleavable complexes could confer drug resistance. In agreement with this, a decreased expression of topo IIα occurs under glucose-regulated stress conditions and correlates well with induction of drug resistance (Shen *et al.*, 1987; Yun *et al.*, 1995).

The GRP-inducing state of cells is closely associated with growth arrest in the G_1 phase of the cell cycle. For example, G_1 arrest and GRP induction are concomitantly induced at a nonpermissive temperature in a temperature-sensitive, cell-cycle-mutant cell line, K12 (Melero, 1981). Hypoxia also causes G_1 cell cycle arrest in various cancer cell lines (Schmaltz *et al.*, 1998). Furthermore, we have reported that chemical stressors commonly induce cell cycle arrest at the G_1 phase in human cancer cell lines (Tomida *et al.*, 1996). This growth arrest may provide another explanation of drug resistance. Supporting this was the findings that the stressed cells also became resistant to camptothecin, vincristine, and methotrexate (Tomida *et al.*, 1996; Ogiso *et al.*, 2000), which are less active against G_1 phase cells.

3. Potential Targets for Reversal of Stress-Mediated Resistance

Because high-level expression of topo IIα is essential for cell death induced by topo-II-directed drugs, restoration of the decreased topo IIα expression would be important for reversing the stress-induced resistance. Recently, we found that proteasome inhibition attenuated the inducible resistance by inhibiting the topo IIα depletion induced by glucose starvation and hypoxia as well as by the chemical stressor A23187 (Ogiso *et al.*, 2000; Kim *et al.*, 1999). The topo IIα restoration was seen only at the protein levels, indicating that topo IIα protein depletion occurred through a proteasome-mediated degradation mechanism. Furthermore, we found that the stress conditions stimulated nuclear accumulation of proteasome in HT-29 human colon cancer cells (Kim *et al.*, 1999; Ogiso *et al.*, 1999). The nuclear proteasome levels both in amount and in activity were increased approximately 4 and 2 times by glucose starvation and hypoxia, respectively. The stress-induced nuclear proteasome accumulation was also observed in A2780 ovarian cancer cells, suggesting that this response occurred regardless of the cell's origin. No changes were detected in the total expression levels of proteasome. These findings indicate that the expression of topo IIα in stressed cells is down-regulated by proteasome-mediated degradation and suggest that the proteolysis of topo IIα can be facilitated by the nuclear accumulation of proteasome (Fig. 3).

In agreement with the topo IIα restoration, the stress-induced etoposide resistance was effectively prevented *in vitro* by the proteasome inhibitor lactacystin (Ogiso *et al.*, 2000). Furthermore, lactacystin significantly enhanced the antitumor activity of etoposide in the refractory HT-29 xenograft. Thus, lactacystin can serve as a new therapeutic agent to circumvent inducible resistance to topo-II-targeted chemotherapy. In this context, a recently developed proteasome inhibitor, PS-341, which is now in phase I clinical trials, may also be interesting (Adams *et al.*, 2000). However, proteasome is ubiquitously expressed in normal tissues and plays essential roles in various cellular functions, such as proliferation, differentiation, and antigen presentation (Baumeister *et al.*, 1998; Tanaka and Chiba, 1998). Therefore, total inhibition of proteasome might have adverse effects, although the combination of etoposide and lactacystin did not enhance the apparent toxicity in mice. Further studies on the mechanisms of topo IIα degradation and nuclear proteasome accumulation would provide tumor-selective strategies to circumvent the inducible resistance to topo-II-directed drugs.

The stress proteins GRP78 and GRP94, as well as proteins involved in the signaling pathway of the ER stress response, are important for cell survival under stress conditions (Kaufman, 1999). Thus, these proteins would be targets for improving current chemotherapy of solid tumors, although it has not formally been shown whether these proteins are involved in inducible drug resistance under stress conditions. For example, suppression of GRP induction by antisense cDNA has been shown to cause decreased cell survival under stress conditions (Koong *et al.*, 1994; Little and Lee, 1995) and to inhibit tumor formation of murine fibrosarcoma cells injected in mice (Jamora *et al.*, 1996). More recently, GRP94 was shown to undergo calpain-dependent proteolytic cleavage during etoposide-induced apoptosis, and reduction of GRP94 by antisense decreased cell viability in etoposide-treated Jurkat cells (Reddy *et al.*, 1999). We have also shown that GRP78 can be involved in cell cycle arrest at the G_1 phase by forming a stable complex with epidermal growth factor receptor (EGFr) and inhibiting EGFr translocation to the cell surface (Cai *et al.*, 1998). Understanding the mechanisms of ER stress response, therefore, may lead to defining a mechanism of the stress-inducible drug resistance pathway.

4. Targeting DNA Repair Systems

Many anticancer drugs, such as platinum drugs and chloroethylnitrosoureas, cause cell killing by inducing DNA

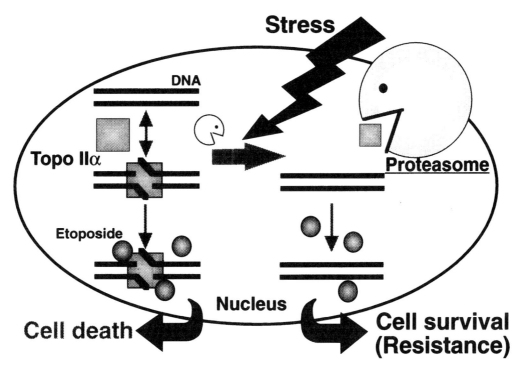

FIGURE 3 Possible mechanisms of stress-induced topoisomerase-II-directed drugs.

damage. Hence, DNA repair can be an important effector of drug sensitivity of tumor cells (Chaney and Sancar, 1996). DNA repair is a somewhat complex process, and more than 50 eukaryotic genes were cloned that are involved in the recognition and elimination of specific DNA lesions thereby leading to restoration of the intact DNA structure (Sancar, 1995). The repair mechanisms can generally be classified as (1) direct repair, (2) base excision repair, (3) nucleotide excision repair, or (4) mismatch repair (Reed, 1998; Buermeyer *et al.,* 1999; Frosina, 2000; Pegg, 2000). These pathways can be involved in resistance to DNA-damaging agents although the importance of base excision repair remains relatively unclear (Chaney and Sancar, 1996). For example, enhanced nucleotide excision repair for bifunctional DNA adducts and enhanced direct repair mediated by O^6-alkylguanine DNA alkyltransferase lead to resistance to platinum drugs and chloroethylnitrosoureas, respectively (Reed, 1998; Pegg, 2000). Tumors with enhanced nucleotide excision repair show an intrinsic resistance to chemotherapy as well as to radiotherapy (Zeng-Rong *et al.,* 1995). In contrast, defects in mismatch repair, which contribute to the development of cancer, confer resistance to DNA-alkylating agents, platinum drugs, doxorubicin, 6-thioguanine, and 5-fluorouracil as well as ionizing radiation (Sedwick *et al.,* 1999). Drug resistance can be associated with the roles of mismatch repair proteins in signaling apoptosis and cell cycle checkpoint or with toxicity arising from futile repair cycling (Jiricny, 1998; Duckett *et al.,* 1999; Li, 1999).

Different steps of DNA repair can be inhibited by several noncytotoxic substances, and this modulation can restore sensitivity to DNA-damaging agents in resistant cancer cells (Heim *et al.,* 2000). For example, O^6-benzylguanine, an inhibitor of O^6-alkylguanine DNA alkyltransferase, has been shown to enhance the antitumor activity of chloroethylnitrosoureas *in vitro* and *in vivo* (Chaney and Sancar, 1996; Pegg, 2000). Phase I clinical trials of O^6-benzylguanine showed that adequate inactivation of O^6-alkylguanine DNA alkyltransferase can be achieved in tumors including malignant gliomas (Friedman *et al.,* 1998; Dolan *et al.,* 1998; Spiro *et al.,* 1999). Although not specific for repair, DNA polymerase inhibitors, such as aphidicolin and cytosine arabinoside, may suppress the nucleotide excision repair by inhibiting the DNA resynthesis step (Chaney and Sancar, 1996). Since DNA repair also protects normal tissue, the selective delivery of such repair inhibitors to the tumor would be necessary. In this context, mismatch repair pathways can be exploited for development of tumor-selective therapeutic modalities (Sedwick *et al.,* 1999). For example, a recent study revealed that aphidicolin in combination with cisplatin is more toxic to mismatch repair-deficient cells than to repair-competent cells (Moreland *et al.,* 1999). More recently, mismatch repair-deficient cells were shown to be more sensitive to both cytotoxicity and mutagenicity of a frameshift-inducing agent, ISR-191, than were repair-competent cells (Chen *et al.,* 2000). Thus, better understanding of the mismatch repair deficiency may provide an opportunity for selective killing of mismatch-repair-defective tumors that are resistant to current chemotherapy.

5. Conclusions

In this chapter, we reviewed drug resistance mechanisms as potential targets for improving current chemotherapy. Cancer cells become resistant to chemotherapeutic agents through various mechanisms, including drug efflux mediated by a wide range of drug transporters, activation of the NF-κB pathway and of the stress response pathway induced by the tumor microenvironment, and altered DNA repair capacity. Other mechanisms, such as alteration in drug metabolism, may also contribute to drug resistance. It is likely that redundant mechanisms of broad drug resistance are present in individual tumors, even in the same cell. The molecular-based understanding of resistance mechanisms has important implications for choice of drugs in cancer treatment and provides opportunities for future therapeutic strategies directed to resistant tumors. Modulation of drug resistance genes or proteins is a promising approach, although we must be very concerned about the physiologic functions in normal tissue. The development of new drugs, which are not substrates of drug transporters, for example, is another way to circumvent drug resistance. Thus, elucidating drug resistance mechanisms can provide useful information for effective cancer chemotherapy.

References

Abolhoda, A., Wilson, A. E., Ross, H., Danenberg, P. V., Burt, M., and Scotto, K. W. (1999). Rapid activation of MDR1 gene expression in human metastatic sarcoma after in vivo exposure to doxorubicin. *Clin. Cancer Res.* **5,** 3352–3356.

Abonour, R., Williams, D. A., Einhorn, L., Hall, K. M., Chen, J., Coffman, J., Traycoff, C. M., Bank, A., Kato, I., Ward, M., Williams, S. D., Hromas, R., Robertson, M. J., Smith, F. O., Woo, D., Mills, B., Srour, E. F., and Cornetta, K. (2000). Efficient retrovirus-mediated transfer of the multidrug resistance 1 gene into autologous human long-term repopulating hematopoietic stem cells. *Nat. Med.* **6,** 652–658.

Adams, J., Palombella, V. J., and Elliott, P. J. (2000). Proteasome inhibition: a new strategy in cancer treatment. *Invest. New Drugs* **18,** 109–121.

Advani, R., Visani, G., Milligan, D., Saba, H., Tallman, M., Rowe, J. M., Wiernik, P. H., Ramek, J., Dugan, K., Lum, B., Villena, J., Davis, E., Paietta, E., Litchman, M., Covelli, A., Sikic, B., and Greenberg, P. (1999). Treatment of poor prognosis AML patients using PSC833 (valspodar) plus mitoxantrone, etoposide, and cytarabine (PSC-MEC). *Adv. Exp. Med. Biol.* **457,** 47–56.

Allen, J. D., Brinkhuis, R. F., Wijnholds, J., and Schinkel, A. H. (1999). The mouse Bcrp1/Mxr/Abcp gene: amplification and overexpression in cell lines selected for resistance to topotecan, mitoxantrone, or doxorubicin. *Cancer Res.* **59,** 4237–4241.

Allikmets, R., Schriml, L. M., Hutchinson, A., Romano-Spica, V., and Dean, M. (1998). A human placenta-specific ATP-binding cassette gene (ABCP) on chromosome 4q22 that is involved in multidrug resistance. *Cancer Res.* **58**, 5337–5339.

Ambudkar, S. V., Dey, S., Hrycyna, C. A., Ramachandra, M., Pastan, I., and Gottesman, M. M. (1999). Biochemical, cellular, and pharmacological aspects of the multidrug transporter. *Annu. Rev. Pharmacol. Toxicol.* **39**, 361–398.

Arceci, R. J., Stieglitz, K., Bras, J., Schinkel, A., Baas, F., and Croop, J. (1993). Monoclonal antibody to an external epitope of the human mdr1 P-glycoprotein. *Cancer Res.* **53**, 310–317.

Atadja, P., Watanabe, T., Xu, H., and Cohen, D. (1998). PSC-833, a frontier in modulation of P-glycoprotein mediated multidrug resistance. *Cancer Metastasis Rev.* **17**, 163–168.

Bargou, R. C., Jurchott, K., Wagener, C., Bergmann, S., Metzner, S., Bommert, K., Mapara, M. Y., Winzer, K. J., Dietel, M., Dorken, B., and Royer, H. D. (1997). Nuclear localization and increased levels of transcription factor YB-1 in primary human breast cancers are associated with intrinsic MDR1 gene expression. *Nat. Med.* **3**, 447–450.

Barkett, M., and Gilmore, T. D. (1999). Control of apoptosis by Rel/NF-κB transcription factors. *Oncogene* **18**, 6910–6924.

Baumeister, W., Walz, J., Zuhl, F., and Seemuller, E. (1998). The proteasome: paradigm of a self-compartmentalizing protease. *Cell* **92**, 367–380.

Beketic-Oreskovic, L., Duran, G. E., Chen, G., Dumontet, C., and Sikic, B. I. (1995). Decreased mutation rate for cellular resistance to doxorubicin and suppression of mdr1 gene activation by the cyclosporin PSC 833. *J. Natl. Cancer Inst.* **87**, 1593–1602.

Bentires-Alj, M., Hellin, A. C., Ameyar, M., Chouaib, S., Merville, M. P., and Bours, V. (1999). Stable inhibition of nuclear factor κB in cancer cells does not increase sensitivity to cytotoxic drugs. *Cancer Res.* **59**, 811–815.

Bentires-Alj, M., Merville, M.-P., and Bours, V. (1999). NF-κB and chemoresistance: could NF-κB be an antitumor target? *Drug Resistance Updates* **2**, 274–276.

Boehm, T., Folkman, J., Browder, T., and O'Reilly, M. S. (1997). Antiangiogenic therapy of experimental cancer does not induce acquired drug resistance. *Nature* **390**, 404–407.

Brock, I., Hipfner, D. R., Nielsen, B. S., Jensen, P. B., Deeley, R. G., Cole, S. P., and Sehested, M. (1995). Sequential coexpression of the multidrug resistance genes MRP and mdr1 and their products in VP-16 (etoposide)-selected H69 small cell lung cancer cells. *Cancer Res.* **55**, 459–462.

Brown, J. M., and Giaccia, A. J. (1998). The unique physiology of solid tumors: opportunities (and problems) for cancer therapy. *Cancer Res.* **58**, 1408–1416.

Buermeyer, A. B., Deschenes, S. M., Baker, S. M., and Liskay, R. M. (1999). Mammalian DNA mismatch repair. *Annu. Rev. Genet.* **33**, 533–564.

Byrne, D., Daly, C., NicAmhlaoibh, R., Howlett, A., Scanlon, K., and Clynes, M. (1998). Use of ribozymes and antisense oligodeoxynucleotides to investigate mechanisms of drug resistance. *Cytotechnology* **27**, 113–136.

Cai, B., Tomida, A., Mikami, K., Nagata, K., and Tsuruo, T. (1998). Downregulation of epidermal growth factor receptor-signaling pathway by binding of GRP78/BiP to the receptor under glucose-starved stress conditions. *J. Cell. Physiol.* **177**, 282–288.

Cai, J. W., Henderson, B. W., Shen, J. W., and Subjeck, J. R. (1993). Induction of glucose regulated proteins during growth of a murine tumor. *J. Cell. Physiol.* **154**, 229–237.

Cai, Z., Korner, M., Tarantino, N., and Chouaib, S. (1997). IκB alpha overexpression in human breast carcinoma MCF7 cells inhibits nuclear factor-κB activation but not tumor necrosis factor-alpha-induced apoptosis. *J. Biol. Chem.* **272**, 96–101.

Chaney, S. G., and Sancar, A. (1996). DNA repair: enzymatic mechanisms and relevance to drug response. *J. Natl. Cancer Inst.* **88**, 1346–1360.

Chatterjee, S., Cheng, M. F., Berger, R. B., Berger, S. J., and Berger, N. A. (1995). Effect of inhibitors of poly(ADP-ribose) polymerase on the in-

duction of GRP78 and subsequent development of resistance to etoposide. *Cancer Res.* **55**, 868–873.

Chen, W. D., Eshleman, J. R., Aminoshariae, M. R., Ma, A. H., Veloso, N., Markowitz, S. D., Sedwick, W. D., and Veigl, M. L. (2000). Cytotoxicity and mutagenicity of frameshift-inducing agent ICR191 in mismatch repair-deficient colon cancer cells. *J. Natl. Cancer Inst.* **92**, 480–485.

Cole, S. P., Bhardwaj, G., Gerlach, J. H., Mackie, J. E., Grant, C. E., Almquist, K. C., Stewart, A. J., Kurz, E. U., Duncan, A. M., and Deeley, R. G. (1992). Overexpression of a transporter gene in a multidrug-resistant human lung cancer cell line. *Science* **258**, 1650–1654.

Cucco, C., and Calabretta, B. (1996). In vitro and in vivo reversal of multidrug resistance in a human leukemia-resistant cell line by mdr1 antisense oligodeoxynucleotides. *Cancer Res.* **56**, 4332–4337.

Cui, Y., Konig, J., Buchholz, J. K., Spring, H., Leier, I., and Keppler, D. (1999). Drug resistance and ATP-dependent conjugate transport mediated by the apical multidrug resistance protein, MRP2, permanently expressed in human and canine cells. *Mol. Pharmacol.* **55**, 929–937.

Cusack, J. C., Liu, R., and Baldwin, A. S. (1999). NF-κB and chemoresistance: potentiation of cancer chemotherapy via inhibition of NF-κB. *Drug Resistance Updates* **2**, 271–273.

Cusack, J. C., Jr., Liu, R., and Baldwin, A. S., Jr. (2000). Inducible chemoresistance to 7-ethyl-10-[4-(1-piperidino)-1-piperidino]-carbonyloxycamptothe cin (CPT-11) in colorectal cancer cells and a xenograft model is overcome by inhibition of nuclear factor-κB activation. *Cancer Res.* **60**, 2323–2330.

Dolan, M. E., Roy, S. K., Fasanmade, A. A., Paras, P. R., Schilsky, R. L., and Ratain, M. J. (1998). O⁶-benzylguanine in humans: metabolic, pharmacokinetic, and pharmacodynamic findings. *J. Clin. Oncol.* **16**, 1803–1810.

Doyle, L. A., Yang, W., Abruzzo, L. V., Krogmann, T., Gao, Y., Rishi, A. K., and Ross, D. D. (1998). A multidrug resistance transporter from human MCF-7 breast cancer cells. *Proc. Natl. Acad. Sci. USA* **95**, 15665–15670.

Duckett, D. R., Bronstein, S. M., Taya, Y., and Modrich, P. (1999). hMutSalpha- and hMutLalpha-dependent phosphorylation of p53 in response to DNA methylator damage. *Proc. Natl. Acad. Sci. USA* **96**, 12384–12388.

Epinat, J. C., and Gilmore, T. D. (1999). Diverse agents act at multiple levels to inhibit the Rel/NF-κB signal transduction pathway. *Oncogene* **18**, 6896–6909.

Ford, J. M., Yang, J. M., and Hait, W. N. (1996). P-glycoprotein-mediated multidrug resistance: experimental and clinical strategies for its reversal. *Cancer Treat. Res.* **87**, 3–38.

Fracasso, P. M., Westerveldt, P., Fears, C. A., Rosen, D. M., Zuhowski, E. G., Cazenave, L. A., Litchman, M., and Egorin, M. J. (2000). Phase I study of paclitaxel in combination with a multidrug resistance modulator, PSC 833 (Valspodar), in refractory malignancies. *J. Clin. Oncol.* **18**, 1124–1134.

Friedman, H. S., Kokkinakis, D. M., Pluda, J., Friedman, A. H., Cokgor, I., Haglund, M. M., Ashley, D. M., Rich, J., Dolan, M. E., Pegg, A. E., Moschel, R. C., McLendon, R. E., Kerby, T., Herndon, J. E., Bigner, D. D., and Schold, S. C., Jr. (1998). Phase I trial of O⁶-benzylguanine for patients undergoing surgery for malignant glioma. *J. Clin. Oncol.* **16**, 3570–3575.

Frosina, G. (2000). Overexpression of enzymes that repair endogenous damage to DNA. *Eur. J. Biochem.* **267**, 2135–2149.

Garrido, C., Ottavi, P., Fromentin, A., Hammann, A., Arrigo, A. P., Chauffert, B., and Mehlen, P. (1997). HSP27 as a mediator of confluence-dependent resistance to cell death induced by anticancer drugs. *Cancer Res.* **57**, 2661–2667.

Gething, M. J., and Sambrook, J. (1992). Protein folding in the cell. *Nature* **355**, 33–45.

Ghosh, S., May, M. J., and Kopp, E. B. (1998). NF-κB and Rel proteins: evolutionarily conserved mediators of immune responses. *Annu. Rev. Immunol.* **16**, 225–260.

Graeber, T. G., Osmanian, C., Jacks, T., Housman, D. E., Koch, C. J., Lowe, S. W., and Giaccia, A. J. (1996). Hypoxia-mediated selection of cells with diminished apoptotic potential in solid tumours. *Nature* **379,** 88–91.

Grant, C. E., Valdimarsson, G., Hipfner, D. R., Almquist, K. C., Cole, S. P., and Deeley, R. G. (1994). Overexpression of multidrug resistance-associated protein (MRP) increases resistance to natural product drugs. *Cancer Res.* **54,** 357–361.

Green, S. K., Frankel, A., and Kerbel, R. S. (1999). Adhesion-dependent multicellular drug resistance. *Anticancer Drug Des.* **14,** 153–168.

Gros, P., Ben Neriah, Y. B., Croop, J. M., and Housman, D. E. (1986). Isolation and expression of a complementary DNA that confers multidrug resistance. *Nature* **323,** 728–731.

Hamada, H., and Tsuruo, T. (1986). Functional role for the 170- to 180-kDa glycoprotein specific to drug-resistant tumor cells as revealed by monoclonal antibodies. *Proc. Natl. Acad. Sci. USA* **83,** 7785–7789.

Hamilton, G. (1998). Multicellular spheroids as an in vitro tumor model. *Cancer Lett.* **131,** 29–34.

Hanania, E. G., Giles, R. E., Kavanagh, J., Fu, S. Q., Ellerson, D., Zu, Z., Wang, T., Su, Y., Kudelka, A., Rahman, Z., Holmes, F., Hortobagyi, G., Claxton, D., Bachier, C., Thall, P., Cheng, S., Hester, J., Ostrove, J. M., Bird, R. E., Chang, A., Korbling, M., Seong, D., Cote, R., Holzmayer, T., Deisseroth, A. B., et al. (1996). Results of MDR-1 vector modification trial indicate that granulocyte/macrophage colony-forming unit cells do not contribute to posttransplant hematopoietic recovery following intensive systemic therapy. *Proc. Natl. Acad. Sci. USA* **93,** 15346–15351.

Harrison, D. J. (1995). Molecular mechanisms of drug resistance in tumours. *J. Pathol.* **175,** 7–12.

Heim, M. M., Eberhardt, W., Seeber, S., and Muller, M. R. (2000). Differential modulation of chemosensitivity to alkylating agents and platinum compounds by DNA repair modulators in human lung cancer cell lines. *J. Cancer Res. Clin. Oncol.* **126,** 198–204.

Hesdorffer, C., Ayello, J., Ward, M., Kaubisch, A., Vahdat, L., Balmaceda, C., Garrett, T., Fetell, M., Reiss, R., Bank, A., and Antman, K. (1998). Phase I trial of retroviral-mediated transfer of the human MDR1 gene as marrow chemoprotection in patients undergoing high-dose chemotherapy and autologous stem-cell transplantation. *J. Clin. Oncol.* **16,** 165–172.

Hinoshita, E., Uchiumi, T., Taguchi, K., Kinukawa, N., Tsuneyoshi, M., Maehara, Y., Sugimachi, K., and Kuwano, M. (2000). Increased expression of an ATP-binding cassette superfamily transporter, multidrug resistance protein 2, in human colorectal carcinomas. *Clin. Cancer Res.* **6,** 2401–2407.

Hipfner, D. R., Deeley, R. G., and Cole, S. P. (1999). Structural, mechanistic and clinical aspects of MRP1. *Biochim. Biophys. Acta* **1461,** 359–376.

Hooijberg, J. H., Broxterman, H. J., Kool, M., Assaraf, Y. G., Peters, G. J., Noordhuis, P., Scheper, R. J., Borst, P., Pinedo, H. M., and Jansen, G. (1999). Antifolate resistance mediated by the multidrug resistance proteins MRP1 and MRP2. *Cancer Res.* **59,** 2532–2535.

Huang, T. T., Wuerzberger-Davis, S. M., Seufzer, B. J., Shumway, S. D., Kurama, T., Boothman, D. A., and Miyamoto, S. (2000). NF-κB activation by camptothecin. A linkage between nuclear DNA damage and cytoplasmic signaling events. *J. Biol. Chem.* **275,** 9501–9509.

Hughes, C. S., Shen, J. W., and Subjeck, J. R. (1989). Resistance to etoposide induced by three glucose-regulated stresses in Chinese hamster ovary cells. *Cancer Res.* **49,** 4452–4454.

Hyafil, F., Vergely, C., Du Vignaud, P., and Grand-Perret, T. (1993). In vitro and in vivo reversal of multidrug resistance by GF120918, an acridonecarboxamide derivative. *Cancer Res.* **53,** 4595–4602.

Israel, A. (2000). The IKK complex: an integrator of all signals that activate NF-κB? *Trends Cell. Biol.* **10,** 129–133.

Izquierdo, M. A., Scheffer, G. L., Flens, M. J., Schroeijers, A. B., van der Valk, P., and Scheper, R. J. (1996). Major vault protein LRP-related multidrug resistance. *Eur. J. Cancer* **32A,** 979–984.

Jamora, C., Dennert, G., and Lee, A. S. (1996). Inhibition of tumor progression by suppression of stress protein GRP78/BiP induction in fibrosarcoma B/C10ME. *Proc. Natl. Acad. Sci. USA* **93,** 7690–7694.

Jiricny, J. (1998). Eukaryotic mismatch repair: an update. *Mutat. Res.* **409,** 107–121.

Johnstone, R. W., Ruefli, A. A., and Smyth, M. J. (2000). Multiple physiological functions for multidrug transporter P-glycoprotein? *Trends Biochem. Sci.* **25,** 1–6.

Kantharidis, P., El-Osta, S., de Silva, M., Lee, G., Hu, X. F., and Zalcberg, J. (2000). Regulation of MDR1 gene expression: emerging concepts. *Drug Resistance Updates* **3,** 99–108.

Karin, M. (1999). How NF-κB is activated: the role of the IκB kinase (IKK) complex. *Oncogene* **18,** 6867–6874.

Karin, M., and Delhase, M. (2000). The IκB kinase (IKK) and NF-κB: key elements of proinflammatory signalling. *Semin. Immunol.* **12,** 85–98.

Kasibhatla, S., Genestier, L., and Green, D. R. (1999). Regulation of fas-ligand expression during activation-induced cell death in T lymphocytes via nuclear factor κB. *J. Biol. Chem.* **274,** 987–992.

Kaufman, R. J. (1999). Stress signaling from the lumen of the endoplasmic reticulum: coordination of gene transcriptional and translational controls. *Genes Dev.* **13,** 1211–1233.

Kerbel, R. S. (2000). Tumor angiogenesis: past, present and the near future. *Carcinogenesis* **21,** 505–515.

Kim, H. D., Tomida, A., Ogiso, Y., and Tsuruo, T. (1999). Glucose-regulated stresses cause degradation of DNA topoisomerase II alpha by inducing nuclear proteasome during G_1 cell cycle arrest in cancer cells. *J. Cell. Physiol.* **180,** 97–104.

Kitazono, M., Sumizawa, T., Takebayashi, Y., Chen, Z. S., Furukawa, T., Nagayama, S., Tani, A., Takao, S., Aikou, T., and Akiyama, S. (1999). Multidrug resistance and the lung resistance-related protein in human colon carcinoma SW-620 cells. *J. Natl. Cancer Inst.* **91,** 1647–1653.

Koc, O. N., Allay, J. A., Lee, K., Davis, B. M., Reese, J. S., and Gerson, S. L. (1996). Transfer of drug resistance genes into hematopoietic progenitors to improve chemotherapy tolerance. *Semin. Oncol.* **23,** 46–65.

Koike, K., Kawabe, T., Tanaka, T., Toh, S., Uchiumi, T., Wada, M., Akiyama, S., Ono, M., and Kuwano, M. (1997). A canalicular multispecific organic anion transporter (cMOAT) antisense cDNA enhances drug sensitivity in human hepatic cancer cells. *Cancer Res.* **57,** 5475–5479.

Konig, J., Nies, A. T., Cui, Y., Leier, I., and Keppler, D. (1999). Conjugate export pumps of the multidrug resistance protein (MRP) family: localization, substrate specificity, and MRP2-mediated drug resistance. *Biochim. Biophys. Acta* **1461,** 377–394.

Kool, M., van der Linden, M., de Haas, M., Scheffer, G. L., de Vree, J. M., Smith, A. J., Jansen, G., Peters, G. J., Ponne, N., Scheper, R. J., Elferink, R. P., Baas, F., and Borst, P. (1999). MRP3, an organic anion transporter able to transport anti-cancer drugs. *Proc. Natl. Acad. Sci. USA* **96,** 6914–6919.

Koong, A. C., Chen, E. Y., Lee, A. S., Brown, J. M., and Giaccia, A. J. (1994). Increased cytotoxicity of chronic hypoxic cells by molecular inhibition of GRP78 induction. *Int. J. Radiat. Oncol. Biol. Phys.* **28,** 661–666.

Krishna, R., and Mayer, L. D. (1997). Liposomal doxorubicin circumvents PSC 833-free drug interactions, resulting in effective therapy of multidrug-resistant solid tumors. *Cancer Res.* **57,** 5246–5253.

Krishna, R., and Mayer, L. D. (1999). The use of liposomal anticancer agents to determine the roles of drug pharmacodistribution and P-glycoprotein (PGP) blockade in overcoming multidrug resistance (MDR). *Anticancer Res.* **19,** 2885–2891.

Kruh, G. D., Chan, A., Myers, K., Gaughan, K., Miki, T., and Aaronson, S. A. (1994). Expression complementary DNA library transfer establishes mrp as a multidrug resistance gene. *Cancer Res.* **54,** 1649–1652.

Lee, A. S. (1992). Mammalian stress response: induction of the glucose-regulated protein family. *Curr. Opin. Cell. Biol.* **4,** 267–273.

Lee, E. J., George, S. L., Caligiuri, M., Szatrowski, T. P., Powell, B. L., Lemke, S., Dodge, R. K., Smith, R., Baer, M., and Schiffer, C. A. (1999). Parallel phase I studies of daunorubicin given with cytarabine and etoposide with or without the multidrug resistance modulator PSC-833 in previously untreated patients 60 years of age or older with acute myeloid leukemia: results of cancer and leukemia group B study 9420. *J. Clin. Oncol.* **17,** 2831–2839.

Li, G. M. (1999). The role of mismatch repair in DNA damage-induced apoptosis. *Oncol. Res.* **11,** 393–400.

Ling, V. (1997). Multidrug resistance: molecular mechanisms and clinical relevance. *Cancer Chemother. Pharmacol.* **40 Suppl,** S3–S8.

Little, E., and Lee, A. S. (1995). Generation of a mamalian cell line deficient in glucose-regulated protein stress induction through targeted ribozyme driven by a stress-inducible promoter. *J. Biol. Chem.* **270,** 9526–9534.

Loo, T. W., and Clarke, D. M. (1997). Correction of defective protein kinesis of human P-glycoprotein mutants by substrates and modulators. *J. Biol. Chem.* **272,** 709–712.

Loo, T. W., and Clarke, D. M. (2000). Blockage of drug resistance in vitro by disulfiram, a drug used to treat alcoholism. *J. Natl. Cancer Inst.* **92,** 898–902.

Maliepaard, M., van Gastelen, M. A., de Jong, L. A., Pluim, D., van Waardenburg, R. C., Ruevekamp-Helmers, M. C., Floot, B. G., and Schellens, J. H. (1999). Overexpression of the BCRP/MXR/ABCP gene in a topotecan-selected ovarian tumor cell line. *Cancer Res.* **59,** 4559–4563.

Mayo, M. W., and Baldwin, A. S. (2000). The transcription factor NF-κB: control of oncogenesis and cancer therapy resistance. *Biochim. Biophys. Acta* **1470,** M55–M62.

Mechetner, E. B., and Roninson, I. B. (1992). Efficient inhibition of P-glycoprotein-mediated multidrug resistance with a monoclonal antibody. *Proc. Natl. Acad. Sci. USA* **89,** 5824–5828.

Melero, J. A. (1981). Identification of the glucose/glycosylation-regulated proteins as those which accumulate in the temperature-sensitive cell line K12. *J. Cell. Physiol.* **109,** 59–67.

Mercurio, F., and Manning, A. M. (1999). NF-κB as a primary regulator of the stress response. *Oncogene* **18,** 6163–6171.

Miyake, K., Mickley, L., Litman, T., Zhan, Z., Robey, R., Cristensen, B., Brangi, M., Greenberger, L., Dean, M., Fojo, T., and Bates, S. E. (1999). Molecular cloning of cDNAs which are highly overexpressed in mitoxantrone-resistant cells: demonstration of homology to ABC transport genes. *Cancer Res.* **59,** 8–13.

Mo, Y. Y., and Beck, W. T. (1999). DNA damage signals induction of fas ligand in tumor cells. *Mol. Pharmacol.* **55,** 216–222.

Moreland, N. J., Illand, M., Kim, Y. T., Paul, J., and Brown, R. (1999). Modulation of drug resistance mediated by loss of mismatch repair by the DNA polymerase inhibitor aphidicolin. *Cancer Res.* **59,** 2102–2106.

Naito, M., Tsuge, H., Kuroko, C., Koyama, T., Tomida, A., Tatsuta, T., Heike, Y., and Tsuruo, T. (1993). Enhancement of cellular accumulation of cyclosporine by anti-P-glycoprotein monoclonal antibody MRK-16 and synergistic modulation of multidrug resistance. *J. Natl. Cancer Inst.* **85,** 311–316.

Naito, M., Watanabe, T., Tsuge, H., Koyama, T., Oh-hara, T., and Tsuruo, T. (1996). Potentiation of the reversal activity of SDZ PSC833 on multidrug resistance by an anti-P-glycoprotein monoclonal antibody MRK-16. *Int. J. Cancer* **67,** 435–440.

Nakamura, T., Oka, M., Aizawa, K., Soda, H., Fukuda, M., Terashi, K., Ikeda, K., Mizuta, Y., Noguchi, Y., Kimura, Y., Tsuruo, T., and Kohno, S. (1999). Direct interaction between a quinoline derivative, MS-209, and multidrug resistance protein (MRP) in human gastric cancer cells. *Biochem. Biophys. Res. Commun.* **255,** 618–624.

Nakanishi, O., and Tsuruo, T. (1996). Multidrug resistance-reversing agents for potential clinical use. *In* "Multidrug Resistance in Cancer Cells: Molecular, Biochemical, Physiological, and Biological Aspects" (S. Gupta and T. Tsuruo, eds.), pp. 375–384. John Wiley & Sons Ltd., Chichester, England.

Newman, M. J., Rodarte, J. C., Benbatoul, K. D., Romano, S. J., Zhang, C., Krane, S., Moran, E. J., Uyeda, R. T., Dixon, R., Guns, E. S., and Mayer, L. D. (2000). Discovery and characterization of OC144-093, a novel inhibitor of P-glycoprotein-mediated multidrug resistance. *Cancer Res.* **60,** 2964–2972.

Oda, Y., Sakamoto, A., Shinohara, N., Ohga, T., Uchiumi, T., Kohno, K., Tsuneyoshi, M., Kuwano, M., and Iwamoto, Y. (1998). Nuclear expression of YB-1 protein correlates with P-glycoprotein expression in human osteosarcoma. *Clin. Cancer Res.* **4,** 2273–2277.

Ogiso, Y., Tomida, A., Kim, H. D., and Tsuruo, T. (1999). Glucose starvation and hypoxia induce nuclear accumulation of proteasome in cancer cells. *Biochem. Biophys. Res. Commun.* **258,** 448–452.

Ogiso, Y., Tomida, A., Lei, S., Omura, S., and Tsuruo, T. (2000). Proteasome inhibition circumvents solid tumor resistance to topoisomerase II-directed drugs. *Cancer Res.* **60,** 2429–2434.

Okochi, E., Iwahashi, T., and Tsuruo, T. (1997). Monoclonal antibodies specific for P-glycoprotein. *Leukemia* **11,** 1119–1123.

Pahl, H. L. (1999). Activators and target genes of Rel/NF-κB transcription factors. *Oncogene* **18,** 6853–6866.

Pearson, J. W., Fogler, W. E., Volker, K., Usui, N., Goldenberg, S. K., Gruys, E., Riggs, C. W., Komschlies, K., Wiltrout, R. H., Tsuruo, T., et al. (1991). Reversal of drug resistance in a human colon cancer xenograft expressing MDR1 complementary DNA by in vivo administration of MRK-16 monoclonal antibody. *J. Natl. Cancer Inst.* **83,** 1386–1391.

Pegg, A. E. (2000). Repair of O(6)-alkylguanine by alkyltransferases. *Mutat. Res.* **462,** 83–100.

Rabindran, S. K., Ross, D. D., Doyle, L. A., Yang, W., and Greenberger, L. M. (2000). Fumitremorgin C reverses multidrug resistance in cells transfected with the breast cancer resistance protein. *Cancer Res.* **60,** 47–50.

Ramachandran, C., and Melnick, S. J. (1999). Multidrug resistance in human tumors—molecular diagnosis and clinical significance. *Mol. Diagn.* **4,** 81–94.

Reddy, R. K., Lu, J., and Lee, A. S. (1999). The endoplasmic reticulum chaperone glycoprotein GRP94 with Ca(2+)-binding and antiapoptotic properties is a novel proteolytic target of calpain during etoposide-induced apoptosis. *J. Biol. Chem.* **274,** 28476–28483.

Reed, E. (1998). Platinum-DNA adduct, nucleotide excision repair and platinum based anti-cancer chemotherapy. *Cancer Treat. Rev.* **24,** 331–344.

Rittmann-Grauer, L. S., Yong, M. A., Sanders, V., and Mackensen, D. G. (1992). Reversal of Vinca alkaloid resistance by anti-P-glycoprotein monoclonal antibody HYB-241 in a human tumor xenograft. *Cancer Res.* **52,** 1810–1816.

Robert, J. (1999). Multidrug resistance in oncology: diagnostic and therapeutic approaches. *Eur. J. Clin. Invest.* **29,** 536–545.

Rofstad, E. K. (2000). Microenvironment-induced cancer metastasis. *Int. J. Radiat. Biol.* **76,** 589–605.

Ross, D. D., Karp, J. E., Chen, T. T., and Doyle, L. A. (2000). Expression of breast cancer resistance protein in blast cells from patients with acute leukemia. *Blood* **96,** 365–368.

Ross, D. D., Yang, W., Abruzzo, L. V., Dalton, W. S., Schneider, E., Lage, H., Dietel, M., Greenberger, L., Cole, S. P., and Doyle, L. A. (1999). Atypical multidrug resistance: breast cancer resistance protein messenger RNA expression in mitoxantrone-selected cell lines. *J. Natl. Cancer Inst.* **91,** 429–433.

Rubin, E. H., Li, T. K., Duann, P., and Liu, L. F. (1996). Cellular resistance to topoisomerase poisons. *Cancer Treat. Res.* **87,** 243–260.

Ryan, K. M., Ernst, M. K., Rice, N. R., and Vousden, K. H. (2000). Role of NF-κB in p53-mediated programmed cell death. *Nature* **404,** 892–897.

Sancar, A. (1995). DNA repair in humans. *Annu. Rev. Genet.* **29,** 69–105.

Scheffer, G. L., Maliepaard, M., Pijnenborg, A. C., van Gastelen, M. A., de Jong, M. C., Schroeijers, A. B., van der Kolk, D. M., Allen, J. D., Ross, D. D., van der Valk, P., Dalton, W. S., Schellens, J. H., and Scheper, R. J. (2000). Breast cancer resistance protein is localized at the plasma membrane in mitoxantrone- and topotecan-resistant cell lines. *Cancer Res.* **60,** 2589–2593.

Schinkel, A. H. (1997). The physiological function of drug-transporting P-glycoproteins. *Semin. Cancer Biol.* **8**, 161–170.

Schinkel, A. H. (1998). Pharmacological insights from P-glycoprotein knockout mice. *Int. J. Clin. Pharmacol. Ther.* **36**, 9–13.

Schmaltz, C., Hardenbergh, P. H., Wells, A., and Fisher, D. E. (1998). Regulation of proliferation-survival decisions during tumor cell hypoxia. *Mol. Cell. Biol.* **18**, 2845–2854.

Sedwick, W. D., Markowitz, S. D., and Veigl, M. L. (1999). Mismatch repair and drug responses in cancer. *Drug Resistance Updates* **2**, 295–306.

Sethi, T., Rintoul, R. C., Moore, S. M., MacKinnon, A. C., Salter, D., Choo, C., Chilvers, E. R., Dransfield, I., Donnelly, S. C., Strieter, R., and Haslett, C. (1999). Extracellular matrix proteins protect small cell lung cancer cells against apoptosis: a mechanism for small cell lung cancer growth and drug resistance in vivo. *Nat. Med.* **5**, 662–668.

Shen, D. W., Fojo, A., Roninson, I. B., Chin, J. E., Soffir, R., Pastan, I., and Gottesman, M. M. (1986). Multidrug resistance of DNA-mediated transformants is linked to transfer of the human mdr1 gene. *Mol. Cell. Biol.* **6**, 4039–4045.

Shen, J., Hughes, C., Chao, C., Cai, J., Bartels, C., Gessner, T., and Subjeck, J. (1987). Coinduction of glucose-regulated proteins and doxorubicin resistance in Chinese hamster cells. *Proc. Natl. Acad. Sci. USA* **84**, 3278–3282.

Shim, H., Chun, Y. S., Lewis, B. C., and Dang, C. V. (1998). A unique glucose-dependent apoptotic pathway induced by c-Myc. *Proc. Natl. Acad. Sci. USA* **95**, 1511–1516.

Sikic, B. I., Fisher, G. A., Lum, B. L., Halsey, J., Beketic-Oreskovic, L., and Chen, G. (1997). Modulation and prevention of multidrug resistance by inhibitors of P-glycoprotein. *Cancer Chemother. Pharmacol.* **40**, S13–S19.

Silverman, J. A. (1999). Multidrug-resistance transporters. *Pharm. Biotechnol.* **12**, 353–386.

Spiro, T. P., Gerson, S. L., Liu, L., Majka, S., Haaga, J., Hoppel, C. L., Ingalls, S. T., Pluda, J. M., and Willson, J. K. (1999). O^6-benzylguanine: a clinical trial establishing the biochemical modulatory dose in tumor tissue for alkyltransferase-directed DNA repair. *Cancer Res.* **59**, 2402–2410.

St. Croix, B., Man, S., and Kerbel, R. S. (1998). Reversal of intrinsic and acquired forms of drug resistance by hyaluronidase treatment of solid tumors. *Cancer Lett.* **131**, 35–44.

Starling, J. J., Shepard, R. L., Cao, J., Law, K. L., Norman, B. H., Kroin, J. S., Ehlhardt, W. J., Baughman, T. M., Winter, M. A., Bell, M. G., Shih, C., Gruber, J., Elmquist, W. F., and Dantzig, A. H. (1997). Pharmacological characterization of LY335979: a potent cyclopropyldibenzosuberane modulator of P-glycoprotein. *Adv. Enzyme Regul.* **37**, 335–347.

Sugimoto, Y., Gottesman, M. M., Pastan, I., and Tsuruo, T. (1998). Construction of MDR1 vectors for gene therapy. *Methods Enzymol.* **292**, 523–537.

Sugiyama, Y., Kato, Y., and Chu, X. (1998). Multiplicity of biliary excretion mechanisms for the camptothecin derivative irinotecan (CPT-11), its metabolite SN-38, and its glucuronide: role of canalicular multispecific organic anion transporter and P-glycoprotein. *Cancer Chemother. Pharmacol.* **42**, S44–S49.

Sutherland, R. M. (1988). Cell and environment interactions in tumor microregions: the multicell spheroid model. *Science* **240**, 177–184.

Tanaka, K., and Chiba, T. (1998). The proteasome: a protein-destroying machine. *Genes Cells* **3**, 499–510.

Tidefelt, U., Liliemark, J., Gruber, A., Liliemark, E., Sundman-Engberg, B., Juliusson, G., Stenke, L., Elmhorn-Rosenborg, A., Mollgard, L., Lehman, S., Xu, D., Covelli, A., Gustavsson, B., and Paul, C. (2000). P-Glycoprotein inhibitor valspodar (PSC 833) increases the intracellular concentrations of daunorubicin in vivo in patients with P-glycoprotein-positive acute myeloid leukemia. *J. Clin. Oncol.* **18**, 1837–1844.

Tomida, A., Suzuki, H., Kim, H.-D., and Tsuruo, T. (1996). Glucose-regulated stresses cause decreased expression of cyclin D1 and hypophosphorylation of retinoblastoma protein in human cancer cells. *Oncogene* **13**, 2699–2705.

Tomida, A., and Tsuruo, T. (1999). Drug resistance mediated by cellular stress response to the microenvironment of solid tumors. *Anti-Cancer Drug Design* **14**, 169–177.

Tomida, A., Yun, J., and Tsuruo, T. (1996). Glucose-regulated stresses induce resistance to camptothecin in human cancer cells. *Int. J. Cancer* **68**, 391–396.

Tsuruo, T. (1988). Mechanisms of multidrug resistance and implications for therapy. *Jpn. J. Cancer Res.* **79**, 285–296.

Tsuruo, T., Hamada, H., Sato, S., and Heike, Y. (1989). Inhibition of multidrug-resistant human tumor growth in athymic mice by anti-P-glycoprotein monoclonal antibodies. *Jpn. J. Cancer Res.* **80**, 627–631.

Tsuruo, T., Iida, H., Tsukagoshi, S., and Sakurai, Y. (1981). Overcoming of vincristine resistance in P388 leukemia in vivo and in vitro through enhanced cytotoxicity of vincristine and vinblastine by verapamil. *Cancer Res.* **41**, 1967–1972.

Ueda, K., Cardarelli, C., Gottesman, M. M., and Pastan, I. (1987). Expression of a full-length cDNA for the human "MDR1" gene confers resistance to colchicine, doxorubicin, and vinblastine. *Proc. Natl. Acad. Sci. USA* **84**, 3004–3008.

Waddick, K. G., and Uckun, F. M. (1999). Innovative treatment programs against cancer: II. Nuclear factor-κB (NF-κB) as a molecular target. *Biochem. Pharmacol.* **57**, 9–17.

Wang, C. Y., Cusack, J. C., Jr., Liu, R., and Baldwin, A. S., Jr. (1999). Control of inducible chemoresistance: enhanced anti-tumor therapy through increased apoptosis by inhibition of NF-κB. *Nat. Med.* **5**, 412–417.

Wang, C. Y., Mayo, M. W., and Baldwin, A. S., Jr. (1996). TNF- and cancer therapy-induced apoptosis: potentiation by inhibition of NF-κB. *Science* **274**, 784–787.

Watanabe, T., Naito, M., Kokubu, N., and Tsuruo, T. (1997). Regression of established tumors expressing P-glycoprotein by combinations of adriamycin, cyclosporin derivatives, and MRK-16 antibodies. *J. Natl. Cancer Inst.* **89**, 512–518.

Wijnholds, J., Mol, C. A., van Deemter, L., de Haas, M., Scheffer, G. L., Baas, F., Beijnen, J. H., Scheper, R. J., Hatse, S., De Clercq, E., Balzarini, J., and Borst, P. (2000). Multidrug-resistance protein 5 is a multispecific organic anion transporter able to transport nucleotide analogs. *Proc. Natl. Acad. Sci. USA* **97**, 7476–7481.

Yun, J., Tomida, A., Nagata, K., and Tsuruo, T. (1995). Glucose-regulated stresses confer resistance to VP-16 in human cancer cells through a decreased expression of DNA topoisomerase II. *Oncol. Res.* **7**, 583–590.

Zaman, G. J., Flens, M. J., van Leusden, M. R., de Haas, M., Mulder, H. S., Lankelma, J., Pinedo, H. M., Scheper, R. J., Baas, F., Broxterman, H. J., and Borst, P. (1994). The human multidrug resistance-associated protein MRP is a plasma membrane drug-efflux pump. *Proc. Natl. Acad. Sci. USA* **91**, 8822–8826.

Zaman, G. J., Lankelma, J., van Tellingen, O., Beijnen, J., Dekker, H., Paulusma, C., Oude Elferink, R. P., Baas, F., and Borst, P. (1995). Role of glutathione in the export of compounds from cells by the multidrug-resistance-associated protein. *Proc. Natl. Acad. Sci. USA* **92**, 7690–7694.

Zeng-Rong, N., Paterson, J., Alpert, L., Tsao, M. S., Viallet, J., and Alaoui-Jamali, M. A. (1995). Elevated DNA repair capacity is associated with intrinsic resistance of lung cancer to chemotherapy. *Cancer Res.* **55**, 4760–4764.

ROLE OF MATRIX METALLOPROTEINASES AND PLASMINOGEN ACTIVATORS IN CANCER INVASION AND METASTASIS: THERAPEUTIC STRATEGIES

Stanley Zucker*,†
Jian Cao†
Christopher J. Molloy‡

*Department of Veterans Affairs Medical Center, Northport, New York;
†School of Medicine, State University of New York, Stony Brook, New York;
and ‡3-Dimensional Pharmaceuticals, Inc., Exton, Pennsylvania

Summary

Cancer progression is a multistage process in which cancer cells undergo genetic changes that lead to phenotypic alterations, including the capacity to metastasize. An overwhelming amount of experimental evidence has been accumulated to implicate a role for matrix metalloproteinases (MMPs) and plasminogen activators (PAs) in invasion and metastasis. However, specific MMPs appear to have different functions depending on the experimental model and the stage of cancer. The fact that most MMPs and PAs in human cancers are produced by reactive stromal cells (fibroblasts, endothelial cells, inflammatory cells) surrounding the tumor rather than the cancer cells themselves needs to be better understood. Proteases may be good anticancer targets in that they appear to be required for the stromal tissue remodeling associated with angiogenesis and tumor metastasis. However, true clinical efficacy may require combination therapy (with cytotoxic agents) as well as long-term administration, possibly at earlier stages of cancer. Numerous highly effective hydroxamic-acid-based MMP inhibitors (MMPIs) have been developed; three of these agents are in clinical trials in patients with advanced cancer. Results of these clinical trials will be critical to future development of this class of drugs.

91

It must be emphasized that the clinical testing of MMPIs in advanced human cancer is not the best trial design since the pathogenic effects of MMPs probably occur earlier in the disease. Potential side effects have been identified for MMPIs related to broad specificity of certain agents in interfering with normal tissue remodeling. Nonetheless, these agents are much better tolerated than standard chemotherapy. It is possible that MMPIs and/or PA inhibitors might be viewed in the future in a more chemopreventive role (promoting "tumor dormancy") rather than a chemotherapeutic role.

1. Introduction

Cancer is on its way to becoming the leading cause of death in the United States. In the vast majority of patients, metastasis and uncontrolled local invasion lead to the patient's demise. Despite the advent of better cancer treatment in the form of surgery, radiotherapy, and systemic chemotherapy, the clinical challenge to oncology remains that of combating metastatic spread. Tumor progression is recognized to be a complex, multistage process by which normal cells undergo genetic changes that result in phenotypic alterations, including acquisition of the ability to disseminate to distant sites in the body. Experimental evidence has shown that tumors are enriched with an array of proteolytic enzymes that appear to be essential for cancer dissemination (Liotta, 1992; Mareel *et al.,* 1993; Nelson *et al.,* 2000; Price *et al.,* 1997; Stetler-Stevenson, 1999). Tumor cell adhesion, motility, and cell receptors also have important roles in cancer invasion (Nelson *et al.,* 2000; Nicolson, 1991; Poste and Fidler, 1980; Price *et al.,* 1997). None of the functions of metastatic cells are unique to cancer since they can be demonstrated during trophoblast implantation, mammary gland involution, embryonic morphogenesis, inflammation, and tissue remodeling. The difference between the normal processes and the pathogenic nature of cancer invasion is therefore one of regulation. Cancer cell invasion cannot be effectively regulated by the host, whereas inflammatory cell invasion is under physiologic control.

The purpose of this chapter is to present current views on the metastatic process with an emphasis on MMPs and PAs. The use of MMPIs in cancer treatment of humans will be discussed in detail. It should be pointed out that with the completion of the human genome project, our understanding of the metastatic process is likely to expand markedly and new therapeutic approaches will invariably be introduced. The use of drugs that will interfere with biological aspects of tumor dissemination is just beginning, and we need to keep an open mind to unique developments and approaches. The combining of cytotoxic chemotherapy with inhibitors of biological processes unique to cancer is just beginning. Other comprehensive reviews of various aspects of cancer metastasis are available for the interested reviewer (Chambers and Matrisian, 1997; Coussens and Werb, 1996; Curran and Murray, 1999; Greenwald *et al.,* 1999; Liotta, 1992; Mareel *et al.,* 1993; McCawley and Matrisian, 2000; Nelson *et al.,* 2000; Noel *et al.,* 1997; Parks and Mecham, 1998; Price *et al.,* 1997; Stetler-Stevenson, 1999; Welch, 1997). Selected topics with therapeutic potential that have been overlooked in other review articles will be presented here with the hope of encouraging renewed interest in these areas.

2. The Extracellular Matrix

Invading cancer cells must breach barriers opposing their movement. These barriers include basement membranes, the extracellular matrix (ECM), and normal cell–cell junctions. The mature ECM, produced by a variety of mostly mesenchymal cells, consists of a supramolecular aggregate of connective tissue proteins, including fibrillar and nonfibrillar collagens, elastin, glycoproteins (laminin, fibronectin, enactin, nidogen), and glycosaminoglycans (ground substances, such as heparan sulfate proteoglycans), which interact with one another through covalent and noncovalent bonds to form highly insoluble materials. Initially, it was thought that the function of the ECM was to create an inert structural barrier or an active antagonist to cancer cell invasion. More recent evidence suggests that the specialized tumor stroma associated with growing neoplasms, especially of epithelial origin, provides enhancing factors for tumor progression (Iozzo, 1995). Embedded in this ECM is a myriad of biological signals, nutrients, and growth factors, in which tumor cells thrive and proliferate at the expense of the host. A causal role of tumor-associated hyaluronan in the spread of cancer has been proposed (Auvinen *et al.,* 2000). The presence of high levels of fibrinogen in the interstitium of tumors led Dvorak to propose that tumors are "wounds that do not heal" (Dvorak, 1986). Connective tissue around carcinoma cells contains increased levels of decorin (a protoglycan involved in cell growth), increased levels of perlecans (which bind fibroblast growth factor), and express spliced variants of tenascin and fibronectin (two matrix molecules directly involved in control of cell proliferation and metastasis) (Iozzo, 1995). Therapeutic approaches in cancer that exploit differences between cancer ECM and normal ECM remain to be developed.

3. Cancer Invasion and Metastasis

A. Basic Concepts of Cancer Dissemination

A major emphasis of research on cancer dissemination has focused on model systems characterizing the sequence of events making up the metastatic cascade. Small animals, primarily mice and rats, were employed initially due to cost, convenience, and availability. Mice are valuable in identifying function of human genes because genome organization corresponds closely between the two species. In a complicated disease such as cancer, investigators must be wary not to overinterpret similarities between rodents and humans. Mice are 3000 times smaller, grow after birth 100 times faster, and age after maturity about 30 times faster; thus, the mouse's life cycle may make it a less than perfect model for cancer in humans.

The gold standard by which cancer dissemination has been assessed consists of an *in vivo* metastasis model in which tumor cells are injected intravenously or subcutaneously in mice, which are later sacrificed to determine the number of lung metastases (Welch, 1997). These studies require awareness of critical technical details (Fidler, 1991). The term "lung colonization" has been applied to the nodules that develop on the surface of the lung after intravenous injection of tumor cells since it was recognized that bypassing spread from the original cancer focus created an artificial system. This model is based on empowering the cancer cell with all of the components required in autonomous proliferation, invasion, migration, and metastasis. Cell adhesion factors and the ability of tumor cells to grow at the site where arrested ultimately determine whether a metastatic colony develops at that site (Rusciano and Burger, 1992). As will be discussed later, cancer cells are not solely responsible for all of the events involved in dissemination. Other *in vivo* approaches currently being employed to better understand the metastatic process make use of transgenic mice or knockout mice that by virtue of over/underexpression of genes develop spontaneous tumors that eventually disseminate (Kerbel, 1999). Numerous *in vitro* models that examine specific steps in metastasis have also been described.

B. Steps in Metastasis

The following steps or stages of the metastatic process have been described (Fig. 1): (1) the initial transforming event involving genetic alterations in gatekeeper genes and caretaker genes (oncogene activation); (2) proliferation of transformed cells as balanced with cell death (apoptosis); (3) the ability of cancer cells to avoid destruction by immune mechanisms; (4) recruitment of a nutritional supply to the tumor mass, which involves the release of tumor angiogenesis factors and the ingrowth of new blood vessels (tumor neovascularization); (5) local invasion and destruction of ECM components and parenchymal cells; (6) migration of tumor cells away from the primary tumor mass; (7) penetration of cancer cells through the blood vessel wall (intravasation); (8) embolization of cancer cells (single cells and aggregates) to distant organs; (9) interaction of cancer cells with platelets, neutrophils, erythrocytes, and plasma coagulation factors in the bloodstream; (10) arrest of cancer cells in the lumen of small blood vessels or lymphatics and adhesion to endothelial cells; (11) reverse penetration of blood vessels (extravasation) at a metastatic site; (12) repetition of the process beginning at step 2 resulting in the formation of secondary tumors (metastases). It should be recognized that the order and importance of these steps might vary with different types

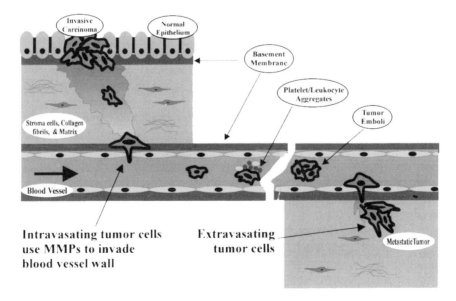

FIGURE 1 Schematic illustration of invasive carcinoma cells penetrating through their underlying basement membrane, migrating through the extracellular matrix, penetrating the blood vessel wall (intravasation), forming tumor emboli, adhering to the endothelium in a distant organ, extravasating, and proliferating at the metastatic site.

of cancer. An example of our uncertainty of key factors in human metastasis comes from a recent report indicating that lung metastases in experimental mice originate from the proliferation of attached intravascular tumor cells rather than from extravascular cells (Al-Medhi *et al.,* 2000).

C. Replacement of Parenchymal Cells by Cancer Cells

It is well recognized that cancer cell replacement of normal parenchymal cells in vital organs, such as liver and bone marrow, can seriously compromise organ function. The mechanism by which normal parenchymal cells become replaced by cancer cells during the process of invasion is an important aspect of tumor biology that has been overlooked. Older morphologic studies led to the suggestion that cancer cells damage normal cells *in situ* by a cell contact mechanism (see review by Zucker, 1988). Studies of numerous human and animal tumor models have demonstrated that the plasma membranes of cancer cells are enriched with hemolytic factors that lyse erythrocytes through proteinase-independent a cell contact (DiStefano, 1986; Zucker *et al.,* 1993a). A potent tumor cytotoxic protein with an apparent molecular weight of 62,000 has been purified from tumor cell membranes which, at higher concentrations, lysed normal nucleated cells (fibroblasts and erythroblasts) (Zucker *et al.,* 1993a). The role of TCP in human cancer invasion remains to be elucidated.

D. Genetics of Metastasis

To develop metastases to different organs, tumor cells must possess or develop at different times many highly differentiated characteristics that define the metastatic phenotype. The development of considerable biological diversity by cancer cells has been attributed to their high mutation rate and genetic instability leading to a heterogeneous population of cells that undergo continual change. This high mutation rate enhances the ability of cancer cell populations to continuously develop clones with metastatic capabilities. For most tumors, the neoplastic population must expand considerably before invasion and metastasis occur. This expansion may be clonal and mainly limited to more aggressive subpopulations of neoplastic cells (clonal dominance theory) (Theodorescu *et al.,* 1991).

Several genes have been implicated in suppression or enhancement (Ree *et al.,* 1999) of cancer dissemination, and their number is likely to increase considerably with the widespread implementation of differential display analysis and DNA microarray technology. The ultimate discovery of the master switch(es) controlling tumorigenesis and metastasis is awaited. Distinguishing between suppression of primary tumor formation/growth and metastasis in animal models requires carefully designed experiments. Loss of gene expression, resulting in increased invasiveness, has been demonstrated for nm23 (Freije *et al.,* 1994) and E-cadherin (Mareel *et al.,* 1993). Using the subtraction hybridization technique, the *KiSS-1* gene, located on chromosome 1q, was identified as a suppressor of metastasis in human melanoma and breast cancer cells (Lee and Welch, 1997). Differential display reverse transcriptase polymerase chain reaction (RTPCR) was employed to identify a gene on human chromosome 11 that was designated breast cancer metastasis suppressor 1 (*BRMS1*). Growth of the local tumor at the primary site of injection in nude mice was slightly delayed in *BRMS1*-transfected breast cancer cells, but metastases were profoundly suppressed (Seraj *et al.,* 2000). Maspin, a gene/protein that contains sequence homology with serine protease inhibitors (Serpins) including plasminogen activator inhibitors (PAIs), suppressed the invasive phenotype of carcinoma cells; this effect may result from maspin-induced alteration of the integrin profile (increased α_5) of cancer cells and subsequent altered cell adherence and signaling (Seftor *et al.,* 1998). A membrane-anchored glycoprotein termed *RECK,* also containing Serpin-like domains, has been found to specifically bind and inhibit the proteolytic activity of MMP-9, as well as suppress the invasive and metastatic potential of cDNA-transfected tumor cells in nude mice (Takahashi *et al.,* 1998). *Kai1, MKK4,* and tissue inhibitors of metalloproteinases (TIMPs) have also been labeled as metastasis suppressor genes (Seraj *et al.,* 2000). CD44, a widely expressed cell surface glycoprotein that serves as an adhesion molecule, appears to have a variety of both positive and negative functions in cancer dissemination (Price *et al.,* 1997).

4. Cell Adhesion in Cancer

Cell–cell adhesion in normal cells involves interactions between numerous surface proteins. Adhesion can function positively to stabilize tissue structure or negatively to facilitate cell dissemination. In the context of cancer, adhesion can be separated into three components: attachment, spreading, and detachment (see reviews by Mareel *et al.,* 1993; Price *et al.,* 1997). Calcium adhesion molecules (CAM) of the cadherin family (E-cadherin, P-cadherin, and N-cadherin) mediate cell–cell binding and generally display an inhibitory effect on the process of metastasis. Cadherin proteins are diminished in cancer cells, leading to a loss of intercellular adhesion. The intracellular domain of cadherins are connected to a group of proteins coined catenins, which function as a link to the actin cytoskeleton. These connections not only reinforce the cell-adhesive capacity of cadherins but also indicate that cadherins are integrated in signal response circuits. The ectodomain of E-cadherin is proteolytically cleaved from some cancer cells by an unidentified membrane-bound metalloprotease to yield a soluble form, and the residual membrane-tethered cleavage product is degraded by an intracellular mechanism (Ito *et al.,* 1999). Transfection studies have demonstrated that E-cadherin functions as an invasion suppressor molecule. In contrast, transfected cancer cells expressing both E- and N-cadherin display enhanced migration, invasion, growth-factor-induced MMP-9 synthesis, and metastatic potential (Hazan *et al.,* 2000). Abnormalities, including mutations of catenins, have also been identified in cancer cells, suggesting that these proteins can act as oncogenes. In addition, members of the immunoglobulin (Ig) superfamily that have been studied for their putative role in invasion-related homotypic cell–cell adhesion include N-CAM, DCC (deleted in colon cancer), and carcinoembryonic antigen (CEA).

Recent studies indicate that tumor cell attachment to endothelial cells by galactoside-mediated adhesion and homotypic aggregation is required for experimental hematogenous metastasis (Al-Medhi *et al.,* 2000; Glinsky *et al.,* 2000). Clustering of galectin-3 on endothelial cells at sites of contact with tumor cell T antigen (a cancer-associated carbohydrate rich in galectin-1) was demonstrated. These data support the possibility of preventing cancer metastasis by antiadhesive therapy (Glinsky *et al.,* 2000).

A. Cancer Cell Integrins

Attachment of cancer cells to specific glycoproteins of the ECM, such as fibronectin, collagen, and laminin, is mediated through surface receptors of the integrin and nonintegrin variety. Integrins are a large class of $\alpha\beta$ heterodimer receptors for adhesion molecules with broad specificity and low binding affinity. Numerous different α and β subunits have been identified that noncovalently associate to produce more than 20 integrin types. Individual cell receptors can bind to more than one type of adhesive molecule, creating structural links between components of the ECM and cytoskeleton by proteins such as talin, vinculin, and actin microfilaments. A reduction or change in the distribution of integrin receptors for laminin and collagen has been found in some cancers, suggesting that loss of attachment to the basement membrane is important for facilitating tumor development. Signaling between integrin and proteinases occurs in cells. The increased expression of selected integrins ($\alpha_v\beta3$, $\alpha_v\beta5$) in tumor-associated blood vessels has been an impetus to develop selective inhibitors of these integrins (humanized monoclonal antibodies and cyclic peptides) as new treatment approaches in cancer (Gutheil *et al.,* 2000).

5. Cancer Cell Motility

Directed movement of cells along a concentration gradient of chemical attractants is an essential characteristic of neoplastic and specialized normal cells; recent progress in understanding the general signaling pathway has been made (Dekker and Segal, 2000). Many motility factors for cancer cells and nonmalignant cells were described initially as growth factors. A motility factor converts a cell from a static to a motile status, a transition that is characterized by the appearance of membrane ruffling, lamellae, and pseudopodia. Several motility factors have been described for cancer cells (for a review, see Mareel *et al.,* 1993; Price *et al.,* 1997), including (1) autocrine motility factor (AMF; neuroleukin/phosphohexose isomerase), which stimulates chemokinesis and chemotaxis of metastatic melanoma cells via an AMF receptor in an autocrine fashion; (2) autotaxin, a basic glycoprotein of 125 kDa with pyrophosphatase, phosphodiesterase, and kinase activity; (3) scatter factor/hepatocyte growth factor (ligands for the c-met oncogene product, a receptor tyrosine kinase family member), which may act as a positive or negative growth factor; (4) the EGF receptor ligands transforming growth factor (TGFβ) and epidermal growth factor (EGF); and (5) insulin-like growth factors that stimulate chemokinesis and chemotaxis. In addition, both intact and degraded ECM proteins act as motility factors for tumor cells, including vitronectin, fibronectin, laminin, collagens, CD44, and thrombospondin.

6. Inflammatory Response to Cancer

The function of inflammatory cell infiltrates in cancer tissue has puzzled pathologists for more than a century. Proponents of the theory of immune surveillance as a means of controlling cancer have suggested that the degree of leukocyte infiltration in a tumor is a measure of the host immune response. These studies were focused primarily on T lymphocytes and killer cells interfering with tumor progression. Other investigators have determined that tumor-associated leukocytes are functionally paralyzed and correlated with poor prognosis. In invasive breast carcinomas, the neoplastic cell population is sometimes outnumbered by tumor-associated macrophages. It is thought that monocytes in peripheral blood are recruited to the tumor site by the release of the chemotactic cytokines, monocyte chemotactic protein-1, colony-stimulating factor (CSF-1), granulocyte macrophage CSF, and vascular endothelial growth factor (VEGF) by such tumors (Leek *et al.,* 1996). Conversely macrophages, which are terminally differentiated monocytes, produce a number of potent angiogenic cytokines and growth factors, such as VEGF, tumor necrosis factor (TNF-α), interleukin-8 (IL-8), and basic fibroblast growth factor (bFGF). Moderate or dense lymphoplasmacytic infiltrates of tumors have been correlated with some independent prognostic indicators (tumor size, stage, grade, oncogene expression), but not prognosis (Pupa *et al.,* 1996). Other studies identified a significant positive correlation between high vascular grade (angiogenesis) of a tumor and increased macrophage index; increased macrophage counts were associated with reduced relapse-free survival (Leek et al., 1996). Since tumor macrophages produce high levels of proteolytic enzymes, the role of these proteases in cancer dissemination needs more intensive study.

7. Proteolytic Enzymes Implicated in Cancer Invasion

Although considerable information is available on the breakdown of connective tissue proteins by soluble tumor enzymes in vitro, less is known about the mechanisms by which tumor cells digest highly complex mixtures of fibrillar proteins in vivo. It appears that several hydrolytic enzymes collaborate to degrade the ECM efficiently. The degree to which the ECM has to be degraded to accommodate invasion by tumor cells is unknown; thus, it is a matter of speculation as to the amount of proteolytic activity required for the process. Morphologic studies suggested that the degradation of the ECM occurs in close proximity to the cell surface.

All four categories of proteinases (serine, cysteine, aspartic proteinases, and metalloproteinases) have been implicated in the invasive process (Zucker, 1988). Some of the matrix-degrading enzymes serve as activators for others and trigger a digestion cascade. It must be emphasized that the evidence supporting the role of these enzymes in invasion is primarily circumstantial and opposing views have been expressed (Della Porta et al., 1999; Noel et al., 1997; Zucker et al., 1992), although not seriously considered.

One important experimental approach that has been used to support the role of proteinases in cancer dissemination has been to show a positive correlation between tumor cell secretion of specific proteinases in vitro or extraction of proteinases from tumor homogenates and the measurement of invasiveness and metastasis in experimental systems (Mignatti and Rifkin, 1993; Zucker, 1988). However, a major limitation to these types of experiments is that only a minute fraction of the tumor cell population chosen for study actually has the potential to metastasize. Hence, the conclusions drawn from the entire tumor population may not accurately reflect the phenotype of the putative "supercharged" tumor cell that is uniquely endowed with the specific characteristics required to complete the metastatic cascade. The proteinase theory of cancer invasion is also supported by the finding that nonmalignant invasive cells, such as activated macrophages and trophoblast cells, produce proteinases. In addition to their effects on invasion, some proteases may affect tumor growth. Cathepsins are aspartyl or cysteine proteases that function primarily at low pH within the lysosomes of cells but are released in high levels by many types of cancer cells and are prominently displayed in some human cancers (Campo et al., 1994; Sloane et al., 1994). The limited support for an impor-

tant role of cathepsins B and L in tumor invasion is due to the limited function of these enzymes at physiologic pH. Tumor enzymes that hydrolyze other extracellular matrix components (glycosidases, hyaluronidase, heparinase) have also been described but will not be discussed further (Nicolson, 1991).

A. Cell Surface Protrusions (Invadopodia) and Vesicles

Invadopodia (podosomes) are specialized cell surface structures composed of a meshwork of microfilaments that have been identified on transformed cells. Invadopodia are involved in the growth of cells on collagen-like matrices and invasion of the underlying matrix. Invadopodia utilize proteases to degrade a variety of immobilized substrates, including fibronectin, laminin, type I and IV collagens, and ECM components. Several integral membrane enzymes of different classes have been identified as important functional components of invadopodia (Nakahara et al., 1998b). These include the serine proteases seprase (surface-expressed proteases) and dipeptidyl peptidase IV, which must form oligomeric structures for expression of proteolytic activity and membrane-type MMP (Nakahara et al., 1998). Various integrins and extracellular matrix metalloproteinase inducer (EMMPRIN) have also been identified in invadopodia. Integrin signaling regulating tyrosine phosphorylation of Rho family members is involved in invadopodia degradative function (Nakahara et al., 1998b). Although not yet explored, inhibition of invadopodia function provides an attractive target for development of anticancer drugs.

Shedding of components of the plasma membrane as vesicles (possibly originating from invadopodia) into the extracellular space is a widespread, energy-requiring event observed both in vitro and in vivo that is more exaggerated in tumor cells than in normal cells (Dollo et al., 1999; Zucker et al., 1987). Membrane vesicles contain densely clustered MMP-9 (Nguyen et al., 1998), MMP-2, β_1 integrins, and urinary plasminogen activator (uPA), which may facilitate directional proteolysis of the ECM during cell migration and especially during cancer invasion. Adhesion of tumor membrane vesicles to ECM fibrils may provide a reservoir for slow release of proteases and growth factors from the ECM (Dollo et al., 1999). The function of vesicle shedding in cancer remains to be determined.

B. Matrix Metalloproteinases: Basic Concepts

MMPs were originally discovered as part of a series of experiments designed to explain how a metamorphosing tadpole of a frog sheds its tail, particularly the collagenous components, which were known to be resistant to established proteolytic degradation (Gross and Lapiere, 1962). Since collagen represents the major structural protein of all tissues and the chief obstacle of the migration of tumor cells, it has long been postulated that collagenolytic enzymes, primarily MMPs, play a pivotal role in facilitating the dissemination of cancer.

MMPs belong to the family of zinc endopeptidases collectively referred to as metzincins. Once activated, MMPs degrade a variety of ECM components (Birkedal-Hansen, 1995; Birkedal-Hansen *et al.*, 1993; Nagase and Woessner, 1999; Stetler-Stevenson, 1999; Woessner, 1991). There are now more than 20 enzymes that are classified as MMPs. These enzymes have both a descriptive name typically based on a preferred substrate (e.g., interstitial collagenase) and an MMP number. Because of uncertainty concerning relevant substrates for many of these enzymes, the number system will be used in this chapter except for the membrane-type MMP subfamily, where the designation MT-MMP is universally employed. Another approach to MMP classification is based on structure (Fig. 2). All MMPs share several highly conserved domains, including an activation locus [PRCGXPD][1] in the amino-terminal "pro" domain and a zinc atom binding domain [VAAHExGHxxGxxH] in the active site (catalytic domain), with the three histidines coordinating the zinc (Fig. 3) (Birkedal-Hansen *et al.*, 1993). A second structural zinc ion and a calcium ion are also present elsewhere in the catalytic domain of MMPs. A "pre" region (signal peptide) targets the proteins for secretion or insertion into the plasma membrane.

The N-terminal prodomain acts as an internal inhibitor of MMP activity and maintains the enzyme in an inactive state until proteinase activity is required. The cysteine residue in the activation locus coordinates the active site zinc atom, thereby conferring latency to the enzyme. The amino acids surrounding the cysteine are also involved in maintaining latency. This link must be broken by proteolytic cleavage or conformational modification before the metalloproteinase can degrade substrates. The majority of MMPs have additional domains, such as a hemopexin-like C-terminal domain (shaped like a β propeller fold with pseudo-fourfold symmetry) or a fibronectin-like region, which are important in substrate recognition and in inhibitor binding. The hinge region, which links the hemopexin and catalytic domains, may be important in determining substrate specificity (Parks and Mecham, 1998). The molecular weights of proMMPs vary between 28,000 and 92,000.

The three-dimensional structures of the catalytic domains of several matrixins have been determined in the past few years (Lovejoy *et al.*, 1999). Superposition of these structures on the more distally related thermolysins and other bacterial metalloproteinases reveals a remarkable similarity in their overall folding. Three interstitial collagenases have been identified: MMP-1 (collagenase-1), MMP-8 (collagenase-2), and MMP-13 (collagenase 3). Collagenases characteristically produce a single cleavage in the collagen molecule at 25°C, resulting in three-fourths and one-fourth size triple-helical fragments. There are two type IV collagenases—MMP-2 (gelatinase A) and MMP-9 (gelatinase B)—which were renamed gelatinases because they function far better in cleaving gelatin (denatured collagen). The gelatinases are responsible for further degradation of the large three-fourths and one-fourth collagen fragments and other proteins, such as fibronectin, laminin, and native elastin. Three MMPs have been identified as stromelysins. MMP-3 (stromelysin-1) and MMP-10 (stromelysin-2) are closely related functionally, degrading various proteoglycan components of the extracellular matrix, as well as fibronectin, laminin, and gelatin. MMP-11 (stromelysin-3) does not appear to degrade ECM proteins but is effective in degrading the serine proteinase inhibitor (serpin), α_1-antiproteinase inhibitor (antitrypsin), and thus may potentiate the action of serine proteinases. Serpinase activity is displayed by other MMPs as well, and supports the hypothesis that metalloproteinases and serine proteinases act in an interdependent manner. Furthermore, since plasminogen activators and other serine proteinases have been shown to be capable of activating latent tumor collagenases, an interaction between these enzymes may be required to bring about collagen breakdown *in vivo* (Birkedal-Hansen *et al.*, 1993).

MMP-7 (matrilysin, formerly known as PUMP) is a short, truncated proteinase that can degrade nonfibrillar collagen, fibronectin, and laminin. MMP-12 (metalloelastase), as implied by the name, is capable of degrading elastin (Shapiro, 1998). A subset of MMPs, known as membrane-type MMPs (MT-MMPs), contains a transmembrane domain of approximately 20 amino acids that attaches the enzyme to the cell surface. It also contains a short cytoplasmic domain (Sato *et al.*, 1994) that is involved in trafficking MT-MMPs to the leading edge of the cell (Lehti *et al.*, 2000; Nakahara *et al.*, 1998a). The most prominent and active member of this category is a 63-kDa matrix metalloproteinase, MT1-MMP (MMP-14). Expression of the gene product of MT1-MMP on tumor cell surface has been shown to cause activation of proMMP-2, leading to enhanced cellular invasion *in vitro* (Sato *et al.*, 1994). Homology screening for MMPs has revealed five other membrane-spanning MMPs sharing considerable homology with MT1-MMP, but different tissue distribution. MT4-MMP is unique in having a glycosylphosphatidylinositol linkage to the plasma membrane (Ito *et al.*, 1999). Recombinant soluble MT1-MMP hydrolyzes type I collagen more effectively than type III collagen and digests cartilage proteoglycan, fibronectin, fibrinogen, vitronectin, laminin, and α_1-antiproteinase. Recently, it has been demonstrated that in the absence of plasminogen, endothelial cell surface MT1-MMP is capable of degrading fibrin and facilitating cell migration through a fibrin clot (Hiraoka *et al.*, 1998). These data support the hypothesis that endothelial

---

[1]Amino acid sequences are referred to by single-letter designations; X indicates any amino acid.

Matrix Metalloproteinase	Enzyme Commission Nomenclature	Domain Structure	Substrates
		Sig. Pro.　　Cat. Hinge HemoTM/Cyto.	
Minimal domain MMP		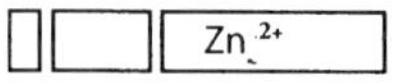	
Matrilysin	MMP-7		Proteoglycans, laminin, gelatins, elastin, enactin, tenascin
Hemopexin/Vitronectin domain MMPs			
Simple-type		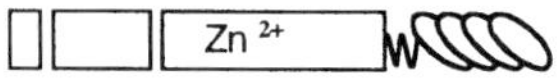	
Collagenase-1(interstitial)	MMP-1		Collagens I, II, III, VII, X
Collagenase-2 (neutrophil)	MMP-8		Collagens I, II, III
Collagenase-3	MMP-13		Collagens I, II, III, aggrecan
Metalloelastase	MMP-12		Elastin, fibrinogen, fibronectin
Stromelysin-1(transin)	MMP-3		Proteoglycans, laminin, gelatins, collagens, III, IV, V, IX, SPARC, proMMP-9, proMMP-1, fibronectin
Stromelysin-2	MMP-10		Proteoglycans, laminin, gelatins, collagens I, III, IV, V, IX, fibronectin
Furin activated-type			
Stromelysin-3	MMP-11	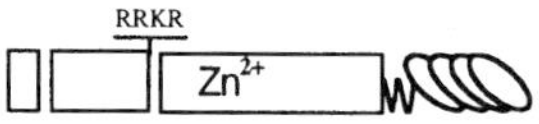 RRKR	Laminin, fibronectin, α1-proteinase inhibitor
Membrane type 1-MMP	MMP-14	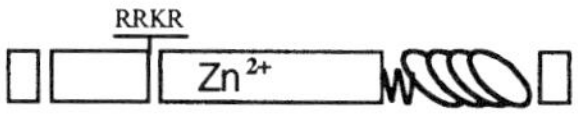 RRKR	Collagens I, II, III, fibronectin, vitronectin, proteoglycans, proMMP-2, proMMP-13
Membrane type 2-MMP	MMP-15		ProMMP-2
Membrane type 3-MMP	MMP-16		ProMMP-2
Membrane type 4-MMP	MMP-17		ProMMP-2
Membrane type 5-MMP	MMP-24		ProMMP-2
Fibronectin-type		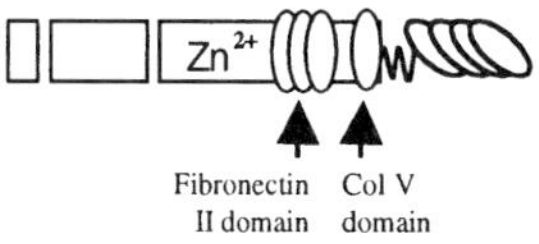	
Gelatinase-A(72 kDa type IV collagenase)	MMP-2	Fibronectin II domain / Col V domain	Gelatins, collagens I, IV, V, VII, X, fibronectin, elastin, proMMP-13, proMMP-9
Gelatinase-B(92 kDa type IV collagenase)	MMP-9		Gelatins, collagens IV, V, elastin

FIGURE 2 Members of the matrix metalloproteinase multigene family implicated in cancer. The commonly employed nomenclature is listed, as are well-known substrates.

Domain Structure of Human Matrix Metalloproteinases

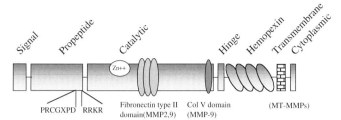

FIGURE 3 The domain structures of matrix metalloproteinases (MMPs) implicated in cancer. The basic structure of MMPs consists of five domains. These include (from the N terminus): a signal peptide domain, a propeptide domain containing a "cysteine switch," a catalytic domain, a hinge region, and a hemopexin-like domain at the C terminus. The exceptions are as follows: MMP-7 lacks a hemopexin-like domain; MT-MMPs have two additional inserts: a transmembrane domain and a cytoplasmic domain at the C terminus; the furin-consensus sequence is present only in MT-MMPs and MMP-11; a fibronectin-like domain is present in MMP-2 and MMP-9; a collagen-V-like domain is present in MMP-9.

MT1-MMP may be important in an early phase of tumor angiogenesis.

1. MMP Regulation

MMP activity is tightly regulated both intracellularly at the level of gene expression and following secretion by actions of activators of proenzymes and inhibitors. In general, MMPs are produced at very low levels; however, cellular expression is rapidly induced at times of active tissue remodeling. The promoter regions of inducible MMP genes show remarkable conservation of regulatory elements. (Interested readers are referred to Vincenti *et al.,* 1996 for a detailed discussion.) MMP proteins are transcribed and secreted by the constitutive secretory pathway, except in the case of neutrophils and macrophages where MMPs can be stored in and released from secretory granules and MT-MMPs (Birkedal-Hansen *et al.,* 1993; Woessner, 1991). The MMP genes are transcriptionally responsive to a wide variety of oncogenes, growth factors, cytokines, and hormones (Birkedal-Hansen *et al.,* 1993). Cytokines, chemokines, and growth factors appear to play an important role in modulation of MMP secretion in different tissues, especially during inflammation, wound healing, and cancer (Crawford and Matrisian, 1996). For example, interleukin 1α (IL-1α) and tumor necrosis factor-α (TNF-α), generally stimulate cellular production of MMP-1, MMP-3, and MMP-9. Interferon-α (IFN-α), IL-4, IL-6, and IL-10 suppress the production of MMP-9 induced by TNF-α and IL-1α in monocyte-derived macrophages (Saren *et al.,* 1996). However, in cell types other than macrophages, INF-α up-regulates MMP expression. A role for mitogen-activated protein kinases, AP-1, and ETS transcription factors in regulation of MMP gene expression during cancer invasion has been proposed (Westermarck and Kahari, 1999). In contrast,

MMP-2 is reported to be constitutively produced and is not enhanced by most cytokines except for possible induction by TGF-α, IL-8, and insulin-like growth factor receptor (Long *et al.,* 1998). There is also evidence about modulation of mRNA stability in response to growth factors and cytokines (Westermarck and Kahari, 1999).

The MMPs are often sequestered as inactive zymogens in the ECM after secretion, thereby providing a reservoir of latent enzyme positioned for activation and proteolytic attack at focal sites. The most likely docking molecules for MMPs (especially MMP-7) are heparan sulfate proteoglycans on and around epithelial cells and in underlying basement membranes (Yu and Woessner, 2000). Proteolytic processing is required to release the catalytically active enzyme.

2. Activation of MMPs

Classical activation of MMPs is achieved by removal of the N-terminal prosequence of approximately 80 amino acids, which dissociates the single cysteine residue in the propeptide domain from the complex ("Velcro" or "cysteine switch" mechanism) to yield mature enzyme (Birkedal-Hansen *et al.,* 1993). Limited proteolysis of the propeptide destabilizes the cysteine–zinc bond, resulting in opening of the switch. Following opening, autocatalytic or proteolytic cleavage of the remainder of the propeptide yields a truncated and catalytically competent enzyme. Although the physiologic activators of specific MMPs are unknown, the initial cleavage event can be carried out *in vitro* by a variety of serine proteinases, including trypsin, plasma kalekirein, and neutrophil elastase. ProMMP-2 may be an exception to direct serine proteinase activation of MMPs. Plasmin generation at the cell surface is cited as a potential mechanism for the physiologic activation of latent MMP-1, MMP-3, and MMP-9 (Fig. 4). However, data derived from urokinase plasminogen activator (uPA) and tissue plasminogen activator (tPA) knockout mice have not shed evidence on the physiologic significance of this pathway (Lijnen *et al.,* 1998). Some of the activated MMPs can further activate other proMMPs. For example, MMP-3 has been shown to activate proMMP-1 and proMMP-9 (Fig. 4).

MMPs containing a furin-like recognition domain in their propeptides [MMP-11, MMP-23 (Velasco *et al.,* 1999) and MT-MMPs (Sato *et al.,* 1994)] are activated intracellularly in the trans-Golgi network by a group of calcium-dependent transmembrane serine proteinases of the subtilisin group termed furin/PACE/kex-2-like proteinases. In some types of transfected cells, cleavage of the propeptide of MT1-MMP is not required for function as an active enzyme at the cell surface (Cao *et al.,* 1998). The physiologic relevance of this process remains uncertain.

3. Naturally Occurring MMP Inhibitors

Once activated, MMPs are modulated by endogenous proteinase inhibitors, which include TIMPs and α_2-macroglobu-

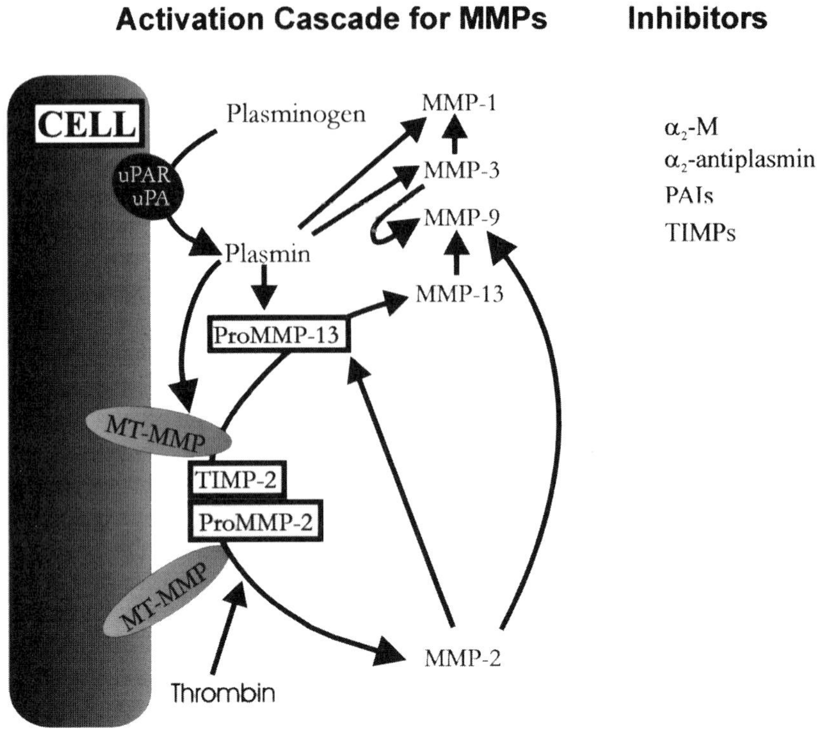

Activation Cascade for MMPs   **Inhibitors**

FIGURE 4   Activation cascade of MMPs on the cell surface.

lin (α_2-M) (Birkedal-Hansen *et al.,* 1993; Stetler-Stevenson, 1999). These negative regulators are important for control of MMP activity with destructive potential. TIMP-1 was first noted in conditioned medium of cultured fibroblasts and in serum where it appeared as a β_1-serum protein that was purified and sequenced. TIMP-2, 3, and 4 were subsequently discovered by protein purification and sequencing methods. These four TIMPs exhibit 44–52% sequence identity and are cross-connected by six disulfide bridges. All of the TIMPs are capable of inhibiting all of the MMPs following formation of tight noncovalent 1:1 complexes. The exception to the general rule is that TIMP-1 appears to be a very poor inhibitor of MT-MMPs attached to the cell surface. All of the TIMPs are soluble proteins that are widely distributed in body fluids except for TIMP-3, which is insoluble and bound to the ECM.

Based on the crystal structure of the MMP-3/TIMP-1 complex, it was demonstrated that TIMP-1 acts as a chelator with the amino N and carbonyl oxygen of Cys-1 chelating the zinc of the active site, while Thr-2 and Val-4 of TIMP-2 access the binding pockets at S1' and S2' (Gomis-Ruth *et al.,* 1997). In addition to binding to the active site of MMPs, the C-terminal domains of TIMP-1 and TIMP-2 form complexes with the C-terminal domains of proMMP-9 and proMMP-2, respectively. These complexes preserve the inhibitory activity of the TIMPs and dampen the activity of the bound MMP. Another consideration in cancer is that TIMPs possess growth-

potentiating activity with several cell types (Corcoran and Stetler-Stevenson, 1995); however, the clinical relevance of these observations remains to be determined. TIMPs also confer resistance to programmed cell death (apoptosis) in malignant B cells through a non-MMP inhibitory pathway (Guedez *et al.,* 1998).

$\alpha 2M$ is a large protein (750 kDa) produced by the liver and present in high concentrations in normal serum. $\alpha 2M$ inhibits all four classes of proteases (serine, cysteine, metallo, aspartyl). Following cleavage by a proteinase, $\alpha 2M$ undergoes a conformational change, trapping the enzyme and sterically blocking its access to protein substrates. $\alpha 2M$ functions primarily in blood where it probably is of less consequence to MMPs since these enzymes are inactive in this location (Zucker *et al.,* 1999).

Finely regulated MMP activity is associated with physiologic processes such as ovulation, trophoblast invasion, mammary involution, and embryonic development. Substantial evidence indicates that inappropriate overexpression of MMPs or underexpression of TIMPs constitutes part of the pathogenic mechanism in several diseases, not limited to cancer. These include destruction of cartilage and bone in rheumatoid arthritis and osteoarthritis, degradation of myelin basic protein in neuroinflammatory diseases (Kieseier *et al.,* 1999), opening of the blood–brain barrier following brain injury (Rosenberg *et al.,* 1998), loss of aortic wall strength in aneurysms, increased matrix turnover in arterial restenonsis lesions (Libby, 1995), and tissue destruction in bullous skin disorders (Liu *et al.,* 1998).

4. Pericellular Activation of MMPs

A pathophysiologically relevant type of MMP activation has been demonstrated for proMMP-2. This mechanism involves stoichiometric binding of TIMP-2 to MT1-MMP on the cell surface followed by the binding of the C-terminal domain of proMMP-2 to the C terminus of TIMP-2, resulting in a trimolecular complex. A second MT1-MMP molecule on the cell surface then cleaves proMMP-2, leaving highly focused active MMP-2 available for efficient substrate degradation and participation in other events (Sato *et al.,* 1994; Strongin *et al.,* 1995; Zucker *et al.,* 1998a). Intermediate-activated MMP-2 can further bind to $\alpha_v\beta_3$ integrin on the cancer or endothelial cell surface (Brooks *et al.,* 1996) and facilitate full autocatalytic maturation of MMP-2. It has been proposed that cross-talk between MT1-MMP and $\alpha_v\beta_3$ integrin enhances proMMP-2 activation at the cell surface and subsequent directional migration of cells. Synthetic MMP inhibitors alter this mechanism by interfering with cleavage and activation of the β_3 integrin subunit (Deryugina *et al.,* 2000). Excess TIMP-2, but not TIMP-1, interferes with this activation mechanism. Pro-MMP-2 associated with integrin-bound collagen may act as a store of enzyme that can feed into the MT1-MMP pathway upon release from the ECM (Ellerbroek and Stack, 1999).

5. Participation of MMPS in Cancer Metastasis

The increased expression of MMPs in advanced tumors and their ability to degrade ECM barriers provided a logical role for these enzymes in cancer dissemination. Most experts in the field have concluded that proteolysis by MMPs is clearly linked to tumor progression (Nelson *et al.,* 2000). However, it cannot be overemphasized that the role of MMPs in human cancer is inferred from model systems. Experimental studies have implicated MMP-2, MMP-9, MT1-MMP, MMP-1, MMP-3, and MMP-7 in cancer invasion and metastasis. Additional support for this concept came from the demonstration that TIMPs were capable of interfering with metastasis in experimental models (Montgomery *et al.,* 1994b).

Because the experimental metastasis assay is dependent on extravasation of tumor cells from the bloodstream and the growth of detectable nodules, it was generally assumed that MMPs were required for the degradation of endothelial cell basement membrane to allow tumor cells to infiltrate lung parenchyma. This view was challenged in studies that used intravital microscopy and quantitative analysis of tumor cell extravasation (Cameron *et al.,* 2000). Mouse melanoma cells transfected with TIMP-1 cDNA resulted in fewer metastatic nodules than control cells but were equally effective at exiting the bloodstream in the chick chorioallantoic membrane. However, the ability of the extravasated cells to grow into

visible tumor nodules was altered by the presence of TIMP-1. These results suggest that MMPs act primarily to alter the extracellular environment to allow sustained growth in an ectopic site as opposed to having a specific role in allowing the cells to extravasate from the blood (Cameron *et al.,* 2000; Chambers and Matrisian, 1997; Nelson *et al.,* 2000). Of interest, normal embryonic fibroblasts can also extravasate from blood vessels, which may not be that surprising considering the other established similarities between embryonic cells and cancer cells. Recent studies support a role for MMPs in tumor cell intravasation (Kim *et al.,* 1998). Using the chick chorioallantoic membrane, human cells capable of invading the bloodstream and circulating to distant sites were quantitated and characterized. The intravasation of human carcinoma cells in a chick embryo model was observed to be dependent on the production of MMP-9 as well as the plasminogen activator system (uPAR). A synthetic inhibitor of MMPs was capable of inhibiting metastasis in this model.

In addition to their effects at metastatic sites, MMPs also contribute to the establishment and growth of primary tumors in their normal environment (orthotopic implantation). For example, human colon cancer cells transfected with MMP-7 cDNA were more tumorigenic when injected into the cecum of nude mice (Nelson *et al.,* 2000); likewise, higher tumorigenicity occurred when human breast cancer cells overexpressing MMP-11 were injected into the mammary fat pad of mice. These experiments further support the concept that MMPs are capable of altering the extracellular environment in a way that enhances experimental cancer cell proliferation and expansion of the tumor. One growth-promoting mechanism could involve the release of latent growth factors from the ECM.

A basic issue in many studies performed to date is the uncertainty of the role of MMPs in the initiation of tissue damage versus their role in the repair mechanisms in disease processes such as inflammation and cancer. Recent data from patients with systemic lupus erythematosus suggest that high blood levels of MMP-3 reflect the repair process rather than the disease process (Zucker *et al.,* 1998b). These data raise the possibility that at certain times the host's MMP response to cancer cell invasion may be an attempt at tissue repair. At that point in the disease, theoretically, the use of an MMP inhibitory drug may have a negative effect. Likewise, it is unclear whether TIMPs are produced in response to increased MMP production or whether they are independently controlled. In this regard, we are only beginning to understand the temporal relationships between MMPs and TIMPs in different diseases.

Another important aspect of MMP and TIMP production in cancer is whether these proteins are produced early or late in the disease. MMP-11 and MMP-7 are present early in tumor development (colon adenomas) at a time when tumors are not known to be invasive or metastatic; this observation suggests that these MMPs may not be involved in metastasis.

6. Stromal Cells Produce Most of the MMPs in Cancer

Based on studies of oncogene-transformed cells, cancer cell lines, and experimental tumors, it has been assumed that cancer cells were responsible for producing the MMPs in human tumors (Liotta, 1992; Nicolson, 1991). However, the seminal report of Basset et al. (1990) in 1990 changed our way of thinking about MMPs in cancer. They reported that MMP-11 was produced by stromal fibroblasts surrounding tumor cell foci, not by tumor cells in human breast cancers. MMP-11 expression was detected in the stromal compartment of epithelial carcinomas of both glandular and stratified origin. Furthermore, MMP-11 knockout mice demonstrated reduced tumor formation in a skin model of tumor progression, which confirms the importance of stromal MMPs.

Using *in situ* hybridization to identify messenger RNA (mRNA) in tissue, most investigators have described human tumor localization (breast, colorectal, lung, prostate, and ovarian) of MMP-1, MMP-2, MMP-3, MMP-7, MMP-11, and MT1-MMP primarily in stromal fibroblasts, especially in proximity to invading cancer cells, but not in the cancer cells themselves (Nelson et al., 2000). The expression pattern of the MT1-MMP gene was similar to that of the MMP-2 gene, which is consistent with the role of MT1-MMP as the activator for proMMP-2 (Polette and Birembaut, 1998). MMP-9 has often been localized to inflammatory cells (macrophages and neutrophils), rather than fibroblasts or tumor cells in colorectal cancer tissue. However, related studies by other groups have reported localization of these MMP mRNAs in pancreatic and prostatic cancer cells (Still et al., 2000) and brain cancer cells rather than stromal cells. It has also been pointed out that MMPs are expressed in the malignant epithelium of tumors that have undergone an epithelial to mesenchymal transformation (Nelson et al., 2000).

Subtypes of TIMPs are expressed in a different spatial pattern than MMPs. TIMP-1 mRNA has been detected in both cancer and surrounding stromal cells in several tumors. The pattern of TIMP-2 expression seems to be similar to that of MMP-2 and found only in limited numbers of stromal cells near invasive cancer cells and not in tumor cells. However, immunolocalization studies that identify proteins using specific antibodies, rather than mRNA expression, have generally identified MMP-2 and MMP-9 protein in cancer cells. These data reinforce the concept that tumor cells have receptors that bind stromal-cell-secreted MMPs. In this regard, MMP-9 was reported to bind with moderate affinity to collagen type IV components on the surface of cells (Olson et al., 1998) and to CD-44 (Yu and Stamenkovic, 2000). However, the issue of whether neoplastic epithelial cells produce low levels (not detected by *in situ* hybridization) of MMP-2 and MT1-MMP in human cancer tissue remains incompletely resolved. Discrepancies between immunohistochemistry and *in situ* hybridization studies may be related to the specificity of the reagents employed.

MMP-7 represents the major exception to the generalization that fibroblasts and inflammatory cells produce the MMPs in a tumor as its expression and protein localization have been identified in neoplastic epithelial cells in human colorectal cancer tissue and not in stromal cells (Nelson et al., 2000). MMP-7 has also been identified in reactive tissues unrelated to cancer, which emphasizes the clinical limitations of MMP measurements. Recent data suggest that MMP-7 cleavage of Fas ligand is an important mediator of epithelial cell apoptosis (Powell et al., 1999). Extrapolation of this information to prostate cancer cells suggests that MMP-7 may exert an anticancer effect.

7. Stromal Cell–Tumor Cell Cross-talk: Role of EMMPRIN

An explanation for the dominant production of MMPs by reactive stromal cells in a tumor rather than the tumor cells themselves comes from the discovery by Biswas et al. (1995) of *e*xtracellular *m*atrix *m*etallo*p*roteinase *in*ducer, EMMPRIN. EMMPRIN is an intrinsic plasma membrane glycoprotein purified initially from cancer cells that stimulates fibroblasts to synthesize and secrete MMP-1, MMP-2, and MMP-3. Tumor cell interactions with fibroblasts via EMMPRIN leads to fibroblast-induced local degradation of interstitial and basement membrane matrix components, thus facilitating tumor cell invasion. On examination of human lung and breast cancer tissue, EMMPRIN expression in cancer cells far exceeds that of normal epithelial cells (Polette et al., 1997). Recently, it has been demonstrated that MMP-1 can bind to EMMPRIN on the cell surface, thus indicating that following EMMPRIN stimulation of MMP synthesis in fibroblasts, a surface localized MMP-1/EMMPRIN complex arms the cancer cell for degradation of the ECM (Guo et al., 2000a) (Fig. 5).

Cell–cell contacts have also been shown to result in MMP-9 activation. Fibroblasts cocultured with carcinoma cells show induction of MMP-9 synthesis in the fibroblasts. This effect required direct cell–cell contacts implicating a cell surface factor (Segain et al., 1996). In a mouse tumor model, metastatic tumors originating from non-MMP-9-producing transformed cells induced MMP-9 synthesis in the tumor stroma (Himelstein et al., 1994). Soluble stimulators of MMP-9 production have also been described but not purified.

Bidirectional signaling pathways between cancer cells and stromal cells leading to enhanced MMP synthesis have been described. The intercellular adhesion molecule-1/LFA-1 interaction by direct cell contact with endothelial cells induces MMP-9 production by T-lymphoma cells (Aoudjit et al., 1998).

A novel host–tumor cell interaction which requires activation of MMP-1 by a proteolytic cascade involving serine proteinases and MMP-3 has also been described (Benbow et al., 1999). Degradation of collagen types I and III in the ECM and tumor cell invasion follows thereafter.

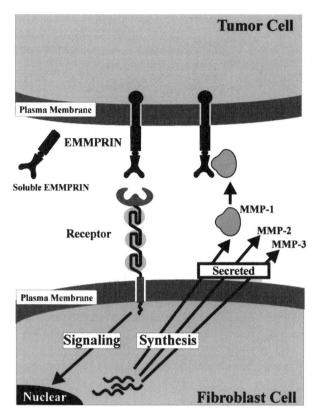

FIGURE 5 EMMPRIN enhances cellular expression of MMPs.

8. MMPs Involved in Tumor Angiogenesis

A role for MMPs in tumor neoangiogenesis has been established for both growth of the initial tumor and distant metastases. MMPs are required for vascular endothelial cells to penetrate their underlying basement membrane in order to produce new capillary sprouts (Haas and Madri, 1999; Stetler-Stevenson, 1999). Based on studies in knockout mice, MT1-MMP appears to be important in selected aspects of neonatal angiogenesis (Holmbeck *et al.,* 1999; Zhou *et al.,* 2000). MMP-2 angiogenic activity is involved in later life. The requirement of MMP-2 activity for tumor angiogenesis has been demonstrated by studies using MMP-2 knockout mice. Tumor cells that are injected into these mice have reduced growth rates, and the tumors that develop are less vascularized than tumors derived from cells introduced in control animals (Itoh *et al.,* 1998). Furthermore, application of a blocking peptide that prevents the interaction of MMP-2 with its substrates has been shown to reduce angiogenesis (Brooks *et al.,* 1998). Suppression of MMP-2 activity by antisense oligonucleotides resulted in loss of angiogenic potential in the chick chorioallantoic membrane assay and decreased tumor growth in a rat tumor model (Fang *et al.,* 2000). In addition, VEGF can indirectly activate MMP-2 in endothelial cells (in the presence of coagulation factors) by the mechanism

of induction of tissue factor synthesis leading to thrombin-induced activation of pro-MMP-2 on the cell surface (Zucker *et al.,* 1995a, 1998c) (Fig. 4).

9. MMP Interaction with Integrins and Growth Factors

Interactions between cell integrins and the ECM trigger signal transduction cascades that affect a variety of cellular functions, including cell survival, proliferation, differentiation, and migration. Thus, the ECM is not static; cells receive cues about their external environment through their attachments to the matrix in order to modulate their response to environmental fluctuations (McCawley and Matrisian, 2000). Degradation of the ECM perturbs some of these signals by destroying the attachment site. Certain attachment sites are hidden or cryptic in the full-length, uncleaved molecule. These sites may become unmasked by loosening the tightly embedded ECM to reveal a site previously prevented from interacting with cell-surface integrin receptors. One such attachment site has been experimentally revealed on melanoma cells by MMP-2 degradation of the collagen matrix (McCawley and Matrisian, 2000; Montgomery *et al.,* 1994a). Likewise, the β_4 integrin was shown to be fragmented in response to MMP-7 activity, indicating that MMPs can cleave matrix receptors in addition to matrix itself (McCawley and Matrisian, 2000).

Cleavage of matrix components also releases polypeptide fragments with new biological properties, as well as releasing signaling components embedded within the matrix. For example, cleavage of full-length laminin-5 (a component of the ECM that promotes cell attachment) by MMP-2 promotes migration of cells (Giannelli *et al.,* 1997). A number of soluble growth factors are secreted and stored in an inactive form bound to ECM molecules. During enhanced proteolysis, these factors are then freed to act on their target receptors. MMP-3 has been shown to cleave the matrix molecule decorin, resulting in the release of TGF-β in its more biologically active form (Imai *et al.,* 1997). MMP-3 also cleaves and releases the soluble-heparin-binding EGF that has proliferative and angiogenic properties. Furthermore, receptors for growth factors are targeted for proteolysis by MMPs; these include FGF type I receptor, which mediates the effects of fibroblast growth factor, IL-1β, and insulin-like growth factor (IGF)–binding proteins (for review, see McCawley and Matrisian, 2000). IGF-binding protein-1 has also been identified as a potential physiologic substrate for MMP-11. Although IGF-binding proteins can confer latency on IGF-I and IGF-II, their degradation can restore the activity of these growth factors, thereby affecting tumor growth (Noel *et al.,* 1997).

10. Metastasis Explored by Gene-Targeting Experiments

Gene-targeting experiments in mice provide an unique *in vivo* model system to study both tumor and tumor–stromal interactions affecting various stages of tumor progression. Studies with transgenic mice that overexpress individual MMPs have revealed an effect of MMPs on initial tumor establishment and growth. For example, a transgenic mouse model with overexpression of MMP-3 was reported to exhibit enhanced breast tumorigenesis resulting from alterations at multiple stages of tumor progression (Sternlicht *et al.,* 1999). Overproduction of MMP-3 led to cleavage of E-cadherin and thus to breakdown of interactions between epithelial cells. Loss of E-cadherin function allows transcriptional activation of MMP-7, which sets in motion additional remodeling events (Lochter *et al.,* 1997). Conversely, rates of tumorigenesis are reduced in certain genetic backgrounds by deletion of MMP-3. Furthermore, in some cases, the effects of MMPs on growth extends to benign as well as malignant tumors. Overexpression of MMP-7 in transgenic mice led to enhanced tumorigenesis in a mouse breast cancer model (Nelson *et al.,* 2000). Likewise, overexpression of MMP-13 led to enhanced tumor formation in a chemically induced model of skin tumorigenesis (D'Armiento *et al.,* 1995). In other experiments, the number of developing adenomas was reduced in MMP-7-null mice that were crossed with mice carrying a mutation in the adenomatous polyposis coli gene that predisposed them to multiple intestinal neoplasms (multiple intestinal neoplasm mutation APC^{min}) (Nelson *et al.,* 2000). Similarly, MMP-11-deficient mice demonstrate impaired tumor formation in response to chemical carcinogenesis. It was concluded that although MMP-11 is made by surrounding stromal fibroblasts, it contributes to the establishment and growth of breast cancer cells (Masson *et al.,* 1998). The importance of MMP-12 in limiting lung metastasis has been confirmed by the use of mice rendered deficient in MMP-12. These experimental models suggest that MMP inhibitors may be effective at inhibiting early stages of tumor progression and possibly may be useful as chemoprotective agents (see discussions by Nelson *et al.,* 2000; Shapiro, 1998). Furthermore, MMP activity appears to influence tumor progression whether the source of the MMP is the tumor or the stroma. An interesting observation requiring further study is that local expression of MMP-12 in macrophages surrounding secondary lung metastasis actually limits growth, in part through generation of angiostatin, the plasminogen degradation product inhibitor of angiogenesis (Shapiro, 1998).

Knockout mice that lack MMP-9 show a failure of vascularization and apoptosis in the skeletal growth plate early in development. When these mice are crossed with animals in which expression of MMP-9 coincides with activation of an angiogenic switch during tumor formation, loss of MMP-9 results in suppression of tumorigenesis (Vu *et al.,* 1998).

Knockout mice lacking MT1-MMP have profound skeletal deformities, including craniofacial dysmorphism, osteopenia, dwarfism, and fibrosis of soft tissues due to ablation of a collagenolytic activity that is essential for modeling of connective tissues; a role for MT1-MMP in skeletal angiogenesis is suspected (Holmbeck *et al.,* 1999; Zhou *et al.,* 2000). Future studies of tumorigenesis and metastasis in MT1-MMP-deficient mouse models will be of considerable interest in terms of defining the role of stromal MT1-MMP in cancer.

11. MMP and TIMP Levels as Prognostic Markers of Tumors

A positive correlation between tumor progression and the expression of multiple MMP family members (MMP-11, MMP-2, MMP-9, MMP-7, MMP-1, MT1-MMP) in tumor tissues has been demonstrated in numerous human and animal studies. For example, MT1-MMP mRNA and protein were not present in normal human brain but were readily detected in malignant astrocytomas. MT1-MMP expression functions as an independent prognostic factor in patients with gastric cancer and cervical carcinoma (see Ellerbroek and Stack, 1999) for discussion. The ratio of activated to total MMP levels, especially MMP-2, has also been correlated with tumor aggressiveness (Brown *et al.,* 1993; Davies *et al.,* 1993). If confirmed in carefully controlled clinical studies, these observations may provide important prognostic information (Michael *et al.,* 1999) that could help direct therapeutic recommendations, including the possibility of targeting drugs that inhibit MMPs for specific patients who display high levels of MMPs. It is of interest that in human cancer tissue increased TIMP-1 levels have been associated with poor prognosis (Lu *et al.,* 1991).

Several years ago, Zucker *et al.* (1993b) proposed that tissue MMPs may leach into the bloodstream in increased amounts in patients with aggressive cancer and thereby provide unique markers for metastatic disease. They demonstrated that MMP-9 and MMP-9:TIMP-1 complexes are increased in the plasma of patients with colorectal cancer and breast cancer as compared with healthy controls. When results from both plasma MMP-9 and MMP-9:TIMP-1 complexes were combined in patients with stage IV colorectal cancer, patients with increased levels of either or both tests had significantly shorter mean survival than patients with normal levels (4 months vs. 20 months, respectively) (Zucker *et al.,* 1995b). It was proposed that these assays may be clinically useful in predicting prognosis in patients with gastrointestinal cancer. However, it is important to note that a major limitation to clinical measurement of MMPs in cancer is that plasma and tissue levels of MMPs are increased in some benign conditions (e.g., inflammatory diseases) and normal physiologic states (e.g., pregnancy) (Zucker *et al.,* 1999).

8. MMPIs as Novel Anticancer Agents

Insight into the pathophysiology of cancer metastasis and rapid advances in our general understanding of the molecular biology of cancer have encouraged the pharmaceutical industry to begin to design new classes of drugs that interfere with specific aspects of cancer progression. Commercial concerns have risen to deliver candidate drugs for clinical development faster than ever before. Based on the principle that local cancer invasion and distant metastasis require cancer cells to release proteolytic enzymes that digest surrounding connective tissues, the pharmaceutical industry has invested hundreds of millions of dollars in trying to develop safe and effective protease inhibitors as treatment for metastasis. A primary focus for this effort has been the MMP class. Industrial interest in inhibition of the plasminogen activator system as a cancer treatment modality has lagged behind because of the uncertainty of the role of plasmin in cancer (see Section 10).

A. Design of MMPIs

Modern cancer drug development is moving beyond cytotoxic compounds detected by random screening to identifying small molecules and genes targeted to the specific molecular abnormalities that create and drive the malignant phenotype. The rational design of potent MMP inhibitors is an example of this process. Initially, drugs were targeted to the chemical functional group that chelates the active site zinc(II) ion, which is a ubiquitous feature of MMPs. Biochemical studies using collagen-like substrates have shown that six amino acids are required for the proteolytic activity of MMPs. The MMP catalytic domain consists of six subsites spanning locations S3 to S3'. Peptide and peptide-like compounds have been designed that combine backbone features (P1, P1', P2', P3' regions) that would favorably interact with the enzyme subsites (S1, S1', S2', S3' pockets) and functionality capable of binding zinc (chelator) in the catalytic site (Borkakoti, 1998; Gomis-Ruth et al., 1997; Grams et al., 1995). The S1' site is the most prominent pocket in the MMP catalytic domain. These drugs essentially mimic the collagen substrate of MMPs and thereby work as competitive, potent, but reversible inhibitors of enzyme activity (Fig. 6).

Early MMPIs were peptide derivatives designed on the basis of the sequence around the glycine-isoleucine and glycine-leucine in the collagen α chain which is cleaved by collagenases. Typically, the zinc-binding group was incorporated into peptide analogues of the sequence on either the left side or right side ("primed binding region") or both sides of the cleavage site (Fig. 6). Other workers followed the approach of screening compound libraries and/or natural products, and identified novel compounds that are structurally related to inhibitors obtained by substrate-based design (Brown and Whittaker, 1999).

1. Broad- vs. Narrow-Spectrum MMP Inhibitors

Medicinal chemists have been faced with the decision of whether to design broad-spectrum or selective inhibitors of MMPs. Selective inhibitors should provide greater specificity and therefore more safety than broad-spectrum MMP inhibitors. On the other hand, experimental studies have revealed that several of the MMP family members are coexpressed in different types of cancer, thereby making it difficult to identify a single MMP as being critical to the disease process. It has been found that acceptable pharmacokinetics can be more readily obtained for nonpeptidic compounds than pseudopeptide MMPIs (Brown and Whittaker, 1999). The structures of some of the more important compounds of current interest are shown in Fig. 7. A detailed description of

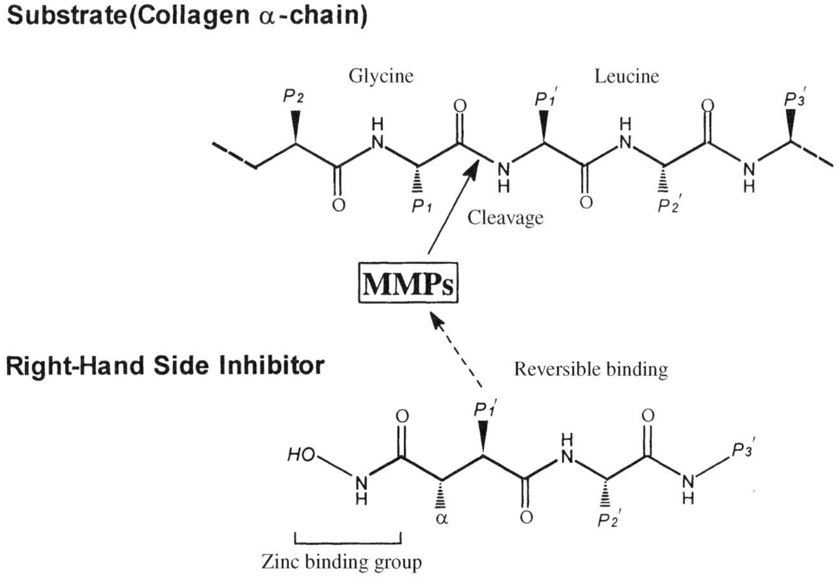

FIGURE 6 Structure of a generic right-hand-side inhibitor of MMPs.

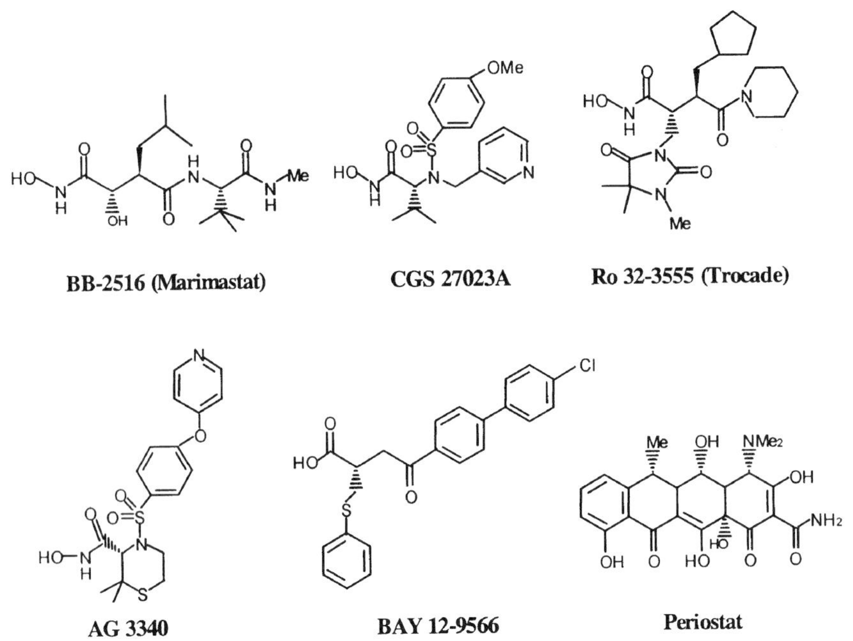

BB-2516 (Marimastat)   **CGS 27023A**   **Ro 32-3555 (Trocade)**

AG 3340   **BAY 12-9566**   **Periostat**

FIGURE 7   Structures of MMP inhibitors that have reached the clinic.

inhibitor-binding characteristics has been published (Borkakoti, 1998).

MMPIs that featured a hydroxamic acid zinc-binding group were initially identified as highly potent compounds in *in vitro* studies. Based on this finding, the majority of inhibitors currently in clinical testing have been designed with this functional group. X-ray crystallography studies have demonstrated that the hydroxamate acts as a bidentate ligand, with each oxygen an optimal distance from the active site zinc(II) ion. The position of the hydroxamate nitrogen suggests that it is protonated and forms a hydrogen bond with a carbonyl oxygen of the enzyme backbone in several MMPs (Grams *et al.*, 1995). The moderate pK_a of the hydroxamic acid moiety ($pK_a \sim 8$) helps maintain key H-bonding interactions with a critical glutamic acid moiety in the catalytic domain of MMPs.

Early examples of these compounds included the pseudopeptide hydroxamic acid MMP inhibitors Galardin Glycomed) and Batimastat (British Biotech), which showed broad specificity in their inhibition of members of the MMP family while displaying minimal activity against other classes of metalloproteinases, such as angiotensin-converting enzyme and enkephalinase (Brown and Whittaker, 1999). Concerns about the unfavorable pharmacokinetics (poor oral bioavailability and rapid clearance) of early designed hydroxamates, as well as concerns over the potential for chronic toxicities arising from metabolic activation of the hydroxamate group, instigated extensive investigation into alternative zinc ligands (carboxylate, phosphinate, sulfodiimine, and thiolate groups) (Babine and Bender, 1997).

It was later found that specific enzyme recognition and thus selectivity (e.g., MMP-3 vs. MMP-1) could be obtained by structural modification of the P1′ (primary) and P2′/P3′ region(s), taking advantage of distinctions in the depth and composition of the S1′, S2′, and S3′ pockets of individual MMPs. The nature, extent, position, and orientation of these backbone modifications exert a substantial effect on enzyme recognition (Beckett and Whittaker, 1998). Structural modification of the pseudopeptide hydroxamic acid derivatives resulted in the discovery by Celltech scientists that a degree of enzyme selectivity could be obtained with the introduction of large P1′ substituents (Porter *et al.*, 1994). The British Biotech group discovered that the combination of certain substituents gave orally active, broad-spectrum compounds. The combination of an α-hydroxy group with *tert*-butylglycine at P2′ as in Marimastat (Fig. 7) was particularly advantageous since it likely reduced the compound's susceptibility to peptidases leading to improved bioavailability (Brown and Whittaker, 1999). A structurally distinct series of nonpeptide MMP-3-directed inhibitors was developed by Novartis, resulting in the orally active compound CGS 27023 (Chin *et al.*, 1998). This series of compounds led to a flurry of activity marking the genesis of a new era of MMPI design (Skotnicki *et al.*, 1999). In this regard, workers at Agouron used a structure-based inhibitor design program that employed high-resolution x-ray crystallography. Crystallography of MMP inhibitor–enzyme complexes has confirmed the binding modes for inhibitors, and together with homology modeling, provided insight into differences in the active site for the different MMPs. Further exploration of the P1′ pocket by the

Agouron team led to the discovery of potent inhibitors that are selective for deep-pocket (MMP-2, MMP-3, MMP-8, MMP-9, MMP-13, and MT1-MMP) over the shallow-pocket enzymes (MMP-1 and MMP-7). Orally active AG3340 was developed using this approach with the hope that sparing MMP-1, which may be responsible for the side effect of arthralgias, would increase the therapeutic index of MMPIs (Shalinsky *et al.*, 1999). Another approach to lessen arthralgias has been to spare the inhibition of sheddases by MMPIs; BMS-275291 (also known as D-2163; Chiroscience R&D Ltd.) was designed to test this hypothesis. These hypotheses are controversial, and supportive preclinical data are sparse.

In related studies, a group at Roche found that the P2′ amino acid could be replaced by a nitrogen heterocycle, and potent activity against MMP-1 and MMP-8 could be maintained if a cyclic imide group was introduced at P1. The orally active hydantoin derivative Ro 32-3555 was identified for treatment of arthritis by this approach (Brown and Whittaker, 1999). Roche scientists have recently demonstrated selectivity of a diphenylether series of inhibitors that are largely determined by their affinity for the preformed S1′ pocket of MMP-13 as compared to the induced fit in MMP-1 (Lovejoy *et al.*, 1999).

2. Nonhydroxamic Acid Inhibitors

The search for alternative zinc-binding groups other than the hydroxamic acid moiety has been driven by considerations of toxicity and intellectual property (Brown and Whittaker, 1999). It was felt that introduction of appropriate high-affinity (P1′ to S1′; P2′ to S2′) substituents on the peptide backbone might compensate for the resulting diminished chelating capacity and yield potent compounds. A comparative study of different zinc-binding groups has suggested the following preference in terms of inhibition of MMP-1: hydroxamate > formylhydroxlamine > sulfhydryl > phosphinate > aminocarboxylate > carboxylate structural types. Scientists at Affymax and Wyeth-Ayerst described the rationale for the design and synthesis of peptide-like mercaptoalcohols and mercaptoketones as the replacement for the hydroxamic acid group. The inhibitory potency of these analogues versus MMP-1 proved to be relatively independent of the size of the P1′ group, while MMP-3 inhibitory activity was significantly improved for the longer heptyl side chain analogues. The isobutyl derivatives are potent and selective MMP-1 inhibitors, while the heptyl series provides more broad-spectrum inhibition of MMPs (Skotnicki *et al.*, 1999). The impact of combinatorial chemistry technology on future MMPI design is anxiously awaited (Szardenings *et al.*, 1999).

B. Preclinical Trials of MMPIs in Cancer

Preclinical studies must demonstrate that a candidate agent selected for clinical development acts by the desired molecular mechanism (inhibition of MMPs) to produce the desired biological effect (delay or reverse cancer progression). Therefore, traditional end points, such as simple tumor cell killing or tumor growth delay, are not sufficient for contemporary needs. Replacing "black box" approaches with suitable surrogate markers has put greater demands on tumor biologists and pharmacologists (Gelmon *et al.*, 1999).

One attractive aspect of inhibiting MMP activity in cancer is that the target of the anticancer therapy will include components produced by nonmalignant cells in the tumor stroma; these cells presumably will not mutate and develop drug resistance. In contrast, malignant cells are highly genetically unstable, so the therapies that target these cells can result in tumor cell modifications that render them resistant to therapy (McCawley and Matrisian, 2000).

In the next section, preclinical studies of selected MMPIs will be described in greater detail. Other effective MMPIs (i.e., Ro 32-3555), which were designed with selectivity for treatment of arthritis (MMP-1, MMP-8, MMP-13 rather than MMP-3, MMP-2, MMP-9), will not be described further (Brewster *et al.*, 1998).

1. Batimastat and Marimastat (British Biotech Pharmaceuticals, Ltd.)

Numerous studies with MMPIs as drugs in cancer models have examined their ability to block experimental metastasis using the organ colonization approach. It is still too early to tell whether syngeneic (tumor and host are from the same species) or human tumor xenografts (human cells implanted in mice) will be predictive of MMPI responses in human cancer.

Batimastat, the most widely studied MMPI in animal models, and the orally effective marimastat have IC_{50} for MMP-1, MMP-2, MMP-7, MMP-9, and MMP-12 ranging between 3 and 16 nM. Marked inhibition of metastasis was demonstrated initially using batimastat in the treatment of mice inoculated with B16 murine melanoma or transformed rat fibroblasts. Animals treated with a short (7-day) course of batimastat developed significantly fewer lung metastases than mice receiving a vehicle control, but approximately half of these animals eventually developed local and distant lymph node metastases (Brown and Whittaker, 1999). Studies in syngeneic murine models suggested that the initiation of batimastat when tumor burden was minimal has a more profound effect on tumor growth inhibition than initiation of treatment at the time of large tumor bulk (Eccles *et al.*, 1996). Thus, early and prolonged treatment with MMPIs may result in sustained tumor-free survival. Batimastat also inhibited endothelioma cell invasion *in vitro* through an ECM substrate (Matrigel), which suggested an inhibitory effect on tumor angiogenesis (Taraboletti *et al.*, 1995).

The use of concurrent versus sequential administration of synthetic MMPIs with cytotoxic agents in early-stage tumors has also been addressed. Survival after implantation of human ovarian xenografts in nude mice was extended threefold in mice treated sequentially with cisplatin followed by batimastat, whereas survival was considerably shorter in mice treated with each single agent. The most dramatic effect was seen in mice treated with a combination of cisplatin and batimastat (Giavazzi *et al.*, 1998). The synergistic effect of combining MMP inhibition (batimastat) with cytotoxic chemotherapy (gemcitabine) has been demonstrated in a murine model of human pancreatic cancer (Haq *et al.*, 2000). Other studies demonstrated that batimastat inhibited the growth of human carcinomas established as xenografts in nude mice by orthotopic implantation in the organ equivalent to the human primary site, i.e., colorectal cancer cells injected into the spleen of mice (An *et al.*, 1997; Brown and Whittaker, 1999). Effects on tumor angiogenesis have varied depending on the experimental model (Sledge *et al.*, 1995).

Batimastat has also been tested in a mouse model of pancreatic islet cell angiogenesis and multistage tumor progression. Three trials were performed, including (1) a prevention trial in which the MMPI was given when tumor nodules had not progressed beyond the stage of carcinoma *in situ*, (2) an intervention trial in which treatment was given when small tumors were present, and (3) a regression trial in which the ability of the drug to extend life span by inducing the regression of large tumors was determined. Batimastat produced a 49% reduction in angiogenesis in the prevention trial and an 83% reduction in tumor burden in the intervention trial, but demonstrated no effect on large, invasive tumors (Bergers *et al.*, 1999). This latter observation needs to be invoked in analyzing clinical trial results of MMPIs employed in advanced human malignancies (see Section 8.D below).

2. CT1746 (Celltech Inc.)

CT1746 is a relatively selective MMPI with enhanced activity against MMP-2 (K_i = 0.04 nM), MMP-9, and MT-MMPs. This compound reduced primary tumor growth rates and localized both spread and spontaneous metastasis even when the treatment was commenced several days after tumor implantation. The requirement for administering the MMPI early in the protocol was proposed to be consistent with an MMP-2/MMP-9 requirement in early metastatic events. CT1746 had a modest effect as a single agent in inhibiting the growth and metastasis of murine Lewis lung carcinoma but provided marked additive effects when used in combination with cisplatin or cyclophosphamide (Anderson *et al.*, 1996). In another study, CT1746 had no effect on spontaneous metastasis in tumors in which inhibitor treatment caused modest reduction in primary tumor growth. These data argue against an obligatory role of MMPs in this spontaneous metastasis model, as compared to the experimental metastasis model (Conway *et al.*, 1996). Clinical trials using CT1746 have not been initiated.

3. AG3340 (Agouron Pharmaceuticals)

Workers at Agouron have reported extensive testing of the effects of AG3340 (Prinomastat) in various tumor models. AG3340 was developed with selective specificity and potency (K_i values of 0.05–0.3 nM) for MMP-2, MMP-3, MMP-9, MMP-13, and MT1-MMP because these MMPs were considered the most relevant targets for oncology indications. In comparison, AG3340 inhibited the enzymatic activities of MMP-1 and MMP-7 approximately 150- and 1000-fold less potently, respectively, than MMP-2 (Shalinsky *et al.*, 1999). AG3340 was active against many human tumors in immunodeficient mice, as well as the Lewis lung carcinoma and murine B16-F10 melanoma (in combination with chemotherapy) in syngeneic metastasis models. In studies employing colon tumors, oral AG3340 (administered twice daily beginning 5 days after tumor implantation and continued for about 50 days) resulted in approximately 80% lower tumor volumes; profound tumor growth delays of about 10–30 days were noted. Similar effectiveness of AG3340 was noted with non-small cell lung cancer, gliomas, breast cancer, and prostate cancer (Shalinsky *et al.*, 1999). In two of these models, AG3340 administration resulted in increased animal survival. AG3340 treatment also increased the extent of apoptosis in tumors. Human xenograft tumors retained sensitivity to AG3340 after extended treatment and serial passage *in vivo*. In gastric cancer, AG3340 did not inhibit tumor growth but potentiated the efficacy of paclitaxel. Of importance in planning human drug trials, the antitumor efficacy of AG3340 in mice was associated with maintaining minimum effective plasma concentrations of AG3340 and was independent of the total daily dose, peak plasma concentration, and drug exposure (Shalinsky *et al.*, 1998, 1999).

Histologic examination of cancer tissues of animals treated with MMPIs has revealed varied results ranging from increased fibrotic stroma or capsule formation to little evidence of change other than the tumors being smaller in treated animals; other tumors have shown enlarged necrotic centers, which may be an indication of increased hydrostatic pressure (Brown and Whittaker, 1999). Importantly, AG3340 markedly decreased tumor angiogenesis and cell proliferation by more than 50% and increased tumor necrosis and apoptosis more than twofold. It was therefore concluded that the antitumor efficacy of AG3340 was due, at least in part, to an inhibition in tumor blood supply. The lack of permanent suppression of tumor growth across animal models and the recognition that other factors are involved in neoplastic progression support the use of AG3340 in combination chemotherapy (Shalinsky *et al.*, 1999).

4. BAY12-9566 (Bayer Corporation)

BAY12-9566 is a novel, nonpeptidic biphenyl MMPI with a zinc-binding carboxyl group that is structurally distinct from other MMPIs (Fig. 7). BAY12-9566 is more selective for MMP-2, MMP-9, MMP-11, MMP-13, and MT1-MMP with IC_{50} ranging between 6 and 13 nM and has a very long terminal plasma half-life (90–100 h), but also has an extremely high plasma protein binding fraction ($>$99.99%). By contrast, AG3340 and marimastat are 70–80% protein bound. BAY 12-9566 has shown anti-invasive, antimetastatic, and antiangiogenic activity (Gatto et al., 1999) in several experimental tumor models, including murine melanoma and lung cancer. After removal of the primary human breast cancer in nude mice, BAY12-9566 resulted in inhibition of tumor regrowth, reduction in pulmonary metastasis, and decrease in volume of metastasis. Initiation of BAY12-9566 5 days after implantation of a human colon cancer cell line resulted in a decrease in both tumor growth and metastasis (see Nelson et al., 2000).

5. Tetracycline Derivatives as MMPIs

Another category of anticancer agents that function in part as inhibitors of MMPs are tetracycline derivatives (Golub et al., 1994). The activity of MMP-8 and MMP-13 in degrading type II collagen was recently shown to be inhibited by more than 50% by 30 μM doxycycline, a concentration achievable in serum after oral dosing (Smith et al., 1999). Tetracyclines may function by disrupting the hemopexin domain of MMP-13 and the catalytic domain of MMP-8. Chemically modified tetracyclines (CMTs) that lack antibacterial activity, especially CMT-3 (6-deoxy, 6-methyl, 4-dedimethylaminotetracycline), have demonstrated activity against prostate cancer in animal models. CMT-3 also inhibits tumor cell invasion in vitro and interferes with cell proliferation by a poorly understood mechanism. When tested in a rat prostate cancer model, oral CMT-3 and doxycycline reduced lung metastasis by more than 50% (Lokeshwar, 1999). Tetracyclines (e.g., Periostat) also interfere with MMP expression in endothelial cells and, hence, may exert an antiangiogenic effect (Hanemaaijer et al., 1998). The effect of tetracyclines in vivo also involves down-regulation of MMP mRNA and protein expression.

C. Potential Negative Effects of MMPIs in Cancer

There are aspects of MMP function that are potentially beneficial in slowing tumor progression. In such cases, MMPIs may be potentially harmful if they interfere with the body's natural mechanism to thwart cancer. For example, it has been observed in integrin α_1-null mice, as a result of a deficiency in the activation of the Ras/Shc/MAPK pathway, the synthesis of MMP-7 and MMP-9 in endothelial cells was markedly increased. Based on the capacity of these MMPs to cleave plasminogen and produce the angiogenesis inhibitor angiostatin, tumors implanted in mice producing high levels of MMPs showed decreased tumor vascularity and smaller tumors in comparison with their wild-type counterparts (Pozzi et al., 2000).

D. Design of Clinical Trials

The development and clinical testing of new drugs by the pharmaceutical industry is a long and challenging process, especially with regard to MMPIs. Since MMPIs do not kill cancer cells, the traditional cytotoxic developmental and testing strategy is inappropriate. Clinical trials will likely require long-term treatment with MMPIs; minimal side effects and easy administration schedules will be needed so as not to limit drug compliance.

A key issue that medical scientists have yet to address is whether spontaneous cancers developing in humans will respond to antimetastatic/antiangiogenic drugs in a similar way to drug responses in experimental models. In other words, do experimental models of cancer dissemination accurately reflect human pathophysiology?

Guidelines for development of human trials for testing MMPIs in cancer were published in 1994 (Zucker, 1994). These included (1) selecting cancer types that have a high probability of metastasis in spite of standard local treatment (surgery/radiotherapy) directed at the primary tumor; (2) selecting cancer types with high levels of MMPs (in situ hybridization or immunohistochemistry of human tumors); (3) treating patients with the best standard treatment modality (chemotherapy/radiotherapy/surgery) prior to or simultaneously with an MMPI; (4) initiating treatment soon after diagnosis, prior to the development of metastases, and continuing treatment until the likelihood of metastasis is diminished (a difficult end point to estimate); (5) monitoring and tailoring drug dosage and schedule to achieve tissue levels that have been demonstrated to have the desired inhibitory effect on MMPs. It should be recognized that lack of an effect of an MMPI in advanced cancer may not be indicative of results achievable in earlier disease. Experimental data implicating an MMP requirement for the switch to an angiogenic tumor phenotype emphasizes the need for early intervention with an MMPI (Fang et al., 2000).

The first MMPIs began animal trials in 1993 and clinical trials in patients in 1997. Four of these MMPIs (marimastat, AG3340, CSG27023A, and Bay 12-9566) are currently being evaluated as treatment for patients with advanced cancers with the hope of controlling cancer progression. Phase I trial design incorporates the evaluation of safety and toxicity with some measure of potential outcome. It is recognized that the only way to demonstrate disease-modifying activity is with large, well-designed, randomized clinical trials, using end points of increased overall survival, progression-free survival, and/or time to disease progression (Rasmussen, 1999).

The pharmaceutical industry has worked to develop guidelines for phase II trials with an attempt at identification of biological markers that could be used to assess the therapeutic potential of a drug as well as being able to identify the optimal biological dose (Rasmussen, 1999). With MMPIs, once complete enzyme inhibition is achieved, no further activity would be expected and it would be inappropriate to continue to increase the dose with the likelihood of additional toxicity with no added benefit. Consequently, the purpose of the phase I–II program with a drug of this class should be to identify the optimal biological dose rather than the maximal tolerable dose. Furthermore, in a traditional cytotoxic developmental program, tumor responses in terms of complete response, partial response, stable disease, and progressive disease are the measurement cornerstones. Although preclinical models have demonstrated that MMPIs can delay growth and metastasis of the primary tumor, the primary impact of MMPIs has not been substantial regression of primary tumors. Given the limitation of secondary end points of response, clinical development of MMPIs has rapidly proceeded to phase III trial design with the end point of survival.

E. Phase I–III trials

Batimastat, which is poorly soluble and consequently has poor bioavailability when administered orally or parenterally, was the first MMPI tested in phase I studies. Blood levels of batimastat in patients with ovarian cancer, many with malignant ascites, remained within the predicted therapeutic range for 1 month after intraperitoneal administration. However, batimastat caused substantial local toxicity in patients without ascites, including peritoneal irritation and severe abdominal pain (Rasmussen, 1999). This compound was superseded by marimastat, an orally active agent. Since marimastat is not a cytotoxic agent, the initial pharmacokinetic work was done in healthy volunteers. A linear dose–plasma concentration relationship was found up to a dose of 200 mg. The elimination half-life showed some variability but was not dose dependent, with a mean half-life of 8–10 h. Plasma concentrations at all dose levels studied were well in excess of inhibitory concentrations, indicating that oral administration of the drug produces pharmacologically active drug levels. It was estimated that trough plasma concentrations of 30–40 ng/ml would result in approximately 90% enzyme inhibition (Rasmussen, 1999).

Three different approaches have been taken in phase II–III MMPI trials. The first approach involves direct comparison of the MMPI with standard chemotherapy; these trials include either marimastat or Bay 12-9566 versus gemcitabine in pancreatic cancer. The second strategy involves concomitant administration of the MMPI with chemotherapy compared with chemotherapy alone. These trials include (1) marimastat plus gemcitabine in pancreatic cancer, (2) AG3340 in

combination with paclitaxel and carboplatin in non-small cell lung cancer, (3) AG3340 in combination with cisplatin and gemcitabine in non-small cell lung cancer, and (4) AG3340 in combination with mitoxantrone and prednisone in hormone-refractory prostate cancer. The third strategy compares an MMPI with placebo in patients with low-volume disease or no evidence of disease after standard chemotherapy. These trials include (1) marimastat in pancreatic cancer, (2) marimastat in unresectable glioblastoma, (3) marimastat in advanced gastric cancer, (4) marimastat in small cell lung cancer, (5) marimastat in non-small cell lung cancer, (6) marimastat in breast cancer, (7) Bay 12-9566 in small cell lung cancer, (8) Bay 12-9566 in non-small cell lung cancer, and (9) Bay 12-9566 in ovarian cancer (Nelson *et al.,* 2000).

1. Results of Early Phase II–III Trials of MMPIs

Marimastat has been tested in phase II dose ranging studies (5–75 mg twice daily) in more than 400 patients with pancreatic, ovarian, colorectal, and prostate cancer. All patients had advanced, mostly metastatic cancer, and had already failed conventional treatment. Cancer-specific antigens were used as surrogate markers for biological activity (CA 19/9 in pancreatic cancer, CA 125 in ovarian cancer, carcinoembryonic antigen in colorectal cancer, and prostate-specific antigen in prostate cancer). Eligibility for this study required that patients exhibit more than a 25% increase in cancer-specific antigen in the month prior to study entry. The rate of rise in cancer-specific antigen was then compared with an equivalent time interval on study drug. Analysis of these studies indicated that marimastat treatment significantly reduced rates of rise of all four cancer-specific antigens in a dose-dependent fashion suggesting an antitumor effect. Histologic examination of tumor tissues in these clinical trials revealed an increase in peritumoral as well as intratumoral fibrosis, consistent with the expected drug effect (Rasmussen, 1999). These data were then used to identify the optimal drug dose for randomized phase III studies.

British Biotech has released the results of several phase III trials. These studies included more than 700 patients with unresectable pancreatic cancer and postchemotherapy progressing gastric cancer. The results do not demonstrate therapeutic superiority of marimastat over gemcitabine in pancreatic cancer. In a randomized double-blind placebo-controlled study of marimastat in patients with inoperable gastric adenocarcinoma following achievement of stable disease with chemotherapy, 369 patients were randomized to oral marimastat versus placebo. Median survival was 167 days for marimastat versus 135 days for placebo ($p = 0.07$). Exclusion of patients who did not receive any study treatment accentuated the differences ($p = 0.046$). Progression-free survival was also significantly improved by marimastat. The authors concluded that this is the first definitive clinical data supporting the use of MMPIs in cancer (Fielding *et al.,* 2000).

A recent trial of marimastat in glioblastomas revealed a lack of efficacy of the drug. The Eastern Cooperative Oncology Group is the first cooperative group to initiate a randomized clinical trial of an MMP inhibitor; marimastat or placebo is being administered to patients with metastatic breast cancer. Three hundred patients with progressive adenocarcinoma of the breast who have received one prior systemic chemotherapy regimen and now have stable or responding disease were eligible for inclusion in this protocol; results are awaited.

Bayer has reported the results of several ongoing clinical trials. In advanced solid tumors, the use of Bay12-9566 has resulted in stable disease for more than 4 years in 40% of patients treated on a phase I study (Nelson *et al.,* 2000). However, in a large pancreatic cancer trial, gemcitabine alone resulted in significantly prolonged overall survival (6.4 months) and progression-free survival as compared to Bay 12-9566 alone (3.2 months) (Moore *et al.,* 2000). Interim analysis of a drug trial of Bay12-9566 versus placebo in patients with stable disease following cytoreductive chemotherapy for advanced small cell lung cancer resulted in shorter survival in drug-treated patients. Based on these results, all clinical trials of Bay 12-9566 were suspended in September 1999 (communication from Bayer Corporation). Additional preclinical models are in progress to investigate the possible reasons for this unexpected result.

In terms of safety, the only clear-cut drug-related toxicity identified so far with hydroxamate MMPIs is a characteristic musculoskeletal syndrome consisting of tendonitis manifested by joint pain, stiffness, edema, reduced mobility, and skin discoloration. These symptoms, which are dose-related, usually start in the small joints in the hands, spreading to the arms and shoulder girdle, often on the dominant side. If dosing is not reduced, the symptoms spread to include other joints. These symptoms respond poorly to nonsteroidal anti-inflammatory drugs. For example, after 3–5 months of treatment with marimastat 10 mg twice per day, approximately 30% of patients required dose reduction. In contrast, AG3340 caused fewer musculoskeletal symptoms at the lower doses in patients with advanced malignancy. CSG27023A has also been associated with arthralgias, myalgias, and a self-limiting maculopapular rash (Giavazzi *et al.,* 1998). Bay 12-9566 has a different side-effect profile, which included asymptomatic elevation of hepatic enzymes and mild thrombocytopenia. Interestingly, no drug-related arthralgias were associated with Bay 12-9566.

In terms of the therapeutic use of MMPIs in other diseases, Roche recently discontinued trials of Ro 32-3555 in rheumatoid arthritis because of lack of efficacy in a well-controlled clinical study. Needless to say, the failure of the initial Bayer and Roche MMPI clinical trials has put a damper on initiation of new trials of MMPIs in the management of cancer and arthritis. The outcome of the ongoing Agouron and British Biotech trials of MMPIs in cancer is anxiously awaited.

F. New Approaches to Development of MMPIs

An exciting new approach in the development of more specific MMPIs involves the use of phage display random peptide libraries to isolate selective enzyme inhibitors. Peptides containing the sequence cyclic HWGF (especially the cyclic decapeptide CTTHWGFTLC) are potent and selective inhibitors of MMP-2 and MMP-9, but not of other MMPs (MMP-8, MMP-13, MT1-MMP). The prototype synthetic peptide inhibited the migration of human endothelial cells and tumor cells, prevented tumor growth and invasion in animal models, targeted angiogenic blood vessels *in vivo,* and improved survival of mice bearing human tumors (Koivunen *et al.,* 1999). The potential of these cyclic peptides as anticancer agents is currently being explored.

9. Sheddases

In the mid-1990s it was reported that the production of soluble TNF-α was dependent on the action of a MMP-like enzyme. Some synthetic MMPIs, but not TIMPs, were found to be powerful inhibitors of TNF-α release in cells, tissues, and animals examined both *in vitro* and *in vivo.* Subsequently, workers at Immunex and Glaxo Wellcome reported that this enzyme (named TNF-α-converting enzyme, TACE, ADAM-17) is a member of the reprolysin family of metzincins, the closest known analogues of MMPs (Black and White, 1998). A range of other membrane proteins (TGF, macrophage colony-stimulating factor, EGF, stem cell factor) are known to be hydrolyzed by uncharacterized proteinases, some being metalloproteinases. This group of enzymes has been designated as "sheddases." A role for sheddases in inflammatory diseases is being actively explored, and their role in cancer remains to be examined.

10. The uPA System: Proteolytic Control of MMP Activation

From a historical perspective, much of the initial interest in tumor proteases centered around the observations by Fischer in 1925 that explants of virally induced tumors caused plasma clot lysis, whereas explants of normal connective tissues did not (Fischer, 1925). Studies by Reich and his colleagues subsequently demonstrated that this effect was mediated by the serine protease PA, which is produced in large amounts by viral and chemically transformed cells (Ossowski *et al.,* 1973). An important feature of the tumor fibrinolytic system is the catalytic nature of PA, which when in the presence of high concentrations of substrate plasminogen in the serum or tissues yields much higher levels of local plasmin (a broad-spectrum serine proteinase) at the leading edge of cancer invasion than could be achieved by the release of enzyme directly from the cancer cell. This section of the chapter will focus on the uPA system as a key plasminogen activator in tumor progression with discussion of new therapeutic approaches that modulate the activity of this system.

A. Urokinase Plasminogen Activator

Plasminogen activators, including tissue plasminogen activator (tPA) and uPA, are secreted serine proteases that convert plasminogen to plasmin. Plasmin, in turn, is a broad-spectrum serine-protease capable of degrading fibrin and other ECM components such as laminin and non-helical components of collagen. Plasmin also activates other matrix proteases, including a subset of MMPs, as well as latent TGF-β (Dano et al., 1999; Rabbani et al., 1995; Wilhelm et al., 1994). While similar in their abilities to activate plasmin, tPA and uPA have different tissue and cellular distributions. Thus, tPA is the principal PA in circulating plasma where it plays a crucial role in fibrinolysis. On the other hand, uPA is a tissue-localized PA that is involved in cell-mediated proteolysis during macrophage invasion, wound healing, tissue remodeling, tumor cell invasion/metastasis, and angiogenesis (for recent reviews, see Andreasen et al., 1997; Conese and Blasi, 1995; Dano et al., 1999; de Vries et al., 1996; Mignatti and Rifkin, 1996; Rabbani et al., 1995; Schmitt et al., 1995; Wilhelm et al., 1994). Differences in the physiologic roles of the PAs have been characterized in elegant gene inactivation studies in mice (Carmeliet et al., 1994). Mice with a deficiency of tPA exhibited impaired thrombolysis. In contrast, uPA-deficient mice developed normally, were fertile, and showed no significant clotting abnormalities under normal conditions. However, experimental vascular remodeling (responses such as arterial-injury-induced neointimal formation and cardiac rupture following myocardial infarction) were markedly reduced in mice lacking uPA, confirming a role for uPA in these processes (Carmeliet et al., 1994, 1997; Heymans et al., 1999).

uPA is expressed by a variety of normal and malignant cells as a single-chain zymogen of 411 amino acids (pro-uPA) that can be converted to an active form (high-molecular-weight uPA, HMW-uPA, two-chain uPA) of approximately 52 kDa following proteolytic cleavage by plasmin and other proteases (e.g., cathepsins B/L, kallikrein; Fig. 8) (Andreasen et al., 1997; Magill et al., 1999; Schmitt et al., 1995; Wilhelm et al., 1994). Pro-uPA consists of three domains: an amino-terminal EGF-like domain (GFD, a.a. 1–44) which contains the binding site for the uPA receptor (uPAR); a kringle domain containing a heparin binding site; and a serine protease domain containing the typical catalytic triad His204, Asp255, and Ser356. Activation of pro-uPA involves cleavage of the Lys158-Ile159 peptide bond resulting in HMW-uPA, a multimeric protein in which the amino-terminal A chain (20 kDa) and the carboxy-terminal catalytic B chain (34 kDa) are linked by a single disulfide bond. HMW-

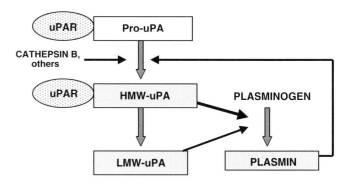

FIGURE 8   Schematic illustration of uPA activation of plasminogen.

uPA may be further degraded to a more enzymatically active low-molecular-weight form of uPA (LMW-uPA, 34 kDa). Both forms of uPA (HMW-uPA, LMW-uPA) cleave plasminogen to form plasmin. In addition, uPA has been reported to cleave fibronectin (a component of the ECM) as well as directly activate hepatocyte growth factor/scatter factor, the polypeptide ligand for cells expressing the c-met tyrosine kinase receptor (Mars et al., 1993; Naldini et al., 1992, 1995).

B. Urokinase Receptor and Endogenous PA Inhibitors

A key feature of the uPA mechanism is the cell surface localization of active enzyme. This is achieved by the interaction of the GFD of secreted uPA (either pro-uPA or HMW-uPA) with the membrane-bound uPA receptor (uPAR). This protein is a cysteine-rich glycoprotein of about 55 kDa consisting of three homologous internal domains linked to the cell surface by a glycosylphosphatidylinositol (GPI) anchor (Behrendt et al., 1995; Frankenne et al., 1999). Localization of pro-uPA greatly facilitates its conversion to active high-molecular-weight uPA, likely through its proximity to surface-localized plasmin. Consequently, uPA promotes a cascade of proteolytic events through the localization of activity for the leading edge of a migrating cell. It also liberates ECM-bound growth factors that further promote angiogenic responses (Mignatti and Rifkin, 1996).

Like TIMPs for the MMPs, specific protein inhibitors of the serpin family, PAI-1, PAI-2, and protease nexin-1 (PN-1), modulate endogenous uPA activity (for reviews, see Frankenne et al., 1999; Reuning et al., 1998; Wilhelm et al., 1994). The interaction between uPA and these molecules results in inactivation of uPA and cleavage of the serpin. PAI-1 is the major PAI present in circulating plasma and is primarily expressed by endothelial cells, platelets, and some other types of cells. PAI-1 inhibits high-molecular weight and low-molecular-weight uPA, but not pro-uPA. It also inhibits active forms of tPA. PAI-1 is produced as an active protease inhibitor but is rapidly converted to a latent form unless it is stabilized by protein binding (e.g., plasma or matrix vitronectin; for recent reviews, see Frankenne *et al.,* 1999; Reuning *et al.,* 1998). Matrix-bound PAI-1 remains active and can inhibit uPA-dependent activation of plasminogen.

PAI-2 is produced mainly by macrophages and placenta, and is not efficiently secreted; thus, a clear physiologic role for this molecule in extracellular proteolysis remains to be defined. It has been suggested that PAI-2 may serve as an intracellular protease inhibitor involved in TNF-mediated cytolysis (Kumar and Baglioni, 1991). Protease nexin 1 (PN-1) inhibits thrombin, plasmin, and trypsin in addition to uPA. This molecule is generally not present in plasma but is expressed by several types of cells, including smooth muscle cells, fibroblasts, and astrocytes. PN-1 has been postulated to play a role in reproductive function and embryonic development.

C. Role of uPA/uPAR in Cancer Growth and Metastasis

The association of uPA expression with poor clinical outcome has been shown in a variety of cancers, including gastric, colorectal, ovarian, and bladder cancers (for reviews, see (Andreasen *et al.,* 1997; Carroll and Binder, 1999; Conese and Blasi, 1995; de Vries *et al.,* 1996; Rabbani, 1998; Reuning *et al.,* 1998). Elevated tissue uPA levels are an independent prognostic factor for overall mortality in breast cancer and in patients with recurrent breast cancer who respond poorly to tamoxifen (Xing *et al.,* 1997). Validation of the therapeutic hypothesis for uPA in malignancy, at least in cell-based and/or animal models, has been provided by a variety of studies. For example, uPA-deficient mice have been reported to be resistant to the progression of several tumor types in multistage chemical carcinogenesis models (Shapiro *et al.,* 1996). Furthermore, in a report by Evans and colleagues (Evans *et al.,* 1997), inhibition of uPAR binding resulted in tumors with smaller size, less vascularization, and

less metastatic potential in a rat prostate carcinoma model. In this study, metastatic MatLyLu cells were induced to overexpress a catalytically inactive uPA mutant that competed for uPAR binding sites, functionally antagonizing cell-surface-localized uPA activity.

Of particular note in many of these recent studies is the association of uPA antagonism with a reduction in angiogenesis. These results therefore correlate with other studies that have linked uPA to neovascularization, including the observations that uPA is associated with migrating endothelial cells *in vitro* (Koolwijk *et al.,* 1996; Pepper *et al.,* 1987; Schnaper *et al.,* 1995; van Hinsbergh *et al.,* 1997) and that uPAR-blocking monoclonal antibodies completely block the formation of capillary microvascular structures in fibrin matrices *in vitro* (Kroon *et al.,* 1999). Therefore, inhibitors of the uPA pathway may exhibit significant antiangiogenic effects, which may be useful in the treatment for cancer as well as other fibroproliferative diseases (for a review, see Dano *et al.,* 1999). Taken together, these observations strongly support the hypothesis that uPA inhibitors may address an unmet medical need for nontoxic agents that control the spread or recurrence of cancer after primary therapy.

D. Development of Novel Therapeutic Agents in the PA Pathway

Effective therapeutic intervention of the pericellular uPA system can be achieved in several ways (Table 1). These include regulation of uPA expression by antisense oligonucleotides, neutralization with specific uPA- or uPAR-directed antibodies, forced expression/delivery of recombinant PAIs, as well as peptide/small molecules that block uPA-uPAR binding or act as direct uPA (enzyme) inhibitors. In this regard, in recent studies, antisense oligodeoxynucleotides to uPA have been reported to decrease uPA expression in rat and

TABLE 1
Potential Sites for Inhibition of uPA Action

Molecular activity	Inhibitor type	Examples (references)
uPA expression	• Antisense oligonucleotides (uPA)	(Wilhelm *et al.,* 1995)
Cell surface localization (uPA-uPAR binding)	• Antisense oligonucleotides (uPAR)	(Fibbi *et al.,* 1998; Yu *et al.,* 1997)
	• Recombinant inactive uPA	(Evans *et al.,* 1997; Guo *et al.,* 2000; Ignar *et al.,* 1998)
	• Synthetic peptides—competitive uPAR antagonists	(Burgle et al., 1997; Tressler et al., 1999)
		(Fibbi *et al.,* 1998)
	• Blocking antibodies	
uPA (serine protease) activity	• Neutralizing antibodies	(Abaza *et al.,* 1998; Kobayashi *et al.,* 1994)
	• Endogenous PAIs	(Mueller *et al.,* 1995; Soff et al., 1995)
	• Polypeptide inhibitors	(Ke *et al.,* 1997; Molloy *et al.,* 1999; Nienaber *et al.,* 2000; Rabbani *et al.,* 1995; Speri *et al.,* 2000; Subasinghe *et al.,* 1999; Tamura *et al.,* 2000; Towle *et al.,* 1993)
	• Small-molecule proteinase inhibitors	

human glioma cells *in vitro* (Engelhard *et al.,* 1996). The tumor cells absorbed the agents *in vivo* with no detectable toxicity at concentrations exceeding expected therapeutic levels. Antisense oligonucleotides directed to uPA have been reported to be effective in reducing the spread of human ovarian cancer in mice (Wilhelm *et al.,* 1995).

Specific uPA-neutralizing antibodies were reported to inhibit metastasis of Hep3 human carcinoma cells to chick embryo lymph nodes (Ossowski and Reich, 1983), and similar studies have shown that these antibodies reduce the progression of lung metastases in the murine B16 melanoma cell model (Hearing *et al.,* 1988) and in the Lewis lung carcinoma cell model (Kobayashi *et al.,* 1994). More recently, neutralizing monoclonal antibodies against uPA have been shown to display a potent cytolytic effect on human breast cancer cells (Abaza *et al.,* 1998). Monoclonal blocking antibodies directed against the ligand binding domain of uPAR also have been described, leading to diminished tumor growth, metastasis, and angiogenesis (Fibbi *et al.,* 1998). In related pharmaceutical research programs, scientists have identified polypeptides and small molecules directed at uPAR that block uPA binding and effectively reduce cell surface localization of uPA. Examples include a peptide derived from uPA (A6, Angstrom Pharmaceuticals; Guo *et al.,* 2000) as well as novel inhibitors from Boehringer Mannheim GmbH Roche (Burgle *et al.,* 1997) and Chiron (for recent review, see Tressler *et al.,* 1999). Although some of these projects are still active, to date there are no published clinical studies for any specific compound.

As stated above, forced expression of endogenous PAIs is another possible approach to inhibiting PA pathways. In studies by Soff and colleagues (Soff *et al.,* 1995), overexpression of PAI-1 in PC-3 human prostate carcinoma cells reduced tumor metastasis and resulted in a less aggressive phenotype, presumably by inhibition of uPA activity. Similar results were obtained in a study by Mueller and colleagues (Mueller *et al.,* 1995) in which forced overexpression of PAI-2 in a metastatic human melanoma cell line correlated positively with a reduction in tumor metastasis *in vivo.* Taken together, these data provide additional support for PA activity as a therapeutic target in tumor invasion and metastasis.

E. Design of Direct-Acting, Small-Molecule uPA Inhibitors

Unlike the MMPs discussed above, the serine protease activity of uPA was not an actively pursued target for small-molecule drug discovery until recently, possibly as a result of reports of the relatively benign phenotype of uPA-deficient mice (Carmeliet *et al.,* 1994; see Section 10A). A number of companies have now established programs aimed at developing small molecules designed to interfere with the catalytic activity of the enzyme (for examples, see Table 1, bottom). An early example of a uPA inhibitor was the potassium-sparing diuretic amiloride,

which was shown to inhibit angiogenesis *in vivo* (Swiercz *et al.,* 1999) (Fig. 9). A relatively weak small-molecule inhibitor of uPA, *p*-aminobenzamidine ($K_i = 82 \ \mu M$), inhibited growth of a human prostate tumor in SCID mice (Billstrom *et al.,* 1995). Small-molecule inhibitors of the benzo[*b*]thiophene-2-carboxamidine class have also shown uPA inhibitory activity and inhibition of fibronectin degradation *in vitro* (Towle *et al.,* 1993). In animal models, one of these agents (B-428) induced a marked decrease in primary tumor volume and weight as well as in the development of tumor metastases in a rat model of prostate cancer (Rabbani *et al.,* 1995). More recently, companies such as Abbott Laboratories, Axys, Corvas, Three-Dimensional Pharmaceuticals, Pfizer, and Wilex have revealed preclinical results on more potent uPA inhibitors (Table 1; (Nienaber *et al.,* 2000a; Speri *et al.,* 2000; Subasinghe *et al.,* 1999; Tamura *et al.,* 2000).

Many of these recent discovery efforts have been aided by advanced structure-based drug design approaches utilizing the three-dimensional crystal structure of uPA or related engineered protein constructs (Nienaber *et al.,* 2000; Renatus *et al.,* 1998; Speri *et al.,* 2000; Spraggon *et al.,* 1995). Experimental results show that uPA has an S1 specificity pocket similar to that of trypsin, with a restricted, less accessible, hydrophobic S2 pocket and a solvent-accessible S3 pocket that is capable of accommodating a wide range of residues. While the overall structure is similar to that of related serine proteases, at six positions the insertion of extra residues in loop regions create unique surface areas. One of these loop regions is highly mobile despite being anchored by the disulfide bridge present in a small subset of serine proteases (i.e., tPA, factor XII and complement factor I (Spraggon *et al.,* 1995). Studies of specific uPA–inhibitor complexes have revealed that the primary binding force resides in hydrogen bonds between the inhibitor's basic group (e.g., amidine or guanidine) and Asp189 in the S1 pocket. In addition, hydrophobic packing between the small-molecule core scaffold and the S1 pocket may also contribute to overall binding. Urokinase–inhibitor complex studies also have revealed additional binding sites adjacent to the S1 pocket, composed of the disulfide bridge at Cys191-Cys220, residues Ser146 and Gly218, and Lys214. Interactions with this "S1b subpocket" result in increased compound potency, as evidenced by the binding of B-248 and amiloride, whereas phenylguanidine lacks a halogen necessary for this type of interaction (Nienaber *et al.,* 2000b). Taken together, these studies have suggested possible means to develop more potent and specific uPA inhibitors.

F. Potential Therapeutic Strategies Involving uPA Inhibitors: Combination Strategies— Therapeutic Synergy?

It should be noted that despite the extensive experimental evidence that uPA is associated with metastasis, angiogenesis, and tumor progression, to date there is no reported hu-

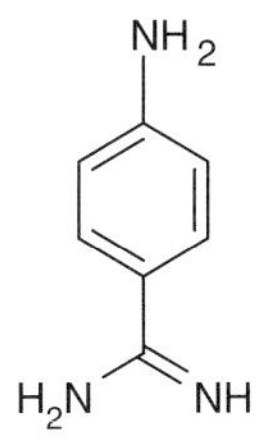

Benzamidine
uPA Ki ~ 80 μM

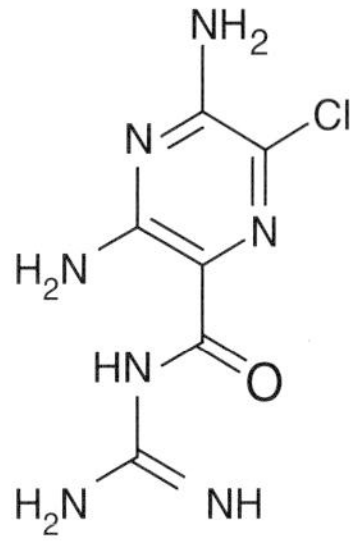

Amiloride
uPA Ki ~ 6 μM

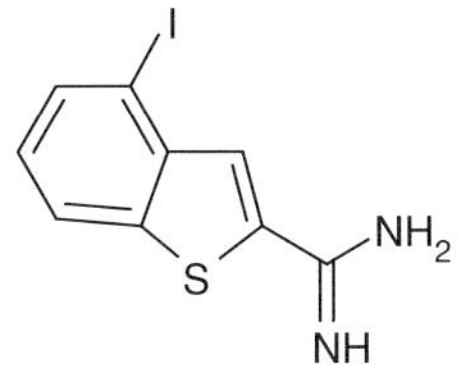

B-428 (Eisai)
uPA Ki ~ 0.3 μM

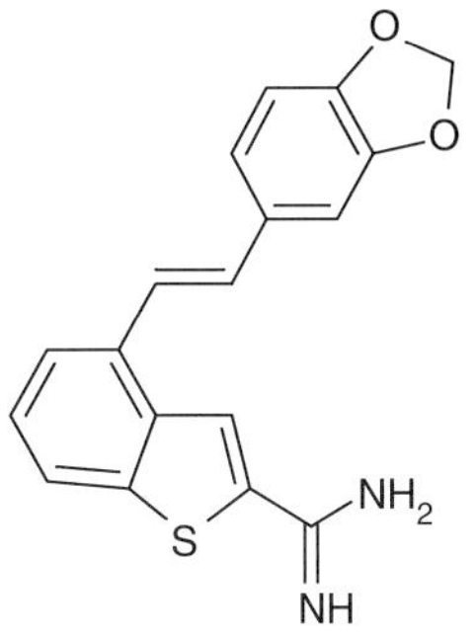

B-623 (Eisai)
uPA Ki ~ 0.07 μM

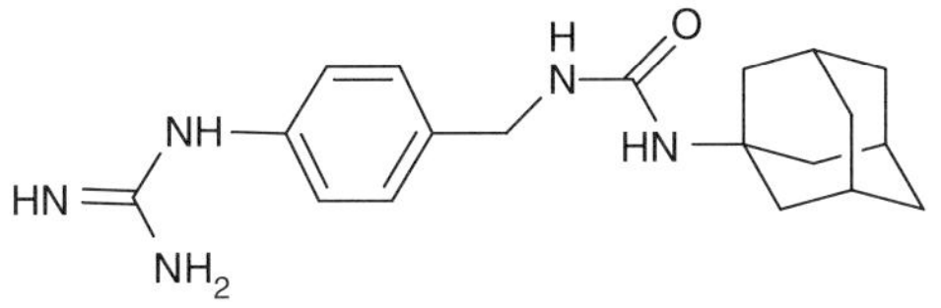

WX-293T (Wilex)
uPA Ki ~ 2.4 μM

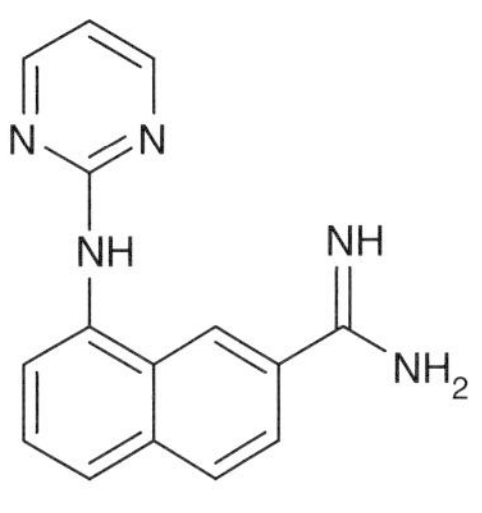

Abbott
uPA Ki ~ 0.03 μM
(Nienaber *et al.*, 2000)

FIGURE 9 Structure of some uPA inhibitors.

man clinical experience with uPA inhibitors. However, it is likely that one or more studies may begin in the next couple of years as compounds in preclinical evaluation enter phase I clinical trials. In this regard, it is expected that uPA inhibitors, like some of their MMP inhibitor predecessors, may be evaluated as adjunctive agents to standard chemotherapy in a variety of cancers, with a focus on those associated with excess uPA expression (e.g., breast, colon, prostate cancer). How-

ever, it is not yet clear that a uPA inhibitor will provide clinically significant benefit in any regimen.

Of possible relevance to the clinical evaluation of uPA inhibitors is the concept that the PA system, along with the MMPs and perhaps other proteases, may be viewed as redundant mechanisms involved in adverse tissue remodeling. It is therefore possible that therapeutic agents targeting specific proteases might be best used in combination to achieve significant interruption of the remodeling associated with increased tumor neovascularization and metastasis. A few notable studies have recently been published supporting this concept (Kim *et al.*, 1998; Lund *et al.*, 1999). One is the previously discussed study by Kim *et al.* demonstrating a requirement for MMP activity as well as uPA activity in an *in vivo* model of human cancer cell intravasation. Inhibition of MMP-9 or the uPA pathway markedly reduced tumor invasion in this model system. Lund and colleagues (Lund *et al.*, 1999) described the functional overlap between plasminogen activation and MMPs in epidermal wound healing, a tissue-remodeling mechanism that in many ways mimics pathologic remodeling associated with cancer invasion and neovascularization (for a review, see Dano *et al.*, 1999). In this study, plasminogen-deficient mice were used to evaluate the role of the PA system. Previous studies have shown that epidermal wound healing is significantly delayed in plasminogen-deficient mice (about 60 days vs. about 14 days in wild-type mice; Romer *et al.*, 1996). The authors treated wild-type mice with galardin, a broad-spectrum MMP inhibitor, and observed a similar pronounced delay in wound closure. However, when galardin was administered to plasminogen-deficient mice, wound healing was completely arrested (>100 days), demonstrating that protease activity is essential for skin wound healing. This requirement for plasminogen activation and MMP activity in the healing process supports the functional overlap of these two classes of matrix-degrading proteases in tissue remodeling. Furthermore, since uPA is the principal PA involved in tissue remodeling, related pathologic remodeling conditions, such as angiogenesis or tumor metastasis, might be optimally treated using a combination of agents blocking these redundant pathways (i.e., uPA inhibitor + MMP inhibitor). This type of "polydrug" combination therapy is well accepted in chemotherapeutic regimens aimed at reducing tumor cell burden directly. In the present scenario, stromal tissues associated with tumor vascularization and metastasis would be targeted as well. Conceptually, additional novel antiangiogenic agents (e.g., integrin antagonists, growth factor antagonists) may also be added to further broaden target coverage for these remodeling conditions. This approach has been discussed in related reviews (Kerbel, 2000).

Acknowledgments

Supported by a Research Enhancement Award Program (REAP) and a Merit Review Grant from the Veterans Administration, a grant from the NIH (CA 79866), and a Postdoctoral Traineeship Award from the U.S. Army Medical Research and Materiel Command Breast Cancer Research Project.

References

Abaza, M. S., Narayan, R. K., and Atassi, M. Z. (1998) Anti-urokinase-type plasminogen activator monoclonal antibodies inhibit the proliferation of human breast cancer cell lines in vitro. *Tumour Biol* **19**, 229–237.

Al-Medhi, A. B., Tozawa, K., Fisher, A. B., Shientag, L., Lee, A., and Muschel, R. J. (2000). Intravascular origin of metastasis from the proliferation of endothelium-attached tumor cells: a new model of metastasis. *Nat. Med.* **6**, 100–102.

An, Z., Wang, X., Willmott, N., Chander, S. K., Tickle, S., and Docherty, A. J. P. (1997). Conversion of a highly malignant colon cancer from an aggressive to a controlled disease by oral administration of a metalloproteinase inhibitor. *Clin. Exp. Metastasis* **15**, 184–195.

Anderson, I. C., Shipp, M. A., Docherty, A. J. P., and Teichner, B. A. (1996). Combination therapy including a gelatinase inhibitor and cytoxic agent reduces local invasion and metastasis of murine Lewis lung carcinoma. *Cancer Res.* **56**, 710–715.

Andreasen, P. A., Kjoller, L., Christensen, L., and Duffy, M. J. (1997). The urokinase-type plasminogen activator system in cancer metastasis: a review. *Int. J. Cancer* **72**, 1–22.

Aoudjit, F., Potworowski, E. F., and St-Pierre, Y. (1998). Bi-directional induction of matrix metalloproteinase-9 and tissue inhibitor of matrix metalloproteinase-1 during T lymphoma/endothelial cell contact: Implication of ICAM-1. *J. Immunol.* **160**, 2967–2973.

Auvinen, P., Tammi, R., Parkkinen, J., Tammi, M., Agren, U., Johansson, R., Hirvikoski, P., Eskelinen, M., and Kosma, V.-M. (2000). Hyaluronan in peritumoral stroma and malignant cells associated with breast cancer spreading and predicts survival. *Am. J. Pathol.* **156**, 529–536.

Babine, R. E., and Bender, S. L. (1997). Molecular recognition of protein-ligand complexes: Applications to drug design. *Chem. Rev.* **97**, 1359–1472.

Basset, P., Bellocq, J. P., Wolf, C., Stoll, I., Hutin, P., Limacher, J. M., Podhajcer, O. L., Chenard, M. P., Rio, M. C., and Chambon, P. (1990). A novel metalloproteinase gene specifically expressed in stromal cells of breast carcinomas. *Nature* **348**, 699–704.

Beckett, R. P., and Whittaker, M. (1998). Matrix metalloproteinase inhibitors 1998. *Exp. Opin. Ther. Patents* **8**, 259–282.

Behrendt, N., Ronne, E., and Dano, K. (1995). The structure and function of the urokinase receptor, a membrane protein governing plasminogen activation on the cell surface. *Biol Chem Hoppe Seyler* **376**, 269–279.

Benbow, U., Schoenermark, M. P., Mitchell, T. I., Rutter, J. I., Shimokawa, K.-I., Nagase, H., and Brinkerhoff, C. E. (1999). A novel host/tumor cell interaction activates matrix metalloproteinase 1 and mediates invasion through type I collagen. *J. Biol. Chem.* **274**, 25371–25378.

Bergers, G., Javaherian, K., Lok, M., Folkman, J., and Hanahan, D. (1999). Effect of angiogenesis inhibitors on multistage carcinogenesis in mice. *Science* **284**, 808–812.

Billstrom, A., Hartley-Asp, B., Lecander, I., Batra, S., and Astedt, B. (1995). The urokinase inhibitor p-aminobenzamidine inhibits growth of a human prostate tumor in SCID mice. *Int. J. Cancer* **61**, 542–547.

Birkedal-Hansen, H. (1995). Proteolytic remodeling of extracellular matrix. *Curr. Opin. Cell Biol.* **7**, 728–735.

Birkedal-Hansen, H., Moore, W. G. I., Bodden, M. K., Windsor, L. J., Birkedal-Hansen, B., DeCarlo, A., and Engler, J. A. (1993). Matrix metalloproteinases: A review. *Crit. Rev. Oral Biol. Med.* **42**, 197–250.

Biswas, C., Zhang, Y., DeCastro, R., Guo, H., Nakamura, T., Kataoka, H., and Nabeshima, K. (1995). The human tumor cell-derived collagenase stimulating factor (renamed EMMPRIN) is a member of the immunoglobulin superfamily. *Cancer Res.* **55**, 434–439.

Black, R. A., and White, J. M. (1998). ADAMs: focus on the protease domain. *Curr. Opin. Cell Biol.* **10**, 654–659.

Borkakoti, N. (1998). Matrix metalloproteases: variations on a theme. *Prog. Biophys. Molec. Biol.* **70**, 73–94.

Brewster, M., Lewis, E. J., Wilson, K. L., Greenham, A. K., and Bottomley, K. M. K. (1998). Ro 32-3555, an orally active collagenase selective inhibitor, prevents structural damage in the STR/ORT mouse model of osteoarthritis. *Arthritis Rheum.* **41,** 1639–1644.

Brooks, P. C., Silletti, S., von Schalscha, T. L., Friedlandwe, M., and Cheresh, D. A. (1998). Disruption of angiogenesis by PEX, a noncatalytic metalloproteinase fragment with integrin binding capacity. *Cell* **92,** 391–400.

Brooks, P. C., Stromblad, S., Sanders, L. C., von Schalscha, T. L., Aimes, R. T., Stetler-Stevenson, W. G., Quigley, J. P., and Cherish, D. A. (1996). Localization of matrix metalloproteinase MMP-2 to the surface of invasive cells by interaction with integrin avb3. *Cell* **85,** 683–693.

Brown, P. D., Bloxidge, R. E., Anderson, E., and Howell, A. (1993). Expression of activated gelatinase in human invasive breast cancer. *Clin. Exp. Metastasis* **11,** 183–189.

Brown, P. D., and Whittaker, M. (1999). Matrix metalloproteinase inhibitors. *In* "Antiangiogenic Agents in Cancer Therapy" (B. A. Teicher, ed.) pp. 205–223. Humana Press, Totowa, NJ.

Burgle, M., Koppitz, M., Riemer, C., Kessler, H., Konig, B., Weidle, U. H., Kellermann, J., Lottspeich, F., Graeff, H., Schmitt, M., Goretzki, L., Reuning, U., Wilhelm, O., and Magdolen, V. (1997). Inhibition of the interaction of urokinase-type plasminogen activator (uPA) with its receptor (uPAR) by synthetic peptides. *Biol. Chem.* **378,** 231–237.

Cameron, M. D., Schmidt, E., Kerkvliet, N., Nadkarni, K. V., Morris, V. L., Groom, A. C., Chambers, A. F., and MacDonald, I. C. (2000). Temporal progression of metastasis in lung: cell survival, dormancy, and location dependence of metastatic inefficiency. *Cancer Res.* **60,** 2541–2546.

Campo, E., Munoz, J., Miquel, R., Palacin, A., Cardesa, A., and Emmert-Buck, M. R. (1994). Cathepsin B expression in colorectal carcinomas correlates with tumor progression and shortened patient survival. *Am. J. Pathol.* **145,** 301–309.

Cao, J., Drews, M., Lee, H. M., Conner, C., Bahou, W. F., and Zucker, S. (1998). The propeptide domain of membrane type I matrix metalloproteinase is required for binding of tissue inhibitor of metalloproteinases and for activation of pro-gelatinase A. *J. Biol. Chem.* **273,** 34745–34752.

Carmeliet, P., Moons, L., Dewerchin, M., Mackman, N., Luther, T., Breier, G., Ploplis, V., Muller, M., Nagy, A., Plow, E., Gerard, R., Edgington, T., Risau, W., and Collen, D. (1997). Insights in vessel development and vascular disorders using targeted inactivation and transfer of vascular endothelial growth factor, the tissue factor receptor, and the plasminogen system. *Ann. NY. Acad. Sci.* **811,** 191–206.

Carmeliet, P., Schoonjans, L., Kieckens, L., Ream, B., Degen, J., Bronson, R., De Vos, R., van den Oord, J. J., Collen, D., and Mulligan, R. C. (1994). Physiological consequences of loss of plasminogen activator gene function in mice. *Nature* **368,** 419–424.

Carroll, V. A., and Binder, B. R. (1999). The role of the plasminogen activation system in cancer. *Semin. Thromb. Hemost.* **25,** 183–197.

Chambers, A. F., and Matrisian, L. M. (1997). Changing views of the role of matrix metalloproteinases in metastasis. *J. Natl. Cancer Inst.* **89,** 1260–1270.

Chin, Y.-C., Zhang, X., Melton, R., Ganu, V., and Gonnella, N. C. (1998). Solution structure of the catalytic domain of human stromelysin-1 complexed to a potent, nonpeptide inhibitor. *Biochemistry* **37,** 14048–14056.

Conese, M., and Blasi, F. (1995). The urokinase/urokinase-receptor system and cancer invasion. *Baillieres Clin. Haematol.* **8,** 365–388.

Conway, J. G., Trexler, S. J., Wakefield, J. A., Dockerty, A. J. P., and McGeehan, G. M. (1996). Effect of matrix metalloproteinase inhibitors on tumor growth and spontaneous metastasis. *Clin. Exp. Metastasis* **14,** 115–124.

Corcoran, M. L., and Stetler-Stevenson, W. G. (1995). Tissue inhibitor of metalloproteinase-2 stimulates fibroblast proliferation via a cAMP-dependent mechanism. *J. Biol. Chem.* **270,** 13454–13459.

Coussens, L. M., and Werb, Z. (1996). Matrix metalloproteinases and the development of cancer. *Chem. Biol.* **3,** 895–904.

Crawford, H. C., and Matrisian, L. M. (1996). Mechanisms controlling the transcription of matrix metalloproteinase genes in normal and neoplastic cells. *Enzyme Protein* **49,** 20–37.

Curran, S., and Murray, G. I. (1999). Matrix metalloproteinases in tumour invasion and metastasis. *J. Pathol.* **189,** 300–308.

D'Armiento, J., DiColandrea, T., Dalal, S. S., Okada, Y., Huang, M. T., Conney, A. H., and Chada, K. (1995). Collagenase expression in transgenic mouse skin causes hyperkeratosis and increases susceptibility to tumorigenesis. *Mol. Cell. Biol.* **15,** 5732–5739.

Dano, K., Romer, J., Nielsen, B. S., Bjorn, S., Pyke, C., Rygaard, J., and Lund, L. R. (1999). Cancer invasion and tissue remodeling-cooperation of protease systems and cell types. *Acta Pathologica Microbiologica et Immunologica Scandinavia* **107,** 120–127.

Davies, B., Miles, D. W., Haperfield, L. C., Naylor, M. S., Bobrow, L. G., Rubens, R. D., and Balkwill, F. R. (1993). Activity of type IV collagenases in benign and malignant breast disease. *Br. J. Cancer* **67,** 1126–1131.

de Vries, T. J., van Muijen, G. N. P., and Ruiter, D. J. (1996). The plasminogen activation system in tumour invasion and metastasis. *Pathol. Res. Pract.* **192,** 718–733.

Dekker, L. V., and Segal, A. W. (2000). Signals to move cells (Perspectives: Signal transduction). *Science* **287,** 982–985.

Della Porta, P., Soeltl, R., Krell, H. W., Collins, K., O'Donoghue, M., Schmitt, M., and Kruger, A. (1999). Combined treatment with serine protease inhibitor aprotinin and matrix metalloproteinase inhibitor Batimastat (BB-94) does not prevent invasion of human esophageal and ovarian carcinoma cells in vitro. *Anticancer Res.* **19,** 3809–3816.

Deryugina, E. I., Bourdon, M., Jungwirth, K., Smith, J. W., and Strongin, A. Y. (2000). Functional activation of integrin avb3 in tumor cells expressing membrane-type 1 matrix metalloproteinase. *Int. J. Cancer* **86,** 15–23.

DiStefano, J. F. (1986). Role of proteases in red blood cell target cell destruction by cells transformed by Rous sarcoma virus mutants. *Cancer Res.* **46,** 1114–1119.

Dollo, V., D'Ascenzo, S., Violini, S., Pompucci, L., Festuccia, C., Ginestrea, A., Vittorelli, M. L., Canevari, S., and Pavan, A. (1999). Matrix-degrading proteinases are shed in membrane vesicles by ovarian cancer cells in vivo and in vitro. *Clin. Exp. Metastasis* **17,** 131–140.

Dvorak, H. F. (1986). Tumors: wounds that do not heal. Similarities between tumor stroma generation and wound healing. *N. Engl. J. Med.* **315,** 1650–1659.

Eccles, S. A., Box, G., Court, W. J., Bone, E. A., Thomas, W., and Brown, P. D. (1996). Control of lymphatic and hematogenous metastasis of a rat mammary carcinoma by the matrix metalloproteinase inhibitor batimastat (BB94). *Cancer Res.* **56,** 2815–2822.

Ellerbroek, S., and Stack, M. S. (1999). Membrane associated matrix metalloproteinase in metastasis. *Bioessays* **21,** 940–949.

Engelhard, H., Narang, C., Homer, R., and Duncan, H. (1996). Urokinase antisense oligodeoxynucleotides as a novel therapeutic agent for malignant glioma: in vitro and in vivo studies of uptake, effects and toxicity. *Biochem. Biophys. Res. Commun.* **227,** 400–405.

Evans, C. P., Elfman, F., Parangi, S., Conn, M., Cunha, G., and Shuman, M. A. (1997). Inhibition of prostate cancer neovascularization and growth by urokinase plasminogen receptor blockade. *Cancer Res.* **57,** 3594–3599.

Fang, J., Shing, Y., Wiederschain, D., Yan, L., Butterfield, C., Jackson, G., Harper, J., Tamvakopoulos, G., and Moses, M. A. (2000). Matrix metalloproteinase-2 is required for the switch to the angiogenic phenotype in a tumor model. *Proc. Natl. Acad. Sci.* **97,** 3884-3889.

Fibbi, G., Caldini, R., Chevanne, M., Pucci, M., Schiavone, N., Morbidelli, L., Parenti, A., Granger, H. J., Del Rosso, M., and Ziche, M. (1998). Urokinase-dependent angiogenesis in vitro and diacylglycerol production are blocked by antisense oligonucleotides against the urokinase receptor. *Lab. Invest.* **78,** 1109–1119.

Fidler, I. J. (1991). Orthotopic implantation of human colon carcinomas into nude mice provides a valuable model for the biology and therapy of metastasis. *Cancer Metastasis Rev.* **10**, 229–243.

Fielding, J., Scholefield, J., Stuart, J., Hawkins, R., McCulloch, P., Maughan, T., Seymour, M., Van Cutsem, E., Thorlacius-Ussing, C., and Hovendal, C. (2000). A randomized double-blind placebo-controlled study of marimastat in patients with inoperable gastric adenocarcinoma. *Proc. Am. Soc. Clin. Oncol.* **19**, 240a (abstract 929).

Fischer, A. (1925). Beitrag zur gewebezellen eine vergleichendbiologische stadie der normalen und malignen gewbezellen in vitro. *Arch. Entwicklungsmech. Org. (Wilhelm Roux)* **104**, 210.

Frankenne, F., Noel, A., Bajou, K., Sounni, N. E., Goffin, F., Masson, V., Munaut, C., Remacle, A., and Foidart, J. M. (1999). Molecular interactions involving urokinase plasminogen activator (uPA), its receptor (uPAR) and its inhibitor, plasminogen activator inhibitor-1 (PAI-1), as new targets for tumour therapy. *Emerg. Ther. Targets* **3**, 469–481.

Freije, J. M. P., Diez-Itza, I., Balbin, M., Sanchez, L. M., Blasco, R., Tolwa, J., and Lopez-Otin, C. (1994). Molecular cloning and expression of collagenase-3, a novel human matrix metalloproteinase produced by breast carcinomas. *J. Biol. Chem.* **269**, 16766–16773.

Gatto, C., Rieppi, M., Borsotti, P., Innocenti, S., Ceruti, R., Drudis, T., Scanziani, E., Casazza, A. M., Taraboletti, G., and Giavazzi, R. (1999). BAY 12-9566, a novel inhibitor of matrix metalloproteinases with antiangiogenic activity. *Clin. Cancer Res.* **5**, 3603–3607.

Gelmon, K. A., Eisenhauer, E. A., Harris, A. L., Ratain, M. J., and Workman, P. (1999). Anticancer agents targeting signaling molecules and cancer cell environment: challenges for drug development. *J. Natl. Cancer Inst.* **91**, 1281–1287.

Giannelli, G., Falk-Marzillier, J., Schiraldi, O., Stetler-Stevenson, W. G., and Quaranta, V. (1997). Induction of cell migration by matrix metalloproteinase-2 cleavage of laminin-5. *Science* **277**, 225–228.

Giavazzi, R., Garofalo, A., Ferri, C., Lucchini, V., Bone, E.A., Chiari, S., Brown, P.D., Nicoletti, M.I., and Tara Boletti, G. (1998). Batimastat, a synthetic inhibitor of matrix metalloproteinases, potentiates the antitumor activity of cisplatin in ovarian carcinoma xenografts. *Clin. Cancer Res.* **4**, 985–992.

Glinsky, V. V., Huflejt, M. E., Glinsky, G. V., Deutscher, S. L., and Quinn, T. P. (2000). Effect of Thomsen-Friedenreich antigen-specific peptide P-30 on b-galactoside-mediated homotypic aggregation and adhesion to the endothelium of MDA-MB-435 human breast carcinoma cells. *Cancer Res.* **60**, 2584–2588.

Golub, L. M., Evans, R. T., McNamara, T. F., Lee, H. M., and Ramamurthy, N. S. (1994). A non-antimicrobial tetracycline inhibits gingival matrix metalloproteinases and bone resorption. *Ann. NY. Acad. Sci.* **732**, 96–111.

Gomis-Ruth, F. X., Maskos, K., Betz, M., Bergner, A., Huber, R., Suzuki, K., Yoshida, N., Nuguse, H., Brew, K., Bourenkov, G. P., Burtunik, H., and Bode, W. (1997). Mechanism of inhibition of the human matrix metalloproteinase stromelysin-1 by TIMP-1. *Nature* **389**, 77–81.

Grams, F., Crimmin, M., Hinnes, L., Huxley, P., Tschesche, H., and Bode, W. (1995). Structure determination and analysis of human neutrophil collagenase complexed with a hydroxamate inhibitor. *Biochemistry* **34**, 14012–14020.

Greenwald, R. A., Zucker, S., and Golub, L. M. (1999). Inhibition of Matrix Metalloproteinase. Therapeutic Implications. *Ann. NY. Acad. Sci.* **878**, 1–761.

Gross, J., and Lapiere, C. M. (1962). Collagenolytic activity in amphibian tissues; a tissue culture assay. *Proc. Natl. Acad. Sci. USA* **48**, 1014–1022.

Guedez, L., Stetler-Stevenson, W. G., Wolff, L., Wang, J., Fukushima, P., Mansor, A., and Stetler-Stevenson, M. (1998). In vitro suppression of programmed cell death of B cells by tissue inhibitor of metalloproteinases-1. *J. Clin. Invest.* **102**, 2002–2010.

Guo, H. L. R., Zucker, S., and Toole, B. P. (2000a). EMMPRIN (CD147),

an inducer of matrix metalloproteinase synthesis, also binds interstitial collagenase to the tumor cell surface. *Cancer Res.* **60**, 888–891.

Guo, Y., Higazi, A. A., Arakelian, A., Sachais, B. S., Cines, D., Goldfarb, R. H., Jones, T. R., Kwaan, H., Mazar, A. P., and Rabbani, S. A. (2000b). A peptide derived from the nonreceptor binding region of urokinase plasminogen activator (uPA) inhibits tumor progression and angiogenesis and induces tumor cell death in vivo. *FASEB J.* **14**, 1400–1410.

Gutheil, J. C., Campbell, T. N., Pierce, P. R., Watakins, J. D., Huse, W. D., Bodkin, D. J., and Cheresh, D. A. (2000). Targeted anti-angiogenic therapy for cancer using vitaxin: A humanized monoclonal antibody to the integrin avb3. *Clin. Cancer Res.* **6**, 3056–3061.

Haas, T. L., and Madri, J. A. (1999). Extracellular matrix-driven matrix metalloproteinase production in endothelial cells: Implications for angiogenesis. *Trends Cardiovasc. Med.* **9**, 70–77.

Hanemaaijer, R., Visser, H., Koolwijk, P., Sorsa, T., Salo, T., Golb, L. M., and van Hinsbergh, V. W. M. (1998). Inhibition of MMP synthesis by doxycycline and chemically modified tetracyclines (CMT) in human endothelial cells. *Adv. Dent. Res.* **12**, 114–118.

Haq, M., Shafii, A., Zervos, E. E., and Rosemurgy, A. S. (2000). Addition of matrix metalloproteinase inhibition to conventional cytotoxic therapy reduces tumor implantation and prolongs survival in a murine model of human pancreatic cancer. *Cancer Res.* **60**, 3207–3211.

Hazan, R. B., Phillips, G. R., Qiao, R. F., and Aaronson, S. A. (2000). Exogenous expression of N-cadherin in breast cancer cells induces cell migration, invasion, and metastasis. *J. Cell Biol.* **148**, 779–790.

Hearing, V. J., Law, L. W., Corti, A., Appella, E., and Blasi, F. (1988). Modulation of metastatic potential by cell surface urokinase of murine melanoma cells. *Cancer Res.* **48**, 1270–1278.

Heymans, S., Luttun, A., Nyyens, D., Theilmeier, G., Creemers, E., Moons, C. L., Dyspersin, G. D., Cleutjens, J. P. M., Shipley, M., Angellilo, A., Levi, M., Nobe, O., Baker, A., Kehet, E., Lupu, P., Herbert, H.-M., Smits, J. F. M., Shapiro, S. D., Baes, M., Borgers, M., Collen, D., Daemen, M. J. A. P., and Carmeliet, P. (1999). Inhibition of plasminogen activators or matrix metalloproteinases prevents cardiac rupture but impairs therapeutic angiogenesis and causes cardiac failure. *Nat. Med.* **5**, 1135–1142.

Himelstein, B. P., Canete-Soler, R., Bernhard, E. J., and Muschel, R. J. (1994). Induction of fibroblast 92 kDa gelatinase/type IV collagenase expression by direct contact with metastatic tumor cells. *J. Cell Physiol.* **107**, 477–486.

Hiraoka, N., Allen, E., Apel, I. J., Gyetko, M. R., and Weiss, S. J. (1998). Matrix metalloproteinases regulate neovascularization by acting as pericellular fibrinolysins. *Cell* **95**, 365–377.

Holmbeck, K., Bianco, P., Caterina, J., Yamada, S., Kromer, M., Kuznetsov, S. A., Mankani, M., Robey, P. G., Poole, R., Pidoux, I., Ward, J. M., and Birkedal-Hansen, H. (1999). MT1-MMP deficient mice develop dwarfism, osteopenia, arthritis, and connective tissue disease due to inadequate collagen turnover. *Cell* **99**, 81–92.

Ignar, D. M., Andrews, J. L., Witherspoon, S. M., Leray, J. D., Clay, W. C., Kilpatrick, K., Onori, J., Kost, T., and Emerson, D. L. (1998). Inhibition of establishment of primary and micrometastatic tumors by a urokinase plasminogen activator receptor antagonist. *Clin. Exp. Metastasis* **16**, 9–20.

Imai, K. et al. (1997). Degradation of decorin by matrix metalloproteinase: identification of the cleavage sites, kinetic analysis and transforming growth factor beta-1 release. *Biochem. J.* **322**, 809–814.

Iozzo, R. V. (1995). Tumor stroma as a regulator of neoplastic behavior. *Lab. Invest.* **73**, 157–160.

Ito, K., Okamoto, I., Araki, N., Kawano, Y., Nakao, M., Fujiyama, S., Tomita, K., Mimori, T., and Saya, H. (1999). Calcium influx triggers the sequential proteolysis of extracellular and cytoplasmic domains of E-cadherin, leading to loss of b-catenin from cell-cell contacts. *Oncogene* **18**, 7080–7090.

Itoh, T., Tanioka, M., Yoshida, H., Nishimoto, H., and Itohara, S. (1998). Reduced angiogenesis and tumor progression in gelatinase A-deficient mice. *Cancer Res.* **58,** 1048–1051.

Jankun, J., and Skrzypczak-Jankun, E. (1999). Molecular basis of specific inhibition of urokinase plasminogen activator by amiloride. *Cancer Biochem Biophys* **17,** 109–123.

Ke, S. H., Coombs, G. S., Tachias, K., Corey, D. R., and Madison, E. L. (1997). Optimal subsite occupancy and design of a selective inhibitor of urokinase. *J Biol Chem* **272,** 20456–20462.

Kerbel, R. S. (1999). What is the optimal rodent model for anti-tumor drug testing? *Cancer Metastasis Rev.* **17,** 301–304.

Kerbel, R. S. (2000). Tumor angiogenesis: past, present and the near future. *Carcinogenesis* **21,** 505–515.

Kieseier, B. C., Seifert, T., Giovannoni, G., and Hartung, H. P. (1999). Matrix metalloproteinases in inflammatory demyelination: targets for treatment. *Neurology* **53,** 20–25.

Kim, J., Yu, W., Kovalski, K., and Ossowski, L. (1998). Requirement for specific proteases in cancer cell intravasation as revealed by a novel semiquantitative PCR-based assay. *Cell* **94,** 353–362.

Kobayashi, H., Gotoh, J., Fujie, M., Shinohara, H., Moniwa, N., and Terao, T. (1994). Inhibition of metastasis of Lewis lung carcinoma by a synthetic peptide within growth factor-like domain of urokinase in the experimental and spontaneous metastasis model. *Int. J. Cancer* **57,** 727–733.

Koivunen, E., Arap, W., Valtanen, H., Rainisalo, A., Medina, O. P., Heikkila, P., Kantor, C., Gahmberg, C. G., Salo, T., Konttinen, Y. T., Sorsa, T., Ruoslahti, E., and Pasqualini, R. (1999). Tumor targeting with a selective gelatinase inhibitor. *Nat. Biotech.* **17,** 768–774.

Koolwijk, P., van Erck, M. G., de Vree, W. J., Vermeer, M. A., Weich, H. A., Hanemaaijer, R., and van Hinsbergh, V. W. (1996). Cooperative effect of TNF-α, bFGF, and VEGF on the formation of tubular structures of human microvascular endothelial cells in a fibrin matrix. Role of urokinase activity. *J. Cell Biol.* **132,** 1177–1188.

Kroon, M. E., Koolwijk, P., van Goor, H., Weidle, U. H., Collen, A., van der Pluijm, G., and van Hinsbergh, V. W. (1999). Role and localization of urokinase receptor in the formation of new microvascular structures in fibrin matrices. *Am. J. Pathol.* **154,** 1731–1742.

Kumar, S., and Baglioni, C. (1991). Protection from tumor necrosis factor-mediated cytolysis by overexpression of plasminogen activator inhibitor type-1. *J. Biol. Chem.* **266,** 20960–20964.

Lee, J.-H., and Welch, D. R. (1997). Suppression of metastasis in human breast carcinoma MDA-MB-435 cells after transfection with the metastasis suppressor gene, KiSS-1. *Cancer Res.* **57,** 2384–2387.

Leek, R. D., Lewis, C. E., Whitehouse, T., Greenall, M., Clarke, J., and Harris, A. L. (1996). Association of macrophage infiltration with angiogenesis and prognosis in invasive breast carcinoma. *Cancer Res.* **56,** 4625–4629.

Lehti, K., Valtanen, H., Wickstrom, S., Lohi, J., and Keski-Oja, J. (2000). Regulation of membrane-type-1 matrix metalloproteinase activity by its cytoplasmic domain. *J. Biol. Chem.* **275,** 15006–15013.

Libby, P. (1995). Molecular basis of acute coronary syndromes. *Circulation* **91,** 2844–2850.

Lijnen, H. R., Van Hoef, B., Lupu, F., Moons, L., Carmeliet, P., and Collen, D. (1998). Function of the plasminogen/plasmin and matrix metalloproteinase systems after vascular injury in mice with targeted inactivation of fibrinolytic system genes. *Thromb. Vasc. Biol.* **18,** 1035–1045.

Liotta, L. A. (1992). Cancer cell invasion and metastasis. *Sci. Am.* **2,** 34–41.

Liu, Z., Shipley, J. M., Zhou, X., Diaz, L. A., Werb, Z., and Senior, R. M. (1998). Gelatinase B-deficient mice are resistant to experimental bullous pemphigoid. *J. Exp. Med.* **188,** 475–482.

Lochter, A., Galosy, S., Muschler, J., Freedman, N., Werb, Z., and Bissell, M. J. (1997). Matrix metalloproteinase stromelysin-1 triggers a cascade of molecular alterations that leads to stable epithelial-to-mesenchymal conversion and a premalignant phenotype in mammary epithelial cells. *J. Cell Biol.* **139,** 1861–1872.

Lokeshwar, B. L. (1999). MMP inhibition in prostate cancer. *Ann. NY Acad. Sci.* **878,** 271–289.

Long, L., Navab, R., and Brodt, P. (1998). Regulation of Mr 72,000 type IV collagenase by the type I insulin-like growth factor receptor. *Cancer Res.* **58,** 3243–3247.

Lovejoy, B., Welch, A. R., Carr, S., Luong, C., Broka, C., Hendricks, T., Campbell, J. A., Walker, K. A. M., Martin, R., Van Wart, H., and Browner, M. F. (1999). Crystal structures of MMP-1 and -13 reveal the structural basis for selectivity of collagenase inhibitors. *Nat. Struct. Biol.* **6,** 217–221.

Lu, X., Levy, M., Weinstein, I. B., and Santella, R. M. (1991). Immunologic quantification of levels of tissue inhibitor of metalloproteinase-1 in human colon cancer. *Cancer Res.* **51,** 6231–6235.

Lund, L. R., Romer, J., Bugge, T. H., Nielsen, B. S., Frandsen, T. L., Degen, J. L., Stephens, R. W., and Dano, K. (1999). Functional overlap between two classes of matrix-degrading proteases in wound healing. *EMBO J.* **18,** 4645–4656.

Magill, C., Katz, B. A., and Mackman, R. L. (1999). Emerging therapeutic targets in oncology: urokinase-type plasminogen activator system. *Emerg. Ther. Targets* **3,** 109–133.

Mareel, M. M., Van Roy, F. M., and Bracke, M. E. (1993). How and when do tumor cells metastasize. *Crit. Rev. Oncog.* **4,** 559–594.

Mars, W. M., Zarnegar, R., and Michalopoulos, G. K. (1993). Activation of hepatocyte growth factor by the plasminogen activators uPA and tPA. *Am. J. Pathol.* **143,** 949–958.

Masson, R., Lefebvre, O., Noel, A., Fahime, M. E., Chenard, M. P., Wendling, C., Kebers, F., LeMeur, M., Dierich, A., Foidart, J. M., Basset, P. and Rio, M. C. (1998). In vivo evidence that the stromelysin-3 metalloproteinase contributes in a paracrine manner to epithelial cell malignancy. *J. Cell Biol.* **140,** 1535–1541.

McCawley, L. J., and Matrisian, L. M. (2000). Matrix metalloproteinases: multifunctional contributors to tumor progression. *Mol. Med. Today* **6,** 149–156.

Michael, M., Babic, B., Khokha, R., Tsao, M., Ho, J., Pintilie, M., Leco, K., Chamberlain, D., and Shepherd, F. A. (1999). Expression and prognostic significance of metalloproteinases and their tissue inhibitors in patients with small-cell lung cancer. *J. Clin. Oncol.* **17,** 1802–1808.

Mignatti, P., and Rifkin, D. B. (1993). Biology and biochemistry of proteinases in tumor invasion. *Physiol. Rev.* **73,** 161–195.

Mignatti, P., and Rifkin, D. B. (1996). Plasminogen activators and matrix metalloproteinases in angiogenesis. *Enzyme Protein* **49,** 117–137.

Molloy, C. J., Sharp, C., Manthey, C. L., Zhou, Z., Randle, T., Green, D., Hoffman, J., N. S., Rudolph, J., Wilson, K., Deckman, I., Bone, R., and Illig, C. (1999). Inhibition of pericellular urokinase plasminogen activator activity and basement membrane cell invasion by novel small molecule urokinase inhibitors. *Clin. Cancer Res.* 5 (Suppl.), **3740s.**

Montgomery, A. M. P., Reisfeld, R.A., and Cheresh, D.A. (1994a). Integrin a3b1 rescues melanoma cells from apoptosis in a three-dimensional dermal collagen. *Proc. Natl. Acad. Sci. U.S.A.* **91,** 8856–8860.

Montgomery, A. M. P., Mueller, B. M., Reisfeld, R. A., Taylor, S. M., and DeClerck, Y. A. (1994b). Effect of tissue inhibitor of the matrix metalloproteinases-2 expression on the growth and spontaneous metastasis of a human melanoma cell line. *Cancer Res.* **54,** 5467–5473.

Moore, M. J., Hamm, H., Eisenberg, P., Dagenais, M., Hagan, K., Fields, A., Greenberg, B., Schwartz, B., Ottaway, J., Zee, B., and Seymour, L. (2000). A comparison between gemcitabine and the matrix metalloproteinase inhibitor BAY 12-9566 in patients with advanced pancreatic cancer. *Proc. Am. Soc. Clin. Oncol.* **19,** 240a (abstract 930).

Mueller, B. M., Yu, Y. B., and Laug, W. E. (1995). Overexpression of plasminogen activator inhibitor 2 in human melanoma cells inhibits spontaneous metastasis in scid/scid mice. *Proc. Natl. Acad. Sci. USA* **92,** 205–209.

Nagase, H., and Woessner, F. (1999). Matrix metalloproteinases. *J. Biol. Chem.* **274,** 21491–21494.

Nakahara, H., Howard, L., Thompson, E. W., Sato, H., Seiki, Y., Yeh, Y., and

Chen, W. T. (1998a). Transmembrane/cytoplasmic domain-mediated membrane type 1-matrix metalloproteinase docking to invadopodia is required for cell invasion. *Proc. Natl. Acad. Sci. USA* **94**, 7959–7964.

Nakahara, H., Mueller, S. C., Nomizu, M., Yamada, Y., Yeh, Y., and Chen, W.T. (1998b). Activation of b1 integrin signaling stimulates tyrosine phosphorylation of p190RhoGAP and membrane-protrusive activities at invadopodia. *J. Biol. Chem.* **273**, 9–12.

Naldini, L., Tamagnone, L., Vigna, E., Sachs, M., Hartmann, G., Birchmeier, W., Daikuhara, Y., Tsubouchi, H., Blasi, F., and Comoglio, P. M. (1992). Extracellular proteolytic cleavage by urokinase is required for activation of hepatocyte growth factor/scatter factor. *EMBO J.* **11**, 4825–4833.

Naldini, L., Vigna, E., Bardelli, A., Follenzi, A., Galimi, F., and Comoglio, P. M. (1995). Biological activation of pro-HGF (hepatocyte growth factor) by urokinase is controlled by a stoichiometric reaction. *J. Biol. Chem.* **270**, 603–611.

Nelson, A. R., Fingleton, B., Rothenberg, M. L., and Matrisian, L. M. (2000). Matrix metalloproteinases: Biologic activity and clinical implications. *J. Clin. Oncol.* **18**, 1135–1139.

Nguyen, M., Arkell, J., and Jackson, C. J. (1998). Active and tissue inhibitor of matrix metalloproteinase-free gelatinase B accumulates within microvascular endothelial vesicles. *J. Biol. Chem.* **273**, 5400–5404.

Nicolson, G. L. (1991). Tumor and host molecules important in the organ preference of metastasis. *Semin. Cancer Biol.* **2**, 143–154.

Nienaber, V., Wang, J., Davidson, D., and Henkin, J. (2000a). Re-engineering of human urokinase provides a system for structure-based drug design at high-resolution and reveals a novel structural subsite. *J. Biol. Chem.* **275**, 7239–7248.

Nienaber, V. L., Davidson, D., Edalji, R., Giranda, V. L., Klinghofer, V., Henkin, J., Magdalinos, P., Mantei, R., Merrick, S., Severin, J. M., Smith, R. A., Stewart, K., Walter, K., Wang, J., Wendt, M., Weitzberg, M., Zhao, X., and Rockway, T. (2000b). Structure-directed discovery of potent nonpeptidic inhibitors of human urokinase that access a novel binding subsite. *Structure* **8**, 553–563.

Noel, A., Gilles, C., Bajou, K., Devy, L., Kebers, F., Lewalle, J. M., Manquoi, E., Munaut, C., Remacle, A., and Foidart, J. M. (1997). Emerging roles for proteinases in cancer. *Invasion Metastasis* **17**, 221–239.

Olson, M. W., Toth, M., Gervasi, D. C., Sado, Y., Ninomiya, Y., and Fridman, R. (1998). High affinity binding of latent matrix metalloproteinase-9 to the a2(IV) chain of collagen IV. *J. Biol. Chem.* **273**, 10672–10681.

Ossowski, L., Quigley, J. P., Kellerman, G. M., and Reich, E. (1973). Fibrinolysis associated with oncogenic transformation. Requirement of plasminogen for correlated changes in cellular morphology, colony formation in agar, and cell migration. *J. Exp. Med.* **138**, 1056–1064.

Ossowski, L., and Reich, E. (1983). Antibodies to plasminogen activator inhibit human tumor metastasis. *Cell* **35**, 611–619.

Parks, W. C., and Mecham, R. P. (1998). "Matrix Metalloproteinases." Academic Press, San Diego.

Pepper, M. S., Vassalli, J. D., Montesano, R., and Orci, L. (1987). Urokinase-type plasminogen activator is induced in migrating capillary endothelial cells. *J. Cell. Biol.* **105**, 2535–2541.

Polette, M., and Birembaut, P. (1998). Membrane-type metalloproteinases in tumor invasion. *Int. J. Biochem. Cell Biol.* **30**, 1195–1202.

Polette, M., Toole, B., Tournier, J.-M., Zucker, S., and Birembaut, P. (1997). TCSF expression and localization in human lung and breast cancers. *J. Histochem. Cytochem.* **45**, 703–709.

Porter, J., Beeley, N. R. A., Boyce, B. A., Mason, B., Millican, A., and Millar, K. (1994). Potent and selective inhibitors of gelatinase A. *Bioorg. Med. Chem. Lett.* **4**, 2741–2746.

Poste, G., and Fidler, I. J. (1980). The pathogenesis of cancer metastasis. *Nature* **283**, 139–146.

Powell, W. C., Fingleton, B., Wilson, C. L., Boothby, M., and Matrisian, L. M. (1999). The metalloproteinase matrilysin proteolytically generates active soluble Fas ligand and potentiates epithelial cell apoptosis. *Current Biol.* **9**, 1441–1447.

Pozzi, A., Moberg, P. E., Miles, L. A., Wagner, S., Soloway, P., and Gardner, H. A. (2000). Elevated matrix metalloprotease and angiostatin levels in integrin a1 knockout mice cause reduced tumor vascularization. *Proc. Natl. Acad. Sci.* **97**, 2202–2207.

Price, J. T., Bonovich, M. T., and Kohn, E. C. (1997). The biochemistry of cancer dissemination. *Crit. Rev. Biochem. Mol. Biol.* **32**, 175–253.

Pupa, S., Bufaino, P., Invernizzi, A. M., Andreola, S., Rilke, F., Lombardi, L., Colnaghi, M. I., and Menard, S. (1996). Macrophage infiltrate and prognosis in c-erbB-2- overexpressing breast carcinomas. *J. Clin. Oncol.* **14**, 85–94.

Rabbani, S. A. (1998). Metalloproteases and urokinase in angiogenesis and tumor progression. *In Vivo* **12**, 135–142.

Rabbani, S. A., Harakidas, P., Davidson, D. J., Henkin, J., and Mazar, A. P. (1995). Prevention of prostate-cancer metastasis in vivo by a novel synthetic inhibitor of urokinase-type plasminogen activator (uPA). *Int. J. Cancer* **63**, 840–845.

Rasmussen, H. S. (1999). Batimastat and Marimastat in cancer. Summary of early clinical data. *In* "Antiangiogenic Agents in Cancer Therapy" (B.A. Teicher, ed.) pp. 399–405. Humana Press, Totowa, NJ.

Ree, A. H., Tvermyr, M., Engebraaten, O., Rooman, M., Rosok, O., Hovig, E., Meza-Zepeda, L. A., Bruland, O. S., and Fodstad, O. (1999). Expression of a novel factor in human breast cancer cells with metastatic potential. *Cancer Res.* **59**, 4675–4680.

Renatus, M., Bode, W., Huber, R., Sturzebecher, J., and Stubbs, M. T. (1998). Structural and functional analyses of benzamidine-based inhibitors in complex with trypsin: implications for the inhibition of factor Xa, tPA, and urokinase. *J Med Chem* **41**, 5445–5456.

Reuning, U., Magdolen, V., Wilhelm, O., Fischer, K., Lutz, V., Graeff, H., and Schmitt, M. (1998). Multifunctional potential of the plasminogen activation system in tumor invasion and metastasis (review). *Int. J. Oncol.* **13**, 893–906.

Romer, J., Bugge, T. H., Pyke, C., Lund, L. R., Flick, M. J., Degen, J., and Dano, K. (1996). Impaired wound healing in mice with a disrupted plasminogen gene. *Nat. Med.* **2**, 287–292.

Rosenberg, G. A., Estrada, E. Y., and Dencoff, J. E. (1998). Matrix metalloproteinases and TIMPs are associated with blood-brain barrier opening after reperfusion in rat brain. *Stroke* **29**, 2189–2195.

Rusciano, D., and Burger, M. (1992). Why do cancer cells metastasize into particular organs? *BioEssays* **14**, 185–194.

Saren, P., Welgus, H. G., and Kovanen, P. T. (1996). TNF-a and IL-1b selectively induce expression of 92-kDa gelatinase by human macrophages. *J. Immunol.* **157**, 4159–4165.

Sato, H., Takino, T., Okada, Y., Cao, J., Shinagawa, A., Yamamoto, E., and Seiki, M. (1994). A matrix metalloproteinase expressed on the surface of invasive tumor cells. *Nature* **370**, 61–65.

Schmitt, M., Wilhelm, O., Janicke, F., Magdolen, V., Reuning, U., Ohi, H., Moniwa, N., Kobayashi, H., Weidle, U., and Graeff, H. (1995). Urokinase-type plasminogen activator (uPA) and its receptor (CD87): a new target in tumor invasion and metastasis. *J. Obstet. Gynecol.* **21**, 151–165.

Schnaper, H. W., Barnathan, E. S., Mazar, A., Maheshwari, S., Ellis, S., Cortez, S. L., Baricos, W. H., and Kleinman, H. K. (1995). Plasminogen activators augment endothelial cell organization in vitro by two distinct pathways. *J Cell Physiol* **165**, 107–118.

Seftor, R. E. B., Seftor, E. A., Sheng, S., Pemberton, P. A., Sager, R., and Hendrix, M. J. C. (1998). Maspin suppresses the invasive phenotype of human breast carcinoma. *Cancer Res.* **58**, 5681–5685.

Segain, J. P., Harb, J., Gregoire, M., Meflah, K., and Menaanteau, J. (1996). Induction of fibroblast gelatinase B expression by direct contact with cell lines derived from primary tumor but not from metastases. *Cancer Res.* **56**, 5506–5512.

Seraj, M. J., Samant, R. S., Verderame, M. F., and Welch, D. R. (2000). Functional evidence for a novel human breast carcinoma metastasis suppressor, BMRS1, encoded at chromosome 11q13. *Cancer Res.* **60**, 2764–2769.

Shalinsky, D. R., Brekken, J., Zou, H., Kolis, S., Wood, A., Webber, S., and Appelt, K. (1998–1999). Antitumor efficacy of AG3340 associated with maintenance of minimum effective plasma concentrations and not total daily dose, exposure or peak plasma concentrations. *Invest. New Drugs* **16**, 303–313.

Shalinsky, D. R., Brekken, J., Zou, H., McDermott, C. D., Forsyth, P., Edwards, D., Margosiak, S., Bender, S., Truitt, G., Wood, A., Varki, N. M., and Appelt, K. (1999). Broad antitumor and antiangiogenic activities of AG3340, a potent and selective MMP inhibitor undergoing advanced oncology clinical trials. *In* "Annals of the New York Academy of Science, Vol. 878. Inhibition of Matrix Metalloproteinase. Therapeutic Applications." R. Greenwald, S. Zucker, and L. Golub, eds.), pp. 236–270.

Shapiro, R. L., Duquette, J. G., Roses, D. F., Nunes, I., Harris, M. N., Kamino, H., Wilson, E. L., and Rifkin, D. B. (1996). Induction of primary cutaneous melanocytic neoplasms in urokinase-type plasminogen activator (uPA)-deficient and wild-type mice: cellular blue nevi invade but do not progress to malignant melanoma in uPA-deficient animals. *Cancer Res.* **56**, 3597–3604.

Shapiro, S. D. (1998). Matrix metalloproteinase degradation of extracellular matrix: biological consequences. *Curr. Biol.* **10**, 602–608.

Skotnicki, J. S., Zask, A., Nelson, F. C., Albright, J. D., and Levin, J. I. (1999). Design and synthetic considerations of matrix metalloproteinase inhibitors. *In* "Annals of New York Academy of Science, Vol. 878, Inhibition of Matrix Metalloproteinase. Therapeutic Applications." (R. A. Greenwald, S. Zucker, and L. M. Golub, eds.) pp. 61–72.

Sledge, G. W. J., Qulali, M., Goulet, R., Bone, E. A., and Fife, R. (1995). Effect of matrix metalloproteinase inhibitor batimastat on breast cancer regrowth and metastasis in athymic mice. *J. Natl. Cancer Inst.* **87**, 1546–1550.

Sloane, B. F., Moin, K., and Lah, T. T. (1994). Regulation of lysosomal endopeptidases in malignant neoplasia. *In* "Biochemical and Molecular Aspects of Selected Cancers (T. G. Pretlow III and T. P. Pretlow, eds.), Vol. 2, pp. 411–466. Academic Press, San Diego.

Smith, G. N., Mickler, E. A., Hasty, K. A., and Brandt, K. D. (1999). Specificity of inhibition of matrix metalloproteinase activity by doxycycline. Relation to structure of the enzyme. *Arthritis Rheum.* **42**, 1140–1146.

Soff, G. A., Sanderowitz, J., Gately, S., Verrusio, E., Weiss, I., Brem, S., and Kwaan, H. C. (1995). Expression of plasminogen activator inhibitor type 1 by human prostate carcinoma cells inhibits primary tumor growth, tumor-associated angiogenesis, and metastasis to lung and liver in an athymic mouse model. *J. Clin. Invest.* **96**, 2593–2600.

Speri, S., Jacob, U., Arroyo de Prada, N., Sturzebecher, J., Wilhelm, O. G., Bode, W., Magdolen, V., Huber, R., and Moroder, L. (2000). (4-Aminomethyl)phenylguanidine derivatives as nonpeptidic highly selective inhibitors of human urokinase. *Proc. Nat. Acad. Sci.* **97**, 5113–5118.

Spraggon, G., Phillips, C., Nowak, U. K., Ponting, C. P., Saunders, D., Dobson, C. M., Stuart, D. I., and Jones, E. Y. (1995). The crystal structure of the catalytic domain of human urokinase-type plasminogen activator. *Structure* **3**, 681–691.

Sternlicht, M. D., Lochter, A., Sympson, C. J., Huey, B., Rougier, J. P., Gray, J. W., Pinkel, D., Bissell, M. J., and Werb, Z. (1999). The stromal proteinase MMP3/stromelysin-1 promotes mammary carcinogenesis. *Cell* **98**, 351–358.

Stetler-Stevenson, W. G. (1999). Matrix metalloproteinases in angiogenesis: a moving target for therapeutic intervention. *J. Clin. Invest.* **103**, 1237–1241.

Still, K., Robson, C. N., Autzen, P., Robinson, M. C., and Hamby, F. C. (2000). Localization and quantification of mRNA for matrix metalloproteinase-2 (MMP-2) and tissue inhibitor of matrix metalloproteinase-2 (TIMP-2) in human benign and malignant prostatic tissue. *Prostate* **42**, 18–25.

Strongin, A. Y., Collier, I., Bannicov, G., Marmer, B. L., Grant, G. Z., and Goldberg, G. I. (1995). Mechanism of cell surface activation of 72-kDa type IV collagenase. Isolation of the activated form of the membrane metalloproteinase. *J. Biol. Chem.* **270**, 5331–5338.

Subasinghe, N., Hoffman, J., Rudolph, J., Soll, R., Wilson, K., Randle, T., Green, D., Lewandowski, F., Zhang, M., Bone, R., Spurlino, J., Deckman, I., Manthey, C., Zhou, Z., Sharp, C., Kratz, D., Grasberger, B., Des-Jarlais, R., Molloy, C. J., and C. I. (1999). Structure-based drug design of novel urokinase plasminogen activator inhibitors. *Clin. Cancer Res.* **5 (Suppl.)**, 3841s.

Swiercz, R., Skrzypczak-Jankun, E., Merrell, M.M., Selman, S.H., and Jankun, J. (1999). Angiostatic activity of synthetic inhibitors of urokinase type plasminogen activator. *Oncol. Rep.* **6**, 523–526.

Szardenings, A. K., Antonenko, V., Campbell, D. A., DeFrancisco, N., Ida, S., Shi, L., Sharkov, N., Tien, D., Wang, Y., and Mavre, M. (1999). Identification of highly selective inhibitors of collagenase-1 from combinatorial libraries of diketopiperazines. *Med. Chem.* **42**, 1348–1357.

Takahashi, C., Sheng, Z., Horan, T. P., Kitayama, H., Maki, M., Hitomi, K., Kitaura, Y., Takai, S., Sasahara, R. M., Horimoto, A., Ikawa, Y., Ratzkin, B. J., Arakawa, T., and Noda, M. (1998). Regulation of matrix metalloproteinase-9 and inhibition of tumor invasion by the membrane-anchored glycoprotein RECK. *Proc. Natl. Acad. Sci. USA* **95**, 13221–13226.

Tamura, S. Y., Weinhouse, M. I., Roberts, C. A., Goldman, E. A., Masukawa, K., Anderson, S. M., Cohen, C. R., Bradbury, A. E., Bernardino, V. T., Dixon, S. A., Ma, M. G., Nolan, T. G., and Brunck, T. K. (2000). Synthesis and biological activity of peptidyl aldehyde urokinase inhibitors. *Bioorg. Med. Chem. Lett.* **10**, 983–987.

Taraboletti, G., Garofalo, A., Belotti, B., Drudis, T., Borsotti, P., Scanziani, E., Brown, P. D., and Giavazzi, R. (1995). Inhibition of angiogenesis and murine hemangioma growth by Batimastat, a synthetic inhibitor of matrix metalloproteinases. *J. Natl. Cancer Inst.* **87**, 293–298.

Theodorescu, D., Cornil, I., Sheehan, C., and Kerbel, R. B. (1991). Dominance of metastatically competent cells in primary murine breast neoplasms is necessary for distant metastasis. *Int. J. Cancer* **47**, 118–123.

Towle, M. J., Lee, A., Maduakor, E. C., Schwartz, C. E., Bridges, A. J., and Littlefield, B. A. (1993). Inhibition of urokinase by 4-substituted benzo[b]thiophene-2-carboxamidines: an important new class of selective synthetic urokinase inhibitor. *Cancer Res.* **53**, 2553–2559.

Tressler, R. J., Pitot, P. A., Stratton, J. R., Forrest, L. D., Zhuo, S., Drummond, R. J., Fong, S., Doyle, M. V., Doyle, L. V., Min, H. Y., and Rosenberg, S. (1999). Urokinase receptor antagonists: discovery and application to in vivo models of tumor growth. *Acta Pathologica Microbiologica et Immunologica Scandinavia* **107**, 168–173.

van Hinsbergh, V. W., Koolwijk, P., and Hanemaaijer, R. (1997). Role of fibrin and plasminogen activators in repair-associated angiogenesis: in vitro studies with human endothelial cells. *EXS* **79**, 391–411.

Velasco, G., Pendas, A. M., Fueyo, A., Knauper, V., Murphy, G., and Lopez-Otin, C. (1999). Cloning and characterization of human MMP-23, a new matrix metalloproteinase predominantly expressed in reproductive tissues and lacking conserved domains in other family members. *J. Biol. Chem.* **274**, 4570–4576.

Vincenti, M. P., White, L. A., Schroen, D. J., Benbow, U., and Brinckerhoff, C. E. (1996). Regulating expression of the gene for matrix metalloproteinase-1 (collagenase): Mechanisms that control enzyme activity, transcription, and mRNA stability. *Crit. Rev. Eukaryot. Gene Expr.* **6**, 391–411.

Vu, T. H., Shipley, J. M., Bergers, G., Berger, J. E., Helms, J. A., Hanahan, D., Shapiro, S. D., Senior, R. M., and Werb, Z. (1998). MMP-9/gelatinase B is a key regulator of growth plate angiogenesis and apoptosis of hypertrophic chondrocytes. *Cell* **93**, 411–422.

Welch, D. R. (1997). Technical considerations for studying cancer metastasis in vivo. *Clin. Exp. Metastasis* **15**, 272–306.

Westermarck, J., and Kahari, V.-M. (1999). Regulation of matrix metalloproteinase expression in tumor invasion. *FASEB J.* **13**, 781–792.

Wilhelm, O., Reuning, U., Janicke, F., Schmitt, M., and Graeff, H. (1994). The role of proteases in tumor invasion and metastasis: prognostic impact and therapeutic challenge? *Onkologie* **17**, 358–366.

Wilhelm, O., Schmitt, M., Hohl, S., Senekowitsch, R., and Graeff, H. (1995). Antisense inhibition of urokinase reduces spread of human ovarian cancer in mice. *Clin Exp Metastasis* **13**, 296–302.

Woessner, J. F. (1991). Matrix metalloproteinases and their inhibitors in connective tissue remodeling. *FASEB J.* **5,** 2145–2154.

Xing, R. H., Mazar, A., Henkin, J., and Rabbani, S. A. (1997). Prevention of breast cancer growth, invasion, and metastasis by antiestrogen tamoxifen alone or in combination with urokinase inhibitor B-428. *Cancer Res.* **57,** 3585–3593.

Yu, Q., and Stamenkovic, I. (2000). Cell surface-localized matrix metalloproteinase-9 proteolytically activates TGF-b and promotes tumor invasion and angiogenesis. *Genes Dev.* **14,** 163–176.

Yu, W., Kim, J., and Ossowski, L. (1997). Reduction in surface urokinase receptor forces malignant cells into a protracted state of dormancy. *J. Cell Biol.* **137,** 767–777.

Yu, W.-H., and Woessner, J. F., Jr. (2000). Heparan sulfate proteoglycans as extracellular docking molecules for matrilysin (Matrix Metalloproteinase 7). *J. Biol. Chem.* **275,** 4183–4191.

Zhou, A., Apte, S. S., Soininen, R., Cao, R., Baaklin, G. Y., Rauser, R. W., Wang, J., Cao, Y., and Tryggvason, K. (2000). Impaired endochondral ossification and angiogenesis in mice deficient in membrane-type matrix metalloproteinase-1. *Proc. Natl. Acad. Sci.* **97,** 4052–4057.

Zucker, S. (1988). A critical appraisal of the role of proteolytic enzymes in cancer invasion: emphasis on tumor surface proteinases. *Cancer Invest.* **6,** 219–231.

Zucker, S., Conner, C., DiMassimo, B. I., Ende, H., Drews, M., Seiki, M., and Bahou, W. F. (1995a). Thrombin induces the activation of progelatinase A in vascular endothelial cells: Physiologic regulation of angiogenesis. *J. Biol. Chem.* **270,** 23730–23738.

Zucker, S., DiMassimo, B. I., Lysik, R. M., and Lyubsky, S. (1993a). Purification and characterization of a novel cytotoxic protein from transformed fibroblasts. *Cancer Res.* **53,** 1195–1203.

Zucker, S., Drews, M., Conner, C., Foda, H. D., DeClerck, A., Langley, K. E., Bahou, W. F., Docherty, A. J. P., and Cao, J. (1998a). Tissue inhibitor of metalloproteinase-2 (TIMP-2) binds to the catalytic domain of the surface receptor, membrane type 1-matrix metalloproteinase 1 (MT1-MMP). *J. Biol. Chem.* **273,** 1216–1222.

Zucker, S., Hymowitz, M., Conner, C., Zarrabi, H. M., Hurewitz, A. N., Matrisian, L., Boyd, D., Nicholson, G., and Montana, S. (1999). Measurement of matrix metalloproteinases (MMPs) and tissue inhibitors of metalloproteinases (TIMPs) in blood and tissues. *Ann. NY. Acad. Sci.* **878,** 212–227.

Zucker, S., Lysik, R. M., DiMassimo, B. I., Zarrabi, H. M., Moll, U. M., Grimson, R., Tickle, S. P., and Docherty, A. J. P. (1995b). Plasma assay of gelatinase B: tissue inhibitor of metalloproteinase (TIMP) complexes in cancer. *Cancer* **76,** 700–708.

Zucker, S., Lysik, R. M., Malik, M., Bauer, B. A., Caamano, J., and Kleinszanto, A. J. P. (1992). Secretion of gelatinases and tissue inhibitors of metalloproteinases by human lung cancer cell lines and revertant cell lines: Not an invariant correlation with metastasis. *Int. J. Cancer* **52,** 1–6.

Zucker, S., Lysik, R. M., Zarrabi, M. H., and Moll, U. (1993b). Mr 92,000 type IV collagenase is increased in plasma of patients with colon cancer and breast cancer. *Cancer Res.* **53,** 140–146.

Zucker, S., Mian, N., Drews, M., Conner, C., Davidson, A., Greenwald, R., Docherty, A. J. P., and Barland, P. (1998b). Increased serum stromelysin-1 in systemic lupus erythematosus: Implications in pathogenesis. *J. Rheumatol.* **26,** 78–80.

Zucker, S., Mirza, H., Conner, C., Lorenz, A., Drews, M., Bahou, W. F., and Jesty, J. (1998c). Vascular endothelial growth factor and matrix metalloproteinase production in endothelial cells: Conversion of prothrombin to thrombin results in progelatinase A activation and cell proliferation. *Int. J. Cancer* **75,** 780–786.

Zucker, S., Wieman, J. M., Lysik, R. M., Wilkie, D., Ramamurthy, N. S., Golub, L. M., and Lane, B. (1987). Enrichment of collagen and gelatin degrading activities in the plasma membrane of human cancer cells. *Cancer Res.* **47,** 1608–1614.

Zucker, S. G. (1994). Guidelines for clinical trial design for evaluation of MMP inhibitors. *Ann. NY. Acad. Sci.* **732,** 273–279.

CHAPTER 7

TUMOR VASCULATURE AS A TARGET

Elianne A. Koop
Emile E. Voest

Laboratory of Medical Oncology
Division of Medical Oncology
University Medical Centre Utrecht
Utrecht, The Netherlands

Summary

Angiogenesis, the formation of new blood vessels from preexisting ones, is thought to be obligatory for tumor growth and the formation of metastasis. The angiogenic switch—the change from an avascular tumor to an abundantly vascularized tumor—is coordinated by both positive and negative regulators. Furthermore, migration and proliferation of the endothelial cells and remodeling of the extracellular matrix are both essential events in angiogenesis. During the last three decades effort has been made to further identify and characterize all of the proteins that have an important role in angiogenesis. Groups of proteins that are known to have a role in angiogenesis are the angiogenic factors, the integrins, the plasminogen activation system, and the matrix metalloproteinases and their inhibitors. The function, interaction, regulation and clinical relevance of these proteins and their receptors have been extensively investigated. Strategies interfering with different stages in the process of angiogenesis have been designed to inhibit tumor growth. Several biological and chemical compounds that interfere with the process of angiogenesis were developed. Furthermore, in the last decade, endogenous inhibitors of angiogenesis and peptides or antibodies that target the tumor's vasculature have also been identified and characterized. Clinical trials with proteins or compounds interfering with the process of angiogenesis are currently under way. In the next decade these clinical trials will provide answers to the question of whether or not antivascular agents will be a valuable addition to the current anticancer armamentarium.

1. Introduction

Angiogenesis is a complex process that is essential in physiologic and pathologic processes. During development angiogenesis is preceded by vasculogenesis, the formation of blood vessels from progenitor cells. In adults the vasculature is normally quiescent, except for processes in the female reproductive cycle. Outside this, angiogenesis is mainly controlled by pathologic conditions, such as wound healing, arthritis, psoriasis, diabetic retinopathy, and cancer. The first suggestion that angiogenesis is essential for tumor growth and metastasis was made by Dr. Folkman about 30 years ago (Folkman, 1972). Since then, the research activity in the field of angiogenesis has increased immensely. It is now generally accepted that tumors do not grow beyond 1–2 mm unless there is a supply of oxygen and nutrients (Folkman, 1995a). At this critical size, tumor growth is balanced on one hand by continuous cell proliferation and on the other hand by apoptotic

processes. In this way, the tumor may remain clinically undetectable for years, a stage called tumor dormancy. The passage from the avascular tumor, a carcinoma *in situ,* to a vascularized tumor, is the result of disequilibrium between
positive and negative regulators of angiogenesis. This is called
the angiogenic switch.

A. The Angiogenic Switch

Different transgenic mouse models have shown that an angiogenic switch becomes activated during early stages of tumor development, suggesting that regulation of angiogenesis
is a discrete, rate-limiting step in tumor growth and development (Hanahan and Folkman, 1996) (Fig. 1, see color insert).
Characterization of the angiogenic switch has been a major
research focus.

First of all it has been shown that prior to tumorigenicity,
different genetic changes are detected. This can involve either
the loss of a tumor suppressor gene or the activation of an
oncogene, which leads to increased secretion of angiogenic
stimulators or decreased secretion of angiogenic inhibitors.
For example, a mutation in the von Hippel–Lindau tumor
suppressor gene leads to formation of vascular tumors in the
central nervous system and eyes and highly vascularized tumors in the kidney. It has been suggested that the loss of the
VHL protein leads to a decrease in the ubiquitination of hypoxia inducible factor 1α (HIF-1α) and a resulting increase
in vascular endothelial growth factor production (Kibel *et al.,*
1995; Conaway *et al.,* 1998; Ohh *et al.,* 2000). Another example is provided by loss of p53 protein function, which
leads to a decreased secretion of the angiogenic inhibitor
thrombospondin-1 (Dameron *et al.,* 1994). Moreover, changes
in the microenvironment, such as hypoxia, inflammation, or
tissue injury, can lead to increased expression of angiogenic
factors, leading to vascularization of the tumor.

B. Angiogenesis in Four Stages

Angiogenesis is a complex process that can be divided
into four stages: (1) establishment of vascular discontinuity;
(2) breakdown of the extracellular matrix (ECM); (3) endothelial cell migration and proliferation; (4) tube formation
and structural reorganization (Hanahan and Folkman, 1996)
(Fig. 2, see color insert). Initiation of the process of angiogenesis requires that endothelial cells be freed from the
contact-inhibited state. This may occur by mechanical disruption as in wounding or by dissolution of the basement membrane which causes discontinuity of the architectural matrix of
the vasculature. For this purpose, proteolytic enzymes, serine
proteases, and matrix metalloproteinases (MMPs) are produced by endothelial cells, tumor cells, and inflammatory
cells (Schmitt *et al.,* 1997). The changes in the ECM composition create a microenvironment in which activated en-

dothelial cells can proliferate, invade, and migrate away from
the preexisting parental vessels. Proliferation and migration
is dependent on the ability of endothelial cells to temporarily
move along their basement membrane. The migration of endothelial cells is initiated by angiogenic factors. Two of the
best characterized angiogenic factors are the basic fibroblast
growth factor (bFGF) and the vascular endothelial growth
factor (VEGF) (Senger *et al.,* 1983; Shing *et al.,* 1984). These
angiogenic factors activate specific cell surface receptor tyrosine kinases. VEGF induces hyperpermeability resulting in
the deposition of plasma proteins including plasminogen, fibrinogen, and vitronectin. This leads to the formation of an angiogenic matrix which supports the invasion and proliferation
of endothelial cells (Dvorak *et al.,* 1995). The integrin $\alpha_v\beta_3$
(and $\alpha_v\beta_5$) plays an essential role in the migration of endothelial cells (Brooks *et al.,* 1996). Cell motility requires the
intracellular domain of the integrin receptors and is dependent on tyrosine-kinase-dependent intracellular signaling
(Klemke *et al.,* 1994). The final step is characterized by structural reorganization and tube formation. Two characteristics
of endothelial cells are essential for three-dimensional
reorganization:

1. Endothelial cells have intrinsic polarity, which is manifested by the formation of a closed loop.
2. Endothelial cells have the ability to form tight junctions
   with other endothelial cells.

Cell matrix interactions are vital to structural integrity and
vascular patterning. As angiogenesis proceeds, secondary
sprouting occurs, following the same rules as the initial angiogenic response. A network of new blood vessels is formed.

C. Angiogenic Factors

I. Fibroblast Growth Factors

Since 1971, extensive research has been undertaken to
identify and characterize angiogenic factors. Basic fibroblast
growth factor (FGF-2) was the first to be discovered (1982),
followed by its relative, acidic fibroblast growth factor (FGF-
1). The FGF-family induces cellular migration, proliferation,
and differentiation (Kanda *et al.,* 1997). FGF-2 is synthesized
mainly by stromal fibroblasts and functions in growth and
differentiation, affecting various mammalian cells and organ
systems. FGF-2 lacks a signal sequence and is therefore not
secreted by classical pathways. The passive secretion of FGF-
2 from the cell may be due to cell death, wound injury, chemical injury, irradiation, or infection (McNeil *et al.,* 1989).
Several suggestions have been made to explain the active secretion of FGF-2, including the involvement of an ATP-
driven protein pump (Klionsky *et al.,* 1992), the involvement
of a complex between FGF-2 and a carrier protein (Piotrowicz *et al.,* 1997), and an exocytosis-independent process of
the endoplasmic reticulum–Golgi pathway (Mignatti *et al.,*

1992). The exact mechanism remains to be determined. Binding of FGF-2 to its receptor requires binding either to the heparan sulfate side chains of a proteoglycan or to free heparin (Yayon et al., 1991). In spite of the fact that FGF-2 is not a secreted protein, levels of FGF-2 mRNA are tightly regulated by factors such as transforming growth factor β_1 (TGF-β_1), plasminogen activator inhibitor 1 (PAI-1), and antithrombin III (Ku and D'Amore, 1995). FGF-2 stimulates wound healing, tissue repair, hematopoiesis, proper functioning of the nervous system, and angiogenesis (Allouche and Bikfalvi, 1995). During angiogenesis, FGF-2 regulates the activities of extracellular molecules, including collagenase, proteases, urokinase plasminogen activator (uPA), and integrins to form new capillary cord structures. FGFs confer their proangiogenic signal through an autocrine signaling loop to the cell nucleus via a family of transmembrane receptor tyrosine kinases. In tumor angiogenesis, VEGF stimulates endothelial cells to produce FGF-2, which further enhances angiogenic activity through both autocrine and paracrine mechanisms (Ferrara et al., 1992).

2. Vascular Endothelial Growth Factor

VEGF is a specific mitogen for endothelial cells and was first identified as vascular permeability factor (VPF) because of its strong effect on vascular permeability (Senger et al., 1986). In contrast with bFGF, VEGF is endothelial specific and plays an essential role in both physiologic and pathologic blood vessel formations (Ferrara and Davis-Smyth, 1997). Mouse embryos lacking one single allele of VEGF are lethal early in development (Carmeliet et al., 1996; Ferrara et al., 1996). VEGF expression is mainly regulated by oxygen tension and oxidative stress leads to an increased VEGF secretion, possibly under the control of hypoxia-inducible factor 1α (HIF-1α) (Iyer et al., 1998). VEGF mRNA expression is also up-regulated by several cytokines, like EGF, TGF-β, or keratinocyte growth factor 1 (KGF-1) (Levy et al., 1996). VEGF (also known as VEGF-A) consists of different isoforms, which are a result of alternative splicing from a single VEGF gene located on chromosome 6 (Mattei et al., 1996). VEGF-A, together with VEGF-B, VEGF-C, and VEGF-D, belongs to the VEGF/PDGF superfamily (Joukov et al., 1996; Olofsson et al., 1996; Yamada et al., 1997). VEGF-C is also involved in angiogenesis of lymphatic endothelial cells (Jeltsch et al., 1997). Two VEGF receptor tyrosine kinases have been identified. The VEGF-R1 and VEGF-R2 receptors bind VEGF with high affinity, and expression of both receptors is mainly restricted to the vascular endothelium. Like VEGF, the expression of the VEGF receptors is mainly regulated by hypoxia. Exposure to acute or chronic hypoxia led to an up-regulation of both VEGF-R1 and VEGF-R2 genes (Tuder et al., 1995).

A variety of functions are known for VEGF. It is known to be a survival protein for endothelial cells cultured under serum-free conditions (Gerber et al., 1998). It induces expression of the serine proteases uPA and tissue plasminogen activators (tPA) and also plasminogen activator inhibitor 1 (PAI-1) (Pepper et al., 1991). It promotes expression of several adhesion molecules (ICAM-1 and VCAM-1) in endothelial cells (Melder et al., 1996). Direct evidence for involvement of VEGF in tumor progression was first demonstrated by Kim et al. (1993) who showed that a specific monoclonal antibody directed against VEGF could suppress tumor growth. In situ hybridization has shown VEGF mRNA in several tumors, with the highest expression of VEGF mRNA found in hypoxic tumor cells near necrotic areas (Philips et al., 1993). More recent studies have shown that VEGF is also produced in tumor stromal cells (Fukumura et al., 1998). Several studies have shown that inhibition of VEGF leads to suppression of tumor growth both in mice and in human models.

3. Angiopoietins

The angiopoietins have been identified as another family of endothelial-cell-specific growth factors. Both angiopoietin-1 and angiopoietin-2 are ligands for the tyrosine kinase receptor Tie-2 (Davis et al., 1996; Suri et al., 1996; Maisonpierre et al., 1997), but a ligand for Tie-1 has not yet been identified. It has been suggested that angiopoietin-1 and angiopoietin-2 have opposing effects on the Tie-2 receptor. Angiopoietin-1 is an agonist of the Tie-2 receptor, whereas angiopoietin-2 is an antagonist of angiopoietin-1 that competes for binding to Tie-2 and blocks angiopoietin-2 induced Tie-2 autophosphorylation (Maisonpierre et al., 1997). While Tie-1 plays a role in endothelial cell differentiation and the establishment of blood vessel integrity, Tie-2 does not participate in the initial vasculogenesis phase but rather in angiogenic outgrowth, vessel remodeling, and maturation. The angiopoietins and Tie-2 receptor appear to be required for the communication of the endothelial cells with the surrounding mesenchyme in order to establish stable cellular and biochemical interactions (Maisonpierre et al., 1997). The angiopoietin/Tie-2 pathway seems to modulate the VEGF-induced postnatal neovascularization (Asahara et al., 1998), and it has been shown that blockage of this pathway by antiangiogenic gene therapy results in inhibition of tumor growth and metastasis (Lin et al., 1998).

D. Role of Integrins during Angiogenesis

Angiogenesis depends on the specific molecular interactions between vascular cells and components of the extracellular matrix. Cellular adhesion is mediated by integrins, which are heterodimeric transmembrane proteins containing one α and one β domain. Integrin-mediated adhesion leads to intracellular signaling that controls all kinds of cellular events, such as cell survival, proliferation, and migration (Aplin et al., 1998). During angiogenesis, integrins that are expressed on the cell surface of activated endothelial cells regulate critical adhesive interactions between the endothelial cells and the ECM-proteins, including fibronectin, vitronectin, different types of collagen, and von Willebrand factor. Of the different integrins, $\alpha_v\beta_3$ has been identified as the most important one in angiogenesis. Containing the RGD adhesive motif, integrin $\alpha_v\beta_3$ is a receptor for a broad range of ECM proteins. Endothelial cells undergoing angiogenesis express high levels of $\alpha_v\beta_3$ (Brooks et al., 1994a). Moreover, the integrin $\alpha_v\beta_3$ can bind matrix metalloproteinases, thereby controlling remodeling of the ECM and enabling endothelial cell invasion of the ECM (Brooks et al., 1996).

E. Breakdown and Remodeling of the Extracellular Matrix

The ECM provides signals that control viability of the endothelial cells. It communicates essential information to the endothelial cells to control processes, such as morphogenesis, apoptosis or survival, gain or loss of tissue-specific functions, cell migration, or tissue repair. During tumor progression the microenvironment of the stroma surrounding the tumor changes. There are parallels between the tumor stroma and wound healing (Dvorak, 1986), since both conditions are characterized by increased fibrinogen deposition, increased permeability of the vessels, and inflammatory responses (Brown et al., 1988; Yeo et al., 1991). In addition, angiogenic factors, including VEGF, which are produced by the tumor cells, induce tissue factor expression on the endothelial cells (Zucker et al., 1998). Exposure of tissue factor, which is also present on matrix components and on the tumor cells (Folkman, 1996; Ruf and Mueller, 1996), leads to thrombin activation resulting in fibrin formation. Together with other proteins, such as vitronectin and fibronectin, a provisional matrix is formed. The continuous formation and remodeling of the ECM is essential for angiogenesis (Fig. 3, see color insert). The major enzymes that control the ECM degradation and remodeling are the matrix metalloproteinases and the tissue serine proteases.

1. The Plasminogen Activator

During the process of angiogenesis a cascade of proteases, called the plasminogen activator (PA system), plays an important role. The PA system consists of the serine proteases, the serine protease inhibitors, and the protease receptors. Angiogenic growth factors induce the expression of uPA and tPA on endothelial cells (Pepper et al., 1991; Flaumenhaft et al., 1992; Ruf and Mueller, 1996). Antibodies against uPA block angiogenesis and tumor growth in both the chorioallantoic membrane assay (CAM assay) and various mouse models (Ossowski and Reich, 1983; Ossowski et al., 1991; Kobayashi et al., 1994). UPA is released from tumor cells or stroma cells and binds to surrounding tumor cells containing

the uPA receptor (uPA-R), which focuses the proteolytic action to the surface of the tumor cells (Ploug et al., 1991; Ruf and Mueller, 1996). High levels of uPA, PAI-1, and uPA-R are associated with poor clinical prognosis. TPA plays a primary role in fibrinolysis and angiogenesis during blood clot degradation and wound healing (Mignatti and Rifkin, 1993). Whereas tPA is normally only expressed by endothelial cells, uPA is expressed at many sites and is known to play an important role in migration of cells other than endothelial cells, including epithelial cells, fibroblasts, and tumor cells. Both uPA and tPA can convert plasminogen to plasmin, which subsequently leads to fibrinolysis. The formation of plasmin is essential for the invasion and migration of endothelial cells to the surrounding tissue. Plasmin breaks down fibrin and components of the ECM, including laminin and fibronectin. Furthermore, plasmin activates matrix metalloproteinases and elastases, which further degrade the ECM. Endothelial cells are the only cells that express PAI-1. PAI-1 inhibits tPA and uPA by binding the active domain and is important in the turnover of inactive uPA (Pepper et al., 1992). PAI-1 is released by proteases such as thrombin (Ehrlich et al., 1991). Basic FGF, VEGF, and TGF-β control the PA system, through a feedback mechanism. The Ets family of transcription factors is increased in situations involving extensive cell migration and tissue remodeling. The proto-oncogene c-ets1 expression correlates with invasive processes during tumor development. C-ets1 transcripts are detected in stromal cells surrounding the invasive carcinoma, as well as in endothelial cells of the new blood vessels neighboring the tumor (Wernert et al., 1992, 1994). C-ets1 can regulate the uPA transcription, as well as the transcription of other proteases (Gutman and Wasylyk, 1990; Wasylyk et al., 1991), and it has been suggested that FGF stimulates interaction of c-ets1 with the promoter region of uPA (Besser et al., 1995). VEGF stimulates the expression of transcription factor Ets-1 through binding to the tyrosine kinases VEGF-R1 and VEGF-R2. This leads to enhancement of the invasiveness of the endothelial cells (Sato et al., 2000). In agreement, activation of c-ets1 by EGF induces the expression of uPA, uPAR, collagenase 1, and MMP-1 in endothelial cells (Watabe et al., 1998). Activated TGF-β is capable of inducing expression of PAI-1, whereas PAI-1 blocks the transformation of latent TGF-β to active TGF-β by inhibiting plasmin formation (Sato et al., 1990; Odekon et al., 1994). Binding of uPA to its receptor leads to plasmin formation, which leads to activation of the latent form of TGF-β and to the release of biologically active bFGF from its ECM binding sites on heparan sulfate proteoglycans (Saksela and Rifkin, 1990). A recently identified regulator of the PA system is thrombin-activatable fibrinolysis inhibitor (TAFI), also known as procarboxypeptidase B. It has been suggested that TAFI can enhance tPA-induced thrombolysis (Refino et al., 1999). Studies on uPA or PAI-1 knockout mice showed an inability of tumor cells to grow.

In the uPA knockout mice, angiogenesis was still measurable, possibly due to tPA-induced and PAI-1-controlled plasmin formation. However, in the absence of PAI-1, capillaries failed to sprout into the vicinity of tumor cells and eventually in the tumor mass. This might be explained by the fact that excessive proteolysis prevents the coordinated growth of endothelial cells into capillary sprouts (Bajou *et al.*, 1998). Some of the newer antiangiogenic agents (Gutierrez *et al.*, 2000) might be based on the principle of excessive proteolysis (Reijerkerk *et al.*, 2000).

2. Matrix Metalloproteinases

The family of matrix metalloproteinases degrades almost any component of the ECM, thereby facilitating cell motility and thus angiogenesis. Most commonly, proteinases facilitate tumor progression by acting on the ECM to free cells from their cell cycle arrest, by mediating invasion, or by releasing angiogenic factors (Coussens and Werb, 1996). However, proteinases may also inhibit tumor progression by releasing latent angiogenic inhibitors or releasing inhibitors from the ECM proteins (Werb, 1997). MMPs are identified by their substrate preferences, such as collagenases, gelatinases, stromeolysins, and membrane-type (MT)-MMP. Currently, 17 MMP family members are identified. MMP-1, MMP-8, and MMP-13 preferentially degrade fibrillar collagens, whereas the gelatinases MMP-2 and MMP-9 express their proteolytic activities mainly on the basement membranes. All MMPs are secreted as inactive proMMPs and undergo an activation step, which can involve other MMPs, plasmin, growth factors, or MT-MMPs. MMPs play an important role in this process of proteolysis, by, for example, localizing the enzymes to the receptors where proteolysis takes place (Andreasen *et al.*, 1997; Nakahara *et al.*, 1997). Furthermore, the ability of endothelial cells to invade fibrin gels depends on the expression of MMP *in vitro* and *in vivo* (Hiraoka *et al.*, 1998). In contrast, some MMPs (MMP-7, MMP-9, and MMP-12) may block angiogenesis by converting plasminogen to angiostatin, which is a powerful inhibitor of angiogenesis (Dong *et al.*, 1997). The importance of matrix degradation for tumor metastasis and angiogenesis has been recognized, and a large number of agents blocking MMP activity have been developed. Several of these compounds are now in clinical trials (Brown, 2000) (see below).

2. How to Inhibit Tumor Angiogenesis

Because tumor growth and metastatic spread are dependent on angiogenesis, attacking the tumor by delivering toxic agents selectively to newly formed blood vessels or inhibiting the outgrowth of capillary sprouts should give a therapeutic benefit. There are several advantages in attacking the tumor's vasculature instead of the tumor cells. First, endothelial cells are considered to be genetically more stable then tumor cells, which decreases the development of drug resistance. Second, the tumor's vasculature is easily accessible to agents in the circulation (e.g., specific antibodies). Third, antiangiogenic therapy is in principle suitable for a wide range of different types of tumors. And finally, specific targeting of drugs to tumor areas should minimize the systemic side effects. Interference with angiogenesis may be accomplished by different points of attack, e.g., blocking the angiogenic activators, blocking matrix breakdown, and remodeling or blocking adhesion and migration of endothelial cells (Fig. 2). In the sections below an overview is given of preclinical and clinical studies with antiangiogenic agents. Because the clinical experience is limited and few trials are published as full papers, recent abstracts have been included to illustrate the clinical efforts in this research area.

A. Blocking Angiogenic Factors

1. Strategies to Block VEGF

Different strategies have been designed to inhibit VEGF function. First of all, specific VEGF antibodies have been developed that neutralize the effects of VEGF. These antibodies showed reduction in tumor growth in mouse models and they are now tested in phase I/II trials (Kim *et al.*, 1993; Presta *et al.*, 1997; Borgstrom *et al.*, 1998). RhuMAb (recombinant humanized monoclonal antibody) to VEGF is designed to provide high-affinity blockage of VEGF binding to its receptors on endothelial cells. A phase II trial with breast cancer patients showed that rhuMAb VEGF is well tolerated and has activity in metastatic breast cancer, although all of the activity seen has been in soft-tissue disease (Sledge *et al.*, 2000). A phase II trial comparing fluorouracil/leucovorin (5-FU/LV) plus rhuMAb treatment with 5-FU/LV alone in metastatic colorectal cancer patients showed an increase in response rate and prolonged time to disease progression for the patients treated with 5-FU/LV plus rhuMAb VEGF (Bergsland *et al.*, 2000). Another phase II trial comparing carboplatin/paclitaxel (CP) plus rhuMAb VEGF treatment (respectively 32 patients receiving low-dose rhuMAb VEGF and 35 patients receiving high-dose rhuMAb VEGF) with CP treatment alone (32 patients) in patients with advanced non-small cell lung carcinomas showed that the combination treatment with CP and rhuMAb VEGF resulted in higher response rates (18.8% for the CP without rhuMAb VEGF, 28.1% for the low-dose rhuMAb VEGF group, and 31.4% for the high dose rhuMAb VEGF group) (DeVore *et al.*, 2000). Furthermore, several new anti-VEGF agents are now being tested in xenograft models and phase I pharmacokinetic studies.

Blocking the interaction between VEGF and its receptors is another approach to inhibit angiogenesis. Purified soluble VEGF receptors bind VEGF with high affinity and block

VEGF-induced endothelial cell proliferation (Kendall *et al.*, 1996). Otherwise, new peptides that interfere with the binding of VEGF to its receptors have been found. By binding to an active region of VEGF, involved in receptor recognition, these peptides inhibit VEGF-induced proliferation (Fairbrother *et al.*, 1998). Aplidine is a new compound isolated from the Mediterranean tunicate *Aplidium albicans.* Aplidine down-regulates the VEGF receptor VEGF-R2 and induces a cell cycle arrest in G_1. It is suggested that the drug blocks the autocrine loop between VEGF and VEGF-R2 (Broggini *et al.*, 2000). A phase I and pharmacokinetic study with aplidine showed toxicity consisting of asthenia, nausea/vomiting, muscle cramps, muscular pain, and loss of muscular strength.

A third approach aims at the inhibition of VEGF receptor signaling by blocking the tyrosine kinase autophosphorylation (Sun *et al.*, 1998). For example, SU-5416 decreases VEGF-R2 phosphorylation resulting in inhibition of VEGF-driven neovascularization. A phase I pharmacokinetic study with SU-5416 showed no dose-limiting toxicity. Although some hypersensitivity reactions and mild thrombophlebitis were noted, no treatment was discontinued. SU-5416 was rapidly cleared through the formation of two metabolites. No tumor regression was observed, but 6 of 21 patients showed stable disease (O'Donnel *et al.*, 2000). In a phase I/II study, patients with untreated metastatic colorectal cancer were treated with a combination of 5-FU/LV and SU-5416. No dose-limiting toxicity could be determined. Of the 28 patients who were treated, 6 responded (1 complete regression, 5 partial regressions), 9 had stable disease, and 4 had progressive disease (Rosen *et al.*, 2000a). In contrast, SU-5416 combined with cisplatin-gemcitabine therapy induced an unacceptable toxicity, i.e., vascular events in various organs (Giaccone *et al.*, 2000). Another potent inhibitor of the VEGF-R2 receptor is SU6668, which is discussed in the next paragraph. VEGF is also used as a conjugate with a toxin, thereby creating a toxic agent specific for endothelial cells (Arora *et al.*, 1999). Apoptotic-induced drug delivery (AIDD) is a new approach that offers a biological mechanism of drug delivery. Genetically engineered endothelial cells (GEECs) were designed to express a VEGF-R2:fas fusion protein that would enable the cells to go into apoptosis upon binding to VEGF and subsequent activation of the fas-pathway. The GEECs were administrated either intratumorally or intravenously to the tumor-bearing mice. So growth factors produced by the tumor cells initiate apoptosis of the endothelial cells that surround them (Jianguo and Gallo, 2000).

2. Strategies to Block FGF

Blocking the intrinsic activity of FGF receptors is a promising new strategy for drug development. A selective inhibitor of FGF-1 receptor tyrosine kinase, PD166866, showed inhibition of microvessel outgrowth from cultured human pla-

cental arteries (Panek *et al.*, 1998). Furthermore, the interaction between FGF and its receptor is also a target for therapy mediated by antiangiogenic agent platelet factor 4 (PF-4). PF-4 inhibits binding of FGF-2 to its receptor by inhibiting FGF-2 dimerization (Perollet *et al.*, 1998). A second inhibitor, SU6668, is a small molecule with a high potential in inhibiting the tyrosine phosphorylation of the VEGF-R2 receptor, the PDGF receptor, and the FGF-1 receptor. SU6668 inhibits VEGF and bFGF endothelial mitogenesis *in vitro* and proliferation of many tumor cell lines. SU6668 induces high levels of apoptosis in tumor microvessels, followed by extensive tumor cell apoptotic death in tumor xenografts (Laird *et al.*, 2000a). SU6668 treatment induced striking regression of large established human tumor xenografts (Laird *et al.*, 2000b). A phase I pharmacokinetic study is currently ongoing (Rosen *et al.*, 2000b).

B. Strategies to Inhibit Endothelial Cell Proliferation

1. TNP470

TNP470 is a fumagillin analogue that was originally isolated from a contaminated culture of capillary endothelial cells. Purified fumagillin inhibited endothelial cell proliferation *in vitro* and tumor-induced angiogenesis *in vivo*. Among the fumagillin analogues, TNP470 was one of the most potent angiostatic agents and showed no toxicity such as hair loss, intestinal disturbance, or infection (Ingber *et al.*, 1990). Treatment of tumor-bearing mice with TNP470 doubled the incidence of apoptotic cells, probably because neovascularization was significantly attenuated and could not support rapid tumor growth (Parangi *et al.*, 1996). It has been suggested that excessive production of nitric oxide, which is produced by nitric oxide synthase, may be involved in TNP470-induced apoptosis by causing mitochondrial dysfunction and DNA damage (Yoshida *et al.*, 1998). Conjugation of the TNP470 with water-soluble polymers was shown to prolong the life of TNP470 in the circulation and to increase the accumulation of the drug in tissue with new-vessel formation (Yasukawa *et al.*, 1999). TNP470 is currently being tested in phase I and II clinical trials.

2. Thalidomide

Thalidomide was first introduced in 1953 as an oral sedative-hypnotic. After being withdrawn because of teratogenicity, it was again introduced in 1965 as an immunomodulatory agent. Novel insights into the biological effects of thalidomide revealed that it inhibits angiogenesis and suppresses TNF-α production (Sampaio *et al.*, 1991). Thalidomide inhibits bFGF and VEGF-induced angiogenesis (D'Amato *et al.*, 1994; Kenyon *et al.*, 1997). Furthermore, thalidomide can modulate cytokines and immunologic reactions (reviewed by Thomas and Kantarjian, 2000). A phase I/II study with thalidomide in patients with glioblastoma multiforme (GBM) showed a tolerated dose of 300 mg/ml with limited biological activity in recurrent GBM, 15% partial regression and 32% stable disease (Marx *et al.*, 2000). Thalidomide was also tested as an antiangiogenic agent in patients with hepatocellular carcinoma. Toxicity included somnolence and skin reactions. No significant antitumor activity could be determined (Patt *et al.*, 2000). A phase I study of thalidomide given to 12 patients with progressive metastatic renal cell cancer showed occasional responses (2 patients had a partial response and 3 patients had stable disease) in patients with poor performance status (Minor and Elias, 2000). A phase II trial with 17 patients with squamous cell carcinoma of the head and neck showed progressive disease in 16 patients evaluated and a median survival of 5.4 months (Tseng *et al.*, 2000).

3. Antiproliferative Drugs

Several synthetic antiproliferative agents have been isolated and tested for antitumor activity. Squalamine was isolated from shark liver. It inhibits mitogen-induced proliferation and migration of endothelial cells, thereby preventing tumor neovascularization. A phase I study showed that squalamine is well tolerated up to a dose of 357 mg/m^2 and demonstrates biologically relevant plasma concentrations approaching those required for antiangiogenic effects *in vitro* (Kalidas *et al.*, 2000). Combretastatin was isolated from the South African tree *Combretum caffrum* and appeared to have antiproliferative activity. The combretastatins have been shown to cause destruction of the tumor vasculature in several models (Dark *et al.*, 1997; Grosios *et al.*, 1999).

C. Strategies to Inhibit Integrin Function

Inhibitors of integrin $\alpha_v\beta_3$ showed disruption of angiogenesis in several *in vivo* models (Brooks *et al.*, 1994a; 1994b; Friedlander *et al.*, 1995; Hammes *et al.*, 1996). Furthermore, $\alpha_v\beta_3$ antagonists induced high levels of apoptotic tumor endothelial cells in animal models with tumor angiogenesis (Storgard *et al.*, 1999). These results suggest a critical role for integrin $\alpha_v\beta_3$ in mediating endothelial cell survival. Friedlander et al. defined two distinct angiogenic pathways mediated by integrins (Friedlander *et al.*, 1995). They showed that anti-integrin $\alpha_v\beta_3$ mAb blocked bFGF-induced angiogenesis and that anti-integrin $\alpha_v\beta_5$ mAb blocked VEGF-induced angiogenesis. Recently, it was shown that TNF and interferon-γ inhibit integrin $\alpha_v\beta_3$ function. This abolishes specific adhesion-dependent survival signals and results in endothelial cell apoptosis and disruption of angiogenesis (Ruegg *et al.*, 1998). A phase I trial (Gutheil *et al.*, 2000) with the humanized anti-integrin $\alpha_v\beta_3$ antibody vitaxin was well tolerated with little or no toxicity. Of 17 patients treated in the phase I trial, one showed a partial response and 10 showed stable disease that in one case lasted 22 months.

D. Strategies to Block Extracellular Matrix Breakdown and Remodeling

1. Tissue Inhibitors of Metalloproteinase Inhibitors

The tissue metalloproteinase inhibitors (TIMP) form a family of which four members have been characterized: TIMP-1, TIMP-2, TIMP-3, and TIMP-4. TIMPs are capable of inhibiting the activities of all known MMPs by forming noncovalent complexes with the MMPs. TIMPs therefore play a key role in maintaining the balance between ECM breakdown and remodeling. TIMP-1 and TIMP-2 are multifunctional proteins with diverse actions leading to inhibition of angiogenesis in several bioassays (Takigawa *et al.*, 1990; Johnson *et al.*, 1994). TIMP-3 is exclusively found in the ECM. It is regulated in a cell-cycle-dependent fashion (Wick *et al.*, 1995) and inhibits neovascularization(Anand-Apte *et al.*, 1997). TIMP-4 may function in a tissue specific dependent fashion in matrix hemostasis.

2. Thrombospondin-1

Thrombospondin-1 (TSP-1) belongs to the family of extracellular matrix proteins that have diverse effects on cell adhesion, motility, proliferation, and survival, i.e., the thrombospondins (Bornstein, 1995). TSP-1 inhibits angiogenesis, by inhibiting growth, sprouting, motility of endothelial cells *in vitro* (Good *et al.*, 1990; Taraboletti *et al.*, 1990; Tolsma *et al.*, 1997). TSP-1 also inhibits neovascularization in the rat corneal pocket assay, the chick chorioallantoic membrane assay, and mouse xenografts models (Dameron *et al.*, 1994; Good *et al.*, 1990). The antiangiogenic importance of TSP-1 could be linked to malignant pathology because loss of wild-type p53 gene function resulted in a loss of thrombospondin-1 expression. This finding first established a possible link between the genetic basis of cancer and angiogenesis (Dameron *et al.*, 1994). A smaller (50-kDa) proteolytic fragment of TSP-1 contains the same inhibitory activity as the intact TSP-1. Several peptides originating from this 50-kDa fragment showed inhibition of angiogenesis in the rat corneal assay (Tolsma *et al.*, 1993). Based on the preclinical results, TSP-1 is now being tested in phase I clinical trials.

3. Synthetic Inhibitors of Matrix Metalloproteinases

During the past decades several synthetic inhibitors of matrix metalloproteinases have been developed. Marimastat is a MMP inhibitor that reached phase III trials. Phase I studies defined optimal dose and showed that the main side effects were fatigue and cumulative reversible inflammatory polyarthritis. Marimastat is currently tested in patients with non–small cell lung cancer, breast cancer, small cell lung cancer in phase III, and glioblastomas and gliosarcomas in phase I/II trials. A phase II trial in patients with breast cancer showed that marimastat was well tolerated, but severe musculoskeletal toxicity resulted in dose-limited chronic administration (Miller *et al.,* 2000). A double-blind placebo-controlled study in 369 patients with inoperable gastric adenocarcinomas showed a small but significant increase in survival in the marimastat-treated patients, i.e., 167 days for marimastat versus 135 days for placebo-treated patients (Fielding *et al.,* 2000).

Col-3 is a tetracycline analogue that inhibits both expression and activity of MMP-2 and MMP-9. A phase I pharmacokinetic and pharmacodynamic study showed that Col-3 is well tolerated on a oral schedule. The MMP-2 and MMP-9 levels decreased in most patients (Rowinsky *et al.,* 2000). Neovastat is a multifunctional antiangiogenic agent purified from shark cartilage (Dupont, 1998). Animal studies showed a 50% reduction of the intratumoral vasculature when Neovastat was administered orally (Berger *et al.,* 2000). Neovastat is currently tested in phase III trials.

E. Endogenous Inhibitors of Angiogenesis

During the past few years, several endogenous inhibitors of angiogenesis have been identified. The clinical observation that removal of the primary tumor led to rapid growth of avascular undetectable metastases suggested the generation of endogenous inhibitory factors produced by the primary tumor (O'Reilly *et al.,* 1994; Holmgren *et al.,* 1995). The major advantage of endogenous inhibitors in the treatment of cancer is that they are less likely to cause side effects, such as suppression of hematopoiesis and gastrointestinal systems (Folkman, 1995a).

1. Angiostatin

Angiostatin is a 38-kDa inhibitor, purified from both urine and serum samples of mice bearing Lewis lung carcinomas. Angiostatin is a specific inhibitor of proliferation of several endothelial cell lines, but not of several nonendothelial cell lines tested *in vitro. In vivo,* angiostatin suppressed neovascularization in the chick chorioallantoic membrane assay and in the mouse corneal neovascularization assay (O'Reilly *et al.,* 1994, 1996). Angiostatin is a proteolytic fragment of plasminogen, containing the first four of five kringle domains of plasminogen. The origin of angiostatin *in vivo* is not known. It is unlikely that tumor cells produce angiostatin because they lack a detectable amount of plasminogen mRNA (Folkman, 1995b). However, tumor cells and macrophages in the tumor may express proteases that are capable of cleaving plasminogen into angiostatin (Dong *et al.,* 1997). The exact mechanism by which angiostatin works is still unknown but several mechanisms have been postulated. (Brooks *et al.,* 1994a, 1994b; Holmgren *et al.,* 1995; Cao *et al.,* 1996a; Lucas *et al.,* 1998). Several fragments of plasminogen containing different kringle domains showed functional differences between the kringle domain structures. The disulfide-bond-mediated folding of the kringle structures in angiostatin is es-

sential to maintain its inhibitory activity on endothelial cell growth (Cao *et al.,* 1996b). Although plasminogen contains the same kringle domains, it is inactive in inhibiting endothelial cell proliferation or primary tumor and metastatic tumor growth (O'Reilly *et al.,* 1994, 1996). Amino acid sequence alignment of the kringle domains of plasminogen showed 45–50% homology between kringle 1, 2, 3, and 4 (Sohndel *et al.,* 1996). K1 was first characterized as the most potent inhibitory segment of angiostatin on endothelial cell proliferation, whereas fragments consisting of K4 are comparatively inefficient in suppressing endothelial cell growth (Cao *et al.,* 1996b). K5 has 57.5% sequence homology with K1 and 52.5% with K4, by which K5 lacks two sets of lysine pairs in comparison with K4. It was demonstrated that K5 inhibits bFGF-stimulated endothelial cell proliferation more efficiently then angiostatin (Cao *et al.,* 1997). Angiostatin is currently being tested in phase I clinical trials.

2. Endostatin

In 1997 O'Reilly et al. found another specific angiogenesis inhibitor, endostatin. The N-terminal sequence of this 20-kDa inhibitor revealed identity to the C-terminal fragment of collagen XVIII. Systemic administration of recombinant endostatin showed potent inhibition of angiogenesis, maintenance of metastases at microscopic size, and regression of primary tumors (O'Reilly *et al.,* 1997). Endostatin induces specific endothelial cell apoptosis by different mechanisms in different stages; endostatin increases caspase-3 activity, induces DNA fragmentation, and decreases Bcl-2 levels (Dhanabal *et al.,* 1999). Mutations in endostatin, affecting heparin binding of recombinant endostatin, abolished inhibition of bFGF-induced angiogenesis in a chick chorioallantoic membrane assay (Sasaki *et al.,* 1999). Recently, Reijerkerk and colleagues established that endostatin binds plasminogen and stimulates tPA-mediated plasmin formation in a lysine-dependent manner (Reijerkerk *et al.,* 2000). The exact mechanism by which endostatin inhibits angiogenesis remains to be determined. Recombinant endostatin has been tested in three phase I trials, and little or no toxicity was encountered. RhEndostatin is associated with changes in blood flow through the tumors but not through the heart. Furthermore, serum levels of VEGF and bFGF were decreased in some patients. The effects of rhEndostatin on tumor progression are not yet known (Eder *et al.,* 2000; Herbst *et al.,* 2000; Thomas *et al.,* 2000).

3. Antithrombin III

Another recently identified endogenous antiangiogenic agent is antithrombin III (O'Reilly *et al.,* 1999). Antithrombin normally circulates in a quiescent form, but upon cleavage and mild denaturation antithrombin changes to a locked antiangiogenic form. Compared with the stressed confirmation of antithrombin, this cleaved and locked antiangiogenic antithrombin (aaAT) conformation inhibits bFGF- and VEGF-induced endothelial cell proliferation, inhibits angiogenesis in the chick chorioallantoic membrane assay, and inhibits tumor progression in *in vivo* mouse models.

F. Vascular Targeting

During the past decade several approaches have been used to develop and characterize antibodies or peptides that specifically target the tumor's vasculature. In 1997, Thorpe and coworkers showed that targeting of human tissue factor to the tumor endothelium induced a major initiation of the thrombogenic cascades leading to tumor infarction. To perform these experiments they produced an antibody–tissue factor conjugate. This antibody was directed against major histocompatibility class II antigens. MHC class II antigens were artificially up-regulated on the tumor endothelium by transfecting tumor cells with the interferon-γ gene (Huang *et al.,* 1997). Later, they described the use of an anti-VCAM-1 antibody–tissue factor conjugate to target the tumor vasculature and induce thrombosis (Ran *et al.,* 1998). In the same year, Neri et al. (1997) described the engineering and use of human antibody fragments directed against a fibronectin isoform with the extra domain B (ED-B), using the phage display antibody library. They showed that the use of a dimeric scFv fragment gave the best tumor-targeting results, with good stability to proteolysis and low liver uptake in mice (Neri *et al.,* 1997). Linkage of these purified scFv fragments to liposomes showed a 45–50% tumor regression in nude mice bearing subcutaneous F9 tumors (Marty *et al.,* 2000).

Another type of library used is the phage display peptide library, in which a peptide instead of an antibody fragment is expressed on the surface of a phage. Using this technique *in vivo,* a nine-residue cyclic peptide containing an RGD sequence was discovered. This peptide could distinguish between an angiogenic endothelial cell in the vascular bed of a tumor and nonproliferating endothelial cells elsewhere in the vasculature (Pasqualini *et al.,* 1997). The peptide selectively targeted angiogenic endothelial cells and, when coupled to a cytotoxic agent, induced tumor regression (Arap *et al.,* 1998a, 1998b). Using this peptide, a targeted proapoptotic peptide was designed containing two functional domains (Ellerby *et al.,* 1999). The targeting domain (RGD) was used to induce homing to the tumor vasculature, and the proapoptotic domain (KLAKLAK) was used to disrupt mitochondrial membranes when internalized in the target cells. Using this designed peptide, progressive apoptosis was seen in Kaposi's sarcoma-derived cells (Ellerby *et al.,* 1999). Recently, Pasqualini and colleagues identified a novel cyclic decapeptide MMP inhibitor, using the phage display technology (Koivunen *et al.,* 1999). They show that this peptide has multiple functions in both inhibiting MMP-2 and MMP-9 and in homing to the tumor vasculature. This CTTHWGFTLC peptide showed inhibition of migration of five human tumor cell lines and two endothelial cell lines tested *in vitro;* furthermore, the peptide showed potent antitumor activity in mouse tumor models.

Targeting or homing of antibodies or peptides toward the tumor vasculature is one of the new promising anticancer strategies. A disadvantages of targeting ECM components up-regulated during angiogenesis is the fact that the process of crossing the endothelial layer, which precedes the antibody binding to, say, the FN isoform located in the abluminal site of the vessel, could be slow because of interstitial pressure (Clauss *et al.,* 1990). The challenge is to find surface markers on angiogenic endothelial cells that do not show cross-reactivity with resting endothelial cells. A peptide or antibody with high affinity for such a marker could be used for many therapeutic purposes in anticancer treatment.

3. Concluding Remarks

The conceptual basis of antivascular therapies is now supported by an abundance of preclinical studies. Several early clinical studies have shown that antiangiogenic treatment has biological activity in patients with cancer. In the next decade both vascular targeting approaches and antiangiogenesis strategies will be incorporated in the treatment of cancer patients. This may either be as single agents or in combination with other antiangiogenic agents, chemotherapeutics, immunotherapy, or radiotherapy.

References

Allouche, M., and Bikfalvi, A. (1995). The role of fibroblast growth factor-2 (FGF-2) in hematopoiesis. *Prog. Growth Factor Res.* **6**, 35–48.

Anand-Apte, B., Pepper, M. S., Voest, E., Montesano, R., Olsen, B., Murphy, G., Apte, S. S., and Zetter, B. (1997). Inhibition of angiogenesis by tissue inhibitor of metalloproteinase-3. *Invest Ophthalmol. Vis. Sci.* **38**, 817–823.

Andreasen, P. A., Kjoller, L., Christensen, L., and Duffy, M. J. (1997). The urokinase-type plasminogen activator system in cancer metastasis: a review. *Int. J. Cancer* **72**, 1–22.

Aplin, A. E., Howe, A., Alahari, S. K., and Juliano, R. L. (1998). Signal transduction and signal modulation by cell adhesion receptors: the role of integrins, cadherins, immunoglobulin-cell adhesion molecules, and selectins. *Pharmacol. Rev.* **50**, 197–263.

Arap, W., Pasqualini, R., and Ruoslahti, E. (1998a). Chemotherapy targeted to tumor vasculature. *Curr. Opin. Oncol.* **10**, 560–565.

Arap, W., Pasqualini, R., and Ruoslahti, E. (1998b). Cancer treatment by targeted drug delivery to tumor vasculature in a mouse model. *Science* **279**, 377–380.

Arora, N., Masood, R., Zheng, T., Cai, J., Smith, D. L., and Gill, P. S. (1999). Vascular endothelial growth factor chimeric toxin is highly active against endothelial cells. *Cancer Res.* **59**, 183–188.

Asahara, T., Chen, D., Takahashi, T., Fujikawa, K., Kearney, M., Magner, M., Yancopoulos, G. D., and Isner, J. M. (1998). Tie2 receptor ligands, angiopoietin-1 and angiopoietin-2, modulate VEGF-induced postnatal neovascularization. *Circ. Res.* **83**, 233–240.

Bajou, K., Noel, A., Gerard, R. D., Masson, V., Brunner, N., Holst-Hansen, C., Skobe, M., Fusenig, N. E., Carmeliet, P., Collen, D., and Foidart, J. M. (1998). Absence of host plasminogen activator inhibitor 1 prevents cancer invasion and vascularization. *Nat. Med.* **4**, 923–928.

Berger, F., Jourdes, A. L., and Benadid, A. L. (2000). In vivo antitumoral activity of the multifunctional antiangiogenic agent Neovastat / AE-941 in experimental glioma. Proceedings 11th NCI-EORTC-AACR symposium on new drugs in cancer therapy, abstract 272.

Bergsland, E., Hurwitz, H., Fehrenbacher, L., Meropol, N. J., Novotny, W. F., Gaudreault, J., Lieberman, G., and Kabbinavar, F. (2000). A randomized phase II trial comparing rhuMAb VEGF plus 5-Flourouacil/Leucovorin (5FU/LV) to 5FU/LV alone in patients with metastatic colorectal cancer. *Proc. Am. Soc. Clin. Oncol.* **19**, abstract 939.

Besser, D., Presta, M., and Nagamine, Y. (1995). Elucidation of a signaling pathway induced by FGF-2 leading to uPA gene expression in NIH 3T3 fibroblasts. *Cell Growth Differ.* **6**, 1009–1017.

Borgstrom, P., Bourdon, M. A., Hillan, K. J., Sriramarao, P., and Ferrara, N. (1998). Neutralizing anti-vascular endothelial growth factor antibody completely inhibits angiogenesis and growth of human prostate carcinoma micro tumors in vivo. *Prostate* **35**, 1–10.

Bornstein, P. (1995). Diversity of function is inherent in matricellular proteins: an appraisal of thrombospondin 1 . *J. Cell Biol.* **130**, 503–506.

Broggini, M., Marchini, S., D'Incalci, M., Taraboleeti, G., Giavazzi, R., Faircloth, G., and Jimeno, J. (2000). Aplidine blocks VEGF secretion and VEGF/VEGF-R1 autocrine loop in human leukemic cell line. Proceedings 11th NCI-EORTC-AACR symposium on new drugs in cancer therapy, abstract 214.

Brooks, P. C., Clark, R. A., and Cheresh, D. A. (1994a). Requirement of vascular integrin alpha v beta 3 for angiogenesis. *Science* **264**, 569–571.

Brooks, P. C., Montgomery, A. M., Rosenfeld, M., Reisfeld, R. A., Hu, T., Klier, G., and Cheresh, D. A. (1994b). Integrin alpha v beta 3 antagonists promote tumor regression by inducing apoptosis of angiogenic blood vessels. *Cell* **79**, 1157–1164.

Brooks, P. C., Stromblad, S., Sanders, L. C., von Schalscha, T. L., Aimes, R. T., Stetler-Stevenson, W. G., Quigley, J. P., and Cheresh, D. A. (1996). Localization of matrix metalloproteinase MMP-2 to the surface of invasive cells by interaction with integrin alpha v beta 3. *Cell* **85**, 683–693.

Brown, L. F., Asch, B., Harvey, V. S., Buchinski, B., and Dvorak, H. F. (1988). Fibrinogen influx and accumulation of cross-linked fibrin in mouse carcinomas. *Cancer Res.* **48**, 1920–1925.

Brown, P. D. (2000). Ongoing trials with matrix metalloproteinase inhibitors. *Exp. Opin. Invest. Drugs* **9**, 2167–2177.

Cao, Y., Chen, A., An, S. A., Ji, R. W., Davidson, D., and Llinas, M. (1997). Kringle 5 of plasminogen is a novel inhibitor of endothelial cell growth. *J. Biol. Chem.* **272**, 22924–22928.

Cao, Y., Chen, H., Zhou, L., Chiang, M. K., Anand Apte, B., Weatherbee, J. A., Wang, Y., Fang, F., Flanagan, J. G., and Tsang, M. L. (1996a). Heterodimers of placenta growth factor/vascular endothelial growth factor. Endothelial activity, tumor cell expression, and high affinity binding to Flk-1/KDR. *J. Biol. Chem.* **271**, 3154–3162.

Cao, Y., Ji, R. W., Davidson, D., Schaller, J., Marti, D., Sohndel, S., McCance, S. G., O'Reilly, M. S., Llinas, M., and Folkman, J. (1996b). Kringle domains of human angiostatin. Characterization of the antiproliferative activity on endothelial cells. *J. Biol. Chem.* **271**, 29461–29467.

Carmeliet, P., Ferreira, V., Breier, G., Pollefeyt, S., Kieckens, L., Gertsenstein, M., Fahrig, M., Vandenhoeck, A., Harpal, K., Eberhardt, C., Declercq, C., Pawling, J., Moons, L., Collen, D., Risau, W., and Nagy, A. (1996). Abnormal blood vessel development and lethality in embryos lacking a single VEGF allele. *Nature* **380**, 435–439.

Clauss, M. A., Jain, R. K. (1990). Interstitial transport of rabbit and sheep antibodies in normal and neoplastic tissues. *Cancer Res.* **50**, 3487–3492.

Conaway, J. W., Kamura, T., and Conaway, R. C. (1998). The Elongin BC complex and the von Hippel-Lindau tumor suppressor protein. *Biochim. Biophys. Acta* **1377**, M49–M54.

Coussens, L. M., and Werb, Z. (1996). Matrix metalloproteinases and the development of cancer. *Chem. Biol.* **3**, 895–904.

D'Amato, R. J., Loughnan, M. S., Flynn, E., and Folkman, J. (1994). Thalidomide is an inhibitor of angiogenesis. *Proc. Natl. Acad. Sci. USA* **91**, 4082–4085.

Dameron, K. M., Volpert, O. V., Tainsky, M. A., and Bouck, N. (1994). Control of angiogenesis in fibroblasts by p53 regulation of thrombospondin-1. *Science* **265**, 1582–1584.

Dark, G. G., Hill, S. A., Prise, V. E., Tozer, G. M., Pettit, G. R., and Chaplin, D. J. (1997). Combretastatin A-4, an agent that displays potent and selective toxicity toward tumor vasculature. *Cancer Res.* **57**, 1829–1834.

Davis, S., Aldrich, T. H., Jones, P. F., Acheson, A., Compton, D. L., Jain, V., Ryan, T. E., Bruno, J., Radziejewski, C., Maisonpierre, P. C., and Yancopoulos, G. D. (1996). Isolation of angiopoietin-1, a ligand for the TIE2 receptor, by secretion-trap expression cloning . *Cell* **87**, 1161–1169.

DeVore, R. F., Fehrenbacher, L., Herbst, R. S., Langer, C. J., Kelly, K., Gaudreault, J., Holmgren, E., Novotny, W. F., and Kabbinavar, F. (2000). A randomized phase II trial comparing rhuMAb VEGF plus carboplatin/paclitaxel (CP) to CP alone in patients with stage IIIB/IV NSCLC. *Proc. Am. Soc. Clin. Oncol.* **19**, abstract 1896.

Dhanabal, M., Ramchandran, R., Waterman, M. J., Lu, H., Knebelmann, B., Segal, M., and Sukhatme, V. P. (1999). Endostatin induces endothelial cell apoptosis. *J. Biol. Chem.* **274**, 11721–11726.

Dong, Z., Kumar, R., Yang, X., and Fidler, I. J. (1997). Macrophage-derived metalloelastase is responsible for the generation of angiostatin in Lewis lung carcinoma. *Cell* **88**, 801–810.

Dvorak, H. F. (1986). Tumors: wounds that do not heal. Similarities between tumor stroma generation and wound healing. *N. Engl. J. Med.* **315**, 1650–1659.

Dvorak, H. F., Brown, L. F., Detmar, M., and Dvorak, A. M. (1995). Vascular permeability factor/vascular endothelial growth factor, microvascular hyperpermeability, and angiogenesis. *Am. J. Pathol.* **146**, 1029–1039.

Eder, J. P., Clark, J. W., Supko, J. G., Shulman, L. N., Garcia-Carbonero, R., Roper, K., Proper, J., Keogan, M., Schnipper, L., Connors, S., Butterfield, C., Fogler, W., Xu, G., Gubish, E., Folkman, J., and Kufe, D. W. (2000). Recombinant human endostatin demonstrates safety, linear pharmacokinetics and biological effects on tumor growth factors: Results of a phase I clinical study. Proceedings 11th NCI-EORTC-AACR symposium on new drugs in cancer therapy, abstract 258.

Ehrlich, H. J., Gebbink, R. K., Preissner, K. T., Keijer, J., Esmon, N. L., Mertens, K., and Pannekoek, H. (1991). Thrombin neutralizes plasminogen activator inhibitor 1 (PAI-1) that is complexed with vitronectin in the endothelial cell matrix. *J. Cell Biol.* **115**, 1773–1781.

Ellerby, H. M., Arap, W., Ellerby, L. M., Kain, R., Andrusiak, R., Rio, G. D., Krajewski, S., Lombardo, C. R., Rao, R., Ruoslahti, E., Bredesen, D. E., and Pasqualini, R. (1999). Anti-cancer activity of targeted pro-apoptotic peptides. *Nat. Med.* **5**, 1032–1038.

Fairbrother, W. J., Christinger, H. W. , Cochran, A. G., Fuh, G., Keenan, C. J., Quan, C., Shriver, S. K., Tom, J. Y., Wells, J. A., and Cunningham, B. C. (1998). Novel peptides selected to bind vascular endothelial growth factor target the receptor-binding site. *Biochemistry* **37**, 17754–17764.

Ferrara, N., Carver-Moore, K., Chen, H., Dowd, M., Lu, L., O'Shea, K. S., Powell-Braxton, L., Hillan, K. J., and Moore, M. W. (1996). Heterozygous embryonic lethality induced by targeted inactivation of the VEGF gene. *Nature* **380**, 439–442.

Ferrara, N., and Davis-Smyth, T. (1997). The biology of vascular endothelial growth factor. *Endocr. Rev.* **18**, 4–25.

Ferrara, N., Houck, K., Jakeman, L., and Leung, D. W. (1992). Molecular and biological properties of the vascular endothelial growth factor family of proteins. *Endocrinol. Rev.* **13**, 18–32.

Fidler, I. J., Kumar, R., Bielenberg, D. R., and Ellis, L. M. (1998). Molecular determinants of angiogenesis in cancer metastasis. *Cancer J. Sci. Am.* **4**(Suppl 1):S58–S66.

Fielding, J., Scholefield, J., Stuart, R., Hawkins, P., McCulloch, P., Maughan, T., Seymour, M., Van Cutsem, E., Thorlacius-Ussing, O., and Hovendal, C. (2000). A randomized double-blind placebo-controlled study of Marimastat in patients with inoperable gastric adenocarcinoma. *Proc. Am. Soc. Clin. Oncol.* **19,** abstract 929.

Flaumenhaft, R., Abe, M., Mignatti, P., and Rifkin, D. B. (1992). Basic fibroblast growth factor-induced activation of latent transforming growth factor beta in endothelial cells: regulation of plasminogen activator activity. *J. Cell Biol.* **118,** 901–909.

Folkman, J. (1972). Anti-angiogenesis: new concept for therapy of solid tumors. *Ann. Surg.* **175,** 409–416.

Folkman, J. (1995a). Seminars in Medicine of the Beth Israel Hospital, Boston. Clinical applications of research on angiogenesis. *N. Engl. J. Med.* **333,** 1757–1763.

Folkman, J. (1995b). Angiogenesis in cancer, vascular, rheumatoid and other disease. *Nat. Med.* **1,** 27–31.

Folkman, J. (1996). Tumor angiogenesis and tissue factor. *Nat. Med.* **2,** 167–168.

Friedlander, M., Brooks, P. C., Shaffer, R. W., Kincaid, C. M., Varner, J. A., and Cheresh, D. A. (1995). Definition of two angiogenic pathways by distinct alpha v integrins. *Science* **270,** 1500–1502.

Fukumura, D., Xavier, R., Sugiura, T., Chen, Y., Park, E. C., Lu, N., Selig, M., Nielsen, G., Taksir, T., Jain, R. K., and Seed, B. (1998). Tumor induction of VEGF promoter activity in stromal cells. *Cell* **94,** 715–725.

Gerber, H. P., Dixit, V., and Ferrara, N. (1998). Vascular endothelial growth factor induces expression of the antiapoptotic proteins Bcl-2 and A1 in vascular endothelial cells. *J. Biol. Chem.* **273,** 13313–13316.

Giaccone, G., Rosen, L., Kuenen, B., Ruijter, R., van der Vijgh, W. J. F., Peters, G. J., Huisman, H., Hoekman, K., Scigalla, P., Smit, E. F., and Pinedo, H. M. (2000). Dose finding study of cisplatin, gemcitabine and SU-5416 in patients with advanced malignancies. Proceedings 11th NCI-EORTC-AACR symposium on new drugs in cancer therapy, abstract 263.

Good, D. J., Polverini, P. J., Rastinejad, F., Le Beau, M. M., Lemons, R. S., and Frazier, W. A. B.-N. (1990). A tumor suppressor-dependent inhibitor of angiogenesis is immunologically and functionally indistinguishable from a fragment of thrombospondin. *Proc. Natl. Acad. Sci. USA* **87,** 6624–6628.

Grosios, K., Holwell, S. E., McGown, A. T., Pettit, G. R., and Bibby, M. C. (1999). In vivo and in vitro evaluation of combretastatin A-4 and its sodium phosphate prodrug. *Br. J. Cancer* **81,** 1318–1327.

Gutheil, J. C., Campbell, T. N., Pierce, P. R., Watkins, J. D., Huse, W. D., Bodkin, D. J., and Cheresh, D. A. (2000). Targeted antiangiogenic therapy for cancer using Vitaxin: a humanized monoclonal antibody to the integrin alphavbeta3. *Clin. Cancer Res.* **6,** 3056–3061.

Gutierrez, L. S., Schulman, A., Brito-Robinson, T., Noria, F., Ploplis, V. A., and Castellino, F. J. (2000). Tumor development is retarded in mice lacking the gene for urokinase-type plasminogen activator or its inhibitor, plasminogen activator inhibitor-1. *Cancer Res.* **60,** 5839–5847.

Gutman, A., and Wasylyk, B. (1990). The collagenase gene promoter contains a TPA and oncogene-responsive unit encompassing the PEA3 and AP-1 binding sites. *EMBO J.* **9,** 2241–2246.

Gutman, M., Singh, R. K., Price, J. E., Fan, D., and Fidler, I. J. (1994). Accelerated growth of human colon cancer cells in nude mice undergoing liver regeneration. *Invasion Metastasis* **14,** 362–371.

Hammes, H. P., Brownlee, M., Jonczyk, A., Sutter, A., and Preissner, K. T. (1996). Subcutaneous injection of a cyclic peptide antagonist of vitronectin receptor-type integrins inhibits retinal neovascularization. *Nat. Med.* **2,** 529–533.

Hanahan, D., and Folkman, J. (1996). Patterns and emerging mechanisms of the angiogenic switch during tumorigenesis. *Cell* **86,** 353–364.

Herbst, R., Tran, H., Hess, K., Madden, T., Charnsangavej, C., Gravel, D.,

Terry, K., Guerra, M., Taebel, K., Ellis, L., Pluda, J., Hong, W. K., and Abbruzzese, J. (2000). A phase I clinical trial of recombinant human endostatin (rHE) in patients (PTS) with solid tumors: pharmacokinetic, safety and efficacy analysis. Proceedings 11th NCI-EORTC-AACR symposium on new drugs in cancer therapy, abstract 258.

Hiraoka, N., Allen, E., Apel, I. J., Gyetko, M. R., and Weiss, S. J. (1998). Matrix metalloproteinases regulate neovascularization by acting as pericellular fibrinolysins. *Cell* **95,** 365–377.

Holmgren, L., O'Reilly, M. S., and Folkman, J. (1995). Dormancy of micrometastases: balanced proliferation and apoptosis in the presence of angiogenesis suppression. *Nat. Med.* **1,** 149–153.

Huang, X., Molema, G., King, S., Watkins, L., Edgington, T. S., and Thorpe, P. E. (1997). Tumor infarction in mice by antibody-directed targeting of tissue factor to tumor vasculature. *Science* **275,** 547–550.

Ingber, D., Fujita, T., Kishimoto, S., Sudo, K., Kanamaru, T., Brem, H., and Folkman, J. (1990). Synthetic analogues of fumagillin that inhibit angiogenesis and suppress tumour growth. *Nature* **348,** 555–557.

Iyer, N. V., Kotch, L. E., Agani, F., Leung, S. W., Laughner, E., Wenger, R. H., Gassmann, M., Gearhart, J. D., Lawler, A. M., Yu, A. Y., and Semenza, G. L. (1998). Cellular and developmental control of O2 homeostasis by hypoxia-inducible factor 1 alpha. *Genes Dev.* **12,** 149–162.

Jeltsch, M., Kaipanen, A., Joukov, V., Meng, X., Lakso, M., Rauvala, H., Schwartz, M., Fukumara, D., Jain, R. K., and Alitalo, K. (1997) Hyperplasia of lymphatic vessels in VEGF-C transgenic mice. *Science* **276,** 1423–1425.

Jianguo, M., and Gallo, J. M. (2000). Cells designed to deliver anticancer drugs by apoptosis. Proceedings 11th NCI-EORTC-AACR symposium on new drugs in cancer therapy, abstract 127.

Johnson, M. D., Kim, H. R., Chesler, L., Tsao-Wu, G., Bouck, N., and Polverini, P. J. (1994). Inhibition of angiogenesis by tissue inhibitor of metalloproteinase. *J. Cell Physiol* **160,** 194–202.

Joukov, V., Pajusola, K., Kaipainen, A., Chilov, D., Lahtinen, I., Kukk, E., Saksela, O., Kalkkinen, N., and Alitalo, K. (1996). A novel vascular endothelial growth factor, VEGF-C, is a ligand for the Flt4 (VEGFR-3) and KDR (VEGFR-2) receptor tyrosine kinases. *EMBO J.* **15,** 1751.

Kalidas, M., Hammond, L.A., Patnaik, A., Denis, L. J., Hidalgo, M., Schwartz, G., Stephenson, J. J., Felton, S. A., Hao, D., McCreery, H., Williams, J., Holroyd, K., Mamum, K., Eckhardt, S. G., Von Hoff, D. D., and Rowinsky, E. K. (2000). A phase I and pharmacokinetic study of the angiogenesis inhibitor, squalamine lactate (MSI-1256F). *Proc. Am. Soc. Clin. Oncol.* **19,** abstract 698.

Kanda, S., Hodgkin, M. N., Woodfield, R. J., Wakelam, M. J., Thomas, G., and Claesson-Welsh, L. (1997). Phosphatidylinositol 3′-kinase-independent p70 S6 kinase activation by fibroblast growth factor receptor-1 is important for proliferation but not differentiation of endothelial cells. *J. Biol. Chem.* **272,** 23347–23353.

Kendall, R. L., Wang, G., and Thomas, K. A. (1996). Identification of a natural soluble form of the vascular endothelial growth factor receptor, FLT-1, and its heterodimerization with KDR. *Biochem. Biophys. Res. Commun.* **226,** 324–328.

Kenyon, B. M., Browne, F., and D'Amato, R. J. (1997). Effects of thalidomide and related metabolites in a mouse corneal model of neovascularization. *Exp. Eye Res.* **64,** 971–978.

Kibel, A., Iliopoulos, O., DeCaprio, J. A., and Kaelin, W. G., Jr. (1995). Binding of the von Hippel-Lindau tumor suppressor protein to Elongin B and C. *Science* **269,** 1444–1446.

Kim, K. J., Li, B., Winer, J., Armanini, M., Gillett, N., Phillips, H. S., and Ferrara, N. (1993). Inhibition of vascular endothelial growth factor-induced angiogenesis suppresses tumour growth in vivo. *Nature* **362,** 841–844.

Klemke, R. L., Yebra, M., Bayna, E. M., and Cheresh, D. A. (1994). Receptor tyrosine kinase signaling required for integrin alpha v beta 5-directed cell motility but not adhesion on vitronectin. *J. Cell Biol.* **127,** 859–866.

Klionsky, D. J., Cueva, R., and Yaver, D. S. (1992). Aminopeptidase I of *Sac-*

charomyces cerevisiae is localized to the vacuole independent of the secretory pathway. *J. Cell Biol.* **119**, 287–299.

Kobayashi, H., Gotoh, J., Shinohara, H., Moniwa, N., and Terao, T. (1994). Inhibition of the metastasis of Lewis lung carcinoma by antibody against urokinase-type plasminogen activator in the experimental and spontaneous metastasis model. *Thromb. Haemost.* **71**, 474–480.

Koivunen, E., Arap, W., Valtanen, H., Rainisalo, A., Medina, O. P., Heikkila, P., Kantor, C., Gahmberg, C. G., Salo, T., Konttinen, Y. T., Sorsa, T., Ruoslahti, E., and Pasqualini, R. (1999). Tumor targeting with a selective gelatinase inhibitor. *Nat. Biotechnol.* **17**, 768–774.

Ku, P. T., and D'Amore, P. A. (1995). Regulation of basic fibroblast growth factor (bFGF) gene and protein expression following its release from sublethally injured endothelial cells. *J. Cell Biochem.* **58**, 328–343.

Laird, A. D., Carver, J., Smith, K., Li, G., Mendel, D. B., and Cherington, J. M. (2000a). SU-6668, a broad spectrum angiogenesis inhibitor, induces apoptosis of microvesells in established A431 tumor xenografts, resulting in tumor destruction. Proceedings 11th NCI-EORTC-AACR symposium on new drugs in cancer therapy, abstract 266.

Laird, A. D., Vajkoczy, P., Shawver, L. K., Thurnher, A., Liang, C., Mohammadi, M., Schlessinger, J., Ullrich, A., Hubbard, S. R., Blake, R. A., Fong, T. A., Strawn, L. M., Sun, L., Tang, C., Hawtin, R., Tang, F., Shenoy, N., Hirth, K. P., McMahon, G., and Cherrington, J. M. (2000b). SU6668 is a potent antiangiogenic and antitumor agent that induces regression of established tumors. *Cancer Res.* **60**, 4152–4160.

Levy, A. P., Levy, N. S., and Goldberg, M. A. (1996). Post-transcriptional regulation of vascular endothelial growth factor by hypoxia. *J. Biol. Chem.* **271**, 2746–2753.

Lin, P., Sankar, S., Shan, S., Dewhirst, M. W., Polverini, P. J., Quinn, T. Q., and Peters, K. G. (1998). Inhibition of tumor growth by targeting tumor endothelium using a soluble vascular endothelial growth factor receptor. *Cell Growth Differ.* **9**, 49–58.

Lucas, R., Holmgren, L., Garcia, I., Jimenez, B., Mandriota, S. J., Borlat, F., Sim, B. K., Wu, Z., Grau, G. E., Shing, Y., Soff, G. A., Bouck, N., and Pepper, M. S. (1998). Multiple forms of angiostatin induce apoptosis in endothelial cells. *Blood* **92**, 4730–4741.

Maisonpierre, P. C., Suri, C., Jones, P. F., Bartunkova, S., Wiegand, S. J., Radziejewski, C., Compton, D., McClain, J., Aldrich, T. H., Papadopoulos, N., Daly, T. J., Davis, S., Sato, T. N., and Yancopoulos, G. D. (1997). Angiopoietin-2, a natural antagonist for Tie2 that disrupts in vivo angiogenesis. *Science* **277**, 55–60.

Marty, C., Ballmer, K., Neri, D., Klemenz, R., and Schwendener, R. (2000). Inhibition of tumor groath by specific targeting of anti-ED-B fibronectin scFv antibody modified liposomes in the F9 mouse teratocarcinoma model. Proceedings 11th NCI-EORTC-AACR symposium on new drugs in cancer therapy, abstract 131.

Marx, G. M., McCowatt, S., Boyle, F., Pavlakis, N., Levi, J. A., Bell, D. R., Freilich, R., Cook, R., Biggs, M., Little, N., and Wheeler, H. R. (2000). Phase II study of Thalidomide as an anti-angiogenic agent in the treatment of recurrent glioblastoma multiform (GBM). *Proc. Am. Soc. Clin. Oncol.* **19**, abstract 613.

Mattei, M. G., Borg, J. P., Rosnet, O., Marme, D., and Birnbaum, D. (1996). Assignment of vascular endothelial growth factor (VEGF) and placenta growth factor (PLGF) genes to human chromosome 6p12-p21 and 14q24-q31 regions, respectively. *Genomics* **32**, 168–169.

McNeil, P. L., Muthukrishnan, L., Warder, E., and D'Amore, P. A. (1989). Growth factors are released by mechanically wounded endothelial cells. *J. Cell Biol.* **109**, 811–822.

Melder, R. J., Koenig, G. C., Witwer, B. P., Safabakhsh, N., Munn, L. L., and Jain, R. K. (1996). During angiogenesis, vascular endothelial growth factor and basic fibroblast growth factor regulate natural killer cell adhesion to tumor endothelium. *Nat. Med.* **2**, 992–997.

Mignatti, P., Morimoto, T., and Rifkin, D. B. (1992). Basic fibroblast growth factor, a protein devoid of secretory signal sequence, is released by cells

via a pathway independent of the endoplasmic reticulum-Golgi complex. *J. Cell Physiol* **151**, 81–93.

Mignatti, P., and Rifkin, D. B. (1993). Biology and biochemistry of proteinases in tumor invasion. *Physiol Rev.* **73**, 161–195.

Miller, K. D., Gradishar, W. J., Schuchter, L. M., Sparano, J. A., Cobleigh, M. A., Robert, N. J., Guiney, P., McDonald, A. L., Rasmussen, H., and Sledge, G. W. A randomized phase II trial of adjuvant Marimastat (MAR) in patients with early breast cancer. *Proc. Am. Soc. Clin. Oncol.* **19**, abstract 369.

Minor, D., and Elias, L. (2000). Thalidomide treatment ot metastatic renal cell carcinoma. *Proc. Am. Soc. Clin. Oncol.* **19**, abstract 1384.

Nakahara, H., Howard, L., Thompson, E. W., Sato, H., Seiki, M., Yeh, Y., and Chen, W. T. (1997). Transmembrane/cytoplasmic domain-mediated membrane type 1-matrix metalloprotease docking to invadopodia is required for cell invasion. *Proc. Natl. Acad. Sci. USA* **94**, 7959–7964.

Neri, D., Carnemolla, B., Nissim, A., Leprini, A., Querze, G., Balza, E., Pini, A., Tarli, L., Halin, C., Neri, P., Zardi, L., and Winter, G. (1997). Targeting by affinity-matured recombinant antibody fragments of an angiogenesis associated fibronectin isoform. *Nat. Biotechnol.* **15**, 1271–1275.

O'Donnel, A. E., Trigo, J. M., Banerji, U., Raynaud, F., Padhani, A., Hannah, A., Hardcastle, A., Aherne, W., Workman, P., and Judson, I. R. (2000). A phase I trial of the VEGF inhibitor SU5416, incorporating dynamic contrast MRI assessment of vascular permeability. *Proc. Am. Soc. Clin. Oncol.* **19**, abstract 685.

O'Reilly, M. S., Boehm, T., Shing, Y., Fukai, N., Vasios, G., Lane, W. S., Flynn, E., Birkhead, J. R., Olsen, B. R., and Folkman, J. (1997). Endostatin: an endogenous inhibitor of angiogenesis and tumor growth. *Cell* **88**, 277–285.

O'Reilly, M. S., Holmgren, L., Chen, C., and Folkman, J. (1996). Angiostatin induces and sustains dormancy of human primary tumors in mice. *Nat. Med.* **2**, 689–692.

O'Reilly, M. S., Holmgren, L., Shing, Y., Chen, C., Rosenthal, R. A., Moses, M., Lane, W. S., Cao, Y., Sage, E. H., and Folkman, J. (1994). Angiostatin: a novel angiogenesis inhibitor that mediates the suppression of metastases by a Lewis lung carcinoma. *Cell* **79**, 315–328.

O'Reilly, M. S., Pirie-Shepherd, S., Lane, W. S., and Folkman, J. (1999). Antiangiogenic activity of the cleaved conformation of the serpin antithrombin. *Science* **285**, 1926–1928.

Odekon, L. E., Blasi, F., and Rifkin, D. B. (1994). Requirement for receptor-bound urokinase in plasmin-dependent cellular conversion of latent TGF-beta to TGF-beta. *J. Cell Physiol* **158**, 398–407.

Ohh, M., Park, C. W., Ivan, M., Hoffman, M. A., Kim, T. Y., Huang, L. E., Pavletich, N., Chau, V., and Kaelin, W. G. (2000). Ubiquitination of hypoxia-inducible factor requires direct binding to the beta-domain of the von Hippel-Lindau protein. *Nat. Cell Biol.* **2**, 423–427.

Olofsson, B., Pajusola, K., Kaipainen, A., von Euler, G., Joukov, V., Saksela, O., Orpana, A., Pettersson, R. F., Alitalo, K., and Eriksson, U. (1996). Vascular endothelial growth factor B, a novel growth factor for endothelial cells. *Proc. Natl. Acad. Sci. USA* **19;93**, 2576–2581.

Ossowski, L., and Reich, E. (1983). Antibodies to plasminogen activator inhibit human tumor metastasis. *Cell* **35**, 611–619.

Ossowski, L., Russo-Payne, H., and Wilson, E. L. (1991). Inhibition of urokinase-type plasminogen activator by antibodies: the effect on dissemination of a human tumor in the nude mouse. *Cancer Res.* **51**, 274–281.

Panek, R. L., Lu, G. H., Dahring, T. K., Batley, B. L., Connolly, C., Hamby, J. M., and Brown, K. J. (1998). In vitro biological characterization and antiangiogenic effects of PD 166866, a selective inhibitor of the FGF-1 receptor tyrosine kinase. *J. Pharmacol. Exp. Ther.* **286**, 569–577.

Parangi, S., O'Reilly, M., Christofori, G., Holmgren, L., Grosfeld, J., Folkman, J., and Hanahan, D. (1996). Antiangiogenic therapy of transgenic mice impairs de novo tumor growth. *Proc. Natl. Acad. Sci. USA* **93**, 2002–2007.

Pasqualini, R., Koivunen, E., and Ruoslahti, E. (1997). Alpha v Integrins as receptors for tumor targeting by circulating ligands. *Nat. Biotechnol.* **15**, 542–546.

Patt, Y. Z., Hassan, M. M., Lozano, R. D., Zeldis, J. B., Schnirer, I., Frome, A., Abbruzzese, J. L., Wolff, R. A., Brown, T. D., Ellis, L. M., and Charnsangavej, C. (2000). Phase II trial of Thalidomide for treatment of non-resectable hepatocellular carcinoma (HCC). *Proc. Am. Soc. Clin. Oncol.* **19**, abstract 1035.

Pepper, M. S., Ferrara, N., Orci, L., and Montesano, R. (1991). Vascular endothelial growth factor (VEGF) induces plasminogen activators and plasminogen activator inhibitor-1 in microvascular endothelial cells. *Biochem. Biophys. Res. Commun.* **181**, 902–906.

Pepper, M. S., Sappino, A. P., Montesano, R., Orci, L., and Vassalli, J. D. (1992). Plasminogen activator inhibitor-1 is induced in migrating endothelial cells. *J. Cell Physiol* **153**, 129–139.

Perollet, C., Han, Z. C., Savona, C., Caen, J. P., and Bikfalvi, A. (1998). Platelet factor 4 modulates fibroblast growth factor 2 (FGF-2) activity and inhibits FGF-2 dimerization. *Blood* **91**, 3289–3299.

Phillips, H. S., Armanini, M., Stavrou, D., Ferrara, N., Westphal, M. (1993). Intense focal expression of vascular endothelial growth factor mRNA in human intracranial neoplasms: Association with regions of necrosis. *Int. J. Oncol.* **2**, 913–919.

Piotrowicz, R. S., Martin, J. L., Dillman, W. H., and Levin, E. G. (1997). The 27-kDa heat shock protein facilitates basic fibroblast growth factor release from endothelial cells. *J. Biol. Chem.* **272**, 7042–7047.

Ploug, M., Behrendt, N., Lober, D., and Dano, K. (1991). Protein structure and membrane anchorage of the cellular receptor for urokinase-type plasminogen activator. *Semin. Thromb. Hemost.* **17**, 183–193.

Presta, L. G., Chen, H., O'Connor, S. J., Chisholm, V., Meng, Y. G., Krummen, L., Winkler, M., and Ferrara, N. (1997). Humanization of an anti-vascular endothelial growth factor monoclonal antibody for the therapy of solid tumors and other disorders. *Cancer Res.* **57**, 4593–4599.

Ran, S., Gao, B., Duffy, S., Watkins, L., Rote, N., and Thorpe, P. E. (1998). Infarction of solid Hodgkin's tumors in mice by antibody-directed targeting of tissue factor to tumor vasculature. *Cancer Res.* **58**, 4646–4653.

Refino, C. J., Himber, J., Burcklen, L., Moran, P., Peek, M., Suggett, S., Devaux, B., and Kirchhofer, D. (1999). A human antibody that binds to the gamma-carboxyglutamic acid domain of factor IX is a potent antithrombotic in vivo. *Thromb. Haemost.* **82**, 1188–1195.

Reijerkerk, A., Voest, E. E., and Gebbink, M. F. (2000). No grip, no growth: the conceptual basis of excessive proteolysis in the treatment of cancer. *Eur. J. Cancer* **36**, 1695–1705.

Rosen, P. J., Amado, R., Hecht, J. R., Chang, D., Mulay, M., Parson, M., Laxa, B., Brown, J., Cropp, G., Hannah, A., and Rosen, L. (2000a). A phase I/II study of SU5416 in combination with 5-FU/Leucovorin in patients with metastatic colorectal cancer. *Proc. Am. Soc. Clin. Oncol.* **19**, abstract 5D.

Rosen, L., Hannah, A., Rosen, P., Kabbinavar, F., Mulay, M., Gicanov, N., DePaoli, A., Cropp, G., and Mabry, M. (2000b). Phase I dose-escalating trial of oral SU006668, a novel multiple receptor tyrosine kinase inhibitor in patients with selected advanced malignancies. *Proc. Am. Soc. Clin. Oncol.* **19**, abstract 708.

Rowinsky, E. K., Eckhardt, S. G., Rizzo, J., Kuhn, J., Hammond, L. A., Schwartz, G., Rha, S. Y., Denis, L., Berg, K., Felton, S., Hao, D., Izbicka, E., Patnaik, A., Tolcher, A. W., and Hidalgo, M. (2000). A phase I and pharmacokinetic study of Col-3, an tetracycline analog and selective matrix metalloprotease (MMP) inhibitor. Proceedings 11th NCI-EORTC-AACR symposium on new drugs in cancer therapy, abstract 202.

Ruegg, C., Yilmaz, A., Bieler, G., Bamat, J., Chaubert, P., and Lejeune, F. J. (1998). Evidence for the involvement of endothelial cell integrin alphaV/beta3 in the disruption of the tumor vasculature induced by TNF and IFN-gamma. *Nat. Med.* **4**, 408–414.

Ruf, W., and Mueller, B. M. (1996). Tissue factor in cancer angiogenesis and metastasis. *Curr. Opin. Hematol.* **3**, 379–384.

Saksela, O., Rifkin, D. B. (1990). Release of basic fibroblast growth

factor–heparan sulfate complexes from endothelial cells by plasminogen activator-mediated proteolytic activity. *J. Cell Biol.* **110**, 767–775.

Sampaio, E. P., Sarno, E. N., Galilly, R., Cohn, Z. A., and Kaplan, G. (1991). Thalidomide selectively inhibits tumor necrosis factor alpha production by stimulated human monocytes. *J. Exp. Med.* **173**, 699–703.

Sasaki, T., Larsson, H., Kreuger, J., Salmivirta, M., Claesson-Welsh, L., Lindahl, U., Hohenester, E., and Timpl, R. (1999). Structural basis and potential role of heparin/heparan sulfate binding to the angiogenesis inhibitor endostatin. *EMBO J.* **18**, 6240–6248.

Sato, Y., Abe, M., Tanaka, K., Iwasaka, C., Oda, N., Kanno, S., Oikawa, M., Nakano, T., and Igarashi, T. (2000). Signal transduction and transcriptional regulation of angiogenesis. *Adv. Exp. Med. Biol.* **476**, 109–115.

Sato, Y., Tsuboi, R., Lyons, R., Moses, H., and Rifkin, D. B. (1990). Characterization of the activation of latent TGF-beta by co-cultures of endothelial cells and pericytes or smooth muscle cells: a self-regulating system. *J. Cell Biol.* **111**, 757–763.

Schmitt, M., Harbeck, N., Thomssen, C., Wilhelm, O., Magdolen, V., Reuning, U., Ulm, K., Hofler, H., Janicke, F. , and Graeff, H. (1997). Clinical impact of the plasminogen activation system in tumor invasion and metastasis: prognostic relevance and target for therapy. *Thromb. Haemost.* **78**, 285–296.

Senger, D. R., Galli, S. J., Dvorak, A. M., Perruzzi, C. A., Harvey, V. S., and Dvorak, H. F. (1983). Tumor cells secrete a vascular permeability factor that promotes accumulation of ascites fluid. *Science* **219**, 983–985.

Senger, D. R., Perruzzi, C. A., Feder, J., and Dvorak, H. F. (1986). A highly conserved vascular permeability factor secreted by a variety of human and rodent tumor cell lines. *Cancer Res.* **46**, 5629–5632.

Shing, Y., Folkman, J., Sullivan, R., Butterfield, C., Murray, J., and Klagsbrun, M. (1984). Heparin affinity: purification of a tumor-derived capillary endothelial cell growth factor. *Science* **223**, 1296–1299.

Sledge, G., Miller, W., Novotny, J., Gaudreault, M., Ash, M., and Colbleigh, M. (2000). Phase II trial of single agent rhuMAb VEGF in patients with relapsed metastatic breast cancer. *Proc. Am. Soc. Clin. Oncol.* **19**, abstract 5C.

Sohndel, S., Hu, C. K., Marti, D., Affolter, M., Schaller, J., Llinas, M., and Rickli, E. E. (1996). Recombinant gene expression and 1H NMR characteristics of the kringle (2 + 3) supermodule: spectroscopic/functional individuality of plasminogen kringle domains. *Biochemistry* **35**, 2357–2364.

Storgard, C. M., Stupack, D. G., Jonczyk, A., Goodman, S. L., Fox, R. I., and Cheresh, D. A. (1999). Decreased angiogenesis and arthritic disease in rabbits treated with an alphavbeta3 antagonist. *J. Clin. Invest* **103**, 47–54.

Sun, L., Tran, N., Tang, F., App, H., Hirth, P., McMahon, G., and Tang, C. (1998). Synthesis and biological evaluations of 3-substituted indolin-2-ones: a novel class of tyrosine kinase inhibitors that exhibit selectivity toward particular receptor tyrosine kinases. *J. Med. Chem.* **41**, 2588–2603.

Suri, C., Jones, P. F., Patan, S., Bartunkova, S., Maisonpierre, P. C., Davis, S., Sato, T. N., and Yancopoulos, G. D. (1996). Requisite role of angiopoietin-1, a ligand for the TIE2 receptor, during embryonic angiogenesis. *Cell* **87**, 1171–1180.

Takigawa, M., Nishida, Y., Suzuki, F., Kishi, J., Yamashita, K., and Hayakawa, T. (1990). Induction of angiogenesis in chick yolk-sac membrane by polyamines and its inhibition by tissue inhibitors of metalloproteinases (TIMP and TIMP-2). *Biochem. Biophys. Res. Commun.* **171**, 1264–1271.

Taraboletti, G., Roberts, D., Liotta, L. A., and Giavazzi, R. (1990). Platelet thrombospondin modulates endothelial cell adhesion, motility, and growth: a potential angiogenesis regulatory factor. *J. Cell Biol.* **111**, 765–772.

Thomas, D. A., Kantarjian, H. M. (2000). Current role of thalidomide in cancer treatment. *Curr. Opin. Oncol.* **12**, 564–573.

Thomas, J. P., Schiller, J., Lee, F., Perlman, S., Friedl, A., Winter, T., Marnocha, R., Arzoomanian, R., Alberti, D., Binger, K., Volkman, J.,

Feierabend, F., Tutsch, K., Dresen, A., Auerbach, R., Pluda, J., and Wilding, G. (2000). A phase I pharmacokinetic and pharmacodynamic study of recombinant endostatin. Proceedings 11th NCI-EORTC-AACR symposium on new drugs in cancer therapy, abstract 260.

Tolsma, S. S., Stack, M. S., and Bouck, N. (1997). Lumen formation and other angiogenic activities of cultured capillary endothelial cells are inhibited by thrombospondin-1. *Microvasc. Res.* **54,** 13–26.

Tolsma, S. S., Volpert, O. V., Good, D. J., Frazier, W. A., Polverini, P. J., and Bouck, N. (1993). Peptides derived from two separate domains of the matrix protein thrombospondin-1 have anti-angiogenic activity. *J. Cell Biol.* **122,** 497–511.

Tseng, J. E., Glisson, B. S., Khuri, F. R., Teddy, S. R., Shin, D. M., Gillenwater, A. M., Myers, J. N., Clayman, G. L., El-Naggar, A. K., Fritsche, H. A., Lawhorn, Jr., K. N., Thall, P. F., Liu, D., and Herbst, R. S. (2000). Phase II trial of thalidomide in the treatment of recurrent and/or metastatic squamous cell carcinoma of the head and neck (SCHN). *Proc. Am. Soc. Clin. Oncol.* **19,** abstract 1645.

Tuder, R. M., Flook, B. E., and Voelkel, N. F. (1995). Increased gene expression for VEGF and the VEGF receptors KDR/Flk and Flt in lungs exposed to acute or to chronic hypoxia. Modulation of gene expression by nitric oxide. *J. Clin. Invest* **95,** 1798–1807.

Wasylyk, C., Gutman, A., Nicholson, R., and Wasylyk, B. (1991). The c-Ets oncoprotein activates the stromelysin promoter through the same elements as several non-nuclear oncoproteins. *EMBO J.* **10,** 1127–1134.

Watabe, T., Yoshida, K., Shindoh, M., Kaya, M., Fujikawa, K., Sato, H., Seiki, M., Ishii, S., and Fujinaga, K. (1998). The Ets-1 and Ets-2 transcription factors activate the promoters for invasion-associated urokinase and collagenase genes in response to epidermal growth factor. *Int. J. Cancer* **77,** 128–137.

Werb, Z. (1997). ECM and cell surface proteolysis: regulating cellular ecology. *Cell* **91,** 439–442.

Wernert, N., Gilles, F., Fafeur, V., Bouali, F., Raes, M. B., Pyke, C., Du-pressoir, T., Seitz, G., Vandenbunder, B., and Stehelin, D. (1994). Stromal expression of c-Ets1 transcription factor correlates with tumor invasion. *Cancer Res.* **54,** 5683–5688.

Wernert, N., Raes, M. B., Lassalle, P., Dehouck, M. P., Gosselin, B., Vandenbunder, B., and Stehelin, D. (1992). c-ets1 proto-oncogene is a transcription factor expressed in endothelial cells during tumor vascularization and other forms of angiogenesis in humans. *Am. J. Pathol.* **140,** 119–127.

Wick, M., Haronen, R., Mumberg, D., Burger, C., Olsen, B. R., Budarf, M. L., Apte, S. S., and Muller, R. (1995). Structure of the human TIMP-3 gene and its cell cycle-regulated promoter. *Biochem. J.* **311,** 549–554.

Yamada, Y., Nezu, J., Shimane, M., and Hirata, Y. (1997). Molecular cloning of a novel vascular endothelial growth factor, VEGF-D. *Genomics* **42,** 483–488.

Yasukawa, T., Kimura, H., Tabata, Y., Miyamoto, H., Honda, Y., Ikada, Y., and Ogura, Y. (1999). Targeted delivery of anti-angiogenic agent TNP-470 using water-soluble polymer in the treatment of choroidal neovascularization. *Invest Ophthalmol. Vis. Sci.* **40,** 2690–2696.

Yayon, A., Klagsbrun, M., Esko, J. D., Leder, P., and Ornitz, D. M. (1991). Cell surface, heparin-like molecules are required for binding of basic fibroblast growth factor to its high affinity receptor. *Cell* **64,** 841–848.

Yeo, T. K., Brown, L., and Dvorak, H. F. (1991). Alterations in proteoglycan synthesis common to healing wounds and tumors. *Am. J. Pathol.* **138,** 1437–1450.

Yoshida, T., Kaneko, Y., Tsukamoto, A., Han, K., Ichinose, M., and Kimura, S. (1998). Suppression of hepatoma growth and angiogenesis by a fumagillin derivative TNP470: possible involvement of nitric oxide synthase. *Cancer Res.* **58,** 3751–3756.

Zucker, S., Mirza, H., Conner, C. E., Lorenz, A. F., Drews, M. H., Bahou, W. F., and Jesty, J. (1998). Vascular endothelial growth factor induces tissue factor and matrix metalloproteinase production in endothelial cells: conversion of prothrombin to thrombin results in progelatinase A activation and cell proliferation. *Int. J. Cancer* **75,** 780–786.

GENE-DIRECTED ENZYME PRODRUG THERAPY

Caroline J. Springer
Ion Niculescu-Duvaz

Cancer Research Campaign Centre for Cancer Therapeutics

Institute of Cancer Research

Sutton, United Kingdom

Summary

The efficacy of cancer chemotherapy is frequently hampered by a low therapeutic index. Recently, strategies have been developed to improve this index by selective delivery of highly cytotoxic drugs to the tumor cells themselves. A key advance in this approach has been the principle of conversion of a specially designed nontoxic prodrug to a cytotoxic drug by an enzyme contained within the tumor cells themselves, on the tumor cell surface, or in the tumor cell microenvironment. Activation of prodrugs can be accomplished by antibody-enzyme conjugates targeted to tumor-associated antigens (ADEPT) or by enzymes expressed by exogenous genes in tumor cells (GDEPT). This chapter discusses the state of the art in GDEPT. The focus is on the development of new and improved prodrugs, and includes discussion of physicochemical and biological properties, pharmacokinetics, and clinical trials.

1. Introduction

Cancer chemotherapy encompasses a vast number of established clinical methods for the treatment of persons with malignant diseases. However, the efficacy of such methods is frequently hampered by an insufficient therapeutic index and the emergence of drug-resistant cell subpopulations. One area where progress has been made is the discovery and synthesis of extremely cytotoxic compounds. Recently, efforts have been directed to new concepts that allow the advantages of these highly potent drugs with methods to enhance their selectivity. Immunoconjugates (Frankel *et al.,* 1996), antibody-directed enzyme prodrug therapy (ADEPT) (Niculescu-Duvaz and Springer, 1995; Melton and Sherwood, 1997), and suicide gene therapy (Niculescu-Duvaz *et al.,* 1998b; Springer and Niculescu-Duvaz, 1999) are some of the new routes under investigation. All of these technologies are two-step treatments that avoid the requirements for drugs exhibiting intrinsic selectivity toward cancer cells, since they rely on the conversion of nontoxic prodrugs to toxic drugs within tumor cells themselves, on their surface, or in their close vicinity.

Gene therapy is broadly defined as a technology aimed at modifying the genetic component of cells for therapeutic benefits. In cancer gene therapy, both malignant and nonmalignant cells can be targeted for a therapeutic gain (Zhang *et al.,* 1995). The possibility of rendering cancer cells more sensitive to chemotherapeutics or toxins by introducing "suicide genes" was suggested in the late 1980s. This approach has two alternatives. In toxin gene therapy, genes for toxic proteins are transduced into cancer cells. In gene-directed enzyme prodrug therapy (GDEPT) (Bridgewater *et al.,* 1995) or virus-directed enzyme prodrug therapy (VDEPT) (Huber *et al.,* 1991), genes for foreign enzymes are transduced into cancer cells that can activate specific prodrugs.

This chapter discusses the state of the art in GDEPT. The delivery systems constitute another important aspect of this technology and are discussed in detail elsewhere (Roth and Cristiano, 1997; Bilbao *et al.,* 1998; Miller, 1998; Nguyen *et al.,* 1998; Robbins and Ghivizzani, 1998). A number of reviews cover the qualitative and quantitative aspects of GDEPT technologies (Roth and Cristiano, 1997; Denny and Wilson, 1998; Niculescu-Duvaz *et al.,* 1998b; Encell *et al.,* 1999; Springer and Niculescu-Duvaz, 1999, 2000). The focus here is on the development of new and improved prodrugs.

2. Background

GDEPT and VDEPT are two-step treatments for patients with solid tumors. In the first step, the gene for a foreign enzyme is delivered in a vector that is targeted to the tumor for expression. In the second step, a prodrug is administered that is activated to the drug selectively by the foreign enzyme expressed in the tumor. The enzyme genes should be expressed exclusively, or with a relatively high ratio, in the tumor cells compared with normal tissues and blood.

Current vectors for gene delivery are incapable of conferring expression of the foreign enzyme in all tumor cells. Therefore, a bystander effect (BE) is required whereby the prodrug is cleaved to an active drug that kills neighboring tumor cells that are not expressing the foreign enzyme (Freeman *et al.,* 1993).

The design of GDEPT systems requires prodrugs "tailored" for the use of the foreign enzymes selected. Preferably the enzyme has no human homologue. An alternative is to use a human enzyme that is normally expressed in locations inaccessible to prodrug. Treatment schedules that are clinically feasible are another consideration.

It is useful to compare the efficacy of different GDEPT systems. We have defined two parameters for this purpose: the "potential of activation" and the "degree of activation" of each system (see Table 1) (Springer and Niculescu-Duvaz, 2000). The first parameter represents the maximal possible efficiency of a given enzyme-prodrug system in a cell system. It is defined as the ratio of the IC_{50} of the prodrug divided by the IC_{50} of the released drug in a control nontransduced cell line. The degree of activation demonstrates the actual efficiency of the system in the transduced cell line. It is defined as the IC_{50} of the prodrug in the nontransfected cell line divided by the IC_{50} of the prodrug in an enzyme-transduced cell line.

3. Enzyme-Prodrug Systems

A large number of enzyme-prodrug systems have been developed for GDEPT recently. These are abbreviated and summarized in Table 1. There are specific requirements of the enzymes for GDEPT. It is preferable for them to have high catalytic activity, without the need for cofactors, as these could become rate limiting in the target cells. The enzyme should achieve a concentration sufficient to activate the prodrug under physiologic conditions.

The enzymes proposed for GDEPT can be characterized into two major classes for convenience. The first class comprises enzymes of nonmammalian origin although they may have human counterparts. Examples include viral TK[1] (Culver *et al.,* 1992), bacterial CD (Mullen *et al.,* 1992), CPG2 (Marais *et al.,* 1996), PNP (Sorscher *et al.,* 1994), NR (Bridgewater *et al.,* 1995), XGPRT (Tamiya *et al.,* 1996), PGA (Moore *et al.,* 1997), Met (Miki *et al.,* 2000), β-L (Moore *et al.,* 1997), β-Gal (Ghosh *et al.,* 1999), yeast CD (Kievit *et al.,* 1999), DAAO (Stegman *et al.,* 1998), plant MDAE (Sethna *et al.,* 1997), and insect dNK (Johansson *et al.,* 1999). However, these enzymes all have structural requirements that are different with respect to their substrates in comparison to the human counterparts.

The second class comprises enzymes of human or other mammalian origin that are absent from, or are expressed at a low concentration in, tumor cells. Examples include CE (Kojima *et al.,* 1998a), TP (Patterson *et al.,* 1995), dCK (Hapke *et al.,* 1996), CPA (Hamstra *et al.,* 2000), β-Glu (Weyel *et al.,* 2000), and CYP450 (Chen *et al.,* 1996a). Their major advantage resides in the reduction in the potential for induction of an immune response. Their presence in normal tissues is likely to preclude specific activation of the prodrugs only in tumors unless the transduced enzymes are modified so as to have different substrate specificities. Genes have been constructed to express mutated enzymes with different substrate requirements in comparison with the wild types (Black *et al.,* 1996; Smith *et al.,* 1997; Encell *et al.,* 1999).

The enzyme gene may be engineered for expression either intracellularly or extracellularly in the recipient tumor cells (Marais *et al.,* 1997). There are potential advantages to each approach. With intracellular expression the prodrug must enter the cells for activation and subsequently the active drug must diffuse through the interstitium across the cell membrane to elicit a BE. This is not a requirement in cells where the enzyme is expressed tethered to the outer cell surface or secreted because the enzyme can activate the prodrug extracellularly. A more substantial BE should theoretically be generated in the latter systems. A leak-back of the active drug into the general circulation is a possible disadvantage of these systems.

---

[1]Abbreviations are defined in Table 1.

TABLE 1
Enzyme-Prodrug Systems

Number	Names and codes	Origin	Expression	Mutation	Prodrugs	Released (pro)drugs	Potential of activation fold	Degree of activation fold	Clinical trials
		Enzyme			Prodrug Systems				
1	Carboxyl esterase (CE)	Human, rabbit	Intracellular	No	Irinotecan 7-ethyl-10-[4-(1-piperidino)-1-piperidino]-carbonyloxy-(20S)-camptothecin	SN-38 7-ethyl-10-hydroxy-(20S)-camptothecin	150–3000	7–17	1
2	Carboxypeptidase A (CPA)	Human	Intracellular and extra-cellular secreted	Yes, for secreted or surface tethered expression and modified substrates	MTX-α-peptides	MTX	>1000	>400	—
3	Carboxypeptidase G2 (CPG2) EC 3.4.22.12	Pseudomonas str.	Intracellular and extra-cellular sur-face tethered	Yes, for extra-cellular expression	CMDA ZD-2767 Self-immolative	CMBA phenol-bisiodonitrogen mustard; alkylating agents, anthracycline antibiotics	21–400	11–115	1
4	Cytochrome P450, Human; CYP2B1, 2B6, 2C8, 2C9, 2C18, and 3A Rat: CYP2B1 Rabbit: 4B1 (with or without red-P450)	Human, rat, rabbit	Intracellular	No	Oxazaphosphorines, ipomeanol, 2-amino-anthracene (2-AA); acetaminophen	Alkylating agents, toxic metabolites, N-acetyl-benzoquinone imine (NABQI)	?	5–100	1
5	Cytosine deaminase (CD) EC 3.5.4.1 (with or without uracil-phosphoribosyl transferase, UPRT)	E. coli, yeast	Intracellular and extra-cellular	Yes, for secreted expression	5-Fluorocytosine (5-FC)	5-Fluorouracil (5-FU)	1000–8000	70–1000	1
6	D-Amino acid oxidase (DAAO)	Rodhoto rula gracilis, (yeast)	Intracellular	No	D-Alanine	Hydrogen peroxide	—	—	—
7	Deoxycytidine kinase (dCK), EC.2.7.1.21	Human	Intracellular	No	Cytosine arabinoside	Cytosine arabinoside monophosphate	—	—	—
8	Deoxyribonucleo-tide kinase (DmNK)	Drosophila melanogaster	Intracellular	No	Analogues of pyrimi-dine and purine 2′-deoxynucleosides	Analogues of pyrimidine and purine 2′-deoxynu-cleotide monophosphates	?	?	No
9	DT-Diaphorase (DT-D)	Human, rat?	Intracellular	No	Bioreductive agents: EO9, etc.	Reduced forms?	—	—	No
10	β-Galactosidase (β-Gal) EC 3.2.1.23	E. coli	Intracellular	No	Self-immolative pro-drugs from anthracy-clin antibiotics	Anthracycline antibiotics	—	—	No
11	β-Glucuronidase (β-Glu)	Human	Intracellular and extra-cellular	Yes, for secreted expression	Self-immolative HM-1826	Doxorubicin	235	4–5	No
12	β-Lactamase (β-L)	Bacterial ?	Extracellular, secreted or surface tethered	Yes	Self-immolative (cephem prodrugs)	Alkylating agents, Vinca alkaloids, anthracycline antibiotics	—	—	—
13	Methionine-α,γ-lyase (MET)	Pseudomonas putida	Intracellular	No	Selenomethionine	Methylselenol	?	400	No
14	Multiple drug activating enzyme (MDAE)	Tomato	Intracellular	No	Acetylated 6-TG, MTX, and other purines	6-TG, MTX, cytotoxic purines	—	—	No

(continues)

TABLE 1 *(continued)*

	Enzyme				Prodrug Systems		Potential of activation fold	Degree of activation fold	Clinical trials
Number	Names and codes	Origin	Expression	Mutation	Prodrugs	Released (pro)drugs			
15	Nitroreductase (NR)	*E. coli*	Intracellular	No	CB-1954 and analogues; self-immolative	Alkylating agents, pyrazolidines, enediynes	>50,000	14–10,000	No
16	Penicillin G amidase (PGA)	?	Extracellular	Yes	—	—	—	—	No
17	Purine nucleotide phosphorylase (PNP), EC2.4.2.1	*E. coli*	Intracellular	No	Purine nucleosides	6-Methylpurine, 2-fluoroadenine	25–1000	40	No
18	Thymidine kinase, (TK), EC2.7.1.21	HSV or V2V	Intracellular	Yes, to improve phosphorylation kinetics	Modified pyrimidine nucleosides: GCV, ACV, valacyclovir, etc; FIAU, purine nucleosides	Monophosphate nucleotide analogues		20–1000	>25
19	Thymidine phosphorylase (TP), EC2.4.2.4	Human	Intracellular	No	Pyrimidine analogues, 5'-DFUR	5-Fluorodeoxyuridine monophosphate (5-FdRMP)	7000	165	No
20	Xanthine-guanine phosphoribbosyl transferase (XGPT)	*E. coli*	Intracellular	No	6-Thiopurines	6-Thiopurine nucleoside	—	—	No

ACV, acyclovir; CB1954, 5-aziridinyl-2,4-dinitrobenzamide; CMBA, *N,N*-(2-chloroethyl)(2-mesyloxyethyl)aminobenzoic acid; CMDA, *N,N*-(2-mesyloxyethyl)aminobenzoyl-L-glutamic acid; 59-DFUR, 5'-deoxy-5-fluorouridine; EO9, 3-hydroxy-5-aziridinyl-l-methyl-(1H-indole-4,7-dione)-propenol; FIAU, 1-(2'-deoxy-2'-fluoro-β-D-arabinofuranosyl)-5-iodouracil; GCV, ganciclovir; HM-1826, *N*-(4-β-glucuronyl-3-nitrobenzyloxycarbonyl)-doxorubicin; HSV, herpes simplex virus; MTX, methotrexate; 6-TG, 6-thioguanine; VZV, varicella zoster virus; ZD-2767, 4-[bis(2-iodoethyl)aminophenyl]-oxycarbonyl-L-glutamic acid.

4. Tailored Prodrugs for GDEPT

Prodrug design must address several issues for clinical applicability. These include ease of transport of the prodrugs within the tumor environment. Intracellular transport is required if the enzyme is to be intracellularly expressed. The prodrug should have very limited cytotoxicity whereas the activated drug should be as potent as possible. There should be effective activation of the prodrug by the expressed enzyme with favorable activation kinetics. Ideally, the drugs released should kill both proliferative and quiescent cells and should induce a BE. Prodrugs should be chemically stable under physiologic conditions.

For intracellular activation, prodrugs that are lipophilic or have active transport mechanisms are required to penetrate cell membranes. It appears that many prodrugs in current use, such as nucleoside analogues, 5-FC, CP, CMDA, and CB1954, penetrate cells by passive diffusion. It is crucial that they have minimal cytotoxicity, since they will be taken up by normal and turnover cells. Modifying the lipophilicity of prodrugs is a possibility, especially when passive diffusion is involved in prodrug uptake. For systems in which the enzyme is extracellularly expressed, it is ideal if the prodrug is prevented from crossing the cell membrane, in contrast with the released drug, which should be membrane permeable.

Activation of the prodrugs is a key step. It is an advantage if the expressed enzyme can activate the prodrug directly to the drug, without the requirement for multiple catalysis steps, since it is possible that the needed host endogenous tumor enzymes will become defective or deficient in cancer cells. Alkylating agent prodrugs such as CP and CB1954 have an activation cascade that depends on endogenous enzymes. CYP activates CP to an intermediate that requires 3',5'-exonuclease action to generate the active metabolite (Bielicki *et al.,* 1984; Brock, 1989). NR activates CB1954 to the 5-aziridinyl-4-hydroxylamino-2-nitrobenzamide intermediate, and a further enzymatic step converts it to a powerful electrophile that can alkylate DNA (Knox *et al.,* 1988, 1992, 1993). Alkylating agent prodrugs, such as CMDA and ZD-2767P, have an advantage since the active drug is released by the expressed enzyme directly after prodrug cleavage (Springer *et al.,* 1990, 1995).

There is a requirement for further catalysis by mammalian adenosine monophosphate deaminase AMP and/or GMP kinases with 6-methoxy purine arabinonucleoside, GCV, and ACV following activation by the expressed VZV- or HSV-TK (Huber *et al.,* 1991). 5-FC is converted to 5-FU by CD. The active metabolite is 2'-deoxy-5-fluorouridine-5'-monophosphate (5-FdUMP) or 5-fluorouridine-5'-triphosphate (5-FUTP), which results from 5-FU conversion by a number of mammalian enzymes involving a complicated activation pattern (MacCoss and Robins, 1990). The sophisticated activation pathway and the existence of salvage paths for these antimetabolites are partially responsible for their propensity to induce resistance (Kinsella *et al.,* 1997).

The prodrugs used in GDEPT are commonly antimetabolites that require cycling cells (S phase) for cytotoxicity and are not active against quiescent cells. It has been speculated that resistance to GCV is not acquired but results from tumor cells that are in G_0 at the time of GCV administration, rendering them insensitive to the action of activated GCV. This hypothesis is supported by the fact that the tumors, which grew out following GDEPT treatment, remained sensitive to GCV (Golumbek *et al.*, 1992).

Optimum half-lives are required from the drugs to maximize efficacy. The half-life should be long enough to allow the BE but short enough to prevent the drug leaking out of the tumor (Springer *et al.*, 1995). The use of alkylating agent prodrugs has a potential advantage over purine nucleosides or 5-FC, since they are cytotoxic to noncycling as well as proliferative cells. It has been shown that the NR/CB1954 system was effective in noncycling cells (Bridgewater *et al.*, 1995). Activity against quiescent cells was also claimed for 6-MeP and 2-FA in PNP-transfected cells (Secrist III *et al.*, 1999).

A. Prodrugs

These prodrugs can be defined as pharmacologically inactive derivatives of drugs, which require chemical transformation to release or be converted to the active drug. In a non-self-immolative prodrug the active drug is formed directly following the activation in a one-step process. The non-self-immolative prodrugs used in GDEPT can be activated by different types of enzymatic reactions:

1. Scission reactions (e.g., CPG2, CE, CPA, PNP, PGA, MDAE, TP, β-Gal, β-L, β-Glu)
2. Reductions (e.g., NR, DT-diaphorase)
3. Phosphorylation (e.g., HSV-TK, VZV-TK, dCK)
4. Hydroxylation (e.g., CYP4B1)
5. Functional group substitution ($NH_2 \cdot OH$) (e.g., CD)
6. Deoxyribosylation (e.g., XGPRT)
7. Oxidation (e.g., DAAO)

Most of the prodrugs used to date in clinical trials have been licensed anticancer agents, as their pharmacology, pharmacokinetics, and dosages are understood.

1. Activation of Prodrugs by Scission Reactions

This is the most common mode of activation. A wide range of anticancer compounds can be made less cytotoxic by conversion to esters, amides, ureides, carbamates, or glycosides. When suitably substituted these are often good substrates for the range of enzymes used in GDEPT. For instance, substrates for CPG2 require an L-glutamyl residue coupled to an aromatic nucleus by an amidic (Springer *et al.*, 1990), ureidic, or carbamic bond (Springer *et al.*, 1995; Dowell *et al.*, 1996). The chemical reactivity of the benzoic, phenol or aniline aromatic nitrogen mustards is greatly reduced when they are functionalized as esters, amides, ureas, or carbamates. Coupling with L-glutamic acid results in prodrugs, such as **1**, that are substrates for CPG2 (Scheme 1). A large number of prodrugs have been designed and synthesized (Scheme 1). The degree of activation in a number of cell lines is up to 400-fold (Niculescu-Duvaz *et al.*, 1999a). Also, good *in vivo* results were reported with this system (Marais *et al.*, 1996; Stribbling *et al.*, 2000).

A similar scission reaction occurs by CE on irinotecan (7-ethyl-10-[4-(1-piperidino)-1-piperidino]-carbonyloxy-(20*S*)-camptothecin, **4**, releasing SN-38 (7-ethyl-10-hydroxy-(20*S*)-camptothecin, **5**, that is approximately 1000-fold more cytotoxic than the corresponding prodrug (Scheme 2) (Kojima *et al.*, 1998a; 1998b). Recently, a more active rabbit CE was proposed to enhance the efficiency of the system (Wierdl *et al.*, 2000).

The α-peptides of *N*-{5-[*N*-(3,4-dihydro-2-methyl-4-oxoquinazolin-6-ylmethyl]-*N*-methylamino}-2-thienoyl-L-glutamic acid (ZD1694) (**6**, R = L-Ala, L-Glu) and *N*-{4-[(2-methyl-3,4-dihydro-4-oxo-6-quinazolinyl)methyl]-*N*-prop-2-ynylamino}-benzoyl-L-glutamic acid (ICI 198538) (**7**, R = L-Ala, L-Glu) for activation by CPA have been synthesized. Differentials of up to 100-fold were obtained *in vitro* in cell lines with and without CPA (Springer *et al.*, 1996) (Scheme 3).

Prodrugs of methotrexate (MTX), **8**, have been described in which a blocking amino acid is conjugated to the α-carboxylic group (through an amide linkage) of the L-glutamic acid residue (Smith *et al.*, 1997; Hamstra *et al.*, 2000). These prodrugs cannot be internalized by the reduced folate cofactor (RFC) and are therefore inactive. Removal of the

SCHEME 1 X, Y = Cl, Br, I, OSO_2CH_3; Z = —, O, NH, CH_2, S; W = CO_2H, NH_2, OH, CH_2CO_2H, SH; R_1 = H, 2(3)-CH_3, 2(3)-F, 2(3)-Cl, 3-*i*-C_3H_7, 3-CN.

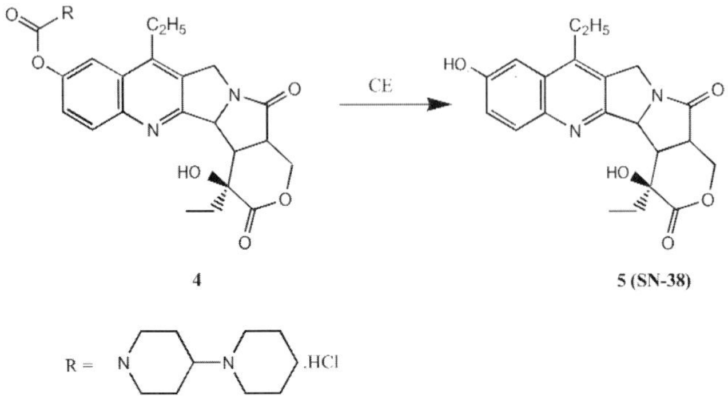

SCHEME 2 Activation of irinotecan by carboxyl esterase C.

amino acid by CPA releases MTX, **9.** However, since these MTX α-amino acid prodrugs are sensitive to endogenous secreted CPA, the enzyme was mutated to allow the design of MTX α-peptides with unnatural blocking amino acid that are not substrates for the wild-type CPA (Scheme 3) (Smith *et al.,* 1997). For instance MTX-α-3-cyclopentyl-Tyr prodrug is 50,000-fold more stable to wild-type CPA (Hamstra *et al.,* 2000). Degrees of activation of up to 400-fold were reported

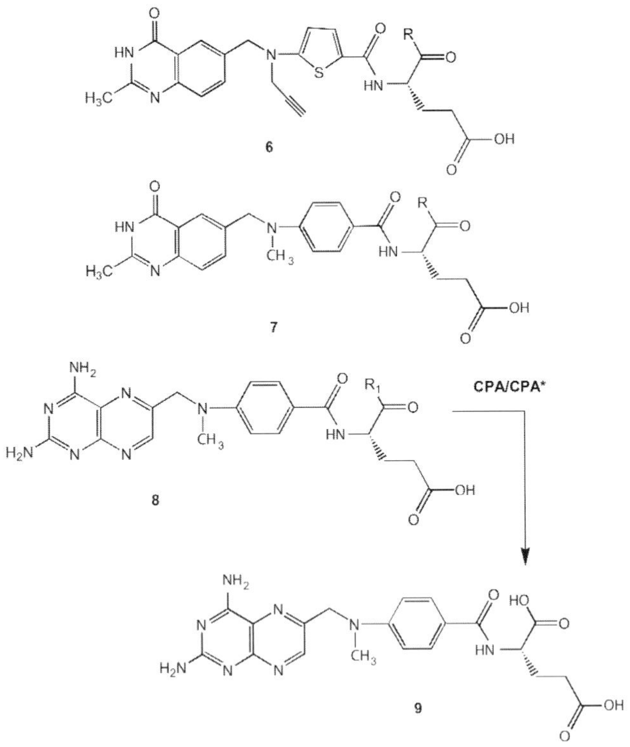

SCHEME 3 Activation of MTX-α-peptides by wild type or mutated CPA. R = L-Ala, L-Glu; R_1 = Glu, Asp, 2-carboxy-Phe, 3-carboxy-Phe, 2-iodo-Phe, 2-cyclopentyl-Phe, 2-cyclohexyl-Phe, 3-cyclobutyl-Phe **(8a),** 3-cyclopentyl-Phe, 2-cyclopentyl-Tyr, 3-cyclobutyl-Tyr, 3-cyclopentyl-Tyr **(8b),** 3-carboxy-Tyr, naphtyl-Ala.

with MTX-α-Phe in this system with secreted CPA *in vitro* (Smith *et al.,* 1997).

A scission reaction of a glycosidic C-N bond by PNP released cytotoxic purines from their corresponding nucleoside prodrugs, **10** (Scheme 4) (Sorscher *et al.,* 1994). Of the purine nucleosides investigated, 6-methyl-9-(2-deoxy-β-D-erythropentafuranosyl)-purine, **10a,** and 2-fluoro-9-β-D-arabinofuranosyladenine, **10b,** proved good substrates. It appeared that both purines were further metabolized to the corresponding nucleoside triphosphates (Parker *et al.,* 1998). Both drugs were also active against quiescent cells (Secrist III *et al.,* 1999).

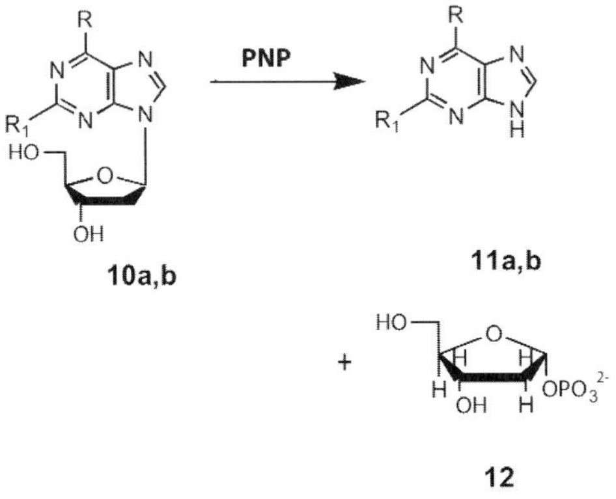

SCHEME 4 Activation of 6-MePdR and 2-FADR by PNP. (a) R = CH_3; R_1 = H; (b) R = NH_2; R_1 = F.

A similar mechanism was suggested for activation of the TP/5′-DFUR system, although there was no demonstration that human TP could cleave the gycosidic bond of 5′-DFUR to yield 5-FU (Patterson *et al.,* 1995; Evrard *et al.,* 1999).

A system based on the use of β-Glu and a glycosylated derivative of doxorubicin was developed. This system has been improved by using a secreted form of the human lysosomal enzyme that converts the doxorubicin prodrug (HMR 1826) to the active drug in the tumor interstitium. The effect is mediated through a BE (Weyel *et al.,* 2000).

Recently, a system based on a gene encoding the glycosidase linamarase was developed using the nontoxic cyanogenic glycoside substrate linamarin (Izquierdo and Corts, 1999). The system released the highly diffusible cyanhydric acid, which had a large BE on neighboring cells.

2. Activation of Prodrugs by Reduction (NR, DT-d)

Reduction of the prodrug CB-1954, **13,** by rat DT-d (k_{cat} = 4.1 min^{-1}) at the 4-nitro group to the hydroxylamine **14** converted the prodrug to a bis-alkylating agent capable of cross-linking DNA (Scheme 5). Human DT-d can also perform this reduction, but at a slower rate (k_{cat} = 0.64 min^{-1}) (Boland *et*

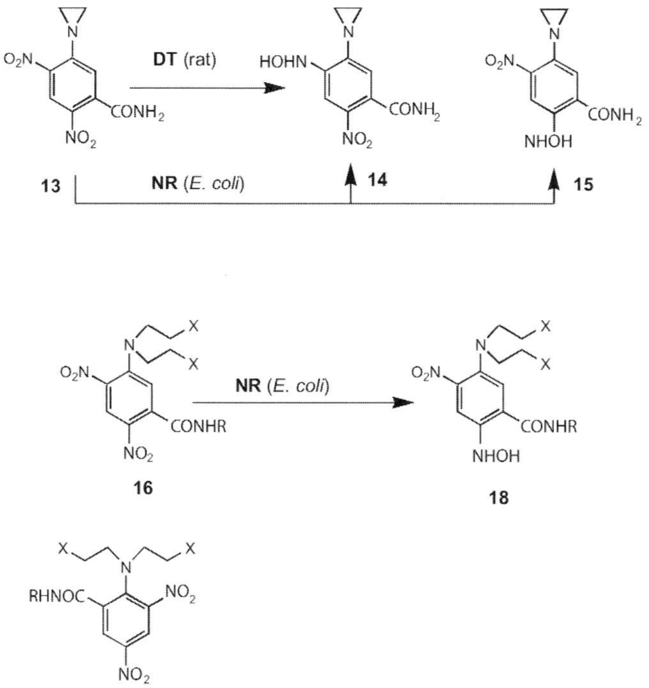

SCHEME 6 Activation of EO9 by DT-diaphorase.

SCHEME 5 Activation of nitroderivatives of alkylating agents by NR (*E. coli*) and DT (rat). X = Cl, Br, I; R = H, CH$_2$CHOHCH$_2$OH.

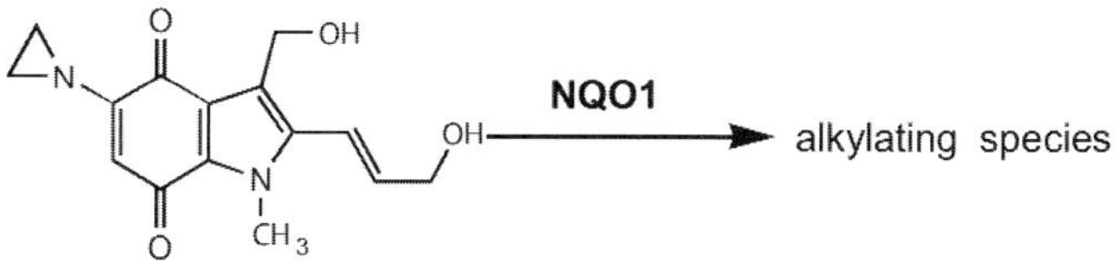

al., 1991). *Escherichia coli* NR was able to reduce either the 2- or the 4-nitro groups in CB-1954 more efficiently (k_{cat} = 360 min^{-1}) (Anlezark *et al.*, 1995; Friedlos *et al.*, 1997). Degrees of activation were reported to be up to 10,000-fold in rodent cell lines, whereas an activation of 670-fold was described in human cell lines (Friedlos *et al.*, 1998).

A similar reduction occurs on aromatic nitrogen mustard analogues, such as **16** or **17** (k_{cat} = 1580 min^{-1}) with *E. coli* NR (Anlezark *et al.*, 1995). Here the activation mechanism is different since the prodrugs already possess a difunctional alkylating moiety. The reduction may be fully activating the aromatic nitrogen mustards, **16** or **17**, by electrons released from the newly formed amino or hydroxylamino groups. The bisiodo- or bisbromo analogues (**16**, X = I, Br, R = CONH$_2$; **17**, X = I, Br, R = CONH$_2$) proved to be superior to CB-1954 from a range of derivatives. Degrees of activation up to 2532-fold were reported *in vitro* for these compounds (Friedlos *et al.*, 1997) (Scheme 5).

The human DT-d (NQO1) has also been suggested for use in GDEPT with bioreductive drugs such as EO9, **19**, mitomycin C, streptonigrine, and diaziquinone (Warrington *et al.*, 1998) (Scheme 6).

3. Activation of Prodrugs by Phosphorylation (Tks)

Phosphorylation is a common reaction in the metabolic pathway of purines and pyrimidines. Nucleosides (or deoxynucleosides) are converted to mono-, di-, and triphosphate analogues by a range of enzymes. The triphosphates are incorporated into DNA or RNA. Therefore, modified purines or pyrimidines can act as fraudulent substrates inhibiting DNA or RNA synthesis, as long as they behave as substrates for the mammalian kinases, DNA or RNA polymerases. Some modified nucleosides, such as GCV, **20**, ACV, **24**, FIAU, **25**, and Ara-M, **26**, are converted to their corresponding monophosphates by endogenous monophosphate kinases with low efficiency. However, viral monophosphate kinases such as herpes simplex virus (HSV)-TK or varicella zoster virus (VZV)-TK are very effective in achieving this conversion. These nucleosides are used as prodrugs with the HSV-TK or VZV-TK enzymes (Scheme 7). Degrees of activation up to 1000 fold were achieved with the HSV-TK/GCV and up to 600 fold with the VZV-TK/araM system. (Averett *et al.*, 1991; Huber *et al.*, 1991; Rubsam *et al.*, 1998).

This approach has led to promising results *in vivo* and more than 30 clinical trials have been initiated with HSV-TK/GCV mainly in glioblastoma. Prodrugs with increased lipophilicity compared to GCV (R = elaidic acid ester) improved the effect *in vitro* (Balzarini *et al.*, 1998). The increased cytotoxicity of this compound is explained by the prolonged intracellular retention of the GCV anabolites in transduced tumor cells. Some clinical advantages were claimed for valaciclovir, the oral form of GCV (Hasenburg *et al.*, 1999). It was considered that the kinetics were not optimal for these substrates. The enzyme was mutated, leading to a TK that compared to wild-type kinase renders the cell 43-fold more sensitive to GCV and 20-fold more sensitive to ACV. The enhanced killing correlates to altered substrate specificity (the K_m of the mutant is 10 mM, 5-fold lower than the K_m of the wild-type enzyme) (Black *et al.*, 1996).

dCK is another enzyme with the ability to activate prodrugs by phosphorylation. The human enzyme is involved in the salvage pathway of deoxyribonucleotide synthesis. The monophophorylation step, catalyzed by dCK, is the rate-limiting step in the conversion of deoxyribonucleosides to deoxyribonucleotides triphosphates. A number of modified nucleosides with anticancer activity, ([1-(β-D-arabinofuranosyl)-cytosine, ara-C, **29**; 2-chloro-2'-deoxyadenosine, CdA, **32**; 2-fluoro-9-(β-D-arabinofuranosyl)-adenine, FaraA, **33**; and

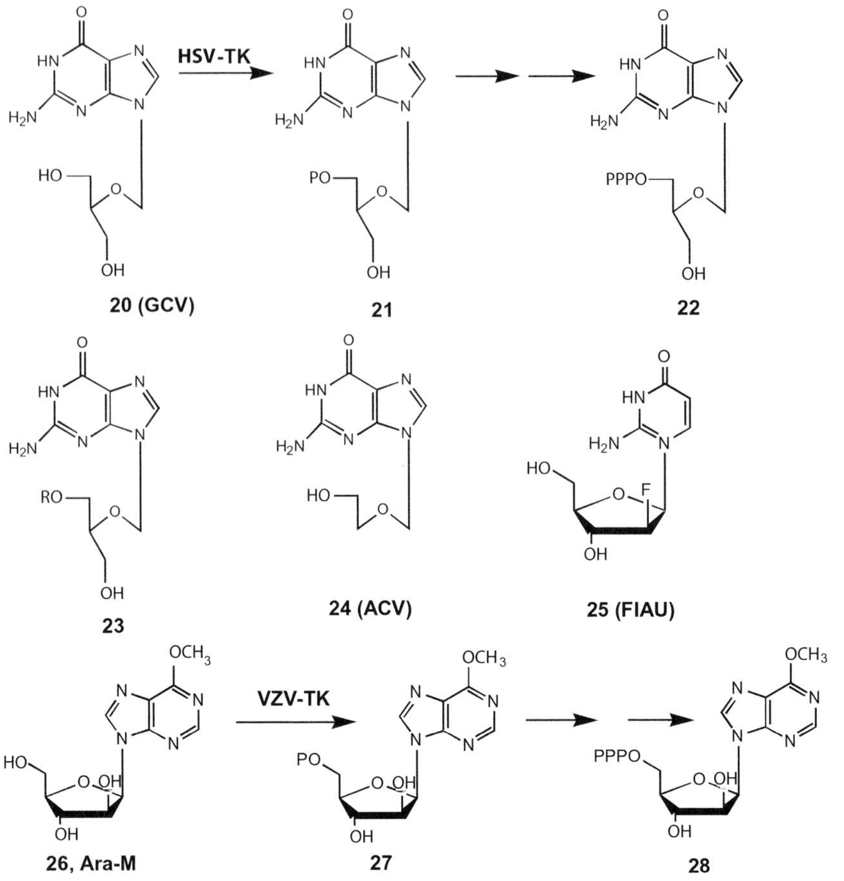

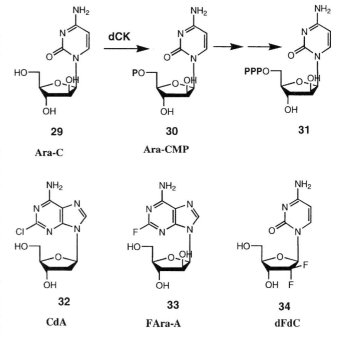

SCHEME 7 Activation of GCV, ACV, FIAU, and Ara-M by viral TK. R = valine ester; elaidic acid ester.

2',2'-difluorodeoxycytosine, dFdC or gemcitabine, **34**) are activated by this mechanism (Scheme 8).

Since tumors express low levels of dCK endogenously, it has been suggested that dCK gene transfer may increase their sensitivity to such modified nucleosides. Ara-C/dCK was proposed for GDEPT (Hapke *et al.,* 1996; Manome *et al.,* 1996).

4. Activation of Prodrugs by C-hydroxylation (Cytochrome P450)

Rabbit cytochrome P450 (CYP4B1) is capable of activating ipomeanol, **35,** efficiently to cytotoxic metabolites (Scheme 9) (Blaise Smith *et al.,* 1995). This combination was recently proposed for GDEPT since the human CYP4B1 isoenzyme possesses only 1% of the rabbit enzyme activity toward ipomeanol (Rainov *et al.,* 1998). CYP4B1/2-aminoanthracene (2-AA) is a similar combination with a degree of activation up to 20-fold in glioma cells expressing CYP4B1 (Rainov *et al.,* 1998).

The human CYP1A2 was shown to be the main isoform responsible for the oxidation of acetaminophen, **36,** to acetyliminoquinone, **37** (NABQI) (Scheme 9). Recently, this system was proposed as a candidate for GDEPT because of the high cytotoxicity of the released NABQI (Tatcher *et al.,* 2000). A BE effect was reported in ovarian- or colon-carcinoma-

SCHEME 8 Activation of analogues of purine and pyridimine nucleotides by dCK.

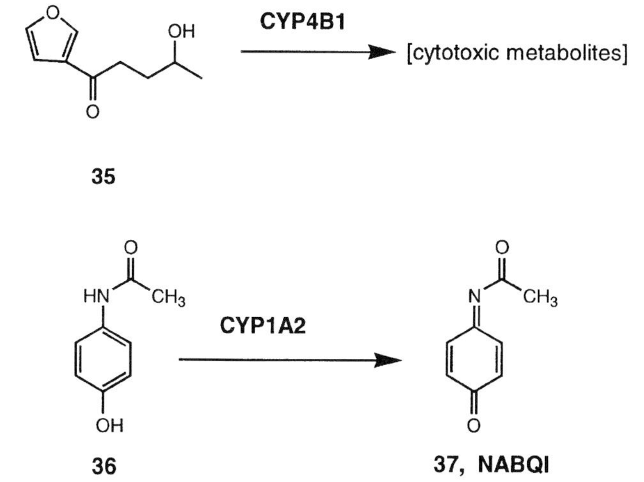

35

36   37, NABQI

SCHEME 9 Activation of ipomeanol by rabbit CYP4B1 and of acetaminophen by CYP1A2.

derived cells transfected with CYP1A2, following acetaminophen treatment.

5. Activation of Prodrugs by Functional Group Substitution (CD)

CD is an enzyme isolated from *E. coli* that can convert the nontoxic antifungal 5-FC, **38,** to the anticancer drug 5-FU, **39.** The latter is converted enzymatically to 5-fluorodeoxyuridine monophosphate (5-FdUMP), **41,** a thymidylate synthase inhibitor, or the triphosphate analogue, **42,** that is incorporated as a fraudulent base in DNA or RNA (Scheme 10) (Huber

et al., 1994). One problem is the low sensitivity for 5-FU of many malignant cells expressing CD due to the absence of uracylphosphoribosyltransferase (UPRT) that catalyzes the conversion of 5-FU to 5-FdUMP in mammalian cells. A hybrid gene for CD and UPRT was transfected into tumor cells to overcome this drawback. The enhanced conversion of 5-FC to 5-FdUMP also has a positive effect on the uptake of the extracellular prodrug. We have calculated that a degree of activation of 70- to 1000-fold was obtained in a number of transfected cell lines (Springer and Niculescu-Duvaz, 2000).

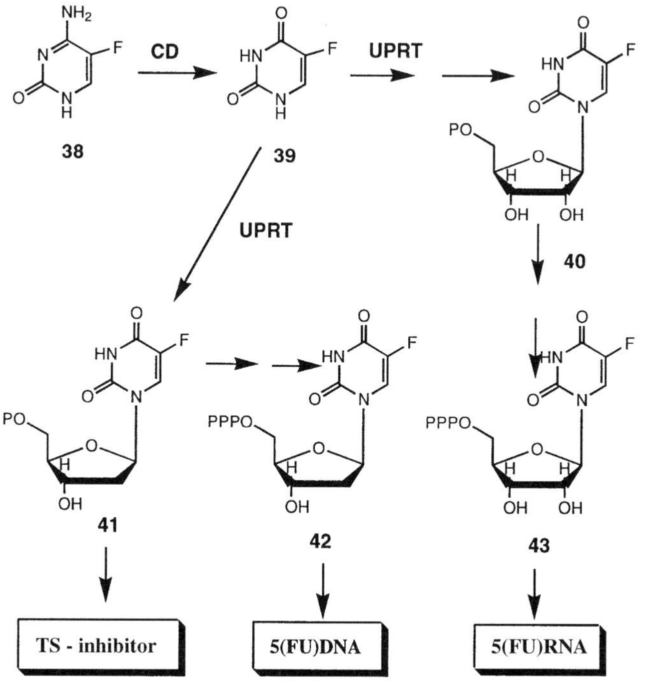

Recently, it was found that CD isolated from yeast has advantages over the bacterial enzyme (Kievit *et al.*, 1999). This GDEPT system was studied extensively. It was found to have a better BE than HSV-TK/GCV and is currently in clinical trials. A phase I clinical trial of suicide therapy with CD/5-FC used with the c-erbB-2 promoter in breast cancer has been described. The approach proved to be safe and resulted in targeted expression in up to 90% of cases (Pandha *et al.*, 1999).

6. Activation of Prodrugs by Deoxyribosylation of Purine Bases (XGPRT)

The bacterial enzyme XGPRT, in contrast to its human counterpart HPRT, can convert xanthine to xanthine monophosphate effectively. XGPRT is also able to transfer the deoxyribose phosphate moiety to 6-mercaptopurine (6-MP), which is further activated to its highly cytotoxic triphosphate analogue (Mulligan and Berg, 1981). 6-Thioguanine (6-TG), **44,** can also be used since it is metabolized to 6-thioxanthine (6-TX), **45,** by endogenous enzymes (Scheme 11). Degrees of activation of 10- to 20-fold were obtained for both prodrugs (Tamiya *et al.*, 1996).

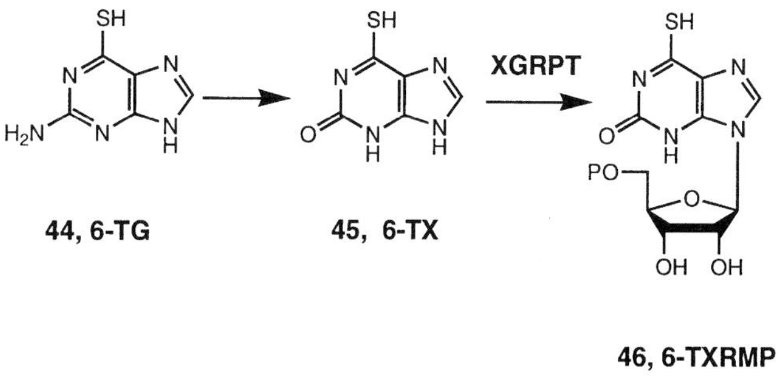

38   39   40

41   42   43

TS - inhibitor   5(FU)DNA   5(FU)RNA

SCHEME 10 Activation of 5-FC by CD.

44, 6-TG   45, 6-TX   46, 6-TXRMP

SCHEME 11 Activation of 6-TG and 6-TX by XGPRT.

7. Production of H_2O_2 by D-Amino Acids Oxidation

H_2O_2 is a relatively stable, membrane-permeable molecule that is cytotoxic to quiescent as well as proliferating cells. Intracellularly generated H_2O_2 can be reduced to hydroxyl radicals via transition-metal-catalyzed Haber–Weiss chemistry (Halliwell and Gutteridge, 1989). The radicals react with DNA, lipids, and protein, resulting in cell death. H_2O_2 was generated selectively in tumor cells by transfection of the DAAO gene from *R. gracilis* and selected amino acids (Scheme 12).

$$\text{D-amino-acid} + H_2O + O_2 \xrightarrow{\textbf{DAAO}} \alpha\text{-keto-acid} + NH_3 + H_2O_2$$
$$(\text{D-alanine})$$

SCHEME 12 Production of H_2O_2 by oxidation of D-amino-acids with DAAO.

The stereoselectivity for D-amino acids appears to be absolute, since L-amino acids are neither substrates nor inhibitors of the enzyme (Pollegioni *et al.*, 1992). The mammalian DAAO enzyme possesses very low activity ($K_M > 6.5$ mM, for D-Ala) and it oxidizes achiral glycine, but this amino acid is a poor substrate for DAAO from *R. gracilis*. The IC_{50} of D-Ala decreased from more than 100 mM to 2.4 mM in DAAO-transfected cells, and a further decrease was obtained when L-buthionine-(S,R)-sulfoximine (BSO, a glutathione transferase inhibitor) was added to the cells. This DAAO/D-Ala combination was suggested as a candidate for GDEPT in the management of the brain tumors (Stegman *et al.*, 1998).

B. Self-Immolative Prodrugs

Many of the enzymes used in GDEPT impose rigid structural requirements for their prodrug substrates. This limits the anticancer agents that can be used in the design of the prodrugs. To overcome this "self-immolative prodrugs" have been synthesized. A self-immolative prodrug can be defined as a compound that generates an unstable intermediate after activation, which then extrudes the active drug in a series of subsequent steps. The activation process is generally enzymatic in nature and is distinct from the extrusion step. The extrusion of the active drug relies on a supplementary spontaneous fragmentation. The mechanism involved can be a 1,6-, 1,4 elimination (Wakselman, 1983; Greenwald *et al.*, 1999) or a cyclization reaction (Sykes *et al.*, 1999). The site of activation is usually separated from the site of extrusion.

The potential advantages of these types of prodrugs is that the range of drugs that can be converted to prodrugs is greatly extended and is unrestricted by the structural substrate requirements for a given enzyme. There is also the possibility of altering the lipophilicity of the prodrugs with minimal effect on the activation kinetics and improving the kinetics of activation by modifying electronic or steric features of the active drug. A number of self-immolative prodrugs have been designed and synthesized based on a range of activation processes.

1. Prodrugs Designed to Be Activated by an Enzymatic Scission Reaction Followed by a 1,6 or 1,4 Elimination

The 1,6-elimination strategy requires the use of a benzylic spacer in the construction of the prodrugs, **47**. The spacer con-

nects the drug to that part of the molecule that is recognized by the enzyme (Niculescu-Duvaz *et al.*, 1999a). A self immolative prodrug designed for activation by CPG2 is described in Scheme 13. As shown, the L-glutamic acid and the active drug are separated by a 4-hydroxy- or 4-amino-substituted benzylic spacer. Activation of these prodrugs involves two steps. First, CPG2 cleaves the oxycarbonyl or carbamoyl L-glutamyl bond. This is followed by the spontaneous decomposition of the carbonic or carbamic acid thus formed, with loss of CO_2. Second, the self-immolative intermediate, **48**, is fragmented by 1,6 elimination, releases a carbonic or carbamic acid, and generates an active drug, **51**, and a quinoneimine, **50**, with loss of CO_2.

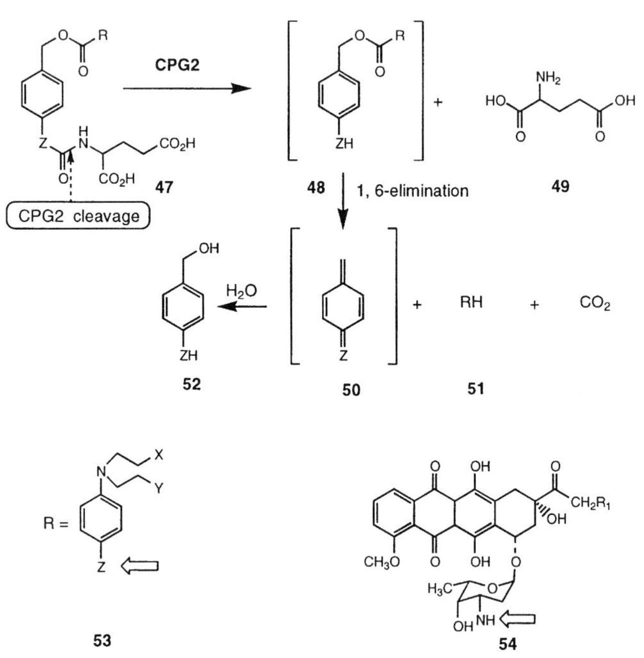

SCHEME 13 Activation of self-immolative drugs by CPG2. X, Y = F, Cl, Br, I, OSO_2CH_3; Z = O, NH; R_1 = H, OH.

Aromatic or aliphatic nitrogen mustards, **53**, and anthracycline antibiotics, **54**, with an amino or hydroxy group were acylated resulting in deactivated molecules. The anthracyclines, such as doxorubicin and daunorubicin, are antitumor drugs with a wide spectrum of activity in human tumors. Their therapeutic efficacy is often limited by toxic side effects, mainly cardiotoxicity and myelosuppression. Several "non-self-immolative" and "self-immolative" anthracycline prodrugs were prepared for activation by different enzymes to overcome these toxicities mainly by derivatization of the amine functionality of the daunosamine (Andrianomenjanahary *et al.*, 1992; Gesson *et al.*, 1994; Farquhar *et al.*, 1998). Unfortunately, CPG2 was unable to activate any of the reported prodrugs. Furthermore, direct addition of L-glutamyl residues to doxorubicin or daunorubicin did not generate a molecule that was a substrate for CPG2. Therefore, prodrugs **47** (R = **54**, R_1 = OH and

R = **54**, R_1 = H) derived from doxorubicin and daunorubicin were based on self-immolative linker strategies with the aim of reducing their intrinsic toxicity (Scheme 14). These prodrugs were activated by CPG2, releasing the active drugs by a 1,6-elimination mechanism (Niculescu-Duvaz et al., 1999b).

Self-immolative prodrugs of nitrogen mustards provided degrees of activation of 12- to 14-fold and a potential of activation of 20- to 33-fold for compounds **47** (R = **53**; Z = NH, O; X = Y = Cl) (Niculescu-Duvaz et al., 1998a). For the doxorubicin prodrug **47** (R = **54**, R_1 = OH), the degree of activation was 11-fold and the potential of activation 21-fold (Niculescu-Duvaz et al., 1999b). Another approach, based on an enzymatic scission reaction catalyzed by E. coli β-Gal, was described. 4(β-D-Galactopyranosyl)benzyl-*N,N,N′,N′*-tetrakis-(2-chloroethyl)phosphorodiamidate was synthesized. The prodrug, **55**, releases by a two-step fragmentation process, the alkylating antitumor agent *N,N,N′,N′*-tetrakis-(2-chloroethyl)phosphorodiamidic acid, **59**, when incubated with β-Gal (Ghosh et al., 1999) (Scheme 14).

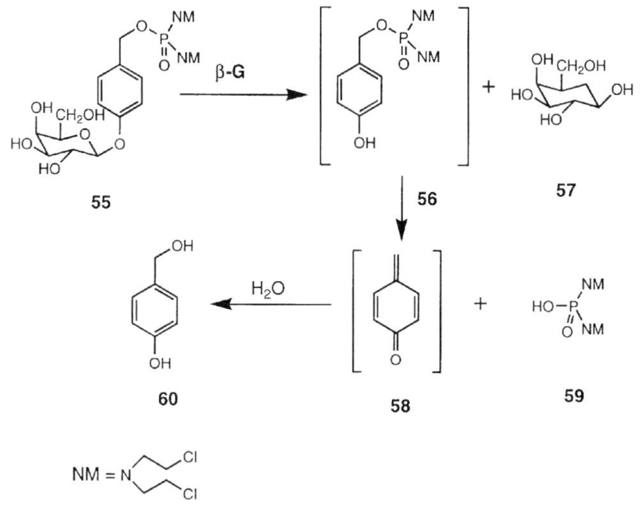

SCHEME 14 Activation of self-immolative alkylating prodrugs by β-G.

Recently, secreted β-lactamase (Moore et al., 1997) was also proposed for GDEPT. There are a number of self-immolative prodrugs, **61,** capable of being activated by this enzyme (Jungheim and Shepherd, 1994). Activation is the result of an enzymatic scission reaction followed by a 1,4-elimination process (Scheme 15).

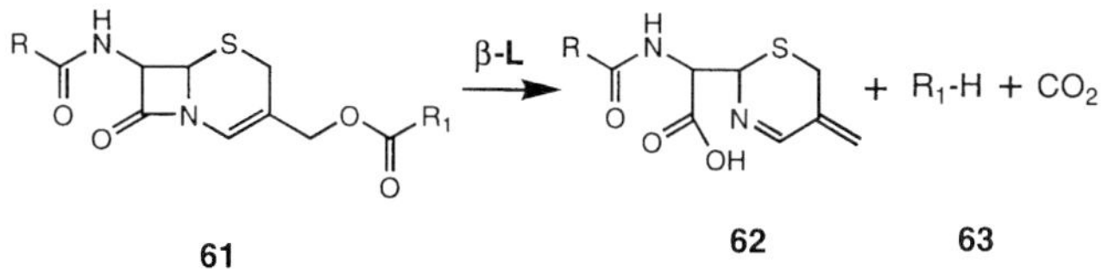

2. Prodrugs Designed to Be Activated by an Enzymatic Reduction Followed by a 1,6 Elimination

Self-immolative prodrugs, including derivatives of aniline nitrogen mustard, enediyne, and amino-*seco*-cyclopropylindolyl, were designed as substrates for *E. coli* NR. Despite different substrate specificities, they were all reduced to the corresponding 4-hydroxylamino derivatives, increasing electron

SCHEME 15 Activation of cephem self-immolative prodrugs by β-lactamase (1, 4-elimination). R = alkyl, aryl, heterocycle, etc.; R_1 = alkylating agent, platinum compound, Vinca alkaloid, anthracycline antibiotics.

density in the π system and stabilizing the positive charge on the benzyl carbon. This triggers a 1,6-elimination process with the extrusion of the active drug (Scheme 16). A prodrug **64** (R = **67**) containing an enediyne residue has been synthesized by this method (Hay et al., 1999b).

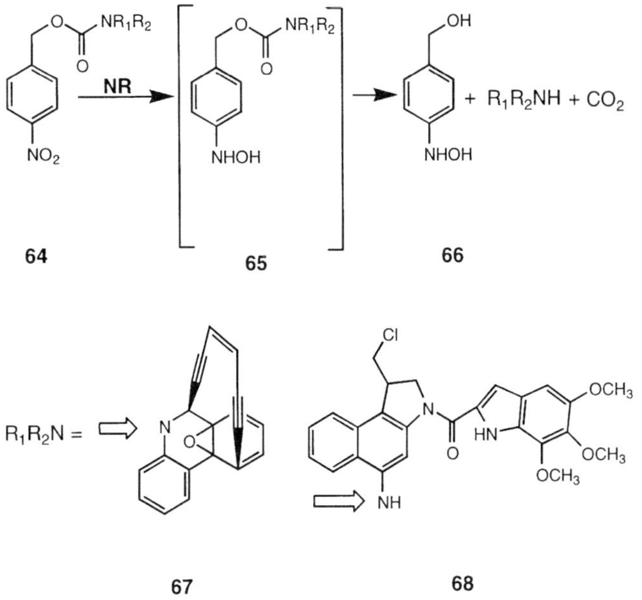

SCHEME 16 Activation of 4-nitrobenzyloxycarbonyl self-immolative prodrugs with NR.

In an effort to extend the range of substrates for NR, the 2-nitroimidazole moiety was considered as a possible substrate. It can fragment after reduction of the nitro group to release the drug. A carbamate prodrug from 5-amino-1-(chloromethyl)-3-(5,6,7-trimethoxyindol-2-ylcarbonyl)-1,2-dihydro-3H-benz[e] indole **69** (R = **68**) has been synthesized and was activated under hypoxic conditions (Hay et al., 1999a) (Scheme 17). Degrees of activation of 21- to 135-fold and 21-fold were reported for compounds **64** (R = **67**) and **69** (R = **68**), respectively (Hay et al., 1999a, 1999b).

3. Prodrugs Designed to Be Activated by an Enzymatic Reduction Followed by Cyclization

A different type of prodrug was prepared based on the reductive release of the amines from 2-(2,6-dinitrophenylamino)-

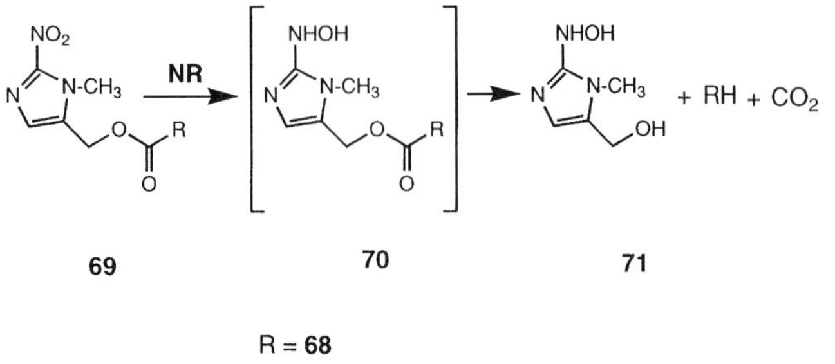

SCHEME 17 Activation of 2-nitro-imidazolylcarbamates self-immolative prodrugs by NR.

propanamide, via hydroxylaminoamide cyclization-extrusion reaction (Sykes *et al.*, 1999). This process is greatly accelerated by an H-bonding "conformational lock" between the anilino NH group and the adjacent 2-(6)-nitro group (Scheme 18).

Prodrug examples containing aniline nitrogen mustard, **72** (R = **75**) or 5-amino-1-(chloromethyl)-3-(5,6,7-trimethoxyindol-2-ylcarbonyl)-1,2-dihydro-3H-benz[e]indole, **72** (R = **68**), have been synthesized but were not activated efficiently by NR (Sykes *et al.*, 1999).

4. Prodrugs Designed to Be Activated by an Enzymatic Hydroxylation Followed by a 1,4 Elimination

Cyclophosphamide (**76**, R = CH$_2$CH$_2$Cl, R$_1$ = H) and ifosfamide (**76**, R = H, R$_2$ = CH$_2$CH$_2$Cl) undergo spontaneous decomposition after hydroxylation by the cytochrome P450 enzyme via the open-form aldophosphamide, **78** (Scheme 19). Aldophosphamide releases a phosphoramidic mustard, **79**, after the 1,4 elimination of acrolein, **80**. This class of prodrug was one of the first types of self-immolative prodrug to be synthesized in cancer chemotherapy, and the mechanism of self-immolation is well known (Brock, 1989).

Human CYT2B6 and CYT3A4 are the most important isoenzymes in liver activation of CP and IF. Rat CYT2B1 is also highly effective. Cytochrome P450 genes (CYT2B1, 2B6, 2C8, 2C9, 2C18 3A) were transfected in tumor cells and investigated in conjunction with oxazaphosphorines (Patterson *et al.*, 1999; Waxman *et al.*, 1999). These studies have also shown that therapeutic benefit is possible despite the contribution of hepatic metabolism to CP and IF activation. Degrees of activation in the range of 10- to 100-fold were reported. An improvement in activation was noticed when a double suicide gene therapy system containing a hybrid gene of *CYP4B1* and *P450-reductase* were transfected to malignant cells (Chen *et al.*, 1997).

5. The Activation Process

A. Kinetic Parameters

The concentration of the drug and the rate at which it is released at the activation site depends on the kinetic parameters of the enzyme-prodrug system. The K_m is an expression of the amount of substrate required to reach half of maximum velocity, V_{max}. The turnover number, k_{cat}, or the V_{max} supplies additional information about the reaction rate, since both are terms to express the rate of drug release. It is impossible to compare enzyme-prodrug systems solely on this basis since these data are not often recorded. It can be hypothesized that low K_m and high V_{max} (or k_{cat}) are associated with more effective systems (Springer and Niculescu-Duvaz, 2000). This hypothesis is exemplified when yeast CD is compared with bacterial CD (Kievit *et al.*, 1999). The yeast enzyme, which proved more effective than its bacterial counterpart, has a lower K_m and a higher V_{max}. An alternative correlation that resulted in the same conclusion was reported when the activity

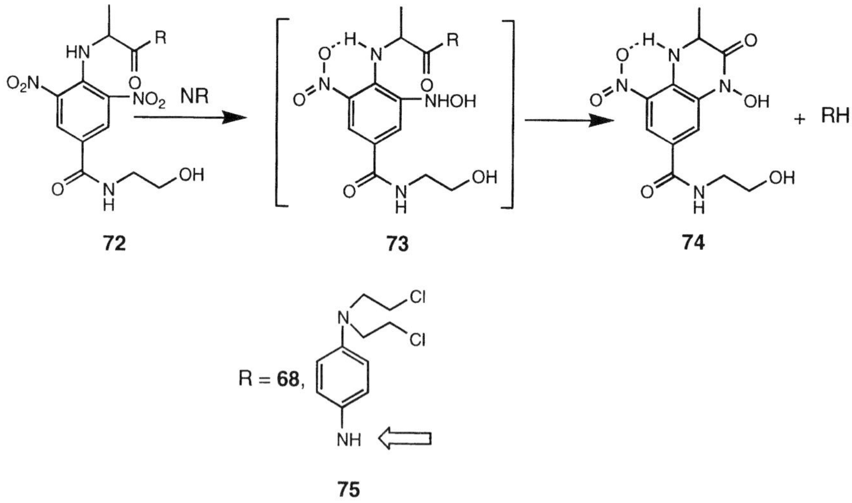

SCHEME 18 Activation of self-immolative 2-(2, 6-dinitro-phenylamino)propionamide by NR.

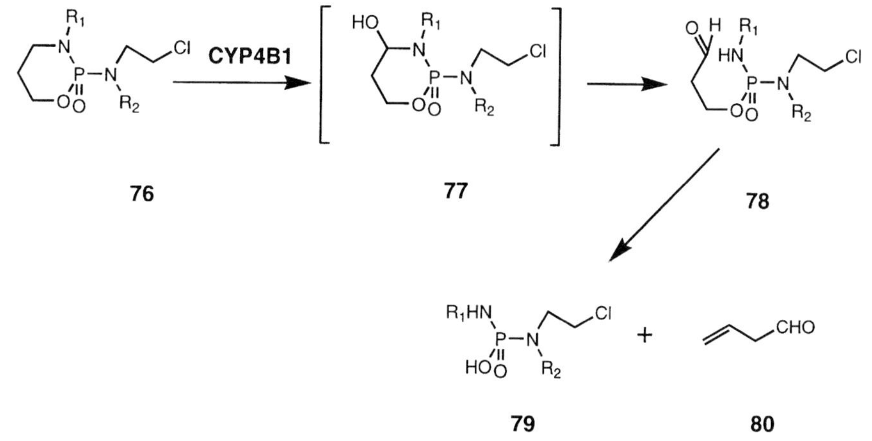

SCHEME 19 Activation of CP and IF by CYP4B1 via aldophosphamide followed by 1,4-elimination. **CP,** R_1 = H; R_2 = CH_2CH_2Cl; **IF,** R_1 = CH_2CH_2Cl; R_2 = H.

of CP (higher k_{cat}, lower IC_{50}) was compared with that of IP (lower k_{cat}, higher IC_{50}) (Chang *et al.*, 1993).

It is not yet known if a slow, constant release of the active drug is preferable to a rapid release. One possibility is that for drugs acting against both quiescent and proliferating cells, the former is likely to be the appropriate choice. By contrast, for drugs acting only against proliferating cells the second alternative may be preferable.

B. Potential of Activation

It is clear that enzyme-prodrug systems should be designed with as large as possible activation potential. However, not all systems can be described in this way since the cytotoxicities of the released drugs are sometimes unavailable. Recently, a new mechanism for the cytotoxicity of GCV was proposed based on the ability of ganciclovir nucleotide triphosphate (GCVTP) to be incorporated into DNA combined with the intrinsic cytotoxicity for ganciclovir nucleotide monophosphate (GCVMP), **21** (Rubsam *et al.*, 1998). Therefore, the potential of activation of this system (as defined here in Section 2) calculated solely on the basis of IC_{50} of GCVTP, **22,** appears to be inaccurate. Another interesting mechanism is for CP activated by CYT P450. A maximum differential of 20- to 25-fold is theoretically achievable based on the IC_{50} values of CP and its corresponding phosphoramide mustard. However, the degree of activation was found to be greater than 100-fold (Springer and Niculescu-Duvaz, 2000), which suggests that the CP phosphoramide mustard is not the final active metabolite.

C. Degree of Activation

The activation process is not always easy to understand. The physicochemical, electronic, and steric parameters in-

volved directly or indirectly influence this process. It is therefore useful to define the degree of activation that reflects the efficiency of the system in a transfected cell line (as defined here in Section 2). Theoretically, it will be lower than or at best equal to the potential of activation. This was found to be the case for all the systems analyzed in Table 1.

One of the drawbacks of these parameters is that although they give us an image of the behavior of a GDEPT system *in vitro*, they may not reflect accurately the situation *in vivo*. A number of additional factors, such as pharmacokinetics, biodistribution, and immunologic effects, serve to complicate the overall picture. However, on a rational basis, these parameters are useful for comparing different GDEPT systems and should also be helpful in designing new systems.

There are means to increase the efficacy of a GDEPT system. One is to increase the available concentration of the prodrug. An improved uptake of the prodrug is important for the efficacy of the enzyme expressed intracellularly in GDEPT systems. The concomitant expression of *E. coli* CD and uracil phosphoribosyltransferase (UPRT) significantly improved the cytotoxicity of 5-FC. It was shown that the combination of the two genes facilitated the uptake of 5-FC by direct channeling of 5-FU (the product of CD activation) to 5-fluorouridine monophosphate by the second enzyme in the cascade, UPRT (Tiraby *et al.*, 1996).

6. Augmenting the Effect

One way of increasing the efficiency of a GDEPT system is to mutate the enzyme for surface-tethered or external expression. The potential advantages of extracellular expression are twofold. It should give an improved BE since the drug will be generated in the tumor interstitium rather than inside the cell. Also, the prodrug need not enter the cell to became activated, and therefore prodrugs that are excluded from cells can be exploited.

CPG2 was the first enzyme mutated for expression tethered to the outer cell membrane (Marais *et al.*, 1997). Mutation of three glycosylation sites (Asn222, Asn264, and Asn272) to the conserved amino acid Gln was required to produce a protein stCPG2(Asn222Gln, Asn264Gln, Asn272Gln) capable of activating CMDA, **1**(R = H, Z = —, X = Cl, and Y = mesyl). The mutated enzyme exhibits the same substrate requirements compared to the wild-type (K_m = 7 μM for MTX), with a somewhat lower but still effective turnover (k_{cat} = 3500 min^{-1}). The system based on external expressed enzyme showed advantages in term of BE (Marais *et al.*, 1997).

Enzyme such as secreted β-Glu (Weyel *et al.*, 2000) has recently been described. Abstracts but not publications illustrating other secreted enzymes as β-L (Moore *et al.*, 1997), CD (Rehemtulla *et al.*, 1997), and PGA (Moore *et al.*, 1997) have been published.

CPA is an enzyme that was expressed in a secretory form to improve its BE. The secretory CPA$_{ST3}$ was constructed by introducing a decapeptide (GLSARNRQKR) between the prodomain and the mature domain of rat CPA (Smith *et al.*, 1997). The expression of this mutated enzyme in cancer cells is responsible for their sensitization to MTX-α-substituted prodrugs, **6**. An externally expressed CPA$_{DAF}$, tethered to the cell, was also reported (Hamstra *et al.*, 2000).

A problem with the CPA/MTX-α-substituted prodrugs system is that the prodrugs are not stable *in vivo* as they are hydrolyzed by endogenous CPA. New bulky phenylalanine and tyrosine (substituted in position 2 or 3 with *t*-butyl, cyclopropyl-, cyclobutyl-, or cyclopropyl moieties) of MTX (i.e., MTX-α-3-cyclobutylphenylalanine, **8a**, or MTX-α-3-cyclopentyltyrosine, **8b**) were synthesized. These compounds are not substrates for the wild-type enzyme and therefore are stable *in vivo*. A mutant of the hCPA1 was produced in which Thr268 was changed with Gly (hCPA1-T268G) to make more room for the substrate (Smith *et al.*, 1997). This mutant can hydrolyze the bulky prodrugs **8a** and **8b** with good kinetics (k_{cat}/K_m are 1.8 and 0.16 μM^{-1}s^{-1} for **8a** and **8b**, respectively).

Using similar techniques, mutants of HSV-TK were obtained with improved kinetic parameters for GCV and ACV (Black *et al.*, 1996). Another way to enhance GDEPT efficiency is by using two or more suicide genes expressed separately or as a fusion gene. "Double-suicide gene therapy" has been reported wherein a combination of suicide genes is introduced simultaneously to augment the effects. The rationale is that the released active drugs act by different mechanisms leading to a synergistic cell kill (Aghi *et al.*, 1999; Blackburn *et al.*, 1999).

Resistant cell populations are less likely to occur when drugs with different mechanisms of action are used. It was

demonstrated that double-suicide gene therapy (HSV-TK+CD), but not transfer of either gene individually, allowed the elimination of human carcinoma cell lines *in vitro* and *in vivo* (Uckert *et al.*, 1998). Generally, such strategies have led to therapeutic improvements *in vivo* (Rogulski *et al.*, 1997).

7. Exploiting the Bystander Effect and Acquired Immunity

A crucial component of GDEPT is that the released drug should be capable of inducing a BE. Most of the systems reported exhibit a significant BE, at least *in vivo*. The mechanisms of the BE have been intensively investigated and include the generation of active metabolites, gap junction transport, and export of cytotoxic metabolites able to kill nontransfected neighboring cells as well as immune responses.

It is difficult to compare the BE from different systems due to the different conditions employed. A quantitative expression of the BE was proposed using the NR/CB1954 system in a range of human tumor cell types. The IC$_{50}$ values of non-NR-expressing cells were measured in the presence of differing proportions of NR-expressing cells. The shift in IC$_{50}$ was used to calculate a value for the BE, termed the transmission efficiency (TE), which is the decrease in IC$_{50}$ due to the BE as the percentage of the maximum decrease possible. The percentage of NR-expressing cells for which the TE was 50% (TE$_{50}$) is a single datum point for the BE. The TE50 in the cell lines ranged from 0.3% to approximately 2% (Friedlos *et al.*, 1998).

The toxic nucleoside phosphates resulting from the activation of purine (GCV, ACV, etc.) or pyrimidine (Ara-C, 5-FDUR, etc.) nucleosides are nondiffusible across cell membranes and require a cell-to-cell contact for a BE (Freeman *et al.*, 1993; Manome *et al.*, 1996). By contrast, for diffusible drugs like aldophosphamide (or phosphoramide mustard), 6-MeP, 2-FA, and CMDB, no such requirement is necessary (Huber *et al.*, 1994; Bridgewater *et al.*, 1995; Chen and Waxman 1995).

The permeable toxic metabolites formed following prodrug activation are released by efflux from dead and dying genetically modified cells. This mechanism is postulated for the metabolites resulting from 5-FC, CP, IP, CMDA, 6-MeP, linamarin, and H$_2$O$_2$ generated by oxidation of D-amino acids. The BE requires different mechanisms with purine and pyrimidine nucleosides since the toxic phosphorylated metabolites cannot diffuse across cell membranes. The HSV-TK/GCV system that releases nonpermeable metabolites requires cell-to-cell contact for the BE. However, the mechanism is complex. The transfer of cytotoxic GCV metabolites from HSV-TK-transfected cells to wild-type tumor cells via gap junctions has been demonstrated as a BE mechanism (Touraine *et al.*,

1998a). When gap junction function was evaluated with a dye transfer technique, tumor cells resistant to the BE did not show dye transfer from cell to cell, whereas BE-sensitive tumor cells did. It was suggested that enhancement of the HSV-TK/GCV BE could be achieved by pharmacologic manipulation of the gap junctions *in vivo*. Dieldrin, **81** (Scheme 20), a drug known to decrease gap junction communications, diminished the dye transfer and also inhibited the BE. Apigenin, **82**, a flavonoid, and lovastatin, **83**, an HMG-CoA reductase inhibitor, were shown to up-regulate gap junction function and dye transfer in tumors expressing gap junctions and to enhance the BE *in vivo* (Touraine *et al.*, 1998a, 1998b).

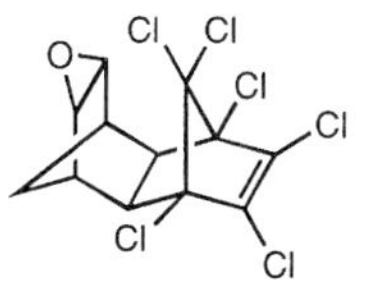

82, dieldrin

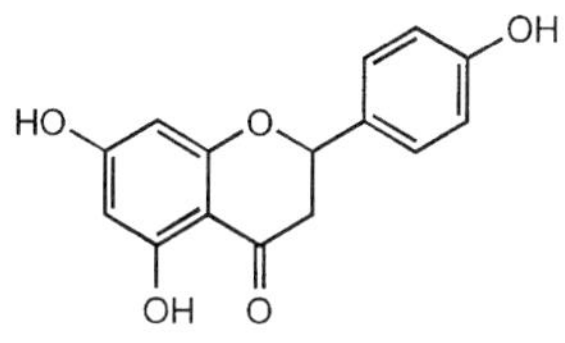

83, apigenin 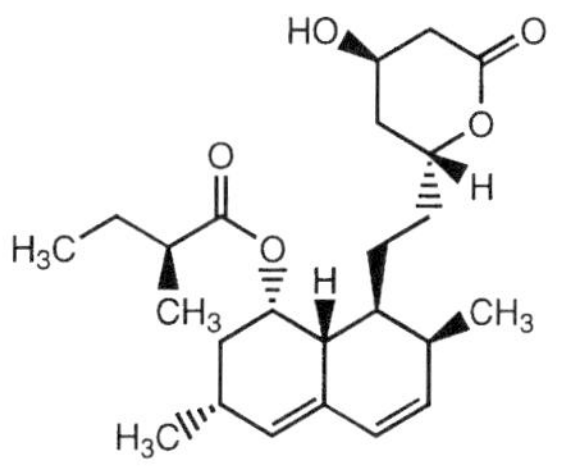   **84, lovastatin**

SCHEME 20 Compounds influencing gap junction communications.

There are data that appear to contradict the gap junction hypothesis and suggest that other mechanisms may be involved. Under different experimental conditions it was found that the BE depended on the concentration of the enzyme, the number of cells expressing HSV-TK, and the overall confluence of the cells, and that the BE did not correlate with gap junction functional communications as determined by the Lucifer yellow assay (Boucher *et al.*, 1998; Imaizumi *et al.*, 1998).

When the enzyme is expressed extracellularly the drug is released outside the cells and an improved BE would be expected. The released drugs should be highly diffusible, and prodrugs releasing permeable metabolites are still favored.

Elicitation of an immune response has been described as a positive factor in GDEPT. Although data are available that show that the BE occurs in immunocompromised animals, other reports show that the BE is mediated through the release of cytokines *in vivo* (Pavlovic *et al.*, 1996; Ramesh *et al.*, 1996; Hall *et al.*, 1998). Beneficial immune effects may

be induced either by stimulation of the host immune system or by the use of additional cytokine gene therapy. Long-lasting immunity in immunocompetent animals has developed as a response to HSV-TK transduction followed by GCV treatment (Pavlovic *et al.*, 1996). These studies suggest that an intact immune system is important for long-term tumor suppression with HSV-TK *in vivo* (Gagandep *et al.*, 1996).

Additional cytokine genes have been examined. Mice treated with both HSV-TK and IL-2 genes developed effective systemic antitumoral immunity against tumorigenic rechallenges. In an attempt to enhance and prolong the immunity, a third vector containing the mouse granulocyte-macrophage colony-stimulating factor (mGM-CSF) gene was employed. The animals treated simultaneously with HSV-TK+IL-2+mGM-CSF vectors followed by administration of GCV developed long-term antitumor immunity and survived for more than 4 months without recurrence (Chen *et al.*, 1995, 1996b)

8. Conclusions

To date GDEPT systems have shown efficacy *in vivo*. There is still room for improvement. The enzyme can be mutated to obtain greater efficiency of activation for a given prodrug. Alternatively, the active site may be mutated to provide greater specificity to the prodrugs as substrates for the transfected genes. The synthesis of new prodrugs, such as self-immolative prodrugs, prodrugs releasing more cytotoxic drugs, drugs able to optimize the BE effect, or prodrugs taking advantage of carrier in order to cross cell membranes, should be also considered. The design of optimized enzyme-prodrug systems and the use of cocktails of prodrugs releasing drugs with different mechanisms of action, which could be activated by the same enzyme, could also lead to improvements.

Additional strategies are being aimed at improving the therapy for solid tumors. For example, combining GDEPT with radiotherapy or immunotherapy has been suggested. Such an approach may involve either a sequential treatment schedule (GDEPT/radiation therapy or GDEPT/immunotherapy) or the transfection of suicide gene(s) together with genes capable of increasing the sensitivity of the tumors to radiation or enhancing the potential of the host immune system with cytokine genes. Ultimately, delivery and targeting are the crux of efficacy in GDEPT.

Acknowledgments

This work was funded by the Cancer Research Campaign (grants SP2330/0201 and SP2330/0102) and the Institute of Cancer Research.

References

Aghi, M., Chou, T. C., Suling, K., Breakefield, X. O., and Chiocca, I. A. (1999). Multimodal cancer treatment mediated by a replicating oncolytic virus that delivers the oxazaphosphorine/rat cytochrome P450 2B1 and ganciclovir/herpes simplex virus thymidine kinase gene therapies. *Cancer Res.* **59**, 3861–3865.

Andrianomenjanahary, S., Dong, X., Florent, J. C., Gaudel, G., Gesson, J. P., Jacquesy, J. C., Koch, M., Michel, S., Mondon, M., Monneret, C., Petit, P., Renoux, B., and Tillequin, F. (1992). Synthesis of novel targeted prodrugs of anthracyclines potentially activated by a monoclonal antibody galactosidase conjugate (Part 1). *Bioorg. Med. Chem. Lett.* **2**(9), 1093–1096.

Anlezark, G. M., Melton, R. G., Sherwood, R. F., Wilson, W. R., Denny, W. A., Palmer, B. D., Knox, R. G., Friedlos, F., and Williams, A. (1995). Bioactivation of dinitrobenzamide mustards by an E. coli B nitroreductase. *Biochem. Pharmacol.* **50**, 609–618.

Averett, D. R., Kozalka, G. A., Fyfe, J. A., Roberts, G. B., Purifoy, D. J. M., and Krenitsky, T. A. (1991). "6-methoxypurine arabinoside as a selective and potent inhibitor of varicella-zoster virus." *Antimicrob. Agents Chemother.* **35**(5), 851–857.

Balzarini, G., Degreve, B., Andrei, G., Neyst, J., Sandvold, M., Myhren, F., and de Clerq, E. (1998). Superior cytostatic activity of the ganciclovir elaidic acid ester due to the prolonged intracellular retention of ganciclovir anabolites in herpes simplex virus type 1 thymidine kinase gene-transfected tumor cells. *Gene Ther.* **5**, 419–426.

Bielicki, L., Voelcker, G., and Hohorst, H. J. (1984). Activated cyclophosphamide: an enzyme-mechanism-based suicide inactivator of DNA polymerase/3′, 5′ exonuclease. *J. Cancer Res. Clin. Oncol.* **107**, 195–198.

Bilbao, G., Contreras, J. L., Gómez-Navarro, J., and Curiel, D. T. (1998). Improving adenoviral vectors for cancer gene therapy. *Tumor Targeting* **3**, 59–79.

Black, M. E., Newcomb, T. G., Wilson, H. M., and Loeb, L. A. (1996). Creation of drug-specific herpes simplex virus type 1 thymidine kinase mutants for gene therapy. *Proc. Natl. Acad. Sci. USA* **93**, 3525–3529.

Blackburn, R. V., Galoforo, S., Corry, P. M., and Lee, Y. J. (1999). Adenoviral transduction of a cytosine deaminase/thymidine kinase fusion gene into prostate carcinoma cells enhances prodrug and radiation sensitivity. *Int. J. Cancer* **82**, 293–297.

Blaise Smith, P., Tiano, H. F., Nesnow, S., Boyd, M. R., Philpot, R. M., and Langenbach, R. (1995). 4-Ipomeanol and 2-aminoanthracene cytotoxicity in C3H/10T1/2 cells expressing rabbit cytochrome P450 4B1. *Biochem. Pharmacol.* **50**, 1567–1575.

Boland, M. P., Knox, R. J., and Roberts, J. J. (1991). The differences in kinetics of rat and human DT-diaphorase result in in a differential sensitivity of cells lines to CB 1954 [5-(aziridin-1-yl)-2,4-dinitrobenzamide. *Biochem. Pharmacol.* **41**, 867–875.

Boucher, P. D., Ruch, R. J., and Shewach, D. S. (1998). Differential ganciclovir-mediated cytotoxicity and bystander killing in human colon carcinoma cell lines expressing herpes simplex virus thymidine kinase. *Human Gene Ther.* **9**(6), 801–814.

Bridgewater, G., Springer, C. J., Knox, R., Minton, N., Michael, P., and Collins, M. (1995). Expression of the bacterial nitroreductase enzyme in mammalian cells renders them selectively sensitive to killing by the prodrug CB1954. *Eur. J. Cancer* **31A**(13/14), 2362–2370.

Brock, N. (1989). Oxazaphosphorine cytostatics: past-present-future. *Cancer Res.* **49**, 1.

Chang, T. K. H., Weber, G. F., Crespi, C. L., and Waxman, D. J. (1993). Differential activation of cyclophosphamide and ifosphamide by cytochromes P450 2B and 3A in human liver microsomes. *Cancer Res.* **53**, 5629–5637.

Chen, L., and Waxman, D. J. (1995). Intratumoral activation and enhanced chemotherapeutic effect of oxazaphosphorines following cytochrome P-450 gene transfer: Development of a combined chemotherapy/cancer gene therapy strategy. *Cancer Res.* **55**, 581–589.

Chen, L., Waxman, D. J., Chen, D., and Kufe, D. C. (1996a). Sensitization of human breast cancer cells to cyclophosphamide and ifosfamide by transfer of a liver cytochrome P-450 gene. *Cancer Res.* **56**, 1331–1340.

Chen, S. H., Kosai, K., Xu, B., Pham-Nguyen, K., Contant, C., Finegold, M. J., and Woo, S. L. C. (1996b). Combination suicide and cytokine gene therapy for hepatic metastases of colon carcinoma: Sustained antitumor immunity prolongs animal survival. *Cancer Res.* **56**, 3758–3762.

Chen, L., Yu, L. J., and Waxman, D. J. (1997). Potentiation of cytochrome P450/cyclophosphamide-based cancer gene therapy by coexpression of the *P450 reductase* gene. *Cancer Res.* **57**, 4830–4837.

Chen, S. H., Li Chen, X. L., Wang, Y., Kosai, K., Finegold, M. J., Rich, S. S., and Woo, S. L. C. (1995). Combination gene therapy for liver metastasis of colon carcinoma in vivo. *Proc. Natl. Acad. Sci. USA* **92**, 2577–2581.

Culver, K. W., Ram, Z., Wallbridge, S., Oldfield, H. E. H., and Blaese, M. R. (1992). In vivo gene transfer with retroviral vector-producer cells for treatment of experimental brain tumors. *Science* **256**, 1550–1552.

Denny, W. A., and Wilson, W. R. (1998). The design of selectively-activated anti-cancer prodrugs for use in antibody-directed and gene-directed enzyme prodrugs therapies. *J. Pharm. Pharmacol.* **50**(4), 387–394.

Dowell, R. I., Springer, C. J., Davies, D. H., Hadley, E. M., Burke, P. J., Boyle, F. T., Melton, R. G., Connors, T. A., Blakey, D. C., and Mauger, A. B. (1996). New mustard prodrug for antibody-directed enzyme prodrug therapy: Alternative to amide link. *J. Med. Chem.* **39**, 1100–1105.

Encell, L. P., Landis, D. M., and Loeb, L. A. (1999). Improving enzymes for gene therapy. *Nat. Biotechnol.* **17**, 143–147.

Evrard, A., Cuq, P., Ciccolini, J., Vian, L., and Cano, J.-P. (1999). Increased cytotoxicity and bystander effect of 5-fluorouracil and 5′-deoxy-5-fluorouridine in human colorectal cancer cells transfected with thymidine phosphorylase. *Br. J. Cancer* **80**(11), 1726–1733.

Farquhar, D., Cherif, A., Bakina, E., and Nelson, G. A. (1998). Intensely potent doxorubicin analogues: Structure-activity relationships. *J. Med. Chem.* **41**, 965–972.

Frankel, A. E., FitzGerald, D., Siegall, C., and Press, O. W. (1996). Advances in immunotoxin biology and therapy: a summary of the Fourth International Symposium on Immunotoxins. *Cancer Res.* **56**, 926–932.

Freeman, S. M., Abboud, C. N., Whartenby, K. A., Packman, C. H., Koeplin, D. S., Moolten, F. S., and Abraham, G. N. (1993). The "bystander effect": Tumor regression when a fraction of the tumor mass is genetically modified. *Cancer Res.* **53**, 5274–5283.

Friedlos, F., Court, S., Ford, M., Denny, W. A., and Springer, C. J. (1998). "Gene-directed enzyme prodrug therapy: quantitative bystander cytotoxicity and DNA damage induced by CB1954 in cells expressing bacterial nitroreductase." *Gene Ther.* **5**(1), 105–112.

Friedlos, F., Denny, W. A., Palmer, B. D., and Springer, C. J. (1997). Mustard prodrugs for activation by *Escherichia coli* nitroreductase in gene-directed enzyme prodrug therapy. *J. Med. Chem.* **40**(8), 1270–1275.

Gagandep, S., Brew, R., Green, B., Christmas, S. E., Klatzmann, D., Poston G. J., and Kinsella, A. R. (1996). Prodrug-activated gene therapy: Involvement of an immunological component in the "bystander effect". *Gene Ther.* **3**(2), 83–88.

Gesson, J. P., Jacquesy, J. C., Mondon, M., Petit, P., Renoux, B., Andrianomenjanahary, S., Dufat-Trinh Van, H., Koch, M., Michel, S., Tillequin, F., Florent, J. C., Monneret, C., Bosslet, K., Czech, J., and Hoffmann, D. (1994). Prodrugs of anthracyclines for chemotherapy via enzyme-monoclonal antibody conjugates. *Anticancer Drug Des.* **9**, 409–423.

Ghosh, A. K., Khan, S., and Farquhar, D. (1999). "A β-galactosidase phosphoramide mustard prodrug for use in conjunction with gene-directed enzyme prodrug therapy." *Chem. Communications* 2527–2528.

Golumbek, P. T., Hamzeh, F. M., Jaffee, E. M., Levitsky, H., Lietman, P. S., and Pardoll, D. M. (1992). Herpes simplex-1 virus thymidine kinase gene is unable to completely eliminatelive, nonimmunogenic tumour cell vaccines. *J. Immunother.* **12**, 224–230.

Greenwald, R. B., Pendri, A., Conover, C. D., Zhao, H., Choe, Y. H., Martinez, A., Shum, K., and Guan, S. (1999). Drug delivery system employing 1,4- or 1,6-elimination: Poly(ethylene glycol) prodrugs of amine-containing compounds. *J. Med. Chem.* **42**, 3657–3667.

Hall, S. J., Sanford, M. A., Atkinson, G., and Chen, S.-H. (1998). Induction of potent antitumor natural killer cell activity by herpes simplex virus-thymidine kinase and ganciclovir therapy in an orthotopic mouse model of prostate cancer. *Cancer Res.* **58**, 3221–3225.

Halliwell, B., and Gutteridge, J. M. (1989). "Free Radicals in Biology and Medicine." Clarendon Press, Oxford.

Hamstra, D. A., Page, M., Maybaum, J., and Rehemtulla, A. (2000). Expression of endogenously activated secreted or cell surface carboxypeptidase A sensitizes tumor cells to methotrexate-a-peptide prodrugs. *Cancer Res.* **60**, 657–665.

Hapke, D. M., Stegmann, A. P. A., and Mitchell, B. S. (1996). Retroviral transfer of deoxycytidine kinase into tumor cell lines enhances nucleoside toxicity. *Cancer Res.* **56**, 2343–2347.

Hasenburg, A., Tong, X. W., Rojas-Martinez, A., Nyberg-Hoffman, C., Kieback, C. C., Kaplan, A. L., Kaufman, R. H., Ramzy, I., Aguilar-Cordova, E., and Kieback, D. G. (1999). Thymidine kinase (TK) gene therapy of solid tumors: Valacyclovir facilitates outpatients treatment. *Anticancer Res.* **19**, 2163–2166.

Hay, M. P., Sykes, B. M., Denny, W. A., and Wilson, W. R. (1999a). A 2-nitroimidazole carbamate prodrug of 5-amino-1-(chloromethyl)-3-[(5,6,7-trimethoxyindol-2-yl)carbonyl]-1,2-dihydro-3H-benz[e]indole (amino-seco-CBI-TMI) for use with ADEPT and GDEPT. *Bioorg. Med. Chem. Lett.* **9**, 2237–2242.

Hay, M. P., Wilson, W. R., and Denny, W. R. (1999b). Nitobenzyl carbamate prodrugs of enediynes for nitroreductase gene-directed enzyme prodrug therapy. *Bioorg. Med. Chem. Lett.* **9**, 3417–3422.

Huber, B. A., Richards, C. A., and Krenitsky, T. A. (1991). Retroviral-mediated gene therapy for the treatment of hepatocellular carcinoma: An innovative approach for cancer therapy. *Proc. Natl. Acad. Sci., USA* **88**, 8039–8043.

Huber, B. E., Austin, E. A., Richards, C. A., Davis, S. T., and Good, S. S. (1994). Metabolism of 5-fluorocytidine to 5-fluorouracil in human colorectal tumor cells transduced with the cytosine deaminase gene: Significant antitumor effects when only a small percentage of tumor cells express cytosine deaminase. *Proc. Natl. Acad. Sci. USA* **91**, 8302–8306.

Imaizumi, K., Hasegawa, Y., Kawabe, T., Emi, N., Saito, H., Naruse, K., and Shimokata, K. (1998). Bystander tumoricidal effect and gap junctional communication in lung cancer cells. *Am. J. Respir. Cell Mol. Biol.* **18**, 205–212.

Izquierdo, M., and Corts, M. L. (1999). Suicide gene therapy system for the treatment of brain tumours. WO 9947653 Boehringer Ingelheim International, 39 pp.

Johansson, M., Van Rompey, A. R., Degreves, B., Balzarini, J., and Karlsson, A. (1999). Cloning and characterization of the multisubstrate deoxyribonucleoside kinase of *Drosophila melanogaster. J. Biol. Chem.* **274**(34), 23814–23819.

Jungheim, L. N., and Shepherd, T. T. (1994). Design of antitumor prodrugs: substrates for antibody targeted enzymes. *Chem. Rev.* **94**, 1553–1566.

Kievit, E., Bershad, E., Ng, E., Sethna, P., Dev, I., Lawrence, T. S., and Rehemtulla, A. (1999). Superiority of yeast over bacterial cytosine deaminase for enzyme/prodrug gene therapy in colon cancer. *Cancer Res.* **59**, 1417–1421.

Kinsella, A. R., Smith, D., and Pickard, M. (1997). Resistance to chemotherapeutic antimetabolites: a function of salvage pathway involvement and cellular response to DNA damage. *Br. J. Cancer* **75**(7), 935–945.

Knox, R. J., Boland, M. P., Friedlos, F., Coles, B., Southan, C., and Roberts, J. J. (1988). The nitroreductase enzyme in Walker cells that activates 5-(aziridin-1-yl)-2,4-dinitrobenzamide (CB 1954) to 5-(aziridin-1-yl)-4-hydroxylamino-2-nitrobenzamide is a form of NAD(P)H dehydrogenase (quinone) (EC 1.6.99.2). *Biochem. Pharmacol.* **44**, 2297–2301.

Knox, R. J., Friedlos, F., Biggs, P. J., Fliter, W. D., Gaskell, M., Goddard, P., Davies, L., and Jarman, M. (1993). Identification, synthesis and properties of 5-(aziridin-1-yl)-2-nitro-4-nitrosobenzamide, a novel DNA cross-linking agent derived from CB 1954. *Biochem. Pharmacol.* **46**, 797–803.

Knox, R. J., Friedlos, F., Sherwood, R. F., Melton, R. G., and Anlezark, G. M. (1992). The bioactivation of 5-(aziridin-1-yl)-2,4-dinitrobenzamide (CB 1954). II. A comparison of an Escherichia coli nitroreductase and Walker DT-diaphorase. *Biochem. Pharmacol.* **44**, 2297–2301.

Kojima, A., Hackett, N. R., and Crystal, R. G. (1998a). Reversal of CPT-11 resistance of lung cancer cells by adenovirus-mediated gene transfer of the human carboxylesterase cDNA. *Cancer Res.* **58**, 4368–4374.

Kojima, A., Hackett, N. R., Ohwada, A., and Crystal, R. G. (1998b). In vivo human carboxylesterase cDNA gene transfer to activate the prodrug CPT-11 for local treatment of solid tumors. *J. Clin. Invest.* **101**, 1789–1796.

MacCoss, M., and Robins, M. J. (1990). Anticancer pyrimidines, pyrimidine nucleosides and prodrugs. In "Chemistry of Antitumour Agents" D. E. V. Wilman, ed., pp. 261–298. Blackie & Son Ltd., Chapman & Hall, London, New York.

Manome, Y., Wen, P. Y., Dong, Y., Tanaka, T., Mitchell, B. S., Kufe, D. W., and Fine, H. A. (1996). Viral vector transduction of the human deoxycytidine kinase cDNA sensitizes glioma cells to the cytotoxic effects of cytosine arabinoside in vitro and in vivo. *Nat. Med.* **2**(5), 567–573.

Marais, R., Spooner, R. A., Light, Y., Martin, J., and Springer, C. J. (1996). Gene-directed enzyme prodrug therapy with a mustard prodrug/carboxypeptidase G2 combination. *Cancer Res.* **56**, 4735–4742.

Marais, R., Spooner, R. A., Stribbling, S. M., Light , Y., Martin, J., and Springer, C. J. (1997). A cell surface tethered enzyme improves efficiency in gene-directed enzyme prodrug therapy. *Nat. Biotechnol.* **15**, 1373–1377.

Melton, R. G., and Sherwood, R. F. (1997). Antibody-enzyme conjugates for cancer therapy. *J. Natl. Cancer Instit.* **88**, 153–160.

Miki, K., Xu., M., An, Z., Wang, X., Yang, M., Al-Refaie, W., Sun, X., Baranov, E., Tan, Y., Chishima, T., Shimada, H., Moossa, A. R., and Hoffman, R. M. (2000). Survival efficacy of the combination of the methioninase gene and methioninase in a lung cancer orthotopic model. *Cancer Gene Ther.* **7**(2), 332–338.

Miller, A. D. (1998). Cationic liposomes for gene therapy. *Angew. Chem. Int. Ed.* **37**, 1768–1785.

Moore, J., Ohmstede, C., Dickerson, S., Chu, L., Sethna, P., Davis, S., and Dev, I. (1997). Gene therapy utilizing enzymes capable of extracellular prodrug conversion of multiple prodrugs. *Proc. Am. Assoc. Cancer Res.* **38**, 379 (abstract 2544).

Mullen, C. A., Kilstrup, M., and Blaese, R. M. (1992). Transfer of the bacterial gene for cytosine deaminase to mammalian cells confers lethal sensitivity to 5-fluorocytosine: A negative selection system. *Proc. Natl. Acad. Sci. USA* **89**, 33–37.

Mulligan, R. C., and Berg, P. (1981). Selection for animal cells that express the Escherichia coli gene coding for xanthine-guanine phosphoribosyltransferase. *Proc. Natl. Acad. Sci. USA* **78**(4), 2072–2076.

Nguyen, J. T., Wu, P., Clouse, M. E., Hlatky, L., and Terwilliger, E. F. (1998). Adeno-associated virus-mediated delivery of antiangiogenic factors as an antitumor stratergy. *Cancer Res.* **58**, 5673–5677.

Niculescu-Duvaz, D., Niculescu-Duvaz, I., Friedlos, F., Martin, J., Spooner, R., Davies, L., Marais, R., and Springer, C. J. (1998). Self-immolative nitrogen mustard prodrugs for suicide gene therapy. *J. Med. Chem.* **41**(26), 5297–5309.

Niculescu-Duvaz, I., Friedlos, F., Niculescu-Duvaz, D., Davies, L., and Springer, C. J. (1999a). "Prodrugs for antibody- and gene-directed enzyme prodrug therapies (ADEPT and GDEPT)." *Anticancer Drug Design* **14**, 517–538.

Niculescu-Duvaz, I., Niculescu-Duvaz, D., Friedlos, F., Spooner, R., Martin, J., Marais, R., and Springer, C. J. (1999b). Self-immolative anthracycline prodrugs for suicide gene therapy. *J. Med. Chem.* **42**(13), 2485–2489.

Niculescu-Duvaz, I., Spooner, R., Marais, R., and Springer, C. J. (1998). Gene-directed enzyme prodrug therapy. *Bioconjug. Chem.* **9**(1), 4–22.

Niculescu-Duvaz, I., and Springer, C. J. (1995). Antibody-directed enzyme prodrug therapy (ADEPT): A targeting strategy in cancer chemotherapy. *Curr. Med. Chem.* **2**, 687–706.

Pandha, H. S., Martin, L. A., Rigg, A., Hurst, H. C., Stamp, G. W. H., Sikora, K., and Lemoine, N. R. (1999). Genetic prodrug activation therapy for breast cancer: A phase I clinical trial of erbB-2-directed suicide gene expression. *J. Clin. Oncol.* **17**, 2180–2189.

Parker, W. B., Allan, P. W., Shaddix, S. C., Rose, L. M., Speegle, H. F., Gillespie, G. Y., and Bennett, L. L. (1998). Metabolism and metabolic actions of 6-methylpurine and 2-fluoroadenine in human cells. *Biochem. Pharmacol.* **55**, 1673–1681.

Patterson, A. V., Zhang, H., Moghaddam, A., Bicknell, R., Talbot, D. C., Stratford, I. J., and Harris, A. L. (1995). Increased sensitivity to the prodrug 5′-deoxy-5-fluorouridine and modulation of 5-fluoro-2′-deoxyuridine sensitivity in MCF-7 cells transfected with thymidine phosphorylase. *Br. J. Cancer* **72**, 669–675.

Patterson, L. H., McKeown, S. R., Robson, T., Gallagher, R., Raleigh, S. M., and Orr, S. (1999). Antitumour prodrug development using cytochrome P450 (CYP) mediated activation. *Anticancer Drug Design* **14**, 473–486.

Pavlovic, J., Nawrath, M., Tu, R., Heinicke, T., and Moelling, K. (1996). Anti-tumor immunity is involved in the thymidine kinase-mediated killing of tumors induced by activated Ki-ras (G12V). *Gene Ther.* **3**, 635–643.

Pollegioni, L., Falbo, B., and Pilone, M. S. (1992). Specificity and kinetics of *Rodotorula gracilis* D-amino-acid oxidase. *Biochim. Biophys. Acta* **120**, 11–16.

Rainov, N. G., Dobberstein, K.-U., Sena-Estevez, M., Herlinger, U., Kramm, C. M., Philpot, R. M., Hilton, J., Chiocca, E. A., and Breakefield, X. O. (1998). New prodrug activation gene therapy for cancer using cytochrome P450 4B1 and 2-aminoanthracene/4-ipomeanol. *Human Gene Ther.* **9**, 1261–1273.

Ramesh, R., Marrogi, A. J., Munshi, A., Abboud, C. N., and Freeman, S. M. (1996). In vivo analysis of the "bystander effect": A cytokine cascade. *Exp. Hematol.* **24**, 829–838.

Rehemtulla, A., Chang, E., Davis, M. A., and Lawrence, T. S. (1997). Extracellular targeting of cytosine deaminase results in prolonged production of 5-fluorouracil compared to intracellular cytosine deaminase. *Proc. Am. Assoc. Cancer Res.* **38**, 381 (abstract 2555).

Robbins, P. D., and Ghivizzani, S. C. (1998). Viral vectors for gene therapy. *Pharmacol Ther.* **80**(1), 35–47.

Rogulski, K. R., Zhang, K., Kolozsvary, A., Kim, J. H., and Freitag, S. O. (1997). Pronounced antitumor effect and tumor radiosensitization of double suicide gene therapy. *Clin. Cancer Res.* **3**, 2081–2088.

Roth, J. A., and Cristiano, R. G. (1997). Gene therapy for cancer: what have we done and where are we going? *J. Natl. Cancer Instit.* **89**, 21–30.

Rubsam, L. Z., Davidson, L., and Shewach, D. S. (1998). Superior cytotoxicity with gancyclovir compared with acyclovir and 1-β-D-arabinofuranosylthymine in herpes simplex virus-thymidine kinase-expressing-cells: a novel paradigm for cell killing. *Cancer Res.* **58**, 3873–3882.

Secrist III, J. A., Parker, W. B., Allan, P. W., Bennett, L. L., Waud, W. R., Truss, J. W., Fowler, A. T., Montgomery, J. A., Ealick, S. E., Gillespie, G. Y., Gadi, V. K., and Sorscher, E. J. (1999). Gene therapy of cancer: Activation of nucleoside prodrugs with *E. coli* purine nucleoside phosphorylase. *Nucleosides Nucleotides* **18**(4, 5), 745–757.

Sethna, P., Talarico, T., Merrill, B., Moore, J., Davis, S., Dikerson, S., and Dev, I. (1997). Cloning of the gene of a multiple drug activation enzyme from tomato for viral-directed enzyme prodrug therapy (VDEPT) for cancer. *Pro. Am. Assoc. Cancer Res.* **38**, 381 (abstract 2554).

Smith, G. K., Banks, S., Blumenkopf, T. A., Cory, M., Humphreys, J., Laethem, A. M., Miller, G., Moxham, C. P., Mullin, R., Ray, P. H., Walton, L. M., and Wolfe III, L. A. (1997). Toward antibody-directed enzyme prodrug therapy with the T268G mutant of human carboxypeptidase A1 and novel *in vivo* stable prodrugs of methotrexate. *J. Biol. Chem.* **272**, 15804–15816.

Sorscher, E. J., Peng, S., Bebock, Z., Allan, P. W., Bennett Jr., L. L., and Parker, W. B. (1994). Tumor cell bystander killing in colonic carcinoma utilizing the Escherichia coli deo-D gene to generate toxic purines. *Gene Ther.* **1**, 233–238.

Springer, C. J., Antoniw, P., Bagshawe, K. D., Searle, F., Bisset, G. M. F., and Jarman, M. (1990). Novel prodrugs which are activated to cytotoxic alkylating agents by carboxypeptidase G2. *J. Med. Chem.* **33**, 677–681.

Springer, C. J., Bavetsias, V., Jackman, A. L., Boyle, T. F., Marshall, D., Pedley, R. B., and Bisset, G. M. F. (1996). Prodrugs of thymidylate synthase inhibitors: potential for antibody-directed enzyme prodrug therapy (ADEPT). *Anticancer Drug Des.* **11**, 625.

Springer, C. J., Dowell, R., Burke, P. J., Hadley, E., Davies, D. H., Blakey, D. C., Melton, R. G., and Niculescu-Duvaz, I. (1995). Optimization of alkylating agent prodrug derived from phenol and aniline mustards: A new clinical candidates prodrug (ZD2767) for antibody-directed prodrug therapy (ADEPT). *J. Med. Chem.* **38**(26), 5051–5065.

Springer, C. J., and Niculescu-Duvaz, I. (1999). Patent property of prodrug involving gene therapy (1996–1999). *Exp. Opin. Ther. Patents.* **9**(10), 1381–1388.

Springer, C. J., and Niculescu-Duvaz, I. (2000). Prodrug-activating systems in suicide gene therapy. *J. Clin. Invest.* **105**(9), 1161–1167.

Stegman, L. D., Zheng, H., Neal, E. R., Ben-Yoseph, O., Pollegioni, L., Pillone, M. S., and Ross, B. D. (1998). Induction of cytotoxic oxidative stress by D-alanine in brain tumor cells expressing *Rhodotorula gracilis* D-amino acid oxidase: A cancer gene therapy strategy. *Human Gene Ther.* **9**, 185–193.

Stribbling, S. M., Friedlos, F., Martin, J., Davies, L., Spooner, R. A., Marais, R., and Springer, C. J. (2000). Regressions of established breast cancer xenografts by carboxypeptidase G2 suicide gene therapy and the prodrug CMDA are due to a bystander effect. *Human Gene Ther.* **11**, 285–292.

Sykes, B. M., Atwell, G. J., Hogg, A., Wilson, W. R., O'Connor, C. J., and Denny, W. R. (1999). N-substituted 2-(2,6-dinitrophenylamino)-propanamides: Novel prodrugs that release a primary amine via nitroreduction and intramolecular cyclization. *J. Med. Chem.* **42**, 346–355.

Tamiya, T., Ono, Y., Wei, M. X., Mroz, P. J., Moolten, F. L., and Chiocca, E. A. (1996). Escherichia coli gpt gene sensitizes rat glioma cells to killing by 6-thioxanthine or 6-thioguanine. *Cancer Gene Ther.* **3**(3), 155–162.

Tatcher, N. J., Edwards, R. J., Lemoine, N. R., Doehmer, J., and Davies, D. S. (2000). The potential of acetaminophen as a prodrug in gene-directed enzyme prodrug therapy. *Cancer Gene Ther.* **7**(4), 521–525.

Tiraby, G., Reynes, J.-P., Tiraby, M., Cazaux, C., and Drocourt, D. (1996). Suicide genes and combinations of pyrimidine nucleoside and nucleobase analogues with suicide genes for gene therapy. WO 9616183 Cayla, France, 47 pp.

Touraine, R. L., Ishii-Morita, H., Ramsey, W. J., and Blaese, R. M. (1998a). The bystander effect in the HSVtk/ganciclovir system and its relation to gap junctional communication. *Gene Ther.* **5**, 1705–1711.

Touraine, R. L., Vahanian, N., Ramsey, W. J., and Blaese, R. M. (1998b). Enhancement of the herpes simplex virus thymidine kinase/ganciclovir bystander effect and its antitumor efficacy in vivo by pharmacologic manipulation of gap junctions. *Human Gene Ther.* **9**(16), 2385–2391.

Uckert, W., Kammertons, T., Haack, K., Qin, Z., Gebert, J., Schendel, D. J., and Blankenstein, T. (1998). Double suicide gene (cytosine deaminase and herpes simplex virus thymidine kinase) but not single gene transfer allows reliable elimination of tumor cells in vivo. *Human Gene Ther.* **9,** 855–865.

Wakselman, M. (1983). 1,4- and 1,6-elimination from hydroxy- and amino-substituted benzyl systems: Chemical and biochemical application. *Nouveau J. Chimie* **7,** 439–447.

Warrington, K. H., Teschendorf, C., Cao, L., Muzyczka, N., and Siemann, D. W. (1998). Developing VDEPT for DT-diaphorase (NQO1) using an AAV vector plasmid. *Int. J. Radiat. Oncol. Biol. Phys.* **42**(4), 909–912.

Waxman, D. J., Chen, L., Hecht, J. E., and Jounaidi, Y. (1999). Cytochrome P450-based cancer gene therapy: Recent advances and future prospects. *Drugs Metab. Rev.* **31**(2), 503–522.

Weyel, D., Sedlacek, H.-H., Muller, R., and Brusselbach, S. (2000). Secreted human β-glucuronidase: a novel tool for gene-directed enzyme prodrug therapy. *Gene Ther.* **7,** 224–231.

Wierdl, M., Morton, C. L., and Potter, P. M. (2000). Development of adenovirus expressing a secreted rabbit liver carboxylesterase for VDEPT with CPT-11. *Proc. Am. Assoc. Cancer Res.* **41,** 671 (abstract 4266).

Zhang, W. W., Fujiwara, T., Grimm, E. A., and Roth, J. A. (1995). Advances in cancer gene theraphy. *Adv. Pharmacol.* **12,** 289–341.

CHAPTER 9

TUMOR ANTIGENS AS TARGETS FOR ANTICANCER DRUG DEVELOPMENT

Mario Sznol

Vion Pharmaceuticals

New Haven, Connecticut

Thomas Davis

Medarex

Annandale, New Jersey

Summary

A vast number of new antigen targets are rapidly being discovered through the efforts of government and industry to sequence the human genome and to identify the expression of all genes in cancer cells. Once the specificity of expression in tumor is determined, the antigens can be used to induce antitumor immune responses or can serve as targets for antibody-based therapeutics. Techniques to generate fully human antibodies are now readily available; therefore, many new antibodies or antibody-based constructs are likely to be introduced into clinical trials in the near future. However, the mechanisms by which the antibodies mediate antitumor activity are not fully understood, and the issues of which antibodies to select for clinical trials, and what approaches are optimal for antitumor activity, have not been resolved. The potential for combinations of therapeutic antibodies against simultaneously expressed antigens will lead to new challenges and hopefully new benefits for patients. Generation of effective antitumor vaccines raises even more complex issues. Rapid and efficient development of cancer vaccines from the wealth of new antigens will require a more thorough understanding of tumor immunobiology and the characteristics of immune responses that are capable of mediating antitumor activity.

1. Introduction

The existence of tumor-specific or tumor-associated antigens, which are the molecular targets of an adaptive immune response, is now well established. Furthermore, in animal tumor models and in patients, there is substantial evidence that immune responses directed against tumor antigens can cause the regression of established tumors. For these reasons, a large effort has been undertaken to develop therapeutic cancer "vaccines" containing tumor antigens that induce antitumor immune responses *in vivo*. An alternative approach has involved the preparation and adoptive transfer of monoclonal antibodies to tumor antigens. The antibodies can be further engineered to carry toxins, radioisotopes, or prodrug-converting enzymes to the tumor. The reengineering of the immune response has even been extended to T lymphocytes, whose specificity can be redirected by introducing genes coding for tumor antigen-specific receptors. Issues in the selection of targets for cancer vaccine and monoclonal-antibody-based therapeutics and the clinical development of these agents will be discussed in this chapter.

2. Antigen Targets for Cancer Vaccines

Much of the recent effort in cancer vaccine development has focused on the induction of T-lymphocyte antitumor responses, based on a greater understanding of antigen presentation to T cells and factors that govern T-cell activation, and animal model data indicating the central role of T lymphocytes in many immunologically mediated antitumor responses. A general scheme for events occurring following immunization with a protein tumor antigen is illustrated in Fig. 1.

T lymphocytes recognize peptides produced from intracellular degradation (processing) of proteins in target or antigen-presenting cells (APCs). Within intracellular compartments, peptides are bound to the groove of self major histocompatibility complex (MHC) molecules, which is determined by certain amino acid binding motifs specific for the MHC molecule. The peptide-MHC complexes are brought to the surface of the cell, where they can be recognized by specific T-lymphocyte receptors (TCRs). $CD8^+$ T cells recognize short peptides from 8 to 10 amino acids in length presented on MHC class I molecules. Upon recognition of a peptide-MHC complex, a $CD8^+$ cell can kill the tumor cell directly or secrete cytokines such as interleukin-2 (IL-2), interferon-γ (IFN-γ), or tumor necrosis factor (TNF). $CD4^+$ T lymphocytes recognize longer peptide fragments bound in the groove of MHC class II molecules. Precursors of mature $CD4^+$ lymphocytes are capable of differentiating into two

types of cytokine-secreting cell: one that produces cytokines important for generating $CD8^+$ cellular responses (the CD4 Th1 phenotype) and the other producing cytokines that help prime B cells for antibody production (the CD4 Th2 phenotype).

Optimal activation of naïve T cells requires the presentation of antigen by professional (APCs) or dendritic cells (DCs) derived from bone marrow precursors. APC take up and present antigens, followed by migration to regional lymph nodes and a maturation process that enables them to present the antigens to T cells. The series of events that lead to full activation of a T cell are complex and depend on the number and duration of MHC-peptide-TCR interactions and costimulatory signals provided by ligands on the APC with receptors on the T cell, as well as cytokines released into the local environment (Fig. 2). Once fully activated, T cells are capable of killing or secreting cytokines by recognition of a small number of peptide-MHC complexes on the tumor. Inadequate or incomplete activation of T cells may compromise their proliferative capacity or end-effector function.

A. Sources and Form of Tumor Antigen

In developing a cancer vaccine, the tumor antigen component can be delivered in the form of a whole tumor cell (Berd *et al.*, 1997; Morton *et al.*, 1992), a tumor cell lysate (Mitchell *et al.*, 1990), an extract or purified fraction of tumor cells (Bystryn *et al.*, 1986, Tamura *et al.*, 1997), or as a defined (recombinant or purified) molecule (Rosenberg *et al.*, 1997, Boon *et al.*, 1997). Vaccines composed of whole tumor cells or cell extracts can be derived from the patient's own tumor (autologous) or from allogeneic cell lines maintained over long periods *in vitro*. For an individual defined protein antigen, several different forms may be used to induce immune responses, including the whole protein, the peptide from the

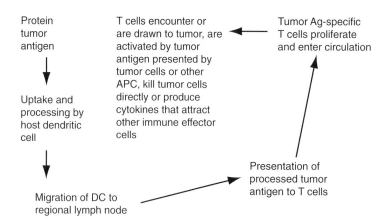

FIGURE 1 Events in vaccine-induced antitumor T-cell immune responses. Interventions may be directed to any or all steps in the process to improve outcome. Interventions include manipulation of the form or source of antigen, the method of administration to the patient, or the addition of cytokines and/or antibodies that enhance dendritic cell (DC) function, T-cell expansion and activation, or T-cell-mediated antitumor effects.

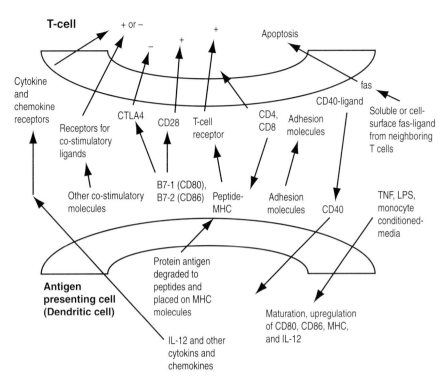

FIGURE 2 The antigen-presenting cell (APC) and T-cell interface. Activation of T cells is a complex process that is the sum of multiple interactions between the T cell, the APC, other T cells, and cytokines in the milieu. Development of a vaccine may involve interventions at one or more of the illustrated interactions, such as an antibody blocking the negative activation signal transmitted by the B7-CTLA4 interaction, thus enhancing T-cell activation.

protein that is actually bound to MHC molecules and presented on the cell surface, or a gene encoded by a DNA plasmid or by various viruses. Individual antigens can also be mimicked by anti-idiotypes, antibodies whose antigen binding domain has a physical resemblance to the tumor antigen (Foon *et al.,* 2000, Livingston, 1998). The proposed advantages and disadvantages of these various approaches are listed in Table 1.

B. Discovery and Selection of Defined Tumor Antigens for Vaccine Development

Similar to targets for small molecules, immunotherapists have sought partially validated targets for cancer vaccine development, which could be defined as tumor antigens targeted by immune responses that are associated with tumor regression or improved survival. Patients with cancer are studied extensively for antibody- or T-cell-mediated responses to their own tumor and to allogeneic tumors of the same histology. Shared antigens between patients that are recognized by these immune responses can then be defined, and the outcome for patients who have the specific immune response can be compared to patients who do not, or the antitumor effect of adoptively transferring T cells or antibodies recognizing the antigen can be determined in clinical trials. If an immune response to a specific antigen is associated with a better prog-

nosis, or if adoptive transfer of an antibody or T cells recognizing the antigen produces tumor regression, then that antigen could be considered an appropriate candidate for development as a "vaccine," particularly if the antigen is uniquely expressed in tumor or overexpressed in comparison with normal tissues (Kawakami *et al.,* 1994; Livingston, 1998).

Alternatively, modern molecular biology techniques have identified, and will continue to identify at a rapidly accelerating pace, molecules that either are tissue specific, e.g., expressed only in prostate or melanocytes, or are overexpressed in certain tumors with limited expression in normal tissues or contain mutations that are found only in tumor. For mutations in particular, the antigen will often be patient specific, requiring determination of the mutation for the individual patient and development of a vaccine applicable only for that patient. Possibly for many other antigens, expression in the tumor will be found in many patients, allowing for the development of an off-the-shelf vaccine (Table 2).

C. Immunologic Concepts Influencing the Selection and Form of Tumor Antigens for Vaccine Development

Although the number of potential tumor antigens discovered by characterizing gene expression in tumors appears to be increasing at a rapid pace, many of these antigens may not

TABLE 1

Sources and Forms of Antigen in Cancer Vaccines

Antigen form or source	Comments and examples	Methods to enhance immunogenicity	Advantages	Disadvantages
Autologous tumor cells	Tumor cells derived from biopsies. Tumor cell suspensions are prepared by enzymatic digestion for future use, or tumor cells are expanded by short-term cultures.	Conjugating tumor cells with foreign protein, administering cells with nonspecific immunologic adjuvants, modifying cells to express cytokine genes, or fusing tumor cells with dendritic cells	Contains multiple potential tumor antigens unique to patient's tumor	Unique preparation for each patient; antigens are difficult to manipulate to increase immunogenicity; low amounts of tumor antigen in vaccine; tumor cells may produce immune suppressive substances; tumor antigens are unknown, therefore monitoring is difficult; possibly greater chance of inducing autoimmunity
Allogeneic tumor cells	Cell lines are maintained in *in vitro* culture	Same as autologous tumor cells	Contains multiple potential shared antigens; same vaccine for multiple different patients	Difficult to fully define the product; foreign antigens may affect response to shared tumor antigens; other disadvantages similar to autologous tumor vaccines
Allogeneic tumor cell lysates	Lysates are prepared from cell lines maintained in *in vitro* culture	Administering with nonspecific adjuvants, presentation by dendritic cells	Same as for allogeneic tumor cells	Same as for allogeneic tumor cells
Extract or purified fraction of tumor cells	Shed antigens from allogeneic melanoma cell lines, or heat shock protein fractions from autologous tumor cells	Same as tumor cell lysates	Same as for allogeneic tumor cells, but the potential tumor antigens are more concentrated, and immune-suppressive substances are possibly removed	Same as for allogeneic tumor cells
Defined antigen (entire molecule)	Recombinant or purified proteins, gangliosides	Administering with nonspecific adjuvants, conjugation with highly immunogenic foreign protein, presentation by dendritic cells	Product well-defined for regulatory purposes; antigen amount not limiting; antigen can be manipulated easily to increase immunogenicity; monitoring facilitated because antigen target is defined; can be off-the-shelf product	Shared antigens may stimulate weaker immune responses; immune responses are directed only to a single antigen; therefore, greater chance of tumor cell escape due to heterogeneity in tumor antigen expression; tolerance to dominant epitopes of full protein, which are the most likely to be presented, may already exist *in vivo*
Fragment of defined antigen	Peptides, several tandem repeats of MUC-1 protein	Same as full defined antigen, also can modify amino acid sequence or add short peptides to enhance presentation on surface of dendritic cells	Same as defined entire molecule, but "competition" from other dominant antigenic epitopes in full molecule eliminated	Immune responses to antigen are narrower, may be limited to only a $CD8^+$ or a $CD4^+$ response; for $CD8^+$ epitopes, lack of $CD4^+$ responses may weaken antitumor effect inside the tumor, or may limit magnitude and potency of response
Gene coding for antigen or antigen fragment	Gene encoding full or part of antigen placed in naked DNA plasmid or in one of several viruses	Viruses or unmethylated CpG sequences of DNA act as immunologic adjuvants, can add other genes to increase Ag presentation, or infect dendritic cells directly	Same as for defined antigens; vectors may amplify amount of antigen available for presentation, some deliver antigen directly to cytoplasm for better presentation to $CD8^+$ T cells; vectors may cause enhanced activation and maturation of antigen-presenting cells	Same as for defined antigens; foreign antigens expressed by vectors may be immunogenic, resulting in increased clearance and decreased Ag presentation with repeat administration; preexisting immunity to viruses may limit Ag presentation; possible toxicity from viral vectors
Anti-idiotypes	Murine polyclonal or monoclonal antibody that contains a physical mimic of tumor antigen	Administer with nonspecific immunologic adjuvants	Anti-idiotype form of antigen presentation may be more immunogenic and capable of breaking tolerance, otherwise similar to defined antigens	Similar to defined antigens; Immune responses limited to single epitope of antigen; often only antibody responses to epitope are induced

TABLE 2
Classes of Defined Tumor Antigen Targets

Pattern of expression	General classes	Examples	Comments
Shared (expressed by tumors from different patients)	Tissue differentiation	MART-1, gp100, tyrosinase, TRP-1, TRP-2	Melanosomal proteins; because of their primary intracellular location, vaccine approaches are directed mostly to T-lymphocyte activation
		Prostate-specific antigen (PSA), prostate-specific membrane antigen (PSMA)	
		MUC-1	Mucin glycoprotein overexpressed in adenocarcinomas; abnormal glycosylation exposes antibody epitopes; tandem repeats of core protein can be recognized by T cells in non-MHC-restricted manner
		sTn	Antibody epitope of MUC-1
		Gangliosides (GM2, GD2, GD3)	Expressed on tissues derived from neural crest, including melanomas, small cell lung cancer, neuroblastoma; induce antibody responses
	Oncofetal antigens	Carcinoembryonic antigen (CEA)	Expressed on several gastrointestinal malignancies and adenocarcinomas
		β-hCG	Expressed on various cancers
	Cancer-testes antigens	Mage 1, 3, 12, NY-ESO, BAGE, GAGE, LAGE, others	Expression found in various tumors and normal testes, perhaps due to hypomethylation of tumor DNA
	Viral antigens	Human papillomavirus 16 E6 and E7 proteins	Involved in pathogenesis of cervical and some anal cancers
	Others	CD55	Complement inhibitor expressed in colon, gastric, ovarian tumors and osteosarcoma
Unique (expressed only by the individual patient's tumor)	Lymphoma and myeloma idiotypes		Antigen binding region of antibody created by recombination serves as unique tumor target
	Chromosomal translocations	Bcr-abl	Expressed in chronic myeloid leukemia, unique peptide formed by fusion may be recognized as unique tumor antigen
	Mutations in individual proteins	p53	In many cancers, mutations spread across the gene but can be determined to create peptide spanning the mutation
		ras	In many cancers, limited number of mutations demonstrated and restricted to defined parts of the protein.

induce effective antitumor immune responses, or perhaps will require manipulation or modification to produce effective antitumor immunity. The concerns arise from the observations of self-tolerance and dominance with regard to many antigen-specific immune responses.

To rationally select tumor antigens for clinical development, consideration must first be given to the characteristics of the immune response that would be effective against human tumors. Unfortunately, only some aspects of effective antitumor immune responses are fully understood, although certain assumptions have been supported by work in experimental animals. Independently, antibody and T-lymphocyte immune responses are capable of mediating antitumor responses, although cell-mediated responses appear to have greater antitumor effects. For either type of effector, outcome may be dependent on quantitative and qualitative aspects of the response. For example, the effectiveness of a vaccine that induces antibody responses may be dependent on the titer of induced antigen-specific antibodies, the affinity for the antigen, the ability to recognize the antigen as expressed on the surface of tumor cells, and the ability to fix complement (complement-dependent cytotoxicity, or CDC) and mediate antibody-dependent cellular cytotoxicity (ADCC). For antigens that induce primarily T-cell responses, effectiveness may be dependent on the frequency of antigen-specific T lymphocytes, the avidity of the T-cell receptor for the antigen-MHC complex on the surface of tumor cells (Zeh *et al.*, 1999), the capacity of the induced T cells to secrete certain cytokines and chemokines (Barth *et al.*, 1991), the cytotoxicity of the T cells (Aebersold *et al.*, 1991), and perhaps the expression by T cells of various adhesion molecules that permit infiltration into tumors. Furthermore, T-lymphocyte responses are complex, and recent evidence indicates the importance of generating both CD4$^+$ and CD8$^+$ T-lymphocyte responses directed against tumor antigens (Pardoll and Topalian, 1998). The cytokine profiles of antigen-specific CD4$^+$ and CD8$^+$ T cells can differ depending on the antigen and method of presentation to the T cells, and certain profiles (Th1, characterized by the production of IFN-γ) appear to be necessary for effective antitumor immunity in some animal tumor models (Hu *et al.*, 1998).

The ability to generate an effective immune response to a tumor antigen in a cancer patient is dependent on the general immune competence of the patient and also on the available repertoire of immune responses specific to the antigen. While still a subject of some debate, most cancer patients, including those with advanced disease, can respond adequately to a challenge with a new foreign antigen and have relatively well-preserved immune function. However, their ability to mount effective immune responses, such as one of sufficient magnitude and quality to cause tumor regression, may not be preserved for all tumor antigens. First, many tumor antigens are self-antigens, and high-avidity responses to the antigen are probably eliminated during neonatal development to prevent autoimmunity (Clarke *et al.*, 1998; Naftzger *et al.*, 1996; Rowse *et al.*, 1998). Second, human tumors have been present in many patients for years before their discovery. During the long period of growth, some evidence suggests that tumors have presented their own antigens to T lymphocytes, either directly or through uptake by the body's professional APCs, in an inefficient manner (Ishida *et al.*, 1998; Staveley-O'Carroll *et al.*, 1998). Suboptimal antigen presentation to T cells may result in the induction of anergy to those antigens. Therefore, at the time of intended vaccination, even against unique tumor antigens, the ability to mount an effective immune response may have been lost or blunted.

The concept of dominance becomes important in selecting the form of antigen to deliver in a vaccine, particularly for T-cell responses. T cells recognize peptides bound to self-MHC molecules on the surface of cells. Intracellular processing of proteins generates the peptides. Both the processing of the protein and the affinity of individual peptides for binding to the MHC molecule determines which of the peptides reaches the surface. Therefore, only certain peptides will be presented on the surface, and the amount of each peptide from a protein that appears on the surface of the cell may vary. Since T-cell activation is in part a function of the number of interac-

tions between the peptide-MHC complex and T-cell receptors of a lymphocyte, the immune response to a protein is directed to only one or a few dominant peptide epitopes. If tolerance has already developed to those epitopes, it may be difficult to induce new effective immune responses if the whole protein (or a tumor cell or lysate containing the antigen) is used for immunization.

It may still be possible to overcome anergy or induce new T-cell responses to the dominant epitopes of proteins by immunizing with a particularly strong stimulus, such as a dendritic cell (see Section 2.D). However, an alternative approach has been to determine subdominant peptide epitopes that are still present on the tumor cell surface but were not presented sufficiently either in neonatal development or during tumor growth to induce T-cell tolerance (Deng *et al.*, 1997). Immunization with these peptides may result in induction of high-magnitude and high-avidity T-lymphocyte responses. Furthermore, the peptides can be modified at the MHC anchor residues to increase their binding affinity to the MHC molecule and therefore maximize the number of potential peptide-MHC complex and T-cell receptor interactions, thus increasing their ability to activate T cells (Dyall *et al.*, 1998; Overwijk *et al.*, 1998; Rosenberg *et al.*, 1998).

In the selection of peptides for clinical trials, including those peptides that span unique mutations in cellular proteins, some evidence should be obtained that the parent protein is processed correctly inside tumor cells and puts the peptide on the surface bound to an MHC molecule. Within a protein, various peptides that bind to an MHC molecule can sometimes be found, but not all of the peptides are presented on the cell surface. Immune responses directed to irrelevant peptides will have no possibility of causing tumor regression (Zaks and Rosenberg, 1998).

D. Antigen Presentation to the Immune System

An accumulating body of evidence indicates that optimal activation of immune responses, particularly T-lymphocyte responses, requires uptake and presentation of the antigen by mature professional APCs or dendritic cells (DCs) (Banchereau and Steinman, 1998). Although many methods are employed to deliver and present antigens in animal models and clinical trials, it appears fairly certain that for all methods the final common pathway of immune system activation involves DC uptake of the antigen and migration of the DC to a regional lymph node. Table 3 lists the various methods to enhance immune responses to antigens.

The various immunologic adjuvants, such as alum, QS-21, DETOX, BCG, and others, when mixed with the tumor antigen are presumed to elicit a local nonspecific inflammatory response, which in turn produces cytokines that direct local dendritic cells to infiltrate the area, take up the tumor antigen, then mature and migrate to draining lymph nodes. Maturation

TABLE 3
Methods to Enhance Immune Responses to Antigens

Approach	Comments
Admixing antigen or tumor cell with nonspecific adjuvants	Commonly used adjuvants: BCG, QS-21, DETOX, alum, and others, produce local inflammation to enhance antigen uptake and presentation by DC
Conjugating antigen to immunogenic foreign protein or substance	Foreign antigen causes local inflammation, also induces helper CD4[+] T-cell responses which provide maturation signals to DC and cytokines for activation, expansion, and function of B cells and other T cells; examples include KLH, dinitrophenyl
Local expression or administration of cytokines or costimulatory molecules	To attract DC and enhance antigen uptake and presenting capacity of DC (GM-CSF, flt3-ligand, CD40 ligand); to enhance T-cell expansion and activation (IL-2; IL-12; CD80 to provide positive costimulatory signal to T cells); to increase tumor cell antigen and MHC expression (IFN-γ)
Systemic administration of cytokines	Systemic expansion of dendritic cell precursors (GM-CSF, flt3-ligand), CD4[+] and CD8[+] T-cell responses (IL-2), expand natural killer lymphocytes to enhance antibody effects
Manipulating the antigen to increase its ability to be recognized by the immune system	Examples include increasing peptide epitope affinity to MHC molecules by altering anchor amino acids (increases peptide–MHC and TCR interactions), adding insertion signal sequences to peptides to cause entry into the endoplasmic reticulum where peptides are bound to MHC molecules
Encoding the antigen in a DNA plasmid	Results in expression of the antigen gene in the cytoplasm of DC. The unmethylated CpG sequences of DNA are immunostimulatory. DNA plasmids have the capacity to express multiple antigens and cytokines and/or costimulatory signals.
Encoding the antigen in viruses	Viruses express large amounts of antigen within DC or other cells, can infect DC, and enhance DC function; replicating viruses amplify antigen expression; some viruses have the capacity for carrying multiple genes, including multiple antigens and cytokines and/or costimulatory signals; examples include adenoviruses, and replicating and nonreplicating poxviruses (vaccinia, fowlpox)
Encoding the antigen in bacteria	Some bacteria are capable of carrying multiple genes and are taken into antigen-presenting cells
Placing the antigen in a dendritic cell	Examples include fusion of tumor cells with dendritic cells, placing whole tumor cell RNA in DC, adding tumor cell lysates or extracts to DC, pulsing DC with defined protein or peptide antigens
Expanding and enhancing the function of dendritic cells	Cytokines such as flt-3 ligand, or GM-CSF in combination with IL-4 cause expansion of DC *in vivo* or *ex vivo;* the addition of TNF, LPS, CD40 ligand, monocyte-conditioned media causes DC maturation, which increases their expression of MHC, costimulatory molecules, and cytokines
Increasing T-cell activation by blocking negative costimulatory signals	Costimulatory ligands B7-1 and B7-2 (CD80, CD86) transmit negative signals for activation and proliferation to T cells through the CTLA4 receptor; interactions can be blocked by antibodies to CTLA4
Pretreatment with low-dose chemotherapy to eliminate suppressor cells	Antigen-specific immune-suppressive T-cell populations, or other immune suppressive cells, possibly eliminated by low-dose chemotherapy, enhancing response to subsequent immunization
Prime-boost strategies	Presentation of antigen in different forms, e.g., successively by different viruses, or by virus followed by the protein or peptide epitope, results in enhanced immune responses
Expanding the antigen-specific T cells *ex vivo*	Isolation of antigen-specific T cells following vaccination, followed by expansion and further activation *in vitro* and adoptive transfer, produces increased antitumor activity in some animal models

of DC involves various cell processes that diminish antigen uptake capacity but up-regulate certain cell surface molecules that optimize antigen presentation and lymphocyte activation in the lymph node (Steinman *et al.,* 1997). Alternatively or in addition to the nonspecific adjuvants, recombinant cytokines can be administered with the antigen, either locally or systemically, or the tumor cells or bystander cells can be genetically engineered to produce cytokines.

In recognition of the importance of DC in the process of antigen presentation, many vaccines in development are placing antigen directly on or into DC (Kugler *et al.,* 2000; Nair *et al.,* 1998). The development of dendritic cell vaccines required the development of processes to generate large num-

bers of DC and DC precursors *ex vivo.* Various methods of DC preparation are under investigation, and distinct populations of DC have been identified. Some of these DC populations appear to have different functions, including the unintended opposite consequence of inducing tolerance or an ineffective immune response (Adler *et al.,* 1998; Bancereau and Steinman, 1998; Steinbrink *et al.,* 1997). In addition, the optimal route and frequency of DC administration is not known, and may depend on the antigen, the method of loading the DC with antigen, the baseline immune status of the patient, the disease, and perhaps even the type of DC.

The molecular events of antigen presentation to T lymphocytes and T-cell activation have been carefully dissected, although not yet completely defined. Nevertheless, enough is understood to intercede directly at the level of the DC to increase DC capacity to activate T lymphocytes, and at the level of the T cell to enhance T-cell activation and expansion. These additional manipulations may be necessary to optimize vaccine-induced antitumor immune responses and to maintain the responses *in vivo*. Examples include the coadministration of ligands or antibodies that activate CD40 on the surface of DC (Leach *et al.*, 1996), which induce maturation of the DC, or by antibodies that bind the CTLA4 receptor on T cells, thus blocking negative costimulatory signals that inhibit T-cell activation (Hurwitz *et al.*, 1998; Leach *et al.*, 1996).

E. Clinical Considerations for Cancer Vaccine Development

Because of the heterogeneity of tumors, optimal efficacy of a cancer vaccine approach would be predicted to require immunization against multiple tumor antigens and perhaps to induce both cell-mediated and antibody responses. Either multiple defined antigens can be administered, or the vaccine can be derived from autologous or allogeneic tumors. These approaches are likely to be effective only if they can be shown to produce the high-magnitude and high-quality immune responses to multiple antigens necessary to mediate antitumor effects.

Defects in antigen and MHC expression in tumors is well documented (Kageshita *et al.*, 1993; Hicklin *et al.*, 1998), and tumors are capable of expressing cell surface molecules or producing cytokines that would limit the induction of immune responses, prevent the ingress of activated cells, or actively inhibit an infiltrating immune response (Lattime *et al.*, 1995; Torre-Amione *et al.*, 1990). Therefore, future progress in the cancer vaccine area may depend on the coadministration of reagents that modify tumor antigen expression, enhance T-cell infiltration and function within tumors, and blunt the tumor immunosuppressive properties. Careful study of tumor-related characteristics in the target treatment population might provide information on possible means to improve vaccine efficacy.

Similar to other types of anticancer agents, monitoring of the immune response to the cancer vaccine in early trials provides relevant information on which decisions can be based to modify the approach or enter later-stage clinical development, such as phase III trials. An incomplete understanding of the characteristics of effective antitumor immune responses complicates precise monitoring of relevant immune responses to antigen. Furthermore, when to monitor for immune response after immunization and where to monitor, e.g., peripheral blood, draining lymph node, or in the tumor, is not clear.

Assessment of clinical antitumor efficacy in early trials remains a problem. Preclinical models predict optimal efficacy of cancer vaccines in minimal residual disease or minimal tumor volume settings. The usual evidence of tumor regression in advanced disease that is often considered a prerequisite for advancing a therapy into the minimal disease setting may not be obtainable for cancer vaccines. Therefore, the crucial decisions to proceed to later-stage development must rely more heavily on the biological monitoring studies, including the ability to induce the intended immune response and perhaps some evidence that the immune response is manifest within tumors, even if no regression or destruction of tumor cells is observed.

Induction of immune responses to cancer antigens has not caused clinically significant toxicity. The potential for causing autoimmunity remains and may surface as methodology for inducing more potent immune responses advances.

3. Tumor Antigens as Targets for Antibody-Based Therapeutics

In many ways, the field of antibody therapeutics is still in its infancy. The original antitumor antibodies produced for clinical trials were of murine origin. The murine antibodies had relatively short half-lives in patients in comparison with natural human antibodies, and due to the rapid development of neutralizing human antimurine antibody responses (HAMA), most could be administered only once. Furthermore, the ability to increase the antibody binding affinity to antigen was limited. Relatively few antigen targets were available, and the overall clinical experience demonstrated minimal to modest antitumor activity for most unmodified antibodies.

In the latter half of the 1990s, several developments generated renewed interest in antibody-based therapeutics for cancer. First, two antibodies, rituximab and trastuzumab, demonstrated substantial benefit for lymphoma and breast cancer patients, respectively, and were approved for marketing by regulatory agencies around the world. Second, the dramatic advances in genomics promised to provide an ever-increasing number of targets for antibody-based therapies. Finally, technologies were introduced to generate humanized or fully human antibodies to newly discovered antigens within time frames that are feasible for clinical development.

The ability to generate fully human or humanized antibodies appears to have had the greatest impact on the field. The fully human or humanized antibodies are minimally immunogenic in patients; therefore, they can be administered repeatedly, and most have a serum half-life approaching that of naturally produced antibodies. Two particularly promising technologies were recently introduced to produce fully human antibodies. The first involves the development of transgenic mice whose immunoglobulin genes (specific for antibody formation) have been replaced by their human counterparts (Green, 1999). The mice are therefore capable of generating fully human antibodies against human antigens without the limitation of tolerance to self-antigens, except perhaps for molecules that are highly conserved between mouse and man. An alternative technique for generating fully human antibodies employs bacteriophage display libraries. Each bacteriophage contains a unique combination of the human variable heavy (VH) and light (VL) antibody chains that have been cloned from normal human B lymphocytes. The bacteriophage library is then used to screen for binding to a particular antigen. Once a bacteriophage that binds to the antigen of interest is isolated, its VH-VL genes are sequenced and then genetically engineered into a fully human complete antibody. After a lead antibody is identified, site-specific mutagenesis of the antigen binding regions permits further improvements in antigen binding affinity.

The issues for clinical development of an antibody-based therapeutic arise from the antigen target, the potential mechanisms by which an antibody binding to the target could produce antitumor activity, and the type of antibody construct that is chosen for clinical development. Depending on the antigen target, various mechanisms may be involved in antibody-mediated antitumor effects. Furthermore, antibodies may be designed or engineered in various ways to mediate antitumor effects against a particular antigen target (Table 4).

A. Antigen Targets

Theoretically, any cell surface molecule associated with tumor cells, tumor stroma, or tumor vasculature is a potential target for an antibody-based therapeutic approach. Furthermore, antibodies may be used to reduce or block growth factors that are directly or indirectly supporting tumor cell growth or the formation of tumor vasculature. Antibodies may also be employed to modulate antitumor immune responses or to reduce tumor-produced immune suppressive factors. For most applications, potential antigens should be tissue specific or overexpressed on tumor versus normal tissue. Antigens that are equally expressed on tumor versus normal tissue may also be appropriate candidates for an antibody-based therapeutic, if antibody binding to the antigen has a differential effect on the tumor in comparison with normal tissues. Various antigen targets for antibody-based therapeutics are listed in Table 5.

B. Mechanisms of Antibody-Based Antitumor Effect

Certain unmodified antibodies are capable of killing tumor cells by fixing complement or by mediating antibody-dependent cellular cytotoxicity (ADCC) (Clynes et al., 2000). ADCC is dependent on the binding of the Fc portion of the antibody to Fc receptors on natural killer cells, granulocytes, and monocytes. The ability to fix complement and mediate ADCC is dependent on the class and isotype of the antibody. To further enhance or replace the innate antitumor effector function of antibodies, antibodies have been genetically engineered or chemically modified to carry or capture radioisotopes, toxins, or prodrug-converting enzymes.

Unmodified antibodies that target growth factors or growth factor receptors appear to mediate antitumor effects *in vivo*, at least partially, by blocking autocrine or paracrine growth factor loops (Lewis et al., 1993; Shan et al., 1998). In some cases, binding of the antibody to an antigen on the tumor cell surface will induce cell-signaling events that result in cell death through apoptosis. If the target is on tumor neovasculature, antibody binding may block angiogenesis or perhaps induce destruction of the existing tumor vasculature, resulting in hemorrhagic necrosis (Brooks et al., 1995; Gutheil et al., 2000; Huang et al., 1997). Similarly, binding to integrins or other adhesion molecules on tumors or normal tissue could block tumor metastasis and invasion. Various antibodies that block angiogenesis or interact with growth factor receptors or integrins appear to have additive or synergistic effects with standard cytotoxic agents (Baselga et al., 1998).

Several antibodies in clinical development modulate immune responses. The antibodies either block or stimulate signaling in dendritic cells or T lymphocytes, resulting in enhanced presentation of antigen and T-cell activation. Enhancement of antitumor responses is also possible by administering antibodies against immunosuppressive cytokines expressed by tumors, or against tumor cell surface molecules that induce T-cell apoptosis or block complement activation.

TABLE 4
Mechanisms for Antibody-Based Therapeutics

Unmodified antibodies	• Mediate CDC, ADCC • Block circulating growth factors • Block cell surface receptors • Transmit apoptotic or sensitivity signals through cell surface receptors (either directly or through cross-linking) • Modulate immune responses
Modified antibodies (modifications can be added to whole antibody molecule, whole antibody with partial deletion of heavy chain, Fab fragment, or recombinant single chain containing VH-VL antigen binding regions)	• Addition of toxins (calicheamycin, ricin, diphtheria toxin, *Pseudomonas* exotoxin, gelonin, doxorubicin, tubulin toxins) • Radioisotopes (^{131}I, ^{90}Y, and others) • Prodrug-converting enzymes (cytosine deaminase, carboxypeptidase G2, nitroreductase, DT diaphorase, and others) • Pretargeting carrier molecules

TABLE 5
Examples of Antigen Targets for Antibody-Based Therapeutics

Antigen target	Diseases	Examples of antibody approaches
Gangliosides (GD2)	Melanoma, neuroblastoma	Chimeric antibody (ch14.18) in phase 3 trial for neuroblastoma, fusion protein containing IL-2 in clinical trials
GA-733 (EPCAM)	Colon cancer	Antibody 17-1A approved for adjuvant Dukes C colon cancer in Germany, additional phase III trials ongoing
Lewis^y	Multiple adenocarcinomas	*Pseudomonas*-based immunotoxins (whole antibody and single chain) and doxorubicin conjugates (BR96-dox) in clinical trials
Tag 72	Multiple adenocarcinomas	CC49 and CH2 deleted CC49 radiolabeled constructs in clinical trials
CEA	Multiple adenocarcinomas	Radiolabeled antibodies in clinical trials, ADEPT-CPG2 approach in clinical trials
PSMA	Prostate cancer	Phase I trials ongoing
Her2/*neu*	Breast, ovarian, and low percentage of various types of tumors	Trastuzumab approved for treatment of metastatic breast cancer
EGF receptor	Breast, lung, head and neck, renal cell, and others	Chimeric antibody in phase II/III clinical trials, other humanized or fully human antibodies in clinical trials
Histones	Tumors with necrotic areas	Radiolabeled antibody in clinical trials
IL-2 receptor (CD25)	Cutaneous T-cell lymphomas, hairy cell leukemia, others	IL-2 diphtheria fusion toxin approved for treatment of CTCL, immunotoxins containing truncated *Pseudomonas* exotoxin in clinical trial
CD20	B-cell lymphomas	Rituximab approved for follicular NHL, ^{90}Y- and ^{131}I-labeled anti-CD20 have completed phase III clinical trials
CD19, CD22	B-cell lymphomas	Immunotoxins in clinical trials
HLA-DR and variants	B-cell lymphomas	Unmodified and radiolabeled antibodies in clinical trials
CD3	T-cell malignancies	Antibodies in clinical trials
CD33	Myeloid leukemias	Unmodified antibody in clinical trials, calicheamycin immunotoxin approved for treatment of relapsed AML, radiolabeled Ab under investigation
VEGF/VEGF receptor	Tumor neovasculature	Antibody to the growth factor and the receptor in clinical trials
Integrin $\alpha_v\beta_3$	Tumor vasculature	Antibody (Vitaxin) in clinical trials

CEH, carcinoembryonic antigen; PSMA, prostate-specific membrane antigen; EGF, epidermal growth factor; IL, interleukin; VEGF, vascular endothelial-derived growth factor; CTCL, cutaneous T-cell leukemia; AML, acute myelogenous leukemia.

C. General Toxicities of Antibody Infusions

Antibody administration to humans can produce fevers, chills, low blood pressure, shortness of breath, and an assortment of other symptoms. The syndrome is most often observed with the initial infusion of an antibody, but it can be observed with second and subsequent infusions of murine antibodies. Supportive care with common medications such as Tylenol or antihistamines can minimize the manifestations of the initial infusion reaction.

Antibodies reactive with immune cells can induce a more severe infusion-related syndrome. The cause is suspected to be the rapid release of cytokines in response to antibody binding. The syndrome can be partially controlled by slowing or delaying the infusion, administering standard prophylactic medications, or splitting the dose. Furthermore, the in-

fusional syndrome is reduced or eliminated with subsequent dosings, presumably because the target cells have been depleted, or their cytokine load has been reduced.

D. Issues in Clinical Development of Antibody-Based Therapeutics

The introduction of chimeric and humanized or fully human antibodies appears to have overcome some of the early limitations in antibody-based therapeutics, but various challenges to successful therapy remain. Antigen expression in tumors is heterogeneous, leading to escape by antigen loss variants. Preclinical studies have demonstrated that tumors exclude large macromolecules, such as unmodified and modified antibodies, at least in part due to high intratumoral pressures (Jain *et al.*, 1988). In recent years, tumors have also been shown to express various immunosuppressive substances, including cytokines that inhibit the entry and function of cellular effectors (Chen *et al.*, 1998), and tumor cell surface inhibitors of complement activation (Schmitt *et al.*, 1999). The blunting of mechanisms involved in antibody-mediated cytotoxicity probably accounts for some of the ineffectiveness of unmodified antibodies observed in clinical trials. Several approaches to improve antitumor activity of antibody-based therapeutics, including better patient selection, selection of novel targets and mechanisms of action, combination with chemotherapy, and modification of the antibody molecule, have been made and are undergoing evaluation in preclinical and clinical trials.

1. Patient Selection

The first consideration for clinical development of an antibody is choosing a patient population whose tumors express the antigen target. Despite the simplicity of the concept, application into practice is much more difficult. For example, outcome may depend on the extent of antigen expression by tumor, assessed as both the fraction of cells containing the antigen and the intensity of expression per cell. Furthermore, efficacy and toxicity may be influenced by the amount of circulating antigen, dictating a different dose and schedule strategy. Optimal patient selection depends on the development and availability of a reliable and valid diagnostic test for tumor antigen expression, and in some cases, for determining the biological consequences of antigen expression within that particular tumor. For example, both preclinical and clinical studies suggested that the antitumor effects of the trastuzumab antibody are correlated with the intensity of expression of Her2/*neu* by tumor cells. However, the definition of Her2/*neu* overexpression is not clear, and the most appropriate test for detecting overexpression that would predict for clinical response has not been fully defined (Jimenez *et al.*, 2000; Johnson *et al.*, 2000).

A second issue in patient selection is the tumor bulk prior to treatment. Although some antibodies clearly produce tumor regression in advanced disease, many antibodies would be predicted to have optimal antitumor activity in a minimal residual disease setting. The lack of activity in advanced disease in phase II trials does not necessarily preclude activity in a surgical adjuvant setting. An example can be found with the murine monoclonal 17-1A, which had limited activity in advanced disease but demonstrated an improvement in survival in surgically resected high-risk colorectal cancer patients when tested in a modest-size randomized trial (Riethmuller *et al.*, 1998). Although the results need to be confirmed in larger studies that are ongoing, the results provide reason to reconsider the traditional drug development paradigms, which require antitumor activity in advanced disease before clinical trials can be conducted in the adjuvant setting.

2. Determination of Optimal Dose and Schedule in Early Trials

Traditionally phase I trials of antibodies are conducted in advanced disease. Besides toxicity, a relevant end point appears to be saturation of antigen binding within tumors, as it is presumed that increasing the dose beyond this point would not increase the therapeutic effect. However, obtaining tumor tissue both pre-treatment and after treatment is often difficult. Since the half-life of the antibody is expected to increase at the dose at which all binding sites *in vivo* have been saturated, the dose at which the $T_{1/2}$ increases has been used as a surrogate for antibody saturation of available binding sites (Baselga *et al.*, 2000). Tumor biopsies and novel noninvasive imaging methodologies may be needed to assess antibody penetration into the tumor and the biological consequences that follow.

With most antibodies that have cross-reactivity with some normal tissues, caution should be taken in applying pharmacokinetic and safety data from patients with large bulk disease or high circulating antigen levels to those with minimal disease. Theoretically, large amounts of tumor may serve as a sink for the antibody, thus obscuring potential toxicity of antibody binding to normal tissues. Similarly, the safety and efficacy of antibodies in a xenograft mouse model underestimates toxicity and overestimates efficacy in humans, since in many cases the antibodies do not cross-react with normal tissues of the mouse.

3. Considerations for Radiolabeled Antibodies

Radiolabeled antibodies have the advantage of killing both the cells bound by the antibody and also bystander tumor cells that might not express the targeted antigen (Buchsbaum, 2000, DeNardo *et al.*, 1999; Knox and Meredith, 2000). For this approach, the antigen target is preferably not subject to internalization, since cellular processing may diminish the effect of bound radioisotopes. The selection of the radioisotope is based on availability and cost, radioactive half-life, and type and energy of the emitted particle, which affects path length.

In general, few objective responses have been observed in trials of radiolabeled antibodies, when administered either as single agents or in combination with cytokines, such as IFN-γ, that up-regulate expression of the surface antigen target. A notable exception is the administration of radiolabeled antibodies against lymphoma surface antigens, which are reported to produce high remission rates (Kaminski *et al.*, 1996; Press, 1999; Wiseman *et al.*, 1999). The low response rates in solid tumors have been attributed to the radioresistance of tumors and the relatively small doses of radiotherapy that can be delivered to tumors with acceptable toxicity. Many of the initial trials were also conducted with murine antibodies; thus, retreatment was not possible due to formation of HAMA.

Recently investigators have introduced humanized antibody constructs that have smaller molecular weights to enhance penetration to tumors (Safavy *et al.,* 1999; Slavin-Chiorini *et al.,* 1997). The reduction in size was accomplished by deleting the second constant region of the heavy chain. The latter construct was also found to have a relatively short circulating half-life compared with full-sized antibodies in animal models, resulting in more rapid clearance from non-antigen-binding normal tissues and producing high tumor-to-normal-tissue radiation ratios.

4. Immunotoxins

Antibodies can be coupled chemically to carry certain toxins, which might include a standard chemotherapy agent, or engineered by recombinant DNA techniques as a single molecule with a biological toxin attached to the targeting aspect. The choice of antigen is critical, since toxins often require internalization into the cell. Thus, the antigen must internalize after binding of the immunotoxin. In many cases, the toxin's own mechanism of entry into cells is removed, thus markedly reducing its potential for nonspecific toxicity to normal tissues (Pastan, 1997).

Two immunotoxins have been approved for use in the United States (Bernstein, 2000; Saleh *et al.,* 1998; Sievers *et al.,* 1999), several others have been extensively evaluated, and many others are in preclinical or early clinical development. The major toxicity has been a nonspecific vascular leak syndrome (Kuan *et al.,* 1995). A major limitation to efficacy has been the inability to administer more than one cycle of treatment, due to the neutralizing immune response against both the murine antibody and toxin components of the immunotoxin (Pai *et al.,* 1996). The toxins are highly immunogenic molecules that are often derived from bacteria or marine organisms.

Several approaches have been taken to improve the efficacy of the immunotoxins against solid tumors. The toxins can be engineered to eliminate nonspecific toxicity, and new agents that temporarily suppress the immune response are being evaluated in combination with the immunotoxins. The immunotoxins can also be made smaller by recombinant DNA techniques to improve penetration into tumors.

5. Pretargeting Approaches

During the time that antibody conjugates circulate in the blood, they cause damage to the normal tissues and organs through which they circulate. A novel approach to improve the therapeutic ratio is to pretarget the antibody, such as by attaching the antibodies to a nontoxic prodrug converting enzyme (Springer and Niculescu-Duvaz, 1997). Nonspecific antibody binding is allowed to clear over a specified period of time, or a reagent is given to remove nonspecifically bound antibody from normal tissues and blood, thus producing high tumor-to-normal-tissue ratios. The prodrug is subsequently administered. Theoretically, the nontoxic prodrug will be converted to a toxic species specifically in the tumor. As a result, high local concentrations of toxic drug are generated within the tumor, which are expected to kill both antigen-positive and antigen-negative tumor cells. Ideally, the prodrug will undergo minimal conversion in normal tissues, will be trapped in the tumor to avoid leak into the systemic circulation, and, if released systemically from the tumor, will be cleared quickly. The general approach has been termed antibody-directed prodrug enzyme therapy, or ADEPT. Enzymes being investigated in preclinical systems include carboxypeptidase G2 (CPG2), nitroreductase, cytosine deaminase, and DT diaphorase. A CPG2-based ADEPT approach to activate an alkylating agent prodrug is currently under clinical evaluation (Bhatia *et al.,* 2000; Martin *et al.,* 1997).

Similar approaches involve pretargeting of radiolabeled compounds or toxins. As an example, the antibody is attached to one of two molecular binding partners. The toxin is attached to the other of the two binding partners. This latter construct has a small molecular weight for penetration into tumors and a relatively short half-life for rapid clearance. Similar to the ADEPT system, the antibody-ligand is administered first, and after clearance from normal tissues, the binding partner for the ligand containing the toxin is administered. Some pretargeting antibody constructs are in development.

References

Adler, A. J., Marsh, D. W., Yochum, G. S., Guzzo, J. L., Nigam, A., Nelson, W. G., and Pardoll, D. M. (1998). CD4+ T cell tolerance to parenchymal self-antigens requires presentation by bone marrow-derived antigen-presenting cells. *J Exp Med* **187,** 1555–1564.

Aebersold, P., Hyatt, C., Johnson, K., Hines, L., Korcak, L., Sanders, M., Lotze, M., Topalian, S., Yang, J., and Rosenberg, S. A. (1991). Lysis of autologous melanoma cells by tumor-infiltrating lymphocytes: association with clinical response. *J. Natl. Cancer. Inst.* **83,** 932–937.

Banchereau, J., and Steinman, R. M. (1998). Dendritic cells and the control of immunity. *Nature* **392,** 245–252.

Barth, R. J., Jr., Mule, J. J., Spiess, P. J., and Rosenberg, S. A. (1991). Interferon gamma and tumor necrosis factor have a role in tumor regressions mediated by murine CD8+ tumor-infiltrating lymphocytes. *J. Exp. Med.* **173,** 647–658.

Baselga, J., Norton, N., Albanell, J., Kim, Y. M., and Mendelsohn, J. (1998). Recombinant humanized anti-HER2 antibody (Herceptin) enhances the antitumor activity of paclitaxel and doxorubicin against HER2/neu overexpressing human breast cancer xenografts. *Cancer Res.* **58,** 2825–2831.

Baselga, J., Pfister, D., Cooper, M. R., Cohen, R., Burtness, B., Bos, M., D'Andrea, G., Seidman, A., Norton, L., Gunnett, K., Falcey, J., Anderson, V., Waksal, H., and Mendelsohn, J. (2000). Phase I studies of anti-epidermal growth factor receptor chimeric antibody C225 alone and in combination with cisplatin. *J. Clin. Oncol.* **18,** 904–914.

Berd, D., Morton, D. L., Foshag, L. J., Hoon, D. S., Nizze, J. A., Famatiga, E., Wanek, L. A., Chang, C., Davtyan, D. G., Gupta, R. K., Elashoff, R., et al. (1992). Prolongation of survival in metastatic melanoma after active specific immunotherapy with a new polyvalent melanoma vaccine. *Ann Surg.* **216,** 463–482.

Bernstein, I. D. (2000). Monoclonal antibodies to the myeloid stem cells: therapeutic implications of CMA-676, a humanized anti-CD33 antibody calicheamicin conjugate. *Leukemia* **14**, 474–475.

Bhatia, J., Sharma, S. K., Chester, K. A., Pedley, R. B., Boden, R. W., Read, D. A., Boxer, G. M., Michael, N. P., and Begent, R. H. (2000). Catalytic activity of an in vivo tumor targeted anti-CEA scFv::carboxypeptidase G2 fusion protein. *Int. J. Cancer* **85**, 571–577.

Boon, T., Coulie, P. G., and Van den Eynde, B. (1997). Tumor antigens recognized by T cells. *Immunol. Today* **18**, 267–268.

Brooks, P. C., Stromblad, S., Klemke, R., Visscher, D., Sarkar, F. H., and Cheresh, D. A. (1995). Antiintegrin alpha v beta 3 blocks human breast cancer growth and angiogenesis in human skin. *J. Clin. Invest.* **96**, 1815–1822.

Buchsbaum, D. J. (2000). Experimental radioimmunotherapy. *Semin. Radiat. Oncol.* **10**, 156–167.

Bystryn, J. C., Jacobsen, S., Harris, M., Roses, D., Speyer, J., and Levin, M. (1986). Preparation and characterization of a polyvalent human melanoma antigen vaccine. *J. Biol. Response Mod.* **5**, 211–224.

Caux, C., Massacrier, C., Vanbervliet, B., Dubois, B., Van Kooten, B., Durand, I., and Banchereau, J. (1994). Activation of human dendritic cells through CD40 cross-linking. *J. Exp. Med* **180**, 1263–1272.

Chen, J. J., Sun, Y., and Nabel, G. J. (1998). Regulation of the proinflammatory effects of Fas ligand (CD95L). *Science* **282**, 1714–1717.

Clarke, P., Mann, J., Simpson, J. F., Rickard-Dickson, K., and Primus, F. J. (1998). Mice transgenic for human carcinoembryonic antigen as a model for immunotherapy. *Cancer Res.* **58**, 1469–1477.

Clynes, R. A., Towers, T. L., Presta, L. G., and Ravetch, J. V. (2000). Inhibitory Fc receptors modulate in vivo cytoxicity against tumor targets . *Nat. Med.* **6**, 443–446.

DeNardo, G. L., O'Donnell, R. T., Kroger, L. A., Richman, C. M., Goldstein, D. S., Shen, S., and DeNardo, S. J. (1999). Strategies for developing effective radioimmunotherapy for solid tumors. *Clin. Cancer Res.* **5**, 3219s–3223s.

Deng, Y., Yewdell, J. W., Eisenlohr, L. C., and Bennink, J. R. (1997). MHC affinity, peptide liberation, T cell repertoire, and immunodominance all contribute to the paucity of MHC class I-restricted peptides recognized by antiviral CTL. *J. Immunol.* **158**, 1507–1515.

Dyall, R., Bowne, W. B., Weber, L. W., LeMaoult, J., Szabo, P., Moroi, Y., Piskun, G., Lewis, J. J., Houghton, A. N., and Nikolic-Zugic, J. (1998). Heteroclitic immunization induces tumor immunity. *J. Exp. Med.* **188**, 1553–1561.

Foon, K. A., Lutzky, J., Baral, R. N., Yannelli, J. R., Hutchins, L., Teitelbaum, A., Kashala, O. L., Das, R., Garrison, J., Reisfeld, R. A., and Bhattacharya-Chatterjee, M.. (2000). Clinical and immune responses in advanced melanoma patients immunized with an anti-idiotype antibody mimicking disialoganglioside GD2. *J. Clin. Oncol.* **18**, 376–384.

Foon, K. A., John, W. J., Chakraborty, M., Das, R., Teitelbaum, A., Garrison, J., Kashala, O., Chatterjee, S. K., and Bhattacharya-Chatterjee, M. (1999). Clinical and immune responses in resected colon cancer patients treated with anti-idiotype monoclonal antibody vaccine that mimics the carcinoembryonic antigen. *J. Clin. Oncol.* **17**, 2889.

Green, L. L. (1999). Antibody engineering via genetic engineering of the mouse: XenoMouse strains are a vehicle for the facile generation of therapeutic human monoclonal antibodies. *J. Immunol. Methods* **231**, 11–23.

Gutheil, J. C., Campbell, T. N., Pierce, P. R., Watkins, J. D., Huse, W. D., Bodkin, D. J., and Cheresh, D. A. (2000). Targeted antiangiogenic therapy for cancer using Vitaxin: a humanized monoclonal antibody to the integrin $\alpha v \beta 3$. *Clin. Cancer Res.* **6**, 3056–3061.

Hicklin, D. J., Wang, Z., Arienti, F., Rivoltini, L., Parmiani, G., and Ferrone, S. (1998). beta2-Microglobulin mutations, HLA class I antigen loss, and tumor progression in melanoma. *J. Clin. Invest.* **101**, 2720–2729.

Hu, H. M., Urba, W. J., and Fox, B. A. (1998). Gene-modified tumor vaccine with therapeutic potential shifts tumor-specific T cell response from a type 2 to a type 1 cytokine profile. *J. Immunol.* **161**, 3033–3041.

Huang, X., Molema, G., King, S., Watkins, L., Edgington, T. S., and Thorpe, P. E. (1997). Tumor infarction in mice by antibody-directed targeting of tissue factor to tumor vasculature. *Science* **275**, 547–550.

Hurwitz, A. A., Yu, T. F., Leach, D. R., and Allison, J. P. (1998). CTLA-4 blockade synergizes with tumor-derived granulocyte-macrophage colony-stimulating factor for treatment of an experimental mammary carcinoma. *Proc. Natl. Acad. Sci. USA* **95**, 10067–10071.

Ishida, T., Oyama, T., Carbone, D. P., and Gabrilovich, D. I. (1998). Defective function of Langerhans cells in tumor-bearing animals is the result of defective maturation from hemopoietic progenitors. *J. Immunol.* **161**, 4842–4851.

Jain, R. K., and Baxter, L. T. (1988). Mechanisms of heterogeneous distribution of monoclonal antibodies and other macromolecules in tumors: significance of elevated interstitial pressure. *Cancer Res.* **48**, 7022–7032.

Jimenez, R. E., Wallis, T., Tabasczka, P., and Visscher, D. W. (2000). Determination of Her-2/*neu* status in breast carcinoma: comparative analysis of immunohistochemistry and fluorescent in situ hybridization. *Mod. Pathol.* **13**, 37–45.

Johnson, R. C., Ricci, A., Jr., Cartun, R. W., Ackroyd, R., and Tsongalis, G. J. (2000). p185HER2 overexpression in human breast cancer using molecular and immunohistochemical methods. *Cancer Invest.* **18**, 336–342.

Kageshita, T., Wang, Z., Calorini, L., Yoshii, A., Kimura, T., Ono, T., Gattoni-Celli, S., and Ferrone, S. (1993). Selective loss of human leukocyte class I allospecificities and staining of melanoma cells by monoclonal antibodies recognizing monomorphic determinants of class I human leukocyte antigens. *Cancer Res.* **53**, 3349–3354.

Kaminski, M. S., Zasadny, K. R., Francis, I. R., Fenner, M. C., Ross, C. W., Milik, A. W., Estes, J., Tuck, M., Regan, D., Fisher, S., Glenn, S. D., and Wahl, R. L. (1996). Iodine-131-anti-B1 radioimmunotherapy for B-cell lymphoma. *J. Clin. Oncol.* **14**, 1974–1981.

Kawakami, Y., Eliyahu, S., Delgado, C. H., Robbins, P. F., Sakaguchi, K., Appella, E., Yannelli, J. R., Adema, G. J., Miki, T., and Rosenberg, S. A. (1994). Identification of a human melanoma antigen recognized by tumor-infiltrating lymphocytes associated with in vivo tumor rejection. *Proc. Natl. Acad. Sci. USA* **91**, 6458–6462.

Knox, S. J., and Meredith, R. F. (2000). Clinical radioimmunotherapy. *Semin. Radiat. Oncol.* **10**, 73–93.

Kuan, C. T., Pai, L. H., and Pastan, I. (1995). Immunotoxins containing Pseudomonas exotoxin that target LeY damage human endothelial cells in an antibody-specific mode: relevance to vascular leak syndrome. *Clin. Cancer Res.* **1**, 1589–1594.

Kugler, A., Stuhler, G., Walden, P., Zoller, G., Zobywalski, A., Brossart, P., Trefzer, U., Ullrich, S., Muller, C. A., Becker, V., Gross, A. J., Hemmerlein, B., Kanz, L., Muller, G. A., and Ringert, R.-H. (2000). Regression of human metastatic renal cell carcinoma after vaccination with tumor cell-dendritic cell hybrids. *Nat. Med.* **6**, 332–336.

Lattime, E. C., Mastrangelo, M. J., Bagasra, O., Li, W., and Berd, D. (1995). Expression of cytokine mRNA in human melanoma tissues. *Cancer Immunol. Immunother.* **41**, 151–156.

Leach, D. R., Krummel, M. F., and Allison, J. P. (1996). Enhancement of antitumor immunity by CTLA-4 blockade . *Science* **271**, 1734–1736.

Lewis, G. D., Figari, I., Fendly, B., Wong, W. L., Carter, P., Gorman, C., and Shepard, H. M. (1993). Differential responses of human tumor cell lines to anti-p185HER2 monoclonal antibodies. *Cancer Immunol. Immunother.* **37**, 255–263.

Livingston, P. (1998). Ganglioside vaccines with emphasis on GM2. *Semin. Oncol.* **25**, 636–645.

Martin, J., Stribbling, S. M., Poon, G. K., Begent, R. H., Napier, M., Sharma, S. K., and Springer, C. J. (1997). Antibody-directed enzyme prodrug therapy: pharmacokinetics and plasma levels of prodrug and drug in a phase I clinical trial. *Cancer Chemother. Pharmacol.* **40**, 189–201.

Mitchell, M. S., Harel, W., Kempf, R. A., Hu, E., Kan-Mitchell, J., Boswell, W. D., Dean, G., and Stevenson, L. (1990). Active-specific immunotherapy for melanoma. *J. Clin. Oncol.* **8**, 856–869.

Morton, D. L., Foshag, L. J., Houn, D. S., Nizze, J. A., Famatiga, E., Wanek, L. A., Chang, C., Davtyan, D. G., Gupta, R. K., Elashoff, R. (1992). Prolongation of survival in metastatic melanoma after active specific immunotherapy with a new polyvalent melanoma vaccine. *Ann. Surg.* **216**, 463–482.

Naftzger, C., Takechi, Y., Kohda, H., Hara, I., Vijayasaradhi, S., and Houghton, A. N. (1996). Immune response to a differentiation antigen induced by altered antigen: a study of tumor rejection and autoimmunity. *Proc. Natl. Acad. Sci. USA* **93**, 14809–14814.

Nair, S. K., Boczkowski, D., Morse, M., Cumming, R. I., Lyerly, H. K., and Gilboa, E. (1998). Induction of primary carcinoembryonic antigen (CEA)-specific cytotoxic T lymphocytes in vitro using human dendritic cells transfected with RNA. *Nat. Biotechnol.* **16**, 364–369.

Overwijk, W. W., Tsung, A., Irvine, K. R., Parkhurst, M. R., Goletz, T. J., Tsung, K., Carroll, M. W., Liu, C., Moss, B., Rosenberg, S. A., and Restifo, N. P. (1998). gp100/pmel 17 is a murine tumor rejection antigen: induction of "self"-reactive, tumoricidal T cells using high-affinity, altered peptide ligand. *J. Exp. Med* **188**, 277–286.

Pai, L. H., Wittes, R., Setser, A., Willingham, M. C., and Pastan, I. (1996). Treatment of advanced solid tumors with immunotoxin LMB-1: an antibody linked to Pseudomonas exotoxin. *Nat. Med* **2**, 350–353.

Pardoll, D. M., and Topalian, S. L. (1998). The role of CD4+ T cell responses in antitumor immunity. *Curr. Opin. Immunol.* **10**, 588–594.

Pastan, I. (1997). Targeted therapy of cancer with recombinant immunotoxins. *Biochim. Biophys. Acta.* **1333**, C1–6.

Press, O. W. (1999). Radiolabeled antibody therapy of B-cell lymphomas. *Semin. Oncol.* **26**, 58–65.

Riethmuller, G., Holz, E., Schlimok, G., Schmiegel, W., Raab, R., Hoffken, K., Gruber, R., Funke, I., Pichlmaier, H., Hirche, H., Buggisch, P., Witte, J., and Pichlmayr, R. (1998). Monoclonal antibody therapy for resected Dukes' C colorectal cancer: seven-year outcome of a multicenter randomized trial. *J. Clin. Oncol.* **16**, 1788–1794.

Rosenberg, S. A. (1997). Cancer vaccines based on the identification of genes encoding cancer regression antigens. *Immunol. Today* **18**, 175–182.

Rosenberg, S. A., Yang, J. C., Schwartzentruber, D. J., Hwu, P., Marincola, F. M., Topalian, S. L., Restifo, N. P., Dudley, M. E., Schwarz, S. L., Spiess, P. J., Wunderlich, J. R., Parkhurst, M. R., Kawakami, Y., Seipp, C. A., Einhorn, J. H., and White, D. E. (1998). Immunologic and therapeutic evaluation of a synthetic peptide vaccine for the treatment of patients with metastatic melanoma. *Nat. Med* **4**, 321–327.

Rowse, G. J., Tempero, R. M., VanLith, M. L., Hollingsworth, M. A., and Gendler, S. J. (1998). Tolerance and immunity to MUC1 in a human MUC1 transgenic murine model. *Cancer Res.* **58**, 315–321.

Safavy, A., Khazaeli, M. B., Safavy, K., Mayo, M. S., and Buchsbaum, D. J. (1999). Biodistribution study of 188Re-labeled trisuccin-HuCC49 and trisuccin-HuCC49deltaCh2 conjugates in athymic nude mice bearing intraperitoneal colon cancer xenografts. *Clin. Cancer Res.* **5**, 2994s–3000s.

Saleh, M. N., LeMaistre, C. F., Kuzel, T. M., Foss, F., Platanias, L. C., Schwartz, G., Ratain, M., Rook, A., Freytes, C. O., Craig, F., Reuben, J.,

Sams, M. W., and Nichols, J. C. (1998). Antitumor activity of DAB389IL-2 fusion toxin in mycosis fungoides. *J. Am. Acad. Dermatol.* **39**, 63–73.

Schmitt, C. A., Schwaeble, W., Wittig, B. M., Meyer zum Buschenfelde, K. H., and Dippold, W. G. (1999). Expression and regulation by interferon-gamma of the membrane-bound complement regulators CD46 (MCP), CD55 (DAF) and CD59 in gastrointestinal tumours. *Eur. J. Cancer* **35**, 117–124.

Shan, D., Ledbetter, J. A., and Press, O. W. (1998). Apoptosis of malignant human B cells by ligation of CD20 with monoclonal antibodies. *Blood* **91**, 1644–1652.

Sievers, E. L., Appelbaum, F. R., Spielberger, R. T., Forman, S. J., Flowers, D., Smith, F. O., Shannon-Dorcy, K., Berger, M. S., and Bernstein, I. D. (1999). Selective ablation of acute myeloid leukemia using antibody-targeted chemotherapy: a phase I study of an anti-CD33 calicheamicin immunoconjugate. *Blood* **93**, 3678–3684.

Slavin-Chiorini, D. C., Kashmiri, S. V., Lee, H. S., Milenic, D. E., Poole, D. J., Bernon, E., Schlom, J., and Hand, P. H. (1997). A CDR-grafted (humanized) domain-deleted antitumor antibody. *Cancer Biother. Radiopharm.* **12**, 305–316.

Springer, C. J., and Niculescu-Duvaz, I. (1997). Antibody-directed enzyme prodrug therapy (ADEPT): a review. *Adv. Drug Deliv. Rev.* **26**, 151–172.

Staveley-O'Carroll, K., Sotomayor, E., Montgomery, J., Borrello, I., Hwang, L., Fein, S., Pardoll, D., and Levitsky, H. (1998). Induction of antigen-specific T cell anergy: An early event in the course of tumor progression. *Proc. Natl. Acad. Sci. USA* **95**, 1178–1183.

Steinbrink, K., Wolfl, M., Jonuleit, H., Knop, J., and Enk, A. H. (1997). Induction of tolerance by IL-10-treated dendritic cells. *J. Immunol.* **159**, 4772–4780.

Steinman, R. M., Pack, M., and Inaba, K. (1997). Dendritic cell development and maturation. *Adv. Exp. Med. Biol.* **417**, 1–6.

Tamura, Y., Peng, P., Liu, K., Daou, M., and Srivastava, P. K. (1997). Immunotherapy of tumors with autologous tumor-derived heat shock protein preparations. *Science* **278**, 117–120.

Torre-Amione, G., Beauchamp, R. D., Koeppen, H., Park, B. H., Schreiber, H., Moses, H. L., and Rowley, D. A. (1990). A highly immunogenic tumor transfected with a murine transforming growth factor type beta 1 cDNA escapes immune surveillance. *Proc. Natl. Acad. Sci. USA* **87**, 1486–1490.

Wiseman, G. A., White, C. A., Witzig, T. E., Gordon, L. I., Emmanouilides, C., Raubitschek, A., Janakiraman, N., Gutheil, J., Schilder, R. J., Spies, S., Silverman, D. H., and Grillo-Lopez, A. J. (1999). Radioimmunotherapy of relapsed non-Hodgkin's lymphoma with zevalin, a 90Y-labeled anti-CD20 monoclonal antibody. *Clin. Cancer Res.* **5**, 3281s–3286s.

Zaks, T. Z., and Rosenberg, S. A. (1998). Immunization with a peptide epitope (p369–377) from HER-2/neu leads to peptide-specific cytotoxic T lymphocytes that fail to recognize HER-2/neu+ tumors. *Cancer Res.* **58**, 4902–4908.

Zeh, H. J., III, Perry-Lalley, D., Dudley, M. E., Rosenberg, S. A., and Yang, J. C. (1999). High avidity CTLs for two self-antigens demonstrate superior in vitro and in vivo antitumor efficacy. *J. Immunol.* **162**, 989–994.

CHAPTER 10

STRUCTURE-BASED DRUG DESIGN AND ITS CONTRIBUTIONS TO CANCER CHEMOTHERAPY

Robert C. Jackson

Cyclacel Limited
Dundee, United Kingdom

Summary

Structure-based drug design (SBDD) has developed as a consequence of the emergence of detailed structural information on drug target molecules, chiefly from advances in protein crystallography. The general principles of SBDD are that the ligand should efficiently fill the space in its binding site, that electrostatic complementarity and hydrogen bond formation between the ligand and its receptor should be maximized, and that the structural water molecules in the active site should be retained. This chapter discusses a number of examples where SBDD has been applied to anticancer drug design, including antimetabolites, protease inhibitors, protein kinase inhibitors, and other targets. The future potential of the SDBB process is most likely to be an iterative one with several cycles of design, synthesis, screening, and structural elucidation, and involving close interaction between medicinal chemists, computational chemists, and biologists.

1. Introduction

Drug discovery has involved a continuing interplay between searching for active compounds among very large numbers of more or less randomly selected candidate compounds ("screening") and "rational" drug design approaches that attempt to preselect compounds based on prior knowledge of the disease process, a putative target macromolecule, or its physiologic substrate or agonist. Anticancer drug development in the past has made use of some of the largest screening exercises in the history of drug discovery, such as that of the U.S. National Cancer Institute. Of course, screening approaches to drug discovery involve an important rational element (particularly in the design of screens), and rational drug design approaches frequently include a serendipitous element (often in the selection of initial leads required to start the optimization process); nevertheless, the distinction between these two contrasting philosophical approaches to drug

171

discovery remains a useful one. When large amounts of detailed structural information about drug target molecules started to become available in the 1980s, chiefly as a result of protein crystallography, there was a widespread assumption in the drug industry that structure-based drug design (SBDD) would become the dominant technology in drug discovery and that screening (often described pejoratively as "random" screening, though it is seldom truly random) would disappear. What has actually happened has been more complex and more interesting: screening approaches have been given a new lease on life as a result of the advent of combinatorial chemistry and of high-throughput screening. The debate over SBDD versus screening approaches thus continues, and even among groups that recognize that both approaches are required for an optimal drug design capability, it is important to question whether SBDD, which remains expensive and technically demanding, is going to earn its keep.

It is not the intention here to provide a detailed technical review of SBDD. This can be obtained from the very comprehensive review article by Babine and Bender (1997), and from the books by Gubernator and Böhm (1998) and Veerapandian (1997). A brief survey of the earlier literature is given in Jackson (1995, 1997) and Kubinyi (1998). The general principles of SBDD have been summarized as follows (Appelt *et al.*, 1991):

1. The ligand should efficiently fill space in its binding site.
2. Electrostatic complementarity between the ligand and its receptor should be maximized.
3. Hydrogen bond formation between ligand and receptor should be maximized.
4. Desolvation penalties should be minimized, i.e., the ligand should be designed around structural water molecules in the active site, unless it is energetically favorable to displace them.
5. Where possible, maintain sufficient structural flexibility of the ligand to permit ready access to the binding site (note, however, that too much flexibility costs binding energy because of the resulting entropic costs of locking the ligand into a single conformation in the bound complex).
6. Approach SBDD as an iterative process, with each structure of a protein-inhibitor complex providing the basis for further refinement in the subsequent design cycle.

There were debates in the past about the relative utility of x-ray crystallography versus high-field nuclear magnetic resonance (NMR). It was suggested that because some proteins were difficult or impossible to crystallize, NMR, being inherently a solution technique, would ultimately prove more useful. There were also concerns that crystal packing forces might induce perturbations in crystal structures, so they might be too different from solution structures to be useful for ligand design. The debate continues: readers should refer to the article by MacArthur *et al.* (1994) for a more detailed discussion of the contributions of the two techniques. Despite advances in magnet design, NMR as a technique for solving structures remains limited to proteins of less than about 40 kDa. The most useful contribution of high-field NMR in drug design is probably in providing information on binding modes of ligands with proteins of known structure.

The difficulties of inducing proteins to crystallize have not entirely gone away, especially when the subject is a hydrophobic or poorly water-soluble protein. For such problem cases, the crystallographer must often enlist the help of a protein engineer, who may mutate one or more amino acid residues to make the target more tractable or cleave off portions of the molecule believed to be structurally distant from the domain that will be used for ligand design. Of course, the molecule being crystallized is then no longer the natural target, and questions may be raised as to whether the relevant portion of the mutated structure is really the same as that of the natural molecule. If deletions or mutations are sufficiently remote from the site of interest, changes to the conformation are probably minimal. The approach is usually justified by its results: when an engineered structure has been used to design a new inhibitor, the inhibitor is tested against the natural enzyme or receptor, as well as against the form used for crystallography, and there is usually no difference in binding potency. Of course, the protein engineering process must involve some preconceptions about the structure; if we want to make a protein more soluble by site-directed mutations that will place more hydrophilic groups on the surface, we must have some idea what the surface residues are (trial and error is possible but likely to be hopelessly laborious for a protein of any size). The structural preconceptions will usually come from sequence comparisons with related proteins of known three-dimensional structure.

Membrane-bound proteins, being inherently lipophilic and often very large, continue to pose special problems for crystallographers, but membrane receptors and ion channels represent more than half of all known drug targets. Some progress has been made with crystallization of intact membrane receptors, but this topic will not be reviewed here. In the cancer field, the membrane receptors that have received most attention have been the tyrosine-kinase-linked receptors, and here the approach has been to work with the isolated, hydrophilic intracellular domains. These partial structures can then be used for design of inhibitors of the tyrosine kinase active site.

It is against this background that this chapter will review the recent contributions of SBDD to cancer chemotherapy, a discussion that will focus on three classes of anticancer agents: antimetabolites, protease inhibitors, and protein kinase inhibitors. Finally, a number of new SBDD techniques will be discussed, along with the extent to which they are likely to expedite the drug design process or to make it more accurate. This chapter will consider the successes and failures of the technique, and ask what can be learned from them to make discovery of new anticancer agents more efficacious, more rapid, and more cost effective.

2. Antimetabolites

It is historically appropriate to begin a survey of the contributions of SBDD to cancer chemotherapy with a discussion of antimetabolites. The first high-resolution x-ray crystal structure of an enzyme with an inhibitor bound to the active site was published by Matthews *et al.* (1977). This was the dihydrofolate reductase (DHFR) of *Escherichia coli* with the anticancer drug methotrexate (an antimetabolite), bound at the active site. Structures of eukaryotic DHFRs were published subsequently (Freisheim and Matthews, 1984), and this information was used in the design of new inhibitors. None of these have as yet become clinically useful drugs. Perhaps this reflects the fact that methotrexate is already an extremely potent inhibitor, with picomolar binding to DHFR, and its limitations as an anticancer drug are issues of selectivity, drug resistance, cellular distribution, and pharmacokinetic properties that cannot be improved by the design of more potent ligands. There is a sense in which SBDD may indirectly address some of these pharmacologic aspects of drug design: by suggesting novel designs for chemically unrelated inhibitors, without loss of binding affinity, it has been possible to generate equipotent inhibitors with different physical and pharmacokinetic properties. The pharmacology of methotrexate is greatly influenced by its anionic glutamate function, which makes it dependent on active transport for entry into cells, and also makes it vulnerable to certain forms of acquired drug resistance. The use of SBDD to design non-glutamate-containing DHFR inhibitors resulted in compounds with very different pharmacology. This topic will be pursued further in the discussion of the thymidylate synthase (TS) inhibitor Thymitaq.

A. Thymidylate Synthase (TS)

TS was of great interest as a target for anticancer drug design. In the 1980s, when these studies began, the most effective drug for treatment of metastatic colorectal carcinoma was 5-fluorouracil (5-FU). Despite being the most active available agent, 5-FU only gave response rates of around 20%. There are believed to be three major reasons for this: First, 5-FU has suboptimal pharmacokinetics, with a very short plasma half-life and extensive first-pass liver metabolism. Second, 5-FU is a prodrug that requires several metabolic activation steps for conversion to its active metabolite, 5-fluorodeoxyuridylate (5-FdUMP). Third, being a pyrimidine base, 5-FU may be incorporated into both RNA and DNA. While it was argued by some that this could contribute to its thera-

peutic effect, it was generally considered that the RNA-directed effect, in particular, might be a major cause of the dose-limiting gastrointestinal toxicity of 5-FU. Interestingly, coadministration of leucovorin (5-formyltetrahydrofolate) with 5-FU increased the response rate of colon cancer (to around 30%). This leucovorin coadministration increased the amount of 5-FdUMP in cells, thus making 5-FU a more effective TS inhibitor (for a recent discussion of 5-FU and leucovorin, see Peters and Köhne, 1999). For all of these reasons, it appeared that a potent antifolate inhibitor of TS should have potential as an anticolon cancer drug. The first-generation antifolate TS inhibitor, CB3717, showed preliminary clinical anticancer activity, but also nephrotoxicity, which was attributed to its low solubility (Calvert *et al.,* 1987). The first crystal structure of TS was of the *E. coli* enzyme bound to CB3717 (Matthews *et al.,* 1990), and this structure was used as the basis for the initial approaches to design of novel TS inhibitors. Because it was believed that the glutamate moiety of CB3717 had contributed to its toxicity and also conferred a requirement for active transport that potentially limited its antitumor spectrum, it was decided to design lipophilic TS inhibitors that did not contain a glutamate moiety. The design story is described in detail by Appelt *et al.* (1991), Varney *et al.* (1992), Webber *et al.* (1993), and Reich and Webber (1993). The structure of human TS was not available at the time of these studies, so a number of multiply mutated *E. coli* TS constructs were engineered in which all the three active site residues that differed between *E. coli* and human were changed to the amino acids found in human TS. Several cycles of iterative crystallography, drug design, and synthesis followed. In outline, removal of the glutamate moiety of CB3717 resulted in a 250-fold decrease in binding potency. This lost binding affinity was restored in the subsequent iterative design cycles in which different heterocyclic ring systems were explored as replacements for the quinazoline or, alternatively, a range of quinazoline substitutions were used that could simultaneously fill space effectively at the active site and retain water solubility. Both of these approaches resulted in inhibitors with inhibitory potency against TS that was comparable to or greater than that of CB3717.

Of the compounds emerging from this project, Thymitaq (AG337; nolatrexed, Fig. 1) progressed furthest in clinical trials. Hughes and Calvert (1999) have recently reviewed the preclinical and clinical studies. Thymitaq, when administered in frequently dosed schedules, was active against several murine tumor systems and human tumor xenografts. In phase II trials it showed clinical activity against hepatocellular carcinoma and against head and neck cancer. Toxicity (myelosuppression and mucositis) was minimal and rapidly reversible. However, Thymitaq had low dose-potency, with the maximum tolerated clinical dose being about 1000 mg/m^2 per day. The plasma half-life was short. As a result, it was necessary to administer the compound by infusion; the plasma

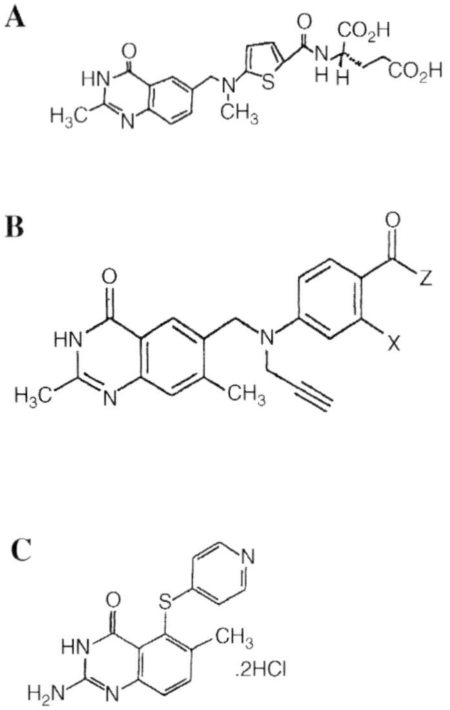

FIGURE 1 Antifolate inhibitors of thymidylate synthase. (**A**) Tomudex (AstraZeneca). (**B**) ZD9331 (AstraZeneca). (**C**) Thymitaq (Agouron).

concentration dropped rapidly after the infusion was stopped. This behavior seems to reflect the fact that the drug is not retained within cells, unlike polyglutamatable antifolates, such as methotrexate and Tomudex. The design of Thymitaq was an early example of SBDD demonstrating its ability to generate potent inhibitors with clinical activity, but because of its pharmacokinetic limitations it seems unlikely that Thymitaq will become an established agent.

The design of Tomudex (raltitrexed, Fig. 1) followed classical medicinal chemical approaches and did not involve SBDD (Hughes *et al.*, 1999). However, as discussed by those authors, subsequent crystallographic studies were used to study the binding mode of Tomudex to TS. At the time of writing, Tomudex is the only member of the new generation of TS inhibitors to have reached the market, when it became the first new drug to be marketed for colorectal carcinoma in 40 years. Unlike Thymitaq, Tomudex is very dose-potent and has favorable pharmacokinetics—properties that are related to its extensive polyglutamylation. These are properties that are not obviously related to inhibition of TS by the parent compound and that could not have been predicted using SBDD. It should be noted, however, that the polyglutamates of Tomudex are much more potent inhibitors of TS than the parent compound, suggesting that the potency advantages of this and related compounds may not be simply a matter of cellular pharmacokinetics. The α-carboxyl of the first glutamate residue contributes to binding to TS by hydrogen-

bonding to Lys48 through a water molecule, and the α-carboxyl of the second glutamate residue in a diglutamate derivative interacts electrostatically with Arg49 (Bavetsias *et al.*, 2000).

Another TS inhibitor related to CB-3717 and Tomudex is ZD-9331 (Jackman *et al.*, 1997; Fig. 1). In this analogue, the γ-carboxyl of the glutamate is replaced by a tetrazole, which makes it chemically incapable of polyglutamylation. Computer graphics modeling indicated that the tetrazole should form an electrostatic interaction with Arg49 at the dipeptide binding region of TS. ZD-9331 requires active transport, which is mediated primarily by the reduced folate carrier. Interestingly, it has dose potency intermediate between that of Tomudex and Thymitaq, consistent with the argument that potency is conferred by concentration within target cells that results partly from active transport and partly from the intracellular trapping of polyglutamates. The contribution of molecular graphics and modeling techniques to the design of this compound was reviewed by Boyle *et al.* (1999). ZD-9331 is now in early clinical trials.

B. Glycinamide Ribonucleotide Formyltransferase

Glycinamide ribonucleotide formyltransferase (GARFT) was shown to be the target enzyme of an antifolate drug lometrexol (Fig. 2), which was developed as an experimental anticancer agent (Moran, 1992). Lometrexol gave clinical activity against a number of hard-to-treat solid tumors but had severe toxicity, prompting a search for new GARFT inhibitors. GARFT is an interesting target for a number of reasons. It forms a rate-limiting step in the purine *de novo* biosynthetic

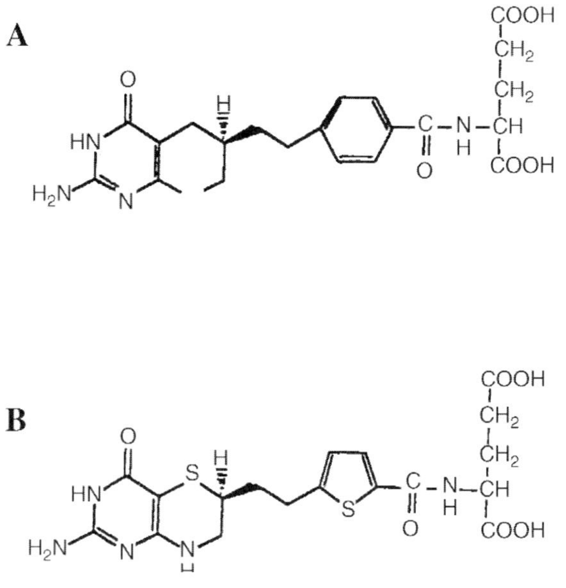

FIGURE 2 Antifolate inhibitors of glycinamide ribonucleotide formyltransferase. (**A**) Lometrexol (Lilly). (**B**) AG2034 (Agouron).

pathway, and a number of older nucleoside or purine-base drugs are believed to act, at least partly, on this pathway, but because of their potential for incorporation into nucleic acids, they were not "clean" drugs, with a single, unequivocal mechanism. Another old anticancer drug, azaserine (a glutamine analogue), also acts on the purine *de novo* pathway. Azaserine was the first drug shown to have curative clinical activity against a human solid tumor, but because it inhibits most glutamine-requiring enzymes, it, too, is not a clean drug. GARFT offers a more selective approach to inhibiting the purine *de novo* pathway.

The structure of *E. coli* GARFT with a bound inhibitor was published several years ago (Almassy *et al.*, 1992), and more recent studies with the human enzyme showed that the folate cofactor binding site was closely homologous (J. Almassy, personal communication). The use of these structures to generate novel GARFT inhibitors through SBDD was described by Varney *et al.* (1997). The GARFT project provides an interesting example of the use of the GRID program (Goodford, 1985) in drug design. GRID is a computational method for exploring which chemical functional groups would be expected to have binding affinity at different parts of a protein molecule. The interactions for chemical groups of interest are systematically calculated over a grid that covers the putative binding region of the protein. A GRID study showed two hot spots at the GARFT active site for affinity to a thioether probe. The compound AG-2034 (Fig. 2) was designed to satisfy the requirement for a sulfur atom at both sites. AG-2034 has a K_i of 28 nM against human GARFT. It is a good substrate for folylpolyglutamate synthetase, and (by analogy with other GARFT inhibitors) it is likely that its polyglutamate derivatives may be more potent GARFT inhibitors than the parent compound. AG-2034 was growth inhibitory to murine and human cells at low nanomolar concentrations. The inhibited cells were blocked at the G_1-S boundary of the cell cycle. Subsequent cell death occurred very slowly and appeared to be associated with the blocked cells moving into S phase, and perhaps for this reason cells (such as cells with mutant p53) that had defective G_1-S checkpoint function appeared to be more sensitive to AG-2034 (Zhang *et al.*, 1998). AG2034 was taken into clinical trials, but the trials have been suspended in favor of a newer analogue, AG-2037 (Fig. 2). A concern with both lometrexol and AG-2034 was that these compounds are extensively transported into cells by the folate receptor; since levels of this receptor are highly sensitive to dietary status, efficacy and toxicity with these compounds can be highly variable. In contrast, AG-2037 is transported exclusively by the reduced folate carrier, whose levels are not highly dependent on nutritional status. Unlike lometrexol and AG-2034, AG-2037 retained antitumor activity in mice fed a low-folate diet and thus is more relevant to the human situation (Bloom *et al.*, 2000).

These pharmacologic and nutritional complexities of drug development are, of course, not addressed by SBDD. However, SBDD makes it possible to work around some of these problems indirectly by facilitating the design of a large number of potent inhibitors with a wide variety of chemical structures. GARFT inhibitors have not yet earned an established place in cancer chemotherapy. However, their preclinical properties are so encouraging, and so distinctively different from that of other classes of antimetabolites, that their continued exploration is surely warranted. The availability of a large collection of GARFT crystal structures with a wide range of ligands should facilitate further research on this target.

C. Other Antimetabolite Targets

Crystal structures have been solved for several other enzymes that are of actual or potential interest as targets for design of anticancer drugs. Inosine 5-monophosphate (IMP) dehydrogenase was shown to be the target of a number of experimental anticancer drugs that for various reasons never made it to market: mycophenolic acid, tiazofurin, selenazofurin, as well as the established anticancer drug and immunosuppressive, 6-mercaptopurine (6-MP). These compounds have in common the interesting property of an unusually wide therapeutic index (for cytotoxic agents). The availability of a crystal structure for IMP dehydrogenase (Colby *et al.*, 1999) has made possible the design of novel inhibitors, which are being developed primarily as immunosuppressives. Mycophenolate mofetil is marketed for this indication, and it is hoped that more potent IMP dehydrogenase inhibitors, with improved pharmacokinetic properties, might be effective in prevention of transplant rejection and management of autoimmune diseases. However, it will also be of interest to explore these new IMP dehydrogenase inhibitors as anticancer agents.

Another immunosuppression target that should also have applications in oncology is purine nucleoside phosphorylase (PNP). The target organ for immunosuppression is the T lymphoblast, but PNP is also present in red blood cells and highly active in liver, and these tissues act as a sink for inhibitors. Inhibition of PNP results in intracellular accumulation of purine nucleosides, including deoxyguanosine, which in turn causes raised levels of dGTP, which is cytotoxic. Many cells contain a dGTP-cleaving enzyme, but T cells lack this activity. The early PNP inhibitors were insufficiently potent to give *in vivo* inhibition to the point where biological activity could be seen. The structure of human erythrocyte PNP was solved several years ago and made possible the design of more potent PNP inhibitors using SBDD approaches (Bugg *et al.*, 1993). The most potent of the new compounds were low nanomolar PNP inhibitors (Niwas *et al.*, 1994), e.g., 9-(3-pyridylmethyl)-9-deazaguanine (Peldesine, BCX-34) is a 35-nM PNP inhibitor. PNP inhibitors are selectively cytotoxic to T lymphocytes and show activity in T-cell-mediated models of immune disease and T-cell malignancies.

3. Protease Inhibitors

Undoubtedly, the therapeutic area where SBDD has had the greatest impact has been antivirals. There are currently five aspartyl protease inhibitors on the market for treatment of persons with HIV infection. SBDD played a major role in the design of these compounds, particularly the newer ones, and the use of these drugs (in combination with reverse transcriptase inhibitors) has resulted in a 70% drop in the death rate from AIDS in developed countries. In this particular case it can be confidently asserted that SBDD has resulted in the creation of life-prolonging drugs. On the heels of this success, structures of several other viral proteases have been solved and are being used in drug design (Kubinyi, 1998). These include serine proteases (e.g., those of hepatitis C virus, and cytomegalovirus and other members of the herpesvirus family) and cysteine proteases (e.g., the 3C protease of rhinovirus).

In the oncology field, proteases are also of great interest: the characteristic malignant properties of invasion and metastasis involve protease cascades, which present possible new drug targets. The most extensively explored protease family in the cancer drug area is the matrix metalloproteases (MMPs), which contain a zinc atom at the active site. This is a family of about 20 extracellular enzymes—some soluble, some membrane-bound—that cleave collagens, gelatins, proteoglycans, and other proteins in the extracellular matrix. MMP activity is frequently elevated around solid tumors and has been linked with the invasive, metastatic, and angiogenic behavior of tumors. MMPs are secreted as inactive proenzymes, so that they themselves require proteolytic cleavage for conversion to their active form. This activation may sometimes be catalyzed by their own active form (autocatalysis), by another MMP, or by a member of another protease family, usually a serine protease. The regulation of MMP activity is further complicated by the presence of a family of endogenous inhibitory proteins, the tissue inhibitors of metalloproteinases (TIMPs). Regulation of MMP activity is thus a complex function involving a balance between proenzymes and active enzymes, and TIMP-inhibited and uninhibited forms. Proteases are dangerous, destructive molecules, and clearly this elaborate regulation is necessary to ensure that they are only active in restricted sites, for a limited time. A recent review of physiologic regulation of MMPs is that of Nagase and Woessner (1999).

The literature on MMP inhibitors as anticancer agents was recently summarized (Clendeninn and Appelt, 2000). Early MMP inhibitors, most notably batimastat and marimastat (Fig. 3) from British Biotech, were designed without the use of protein structure data. They are small peptidic molecules, containing a hydroxamate function, which is a potent zinc chelator. In preclinical test systems, these compounds have antimetastatic and antiangiogenic activity. Marimastat has

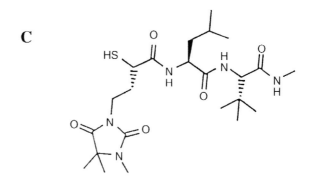

FIGURE 3 Matrix metalloprotease inhibitors. (**A**) Marimastat (British Biotech). (**B**) Prinomastat (Agouron). (**C**) D2163 (Celltech-Chiroscience).

been explored extensively in clinical trials; its dose-limiting toxicity was joint pain (also seen in rats and marmosets), which can be severe but which is reversible on cessation of treatment. Marimastat is a relatively nonspecific inhibitor of the MMP family of enzymes and to a lesser extent inhibits non-MMP members of the zinc protease superfamily. The complex role of the various MMP family members in the biology of invasion, metastasis, and angiogenesis is still being unraveled, but MMPs 2, 9, and 14 appear to be involved in these processes. Some obvious questions arise: (1) Is it necessary or desirable to inhibit multiple members of the MMP family to achieve a biological effect? Would a more selective MMP inhibitor be a better or a worse drug? (2) Of the three possible anticancer mechanisms of MMP inhibitors—invasion, metastasis, and angiogenesis—which is the most profitable to target? Or, again, is a multiple effect desirable? (3) What causes the joint pain? Is this an MMP-related side effect?

An example of the complex proteolytic cascades that occur is shown in Fig. 4. Vascular endothelial growth factor (VEGF), under hypoxic conditions, stimulates expression of $\alpha_v\beta_3$ integrin on the surface of endothelial cells. In the presence of this integrin, MMP-14 on the surface of a tumor cell can activate pro-MMP-2, present in the extracellular fluid, into active MMP-2, which stimulates new angiogenesis. Interestingly, this activation requires both active MMP-14 and TIMP-2-bound MMP-14. The MMP-14 (and other MMPs) are activated from their proenzyme form by urokinase-type plasminogen activator, though soluble plasmin degrades MMPs. Angiogenesis is thus a complex process, stimulated by hypoxia, and involving multiple members of the MMP family, a serine protease cascade, growth factors, and integrins, all of which are potential sites for therapeutic intervention.

High-resolution crystal structures of several members of the MMP family are available, with bound inhibitors (Clendeninn and Appelt, 2000), making possible the design of new inhibitors with greater selectivity against specific members of the MMP family. The active sites of MMPs consist of a trough that accommodates the cleavable region of the polypeptide backbone of the substrate protein. From this trough extend pockets that contain the side chains of the substrate amino acid residues. The size, shape, and charge distribution of these pockets determine the substrate specificity of the particular MMP. The catalytic zinc atom is bound in close proximity to the scissile peptide bond, coordinated to three histidine residues. For example, stromelysin-1 has a deep S1′ pocket, whereas this side-chain pocket is small in collagenase-1 and intermediate in matrilysin. Thus, by designing inhibitors of known binding mode with large P1′ substituents, it is possible to make selective stromelysin-1 inhibitors (Browner et al., 1995). This strategy was adapted in the design of prinomastat (AG-3340, Fig. 3), which is a 270-pM inhibitor of stromelysin-1(MMP-3), but 8

nM against collagenase-1 (MMP-1) and 54 nM against matrilysin (MMP-7). Prinomastat is also a potent inhibitor of gelatinases A and B (MMP-2 and MMP-9), collagenase-3 (MMP-13), and membrane-type MMP-1 (MMP-14). Because the joint pain side effect of the first-generation MMP inhibitors was accompanied by collagen deposition at certain sites, and because MMP-1 (fibroblast collagenase) is the primary enzyme responsible for collagen turnover, it was argued that inhibition of MMP-1 was undesirable and that designing out this feature might avoid the joint pain side-effect. The design philosophy behind prinomastat was thus threefold: (1) build potency against MMPs 2, 3, and 13; (2) minimize potency against MMP-1; (3) minimize peptidic properties. Prinomastat had antimetastatic and antiangiogenic activity against a wide range of preclinical models (Bender and Appelt, 2000). It is now in phase III clinical trials. Some joint pain is observed at high doses, calling into question the theory that inhibition of MMP-1 is the cause of this side effect.

A completely different approach to MMP inhibitor design was described by Baxter et al. (2000). These authors also believed that MMP-2 was a primary therapeutic target but had a completely different hypothesis to account for the joint pain toxicity, to be described below. They elected to retain the peptide-like structure but emphasized the use of a thioamide zinc-chelating function, as an alternative to the hydroxamate used in marimastat and prinomastat or the carboxylate used in some other early MMP inhibitors. Thioamide-substituted peptides had previously been explored as inhibitors of other zinc peptidases, such as angiotensin-converting enzyme (ACE) and neutral endopeptidase. When the project started, the group did not have a crystal structure of a thioamide inhibitor bound to an MMP. As a starting point, they utilized a three-dimensional structure of an early hydroxamate-containing MMP inhibitor bound to the active site of MMP-8 (Stams et al., 1994). Figure 5 shows a molecular model of a simple dipeptide thioamide N-(α-thioacetyl)leuylphenylalanyl-methylamide, bound to MMP-8. It was expected that the thioamide would form a bidentate interaction with the zinc, similar to that formed by a hydroxamate. However, the NH group of the hydroxamate is capable of forming an additional hydrogen bond, and the thioamide structure does not have a hydrogen bond donor at this position, so it cannot form the corresponding hydrogen bond. In addition, the thioamide is an intrinsically less potent zinc chelator than hydroxamate. Thus additional enzyme–inhibitor interactions were required to maintain satisfactory potency. This was achieved partly by optimization of the P2′ residue, and partly by exploring α substituents on the thioamide (Baxter et al., 2000). This latter position provides a site for substitution that is not available with hydroxamates. SBDD provided important insights at this stage of the design process, e.g., modeling suggested that by introducing a hydrogen bond acceptor into the α position, a hydrogen bond could be formed to serine 172 of the

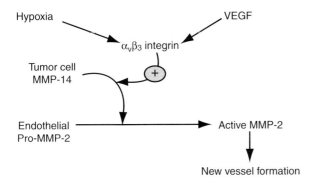

FIGURE 4 The role of MMP-2 and MMP-14 in tumor angiogenesis.

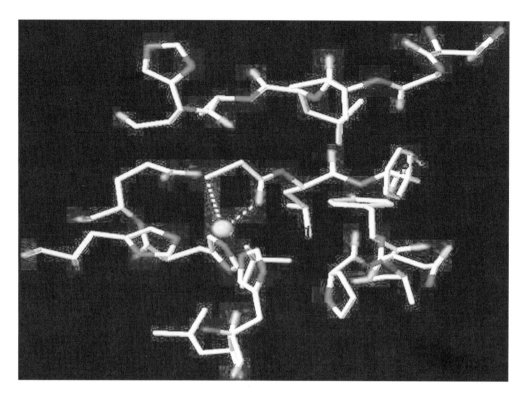

FIGURE 5 A molecular model of a thioamide dipeptide inhibitor docked into the active site of MMP-8. (From Baxter *et al.*, 2000. Reproduced with kind permission of Humana Press, Inc.)

collagenases or tyrosine 172 of the gelatinases. Modeling studies also suggested that this hydrogen bond acceptor should optimally be positioned at the end of a three-carbon chain relative to the backbone (Baxter *et al.*, 1997).

Simultaneous with the use of modeling and of conventional SAR analysis to obtain potency against MMPs, attempts were made to design compounds with less potential for joint pain. The hypothesis being tested in these studies was that this side effect may result from unwanted inhibition of zinc-protease sheddases. These are a class of metalloproteases, distinct from the MMPs, that are involved in the cleavage of membrane-bound precursors of cytokines and their receptors, resulting in shedding of soluble proteins into the extracellular fluid. One such protein that is shed by a metalloprotease-dependent process is soluble receptor for tumor necrosis factor α (TNF-α). To exert its proinflammatory effect, TNF-α must interact with membrane-bound receptors, which then transmit an intracellular signal. It is believed that soluble TNF receptor in the synovial fluid of joints acts as a "decoy" by binding TNF-α and thus lowering the amount of TNF-α available to transmit its inflammatory signal through binding to membrane-bound receptors. Shedding of soluble receptor thus provides a homeostatic, anti-inflammatory function. Conversely, inhibition of this shedding process by broad-spectrum metalloprotease inhibitors causes inflammation and joint pain. This hypothesis is still speculative, but an inverse correlation has been demonstrated between inhibition of TNF-α shedding and arthropathy in rats (J. Bird and A. Baxter,

personal communication). Structural data are not available for sheddases, so this stage of the lead optimization process followed conventional structure–activity approaches.

It was expected that for a therapeutic benefit to result from inhibition of MMPs the target enzymes must be continually inhibited for long periods (months to years). This makes development of compounds with oral activity highly desirable. The physicochemical properties, such as aqueous solubility, of molecules play a major role in determining the degree of oral absorption. In addition to optimizing aqueous solubility to improve oral availability, Baxter *et al.* (1997, 2000) made use of the parameter $\Delta \log P$, which is a measure of the total hydrogen bonding capacity of a molecule. This parameter was described by the Abbott group in the course of their development of endothelin A antagonists, who proposed that a value of $\Delta \log P$ in the range 3.5–4.5 was associated with satisfactory oral availability.

Using these approaches, Baxter *et al.* (1997, 2000) developed the compound D2163 (Fig. 3), which is a low- to mid-nanomolar inhibitor of collagenases and gelatinases (e.g., IC_{50} against MMP-13 was 4 nM and against MMP-2 was 41 nM), and showed high oral bioavailability in rats. D2163 gave activity in rodent models of metastasis and angiogenesis. It did not inhibit shedding of TNF-α or its receptor from whole cells and did not cause arthropathies after long-term treatment in rats and marmosets. D2163 was taken into phase I clinical trial in normal volunteers and gave high blood levels, in a potentially therapeutic range, and no serious adverse effects. The plasma half-life was consistent with once-daily dosing. D2163 is currently in phase II and phase III clinical trials.

Other proteases that are potential targets for anticancer drug design fall into the serine and cysteine protease superfamilies. The serine protease that has been most extensively explored as a subject for SBDD is thrombin (Kubinyi, 1998). The primary therapeutic interest in thrombin inhibitors is as anticoagulants, and based on the thrombin crystal structure, highly selective nanomolar inhibitors have been designed (Obst *et al.,* 1997). Because antithrombotics display antimetastatic activity in preclinical models, this target is potentially of interest in oncology, as are certain cysteine proteases, including caspases and cathepsins (Otto and Schirmeister, 1997).

4. Protein Kinase Inhibitors

The discovery that protein tyrosine kinase (PTK) activity is an essential component of cell signaling pathways emerged from the early work leading to the oncogene concept (Hunter, 1991). As the elucidation of signaling pathways proceeded, the role of protein serine/threonine kinases further down the chain became apparent, and it was clear that mutations in these kinases could also be oncogenic. Although no established anticancer drugs operate by protein kinase inhibition, the link between altered kinases and cancer causation is so compelling that many of these enzymes are considered to be attractive drug design targets, and the development of protein kinase inhibitors is currently one of the liveliest areas of new anticancer drug ideas. An entire issue of the journal *Anti-Cancer Drug Design* was devoted to this topic (Sausville, 2000), and many features are reviewed in Chapter 2 of this book. The first protein kinase structure to be solved was that of the cyclic-AMP-dependent serine/threonine protein kinase PKA (Zheng *et al.,* 1993). Several x-ray crystal structures of protein kinases with bound inhibitors have subsequently been solved, and SBDD techniques have been widely used in this field. Protein kinases constitute a large family of enzymes (probably several hundred in higher eukaryotes), so the question of selectivity looms large. Initially it was expected that ATP binding sites would be highly conserved and that selectivity would reside at the binding site of the protein substrate so that, as with proteases, inhibitors would have to be designed against the substrate site. Perhaps surprisingly it has proved possible to design inhibitors that bind to the ATP site but nevertheless have a considerable degree of selectivity (many orders of magnitude, in some cases). Often the early leads have come from natural products, such as the staurosporines, olomoucine, and flavopyridol, and the role of SBDD has been to design next-generation compounds with improved selectivity and potency.

A. Protein Tyrosine Kinases

These drug design targets (see also Chapter 3 of this book) were the subject of a comprehensive early review (Fry and Bridges, 1995). The first crystal structure of a PTK to be published was of the tyrosine kinase domain of the human insulin receptor (Hubbard *et al.,* 1994). Although not directly relevant to anticancer drug design, this structure was of obvious interest to the entire field of PTK inhibitor development, particularly in facilitating understanding of the geometry of ATP in its binding site. Recent development of PTK-inhibiting anticancer agents has focused on the kinase domains of the epidermal growth factor (EGF) receptor, the platelet-derived growth factor (PDGF) receptor, and the vascular endothelial growth factor (VEGF) receptor.

Work on the PTK domains of EGF receptor and related receptors, the erbB family of receptors, has been summarized by Fry (2000). There are four known members of this receptor family, and they bind several groups of growth factor ligands, some from epithelial or mesenchymal tissues, and some from nerve tissue. The binding specificity of the different members of the receptor family for the various ligands tends to overlap. The receptor molecules may homo- or heterodimerize, and certain tyrosine residues in the intracellular domain, when autophosphorylated, form binding sites for SH2 domains of a variety of signaling proteins. The relationship of the erbB receptor family to cancer, and its potential as a target for drug design, is discussed by Fry (2000).

Currently no crystal structure is available for a PTK of this class. Palmer *et al.* (1997) described a homology model of the ATP binding region of the EGF receptor PTK domain, based on the PKA structure of Zheng *et al.* (1993). This model played an important part in the decision of Fry and colleagues to attempt the development of irreversible PTK inhibitors. It was observed that 2′-thioadenosine was about 400-fold more effective as an inhibitor than adenosine itself, and the model suggested the formation of a disulfide bond with Cys797 of the kinase. The same model also suggested Cys773 as a site for covalent adduct formation, and a potent acrylamide-substituted quinazoline inhibitor, PD168393 (Fig. 6) was shown to bind to this amino acid. A mutant enzyme in which Cys773 was replaced by serine was essentially unaffected. PD-168393 was also inactive against a panel of other protein kinases (Fry *et al.,* 1998). PD-168393 had strong *in vivo* antitumor activity against a panel of human carcinoma xenografts following oral or systemic administration.

B. Vascular Endothelial Growth Factor Receptor

VEGF receptor is another membrane protein whose intracellular PTK domain is of great interest as a target for drug design. In this case the biological objective is inhibition of the process of tumor angiogenesis, which should confer

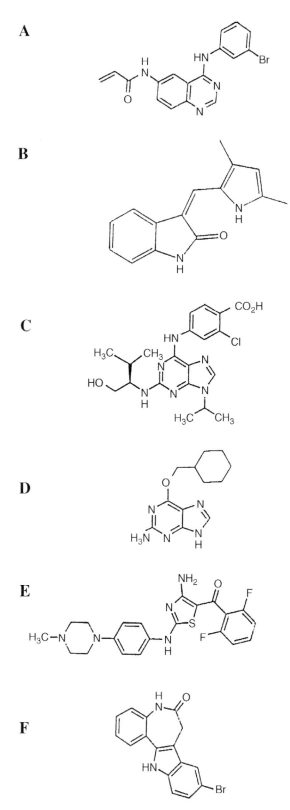

A

B

C

D

E

F

FIGURE 6 Structures of protein kinase inhibitors. (**A**) PD 168393 (Warner-Lambert/Parke-Davis). (**B**) SU5416 (Sugen). (**C**) Purvanolol B (University of California). (**D**) NU-2058 (University of Newcastle upon Tyne). (**E**) AG12275 (Agouron). (**F**) Kenpaullone (National Cancer Institute).

broad-spectrum activity against solid tumors with minimal host toxicity. In fact, VEGF binds to several PTK receptors: VEGFR-1, also known as Flt-1, VEGFR-2, also known as Flk-1 and KDR, and neurophilin-1. Flk-1/KDR appears to be the dominant driver of endothelial cell proliferation. At present, crystal structures have not been published for any of the VEGF receptor PTKs. However, Mendel *et al.* (2000) have made use of homology models based on the published structure for the fibroblast growth factor (FGF) receptor PTK domain (Mohammadi *et al.*, 1997). A number of indolin-2-ones were cocrystallized with the FGF receptor PTK domain, and analysis of these structures showed that the indolin-2-one core occupied the binding pocket in which the adenine of ATP was normally present and formed hydrogen bonds with a number of conserved residues of the protein backbone. Substituents on the indolin-2-one ring system could occupy hydrophobic pockets in the receptor that remained unoccupied when ATP was bound in the active site. Homology models for a number of PTK domains suggested that the ATP binding site was well conserved but that there were differences in the hydrophobic pockets that offered potential for design of selective inhibitors (Mendel *et al.*, 2000).

Combinatorial libraries based on the indolin-2-one structure were screened in a search for selective inhibitors of VEGF receptors. As a result, SU-5416 (Fig. 6) was selected for further development. SU-5416 is a 160-nM inhibitor of Flk-1, a 19-μM inhibitor of FGFR-1, and a 320-nM inhibitor of PDGFR-β (Mendel *et al.*, 2000). It is active in preclinical angiogenesis models and has been selected for clinical development. The modeling work clearly made an important contribution to the design of SU-5416, though the authors note that the homology model of Flk-1/KDR based on the experimental FGF receptor kinase structure was unable to fully account for the unexpected potency of SU5416 against Flk-1/KDR.

C. Cyclin-Dependent Kinases

Protein serine/threonine kinases are a very large family that are of interest as drug design targets in many clinical areas other than oncology. The two subfamilies of serine/threonine kinases that have been of most interest as anticancer drug design targets are protein kinase C (PKC) and the cyclin-dependent kinases (CDKs). To this point, no crystal structure of a PKC-inhibitor complex has been published, and drug design against this target has followed conventional approaches. However, SBDD has been extensively employed in the design of inhibitors of CDKs. A comprehensive review of the design of CDK inhibitors as anticancer agents was recently presented by Fry and Garrett (2000), and this article also provides a concise summary of current understanding of the function of CDKs in control of the cell cycle, and of their regulation. Crystal structures of CDK2 were published by

Schulze-Gahmen *et al.* (1995), in complex with olomoucine or isopentenyladenine, by Russo *et al.* (1996), in complex with the endogenous inhibitory protein, p27/kip-1 and cyclin-A, and by De Azevedo *et al.* (1997) in complex with roscovitine. The crystal structures showed that olomoucine, isopentenyladenine, and roscovitine bound at the ATP site but that the binding orientation of the inhibitors was different from that of the purine ring of ATP (Noble and Endicott, 1999); drug design based on the structural data resulted in low-micromolar inhibitors, based on a 6-amino-substituted purine structure, e.g., NU-2058 (Fig. 6; Newell *et al.,* 1999). A crystal structure of NU-2058 bound to CDK2 showed hydrogen bonding from the 3 and 9 nitrogen atoms and the 2-amino group of the purine to Glu81 and Leu83 of the protein (Grant *et al.,* 1998). Gray *et al.* (1998) describe how CDK2 structural information was used in the design of directed combinatorial libraries, resulting in inhibitors 1000-fold more potent than the original leads. One such compound, purvanolol B (Fig. 6), was a 6-nM inhibitor of CDK2/cyclin A and also a 6-nM inhibitor of CDK1/cyclin B. A 2C structure of the complex of CDK2 with purvanolol B was reported by Gray *et al.* (1998).

The crystal structure of CDK4, which is more hydrophobic and less water soluble than CDK2, has so far not been reported, though SBDD using homology models based on CDK2 structures was reported by the Agouron group. They described a very potent series of 4-aminothiazoles, some of which had broad-spectrum activity against CDK1, CDK2, and CDK4, while others were up to 100-fold selective against CDK4, e.g., AG-12275 (Fig. 6) (Lundgren *et al.,* 1999). This compound caused a G_1-phase block that was dependent on functional Rb-protein, and gave growth delay of human colon carcinoma xenografts, thus proving that a selective CDK4 inhibitor displays the predicted cell cycle properties and possesses *in vivo* anticancer activity.

Homology modeling from the CDK2 structures has also been used in the design of selective CDK1 inhibitors. The best documented example is the description of the development of the paullone series of CDK1 inhibitors by Gussio *et al.* (2000). The initial lead, kenpaullone (Fig. 6), was identified as a cell growth inhibitor by the NCI human cell line screen, and shown by the COMPARE program, a pattern-recognition algorithm that compares inhibition patterns across the 62 cell lines in the panel, to have an inhibition profile similar to that of flavopiridol, suggesting that its mechanism of action might be similar. Kenpaullone was then shown to inhibit CDKs, with IC_{50} of 400 nM against CDK1 and 680 nM against CDK2, but little activity against CDK4. Subsequent analogue development utilized three-dimensional quantitative structure–activity relationship (3D-QSAR) analysis, and SBDD based on a homology model of CDK1 based on the published CDK2 coordinates of Russo *et al.* (1996). The model suggested that potential existed for formation of additional hydrogen bonds between the

enzyme and inhibitor. The 9-cyano derivative is able to form an additional hydrogen bond to a structural water molecule that is hydrogen bonded to the π electron system of Phe80. This substitution resulted in a drop of more than one log in the IC_{50} against CDK1 to 24 nM. Figure 7 (see color insert) shows a stereodiagram of 9-cyanopaullone docked in the ATP binding site of CDK1. The modeling work also suggested that putting an electronegative nitro group at the 9-position should facilitate charge transfer from aliphatic side chains of the binding site. The 9-nitro compound alsterpaullone inhibited CDK1 with an IC_{50} of 35 nM and had IC_{50} in the cell proliferation assay of 460 nM. Interestingly, the 9-cyano analogue, which was slightly more potent than 9-nitro as an enzyme inhibitor, gave an IC_{50} of only 90 μM in the cell proliferation assay (Gussio *et al.,* 2000).

5. Other Targets

A. *Ras*-p21

A number of high-resolution x-ray structures of this critical family of signaling proteins have been solved, and a complete nuclear magnetic resonance (NMR) solution-phase structure is also available. Its mechanism is well understood at the molecular level. Oncogenic mutations in *ras* frequently operate by disabling its GTPase activity, resulting in this molecular switch becoming jammed in the on position (Wittinghofer and Pai, 1991). The presence of a well-defined GDP/GTP binding pocket suggested that it might be possible to design potent ligands that would stabilize the GDP conformation and thus inhibit signaling. It might even be possible to design ligands that would be selective against transformed *ras,* as opposed to wild-type *ras.* These attempts have, to date, proved fruitless. The natural guanine nucleotide ligands bind with nanomolar potency and are present in the cell at millimolar concentration; a ligand that is designed to dislodge GTP must therefore operate against a six-log kinetic disadvantage. *Ras*-p21 continues to present a theoretically appealing target, but the most promising inhibitors currently available operate by inhibiting its farnesylation (Garrett and Workman, 1999), and SBDD has not contributed to their design.

B. Hsp90

The molecular chaperone heat-shock protein 90 (Hsp90) was shown to be inhibited by the antitumor antibiotics radicicol and geldanomycin, and structures of Hsp90 with these antibiotics bound were recently published by Roe *et al.* (1999). Inhibition of Hsp90 results in depletion of a number of growth regulatory proteins, whose correct processing presumably depends on this chaperone: these include cRAF-1, CDK4, steroid receptors, and mutant p53. Roe *et al.* (1999)

suggest that their structure will be useful for the development of improved geldanamycin analogues.

6. Novel Methods in Structure-Based Drug Design

In addition to x-ray crystallography and high-field NMR, other physical techniques are beginning to make contributions to protein structure determination. Atomic force microscopy is providing information on folding patterns of membrane proteins that are difficult to study by more conventional methods (Oesterhelt et al., 2000). Three-dimensional electron microscopy, while capable of much less resolution than x-ray crystallography, has given interesting glimpses of the structures of multimolecular complexes, such as the 38Å native structure of the eukaryotic 80S ribosome (Verschoor et al., 1996). Raman spectroscopy has become sufficiently sensitive to facilitate derivation of structural information. Microcalorimetry can provide accurate binding enthalpies and, in conjunction with accurate binding free-energy estimates, can allow estimation of entropic contributions to ligand binding.

Nevertheless, x-ray crystallography remains the primary tool of structural biologists. Recent technological developments for solving crystal structures include more sensitive detectors (e.g., charge-coupled devices), increased synchrotron access, and techniques such as multiple anomalous dispersion (MAD) that sometimes make possible phasing of x-ray diffraction data without the need for isomorphic heavy-atom derivatives. Of course, bigger NMR magnets are increasing the resolving power of NMR.

Perhaps even more important than hardware developments are new software tools, both for solving structures (e.g., computational similarity searches of the protein data base for trial solutions, improved alignment algorithms, and programs to assist in x-ray data interpretation) and for ligand design (e.g., scoring algorithms, flexible docking programs, de novo design approaches, and computational techniques for predicting "drug-like properties").

A. Predicting Inhibitor Binding Energy

Having designed a novel inhibitor into the active site of our target macromolecule, how can we predict how potent an inhibitor it will be and thus prioritize designs for synthesis? This so-called scoring problem continues to be one of the limiting factors in SBDD. Broadly speaking, there are two main approaches: free-energy calculations, which are comparatively rigorous but computationally expensive, and empirical methods, which are computationally cheaper but require a more extensive training set of existing structural and binding data. A useful review, citing much of the literature to 1998, is that of Hirst (1998).

For systems where a large number of solved crystal structures of protein–ligand complexes are available in the Protein Data Bank (PDB), it is possible to use an empirical-knowledge-based approach. For example, well over 100 structures of HIV protease, with bound inhibitors, have been deposited, and for many of these experimental binding affinities are available (DeWitte and Shakhnovitch, 1996). This method develops a set of interatomic interaction energies, for all pairs of atom types, and sums these energies over each atom in the inhibitor to give an estimate of the total binding free energy. Ideally, all of the experimental binding data should be measured under identical conditions, by the same laboratory, though obviously this is seldom possible. If binding enthalpies are available (e.g., measured by microcalorimetry), then it becomes possible to derive separate estimates of enthalpic and entropic contributions to binding. In principle, this technique could be extended to enable predictions to be made for different target molecules; in practice it works best for sets of closely related ligands to the same receptor, with similar binding geometry.

At the other end of the scale is the more rigorous but laborious technique of free-energy perturbation analysis (Lamb and Jorgenson, 1997). This approach requires that accurate structural and binding data be available for one protein-ligand pair. The binding free energy for the other "unknown" ligand is then estimated by a computational transformation of the "known" ligand (i.e., the one whose binding free energy is known) to the "unknown" ligand, in both bound and unbound states. The technique, though the most rigorous of current methods for predicting binding energies, is computationally intensive and in some cases may literally be slower than synthesizing the novel inhibitor and measuring its binding energy. A brief review of the method is given by Hirst (1998).

B. Homology Modeling

When the structure of a target protein is unknown but a structure exists for a closely related protein, it may be reasonable to assume that their overall fold will be similar, so that the minor details may be modeled using any of the standard molecular graphics programs. To choose a trivial example, if the three-dimensional structure of a certain protein has been solved to high resolution, and we have another protein whose structure is unknown but whose amino acid sequence is identical to that of the known protein except that a particular alanine has been mutated to glycine, it is almost certainly safe to assume that the structures are identical except for the absence of the methyl side chain in the "unknown" protein. In most situations of interest there are likely to be several amino acids that are different; more often, the known and unknown protein have extensive overall differences but contain one particular domain with extensive homology (e.g., an ATP binding site). In such cases, the uncertainties of the homology modeling process become greater. As the database of solved structures becomes greater, the chances that a close relative of the unknown structure of interest has already been solved also become greater; as a result, this technique is becoming more widely used and more accurate. Examples have been given above of the productive use of homology modeling in design of MMP inhibitors and of protein kinase inhibitors. The obvious dangers of the approach are that a change of a nonpolar to a polar group (for example) can cause an unexpectedly large rotation or translation of part of the molecule, or change its hydration state, and for useful drug design atomic positions at the ligand binding site must be known to within a fraction of an angstrom unit.

7. Conclusions and Current Questions

Almost all major drug discovery organizations have now accepted the importance of the contributions of SBDD to their armamentarium. However, these same organizations have also invariably implemented combinatorial chemistry and high-throughput screening, so the day when most drugs will be designed *de novo,* with the medicinal chemist representing only the final stage of the process has not yet arrived. It probably never will; because protein–ligand interactions, though amenable to rational analysis, are matters of immense complexity, the SDBB process is likely to remain an iterative one, with several cycles of design, synthesis, and structural elucidation requiring close interaction between medicinal chemists, computational chemists, and structural biologists.

How cost effective is SBDD? It is still not routine, but x-ray sources and detection systems are becoming smaller and more affordable. How does SBDD fit within the general trend of drug discovery techniques to involve very high throughput? Better trial solutions (and faster data collection) should make experimental structure solving more productive, but whereas it is quite feasible to generate a combinatorial library of many thousands of related compounds, it is not likely that we can generate structural data on this scale, nor is it appropriate to ask for this. Rather, combinatorial chemistry should be regarded as an alternative method of mapping space. Experience so far suggests that SBDD has been more successful at optimizing existing leads than at finding initial leads, and many groups now use combinatorial chemistry, as natural product screening was once used, to generate initial leads. Then once a screening hit has been found, it can be used to generate the first cocrystal structure, thus beginning the iterative design cycle.

So we need both screening and SBDD. The real dilemma is that with all of the expensive new technologies becoming essential, it is difficult for drug discovery groups to remain competitive (the "arms race"). Compounding this is the ex-

pected trend toward greater individualization of therapy, meaning that many more new drugs will be needed. How is this to be achieved without the total cost of drug discovery and development exceeding the gross national product? The answer must be that approaches to individualizing therapy must factor in information on individual structural differences. As the Human Genome Project generates large amounts of data on the several hundred thousand single-nucleotide polymorphisms (SNPs) that determine human individuality, instead of treating hypertension with a "one size fits all" ACE inhibitor, we will need a family of ACE inhibitors, one tailored to each allele of this gene. Homology modeling, coupled with SBDD techniques, should make this affordable, especially if some of the later stages of development could be made higher throughput, e.g., by use of cassette-dosing pharmacokinetics and clinical trial simulations. In the case of oncology (as in infectious diseases) the problem is complicated by the fact that we must consider not only individual differences between patients but also differences between tumors (or pathogens). One of the groups of authors whose work was reviewed above envisaged the SBDD-assisted production of "designer drugs" to address the problem of acquired drug resistance: "One great advantage of the SBDD approach is that if drug-selected resistance occurs due to target mutations, the designer is already strategically positioned to optimize for the mutated target" (Gussio *et al.,* 2000).

In the short term, the first implication of the Human Genome Project for SBDD is that there will huge numbers of newly discovered gene products that must be considered for suitability as drug design targets, which, if selected as targets, will require structural elucidation. Learning more about protein folding rules, and the increasing ability to use knowledge-based expert systems on the growing data base of solved structures will both make this process easier and raise the question of whether it eventually will become possible to solve protein structures through artificial intelligence techniques, without having to do crystallography.

References

Almassy, R. J., Janson, C. A., Kan, C. C., et al. (1992). Structure of apo and complexed *Escherichia coli* glycinamide ribonucleotide transformylase. *Proc. Natl. Acad. Sci. USA* **89**, 6114–6118.

Appelt, K., Bacquet, R. J., Bartlett, C. A., et al. (1991). Design of enzyme inhibitors using iterative protein crystallographic analysis. *J. Med. Chem.* **34**, 1925–1934.

Babine, R. E., and Bender, S. L. (1997). Molecular recognition of protein-ligand complexes: applications to drug design. *Chem. Rev.* **97**, 1359–1472.

Bavetsias, V., Marriott, J. H., Melin, C., Kimbell, R., Matusiak, Z. S., Boyle, F. T., and Jackman, A. L. (2000). Design and synthesis of cyclopentyl[g]quinazoline-based antifolates as inhibitors of thymidylate synthase and potential antitumor agents. *J. Med. Chem.* **43**, 1910–1926.

Baxter, A. D., Bhgal, R., Bird, J. B., Buckley, G. M., Gregory, D. S., Hedger, B. C., Manallack, D. T., Massil, T., Minton, K. J., Montana, J. G.,

Neidle, S., Owen, D. A., and Watson, R. J. (1997). Mercaptoacyl matrix metalloproteinase inhibitors: the effect of substitution at the mercaptoacyl moiety. *Biomed. Chem. Lett.* **7**, 2765–2770.

Baxter, A. D., Bird, J. B., Bannister, R., Bhogal, R., Manallack, D. T., Watson, R. W., Owen, D. A., Montana, J., Henshilwood, J., and Jackson, R. C. (2000). D1927 and D2163: novel mercaptoamide inhibitors of matrix metalloproteinases. *In* "Matrix Metalloproteinase Inhibitors in Cancer Therapy" (N. J. Clendeninn and K. Appelt, eds.). Humana Press, Totowa, NJ.

Bender, S. L., and Appelt, K. (2000). Strategies in designing MMP inhibitors. *In* "Matrix Metalloproteinase Inhibitors in Cancer Therapy" (N. J. Clendeninn and K. Appelt, eds.). Humana Press, Totowa, NJ.

Bloom, L. A., Bartlett, C. A., and Boritzki, T. J. (2000). Assessing the effects of dose and schedule on the in vivo antitumor activity of AG2037 in the low folate mouse using a hazard analysis. *Proc. Am. Assoc. Cancer Res.* **41**, 700.

Boyle, F. T., Stephens, T. C., Averbuch, S. D., and Jackman, A. L. (1999). ZD9331. Preclinical and clinical studies. *In* "Antifolate Drugs in Cancer Therapy" (A. L. Jackman, ed.), pp. 243–260. Humana Press, Totowa, NJ.

Browner, M. F., Smith, W. W., and Castelhano, A. L. (1995). Matrilysin-inhibitor complexes: common themes among metalloproteases. *Biochemistry* **34**, 6602–6610.

Bugg, C. E., Carcon, W. M., and Montgomery, J. A. (1993). Drugs by design. *Sci. Am.* **269**, 92–98.

Calvert, A. H., Newell, D. R., Jackman, A. L., et al. (1987). Recent preclinical and clinical studies with the thymidylate synthase inhibitor 10-propargyl-5,8-dideazafolic acid, CB3717. *NCI Monogr.* **5**, 213–218.

Clendeninn, N. J., and Appelt, K., (eds.) (2000). "Matrix Metalloproteinase Inhibitors in Cancer Therapy." Humana Press, Totowa, NJ.

Colby, T. D., Vanderveen, K., Strickler, M. D., Markham, G. D., and Goldstein, B. M. (1999). Crystal structure of human type II inosine monophosphate dehydrogenase: Implications for ligand binding and drug design. *Proc. Nat. Acad. Sci. USA* **96**, 3531–3536.

DeAzevedo, W. F., LeClerc, S., Meijer, L., Havlicek, L., Strnad, M., and Kim, S. H. (1997). Inhibition of cyclin-dependent kinases by purine analogues: crystal structure of human cdk2 complexed with roscovitine. *Eur. J. Biochem.* **243**, 518–523.

DeWitte, R. S., and Shakhnovitch, E. I. (1996). SMoG: de novo design method based on simple, fast, and accurate free energy estimates. 1. Methodology and supporting evidence. *J. Am. Chem. Soc.* **118**, 11733–11744.

Freisheim, J. H., and Matthews, D. A.(1984). The comparative biochemistry of dihydrofolate reductase. *In* "Folate Antagonists as Therapeutic Agents" (F. M. Sirotnak, J. J. Burchall, W. D. Ensminger, and J. A. Montgomery, eds.), Vol. 1, pp. 69–131. Academic Press, Orlando, FL.

Fry, D. W. (2000). Site-directed irreversible inhibitors of the erbB family of receptor tyrosine kinases as novel chemotherapeutic agents for cancer. *Anticancer Drug Design* **15**, 3–16.

Fry, D. W., and Garrett, M. D. (2000). Inhibitors of cyclin-dependent kinases as therapeutic agents for the treatment of cancer. *Curr. Opin. Oncol. Endocr. Metab. Invest. Drugs* **2**, 40–59.

Fry, D. W., Bridges, A. J., Denny, W. A., Doherty, A., Greis, K., Hicks, J. L., Hook, K.E., Keller, P. R., Leopold, W. R., Loo, J., McNamara, D. J., Nelson, J. M., Sherwood, V., Smail, J. B., Trumpp-Kallmeyer, S., and Dobrusin, E. M. (1998). Specific, irreversible inactivation of the epidermal growth factor receptor and erbB2 by a unique class of tyrosine kinase inhibitor. *Proc. Natl. Acad. Sci. USA* **95**, 12022–12027.

Garrett, M. D., and Workman, P. (1999). Discovering novel chemotherapeutic drugs for the third millennium. *Eur. J. Cancer* **35**, 2010–2030.

Goodford, P. J. (1985). A computational procedure for determining energetically favorable binding sites on biologically important macromolecules. *J. Med. Chem.* **28**, 849–857.

Grant, S., Boyle, F. T., Calvert, A. H., Curtin, N. J., Endicott, J., Golding, B. T., Griffin, R. J., Johnson, L. N., Newell, D. R., Noble, M. E. M., and Robson, C. (1998). Crystal structure-based design of cyclin dependent kinase inhibitors. *Proc. Am. Assoc. Cancer Res.* **39**, 176.

Gray, N. S., Wodicka, L., Thunnissen, A. W. H., Norman, T. C., Kwon, S., Espinoza, F. H., Morgan, D. O., Barnes, G., LeClerc, S., Meijer, L., Kim, S. H., Lockhart, D. J., and Schultz, P. G. (1998). Exploiting chemical libraries, structure, and genomics in the search for kinase inhibitors. *Science* **281**, 533–538.

Gubernator, K., and Böhm, H. J. (eds.) (1998). "Structure-Based Ligand Design." Wiley-VCH, Weinheim.

Gussio, R., Zaharevitz, D. W., McGrath, C. F., Pattabiraman, N., Kellogg, G. E., Schultz, C., Link, A., Kunick, C., Leost, M., Meijer, L., and Sausville, E. A. (2000). Structure-based design modifications of the paullone molecular scaffold for cyclin-dependent kinase inhibition. *Anticancer Drug Design* **15**, 53–66.

Hirst, J. D. (1998). Predicting ligand binding energies. *Curr. Opin. Drug Disc. Dev.* **1**, 28–33.

Hubbard, S. R., Wei, L., Ellis, L., and Hendrickson, W. A. (1994). Crystal structure of the tyrosine kinase domain of the human insulin receptor. *Nature* **372**, 746–754.

Hughes, A., and Calvert, A. H (1999). Preclinical and clinical studies with the novel thymidylate synthase inhibitor nolatrexed dihydrochloride (Thymitaq, AG337). *In* "Antifolate Drugs in Cancer Therapy" (A. L. Jackman, ed.), pp. 229–241. Humana Press, Totowa NJ.

Hughes, L. R., Stephens, T. C., Boyle, F. T., and Jackman, A. L. (1999). Raltitrexed (Tomudex™), a highly polyglutamatable antifolate thymidylate synthase inhibitor. *In* "Antifolate Drugs in Cancer Therapy" (A. L. Jackman, ed.), pp. 147–165. Humana Press, Totowa NJ.

Hunter, T. (1991). Cooperation between oncogenes. *Cell* **64**, 249–270.

Jackman, A. L. (ed). "Antifolate Drugs in Cancer Therapy." Humana Press, Totowa NJ.

Jackman, A. L., Kimbell, R., Aherne, G. W., Brunton, L., Jansen, G., Stephens, T. C., Smith, M. N., Wardleworth, J. M., and Boyle, F. T. (1997). Cellular pharmacology and in vivo activity of a new anticancer agent ZD9331: a water-soluble, non-polyglutamatable, quinazoline-based inhibitor of thymidylate synthase. *Clin. Cancer Res.* **3**, 911–921.

Jackson, R. C. (1995). Update on computer-aided drug design. *Curr. Opin. Biotechnol.* **6**, 646–651.

Jackson, R. C. (1997). Contributions of protein structure-based drug design to cancer chemotherapy. *Semin. Oncol.* **24**, 164–172.

Kubinyi, H. (1998). Structure-based design of enzyme inhibitors and receptor ligands. *Curr. Opin. Drug Discovery Dev.* **1**, 4–15.

Lamb, M. L., and Jorgenson, W. L. (1997). Computational approaches to molecular recognition. *Curr. Opin. Chem. Biol.* **1**, 449–457.

Lundgren, K., Price, S. M., Escobar, J., Huber, A., Chong, W., Li, L., Duvadie, R., Chu, S. S., Yang, Y., Nonomiya, J., Tucker, K., Knighton, D., Ferre, R., and Lewis, C. (1999). Diaminothiazoles: potent, selective cyclin-dependent kinase inhibitors with antitumor efficacy. *Clin. Cancer Res.* **5**, 3755s.

MacArthur, M. W., Driscoll, P. C., and Thornton, J. M. (1994). NMR and crystallography—complementary approaches to structure determination. *Trends Biotechnol.* **12**, 149–153.

Matthews, D. A., Alden, R. A., Bolin, J. T., et al. (1977). Dihydrofolate reductase: x-ray structure of the binary complex with methotrexate. *Science* **197**, 452–455.

Matthews, D. A., Appelt, K., Oatley, S. J., et al. (1990). Crystal structure of *Escherichia coli* thymidylate synthase containing bound 5-fluoro-2'-deoxyuridylate and 10-propargyl-5,8-dideazafolate. *J. Mol. Biol.* **214**, 923–936.

Mendel, D. B., Laird, A. D., Smolich, B. D., Blake, R. A., Liang, C., Hannah, A. L., Shaheen, R. M., Ellis, L. M., Weitman, S., Shawver, L. K., and Cherrington, J. M. (2000). Development of SU5416, a selective small molecule inhibitor of VEGF receptor tyrosine kinase activity, as an antiangiogenesis agent. *Anticancer Drug Design* **15**, 29–41.

Mohammadi, M., McMahon, G., Sun, L., Tang, C., Hirth, P., Yeh, B. K., Hubbard, S. R., and Schlessinger, J. (1997). Structure of the tyrosine kinase domain of fibroblast growth factor receptor in complex with inhibitors. *Science* **276**, 955–957.

Moran, R. G. (1992). Folate antimetabolites inhibitory to purine synthesis. In "New Drugs, Concepts and Results in Cancer Chemotherapy" (F. M. Muggia, ed.), pp. 65–87. Kluwer Academic Publishers, Boston, MA.

Nagase, H., and Woessner, J. F. (1999). Matrix metalloproteases. *J. Biol. Chem.* **274**, 21491–21494.

Newell, D. R., Arris, C. E., Boyle, F. T., Calvert, A. H., Curtin, N. J., Dewsbury, P., Endicott, J. A., Garman, E. F., Gibson, A. E., Golding, B. T., Griffin, R. J., Johnson, L. N., Lawrie, A., Noble, M. E. M., Sausville, E. A., and Schultz, R. (1999). Antiproliferative cyclin-dependent kinase inhibitors with distinct molecular interactions and tumor cell growth inhibition profiles. *Clin. Cancer Res.* **5**, 3755s.

Niwas, S., Chand, P., Pathak, V. P., et al. (1994). Structure-based design of inhibitors of purine nucleoside phosphorylase. 5. 9-Deazahypoxanthines. *J. Med. Chem.* **37**, 2477–2480.

Noble, M. E. M., and Endicott, J. A. (1999). Chemical inhibitors of cyclin-dependent kinases: insights into design from x-ray crystallographic studies. *Pharmacol. Ther.* **82**, 269–278.

Obst, U., Banner, D. W., Weber, L., and Diederich, F. (1997). Molecular recognition at the thrombin active site: structure-based design and synthesis of potent and selective thrombin inhibitors and the x-ray crystal structures of two thrombin-inhibitor complexes. *Chem. Biol.* **4**, 287–295.

Oesterhelt, F., Oesterhelt, D., Pfeiffer, M., Engel, A., Gaub, H. E., and Muller, D. J. (2000). Unfolding pathways of individual bacteriorhodopsins. *Science* **288**, 143–146.

Otto, H. H., and Schirmeister, T. (1997). Cysteine proteases and their inhibitors. *Chem. Rev.* **97**, 133–171.

Palmer, B. D., Trump-Kallmeyer, S., Fry, D. W., Nelson, J. M., Showalter, H. D. H, and Denny, W. A. (1997). Tyrosine kinase inhibitors. 11: Soluble analogues of pyrrolo- and pyrazoloquinazolines as epidermal growth factor receptor inhibitors: synthesis, biological evaluation, modeling of the mode of binding. *J. Med. Chem.* **40**, 1519–1529.

Peters, G. H., and Köhne, C. H. (1999). Fluoropyrimidines as antifolate drugs. In "Antifolate Drugs in Cancer Therapy" (A. L. Jackman, ed.), pp. 101–145. Humana Press, Totowa NJ.

Reich, S. H., and Webber, S. E. (1993). Structure-based drug design (SBDD): every structure tells a story. *Perspect. Drug Discovery Design* **1**, 371–390.

Roe, S. M., Prodromou, C., O'Brien, R., Ladbury, J. E., Piper, P. W., and Pearl, L. H. (1999). Structural basis for inhibition of the Hsp90 molecular chaperone by the antitumor antibiotics radicicol and geldanomycin. *J. Med. Chem.* **42**, 260–266.

Russo, A. A., Jeffrey, P. D., Patten, A. K., Massague, P., and Pavletich, N. P. (1996). Crystal structure of the p27Kip1 cyclin-dependent kinase inhibitor bound to the cyclin A–Cdk2 complex. *Nature* **382**, 325–331.

Sausville, E. A. (2000). Protein kinase antagonists: interim challenges and issues. *Anticancer Drug Design* **15**, 1–2.

Schulze-Gahmen, U., Brandsen, J., Jones, H. D., Morgan, D. O., Meijer, L., Vesely, J., and Kim, S. H. (1995). Multiple modes of ligand recognition: crystal structures of cyclin-dependent protein kinase 2 in complex with ATP and two inhibitors, olomoucine and isopentenyl-adenine. *Proteins Struct. Func. Gen.* **22**, 378–391.

Stams, T., Spurlino, J. C., Smith, D. L., Wahl, R. C., Ho, T. F., Qoronfleh, M. W., Banks, T. M., and Rubin, B. (1994). Structure of human neutrophil collagenase reveals large S1' specificity pocket. *Nat. Struct. Biol.* **1**, 119–123.

Varney, M. D., Marzoni, G. P., Palmer, C. L., et al. (1992). Crystal structure-based design and synthesis of benz[cd]indole-containing inhibitors of thymidylate synthase. *J. Med. Chem.* **35**, 663–676.

Varney, M. D., Palmer, C. L., Romines, W. H., et al. (1997). Protein structure-based design, synthesis, and biological evaluation of 5-thia-2,6-diamino-4-[3H]-oxopyrimidinones: inhibitors of glycinamide ribonucleotide transformylase with potent cell growth inhibition. *J. Med. Chem.* **40**, 2502–2524.

Veerapandian, P. (ed.) (1997). "Structure-Based Drug Design." Marcel Dekker, New York.

Verschoor, A., Srivastava, S., Grassucci, R., and Frank, J. (1996). Native 3D structure of eukaryotic 80S ribosome: morphological homology with the E. coli 70S ribosome. *J. Cell. Biol.* **133**, 495–505.

Webber, S. E., Bleckman, T. M., Attard, J., et al. (1993). Design of thymidylate synthase inhibitors using protein crystal structures: the synthesis and biological evaluation of a novel class of 5-substituted quinazolines. *J. Med. Chem.* **36**, 733–746.

Wittinghofer, A., and Pai, E. F. (1991). The structure of Ras protein: a model for a universal switch. *Trends Biochem. Sci.* **16**, 382–387.

Zhang, C. C., Boritzki, T. J., and Jackson, R. C. (1998). An inhibitor of glycinamide ribonucleotide formyltransferase is selectively cytotoxic to cells that lack a functional G_1 checkpoint. *Cancer Chemother. Pharmacol.* **41**, 223–228.

Zheng, J., Knighton, D. R., Ten Eyck, L. F., Darlsson, R., Xuong, N., Taylor, S. S., and Sowadski, J. M (1993). Crystal structure of the catalytic subunit of the cAMP Ser/Thr-dependent protein kinase complexed with MgATP and peptide inhibitor. *Biochemistry* **32**, 2154–2159.

CHAPTER 11

THE CONTRIBUTION OF SYNTHETIC ORGANIC CHEMISTRY TO ANTICANCER DRUG DEVELOPMENT

William A Denny

Auckland Cancer Society Research Centre

Faculty of Medical and Health Sciences

The University of Auckland

Auckland, New Zealand

Summary

Synthetic organic chemistry has always played a vital role in anticancer drug development, but the nature of its major contributions has varied over time. In the 1950s, knowledge of DNA metabolism allowed the semirational development of nucleotide mimics and antagonists. From about 1960 to 1985, random screening (of natural products and synthetics) was dominant, driven primarily by the large screening program of the U.S. National Cancer Institute. This empirical approach had merit when there were few targets besides DNA to focus on, but it also had drawbacks. The nature of the screens facilitated selection of antiproliferative cytotoxins, and natural products identified were usually too complex to be modified. The main value of natural-product screening is now as lead discovery, since quite complex structures can now be synthesised economically due to improvements in organic synthesis. Better ways of defining molecular structure in terms of numeric parameters allowed the development of quantitative relationships between drug structure and biological activity. Organic chemistry has also contributed many concepts to the rational design of drug classes, such as tumor-activated prodrugs of cytotoxins, especially for methods of deactivating the toxins. Finally, anticancer drug development in the genomics era again focuses on the random screening of massive numbers of compounds, using automated high-throughput screening against pure enzymes. Organic chemistry has responded by the development of combinatorial methods of synthesis, enabling the simultaneous preparation of large numbers of compounds. Initially used to prepare polypeptides, this has been adapted to the preparation of a wide range of compounds, including complex natural products.

1. Introduction

Synthetic organic chemistry has always been a vital part of the highly integrated and multidisciplinary process of anticancer drug development. However, the nature of its major contributions has varied over time. Its relative importance in driving changes in the philosophy of anticancer drug development has also waxed and waned in comparison with other disciplines such as biochemistry, enzymology, and molecular biology. This chapter describes the particular contributions of synthetic organic chemistry to the philosophy of anticancer drug development, using particular drug classes as illustrations.

2. Early Rationality

In the earliest days of chemotherapy, knowledge of DNA metabolism allowed pioneers such as George Hitchings, Gertrude Elion, and Charles Heidelberger to develop nucleotide mimics and antagonists, largely by rational design (Elion, 1989). This led to such drugs as 6-mercaptopurine (I), cytosine arabinoside (II), 5-fluorouracil (III), and methotrexate (IV), which are still widely used in cytotoxic chemotherapy. At about the same time, Haddow, Ross and others were exploring the family of nitrogen mustards, sparked by the initial observation of depression of white cell count in people exposed to the war gas bis(2-chloroethyl)amine (mustard gas; V). This led to the development of mechlorethamine (VI) (Goodman *et al.,* 1946) and the less vesicant analogue chlorambucil (VII), melphalan (VIII), and the still widely used cyclophosphamide (IX) (Colvin, 1999). Chemistry played a leading intellectual role in the development of these drugs. In the case of the mustards, a good understanding was gained of the relationships between structure, reactivity, potency, and efficacy (at least in forming the primary DNA lesions) (Wilman and Connors, 1983).

3. The Random Screening Era: Directly from Screen to Clinic

In the ensuing 25 years, from about 1960 to 1985, there was a great expansion of effort in seeking new anticancer

drugs, with much of this expended in more or less random screening of compounds. These included compounds isolated from natural sources as well as synthetic compounds usually produced for some other purpose. An important impetus to this work was the large screening program of the National Cancer Institute (Zee-Cheng and Cheng, 1988), which during that time evaluated approximately 600,000 materials (both pure compounds and crude extracts from synthetic and natural sources). The primary screen comprised mouse leukemia cell lines, both in culture but primarily implanted intraperitoneally in mice. About 300 compounds from this screen proceeded to some level of evaluation in humans, and 42 were approved by the U.S. Food and Drug Administration as available medicines (Zee-Cheng and Cheng, 1988). However, a much smaller number went on to become useful drugs.

In a time when there were few targets other than DNA to focus on, such an empirical approach had merit, but also drawbacks. Apart from the fact that screens of this nature selected out antiproliferative cytotoxins, whose main therapeutic edge was based on cytokinetics (selectivity for cycling cells rather than cancer cells), it made little creative use of synthetic organic chemistry in the drug development process. While state-of-the-art structural chemistry was required to elucidate the structures of the many cytotoxic natural products revealed by these screens, the compounds were usually so complex that neither the compounds themselves or their analogues could be economically produced by synthesis. This is well illustrated by compounds such as homoharringtonine (X) (Zhou *et al.,* 1995), maytansine (XI) (Issell and Crook, 1978; Hamel, 1992), vincristine (XII) (Zhou and Rahmani, 1992), halichondrin B (XIII) (Hamel, 1992; Munro *et al.,* 1999), and esperamicin A_1 (XIV) (Golik *et al.,* 1987; Smith and Nicolaou, 1996). The structural complexity of these compounds severely limited the development of improved analogues and, in many cases, the production of sufficient quantities of drug to be viable. Thus chemistry could not be utilized to optimize the potencies of these compounds at their cellular target or to improve their pharmacokinetic properties. Hits from the primary screen progressed through a complex eval-

uation pathway to the clinic without chemical modification, and often without knowledge of their mechanism of action, with a heavy emphasis being placed on absolute potency.

4. Organic Synthesis Catches Up: Development of Natural Product Leads

The "random screening" of natural products for their direct use as drugs was successful, introducing compounds such as anthracyclines (Hortobagyi, 1997), *Vinca* alkaloids (Zhou and Rahmani, 1992), epipodophyllotoxins (Damayanthi and Lown, 1998), and taxanes (Wall, 1998) into clinical use. However, its main value is now seen by many more in the discovery of new leads than in the direct procurement of clinical agents. This has come about partly because of a better understanding of the desirable physicochemical requirements of an anticancer drug, such as solubility, distributive properties, pharmacokinetics, and resistance to metabolism. There is no reason to expect that a natural product, evolved over millions of years to fulfill a particular function for its host, will have these properties optimized. This view has also been driven by the increasing power of modern synthetic organic chemistry. It is now much more likely that complex natural-product leads can be synthesized economically and therefore that analogues can be explored in an effort to optimize physicochemical properties. Two recent examples of the relatively rapid development of simpler clinical candidates from a complex natural-product lead are the cyclopropylindolines and the epothilones.

A. Cyclopropylindolines

In 1980, chemists at Upjohn determined the structure of the extraordinarily potent compound CC-1065 (XV) isolated from *Streptomcyes zelensis* (Martin *et al.,* 1980), and others later isolated related analogues (duocarmycins; e.g., XVI) from other *Streptomyces* species (Ichimura *et al.,* 1990). These compounds were shown to be very selective DNA alkylating agents, reacting only at adenine N3 sites in runs of adenines (Boger and Johnson, 1996). They demonstrated extraordinary cytotoxicity in cell culture (IC_{50} values down to 0.02 nM) and good antitumor activity in animal models at extremely low doses (Boger and Johnson, 1995, 1996). This high potency is thought to be due in part to their DNA-binding-induced activation, where a change in the conformation of the molecule as it binds to DNA disrupts its coplanar structure (Boger and Garbaccio, 1999). CC-1065 itself was shown to have chronic toxicity in animal models that prevented its further development (McGovren *et al.,* 1984). However, a large synthetic effort, devoted initially to the synthesis of CC-1065 itself (Kelly *et al.,* 1987; Boger and Coleman, 1988), allowed the preparation of other analogues such as adozelesin (XVII) (Li *et al.*, 1991) and carzelesin (XVIII) (Mealy and Castaner, 1996) which did not have this side effect, and these synthetic compounds went on to clinical trial (Cristofanilli *et al.*, 1999; Pavildis *et al.*, 2000). Many other analogues of the original natural products have now been prepared, including some designed for use in prodrug approaches (Atwell *et al.*, 1998) (see Section 7), by a variety of routes.

B. Microtubule-Stabilizing Agents

The microtubule stabilizing agent paclitaxel (XIX) is a major anticancer drug, originally isolated from the bark of the yew tree *Taxus baccata,* and is still produced from natural sources. More recently, other natural product microtubule-stabilizing agents have been reported, where organic synthesis has played a more important role. The cryptophycins are cyclic depsipeptide metabolites from cyanobacteria (Smith *et al.*, 1994), and their discovery sparked intensive synthetic studies (Liang *et al.*, 2000; Dhokte *et al.*, 1998), so that the first analogue to be tested clinically (cryptophycin-52; LY-355703) (XX) is a synthetic product (Panda *et al.*, 2000). Similarly, discovery (Bollag *et al.*, 1995; Gerth *et al.*, 1996) of the epothilones (e.g., epothilone A; XXI), metabolites from the myxobacterium *Sorangium cellulosum,* has sparked a similarly intensive synthetic effort (Harris and Danishefsky, 1999; Chappell *et al.*, 2000), allowing the development of synthetic analogues (e.g., desoxyepothilone B; XXII) with superior properties (Chou *et al.*, 1998). Comparison of structure–activity relationships for tubulin binding, together with binding models based

on crystal structure data, have allowed postulation of a "common pharmacophore" shared by both paclitaxel and epothilone analogues (Giannakakou *et al.*, 2000; He *et al.*, 2000).

5. Development of Synthetic Compounds: Structure–Activity Relationships

Many cytotoxic synthetic compounds were also discovered during the random screening period. These were usually much less complex molecules than the natural products. There were also substantial advances in synthetic chemistry methodology, especially in mild and selective methods for carbon–carbon bond formation (Luh *et al.*, 2000) and in selective protecting groups. The range of analogues of these leads that could be prepared and tested was thus greatly expanded. Furthermore, advances in physical-organic chemistry led to a better understanding of how to define molecular structure in terms of a series of quantifiable parameters. Properties such as molecular charge distribution, energies of molecular orbitals, and both local (substituent) and global (whole-molecule) electronic, steric, and hydrophobic effects were accurately parameterized (Hansch and Leo, 1979).

These advances provided the impetus for the development of quantitative structure–activity relationships (QSAR) for anticancer drugs, relating drug structure (defined in terms of the above parameters) to measures of biological activity such as cy-

XIX

XX

XXI: R = H
XXII: R = Me

XXIII

XXIV

totoxicity (Panthananickal *et al.*, 1979; Gupta, 1994), using the statistical methods originally developed by Hansch's group (Hansch *et al.*, 1996). For example, studies with aromatic nitrogen mustard alkylating agents (XXIII) quantified relationships between cytotoxicity and the electronic properties of substituents (R) (Panthananickal *et al.*, 1979; Palmer *et al.*, 1990) that were important in the design of hypoxia-selective drugs (Denny and Wilson, 1986) (see also Section 7). Similar QSAR studies with synthetic DNA-intercalating agents, especially the 9-anilinoacridines (XXIV), showed that their potency usually correlated positively with their strength of binding to DNA (Fink *et al.*, 1980; Denny *et al.*, 1982; Hartley *et al.*, 1988), resulting in a search for more tightly binding analogues. However, in this case the discovery that the antitumor activity of these compounds is due primarily to their ability to produce DNA strand breaks by interfering with the normal functioning of topoisomerase enzymes (Zwelling *et al.*, 1981; Drlica and Franko, 1988) showed that this relationship is not simple.

In addition to delineating structure–activity relationships for many individual classes of compounds, QSAR studies also provided more global information, including the likely

optimal lipophilicity for activity in particular cytotoxicity assays (Selassie *et al.*, 1986; Gupta, 1994). Approaches to minimize the effect of induced cellular resistance due to enhanced drug efflux were also suggested (Howbert *et al.*, 1990; Selassie *et al.*, 1990). Overall, the experience gained in this period in the application of QSAR ensured its acceptance as a standard tool in the development of anticancer drugs.

6. Immunotoxins: Synthetic Organic Chemistry Applied to Large Molecules

The first immunotoxins employed polypeptide cytotoxins or radioisotopes such as iodine-125 linked to monoclonal antibodies to improve delivery to tumor cells by antibody binding to tumor-associated antigens (Ghetie and Vitetta, 1994). Problems with this approach include difficulties in the consistent construction of suitable drug-antibody conjugates and the low proportion of toxin delivered (typically 0.001–0.01%), requiring very potent agents. The lack of toxin bystander effects to overcome the heterogeneity of clinical solid tumors (where many cells express little or no target antigen) was also a problem (Bodey *et al.*, 2000). However, this field is undergoing renewed interest, partly because of advances in organic chemistry that have provided more specific methods for stable linking of cytotoxins and antibodies (Carroll *et al.*, 1994). More efficient mechanisms of toxin cleavage in tumor tissue (DeFeo-Jones *et al.*, 2000) and very potent cytotoxins with good bystander effects, such as cyclopropylindoles (Charie *et al.*, 1995) and enediynes (Sievers *et al.*, 1999), have now been used.

7. Organic Synthesis in Rational Design: Tumor-Activated Prodrugs of Cytotoxins

This concept was devised to improve the specificity of the "classical" DNA-targeted systemic cytotoxins that essentially target cycling cell rather than tumor cell populations. Prodrugs can be defined as entities that are acted on in the body, either by chemical reactions or metabolism, resulting in formation of the desired, pharmacologically active species.

Tumor-activated prodrugs are systemic compounds that are activated selectively in tumor tissue by exploiting some unique physiologic, metabolic, or genetic difference between tumor and normal cells. The design of prodrug structures to meet the exacting set of criteria required draws heavily on concepts from synthetic organic chemistry. A modular approach to the design of such prodrugs has been suggested (Denny et al., 1996), where a "trigger" unit is joined to a separate "effector" unit by a "linker," resulting in deactivation of the effector until metabolism of the trigger (Fig. 1). One advantage of this approach is that the properties of the units can be optimized independently for their particular role. One of the main challenges is to learn how to control and thus optimize both the distributive properties of the prodrug and the bystander effects of the activated effector, by modulating their chemical properties. Again, this requires novel chemical approaches.

A. The Trigger Unit

The primary function of the trigger unit is to determine selectivity by undergoing tumor-specific metabolism and (when the activation mechanism is extracellular) by containing functionality that excludes the prodrug from cells. The required properties of the trigger depend on the mechanism of selective activation that is chosen. The main phenomena exploited for selective activation of prodrugs in tumor tissue are discussed below.

1. Tumor Hypoxia

Tumor hypoxia is now recognized as a consistent and unique property of cells in solid tumors, as a result of a disorganized microvascular system in tumors (Vaupel et al., 1991; Brizel et al., 1994). Hypoxic cells in tumors limit response to radiation therapy (and some chemotherapy) and drive key aspects of tumor progression, such as angiogenesis and the selection of p53 mutations (Brown and Giaccia, 1998). Triggers for hypoxia-activated prodrugs are substrates for endogenous one-electron reductases such as cytochrome P450 reductase (Patterson et al., 1998). The initial one-electron adducts formed by these compounds are rapidly back-oxidized by free oxygen in normal tissue to form the parent prodrug in a futile metabolism cycle. However, in hypoxic cells the one-electron adducts undergo further irreversible reduction or rearrangement to give cytotoxic species. Units used as triggers include nitroaromatics (e.g., in CB-

1954; XXV) (Knox et al., 1993), aliphatic N-oxides (e.g., in AQ4N; XXVI) (Patterson et al., 2000), transition metal complexes (e.g., in SN-24771; XXVII) (Ware et al., 1993), anthraquinones (e.g., in porfiromycin; XXVIII) (Haffty et al., 1997), and aromatic di-N-oxides (e.g., in tirapazamine; XXIX) (Brown and Wang, 1998). Compounds using the latter two triggers, porfiromycin and tirapazamine, are in clinical trial as hypoxia-selective drugs, with tirapazamine showing particular promise (Denny and Wilson, 2000).

2. Lower Extracellular pH

Tumor cells in solid tumors consistently have lower extracellular pH levels than normal tissues because of the inefficient clearance of metabolic acids from chronically hypoxic cells (Tannock and Rotin, 1989). However this difference (0.6–0.8 pH unit) is small in chemical terms and has proved difficult to exploit. One interesting approach used releases a phosphoramide mustard from the sugar acetal (XXX) (Tietze et al., 1989).

3. Therapeutic Radiation

In principle, prodrugs can be activated by use of the reducing species produced from the radiolysis of water by ionizing radiation (Wilson et al., 1998b). This obviates the need to rely on what may be variable levels of endogenous activating enzymes. However, a therapeutic dose of radiation (about 2 Gy) generates only a very small amount of reducing equivalents. This requires prodrugs with very efficient trigger units to capture these, substances capable of releasing/activating very potent effectors in an oxygen-inhibited process (Wilson et al., 1998b). The design of such agents requires novel chemistry; for example, heterocyclic quaternary ammonium salts may be suitable triggers (Wilson et al., 1998a).

4. Exogenous Enzymes; ADEPT and GDEPT Strategies

There are methodologies for either specifically locating (antibody-directed enzyme-prodrug therapy; ADEPT) or specifically generating (gene-directed enzyme-prodrug therapy; GDEPT) a nonhuman enzyme on tumor cells, and using this to selectively and catalytically activate a prodrug. In ADEPT, the enzyme is delivered as an antibody-enzyme conjugate that locates preferentially on tumor cells (Syrigos and Epenetos, 1999). In GDEPT, gene therapy methods are used to express the foreign enzyme preferentially in tumor cells (Denny and Wilson, 1998). In these approaches, the selected enzyme must efficiently and selectively metabolize the trigger unit.

B. The Linker Unit

This must deactivate the effector in the intact prodrug yet rapidly transmit an activating signal on metabolism of the trigger (Denny et al., 1996). Several concepts for linkers have been explored, drawn from mechanistic organic chemistry:

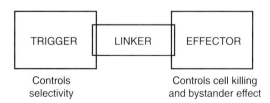

FIGURE 1   Modular design of hypoxia-activated prodrugs.

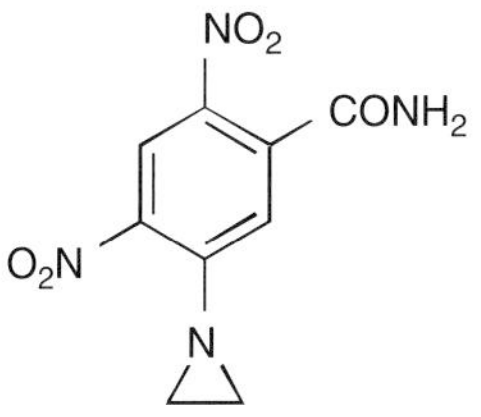

XXV

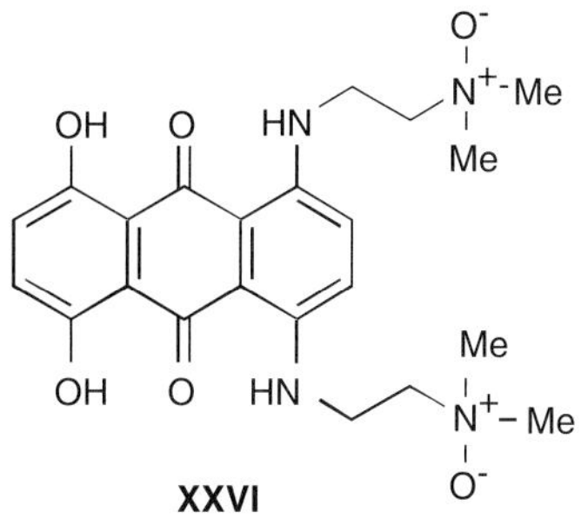

XXVI

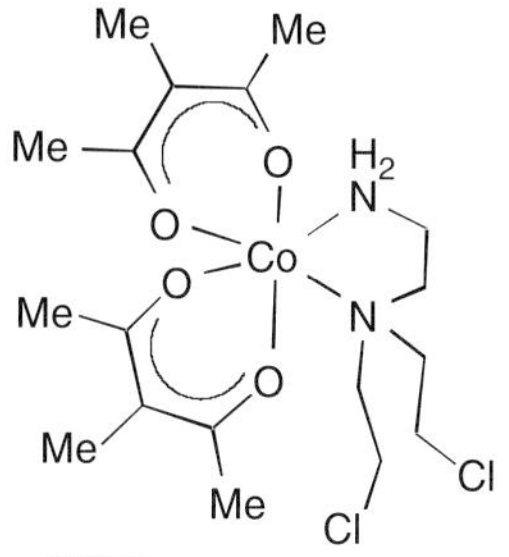

XXVII

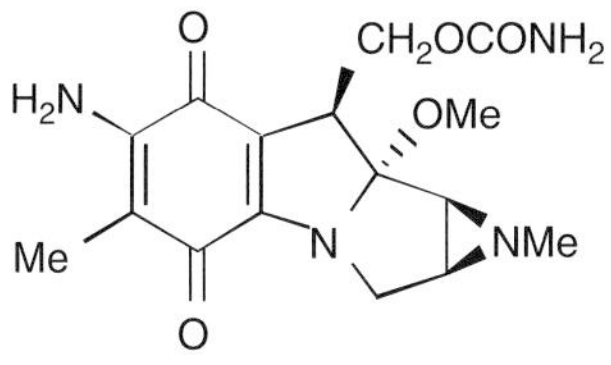

XXVIII

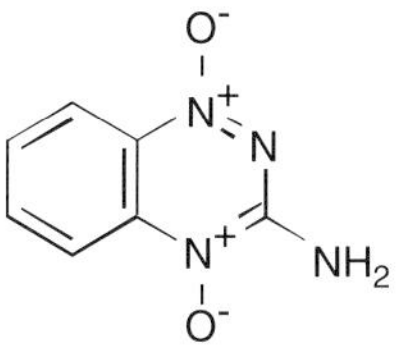

XXIX

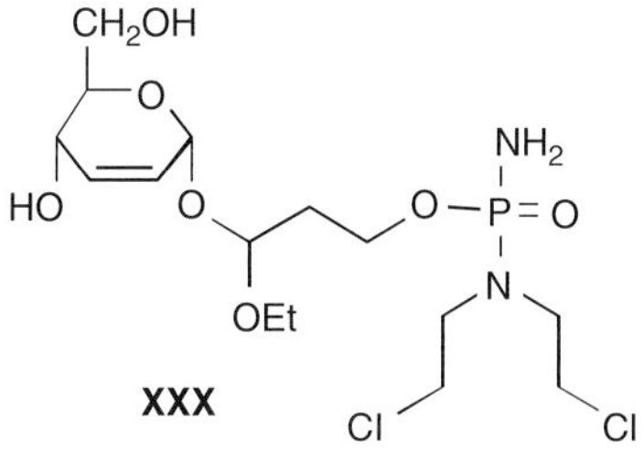

XXX

1. Electron Release through an Aromatic System

Structure–activity relationship studies with aromatic nitrogen mustards have shown the high dependence of cytotoxicity on electron density at the mustard nitrogen (Panthananickal et al., 1979; Palmer et al., 1990). Thus, reduction of an electron-withdrawing nitro group to highly electron-donating hydroxylamine or amine groups on an aromatic system results in very large and instantaneous changes in electron redistribution, which can provide a large increase in the cytotoxicity of prepositioned groups. Thus, the simple 4-aminoaniline mustard (XXXI) is 17,000-fold more cytotoxic (CT_{10} clonogenic assay, UV4 cells) than its 4-nitro precursor (XXXII) (Palmer et al., 1990).

2. Generation of Cationic Species

The concept of cation masking arose from knowledge about the chemical properties of tertiary amine N-oxides, which have much lower pK_a values (up to 5 pK_a units) than the amines themselves. This has led to the development of N-oxide prodrugs of DNA intercalating agents, which are much less toxic due to loss of the DNA binding ability normally conferred by the cationic tertiary amine (Wilson et al., 1992). The hypoxia-selective prodrug AQ4N (XXVI) (Patterson et al., 2000) is of this type.

3. Induced "Through-bond" Fragmentation

Charge-transfer reactions resulting in fragmentation of a molecule are well known in organic chemistry and have been adapted to the development of prodrugs. The best known examples are the 4-nitrobenzyl carbamates, wherein reduction to the corresponding 4-hydroxylamines is followed by fragmentation, because the increased electron release to the π system stabilizes

the developing positive charge on the benzylic carbon (Hay et al., 1999b) (Fig. 2). For example, 4-nitrobenzyl carbamate derivatives (XXXII, XXXIV) of mitomycin C (Mauger et al., 1994) and amino-CBI (Hay et al., 1999a) respectively are substrates for the nitroreductase from E. coli and show higher potencies in cell lines transfected with this enzyme. The kinetics of the fragmentation of the intermediate 4-hydroxylamines has been studied in a model system and can be modulated by additional substituents on the aromatic ring (Hay et al., 1999b).

4. Induced "Through-space" Intramolecular Cyclization

Mechanisms related to the above but whereby the fragmentation is induced by "through-space" electronic interactions also have many parallels in organic chemistry, and allow electronic uncoupling of the trigger and effector units.

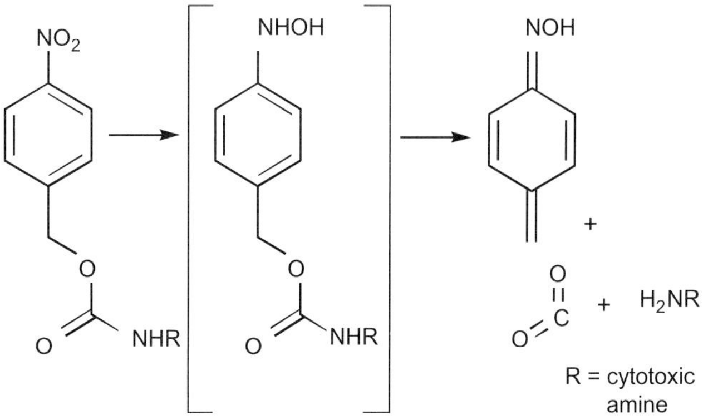

R = cytotoxic amine

FIGURE 2 "Through-bond" fragmentation of reduced 4-nitrobenzyl carbamates.

For example, the prodrug (XXXV) (Sykes *et al.,* 1999), with a *N*-(2,6-dinitrophenyl)amino trigger, is based on a concept used previously for the sequential cleavage of peptide bonds (Kirk and Cohen, 1969). H-bond "locking" by the second nitro group correctly positions the initial hydroxylamine or amine for fast cyclization/extrusion, resulting in facile cyclization even of very electron-deficient amines. Reduction of the nitroquinoline (XXXVI) was postulated to result in a related base-catalyzed through-space rearrangement, releasing a phosphoramide cytotoxin (Firestone *et al.,* 1991).

C. The Effector Unit

This requires a chemistry that allows it to be substantially deactivated in the prodrug form, but in the active form to be a potent cytotoxin capable of killing cells under a variety of pH and oxygen levels, and at all phases of the cell cycle. It is also required to have a substantial bystander effect (the ability to diffuse some distance from the cell where it is generated to kill surrounding tumor cells). This allows for the fact that only a small proportion of cells in a tumor may be capable of activating a particular prodrug. The most widely employed effectors have been DNA-alkylating agents, which

have a well-defined chemistry and fulfill many of the above criteria (Denny and Wilson, 1993).

8. Early Genomics: Inhibitors of Transmembrane Tyrosine Kinases

During the 1990s, the overexpressed or mutated protein products of many oncogenes were identified and characterized, in work that significantly preceded the Human Genome Project. Many of these proteins were enzymes in the growth signal transduction pathways in cells, and particularly the transmembrane tyrosine kinases that initiate these pathways (Sedlacek, 2000). The development of specific small-molecule inhibitors of the intracellular kinase domains of these enzymes has been one of the major anticancer success stories of the second half of the 1990s and represents a major move away from drugs targeted at DNA function (Gibbs, 2000). The rapid development of this new class of agents has been achieved by mass screening in high-throughput isolated enzyme assays for initial leads, followed by optimization of these leads in the same assays. Analogues were prepared by a combination of classical one-at-a-time (singleton) synthesis and combinatorial synthesis methods (see Section 9), with the latter becoming increasingly important. Development has also been greatly assisted by the availability of crystal structures (or derived computer models) of enzyme–inhibitor complexes.

An illustrative example of these points is the development of inhibitors of the epidermal growth factor receptor, a member of the *erbB* family of transmembrane tyrosine kinases (Daly, 1999). Initial leads with moderate potencies in the enzyme assay were rapidly developed into extraordinarily potent and selective inhibitors (e.g., PD-153035; XXXVII; IC$_{50}$ 0.029 nM) (Fry *et al.*, 1994; Bridges *et al.*, 1996). Work in several laboratories led to the development of the clinical agents Iressa (XXXVIII) (Ciardello *et al.*, 2000) and CP-358774 (XXXIX) (Moyer *et al.*, 1997). Later studies of the enzyme binding mode of these compounds led to the development of the irreversible inhibitor CI-1033 (XL) (Smaill *et al.*, 2000; Bridges, 1999), by appropriate positioning of a weak alkylating agent to pick up a unique cysteine residue (cys773) in the enzyme binding site. Another drug resulting from this new approach now in clinical trial is STI-571 (XLI) targeted at *c-abl* kinase (Schindler *et al.*, 2000). Also in development are compounds targeted against later enzymes in these pathways (MEK, ERK) (Gould and Stephano, 2000), and against the cyclin kinases that control the cell cycle checkpoints (Senderowicz and Sausville, 2000).

This work has shown that medicinal chemistry can be used to rapidly refine leads, achieving large increases in potency in isolated enzyme assays. However, it must be remembered that these screens do not provide information on the effectiveness of the compounds in living hosts. Thus, a constant emphasis on "drug-like" structures and early pharmacokinetic screening of representative analogues is important.

9. The Genomics/Proteomics Era: Combinatorial Chemistry

The imminent completion of the Human Genome Project (identification of all human genes) and the subsequent delineation of their function is expected to lead to the addition of a plethora of potential new enzyme targets for anticancer drugs, in addition to those uncovered recently (see Section 8). Rapid exploitation of this multiplicity of targets will require greater use of the various combinatorial methods of drug synthesis that have been developed over the last few years.

Combinatorial synthesis allows the rapid preparation of large numbers (libraries) of related compounds. The concept arose originally from the Merrifield solid-phase synthesis of peptides, and most of the first libraries were of polypeptides or oligonucleotides. However, more recently the technique

XXXVII

XXXVIII

XXXIX

XL

XLI

has expanded to cover many other types of small molecules, particularly heterocycles (Nefzi *et al.,* 1997). In conjunction with high-throughput screening, usually against purified enzyme targets, combinatorial synthesis has greatly influenced the way in which drugs are discovered and developed. Over the period from 1992 to 1999, the synthesis of 975 distinct libraries of compounds was reported in the literature (Dolle, 2000). Of the 240 for which biological data were reported, only a small proportion (less than 14%) were of cytotoxic anticancer drugs, but this proportion will presumably increase as enzyme inhibitors become a major class of anticancer drugs (see Section 8).

The basic idea behind combinatorial synthesis is to rapidly generate libraries of compound with chemical diversity. Two main types of libraries can be distinguished: discovery libraries and optimization libraries. Discovery libraries are large (arbitrarily defined as more than 5000 members) (Dolle, 2000) and not prepared against any preconceived target. The main aims in such libraries, which are used for primary screening for hits against new targets, is that members should be "drug-like" and as chemically diverse as possible. Optimization libraries are smaller, and the main aims are to improve the "drug-like" properties (potency, selectivity, solubility, pharmacokinetics, etc.) of some lead molecule.

While definition of drug-like character is difficult, the simple "rule-of-five" developed by Lipinski *et al.* (1997) is easy to apply as a rough guideline. This states that the lipophilicity (computed by the program CLOGP) should be less than 5, the molecular weight should be less than 500, the number of H-bond donor groups should be less than 5, and the number of H-bond acceptor groups should be less than 10. More sophisticated computer models that compare structure with data parameters constructed from existing drugs are also available (Wang and Ramnarayan, 1999; Frimurer *et al.,* 2000). True diversity in these larger sets is also hard to achieve; while computer programs to maximize this have been devised (Koehler and Villar, 2000), library diversity is often compromised by the availability of starting materials and the scope of the reactions employed.

A. Methods of Combinatorial Chemistry

Combinatorial chemistry is now a huge subject, and much has been written about the various concepts for library generation, as well as their strengths and weaknesses (Thompson and Ellman, 1996; Lam, 1997; Nefzi *et al.,* 1997; Pirrung, 1997). Most of the focus has been on "solid-phase" synthesis, since the concept arose originally from the Merrifield resin-attached approach to the synthesis of peptides. In this, temporary covalent attachment of the first building block to a resin allowed the stepwise construction of long polypeptides in an automatable fashion, with excess reagents being washed away after each step. Cleavage of the initial resin-building block bond allowed easy isolation of a pure, homogeneous product (Fig. 3).

The shift to true combinatorial synthesis (initially of peptides but later of other molecules) came with the "split-and-mix" concept, which allowed the preparation of very large libraries (Furka *et al.,* 1991; Lam *et al.,* 1991). In this method (Fig. 4), the first component is attached to small (100 μm) resin beads by a cleavable linkage, and the beads are divided into n equal portions. Each portion is then reacted with one of n different second components. After the reaction the individual portions are then remixed and redivided for a further round of treatment. After x such split-and-mix reaction cycles the beads will contain n^x different compounds, but each bead will contain only one pure compound (the "one-bead-one-compound" concept; Lam *et al.,* 1991). While peptide libraries built in this way are usually linear in nature, there is more scope with small-molecule libraries, where branched and scaffolded libraries can be constructed (Lam, 1997).

There are many methods for biological screening of the products from combinatorial libraries. For products designed to bind to enzyme receptors, enzyme-linked colorimetric as-

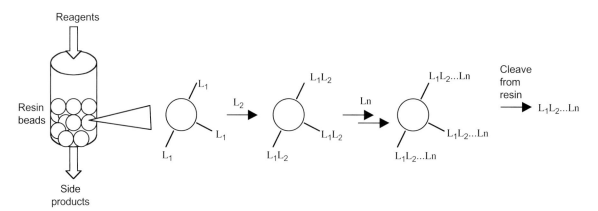

FIGURE 3 Concept of automated solid-phase synthesis.

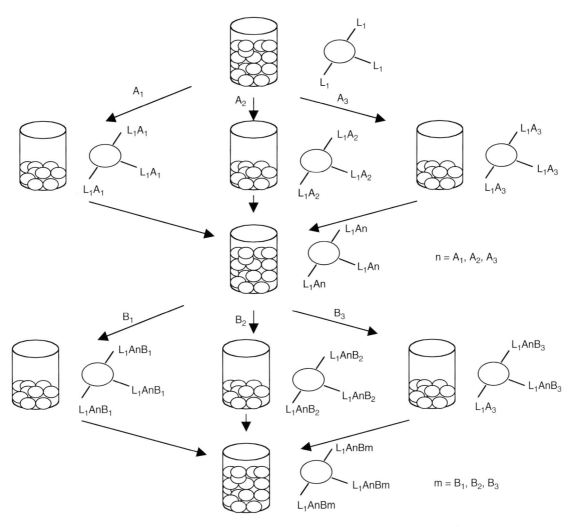

FIGURE 4   Concept of "split and mix, one-bead-one-compound," solid-phase synthesis.

says can be used to pick out individual "active" beads, where the synthesized compounds are still attached to the beads (Lam *et al.*, 1991). An ingenious approach (Salmon *et al.*, 1996) for screening using cellular cytotoxicity assays (of particular value for anticancer drugs) is to attach the compounds to the beads using two different linkers that release the compounds at different pHs. The beads are plated with tumor cells in soft agarose, and one of the linkers is cleaved at the resulting neutral pH, so that any active compounds released cause a zone of lysis around the bead. These beads can then be recovered, and the remaining compound still attached by the second linker can be cleaved and analyzed to determine its structure.

Many other methods of separately "tagging" beads to record their history and thus allow "deconvolution" of the library, allowing determination of the structure of the particular compound attached to a particular bead, have been reported (Lam *et al.*, 1997; Fitch *et al.*, 1999). These include the use of polynucleotides (Needels *et al.*, 1993) and small polypeptides (Kerr

et al., 1993), for which there are routine and sensitive detection methods. Tags more compatible with organic reagents include halocarbons (determined by gas chromatography after silylation) (Burbaum *et al.*, 1995) and alkylamines (recovered by hydrolysis, dansylated and analyzed by high-performance liquid chromatography) (Ni *et al.*, 1996). More recently, radiofrequency transmitting chips have been used to encode the chemical reaction history of each bead (Moran *et al.*, 1995). These have the advantage of nondestructive readout but are expensive. Smaller optimization libraries are often produced by solution-phase parallel synthesis, avoiding the deconvolution problem altogether (Schrieber, 2000).

B. Application of Combinatorial Chemistry to Anticancer Drugs

As for many applications, a good proportion of anticancer agent combinatorial libraries are on-bead libraries of peptides or peptidomimetics. Recent examples include synthetic epitopes for tumor-specific cytotoxic T lymphocytes (Linneman *et al.*, 1998), mimics of the tumor-associated antigen sialyl-Lewis A (Insug *et al.*, 1999), *O*-phosphotyrosyl surrogate-containing p56lck SH2-domain-binding peptides (Broadbridge and Sharma, 1999), peptide aptamers designed for E2F's DNA binding and dimerization domains (Fabrizio *et al.*, 1999), and peptidomimetic ligands for the pp60c-src substrate binding site (Orfi *et al.*, 1999; Maly *et al.*, 2000) and for farnesyl-protein transferase (Wallace *et al.*, 1996).

Smaller libraries of relatively simple nonpeptide compounds have largely been prepared by classical solution-phase parallel synthesis methods. Recent examples include analogues of aspergillamide (XLII) (Beck and Hess, 2000), piperazine-2,5-diones (XLIII) (Loughlin *et al.*, 2000), 2,5-diphenyloxazole-based inhibitors of Cdc25 phosphatase (XLIV) (Ducruet *et al.*, 2000), disulfide inhibitors of the thioredoxin redox system (XLV) (Kirkpatrick *et al.*, 1999), and 2,6,9-trisubstituted purines as CDK inhibitors (Chang *et al.*, 1999). Libraries of paclitaxel C7 esters (Bhat *et al.*, 1998) and benzodiazepines (as c-Src inhibitors) (Ramdas *et al.*, 1999) prepared by this method have also been reported. The technique has also been extended to the synthesis of tetraphenylporphyrins as potential photodynamic anticancer drugs (Berlin *et al.*, 1998).

Libraries of more complex molecules, requiring a greater number of steps to be performed, have been constructed using solid-phase synthesis. A series of 7α-alkylamide estradi-

ols (e.g., XLVI) were prepared as estrogen receptor antagonists derivatives on an aminomethyl resin via a photolabile *o*-nitrobenzyl linker (Tremblay *et al.*, 1999). Finally, the total syntheses by Nicolaou's laboratory of libraries of analogues of the natural-product microtubule-stabilizing agents epothilone (XXI) (Nicolaou *et al.*, 1997a, 1997b) and sarcodictyin (XLVII) (Nicolaou *et al.*, 1998) by solid-phase parallel synthesis, and the recent report by Hecht's group (Leitheiser *et al.*, 2000) of the solid-phase synthesis of two deglycobleomycin analogues, indicate the combined power of this technique and modern organic synthesis to rapidly optimize the activity of very complex molecules.

10. Conclusion

The role of synthetic organic chemistry in the development of anticancer drugs has changed over time as the power of the synthetic techniques has increased and as it has adapted to other changes in drug development. In the random screening era, particularly for natural products, the role of organic chemistry was primarily isolation and structure determination. A great deal of work on the total synthesis of such natural products was carried out, and this greatly helped to develop the power of modern organic synthesis. However, these syntheses were not generally economically competitive with purification from natural sources. The availability of analogues to allow the development of structure–activity relationships was also limited. In contrast, the easier preparation of analogues of the synthetic compounds discovered during this same era allowed the exploration of detailed structure–activity relationship studies, and these served to develop the tools of compound paramerization, molecular diversity, and QSAR modeling that have become standard tools of drug design.

More recently, the increasing power of synthetic organic chemistry has resulted in economic total syntheses of complex natural products, making these (and their possibly improved analogues) available in sufficient quantities to allow their clinical development. Natural products will thus increasingly serve as ideas for the development of anticancer drugs, rather than the drugs themselves. In addition, organic chemistry continues to provide novel concepts for the development of new types of anticancer drugs; a good example is the tumor-activated prodrugs.

The field of organic chemistry has also responded to the molecular biology revolution, which is in the process of identifying many new enzymes as potential targets for anticancer drugs, by the development of combinatorial methods for the simultaneous or parallel preparation of large numbers of compounds to accelerate drug discovery. In the process it is also developing the discrimination tools that will hopefully allow the preparation of compound libraries of diverse but "drug-like" structures. Recent work suggests that even very complex natural products and their analogues (epothilones, bleomycins) can be prepared by combinatorial methods. This will allow the development of much more detailed structure–activity relationships in order to optimize the anticancer activities of these compounds.

References

Atwell, G. J., Tercel, M., Boyd, M., Wilson, W. R., and Denny, W.A. (1998). Synthesis and cytotoxicity of 5-amino-1-(chloromethyl)-3-[(5,6,7-trimethoxyindol-2-yl)carbonyl]-1,2-dihydro-3H-benz[e]indole (amino-seco-CBI-TMI) and related 5-alkylamino analogues: new DNA minor groove alkylating agents. J. Org. Chem. 63, 9414–9420.

Beck, B., and Hess, S. (2000). One-pot synthesis and biological evaluation of aspergillamides. Bioorg. Med. Chem. Lett. 10, 1701–1705.

Berlin, K., Jain, R. K., and Richert, C. (1998). Are porphyrin mixtures favorable photodynamic anticancer drugs? A model study with combinatorial libraries of tetraphenylporphyrins. Biotechnol. Bioeng. 61, 107–118.

Bhat, L., Liu, Y., Victory, S. F., Himes, R. H., and Georg, G. I. (1998). Synthesis and evaluation of paclitaxel C7 derivatives: solution phase synthesis of combinatorial libraries. Bioorg. Med. Chem. Lett. 8, 3181–3186.

Bodey, B., Bodey, B., Jr., Siegel, S. E., and Kaiser, H. E. (2000). Genetically engineered monoclonal antibodies for direct anti-neoplastic treatment and cancer cell specific delivery of chemotherapeutic agents. Curr. Pharm. Des. 6, 261–276.

Boger, D. L., and Coleman, R. S. (1988). Total synthesis of (+)-CC-1065 and ent-(-)-CC-1065. J. Am. Chem. Soc. 110, 1321–1323.

Boger, D. L., and Garbaccio, R. M. (1999). Shape-dependent catalysis: insights into the source of catalysis for the CC-1065 and duocarmycin DNA alkylation reaction. Acc. Chem. Res. 32, 1043–1052.

Boger, D. L., and Johnson, D. S. (1995). CC-1065 and the duocarmycins: unraveling the keys to a new class of naturally derived DNA alkylating agents. Proc. Natl. Acad. Sci. USA 92, 3642–3649.

Boger, D. L., and Johnson, D. S. (1996). CC-1065 and the duocarmycins: understanding their biological function through mechanistic studies. Angew. Chem., Int. Ed. Engl. 35, 1438–1474.

Bollag, D. M., McQueney, P. A., Zhu, J., Hensens, O., Koupal, L., Liesch, J., Goetz, M., Lazarides, E., and Woods, C. M. (1995). Epothilones, a new class of microtubule-stabilizing agents with a taxol-like mechanism of action. Cancer Res. 55, 2325–2333.

Bridges, A. J. (1999). The rationale and strategy used to develop a series of highly potent, irreversible, inhibitors of the epidermal growth factor receptor family of tyrosine kinases. Curr. Med. Chem. 6, 825–843.

Bridges, A. J., Zhou, H., Cody, D. R., Rewcastle, G. W., McMichael, A., Showalter, H. D. H., Fry, D. W., Kraker, A. J., and Denny, W. A. (1996). Tyrosine kinase inhibitors. 8. An unusually steep structure-activity relationship for analogues of 4-(3-bromoanilino)-6,7-dimethoxyquinazoline (PD 153035), a potent inhibitor of the epidermal growth factor receptor. J. Med. Chem. 39, 267–276.

Brizel, D. M., Rosner, G. L., Harrelson, J., Prosnitz, L. R., and Dewhirst, M. W. (1994). Pretreatment oxygenation profiles of human soft tissue sarcomas. Int. J. Radiat. Oncol. Biol. Phys. 30, 635–642.

Broadbridge, R. J., and Sharma, P. P. (1999). p56lck SH2 domain binding motifs from bead binding screening of peptide libraries containing phosphotyrosine surrogates. Lett. Pept. Sci. 6, 335–341.

Brown, J. M., and Giaccia, A. J. (1998). The unique physiology of solid tumors: opportunities (and problems) for cancer chemotherapy. Cancer Res. 58, 1405–1416.

Brown, J. M., and Wang, L. H. (1998). Tirapazamine: laboratory data relevant to clinical activity. Anticancer Drug Des. 13, 529–539.

Burbaum, J. J., Ohlmeyer, M. H. J., Reader, J. C., Henderson, I., Dillard, L. W., Li, G., Randle, T. L., Sigal, N. H., Chelsky, D., and Baldwin, J. J. (1995). A paradigm for drug discovery employing encoded combinatorial libraries. Proc. Natl. Acad. Sci. USA 92, 6027–6031.

Carroll, S. F., Bernhard, S. L., Goff, D.A., Bauer, R. J., Leach, W., and Kung, A. H. C. (1994). Enhanced stability in vitro and in vivo of immunoconjugates prepared with 5 methyl-2-iminothiolane. Bioconjugate Chem. 5, 248–256.

Chang, Y-T., Gray, N. S., Rosania, G. R., Sutherlin, D. P., Kwon, S., Norman, T. C., Sarohia, R., Leost, M., Meijer, L., and Schultz, P. G. (1999). Synthesis and application of functionally diverse 2,6,9-trisubstituted purine libraries as CDK inhibitors. Chem. Biol. 6, 361–375.

Chappell, M. D., Stachel, S. J., Lee, C. B., and Danishefsky, S. J. (2000). A En route to a plant scale synthesis of the promising antitumor agent 12,13-desoxyepothilone B. Org. Lett. 2, 1633–1636.

Charie, R. V. J., Jackel, K. A., Bourret, L. A., Derr, S. M., Tadayoni, B. M., Mattocks, K. M., Shah, S. A., Liu, C. N., Blattler, W. A., and Goldmacher, V. S. (1995). Enhancement of the selectivity and antitumor efficacy of a CC-1065 analogue through immunoconjugate formation. Cancer Res. 55, 4079–4084.

Chou, T. C., Zhang, X. G., Balog, A., Su, D. S., Meng, D., Savin, K., Bertino, J. R., and Danishefsky, S. J. (1998). Desoxyepothilone B: an efficacious microtubule-targeted antitumor agent with a promising in vivo profile relative to epothilone B. Proc. Natl. Acad. Sci. USA 95, 9642–9647.

Ciardiello, F., Caputo, R., Bianco, R., Damiano, V., Pomatico, G., De Placido, S., Bianco, A. R., and Tortora, G. (2000). Antitumor effect and potentiation of cytotoxic drugs activity in human cancer cells by ZD-1839 (Iressa), an epidermal growth factor receptor-selective tyrosine kinase inhibitor. Clin. Cancer Res. 6, 2053–2063.

Colvin, O. M. (1999). An overview of cyclophosphamide development and clinical applications. Curr. Pharm. Des. 5, 555–560.

Cristofanilli, M., Bryan, W. J., Miller, L. L., Chang, A. Y-C, Gradishar, W. J., Kufe, D. W., and Hortobagyi, G. N. (1998). Phase II study of adozelesin in untreated metastatic breast cancer. Anticancer Drugs 9, 779–782.

Daly, R. J. (1999). Take your partners, please—signal diversification by the erbB family of receptor tyrosine kinases. *Growth Factors* **16,** 255–263.

Damayanthi, Y., and Lown, J. W. (1998). Podophyllotoxins: current status and recent developments. *Curr. Med. Chem.* **5,** 205–252.

DeFeo-Jones, D., Garsky, V. M., Wong, B. K., Feng, D-M., Bolyar, T., and Haskel, K. (2000). A peptide-doxorubicin 'prodrug' activated by prostate-specific antigen selectively kills prostate tumor cells positive for prostate-specific antigen in vivo. *Nat. Med.* **6,**1248–1252.

Denny, W. A., Atwell, G. J., Cain, B. F., Leo, A., Panthananickal, A., and Hansch, C. (1982). Potential Antitumor Agents. Part 36. Quantitative relationships between antitumor potency, toxicity and structure for the general class of 9-anilinoacridine antitumor agents. *J. Med. Chem.* **25,** 276–316.

Denny. W. A., Wilson. W. R., and Hay, M. P. (1996). Recent developments in the design of bioreductive drugs. *Br. J. Cancer* **74** (Suppl. 17), 32–38.

Denny, W. A., and Wilson, W. R. (1986). Considerations for the design of nitrophenyl mustards as drugs selectively toxic for hypoxic mammalian cells. *J. Med. Chem.,* **29,** 879–887.

Denny, W. A., and Wilson, W. R. (1993). Bioreducible mustards: a paradigm for hypoxia-selective prodrugs of diffusible cytotoxins (HPDCs). *Cancer Metab. Rev.* **12,** 135–151.

Denny, W. A., and Wilson, W. R. (1998). The design of selectively-activated anti-cancer prodrugs for use in antibody-directed and gene-directed enzyme-prodrug therapies. *J. Pharm. Pharmacol.* **50,** 387–394.

Denny, W. A., and Wilson, W. R. (2000). Tirapazamine: a bioreductive anticancer drug which exploits tumor hypoxia. *Exp. Opin. Inv. Drugs,* **9,** 2889–2901.

Dhokte, U. P., Khau, V. V., Hutchison, D. R., and Martinelli, M. J. (1998). A novel approach for total synthesis of cryptophycins via asymmetric crotylboration protocol. *Tetrahedron Lett.* **39,** 8771–8774.

Dolle, R. E. (2000). Comprehensive survey of combinatorial library synthesis: 1999. *J. Comb. Chem.* **2,** 383–433.

Drlica, K., and Franko, R. J. (1988). Inhibitors of DNA topoisomerases. *Biochemistry* **27,** 2253–2259.

Ducruet, A. P., Rice, R. L., Tamura, K., Yokokawa, F., Yokokawa, S., Wipf, P., and Lazo, J..S. (2000). Identification of new dual specificity phosphatase inhibitors in a targeted small molecule array. *Bioorg. Med. Chem.* **8,** 1451–1466.

Elion, G. B. (1989). Nobel Lecture. The purine path to chemotherapy. *Bioscience Rep.* **9,** 509–529.

Fabrizio, E., Le Cam, L., Polanowska, J., Kaczorek, M., Lamb, N., Brent, R., and Sardet, C. (1999). Inhibition of mammalian cell proliferation by genetically selected peptide aptamers that functionally antagonize E2F activity. *Oncogene* **18,** 4357–4363.

Fink, S. I., Leo, A., Yamakawa, M., Hansch, C., and Quinn, F. R. (1980). The quantitative structure-selectivity relationship of anthracycline antitumor activity and cardiac toxicity. *Farmaco* **35,** 965–979.

Firestone, A., Mulcahy, R. T., and Borch, R.F. (1991). Nitroheterocycle reduction as a paradigm for intramolecular catalysis of drug delivery to hypoxic cells. *J. Med. Chem.* **31,** 2933–2935.

Fitch, W. I , Baer, T. A., Chen, W., Holden, F., Holmes, C. P., Maclean, D., Shah, N., Sullivan, E., Tang, M., and Waybourn, P. (1999). Improved methods for encoding and decoding dialkylamine-encoded combinatorial libraries. *J. Comb. Chem.* **1,** 188–194.

Frimurer, T. M., Bywater, R., Nrum, L., Lauritsen, L. N., and Brunak, S. (2000). Improving the odds in discriminating "drug-like" from "non drug-like" compounds. *J. Chem. Inf. Comput. Sci.* **40,** 1315–1324.

Fry, D. W., Kraker, A. J., McMichael, A., Ambroso, L. A., Nelson, J. M., Leopold, W. R., Connors, R. W., and Bridges, A.J. (1994). A specific inhibitor of the epidermal growth factor receptor tyrosine kinase. *Science* **265,** 1093–1095.

Furka, A., Sebestyen, F., Asgedom, M., and Dibo, G. (1991). General method for rapid synthesis of multicomponent peptide mixtures. *Int. J. Pept. Protein Res.* **37,** 487–493.

Gerth, K., Bedorf, N., Hoefle, G., Irschik, H., and Reichenbach, H. (1996). Antibiotics from gliding bacteria. 74. Epothilons A and B: antifungal and cytotoxic compounds from *Sorangium cellulosum* (Myxobacteria): production, physico-chemical and biological properties. *J. Antibiot.* **49,** 560–563.

Ghetie, V., and Vitetta, E. (1994). Immunotoxins in the therapy of cancer: from bench to clinic. *Pharmacol. Ther.* **63,** 209–234.

Giannakakou, P., Gussio, R., Nogales, E., Downing, K. H., Zaharevitz, D., Bollbuck, B., Poy, G., Sackett, D., Nicolaou, K. C., and Fojo, T. (2000). A common pharmacophore for epothilone and taxanes: molecular basis for drug resistance conferred by tubulin mutations in human cancer cells. *Proc. Natl. Acad. Sci. USA* **97,** 2904–2909.

Gibbs, J. B. (2000). Mechanism-based target identification and drug discovery in cancer research. *Science* **287,** 1969–1973.

Golik, J., Dubay, G., Groenewold, G., Kawaguchi, H., Konishi, M., Krishnan, B., Ohkuma, H., Saitoh, K., and Doyle, T. W. (1987). Esperamicins, a novel class of potent antitumor antibiotics. 3. Structures of esperamicins A1, A2, and A1b. *J. Am. Chem. Soc.* **109,** 3462–3464.

Goodman, L. S., Wintrobe, M. M., Damesheck, W., Goodman, M. J., Gilman, A., and McLennan, M. T. (1946). Nitrogen mustard therapy. Use of methyl-bis(β-chloroethyl)amine hydrochloride and tris-(β-chloroethyl)-amine hydrochloride for Hodgkin's disease, lymphosarcoma, leukemia and certain allied and miscellaneous disorders. *J. Am. Med. Assoc.* **132,** 126–132.

Gould, M. C., and Stephano, J.L. (2000). Inactivation of Ca2+ action potential channels by the mek inhibitor PD 98059. *Exp. Cell Res.* **260,** 175–179.

Gupta, S. P. (1994). Quantitative structure-activity relationship studies on anticancer drugs. *Chem. Rev.* **94,** 1507–1551.

Haffty, B. G., Son, Y. H., Wilson, L. D., Papac, R., Fischer, D., Rockwell, S., Sartorelli, A. C., Ross, D., Sasaki, C. T., and Fischer, J. J. (1997). Bioreductive alkylating agent porfiromycin in combination with radiation therapy for the management of squamous cell carcinoma of the head and neck. *Radiat. Oncol. Inv.* **5,** 235–245.

Hamel, E. (1992). Natural products which interact with tubulin in the vinca domain: maytansine, rhizoxin, phomopsin A, dolastatins 10 and 15 and halichondrin B. *Pharmacol. Ther.* **55,** 31–51.

Hansch, C., Hoekman, D., and Gao, H. (1996). Comparative QSAR: toward a deeper understanding of chemicobiological interactions. *Chem. Rev.* **96,** 1045–1075.

Hansch, C., and Leo, A. J. (1979). "Substituent Constants for Correlation Analysis in Chemistry and Biology." Wiley-Interscience, New York, NY.

Harris, C. R., and Danishefsky, S. J. (1999). Complex target-oriented synthesis in the drug discovery process: a case history in the dEpoB series. *J. Org. Chem.* **64,** 8434–8456.

Hartley, J. A., Reszko, K., Zuo, E. T., Wilson, W. D., Morgan, A. R., and Lown, J. W. (1988). Characteristics of the interaction of anthrapyrazole anticancer agents with deoxyribonucleic acids; structural requirements for DNA binding, intercalation and photosensitisation. *Mol. Pharmacol.* **33,** 265–271.

Hay, M. P., Sykes, B. M., Denny, W. A., and Wilson, W. R. (1999a). A 2-nitroimidazole carbamate prodrug of 5-amino-1-(chloromethyl)-3-[(5,6,7-trimethoxyindol-2-yl)carbonyl]-1,2-dihydro-3H-benz[e]indole (amino-*seco*-CBI-TMI) for use with ADEPT and GDEPT. *Bioorg. Med. Chem. Lett.* **15,** 2237–2242.

Hay, M. P., Sykes, B. M., O'Connor, C. J., and Denny, W. A. (1999b). Substituent effects on the kinetics of reductively-initiated fragmentation of nitrobenzyl carbamates designed as triggers for bioreductive drugs. *J. Chem. Soc. Perkin Trans.* **I,** 2759–2770.

He, L., Jagtap, P. G., Kingston, D. G. I., Shen, H-J., Orr, G. A., and Horwitz, S. B. (2000). A common pharmacophore for taxol and the epothilones based on the biological activity of a taxane molecule lacking a C-13 side chain. *Biochemistry* **39,** 3972–3978.

Hortobagyi, G. N. (1997). Anthracyclines in the treatment of cancer. An overview. *Drugs* **54** (Suppl 4), 1–7.

Howbert, J. J., Grossman, C. S., Crowell, T. A., Rieder, B. J., Harper, R. W., Kramer, K. E., Tao, E. V., Aikins, J., and Poore, G. A. (1990). Novel agents effective against solid tumors: the diarylsulfonylureas. Synthesis, activities, and analysis of quantitative structure-activity relationships. *J. Med. Chem.* **33**, 2393–2407.

Ichimura, M., Ogawa, T., Takahashi, K., Kobayashi, E., Kawamoto, I., Yasuzawa, T., Takahashi, I., and Nakano, H. (1990). Duocarmycin SA, a new antitumor antibiotic from Streptomyces sp. *J. Antibiot.* **43**, 1037–1038.

Insug, O., Kieber-Emmons, T., Otvos, L., and Blaszczyk-Thurin, M. (1999). Peptides mimicking sialyl-Lewis A isolated from a random peptide library and peptide array. *Ann. NY. Acad. Sci.* **886**, 276–279.

Issell, B. F., and Crooke, S. T. (1978), Maytansine. *Cancer Treat. Rev.* **5**, 199–207.

Kelly, R. C., Gebhard, I., Wicnienski, N., Aristoff, P. A., Johnson, P. D., and Martin, D. G. (1987). Coupling of cyclopropapyrroloindole (CPI) derivatives. The preparation of CC-1065, ent-CC-1065, and analogs. *J. Am. Chem. Soc.* **109**, 6837–6838.

Kerr, J. M., Banville, S. C., and Zuckermann, R. N. J. (1993). Encoded combinatorial peptide libraries containing non-natural amino acids. *J. Am. Chem. Soc.* **115**, 2529–2531.

Kirk, K. L., and Cohen, L. A. (1969). Participation of the anilino group in peptide bond cleavage. The use of *t*-butyl 3,5-dinitro-2-fluorocarbanilate as a peptide reagent. *J. Org. Chem.* **34**, 395–397.

Kirkpatrick, D. L., Watson, S., Kunkel, M., Fletcher, S., Ulhaq, S., and Powis, G. (1999). Parallel syntheses of disulfide inhibitors of the thioredoxin redox system as potential antitumor agents. *Anticancer Drug Des.* **14**, 421–432.

Knox, R. J., Friedlos, F., and Boland, M. P. (1993). The bioactivation of CB 1954 and its use as a prodrug in antibody-directed enzyme prodrug therapy (ADEPT). *Cancer Metab. Rev.* **12**, 195–212.

Koehler, R. T., and Villar, H. O. (2000). Design of screening libraries biased for pharmaceutical discovery. *J. Comput. Chem.* **21**, 1145–1152.

Lam, K. S., Salmon, S., Hersh, E., Hruby, V., Kazmierski, W., and Knapp, R. (1991). A new type of synthetic peptide library for identifying ligand-binding activity. *Nature* **354**, 82–84.

Lam, K. S. (1997). Application of combinatorial library methods in cancer research and drug discovery. *Anticancer Drug Des.* **12**, 145–167.

Lam, K. S., Lebl, M., and Krchák, V. (1997). The "One-Bead-One-Compound" combinatorial library method. *Chem. Rev.* **97**, 411–448.

Leitheiser, C. J., Rishel, M. J., Wu, X., and Hecht, S. M. (2000). Solid-phase synthesis of bleomycin group antibiotics. Elaboration of deglycobleomycin A5. *Org. Lett.* **2**, 3397–3399.

Li, L. H., Kelly, R. C., Warpehoski, M. A., McGovern, J. P., Gebhard, I., and DeKoning, T. F. (1991). Adozelesin, a selected lead among cyclopropylpyrroloindole analogs of the DNA-binding antibiotic, CC-1065. *Invest. New Drugs* **9**, 137–148.

Liang, J., Moher, E. D., Moore, R. E., and Hoard, D. W. (2000). Synthesis of Cryptophycin 52 using the Sharpless asymmetric dihydroxylation: diol to epoxide transformation optimized for a base-sensitive substrate. *J. Org. Chem.* **65**, 3143–3147.

Linnemann, T., Brock, C., Sparbier, K., Muche, M., Mielke, A., Lukowsky, A., Sterry, W., Kaltoft, K., Wicsmuller, K. H., and Walden, P. (1998). Identification of epitopes for CTCL-specific cytotoxic T lymphocytes. *Adv. Exp. Med. Biol.* **451**, 231–235.

Lipinski, C. A., Lombardo, F., Dominy, B. W., and Feeney, P. J. (1997). Experimental and computational approaches to estimate solubility and permeability in drug discovery and development settings. *Adv. Drug Delivery Rev.* **23**, 3–25.

Loughlin, W. A., Marshall, R. L., Carreiro, A., and Elson, K. E. (2000). Solution-phase combinatorial synthesis and evaluation of piperazine-2,5-dione derivatives. *Bioorg. Med. Chem. Lett.* **10**, 91–94.

Luh, T. Y., Leung, M. K., and Wong, K. T. (2000). Transition metal-catalyzed activation of aliphatic C-X bonds in carbon-carbon bond formation. *Chem. Rev.* **100**, 3187–3204.

Maly, D. J., Choong, I. C., and Ellman, J. A. (2000). Combinatorial target-guided ligand assembly: Identification of potent subtype-selective c-Src inhibitors. *Proc. Natl. Acad. Sci. USA* **97**, 2419–2424.

Martin, D. G., Chidester, C. G., Duchamp, D. J., and Mizsak, S.A. (1980). Structure of CC-1065 (NSC-298223), a new antitumor antibiotic. *J. Antibiot.* **33**, 902–903.

Mauger, A. B., Burke, P. J., Somani, H. H., Friedlos, F., and Knox, R. J. (1994). Self-immolative prodrugs: candidates for antibody-directed enzyme prodrug therapy in conjunction with a nitroreductase enzyme. *J. Med. Chem.* **37**, 3452–3458.

McGovren, J. P., Clarke, G. L., Pratt, E. A., and DeKoning, T.F. (1984). Preliminary toxicity studies with the DNA-binding antibiotic, CC-1065. *J. Antibiot.* **37**, 63–70.

Mealy, N., and Castaner, J. (1996). Carzelesin. U-80244. NSC-619029. Antineoplastic. Alkylating agent. *Drugs Future* **21**, 245–248.

Moran, E. J., Sarshar, S., Cargill, J. F., Shahbaz, M. M., Lio, A., Mjalli, A. M. M., and Armstrong, R. W. (1995). Radio frequency tag encoded combinatorial library method for the discovery of tripeptide-substituted cinnamic acid inhibitors of the protein tyrosine phosphatase PTP1B. *J. Am. Chem. Soc.* **117**, 10787–10788.

Moyer, J. D., Barbacci, E .G., Iwata, K. K., Arnold, L., Boman, B., Cunningham, A., Diorio, C., Doty, J., Morin, M. J., Moyer, M. P., Neveu, M., Pollack, V. A., Pustilnik, L. R., Reynolds, M. M., Sloan, D., Theleman, A., and Miller P. (1997). Induction of apoptosis and cell cycle arrest by CP-358774, an inhibitor of epidermal growth factor receptor tyrosine kinase. *Cancer Res.* **57**, 4838–4848.

Munro, M. H., Blunt, J. W., Dumdei, E. J., Hickford, S. J., Lill, R. E., Li, S., Battershill, C. N., and Duckworth, A. R. (1999). The discovery and development of marine compounds with pharmaceutical potential. *J. Biotech.* **70**, 15–25.

Needels, M. C., Jones, D. G., Tate, E. H., Heinkel, G. L., Kochersperger, L. M., Dower, W. J., Barrett, R. W., and Gallop, M. A. (1993). Generation and screening of an oligonucleotide-encoded synthetic peptide library. *Proc. Natl. Acad. Sci. USA* **90**, 10700–10704.

Nefzi, A., Ostresh, J. M., and Houghten, R. A. (1997). The current status of heterocyclic combinatorial libraries. *Chem. Rev.* **97**, 449–472.

Ni, Z-J., Maclean, D., Holmes, C. P., Murphy, M. M., Ruhland, B., Jacobs, J. W., Gordon, E. M., and Gallop, M. A. (1996). Versatile approach to encoding combinatorial organic syntheses using chemically robust secondary amine tags. *J. Med. Chem.* **39**, 1601–1608.

Nicolaou, K. C., Vourloumis, D., Li, T., Pastor, J., Winssinger, N., He, Y., Ninkovic, S., Sarabia, F., Vallberg, H., Roschangar, F., King, N. P., Finlay, M. R. V., Giannakakou, P., Verdier-Pinard, P., and Hamel, E. (1997a). Designed epothilones: combinatorial synthesis, tubulin assembly properties, and cytotoxic action against taxol-resistant tumor cells. *Angew. Chem., Int. Ed. Engl.* **36**, 2097–2103.

Nicolaou, K. C., Winssinger, N., Pastor, J., Ninkovic, S., Sarabia, F., He, Y., Vourloumis, D., Yang, Z., Li, T., Giannakakou, P., and Hamel, E. (1997b). Synthesis of epothilones A and B in solid and solution phase. *Nature* **387**, 268–272.

Nicolaou, K. C., Winssinger, N., Vourloumis, D., Ohshima, T., Kim, S., Pfefferkorn, J., Xu, J-Y., and Li, T. (1998). Solid and solution phase synthesis and biological evaluation of combinatorial sarcodictyin libraries. *J. Am. Chem. Soc.* **120**, 10814–10826.

Orfi, L., Waczek, F., Kovesdi, I., Meszaros, G., Idei, M., Horvath, A., Hollosy, F., Mak, M., Szegedi, Z., Szende, B., and Keri, G. (1999). New antitumor leads from a peptidomimetic library. *Lett. Pept. Sci.* **6**, 325–333.

Palmer, B. D., Wilson, W. R., Pullen, S. M., and Denny, W. A. (1990). Hypoxia-selective antitumor agents. 3. Relationships between structure and cytotoxicity against cultured tumor cells for substituted N,N-bis(2-chloroethyl)anilines. *J. Med. Chem.* **33**, 112–121.

Panda, D., Ananthnarayan, V., Larson, G., Shih, C., Jordan, M. A., and Wilson, L. (2000). Interaction of the antitumor compound cryptophycin-52 with tubulin. *Biochemistry* **39**, 14121–14127.

Panthananickal, A., Hansch, C., and Leo, A. (1979). Structure-activity relationship of aniline mustards acting against B-16 melanoma in mice. *J. Med. Chem.* **22,** 1267–1269.

Patterson, A. V., Saunders, M. P., Chinje, E. C., Patterson, L. H., and Stratford, I. J. (1998). Enzymology of tirapazamine metabolism: a review. *Anticancer Drug Des.* **13,** 541–573.

Patterson, L. H., McKeown, S. R., Ruparelia, K., Double, J. A., Bibby, M. C., Cole, S., and Stratford I. J. (2000). Enhancement of chemotherapy and radiotherapy of murine tumors by AQ4N, a bioreductively activated anti-tumor agent. *Br. J. Cancer* **82,** 1984–1990.

Pavlidis, N., Aamdal, S., Awada, A., Calvert, H., Fumoleau, P., Sorio, R., Punt, C., Verweij, J., van Oosterom, A., Morant, R., Wanders, J., and Hanauske A-R. (2000). Carzelesin phase II study in advanced breast, ovarian, colorectal, gastric, head and neck cancer, non-Hodgkin's lymphoma and malignant melanoma: a study of the EORTC early clinical studies group (ECSG). *Cancer Chemother. Pharmacol.* **46,** 167–171.

Pirrung, M. C. (1997). Spatially addressable combinatorial libraries. *Chem. Rev.* **97,** 473–488.

Ramdas, L., Bunnin, B. A., Plunkett, M. J., Sun, G., Ellman, J., Gallick, G., and Budde R. J. A. (1999). Benzodiazepine compounds as inhibitors of the Src protein tyrosine kinase: screening of a combinatorial library of 1,4-benzodiazepines. *Arch. Biochem. Biophys.* **368,** 394–400.

Salmon, S. E., Liu-Steven, R. H., Zhao, Y., Lebl, M., Krchnak, V., Wertman, K., Sepetov, N., and Lam, K. S. (1996). High-volume cellular screening for anticancer agents with combinatorial chemical libraries: a new methodology. *Mol. Diversity* **2,** 57–63.

Schindler, T., Bornmann, W., Pellicena, P., Miller, W.T., Clarkson, B., and Kuriyan, J. (2000). Structural mechanism for STI-571 inhibition of abelson tyrosine kinase. *Science* **289,** 1938–1942.

Schrieber, S. L. (2000). Target-oriented and diversity-oriented organic synthesis in drug discovery. *Science* **287,** 1964–1969.

Sedlacek, H .H. (2000). Kinase inhibitors in cancer therapy: a look ahead. *Drugs* **59,** 435–476.

Selassie, C. D., Strong, C. D., Hansch, C., Delcamp, T. J., Freisheim, J.H., and Khwaja, T. A. (1986). Comparison of triazines as inhibitors of L1210 dihydrofolate reductase and of L1210 cells sensitive and resistant to methotrexate. *Cancer Res.* **46,** 744–756.

Selassie, C. D., Hansch, C., and Khwaja T. A. (1990). Structure-activity relationships of antineoplastic agents in multidrug resistance. *J. Med. Chem.* **33,** 1914–1919.

Senderowicz, A. M., and Sausville E. A. (2000). Preclinical and clinical development of cyclin-dependent kinase modulators. *J. Natl. Cancer Inst.* **92,** 376–387.

Sievers, E. L., Appelbaum, F. R., Spielberger, R. T., Forman, S. J., Flowers, D., Smith, F. O., Shannon-Dorcy, K., Berger, M. S., and Bernstein I. D. (1999). Selective ablation of acute myeloid leukemia using antibody-targeted chemotherapy: A phase I study of an anti-CD33 calicheamicin immunoconjugate. *Blood* **93,** 3678–3684.

Smaill, J. B., Rewcastle, G. W., Bridges, A. J., Zhou, H., Showalter, H. D. H., Fry, D. W., Nelson, J. M., Sherwood, V., Elliott, W. L., Vincent, P. W., DeJohn, D., Loo, J. A., Gries, K. D., Chan, O. H., Reyner, E. L., Lipka, E., and Denny, W. A. (2000). Tyrosine kinase inhibitors. 17. Irreversible inhibitors of the epidermal growth factor receptor: 4-(phenylamino)quinazoline- and 4-(phenylamino)pyrido[3,2-*d*]pyrimidine-6-acrylamides bearing additional solubilizing functions. *J. Med. Chem.* **43,** 1380–1397.

Smith, A. L., and Nicolaou, K. C. (1996). The enediyne antibiotics. *J. Med. Chem.* **39,** 2103–2017.

Smith, C. D., Zhang, X., Mooberry, S. L., Patterson, G. M. L., and Moore, R. E. (1994). Cryptophycin: a new antimicrotubule agent active against drug-resistant cells. *Cancer Res.* **54,** 3779–3784.

Sykes, B. M., Atwell, G. J., Hogg, A., Wilson, W. R., O'Connor, C. J., and Denny, W. A. (1999). N-Substituted 2-(2,6-dinitrophenylamino)-propanamides: novel prodrugs that release a primary amine via nitroreduction and intramolecular cyclization. *J. Med. Chem.* **42,** 346–355.

Syrigos, K. N., and Epenetos, A. A. (1999). Antibody directed enzyme prodrug therapy (ADEPT): a review of the experimental and clinical considerations. *Anticancer Res.* **19,** 605–613.

Tannock, I. F., and Rotin. D. (1989). Acid pH in tumors and its potential for therapeutic exploitation. *Cancer Res.* **49,** 4373–4384.

Thompson, L. A., and Ellman, J. A. (1996). Synthesis and application of small molecule libraries. *Chem. Rev.* **96,** 555–600.

Tietze, L. F., Newman, M., Mollers, T., Fischer, R., Glusenkamp, K-H., Rajewsky, M., and Jahde, E. (1989). Proton-mediated liberation of aldophosphamide from a non-toxic prodrug: a strategy for tumor-selective activation of cytocidal drugs. *Cancer Res.* **49,** 4179–4184.

Tremblay, M. R., Simard, J., and Poirier, D. (1999). Parallel solid-phase synthesis of a model library of 7α-alkylamide estradiol derivatives as potential estrogen receptor antagonists. *Bioorg. Med. Chem. Lett.* **9,** 2827–2832.

Vaupel, P., Schlenger, K., Knoop, C., and Hockel, M. (1991). Oxygenation of human tumors: evaluation of tissue oxygen distribution in breast cancers by computerized O2 tension measurements. *Cancer Res.* **51,** 3316–3322.

Wall, M. E. (1998). Camptothecin and taxol: discovery to clinic. *Med. Res. Rev.,* **18,** 299–314.

Wallace, A., Koblan, K., Hamilton, K., Marquis-Omer, D. J., Miller, P. J., Mosser, S. D., Omer, C. A., Schaber, M. D., Cortese, R., Oliff, A., Gibbs, J. B., and Pessi A. (1996). Selection of potent inhibitors of farnesyl-protein transferase from a synthetic tetrapeptide combinatorial library. *J. Biol. Chem.* **271,** 31306–31311.

Wang, J., and Ramnarayan, K. (1999). Toward designing drug-like libraries: a novel computational approach for prediction of drug feasibility of compounds. *J. Comb. Chem.* **1,** 524–533.

Ware, D. C., Palmer, B. D., Wilson, W. R., and Denny, W. A. (1993). Hypoxia-selective antitumor agents. 7. Metal complexes of aliphatic mustards as a new class of hypoxia-selective cytotoxins. Synthesis and evaluation of cobalt(III) complexes of bidentate mustards. *J. Med. Chem.* **36,** 1839–1846.

Wilman, D. E. V., and Connors, T. A. (1983). Molecular structure and antitumour activity of alkylating agents. In "Molecular Aspects of Anticancer Drug Action" (S. Neidle and M. J. Waring, eds.), pp. 234–282, MacMillan, London.

Wilson, W. R., Ferry, D. M., Tercel, M., Anderson, R. F., and Denny, W. A. (1998a). Reduction of nitroarylmethyl quaternary ammonium prodrugs of mechlorethamine by radiation. *Radiat. Res.* **149,** 237–245.

Wilson, W. R., Tercel, M., Anderson, R. F., and Denny, W. A. (1998b). Radiation-activated prodrugs as hypoxia-selective cytotoxins: model studies with nitroarylmethyl quaternary salts. *Anticancer Drug Des.* **13,** 663–685.

Wilson, W. R., van Zijl, P., and Denny, W. A. (1992). Bis-bioreductive agents as hypoxia-selective cytotoxins: N-oxides of nitracrine. *Int. J. Radiat. Oncol. Biol. Phys.* **22,** 693–697.

Zee-Cheng, R. K-Y., and Cheng, C. C. (1988). Screening and evaluation of anticancer agents. *Methods Find. Exp. Clin. Pharmacol.* **10,** 67–101.

Zhou, D. C., Zittoun, R., and Marie, J. P. (1995). Homoharringtonine: an effective new natural product in cancer chemotherapy. *Bull. Cancer* **82,** 987–995.

Zhou, X. J., and Rahmani, R. (1992). Preclinical and clinical pharmacology of vinca alkaloids. *Drugs* **44** (Suppl. 4), 1–16.

Zwelling, L. A., Michaels, S., Erickson, L. C., Ungerleider, R. S., Nichols, M., and Kohn, K. W. (1981). Protein-associated deoxyribonucleic acid strand breaks in L1210 cells treated with the deoxyribonucleic acid intercalating agents 4'-(9-acridinylamino)methanesulfon-*m*-anisidide and Adriamycin. *Biochemistry* **20,** 6553–6563.

BIOSYNTHETIC PRODUCTS FOR ANTICANCER DRUG DESIGN AND TREATMENT: THE BRYOSTATINS

George R. Pettit
Cherry L. Herald
Fiona Hogan

Cancer Research Institute and Department of Chemistry and Biochemistry

Arizona State University

Tempe, Arizona

Summary

The field of anticancer drug discovery based on natural products is vast and covers many areas, including isolation, chemical identification and synthesis, preclinical evaluation both *in vitro* and *in vivo,* and clinical trials. Rather than try to cover a number of different classes of natural products at a superficial level, this review provides an in-depth examination of the bryostatins as an especially important example, encompassing all steps from its discovery to its advancement to clinical trial as a promising anticancer drug for improving human cancer treatment. The bryostatins are particularly interesting because of the diversity of their chemical structures and the novelty of their molecular action, e.g., stimulation of the enzyme protein kinase C and induction of apoptosis in tumor cells. A variety of preclinical studies have culminated in phase I or phase II clinical trials of bryostatin 1. More than 700 patients have been treated, and results have included complete and partial responses, as well as disease stabilization.

1. Introduction

The biosynthetic products available on our planet are the result of 3.8 billion years of evolutionary biosynthetic organic reactions directed at ever more specific molecular design and targeting. The net result of millions of biosynthetic organic reactions (biosynthetic combinatorial processes) is an astronomical number of exquisitely designed candidates for use as anticancer drugs and as drugs necessary across the medical spectrum of human disease. However, they need to be discovered and developed to the point of clinical efficacy. Some of the extraordinarily exciting potential for discovery of new naturally occurring anticancer drugs can be easily recognized. Consider that the world's flora may number some 800,000 species, and the angiosperms may include 300,000 to some 500,000 species. Furthermore, enormous numbers of marine animal (more than 2 million) and microorganism (more than 30 million) species are available for investigation. Fewer than 10% of the higher plants and fewer than 0.5% of the marine animals have received even a cursory effort to detect antineoplastic constituents. A multitude of animal, microorganism, and plant anticancer drugs still awaits discovery. That assumption is even more obvious considering that one can easily extract several thousand compounds from each animal, microorganism, or plant species, making the total of theoretically available biosynthetic constituents more than 100 billion! Thus, it appears certain the number of potentially useful and very carefully designed biosynthetic products for improving human cancer treatment is huge. And, by use of current molecular targeting bioassays, the probability of locating useful anticancer drugs can be markedly increased.

The U.S. National Cancer Institute (NCI) research programs directed at discovery of new and clinically useful animal, plant, and microorganism anticancer constituents were implemented in September 1957 and quickly demonstrated that 2–4% of plant specimens produce a great variety of anticancer agents. The dramatic discoveries arising from the early NCI research, such as camptothecin and taxol, have stimulated considerable worldwide interest and initiation of analogous programs. Because of this vitally important NCI endeavor, new antineoplastic and/or cytotoxic biosynthetic products are now being discovered worldwide at an increasing rate. Certainly, as just noted, the potential for discovery of new animal, plant, and microorganism biosynthetic products for treatment of human cancer is truly extraordinary and offers great promise of many curative approaches to the cancer problem.

2. Background to the Bryostatins

The development of natural products as anticancer drugs from drug isolation and identification to clinical trial represents a process of great complexity. Since it is impossible to discuss this process in general terms for all anticancer drugs derived from natural products, we have illustrated each step in drug development with regard to a group of natural products called the bryostatins. These were discovered in the early phases of collaborative endeavors with the NCI, and research has continued uninterrupted for the past 33 years.

In 1965–1966, we began the first systematic study of marine invertebrates and vertebrates as potential sources of new and potentially useful cancer chemotherapeutic drugs. By 1969, we found that 9–10% of marine animals yielded extracts with high and reproducible (confirmed active) antineoplastic activity in the NCI's P388 *in vivo* lymphocytic leukemia screening system. From this very high level of confirmed activity it was abundantly clear that such natural products present an unusually good opportunity for the discovery of clinically useful anticancer drugs. To date, we have isolated a large number of new cytotoxic and/or antineoplastic agents from marine animals. However, the focus of this chapter will be the discovery and development of the bryostatins to the present.

By 1968, we had collected (from the upper Gulf of Mexico) a specimen that was found to be *Bugula neritina* (Bryozoa). This bryozoan gave extracts that more than doubled the life span of mice with P388 lymphocytic leukemia. Meanwhile, we were conducting expeditions in the Gulf of California and collected another bryozoan, again powerfully active, which turned out to be *B. neritina*. Research was continued with that specimen, and later we found it again off the coast of California. Extensive bioassay-directed (P388 leukemia) separation of the California *B. neritina* extracts led to isolation of the first milligram of bryostatin 1 (hereinafter referred to simply as bryostatin, unless ambiguity could result) in 1981. We were able to crystallize this substance and complete the x-ray crystallographic structural determination. Bryostatin was found to be a remarkable macrocyclic lactone.

Subsequently, we discovered a total of 20 new bryostatins from *B. neritina* collections that ranged from the Gulf of Mexico, Gulf of California, and coast of California, to Japan (Gulf of Sagami). More recently, we explored *B. neritina* from two more remote areas in the Gulf of Japan and from one of these found bryostatin 10 in fairly abundant amounts (about $10^{-3}\%$). Bryostatin 1 was found in $10^{-6}\%$ yields, and some of the more rare bryostatins in yields of $10^{-8}\%$. The natural production of bryostatin 10 in $10^{-3}\%$ yields is very important for the future development of this structural modification to clinical trials. Among the early biological aspects of bryostatin was the observation that microgram doses (usually around 50 µg/kg) would double survival times against the P388 lymphocytic leukemia and would provide cures against the B16 melanoma in the mouse (particularly the variation that metastasizes to the lungs). Similar activity was found against the M5 ovary system. Subsequently, experiments by Dr. Blumberg in the NCI showed that the potent anticancer activity of bryostatin and the bryostatins was primarily based on modulation (initial activation followed by rapid down-regulation) of protein kinase C (PKC), a very important family of isozymes in the cell transduction pathway involved in regulation of cell growth, differentiation, gene expression, and tumor promotion. In contrast to some PKC interactive substances, bryostatin has proved to be a very potent anti-tumor-promoting agent and a very promising anticancer drug. The discovery and development (preclinical and clinical) of bryostatin nicely illustrates our focus on PKC targeting. Later, bryostatin was found to promote the normal growth of bone marrow progenitor cells. One consequence of the hematopoietic progenitor effects was found when mice, given 1 µg of bryostatin, followed by a lethal dose of radiation, were found to survive. Furthermore, bryostatin was found to be an immune stimulant and also to stimulate the normal production of interleukin-2 (IL-2) and interferon.

Bryostatin has provided curative levels of activity against a variety of murine experimental cancer systems, including those mentioned above, M5076 sarcoma, and L10AB cell lymphoma. Against human cancer models, in the nude or severe combined immunodeficiency (SCID) models, bryostatin evidenced excellent activity against myeloid and lymphoid leukemias, as well as against lymphoma cancer xenografts. Very importantly, bryostatin exhibits immunostimulatory properties, including stimulation of cytokine release and enhancement of T- and B-cell activation and lymphokine-activated killer cell activity. In addition, neutrophil phagocytic activity and degranulation have been demonstrated. Also very important have been observations that bryostatin down-regulates *mdr-1* (multidrug resistance), down-regulates *bcl-2* (resistance to programmed cell death or apoptosis), and up-regulates *bax* (induction of apoptosis). These and a considerable number of other favorable biological aspects of bryostatin activities have been reported in more than 520 scientific and medical research publications.

Clinical development of bryostatin has been ongoing since 1990. In addition to more than 80 human cancer clinical trials of bryostatin either completed (20) or now ongoing in the United States, England, and Canada under the auspices of the NCI, the British Cancer Research Campaign, and the Cancer Institute of Canada, respectively, and involving 178 principal investigators in 148 different institutions, the clinical development of bryostatin is still expanding at the phase I/II levels. To date, well over 700 patients have been treated with bryostatin in phase I or phase II cancer clinical trials, and of these so far a substantial number of patients have received promising benefit ranging from complete response (CR) and partial response (PR) to stable disease (SD). Initial reports from clinical trials combining bryostatin with well-known anticancer drugs, such as paclitaxel, vincristine, fludarabine, cisplatin, 2-chlorodeoxyadenosine (2-CdA), and arabinosinyl cytosine (ara-C), suggest that bryostatin will become an important anticancer drug and in combination with other anticancer drugs such as just noted should lead to useful improvements in human cancer treatment.

Clinical trials of bryostatin are now covering a broad spectrum of human cancer types, and interesting CRs have been observed in patients with chronic lymphocytic leukemia, chronic myelogenous leukemia, pancreatic carcinoma, renal cell carcinoma, relapsed non-Hodgkin's low-grade lymphoma, and esophageal cancer. With patients whose disease is refractory to the better known anticancer drugs, a combination of some of those with bryostatin has given the most promising clinical results. Animal studies had already shown that the combination of bryostatin with certain other anticancer drugs, such as vincristine, paclitaxel, cisplatin, fludarabine, 2-CdA, and ara-C, led to considerably improved efficacy in comparison with either drug individually. Indeed, there is every indication that such combinations will lead to very important clinical roles for bryostatin in improving future cancer treatments. From current clinical trials evidence, bryostatin will eventually qualify for New Drug Application (NDA) status with the U.S. Food and Drug Administration

and may become the first marine invertebrate anticancer constituent to find broad application in human cancer treatments.

Exploratory expeditions have been conducted by our research group and the NCI in areas as diverse as Asian and Western Pacific countries, the North and South American continent, and the African continent including the eastern and western Indian oceans. They have provided a considerable number of new top-priority marine organism, microorganism, and plant leads to new anticancer drugs exhibiting structures that we organic and medicinal chemists would never have devised without the incredibly accurate molecular design of evolutionary biosynthesis. The general background to this work can be obtained from a series of articles (Pettit *et al.*, 1970, 1989, 1993; Carter and Livingston, 1976; Cordell and Farnsworth, 1976, 1977; Douros, 1976; Hartwell, 1976; Kupchan, 1976; Smith *et al.*, 1976; Spjut and Perdue, 1976; Wall *et al.*, 1976; Suffness and Douros, 1979; Bradner, 1980; Cassady and Douros, 1980; Fox, 1991; Baker *et al.*, 1995; Boyd and Paull, 1995; Pettit, 1996; Boyd, 1997; Boyd *et al.*, 1997; Christian *et al.*, 1997; Cragg *et al.*, 1997a, 1997b; Sutherland and Whitfield, 1997; Lawrence, 1999). Different aspects of the field have been reviewed (Pettit, 1991; Zonder and Philip, 1999; Mutter and Wills, 2000).

3. Comprehensive Review of Bryostatin Scientific and Medical Reports

A. Discovery of the Bryostatins and Related Chemistry

The bryostatins comprise a large series of compounds (structures shown in Fig. 1), the discovery of which has occurred over a number of years (Pettit *et al.*, 1982, 1983a, 1983b, 1984, 1985, 1986, 1987a, 1987b, 1991a). The three new 20-desoxybryostatins 16, 17, and 18 showed significant growth inhibitory activity (ED_{50} values) of 9.3, 19, and 3.3 ng/ml, respectively, against murine P388 lymphocytic leukemia (Pettit *et al.*, 1996). *B. neritina* from the Gulf of Aomori, Japan, was found to contain bryostatin-10 in high yield ($10^{-3}\%$) for this class of compounds. The conformation of bryostatin 10 in solution was revealed by nuclear magnetic resonance (NMR) studies (Kamano *et al.*, 1995, 1996). Bryostatin 3 and the corresponding 26-ketone, which represents a new bryostatin, were isolated from the marine bryozoan *B. neritina* (Bugulidae). Bryostatin 3 showed [^{3}H]phorbol dibutyrate (PDBu) receptor displacement activity similar to that of bryostatin, whereas the corresponding 26-ketone was significantly less active. Bryostatin NMR measurements indicated that parts of the published ^{13}C- and ^{1}H-NMR assignments had to be revised, based on extensive homonuclear and heteronuclear one- and two-dimensional NMR techniques performed at 500 MHz (Schaufelberger *et al.*, 1991a, 1991b).

BRYOSTATIN STRUCTURES

Bryostatin 1

Bryostatin 2

Bryostatin 3

R	R₁	
D	C	Bryostatin 4
A	C	Bryostatin 5
A	D	Bryostatin 6
A	A	Bryostatin 7
D	D	Bryostatin 8
D	A	Bryostatin 9
H	C	Bryostatin 10
H	A	Bryostatin 11
B	D	Bryostatin 12
H	D	Bryostatin 13
OH	C	Bryostatin 14
E	A	Bryostatin 15

A =

B =

C =

D =

E =

Bryostatin 16

Bryostatin 17

Bryostatin 18

1. Structural Modifications of the Bryostatins

A series of papers describes the structure–activity relationships (SARs) of the bryostatins (Wender *et al.*, 1988, 1998a, 1998b, 1998c; Wender and Lippa, 2000). Bryostatin 2 has been converted to bryostatin 1 and bryostatin 12 by a selective protection and deprotection involving the C26 hydroxyl group (Pettit *et al.*, 1991b, 1992). 26-Succinylbryostatin 1 has been prepared and shares some but not all of the pharmacologic properties of bryostatin and can activate protein phosphorylation without lowering cytosolic levels of PKC (Bignami *et al.*, 1996).

2. Preclinical and Clinical Supply of Bryostatin

One of the key problems in the development of the bryostatins was to isolate sufficient supplies of drug for preclinical and clinical studies (Newman, 1996; Cragg, 1998; Haygood and Davidson, 1997; Davidson and Haygood, 1999). A novel process was designed for the large-scale isolation of bryostatin from *B. neritina* L to obtain multigram quantities of highly pure material for formulation studies, preclinical toxicology, and clinical trials in cancer patients (Schaufelberger *et al.*, 1991c).

3. High-Performance Liquid Chromatography Assay

High-performance liquid chromatography (HPLC) techniques, including solid-phase extraction techniques, have been developed to detect and quantitate bryostatins 1 and 2 from crude extracts of *B. neritina* (Khan *et al.*, 1998; Baer *et al.*, 1989; Kamano *et al.*, 2000; Schaufelberger *et al.*, 1990).

4. Synthesis of Bryostatins 1, 2, 3, and 7

A particular challenge to the development of the bryostatins has been to synthesize each of the different members of the series (Masamune, 1988a, 1988b; Kageyama *et al.*, 1990; Evans *et al.*, 1991, 1998, 1999; Ohmori *et al.*, 1993, 1995a, 1995b, 2000; Hale *et al.*, 1995; Kerr *et al.*, 1996; Kalesse and Eh, 1996; DeBrabander *et al.*, 1997; Kiyooka and Maeda, 1997; Obitsu *et al.*, 1998; Baxter *et al.*, 1998; Yoshikawa *et al.*, 1999). A practical route to the C1–C9 segment of bryostatin in forms suitable for both synthetic elaboration and biological studies has been achieved via a single disconnection (Roy and Rey, 1990). The construction of the fragments C1–C9 and C17–C27 of the bryostatins in an enantioselective and highly diastereoselective fashion has been described (DeBrabander and Vandewalle, 1996). The C1–C9 segment of bryostatin has been prepared in 11 steps in 21% overall yield (Weiss and Hoffmann, 1997).

B. *In Vitro* Evaluations

1. Human Bone Marrow and Monocytes

Bryostatin activates human neutrophils by binding to the phorbol receptor (Berkow and Kraft, 1985). The coupling of antineoplastic activity to stimulatory growth properties of normal hematopoietic cells makes this an excellent probe to dissect the mechanisms of normal hematopoiesis, with possible use in bone marrow failure (May *et al.*, 1987b). Inactive thymocytes from W/Wv mice in coculture with W/Wv bone marrow showed stimulation of erythropoiesis in the presence of bryostatin, suggesting that bryostatin may in part act by stimulating T lymphocytes to release physiologic concentrations of lymphokines (Leonard *et al.*, 1988). The early mitogenic signals generated by IL-3 and bryostatin may converge at the level of the nuclear envelope, perhaps through a PKC-like activity that mediates phosphorylation of specific nuclear envelope polypeptides such as lamin B (Fields *et al.*, 1989). The results are consistent with the hypothesis that bryostatin has a stimulatory effect on the accessory cell populations to produce either IL-3 or granulocyte-monocyte colony-stimulating factor (GM-CSF). Further support for this notion was obtained by demonstrating that T cells, which are known to produce IL-3 and GM-CSF, are stimulated by bryostatin to express mRNA for specific growth factors including GM-CSF. Thus, bryostatin may be a useful clinical agent to stimulate hematopoiesis *in vivo* (Sharkis *et al.*, 1990).

Leukemic myeloblasts have a different cytoskeletal response to a tumor promoter and an antineoplastic agent despite their common receptor (Sham *et al.*, 1990). Bryostatin inhibits clonogenic leukemia cells at concentrations that stimulate normal hematopoietic progenitors. Its differential effects on normal and abnormal hematopoiesis suggest value in the treatment of leukemias and myelodysplastic syndromes (Jones, R. J. *et al.*, 1990). Treatment of quiescent NIH/3T3 cells with platelet-derived growth factor (PDGF), phorbol 12-myristate 13-acetate (PMA; TPA), or bryostatin leads to rapid translocation of PKC to the nuclear envelope. Rapid nuclear events, including translocation of cytosolic PKC to the nuclear membrane and lamina phosphorylation, may play a role in the transduction of the mitogenic signals of PDGF from the cytoplasm to the nucleus in NIH/3T3 fibroblasts (Fields *et al.*, 1990).

Bryostatin induces rapid down-regulation of the GM-CSF receptor in neutrophils, monocytes, and partially purified myeloid progenitor cells, suggesting an effect at least partially mediated by PKC (Cannistra *et al.*, 1990). PKC activation may play a complex role in regulating the response of normal myeloid progenitors to growth factors such as recombinant GM-CSF. Under some circumstances the phorbol ester PDBu triggers events that inhibit the growth of myeloid progenitors, and this process may be blocked by bryostatin (McCrady *et al.*, 1991). GM-CSF-induced proliferation of MO7 cells was inhibited by two activators of PKC: PMA and bryostatin (Kanakura *et al.*, 1991). Expression of the *jun*-B gene was also affected (Datta *et al.*, 1991). Bryostatin may modulate the *in vitro* response of certain normal and leukemic progenitor cells to recombinant GM-CSF, but the nature of this response differs between the two cell types. It may be particularly effective in limiting the self-renewal capacity of leukemic myeloblasts, an *in vitro* characteristic with potentially important *in vivo* significance (Grant *et al.*, 1991b). Bryostatin stimulated DNA synthesis in HCD-57 cells at subnanomolar concentrations (Spivak *et al.*, 1992). Leukemic cells exposed to bryostatin showed a variable degree of monocytic differentiation as evaluated by α-naphthyl acetate esterase (ANAE) staining and morphology. Bryostatin was also capable of inhibiting the growth of granulocyte-macrophage colony-forming unit (GM-CFU) from myelodysplastic marrow and to shorten the duration of dysplastic hematopoiesis in liquid culture (Gebbia *et al.*, 1992). Pharmacologic interventions by bryostatin at the level of PKC regulated both proliferation and lineage commitment of human hematopoietic progenitors exposed to recombinant GM-CSF and recombinant IL-3 (Li *et al.*, 1992). The presence of G-CSF or IL-6 was required throughout a colony-forming assay for an optimal synergistic effect with bryostatin to be observed; thus, agents that activate PKC may promote the proliferation and development of GM-CFC (colony-forming cells) via a synergistic interaction with G-CSF or IL-6 (Heyworth *et al.*, 1993).

In cytostatic assays, polymorphonuclear neutrophils treated with bryostatin inhibited the growth of the erythroleukemic cell line K562 in a concentration-dependent manner. These findings suggest that the antineoplastic effect of bryostatins may result at least in part from activation of granulocytes and monocytes (Esa *et al.*, 1995). Bryostatin induces tumor necrosis factor (TNF) secretion in human monocytes via a PKC-dependent and CD14-independent pathway and by a mechanism that is most likely based on a strong increase of the TNF mRNA level (Steube and Drexler, 1995). Bryostatin is a powerful activator of human monocytes, suggesting that stimulation of monokine secretion may represent at least one of the mechanisms responsible for its antitumor activity (Bosco *et al.*, 1997). Bryostatin-induced inhibition of clonogenic cell growth is not mediated by a direct effect of bryostatin on CD34 cells but rather is a result of a process involving production of TNF by CD14[+] cells upon bryostatin stimulation together with the induction of secondary factor(s) by TNF, which together with bryostatin is inhibitory toward clonogenic cell growth (Drager *et al.*, 1999).

2. CD34[+] Bone Marrow Cells

The developmental stage-specific module CD34 is a phosphorylation target for activated PKC. Phosphorylation of CD34 may thus play a role in signal transduction during early lymphohematopoiesis (Fackler *et al.*, 1990). The effect of bryostatin on the proliferative capacity and lineage commitment of CD34[+] human bone marrow cells exposed to GM-CSF/IL-3 fusion protein pIXY 321 was studied. In contrast to its effects on committed myeloid progenitors, bryostatin did not increase the growth of erythroid and multipotent prog-

enitors stimulated by pIXY 321 but instead inhibited colony formation at higher concentrations (McCrady *et al.*, 1993). Bryostatin also stimulated differentiation of embryonic stem cells (Kalmaz *et al.*, 1996) and CD34[+] progenitor cells (Kalmaz *et al.*, 1997).

3. Human Cervical Carcinoma

The effects of growth factors on the sensitivity of human cervical carcinoma (HeLa) cells to cisplatin were also investigated. Bryostatin reversed the increase in cisplatin content by PDBu but failed to block the increase in cisplatin accumulation induced by epidermal growth factor (EGF). Therefore, although the mechanism of cisplatin sensitization by both EGF and phorbol ester appears to involve enhanced drug uptake, they may utilize distinct signal transduction pathways (Basu and Evans, 1994). Bryostatin also increased cellular sensitivity to cisplatin. The concentration- and time-dependent enhancement was related to the increase in level of the metabolite *cis*-diethylpropanediol (*cis*-DEP) (Basu and Lazo, 1992).

4. Human Colon Cancer

Several groups have investigated the effect of bryostatin on colon cancer cells (McBain *et al.*, 1988, 1996; Weiss *et al.*, 1997). Since both TPA and bryostatin produce their effects through the activation of members of the PKC class of enzymes, the differentiation state of these colon cancer cells may be regulated by a differential activation of isozymes or a ligand-directed phosphorylation of proteins that are involved in proteoglycan metabolism (McBain *et al.*, 1990).

5. Intestinal Transport

Bryostatin transiently inhibits $Na^+/K^+/Cl^-$ cotransport and Cl^- secretion, possibly through a PKC isoform. Unlike phorbol esters, bryostatin does not impair barrier function, implying that bryostatin and phorbol esters differentially affect a PKC isoform involved in junctional regulation and that epithelial transport and barrier function may be regulated by distinct PKC isoforms (Farokhzad *et al.*, 1998; Soybel *et al.*, 1998).

6. Breast Cancer

A number of studies have investigated cultured breast cancer cells (Martin *et al.*, 1995; Martinez-Lacaci *et al.*, 1995, 1996; Philip *et al.*, 1999). Bryostatin has little effect on transforming growth factor β_1 (TGF-β_1) expression either alone or in combination with estradiol, consistent with the hypothesis that the inhibitory effect of TPA on MCF-7 cells is partly due to autocrine inhibition by TGF-β_1 (Nutt *et al.*, 1991). Bryostatin inhibited growth of only MCF-7 cells, but only at a relatively high dose (100 nM). Differential actions of bryostatin and TPA on PKC activity and α-isoform level in the membrane-associated fraction of MCF-7 and MDA-MB-468 cells may account for the divergent effects of these two agents on cell growth and morphology. The PKC-α isoform may specifically play a role in inhibiting growth of human breast cancer cells (Kennedy *et al.*, 1992). PKC controls eicosanoid synthesis and growth in human breast cancer cells. Although the findings are consistent with bryostatin acting as an antagonist/weak agonist in relation to TPA action, the mechanistic basis for this differential action of TPA and bryostatin is uncertain (Boorne *et al.*, 1998). The data highlight the potential usefulness of bryostatin as an anti-invasive and/or antimetastatic agent (Johnson *et al.*, 1999).

7. Bryostatin and Tamoxifen

The growth inhibitory effects of bryostatin were increased by approximately 200-fold in the presence of noninhibitory concentrations of tamoxifen. Growth inhibition by tamoxifen in the presence of noninhibitory concentrations of bryostatin was also increased by more than 30-fold (McGown *et al.*, 1998).

8. A549 Human Lung Carcinoma

PKC appears to be involved in the mediation of bryostatin-induced growth inhibition of A549 cells, but the relationship between growth arrest and PKC translocation or down-regulation is complex (Dale *et al.*, 1989). The bryostatins not only interfere with A549 cell growth but can also counter the growth inhibitory effect of PKC activators, presumably via interaction with a target separate from the phorbol ester receptor site (Dale and Gescher, 1989). Growth arrest of human-derived A549 lung carcinoma cells caused by bryostatin was equally transitory in serum-supplemented and serum-deprived cells. There was no difference in rate of TPA-induced down-regulation of PKC activity and cytosolic phorbol ester receptor sites between cells grown with or without serum (Bradshaw *et al.*, 1991). Subcellular localization of PKC in A549 cells can be pharmacologically manipulated even under conditions of inhibited kinase function (Bradshaw *et al.*, 1992).

9. Leukemias

a. Acute Lymphoblastic Leukemia

Bryostatin induces a number of responses in cultured leukemia cells (Al-Katib *et al.*, 1992; Mohammad *et al.*, 1996b; Wall *et al.*, 1998b; Varma *et al.*, 1999) and is capable of inducing further differentiation of the Reh cells along the B-cell lineage, effects similar to those of TPA (Al-Katib *et al.*, 1993c).

b. Chronic Myeloid Leukemia

Bryostatin induces macrophage-like differentiation in maturing chronic myeloid leukemia (CML) cells, secretion of GM-CSF by cells in suspension and semisolid medium, and clonal extinction of granulocyte-macrophage progenitors, suggesting a possible therapy agent for CML (Lilly *et al.*,

1990). Bryostatin may produce a cytotoxic effect on chronic myelomonocytic leukemia (CMMol) cells in part by increasing the secretion of, or sensitivity to, tumor necrosis factor (TNF) and may have therapeutic potential in CMMoL (Lilly *et al.*, 1991; Thijsen *et al.*, 1999; Bhatia and Munthe, 1998). Bryostatin selectively inhibits CML at the long-term culture inhibitory cell level, suggesting a role as a purging modality (Thijsen *et al.*, 1999).

c. Acute Promyelocytic Leukemia

The responses of NB4 and HL-60 cells to the biomodulators all-*trans* retinoic acid, vitamin D_3, and bryostatin were analyzed. It is possible that induction of terminal differentiation of leukemic cells by physiologic or pharmacologic modulators may limit the growth of the malignant cells (Hu *et al.*, 1993c). The combination of bryostatin and $1\alpha,25$-dihydroxyvitamin D_3 strongly affects NB4 cell differentiation and proliferation, suggesting a potential therapeutic regimen for APL patients (Song and Norman, 1997; Song *et al.*, 1999).

d. Chronic Lymphocytic Leukemia

Bryostatin is as effective as TPA in inducing further differentiation of chronic lymphocytic leukemia (CLL) cells to a hairy cell stage (Al-Katib *et al.*, 1993a). Combination therapies with fludarabine and new agents such as flavopiridol, IDEC-C2B8, Campath-1H, UCN-01, bryostatin, FR-901228, and melarsoprol will hopefully represent the next advance to improved therapy of CLL (Byrd *et al.*, 1998). The similarity between the membrane lipids in 2-CdA-sensitive CLL cells and the bryostatin-treated WSU-CLL cell line supports the suggestion that membrane lipid alteration might be an important step in the drug resistance mechanism (Liu *et al.*, 1998). Not only is bryostatin capable of inducing apoptosis by itself; it also sensitizes *de novo* resistant WSU-CLL cells to the chemotherapeutic effects of 2-CdA. Bryostatin increases the ratio of deoxycytidine kinase to 5'-nucleotidyltransferase NT activity and increases the ratio of *bax* to *bcl*-2 expression. There are at least two mechanisms through which this natural compound can potentiate the antitumor activity of CdA in otherwise resistant CLL cells (Katato *et al.*, 1996; Mohammad *et al.*, 1998a, 1998d).

e. B-Chronic Lymphocytic Leukemia (B-CLL)

B-chronic lymphocytic leukemia (B-CLL) has been the subject of a number of studies (Liu *et al.*, 1997; Mohammad *et al.*, 1997; Beck *et al.*, 1998; Kitada *et al.*, 1998, 1999; Ning *et al.*, 1996). Bryostatin has effective differentiation-inducing properties on B-CLL cells that can be accentuated by a calcium ionophore (Drexler *et al.*, 1989). Bryostatin stimulated production of PKC and rapidly but temporarily induced production of c-*jun* mRNA in B-CLL cells. Along with other results on the induction of long-term phenotypical cellular changes, such as alteration of morphology and other features of differentiation, this supports the notion that second-messenger (PKC) and third-messenger (proto-oncogene products) pathways are intact in B-CLL cells (Gignac *et al.*, 1990a). In the presence of the calcium ionophore A23187, bryostatin caused morphologic changes indicative of differentiation to plasmacytoid cells. This suggests that as a consequence of maturation, differentiated B-CLL cells down-regulate CD5 expression by analogy with the normal ontogenic process (Gignac *et al.*, 1990b). Stimulation of PKC by bryostatin induces B-CLL cells to convert to hairy cell leukemia (HCL). These observations provide support for the idea that HCL and HCL-like cells might differentiate along a separate branch of B-cell lineage and represent mature end-stage cells (Gignac *et al.*, 1990c). The effects of incubation of adherence purified B-CLL cells with PMA, all-*trans* retinoic acid, and bryostatin were later studied, but none induced a true HCL phenotype (Gartenhaus *et al.*, 1996). Bryostatin increased the sensitivity of WSU-CLL cells to chemotherapeutic agents such as 2-CdA by its action on two cell targets, causing changes in plasma membrane permeability and changes in lipid and DNA content of the mitochondria (Liu *et al.*, 1999; Beck *et al.*, 2000).

f. Human Myeloid Leukemia

The human myeloid leukemia (HL-60) cell line has been the subject of a number of studies (Warren *et al.*, 1987, 1988; Kraft *et al.*, 1987a, 1987b; Kiss *et al.*, 1987a, 1988, 1991a; Stone *et al.*, 1988; William *et al.*, 1988; Cost *et al.*, 1991; Sham *et al.*, 1991; Schwaller *et al.*, 1997; Liou *et al.*, 1997). Specific activation of PKC at the nuclear membrane could explain, at least in part, the divergent effects of bryostatin and phorbol esters on HL-60 cell growth (Fields *et al.*, 1988). Exposure to phorbol esters and bryostatin increases c-*jun* expression, suggesting that the increase in c-*jun* RNA observed during TPA-induced monocytic differentiation is mediated by both transcriptional and posttranscriptional mechanisms (Sherman *et al.*, 1990). Steady-state levels of prothymosin-α mRNA, which are high in exponentially growing HL-60, decrease within hours after induction of HL-60 to differentiate along the neutrophil pathway with dimethylsulfoxide or along the macrophage lineage with either TPA or bryostatin (Smith *et al.*, 1993). Ceramide-related apoptosis was reduced by acute exposure to phorbol esters and bryostatin (Jarvis *et al.*, 1994a). Induction of additional distinct transcription factors, such as AP-1, may contribute to lineage-specific determinants of cell fate (Davis *et al.*, 1997).

g. Leukemias and Lymphomas

Many leukemia and lymphoma lines have been studied (Jones, R. A. *et al.*, 1990; Tilden and Kraft, 1991; Massey *et al.*, 1991; Mohammad *et al.*, 1993; Elgie *et al.*, 1993; Akompong *et al.*, 1995; Adler and Kraft, 1995; Schonhorn *et al.*, 1995; Vrana and Grant, 1996; Li and Chen, 1997). Although

bryostatin inhibits phorbol ester binding in intact Friend erythroleukemia cell clone PS-7, the mechanism for this antagonism cannot be explained by simple competition at the binding site (Dell'Aquila *et al.*, 1987). The addition of TNF to bryostatin in four HL-60 cell lines effected an additive inhibition of growth, suggesting that bryostatin in combination with other biological response modifiers might have a role in the management of human leukemia (Kraft *et al.*, 1989). The immunostimulatory effects of bryostatin on various aspects of B-cell activation and proliferation was also examined using human tonsillar B cells (Drexler *et al.*, 1990). The effects of bryostatin and phorbol esters on topoisomerase-II-mediated events have also been investigated (Zwelling *et al.*, 1991). Bryostatin antagonized TPA-mediated effects on proliferation and morphologic alterations (Steube *et al.*, 1993). Since bryostatin lacks tumor-promoting activity, it has a potential role as a differentiating agent in the therapy of B-cell neoplasms (Hu *et al.*, 1993a). mRNA for annexin VIII, a calcium- and phospholipid-binding protein with anticoagulant activity, is up-regulated by bryostatin but down-regulated by TPA. Annexin VIII gene expression may play a unique role in the proliferation and/or differentiation of leukemic cells and could be associated with abnormal hemostasis of some leukemias (Hu *et al.*, 1993b).

Differentiation induced by TPA and bryostatin-11 by all-*trans* retinoic acid was associated with a decrease in myeloperoxidase (MPO) mRNA in seven initially positive cell lines studied; MPO can be used as an excellent parameter to characterize the various stages of normal and induced differentiation (Hu *et al.*, 1993d). Down-regulation of mRNA for the Wilms' tumor suppressor gene *WT1* is not a generalized phenomenon of growth inhibition and does not occur when TPA-induced differentiation is blocked by bryostatin. This suggests that human K562 erythroleukemia cells will be a valuable system for unraveling signal transduction pathways for *WT1* and for investigating the role of *WT1* in differentiation (Phelan *et al.*, 1994).

A leukemia line resistant to bryostatin has been isolated (Prendiville *et al.*, 1994). Bryostatin, while lacking tumor-promoting activity, induces differentiation in maturation-arrested leukemia cells, exhibits selective antiproliferative properties in normal or malignant hematopoietic cells, and supports growth of multipotent stem cells (Steube and Drexler, 1993). The effects of bryostatin and phorbol esters indicate that PKCβ II plays a role in modulating etoposide-induced DNA binding activity of topoisomerase II in resistant K/VP.5 cells, through a mechanism linked to phosphorylation of topoisomerase II (Ritke *et al.*, 1995). Treatment of four megakaryoblastic cell lines with PKC activators TPA and bryostatin led to terminal differentiation as assessed by morphologic alterations, changes in the surface marker profile, and growth arrest (Hu *et al.*, 1994). Treatment of U937 human leukemic cells with bryostatin caused a 60% reduction in cell growth, and TPA completely inhibited cell growth. Both compounds induced inhibition of cyclin-dependent kinase 2 (cdk2) activity (Asiedu *et al.*, 1995). In a later study, bryostatin induced only a modest degree of U937 growth inhibition and antagonized TPA-stimulated growth arrest (Carey *et al.*, 1996). Enhanced expression and activation of fyn kinases are critical events associated with monocytic differentiation induced by bryostatin in THP-1 cells (Li *et al.*, 1997). Bryostatin increased the susceptibility of U937 cells to taxol-induced apoptosis and inhibition of clonogenicity, raising the possibility of functional alterations in Bcl-2 and/or other proteins involved in regulation of the cell death pathway (Wang *et al.*, 1998). Pretreatment of leukemic cells with certain deoxycytidine analogues interferes with CDKI induction by PMA and bryostatin, possibly contributing to the modulation of apoptosis and differentiation in cells exposed sequentially to these agents. Bryostatin is a considerably weaker stimulus than PMA for U937 cell differentiation, perhaps by its failure to induce p21^{CIP1} and trigger cell cycle arrest (Vrana *et al.*, 1998b, 1999a).

h. Lymphoma Cell Lines

Bryostatin induces a unidirectional change from high-grade lymphoma to intermediate-grade lymphoma and shows similarity to TPA (Al-Katib *et al.*, 1990). In B-lymphocyte cell lines latently infected with Epstein–Barr virus, bryostatin induces the production of transforming virus particles over a wide range of concentrations (Stewart *et al.*, 1993). In human diffuse large cell lymphoma, bryostatin induces α-enolase, which may play a significant role in the differentiation of lymphoma in man (Mohammad *et al.*, 1995b).

C. Antiviral Activity

The antiviral activity of the bryostatins is covered in a series of studies (Matthes *et al.*, 1990; Kinter *et al.*, 1990; Boto *et al.*, 1991; Vlach and Pitha, 1992; Qatsha *et al.*, 1993; Gulakowski *et al.*, 1997; Bodily *et al.*, 1999).

D. Murine *in Vivo* Anticancer Studies

A number of papers are relevant to this topic (Al-Katib *et al.*, 1996; Mohammad *et al.*, 1996c; Ruff *et al.*, 1999). *In vivo* results have extended *in vitro* findings that bryostatin acts as a partial inhibitor of PKC function (Hennings *et al.*, 1987). In a clonogenic assay, bryostatin had a direct antiproliferative effect against B16 melanoma, suggesting an effect on the B16 melanoma pulmonary metastases (Schuchter *et al.*, 1991). The success of *in vivo* administration of bryostatin in mice bearing subcutaneous L10A lymphomas and the observation that 5/6 human B-cell lymphoma cell lines were sensitive to the growth inhibitory effects of bryostatin *in vitro* suggest that bryostatin may be effective in the management

of lymphoid malignancies in humans (Hornung *et al.*, 1992). The ability of bryostatin to stimulate murine haematopoiesis *in vivo* also makes this drug particularly attractive in clinical applications (Gebbia *et al.*, 1993). Bryostatin is capable of activating platelets and neutrophils and modulating PKC *in vivo* (Berkow *et al.*, 1993). 4T1 cells respond *in vivo* to bryostatin therapy, and *in vivo* administration inhibits both primary and secondary tumor growth by 50%. The therapeutic effects of bryostatin in this system do not involve alterations in levels and distribution of PKC but may cause p53-independent up-regulation of *bax/bcl*-2 ratios (Wang, S. *et al.*, 1998). The characterization of a permanent pancreatic cell line (KCI-MOH1), established as a xenograft in severe combined immune-deficient mice, from a 74-year-old African American male patient diagnosed with pancreatic cancer was reported; results show that gemcitabine, ara-C, and bryostatin were active (Mohammad *et al.*, 1998b). The Wayne State University–CLL–severe combined immunodeficiency mouse (WSU-CLL-SCID) model showed an increase in CD11c/CD22 coexpression upon treatment. The results demonstrate the validity of the WSU-CLL-SCID model in predicting biological effects of bryostatin in humans for future translational research and clinical applications (Vaishampayan *et al.*, 1999). The clonal preservation of the human pancreatic cell line KCI-MOH1 has been reported and a KCI-MOH1 xenograft in SCID mice was used for efficacy evaluation of bryostatin alone or in combination with auristatin PE, spongistatin-1, and gemcitabine (Mohammad *et al.*, 1999a).

E. Bryostatin as a Major Anti-Tumor Promoter

Bryostatin as an anti-tumor promoter is a key area of research (Sako *et al.*, 1987; Reeves *et al.*, 1987; Jetten *et al.*, 1989; Hysmith and Gotto, 1989; Tavakkol *et al.*, 1991; Hennings *et al.*, 1991; Dlugosz and Yuspa, 1991; Klein *et al.*, 1992; Grossman *et al.*, 1992; Szallasi *et al.*, 1993a, 1993b, 1995; Saunders *et al.*, 1993; Fisher *et al.*, 1993; Hagerman *et al.*, 1997). Simultaneous treatment with TPA and known inhibitors of skin tumor promotion, such as retinoic acid, fluocinolone acetonide, and bryostatin, blocked colony formation of 308 cells in coculture with normal keratinocytes. The actions of promoters and inhibitors both appear to be mediated by normal keratinocytes (Hennings *et al.*, 1990). Activation of PKC in cultured human keratinocytes is required for differentiation. This is crucial to the analysis of compounds suspected of promoting or inhibiting epidermal tumors (Gschwendt *et al.*, 1992a; Matsui *et al.*, 1993). Earlier it was shown that expression of mutant p21-*ras* confirmed a striking sensitivity to the toxic effects of phorbol esters; in a thyroid tumor line, the effects of the phorbol esters could be separated from that of bryostatin (Dawson *et al.*, 1993). Activation of PKC concurrently enhances expression of mRNAs and proteins for the granular cell markers loricrin and filaggrin. This response does not occur in cells pretreated with bryostatin to inactivate PKC. PKC is thus a fundamental regulator of the coordinate changes in keratinocyte gene expression that occur during the spinous to granular cell transition in epidermis (Dlugosz and Yuspa, 1993). Recombinant human hepatocyte growth factor and anti-IgE may act on human mast cells through a common pathway to increase free cytosolic Ca^{2+} levels, and this effect is similarly modulated by bryostatin (Columbo et al., 1994).

The induction of TG-K gene expression by Ca^{2+} is dependent on PKC, providing further support for PKC's regulation of the late stages of epidermal differentiation (Dlugosz and Yuspa, 1994). Long-term exposure to bryostatin selectively depletes PKC-α (Uberall et al., 1994). The results of a study using bryostatin to block PKC function suggests that ras alters keratinocyte differentiation by altering the PKC signaling pathway and that PKC-α is the specific isozyme involved in down-modulating expression of keratins and upregulating expression of loricrin, filaggrin, and keratinocyte transglutaminase (Dlugosz et al., 1994). PKC-α, -ϵ and -δ, but not PKC-η and -ζ, were down-regulated by treatment of both cell types with bryostatin. Pretreatment of cells with bryostatin inhibited staurosporine-induced protein cross-linking and marker expression, suggesting a necessity for the α, δ, and/or ϵ isoforms in staurosporine-induced differentiation (Stanwell et al., 1996b). In cells pretreated with bryostatin to selectively down-modulate specific PKC isoforms, staurosporine-induced loricrin, filaggrin, and SPR-1 expression was suppressed when PKC-α, -ϵ, and/or -δ were down-regulated, suggesting that these isozymes are necessary for marker expression in response to this agent (Stanwell et al., 1996a). When PKC was either down-regulated with bryostatin 5 or inhibited with Ro 31-8220 or staurosporine, the expression of both uPA and uPA-R was greatly decreased in migrating keratinocytes (Ando and Jensen, 1996). Inhibition of PKC function using bryostatin or GF-109203X blocked the induction of keratinocyte differentiation markers at high cell densities. Thus, endogenous activation of PKC is responsible for cell-density-mediated stimulation of normal human epidermal keratinocytes (NHEKs) differentiation in humans as well as in mice (Lee et al., 1998). The effects of PKC down-regulation on desmoglein (Dsg) isoform expression were evaluated. Long-term treatment with either the phorbol ester TPA or bryostatin inhibited levels of Dsg1 and Dsg3, but not Dsg2 in NHEKs and HaCaT cells. These results identify several regulatory mechanisms by which the differentiation-specific pattern of desmosomal cadherins is established in the epidermis (Denning et al., 1998).

F. Adoptive Immunotherapy

Phase I/II clinical trials currently in progress on AIDS and cancer patients treated with AS101 show significant increases in various immunologic parameters, with minimal toxicity. The synergistic effect of AS101 and a partially purified preparation of bryostatin on the production of several cytokines was confirmed with greatly enhanced cell proliferation, IL-2, TNF, and interferon-γ (IFN-γ) secretion by human mononuclear cells and production of IL-2 and TNF by mouse cells. The absence of tumor-promoting activity of the bryostatins makes them particularly good candidates, in combination with AS101, for immunomodulation in vivo in clinically immunosuppressed conditions (Sredni et al., 1990). The ability of bryostatin plus the calcium ionophore ionomycin to activate lymphocytes obtained from draining popliteal lymph nodes (DLNs) from an MCA-105 footpad tumor was evaluated. Adoptive transfer of bryostatin/ionomycin (B/I)–stimulated DLN cells eradicated MCA-105 pulmonary metastases. B/I-activated DLN cells from MCA-105-tumor-bearing hosts had no therapeutic efficacy against B16 melanoma or MCA-203 sarcoma metastases (Tuttle et al., 1992a, 1992b). DLN cells activated with bryostatin and ionomycin persist for the long term in vivo as functional memory cells after adoptive transfer (Tuttle et al., 1992c). When adoptively transferred to mice with established liver metastases, DLN cells restimulated with B/I-mediated specific tumor regression (Tuttle et al., 1992d). The results suggest that secretion of IFN-γ by adoptively transferred DLN cells also plays an essential role in tumor rejection (Tuttle et al., 1992b, 1993).

Current adoptive immunotherapy strategies in cancer patients require large numbers of activated T cells and are limited by the availability of autologous tumor. In vitro exposure of thawed cells to B/I followed by culture in low-dose IL-2 and restimulation on day 10 resulted in 269- to 28,200-fold expansion in cell numbers, counted 17 days after initial stimulation. B/I-expanded T cells from five out of six patients secreted the cytokines TNF-α and IFN-γ in response to coculture with autologous tumor cells but not with irrelevant tumor cells. The results are analogous to the murine findings and laid the groundwork for a clinical trial of this novel adoptive immunotherapy strategy (Lind et al., 1993). The administration of low-dose cyclophosphamide prior to harvesting DLN cells may improve the success of adoptive immunotherapy in cancer patients (Tuttle et al., 1994). B/I treatment of lymphocytes from antigen-sensitized mice apparently causes preferential activation and expansion of sensitized or memory T cells (Fleming et al., 1994). Adoptive transfer of tumor-sensitized B/I-activated DLN cells confers protection against tumor challenge without prior in vitro expansion of the effector cells. Phenotyping studies demonstrated that donor cells activated with B/I expanded in recipient mice after adoptive transfer and could move to tumor sites. Moreover, these cells could mediate a therapeutic effect on established tumor metastases when combined with chemotherapy (Fleming et al., 1995). Thus, despite rapid disappearance of the drug from plasma, a single dose of bryostatin exhibits significant and sustained effects on normal murine spleen cells, including early lymphocyte activation, prolonged depletion of PKC activity, splenocyte proliferation, and splenomegaly (Bear *et al.*, 1996). A reproducible and sustained eradication of a malignant glioma can also be achieved by adoptive transfer of tumor-sensitized, *ex-vivo*-expanded CTL, and a phase I clinical trial is underway (Merchant *et al.*, 1997). Adoptive transfer of B/I-activated DLN lymphocytes sensitized by inoculation of WT B16-F10, or of IL-4-, GM-CSF-, or IFN-γ-expressing cells significantly reduced pulmonary metastases (Lipshy *et al.*, 1997; Rice *et al.*, 1997). When DLNs were cultured with low-dose IL-2, incubated with B/I, and injected into 3-day intracerebral RT-2 glioma models, tumors were almost always eliminated. Thus, successful expansion of glioma-sensitized DLN lymphocytes is possible, and adoptive immunotherapy using these cells is capable of both effectively limiting the progression of large gliomas and totally eradicating small ones (Baldwin *et al.*, 1997).

G. Bryostatin Mechanisms of Action

1. Protein Kinase C

Work by a number of groups, especially by Blumberg (see Blumberg et al., 1989; Hennings *et al.*, 1987) has established that bryostatin binds to and activates PKC in a manner that mimics, and competes with, the phorbol esters but has different physiologic effects (May *et al.*, 1987a; Kraft *et al.*, 1988; Sako *et al.*, 1988; Gschwendt *et al.*, 1988; Parker *et al.*, 1988; de Vries *et al.*, 1988; Kiss and Anderson, 1989; Membreno *et al.*, 1989; Mond *et al.*, 1990; Parkinson *et al.*, 1994; Steube *et al.*, 1994; Southern *et al.*, 1995; Columbo *et al.*, 1996; Grant and Jarvis, 1996; Racke *et al.*, 1997; Sansbury *et al.*, 1997; Smith *et al.*, 1997; Van Iderstine *et al.*, 1997; Wojtowicz-Praga *et al.*, 1997; Goekjian and Jirousek, 1999; Tan *et al.*, 1999; Watters and Parsons, 1999). Bryostatin may activate polymorphonuclear leukocytes by binding to the PMA receptor (Berkow and Kraft, 1985). Bryostatin potently inhibits the binding of PDBu to a high-affinity receptor in the cells, suggesting that bryostatins and TPA act via the same receptor in these cells (Smith *et al.*, 1985). Activation of PKC by some agents is not sufficient for induction of HL-60 cell differentiation, which implies that some of the biological effects of phorbol esters may occur through a more complex mechanism (Kraft *et al.*, 1986). Different activators of PKC (such as bryostatins 1 and 2) may elicit different cellular responses by altering the substrate specificity or activating multiple forms of the kinase (Ramsdell *et al.*, 1986). Coadminstration of bryostatin at equimolar concentration prevented the PMA inhibitory effect on chondrocytic expression, confirming the other findings that phorbol activation of PKC cannot exclusively account for the activity of phorbol on cell expression (Garrison *et al.*, 1987). The actions of 1-oleoyl-2-acetylglycerol (OAG), TPA, and mezerein were very similar to that of

bryostatin but not fully equivalent; KG-1a cells exhibited altered phosphorylation patterns, perhaps related to the TPA resistance characteristic of this subline of cells (Kiss *et al.*, 1987b). The findings on arachidonic acid metabolite release argue against transient activation of the PKC pathway as the sole explanation of bryostatin action (Dell'Aquila *et al.*, 1988). Time-dependent inhibition of the PKC pathway could account for many of the observed differences between the actions of the phorbol esters and bryostatin (Pasti *et al.*, 1988).

Bryostatin 1 at 5 nM and bryostatin 2 at 100 nM inhibited DNA synthesis as measured by incorporation of [^{3}H]thymidine by SH-SY5Y cells, although to a significantly lesser degree than TPA (Jalava *et al.*, 1990). Transformation of cells by certain oncogenes differentially affects phospholipase-D-mediated hydrolysis of phosphatidylethanolamine induced by PMA and bryostatin, suggesting that the action of PMA might involve two different mechanisms (Kiss *et al.*, 1991b). At least some of the differences in the biological effects induced by bryostatin and PMA may be due to distinct regulation of PKC; thus, although both agents can initially bind to and activate PKC at a later time (approximately 16 h), bryostatin, but not PMA, induces rapid PKC degradation and inhibition of PKC-regulated biological responses that are dependent on the continuous presence and/or activation of the enzyme (Galron *et al.*, 1993).

Bryostatin induces activation of Raf-1 in FDC-P1 cells, suggesting a pathway for promoting hematopoietic cell growth through serine phosphorylation (Carroll and May, 1994). Bryostatin-sensitive PKC is distinct from PMA- or K252a-sensitive kinases and is necessary, but not sufficient, for neurite outgrowth, acting in the nucleus in a manner independent of c-*fos* and c-*jun* transcription (Singh *et al.*, 1994). The effects of a series of protein kinase inhibitors on nerve growth factor dependent and independent neurite outgrowth in PC12 cells have established an ordered relationship among those protein kinases sensitive to down-regulation by bryostatin, stimulation by staurosporine, inhibition by sphingosine, or inhibition by 6-thioguanine (Campbell and Neet, 1995). Viral enzymes not naturally expressed by tumors, such as thymidine kinase, may be induced by PKC activators, thus rendering tumor cells sensitive to killing by ganciclovir (Ambinder *et al.*, 1996). The blocking of PKC function in v-*ras*-H-α-keratinocytes with bryostatin restored RAR-α protein to near normal levels, reflecting the involvement of PKC in RAR-α regulation (Darwiche *et al.*, 1996).

2. PKC Isoforms, Isozymes, and Isotypes

Other articles describe the interactions of bryostatins with PKC isoforms (Levine *et al.*, 1991; Kiss, 1992; Kiss and Deli, 1992; Gschwendt *et al.*, 1992b; Ng and Guy, 1992; Jalava *et al.*, 1993a; Reynolds *et al.*, 1994; Kazanietz *et al.*, 1994a; Zang *et al.*, 1994; Gschwendt *et al.*, 1994; Courage *et al.*, 1995; Geiges *et al.*, 1995; Gschwendt *et al.*, 1995; Walker *et al.*, 1995; Turner *et al.*, 1996; Ekinci *et al.*, 1996; Malarkey *et al.*, 1996; Slater *et al.*, 1996; Sylvia *et al.*, 1996; Keenan *et al.*, 1997; Lorenzo *et al.*, 1997b; Clarke *et al.*, 1999; Haussermann *et al.*, 1999; Kimura *et al.*, 1999; Wang, Q. M. J. *et al.*, 1999; Wender *et al.*, 1999b). Overexpression of PKC-β1 is not sufficient to induce factor independence in the IL-3-dependent myeloid cell line FDC-P1; addition of phorbol esters or bryostatin to these cells markedly decreased the levels of PKC without affecting the ability of these cells to grow in IL-3 (Kraft *et al.*, 1990). Bryostatin did not induce differentiation of HL-60 cells and blocked the cytostatic effect of PDBu; α- and β-II-PKC differed with respect to activator responsiveness, intracellular distribution, and substrate specificity (Hocevar and Fields, 1991); data indicate that the divergent effects of PMA and bryostatin on erythroleukemia cell proliferation and differentiation correspond to differential activation of β-II PKC at the nuclear membrane (Hocevar *et al.*, 1992).

There are six isoforms of PKC (α, β, γ, δ, ε, and ζ) in human prostate adenocarcinoma PC-3 cells, and each of these isozymes reacts distinctively to bryostatin-2, diolein, OAG and PMA, in part due to an altered molecular size and conceivably discrete binding site (Choi and Ahn, 1993). Phosphorylation of PKC substrates and associated functional changes do not require isozyme translocation to the surface membrane, even when these events are induced by a direct activator of PKC (Grabarek and Ware, 1993). It seems that the divergent actions of bryostatin and TPA in SH-SY5Y cells are at least partially due to differential modulation of PKC-α but not of PKC-ε (Jalava *et al.*, 1993b). Bryostatin mediates a faster depletion of the PKC-α isoform in rat nesangial cells than the other PKC activators tested (Huwiler *et al.*, 1994). The susceptibility of adenocarcinoma cells to bryostatin-induced growth delay are determined by cellular levels of PKC-α and/or -ε; however, differences between the abilities of bryostatin and TPA to inhibit cell growth do not seem to be intrinsically related to differences in redistribution or down-regulation of specific PKC isoenzymes (Stanwell *et al.*, 1994). Although PKC-ε was readily translocated by both PMA and bryostatin, the PKC-α originally associated with the particulate fraction showed no down-regulation by either of these agents. Differential regulation of PKC isozymes by PMA and bryostatin may contribute to the different patterns of biological responses (Szallasi *et al.*, 1994a). Bryostatin showed substantially different regulation for PKC-α, PKC-δ, and PKC-ε, whereas PMA distinguished only weakly between these isozymes (Szallasi *et al.*, 1994b). Alterations in the PKC pathway can modulate the "decision" of a breast cancer cell to undergo death or differentiation; in addition, PKC activation can induce expression of gadd45 in a p53-independent fashion (de Vente *et al.*, 1995). Selective down-regulation of PKC isoforms by either 12-deoxyphorbol-13-phenylacetate or bryostatin inhibited Ca^{2+}-induced expression of differentiation markers at doses most specific for

the down-regulation of PKC-α. These observations suggest that the induction of keratinocyte differentiation by Ca^{2+} results in activation of specific PKC isozymes (Denning *et al.*, 1995). The C-terminal portion of the PKC-δ does not appear to be essential for binding, and the loop comprising amino acids 20–28 is implicated in the binding activity (Kazanietz *et al.*, 1995).

Bryostatin inhibits TPA-induced depletion of both insulin receptor substrate 1 and PKC-δ expression in MCF-7 cells (de Vente *et al.*, 1996). Nonmotile lymphocytes recevied long-term treatment with bryostatin and the time courses of induction of motility and down-regulation of PKC isotypes were compared. Induction of motility correlated better with down-regulation of ε, η and θ than with α or β. It was concluded that the data fit best with the involvement of a nonclassical PKC isotype in regulating lymphocyte motility, although no association with a particular isotype was found (Thorp *et al.*, 1996). Evidence for a unique role of PKC-ε in the regulation of tau phosphorylation and neuronal differentiation was obtained, together with the demonstration that bryostatin can function under certain conditions as a selective PKC-ε activator (Ekinci and Shea, 1997). Given the different substrate specificities and modes of activation by various tumor-promoting and non-tumor-promoting agents, such as bryostatin, as well as the different sensitivities to various inhibitors, there is considerable divergence of individual PKC subtypes in signal transduction (Geiges *et al.*, 1997). The down-modulation of PKC-α and PKC-ε occurs principally via the ubiquitin/proteasome pathway (Lee, *et al.*, 1996a, 1996b, 1997). The catalytic domain of PKC-δ confers protection from down-regulation induced by bryostatin or bryostatin plus PMA, suggesting that this domain contains the isotype-specific determinants involved in the unique effect of bryostatin on PKC-δ (Lorenzo *et al.*, 1997a, 1997b). The tumor-promoting effect of phorbol esters may thus be due to depletion of PKC-δ, which has an apparent tumor suppressor function (Lu *et al.*, 1997).

PKC has been implicated in TNF signaling. Activators of PKC, such as PDBu (1 μM), indolactam V (10 μM), and bryostatin (1 μM), decreased the sensitivity of MCF-7 cells to TNF by 5-, 10-, and 1.7-fold, respectively. The novel regulation of PKC-η implicates this isozyme in PDBu-mediated protection of MCF-7 cells against TNF cytotoxicity (Basu, 1998). In a study of the relative interaction of ligands differing in structure and pattern of biological response with the C1a and C1b domains of PKC-δ, selectivity was not observed for bryostatin, which was a partial antagonist. The pattern of response corresponded to the activity of the compounds as complete tumor promoters (Bogi *et al.*, 1998). The regulatory domain of PKC-δ mediates the inhibitory effect of this isoform on the expression of glutamine synthetase. Phosphorylation of PKC-δ on tyrosine residues in the regulatory domain is implicated in this inhibitory effect (Brodie *et al.*, 1998).

Nerve growth factor stimulation of PC12 cells activates signaling pathways, leading to new protein expression and growth of neurites. PMA or bryostatin incubation, followed by NGF, may activate PKC isoforms δ and ε, leading to outgrowth of long neurites (Burry, 1998). Four neural-derived cell lines (C6 rat glioma, N1E-115 mouse, and SK-N-MC and SK-N-SH human neuroblastoma) express different PKC isoforms and respond differentially to β-TPA stimulation of phosphatidyl choline synthesis. β-TPA or bryostatin produced similar enhancement of choline incorporation (Cook *et al.*, 1998). A cellular assay for PKC-β II function was devised based on the finding that in response to bryostatin PKC-β II selectively translocates to the nucleus and phosphorylates nuclear lamin B (Gokmen and Fields, 1998). YT cell cytolytic activity is dependent on PKC-δ, which is selectively down-regulated by bryostatin (Kos and Bear, 1998). Although high- and low-affinity phorbol ester binding sites are found on non-membrane-associated PKC, the phorbol ester binding properties change significantly upon association with membranes (Slater *et al.*, 1998). Studies on the ability of bryostatin to block nerve growth factor–induced differentiation of pheochromocytoma PC12 cells suggest that the phosphorylation state of PKC-δ may regulate its ability to participate in signal coupling and modulation of cell growth and differentiation pathways (Wooten *et al.*, 1998). Bryostatin specifically down-regulated PKC-α *in vitro* in glioblastoma-derived cell lines but without significant growth inhibition. The observed overexpression of PKC-α in glioblastoma-derived cell lines may be an artifact of *in vitro* growth (Zellner *et al.*, 1998). PKC-δ also regulates the activation of caspases, and the biphasic concentration response of bryostatin on cisplatin-induced cell death could be explained by its distinct effect on PKC-δ down-regulation and caspase activation (Basu and Akkaraju, 1999). Treatment of U-937 and HL-60 myeloid leukemia cells with TPA, PDBu, or bryostatin was associated with the induction of stress-activated protein kinase (SAPK), indicating that PKC-β activation is necessary for activation of the MEK-1/SEK1/SAPK cascade in the TPA response of myeloid leukemia cells (Kaneki *et al.*, 1999). The C1 domains of PKC-δ do not have equivalent roles in inducing protection against bryostatin-induced down-regulation, and elucidation of the differential effect of bryostatin on PKC-δ may suggest strategies for the design of novel bryostatin-like compounds (Lorenzo *et al.*, 1999).

3. Protein Kinase D

PKD mediates some of the multiple biphasic biological responses induced by bryostatin in intact cells (Matthews *et al.*, 1997). It is activated by phosphorylation in intact cells stimulated by phorbol esters, cell permeant diacylglycerols, bryostatin, neuropeptides, and growth factors. PKD is activated by phosphorylation of residues Ser744 and Ser748 (Iglesias *et al.*, 1998; Waldron *et al.*, 1999).

4. Human Basophils

Bryostatin modulates the effects of a number of functions of basophils (Columbo *et al.*, 1990; de Paulis *et al.*, 1991). Cyclosporin A had no effect on the release of histamine caused by phorbol myristate and bryostatin (Cirillo *et al.*, 1990). Nimesulide inhibited histamine release from basophils induced by the Ca^{2+} ionophore A23187 and different PKC activators, such as TPA and bryostatins 1 and 5 (Casolaro *et al.*, 1993). Bryostatin was a more potent (approximately 30-fold) inhibitor of IgE-mediated histamine release than was TPA. The heterogeneous effects exerted by bryostatins on human basophils and mast cells are of interest in designing therapeutic trials (Patella *et al.*, 1995; Noll *et al.*, 1997).

5. T Cells

A wide variety of effects on T cells has been reported (Takayama and Sitkovsky, 1987; Esa *et al.*, 1990; Galron *et al.*, 1993, 1994; McFadden *et al.*, 1994; Thoburn and Hess, 1995; Flandina *et al.*, 1996; Curiel *et al.*, 1999; Espinoza-Delgado *et al.*, 1999a). The IL2 and IFN-γ production kinetics of cultures induced with either A23187/bryostatin or A23187/PMA were practically identical (Mohr *et al.*, 1987). Bryostatin has potent immunopotentiating properties that share some similar effects of PMA but offer the additional property of modulating other phorbol ester effects on proliferation (Hess *et al.*, 1988). Bryostatins 1 and 2 synergize with Ca^{2+} ionophores in triggering the exocytosis of cytolytic granules from cytotoxic T lymphocytes at very low concentrations (Trenn *et al.*, 1988). Direct stimulation of PKC with either PDBu or bryostatin substantially overcame dexamethasone's effects, resulting in a recovery of IL-2 production and significant restoration of the T-cell proliferative response; thus, treatment with bryostatin might reduce corticosteroid-induced immunosuppression (McVicar *et al.*, 1992). Bryostatin inhibits PMA-induced T-cell proliferation by causing rapid degradation of PKC, reflecting a requirement of persistent PKC stimulation (lasting approximately 48 h) for the activation of human T cells and progression through the cell cycle (Isakov *et al.*, 1993). Tyrosine phosphorylation and the association of p36-38 with Lck are differentially affected by bryostatin and PMA, suggesting that PKC regulates the interaction of potential signaling molecules with Lck, thereby regulating biochemical events that are relevant to T-cell mitogenesis and/or transformation (Galron *et al.*, 1997). Activation of T cells with bryostatin should be carried out under protection of exogenous IL-2 to ensure survival and expansion of T cells that may exhibit antitumor activity (Kos *et al.*, 2000).

6. Cytokines

In human U937 myeloid cells, sustained expression of pim-1 protein was induced by GM-CSF, G-CSF, and IL-6, but not by bryostatin. The pim-1 kinase may be an important intermediate in transmembrane signaling or response phenotype

induced by IL-3, GM-CSF, and other cytokines whose receptors are structurally similar. Its constitutive expression in some myeloid leukemia cell lines suggests activation of signal cascades utilized by myeloid growth factors (Lilly *et al.,* 1992). In cultured human tumor cells, bryostatin enhances lymphokine-activated killer sensitivity and on the basis of these results the use of bryostatin in combination with immunostimulating cytokines, such as IL-2, in the treatment of human cancer is suggested (Correale *et al.,* 1995). Cyclosporine-resistant proliferative responses induced by direct PKC activators, such as mitogenic concentrations of TPA or bryostatin, were inhibited in a concentration-dependent manner by the non-specific lipoxygenase inhibitor nordihydroguaiaretic acid (Esa and Converse, 1996). The synergistic interaction between IL-1α and bryostatin was dose and schedule dependent, and required simultaneous application for an optimal effect. Bryostatin may promote the release of cytokines from several accessory cell populations, including marrow stromal cells, to accomplish its *in vivo* hematopoietic effects (Lilly *et al.,* 1996). Bryostatin and IFN-· synergize in the induction of NO production as well as *iNOS* gene expression, suggesting the involvement of posttranscriptional mechanisms in the induction of iNOS mRNA (Taylor *et al.,* 1997). Modulation of erythropoiesis has also been reported (Sharkis *et al.,* 1989).

7. Apoptosis and Bcl-2 Phosphorylation

One of the most interesting properties of the bryostatins is the modulation of apoptosis through phosphorylation of Bcl-2 (May *et al.,* 1993; Grant *et al.,* 1997, 1998b; Ito *et al.,* 1997; Wall *et al.,* 1998a, 1999a, 1999b, 2000; Chen and Chen, 1999; Vrana and Grant, 1999; Vrana *et al.,* 1999b; Wang, S. *et al.,* 1999a, b, c; Chen *et al.,* 2000). PKC plays a role in growth-factor-induced Bcl-2 α-phosphorylation as well as in suppression of apoptosis (May *et al.,* 1994). Sphingoid bases have an intrinsic ability to induce apoptosis in HL-60 and U937 cells. The apoptotic capacity of bacterial sphingomyelinase was enhanced either by acute coexposure to highly selective pharmacologic inhibitors of PKC, such as calphostin C and chelerythrine, or by chronic preexposure to bryostatin, which completely down-modulated total assayable PKC activity (Jarvis *et al.,* 1996). Bryostatin may act, through modification of Bcl-2 phosphorylation status, at a distal site in the cell death pathway (Grant, 1997). IL-3 stimulates the net growth of murine-factor-dependent NSF/N1.H7 and FDC-P1/ER myeloid cells by stimulating proliferation and suppressing apoptosis. Treatment of factor-deprived cells with bryostatin dramatically increases the association between PP2A and Bcl-2 (Deng *et al.,* 1998). Treatment of the PKC-α transformants with bryostatin leads to higher levels of mitochondrial PKC-α, Bcl-2 phosphorylation, and REH cell survival following chemotherapy; thus, PKC-α has a functional role in Bcl-2 phosphorylation and in resistance to chemotherapy (Ruvolo *et al.,* 1998). Exposure to cells in the human monocytic leukemia cell line

U937 to bryostatin after (but not before) a 6-h incubation with paclitaxel significantly increases apoptosis and results in an approximately 3-log reduction in clonogenicity. Thus, bryostatin increases the susceptibility of U937 cells to paclitaxel-induced apoptosis and cytotoxicity. This may involve functional alterations in Bcl-2 or other proteins involved in regulation of the cell death pathway (Wang, S. *et al.,* 1998). The functional role of the cyclin-dependent kinase inhibitor p21$^{WAF1/CIP1}$ in leukemic cell G$_1$ arrest, differentiation, and apoptosis induced by PMA and bryostatin was examined using antisense-expressing lines. Following treatment with these agents, dysregulation of p21 prevents leukemic cells from engaging a normal differentiation program through a c-*myc*-independent mechanism and instead directs cells along an apoptotic pathway (Wang, Z. *et al.,* 1998).

H. Multidrug Resistance Studies

The bryostatins have important effects on multidrug resistance (MDR) (Scala *et al.,* 1995; Utz *et al.,* 1995; Basu *et al.,* 1996). Bryostatin down-regulates *mdr-1* overexpression and enhances Adriamycin-induced cytotoxicity in prostatic carcinoma. Therefore, bryostatin would be a useful adjunct to chemotherapy affected by *mdr-1* overexpression (Kamanda and Leese, 1998). Bryostatin interacts with both the mutated *mdr-1*-V185 and the wild-type *mdr-1*-G185, but reverses multidrug resistance and inhibits drug efflux only in PGP-V185 mutants; this effect is not due to an interference of PKC with PGP (Spitaler *et al.,* 1998). Bryostatin-induced down-regulation of *mdr* might be one mechanism by which bryostatin potentiates vincristine activity. The sequential use of both agents resulted in clinically significant antitumor activity in diffuse large cell lymphoma xenograafts (Al-Katib *et al.,* 1998).

I. Preclinical Development of the Bryostatins

The potent antineoplastic actions displayed *in vitro* by bryostatin have led to the introduction of short-term bryostatin infusions in phase I clinical trials. The effects of bryostatin on clonogenic leukemia cell growth are strongly dependent on scheduling and dose varying between and within individual AML samples. The results caution against *in vivo* bryostatin pulse therapy, as currently applied for treatment of AML (van der Hem *et al.,* 1996). The PKC target may also be important in targeting tumor angiogenesis (Harris *et al.,* 1994). Determination of whether agents that target PKC isoforms will be effective anticancer agents is an important objective of pediatric clinical investigations (Smith and Ho, 1996).

1. Bryostatin with ara-C

Bryostatin induces biochemical perturbations in leukemic cells that favor ara-C activation, particularly in high-density cells exhibiting impaired ara-C nucleotide formation (Grant *et al.*, 1991a). Exposure of HL-60 cells to bryostatin renders them more susceptible to ara-C-related DNA damage, contributing to the cytotoxic effects of this drug combination. It is possible that bryostatin, perhaps through modulation of intracellular signaling events in leukemic cells, has the capacity to potentiate ara-C-related apoptosis or programmed cell death (Grant *et al.*, 1992a). While bryostatin exerts a heterogeneous effect on ara-C metabolism in leukemic myeloblasts, it is capable of potentiating ara-C phosphorylation in a subset of patient samples, including some that do not exhibit an increase in response to recombinant GM-CSF. It is possible that bryostatin-induced potentiation of ara-C metabolism in some leukemic cells may contribute, at least in part, to the antileukemic efficacy of this drug combination (Grant *et al.*, 1992b).

Combined exposure *in vitro* to ara-C and bryostatin, both with and without rGM-CSF, effectively inhibits the growth of leukemic cells with self-renewal capacity while sparing a significant fraction of normal committed and primitive hematopoietic progenitors (Grant *et al.*, 1992d). Bryostatin potentiates apoptosis in human myeloid leukemia cells (Grant *et al.*, 1994b). A quantitative basis for assessing the ability of bryostatin and related compounds to potentiate ara-C-induced damage to DNA underscores the complex and pleiotropic effects that modulation of the PKC family exerts on ara-C-related apoptosis in human leukemia cells (Jarvis *et al.*, 1994b). A23187-induced perturbations in intracellular Ca^{2+} homeostasis permit bryostatin to induce differentiation in an unresponsive myeloid leukemia cell line while antagonizing the ability of this agent to augment ara-C-related apoptosis. While A23187 and bryostatin-associated differentiation protects cells from ara-C-induced programmed cell death, this phenomenon is not accompanied by the restoration of leukemic cell clonogenic potential (Grant *et al.*, 1995).

Bryostatin reverses, at least in part, the reduced susceptibility of clonogenic U937 cells to ara-C conferred by c-*jun* dysregulation, further suggesting that this phenomenon proceeds via nonapoptotic mechanisms (Freemerman *et al.*, 1996). Pretreatment of HL-60 cells with bryostatin potentiates ara-C-induced apoptosis. To test the hypothesis that this capacity stems from down-regulation of PKC activity, comparisons were made between the effects of bryostatin and those of the tumor promoter mezerein under conditions favoring either cellular differentiation or drug-induced apoptosis. Down-regulation of total assayable PKC activity and Ca^{2+}-dependent PKC expression by bryostatin appear to be insufficient, by themselves, to account for potentiation of leukemic cell apoptosis, at least under conditions in which differentiation occurs. Evidence is also provided that a reciprocal and highly schedule-dependent relationship exists between leukemic cell differentiation and drug-induced apoptosis (Grant *et al.*, 1996). AS101 partially restores the ability of bryostatin to trigger a differentiation program in an other-

wise unresponsive HL-60 cell line, possibly by facilitating bryostatin-mediated G_1 arrest. AS101 also potentiates the antiproliferative effects of bryostatin administered alone or in combination with ara-C through a mechanism other than, or in addition to, induction of apoptosis (Rao *et al.*, 1996).

The ability of bryostatin to facilitate drug-induced apoptosis in human myeloid leukemia cells involves factors other than quantitative changes in the expression of Bcl-2 family members, suggesting that qualitative alterations in the Bcl-2 protein, such as phosphorylation status, may contribute to this capacity (Bartimole *et al.*, 1997). HL-60 cell apoptosis proceeds by both c-*myc*-dependent and independent pathways, and only the former appears to be involved in the potentiation of ara-C-mediated cell death by bryostatin (Chelliah *et al.*, 1997). Surprisingly, bryostatin and PKC inhibitors (staurosporine and UCN-01) circumvent resistance of Bcl-2-overexpressing leukemic cells to ara-C-induced apoptosis and activation of the protease cascade (Wang, S. *et al.*, 1997). The modulation of ara-C resistance by bryostatin emphasizes the need to optimize treatment regimens for individual patients (Elgie *et al.*, 1998). The cytotoxicity of ara-C was substantially increased by pharmacologic reductions of PKC, including down-regulation of PKC by chronic preexposure to bryostatin or inhibition of PKC by acute coexposure to the dihydrosphingosine analogue safingol (Jarvis *et al.*, 1998). The inability of bryostatin to potentiate apoptosis in ara-C-pretreated HL-60 cells may involve factors other than an inadequate differentiation stimulus (Vrana *et al.*, 1998a).

2. Bryostatin with Auristatin PE

There is a synergistic effect between auristatin PE, dolastatin-10, or vincristine and bryostatin, which is more apparent in the bryostatin/auristatin PE combination. The use of these agents should be further explored clinically in the treatment of lymphoma (Mohammad *et al.*, 1998e). When the drugs were given in combination, animals treated with auristatin PE and bryostatin were all free of tumors for 150 days and considered cured (Mohammad *et al.*, 1998f).

3. Bryostatin with 2-CdA

A few studies have examined this combination (Mohammad *et al.*, 1998a, 1999c; Beck *et al.*, 1999). A xenograft model of CLL in WSU-CLL-bearing mice with severe combined immune deficiency was used. Sequential treatment with bryostatin followed by 2-CdA resulted in higher antitumor activity and improved animal survival (Mohammad *et al.*, 1998c).

4. Bryostatin with Dolastatin 10

TPA- or bryostatin-induced differentiation of AML cells was not affected by the dolastatins. Short-term exposure to the phorbol ester conferred reduced sensitivity of the cell line HL-60 to the antiproliferative effect of these drugs, suggesting that the dolastatins alone or in combination with other drugs might exert a role in the treatment of human myeloid leukemia (Steube *et al.*, 1992). WSU-DLCL2 cells were negative for p53 protein expression, upon treatment with bryostatin or dolastatin 10. The expression of p53 was weak and moderate with the bryostatin/dolastatin 10 combination. The inverse correlation between Bcl-2 and p53 oncoprotein expression seems to be related to induction of apoptosis in this lymphoma cell line (Maki *et al.*, 1995). The combination has also been evaluated in lymphoma xenogratfts (Mohammad *et al.*, 1996a).

5. Bryostatin with Fludarabine

Bryostatin sensitizes WSU-CLL cells to fludarabine and enhances apoptosis. The sequential treatment with bryostatin followed by fludarabine resulted in higher antitumor activity compared with either agent alone, in combination, or the reverse addition of these agents. These results are comparable to those of bryostatin followed by 2-CdA, suggesting common pathways of interaction between bryostatin and purine analogues (Mohammad *et al.*, 1999b).

6. Bryostatin with Interleukin-2

Based on examination using the B16 melanoma system, the combination of bryostatin with low-dose IL-2 is as effective as, but less toxic than, high-dose IL-2 alone (Espinoza-Delgado *et al.*, 1999b).

7. Bryostatin with Vincristine

Vincristine augments the antitumor effect of byostatin (Al-Katib *et al.*, 1993b; Mohammad *et al.*, 1994b, 1994c). Exposure of WSU-DLCL2 cells to bryostatin prior to treatment with vincristine enhances apoptosis (Mohammad *et al.*, 1995a). Bryostatin given 24 h before vincristine or melphalan resulted in the highest tumor growth inhibition, tumor growth delay, and tumor cell kill. Two of five mice receiving the bryostatin/vincristine combination were free of tumors more than 200 days after treatment. Whether bryostatin acts as a differentiating agent or as a direct anti-Waldenström's macroglobulinemia tumor agent remains unclear (Mohammad *et al.*, 1994a).

8. Preclinical Pharmacology

A study of the pharmacokinetics, tissue distribution, metabolism, and elimination of bryostatin in mice was undertaken using (C26-^{3}H)-labeled bryostatin. Bryostatin was relatively stable *in vivo*, widely distributed but concentrated in some major tissues, and rapidly excreted first through urine and at later times through the feces (Zhang *et al.*, 1996).

9. Assay for Bryostatin

A sensitive assay based on platelet activation has been developed (Carr *et al.*, 1995).

10. Formulation of Bryostatin

The formulation of a selected number of agents has been reviewed (Beijnen *et al.*, 1995). Bryostatin can be used for 4-week intravenous administration using polypropylene but not polyvinyl chloride infusion bags (Cheung *et al.*, 1998).

11. Radioprotective Effects of Bryostatin

Bryostatin potentiates the *in vitro* radioprotective effects of rGM-CSF and may also regulate the lineage specificity of this response (Grant *et al.*, 1992c). Induction of c-*jun* expression by x-rays, as well as H_2O_2, is inhibited by prolonged exposure to TPA or bryostatin, and also by H7, a nonspecific inhibitor of PKC-like protein kinases, but not by HA1004, a more selective inhibitor of cyclic-nucleotide-dependent protein kinase activity. Ionizing radiation induces c-*jun* gene transcription through the formation of reactive oxygen intermediates, and a protein kinase, perhaps a PKC isoform distinct from PKC-α and PKC-β, is also involved in this (Datta *et al.*, 1992). Bryostatin is a particularly good candidate in combination with AS101 for treatment *in vivo* in counteracting chemotherapy- or radiation-induced hematopoietic suppression or in generally improving the restoration of immune response under conditions involving hemopoietic damage (Kalechman *et al.*, 1992). GM-CSF/IL-3 fusion protein pIXY 321 exhibits significant *in vitro* radioprotective effects toward normal human bone marrow myeloid progenitors, and coadministration of PKC activators such as bryostatin selectively augments the radioprotective capacity of this hybrid cytokine toward noneosinophilic elements (Grant *et al.*, 1993). Colony-forming assays showed higher colony survival for irradiated T cells stimulated with bryostatin than with PMA. These results support the important role of PKC in T-cell radiation responses and suggest a potential role for bryostatin in enhancing T-lymphocyte survival during radiation therapy (Sung *et al.*, 1994). Bryostatin exhibits intrinsic *in vivo* radioprotective effects in lethally irradiated Balb/c and C3H/HeN mice, and may augment the radioprotective capacity of rmGM-CSF (Grant *et al.*, 1994a). It increases the sensitivity of human myeloid leukemic cells to low radiation doses without enhancing DNA fragmentation or apoptosis, and this capacity may involve factors other than, or in addition to, downmodulation of PKC activity (Watson *et al.*, 1996).

J. Phase I and II Human Cancer Clinical Trials

A number of clinical trials have been conducted (Varterasian *et al.*, 1996, 1998b; Stone *et al.*, 1998; Propper *et al.*, 1998; Gonzalez *et al.*, 1999). A phase I study recommended that bryostatin be used at a dose of 35–50 μg/m^2 every 2 weeks in phase II studies in patients with malignancies, including lymphoma, leukemia, melanoma, and hypernephroma (Prendiville *et al.*, 1993). Two patients with metastatic malignant melanoma had PRs after three or four cycles of therapy; remission lasted 6 weeks and >10 months, respectively. Antitumor activity against malignant melanoma was observed early in the course of treatment (Philip *et al.*, 1993). Intravenous administration of bryostatin increased the potential of IL-2 to induce proliferation and LAK activity in lymphocytes, making bryostatin an interesting candidate for combination studies (Scheid *et al.*, 1994). In a phase I study, responses were seen in four patients, including two PRs (4 months) and two minor responses. The PRs were seen in patients with ovarian carcinoma and low-grade non-Hodgkin's lymphoma. Two patients with ovarian carcinoma, one with a PR and the other with a minor response, were subsequently treated with tamoxifen, a PKC inhibitor; the former patient had a PR (14 months) in response to tamoxifen (Jayson *et al.*, 1995). In some patients, bryostatin treatment increased LAK activity, indicating that bryostatin at doses of 25 μg/m^2 can induce *in vivo* peripheral blood mononuclear cell PKC down-regulation in at least a subset of patients. Higher bryostatin doses might be more effective in achieving this effect (Grant *et al.*, 1998a). Another phase I study defined the MTD and recommended the phase II dose of bryostatin, when administered over 72 h every 2 weeks, to be 120 μg/m^2 (40 μg/m^2 for 3 days). Eleven patients achieved SD for 2–19 months (Varterasian *et al.*, 1998a). In a phase I trial in children with refractory solid tumors, bryostatin infusion was generally well tolerated, and stable disease was observed in several patients. One patient with renal cell carcinoma and another with neuroblastoma were stable while undergoing treatment, and two other patients with microscopic disease (one germ cell, one renal cell) were also stable during the study (Weitman *et al.*, 1999). In a phase II study among melanoma patients receiving 72-h infusion of bryostatin, there was one minor response and one PR. There was one minor response in patients treated with a 24-h infusion (Bedikian *et al.*, 1999). Preliminary results of an ongoing study of bryostatin in relapsed multiple myeloma patients indicated that bryostatin administered at its MTD by continuous infusion over 72 h every 2 weeks was well tolerated in this patient population (Trivedi *et al.*, 1999). In another phase II trial, 9 patients received sequential treatment with bryostatin and vincristine. Bryostatin alone resulted in one CR and two PR (Varterasian *et al.*, 2000). The current results of ongoing clinical trials of bryostatin in combination with certain well-known anticancer drugs (e.g., cisplatin, taxol, vincristine) are very promising for improvement of future human cancer treatments. Some earlier results are summarized below.

1. Myalgia

Myalgia has been noted as a side effect (Brinkmeier and Jockusch, 1987; Hickman *et al.*, 1995). Nifedipine counteracted the vasoconstrictive effect of bryostatin, but because nifedipine itself had an unexpected effect on mitochondrial metabolism, it was not possible to assess whether nifedipine modified bryostatin's effect (Thompson *et al.*, 1996).

K. Clinical Combinations of Bryostatin with Other Anticancer Drugs

1. Bryostatin with ara-C

A phase I trial has been initiated in which patients with refractory/relapsed AML and ALL received escalating doses of bryostatin both before and after a fixed dose of high-dose ara-C. The effects of bryostatin on leukemic blast PKC activity were variable, ranging from significant reductions in activity to essentially no change. Preliminary results indicate that bryostatin can be safely combined with high-dose ara-C in patients with refractory leukemia (Grant *et al.*, 1999a).

2. Bryostatin with 2-CdA

Sequential treatment of chronic lymphocytic leukemia with these agents has been reported (Ahmad *et al.*, 2000).

3. Bryostatin with Cisplatin

Several trials have been reported (Franco *et al.*, 1999). Toxicities of the combination treatment appear to be due to cisplatin administration, although myalgia has not been reported in a trial, still in progress and with one PR, of 13 patients with melanoma (Rosenthal *et al.*, 1999). Studies have demonstrated synergy between bryostatin and cisplatin and reversal of cisplatin resistance with the addition of bryostatin. One patient with esophageal adenocarcinoma had a PR lasting 6 weeks. Most interestingly, two refractory colon cancer patients had a 30% reduction of index lesions and stable disease, and remain on study for six and four cycles, respectively. Future plans include a phase II study dedicated to refractory colon cancer (Bangalore *et al.*, 2000). In another phase I combination trial of bryostatin and cisplatin, 17 evaluable patients with metastatic and/or unresectable carcinoma of the stomach and lung were assigned to receive one of five levels of bryostatin (15–55 μg/m^2) infused over 72 hours followed by cisplatin 50 mg/m^2 infused over 1 h. Of 16 patients evaluable for response, 1 had a CR, 2 a PR, 9 disease stabilization, and 4 progression (Lenz *et al.*, 2000).

4. Bryostatin with Fludarabine

Despite a low initial dose of fludarabine, several objective responses have been obtained in a phase I study. Two patients with previously treated NHL experienced CRs after 4–6 cycles of therapy. An additional three patients obtained objective PR, and six patients had stabilization of disease. One patient with NHL exhibited disappearance of pleural effusions and ascites at the 12.5 mg/m^2 per day dose level when combined with bryostatin. This trial may serve as a prototype for others of its kind in which cytotoxic drugs are combined with agents such as bryostatin that interrupt signal transduction pathways in the treatment of patients with hematologic malignancies (Grant *et al.*, 1999b).

5. Bryostatin with Paclitaxel

In a combined-agent trial, one patient with metastatic esophageal to liver cancer has a PR. Another patient experienced a minor response with pancreatic cancer and is continuing in the study. Sequential paclitaxel and bryostatin is well tolerated (Kaubisch *et al.*, 1999). Bryostatin enhances the activity of paclitaxel and cisplatin, provided paclitaxel precedes bryostatin, and cisplatin follows bryostatin (Koutcher *et al.*, 2000). The MTDs of paclitaxel and bryostatin on this schedule are 90 mg/m^2 and 50 μg/m^2, respectively (Kaubisch *et al.*, 2000).

6. Bryostatin with Vincristine

A phase I trial of 24-h infusion of bryostatin followed immediately by a bolus injection of vincristine was undertaken. Prolonged SD and one PR have been seen in two patients with pretreated (one posttransplantation) non-Hodgkin's lymphoma (6 months with SD and then progressed, 7 months with PR and bone marrow infiltration resolved) and SD in two patients with transplant-failed myeloma (6 and 7 months) (Dowlati et al., 1999, 2000).

L. Evaluation of Other Bryostatins

The area has been reviewed (Wender *et al.*, 1999a). Bryostatin 7 induces aggregation of human platelets and the phosphorylation of specific platelet proteins (Tallant *et al.*, 1987). Bryostatin 4 affects human hematopoietic progenitor cells (Gebbia *et al.*, 1988). Several bryostatins and TPA were used to examine the role of PKC in the regulation of GH-4C-1 rat pituitary tumor cell proliferation, and the results suggest that sustained activation of PKC inhibits GH-4 cell proliferation by blocking G$_1$-phase cells from entering S phase. Bryostatins also show a high degree of selectivity that appears to be due to the acetyl ester linkage in the C7 position (Mackanos *et al.*, 1991). Inversion at the chiral center at C26 of bryostatin 4 caused a dramatic decrease in binding affinity, but binding was competitively inhibited by phorbol 12,13-diacetate, as expected for ligands that interact at the same binding site (Lewin *et al.*, 1991). (26-^{3}H)-Bryostatin 4 was synthesized and its binding to PKC characterized. Little difference was found in its binding affinity to PKC isozymes α, β, and γ, suggesting that differential recognition by these isozymes does not account for the unique biological activity of the bryostatins (Lewin *et al.*, 1992). The unique pattern of biological responses to the bryostatins does not represent a unique pattern of isotype recognition (Kazanietz *et al.*, 1994b). The effects of TPA and bryostatin 5 have been com-

pared (Watters *et al.*, 1992). Exposure to bryostatin 5 leads to a strong macrophage-like cell differentiation in human myeloid leukemia, strengthening the potential of bryostatins as possible antileukemic agents (van der Hem *et al.*, 1993, 1994). Bryostatin 5 exerts an antiproliferative effect on AML cells and counteracts growth-factor-induced leukemic proliferation (van der Hem *et al.*, 1995a). Differential modulation of normal and leukemic myeloid clonogenicity by bryostatin 5 suggests a possible role in the treatment of acute myeloid leukemia (van der Hem *et al.*, 1995b). An adrenocortical hormone production promoter comprising bryostatin 10 derived from *B. neritina* as an active ingredient has been reported (Noriaki *et al.*, 1995). The growth inhibition of the bryostatins, at least in B16/F10 melanoma cells *in vitro*, does not result from interaction with PKC. As exemplified by 26-epibryostatin, this insight permits the design of analogues with growth inhibition comparable to bryostatin but with reduced toxicity (Szallasi *et al.*, 1996). A novel assay to measure the level of all bryostatins in the plasma of patients undergoing treatment is described (Kraft *et al.*, 1996). Bryostatin 5 preferentially regulates PKC-α activity through the second cysteine-rich sequence (CYS2) of C1, while regulation by the diterpene ester mezerein displayed strong preference for the first cysteine-rich sequence (CYS1) of C1 (Shieh *et al.*, 1996). An antiretroviral agent capable of effectively inhibiting HIV infection and spread contained bryostatin 10 as an active ingredient (Noriaki *et al.*, 1996). Bryostatin 10-induced steroidogenesis is caused by PKC activation similar to that of PMA (Kamano *et al.*, 1998).

Acknowledgments

We acknowledge with pleasure the expert contributions of Mrs. Georgia Reimus, Mrs. Theresa Thornburgh, and Professor Bruce Baguley to the preparation of the manuscript. GRP expresses thanks and appreciation to the very capable members of his research group, including Professors Cherry L. Herald, Yoshiaki Kamano, and Jean M. Schmidt and Dr. John E. Leet, as well as the National Cancer Institute and cancer cell biology, oncology, and other colleagues over the past 33 years who contributed to advancing this bryostatin anticancer drug discovery research. Financial support was provided by Outstanding Investigator Grant OIG CA44344-01A1-012 (U.S. National Cancer Institute, DHHS), the Arizona Disease Control Research Commission, and the Robert B. Dalton Endowment Fund.

References

Adler, V., and Kraft, A. S. (1995). Regulation of AP-3 enhancer activity during hematopoietic differentiation. *J. Cell. Physiol.* **164**, 26–34.

Ahmad, I., Al-Katib, A. M., Beck, F. W. J, and Mohammad, R. M. (2000). Sequential treatment of a resistant chronic lymphocytic leukemia patient with bryostatin 1 followed by 2-chlorodeoxyadenosine: case report. *Clin. Cancer Res.* **6,** 1328–1332.

Akompong, T., Inman, R. S., and Wessling-Resnick, M. (1995). Phorbol esters stimulate non-transferrin iron uptake by K562 cells. *J. Biol. Chem.* **270,** 20937–20941.

Al-Katib, A., Mohammad, R. M., Mohamed, A. N., Pettit, G. R., and Sensenbrenner, L. L. (1990). Conversion of high grade lymphoma tumor cell line to intermediate grade with TPA and bryostatin 1 as determined by polypeptide analysis on 2D gel electrophoresis. *Hematol. Oncol.* **8,** 81–89.

Al-Katib, A., Mohammad, R. M., Eliasberg, S., and Sensenbrenner, L. L. (1992). Immunomodulatory effects of recombinant human alpha-interferon (alpha-IFN) in combination with bryostatin 1 on the acute lymphoblastic leukemia (ALL) cell line, Reh. *Exp. Hematol.* **20,** 785.

Al-Katib, A., Mohammad, R. M., Dan, M., Hussein, M. E., Akhtar, A., Pettit, G. R., and Sensenbrenner, L.L. (1993a). Bryostatin 1-induced hairy cell features on chronic lymphocytic leukemia cells *in vitro. Exp. Hematol.* **21,** 61–65.

Al-Katib, A., Mohammad, R. M., Hamdan, M., Pettit, G. R., and Sensenbrenner, L. L. (1993b). Bryostatin 1 augments the antitumor effect of vincristine against human diffuse large cell lymphoma in a SCID mouse xenograft model. *Exp. Hematol.* **21,** 1124.

Al-Katib, A., Mohammad, R. M., Khan, K., Dan, M. E., Pettit, G. R., and Sensenbrenner, L. L. (1993c). Bryostatin 1-induced modulation of the acute lymphoblastic leukemia cell line Reh. *J. Immunother.* **14,** 33–42.

Al-Katib, A., Katato, K., Varterasian, M., Mohamed, A. N., Dugan, M., and Mohammad, R. M. (1996). Antitumor activity of bryostatin 1 against chronic lymphocytic leukemia (CLL) in a SCID mouse xenograft model. *Exp. Hematol.* **24,** 693.

Al-Katib, A. M., Smith, M. R., Kamanda, W. S., Pettit, G. R., Hamdan, M., Mohamed, A. N., Chelladurai, B., and Mohammad, R. M. (1998). Bryostatin 1 down-regulates *mdr*1 and potentiates vincristine cytotoxicity in diffuse large cell lymphoma xenografts. *Clin. Cancer Res.* **4,** 1305–1314.

Ambinder, R. F., Robertson, K. D., Moore, S. M., and Yang, J. (1996). Epstein-Barr virus as a therapeutic target in Hodgkins disease and nasopharyngeal carcinoma. *Semin. Cancer Biol.* **7,** 217–226.

Ando, Y., and Jensen, P. J. (1996). Protein kinase C mediates up-regulation of urokinase and its receptor in the migrating keratinocytes of wounded cultures, but urokinase is not required for movement across a substratum *in vitro. J. Cell. Physiol.* **167,** 500–511.

Asiedu, C., Biggs, J., Lilly, M., and Kraft, A. S. (1995). Inhibition of leukemic cell growth by the protein kinase C activator bryostatin 1 correlates with the dephosphorylation of cyclin-dependent kinase 2. *Cancer Res.* **55,** 3716–3720.

Baer, J. C., Slack, J. A., and Pettit, G. R. (1989). Stability-indicating high-performance liquid chromatography assay for the anticancer drug bryostatin 1. *J. Chromatogr.* **467,** 332–335.

Baker, J. T., Borris, R. P., Carté, B., Cordell, G. A., Soejarto, D. D., Cragg, G. M., Gupta, M. P., Iwu, M. M., Madulid, D. R., and Tyler, V. E. (1995). Natural product drug discovery and development: new perspectives on international collaboration. *J. Nat. Prod.* **58,** 1325–1357.

Baldwin, N. G., Rice, C. D., Tuttle, T. M., Bear, H. D., Hirsch, J. I., and Merchant, R. E. (1997). Ex vivo expansion of tumor-draining lymph node cells using compounds which activate intracellular signal transduction. I. Characterization and *in vivo* antitumor activity of glioma-sensitized lymphocytes. *J. Neurooncol.* **32,** 19–28.

Bangalore, N. S., Baidas, S., Bhargava, P., Rizvi, N., El-Ashry, D., Ness, L., and Marshall, J. L. (2000). Phase I study of bryostatin 1 and cisplatin in patients with advanced cancer. *Proc. Am. Soc. Clin. Oncol.* **19,** 794.

Bartimole, T. M., Vrana, J. A., Freemerman, A. J., Jarvis, W. D., Reed, J. C., Boise, L. H., and Grant, S. (1997). Modulation of the expression of

Bcl-2 and related proteins in human leukemia cells by protein kinase C activators: relationship to effects on 1-[beta-D-arabinofuranosyl]cytosine-induced apoptosis. *Cell Death Different.* **4,** 294–303.

Basu, A. (1998). The involvement of novel protein kinase C isozymes in influencing sensitivity of breast cancer MCF-7 cells to tumor necrosis factor-alpha. *Mol. Pharmacol.* **53,** 105–111.

Basu, A., and Akkaraju, G. R. (1999). Regulation of caspase activation and cis-diamminedichloroplatinum(II)-induced cell death by protein kinase C. *Biochemistry* **38,** 4245–4251.

Basu, A., and Evans, R. W. (1994). Comparison of effects of growth factors and protein kinase C activators on cellular sensitivity to *cis*-diamminedichloroplatinum(II). *Int. J. Cancer* **58,** 587–591.

Basu, A., and Lazo, J. S. (1992). Sensitization of human cervical carcinoma cells to *cis*-diamminedichloroplatinum(II) by bryostatin 1. *Cancer Res.* **52,** 3119–3124.

Basu, A., Weixel, K., and Saijo, N. (1996). Characterization of the protein kinase C signal transduction pathway in cisplatin-sensitive and -resistant human small cell lung carcinoma cells. *Cell Growth Different.* **7,** 1507–1512.

Baxter, J., Mata, E. G., and Thomas, E. J. (1998). An approach to the synthesis of the C(17)-C(27) fragment of bryostatins. *Tetrahedron* **54,** 14359–14376.

Bear, H. D., McFadden, A. W. J., Kostuchenko, P. J., Lipshy, K. A., Hamad, G. G., Turner, A. J., Roberts, J. D., Carr, M., Carr, S., and Grant, S. (1996). Bryostatin 1 activates splenic lymphocytes and induces sustained depletion of splenocyte protein kinase C activity *in vivo* after a single intravenous administration. *Anticancer Drugs* **7,** 299–306.

Beck, F. W. J., Al-Katib, A. M., Liu, K. Z., and Mohammad, R. M. (1998). Bryostatin 1 down-regulation of Es nucleoside transporters is associated with increased 2-Cda influx in a resistant B-CLL cell line. *Blood* **92,** 191B.

Beck, F. W. J., Al-Katib, A. M., Ahmad, I., and Mohammad, R. M. (1999). Bryostatin 1 (bryo) enhances 2-chlorodeoxyadenosine (2CdA) chemotherapeutic activity in human chronic lymphocytic leukemia cells by increasing 2CdA influx and deoxycytidine kinase (dCK) activity. *Blood* **94,** 295b.

Beck, F. W. J., Al-Katib, A. M., Ahmad, I., Wall, N. R., Liu, K. Z., Mantsch, H. H., and Mohammad, R. M. (2000). Bryostatin 1-induced modulation of nucleoside transporters and 2-chlorodeoxyadenosine influx in WSU-CLL cells. *Int. J. Mol. Med.* **5,** 341–347.

Bedikian, A., Plager, C., Papadopulos, N., Eton, O., Ellerhorst, J., and Smith, T. (1999). Phase II trial of bryostatin 1 in patients with melanoma. *Proc. Am. Soc. Clin. Oncol.* **18,** 2051.

Beijnen, J. H., Flora, K. P., Halbert, G. W., Henrar, R. E. C., and Slack, J. A. (1995). CRC/EORTC/NCI joint formulation working party: experiences in the formulation of investigational cytotoxic drugs. *Br. J. Cancer* **72,** 210–218.

Berkow, R. L., and Kraft, A. S. (1985). Bryostatin, a non-phorbol macrocyclic lactone, activates intact human polymorphonuclear leukocytes and binds to the phorbol ester receptor. *Biochem. Biophys. Res. Commun.* **131,** 1109–1116.

Berkow, R. L., Schlabach, L., Dodson, R., Benjamin, W. H., Jr., Pettit, G. R., Rustage, P., and Kraft, A. S. (1993). *In vivo* administration of the anticancer agent bryostatin 1 activates platelets and neutrophils and modulates protein kinase C activity. *Cancer Res.* **53,** 2810–2815.

Bhatia, R., and Munthe, H. (1998). Restoration of integrin-mediated adhesion and signaling in CML progenitors treated with bryostatin 1. *Blood* **92,** 252A.

Bignami, G. S., Wagner, F., Grothaus, P. G., Rustagi, P., Davis, D. E., and Kraft, A. S. (1996). Biological activity of 26-succinylbryostatin 1. *Biochim. Biophys. Acta* **1312,** 197–206.

Blumberg, P. M., Pettit, G. R., Warren, B. S., Szallasi, A., Schuman, L. D., Sharkey, N. A., Nakakuma, H., Dell'Aquila, M. L., and de Vries, D. J.

(1989). The protein kinase C pathway in tumor promotion. *Prog. Clin. Biol. Res.* **298** (skin carcinogenesis), 201–212.

Bodily, J. M., Hoopes, D. J., Roeder, B. L., Gilbert, S. G., Pettit, G. R., Herald, C. L., Rollins, D. N., and Robison, R. A. (1999). The inhibitory effects of bryostatin 1 administration on the growth of rabbit papillomas. *Cancer Lett.* **136,** 67–74.

Bogi, K., Lorenzo, P. S., Szallasi, Z., Acs, P., Wagner, G. S., and Blumberg, P. M. (1998). Differential selectivity of ligands for the C1a and C1b phorbol ester binding domains of protein kinase Cdelta: possible correlation with tumor-promoting activity. *Cancer Res.* **58,** 1423–1428.

Boorne, A. J., Donnelly, N., and Schrey, M. P. (1998). Differential effects of protein kinase C agonists on prostaglandin production and growth in human breast cancer cells. *Breast Cancer Res. Treat.* **48,** 117–124.

Bosco, M. C., Rottschafer, S., Taylor, L. S., Ortaldo, J. R., Longo, D. L., and Espinoza-Delgado, I. (1997). The antineoplastic agent bryostatin 1 induces proinflammatory cytokine production in human monocytes: synergy with interleukin-2 and modulation of interleukin-2Rgamma chain expression. *Blood* **89,** 3402–3411.

Boto, W. M., Brown, L., Chrest, J., and Adler, W. H. (1991). Distinct modulatory effects of bryostatin 1 and staurosporine on the biosynthesis and expression of the HIV receptor protein (CD4) by T cells. *Cell. Regul.* **2,** 95–103.

Boyd, M. R. (1997). The NCI *in Vitro* Anticancer Drug Discovery Screen: Concept, Implementation, and Operation, 1985–1995. *In* "Anticancer Drug Development Guide: Preclinical Screening, Clinical Trials, and Approval" (B. Teicher, ed.), pp. 23–42. Humana Press, Totowa, NJ.

Boyd, M. R., and Paull, K. D. (1995). Some practical considerations and applications of the National Cancer Institute *in vitro* anticancer drug discovery screen. *Drug Dev. Res.* **34,** 91–109.

Boyd, M. R., Gustafson, K. R., McMahon, J. B., Shoemaker, R. H., O'Keefe, B. R., Mori, T., Gulakowski, R. J., Wu, L., Rivera, M. I., Laurencot, C. M., Currens, M. J., Cardellina II, J. H., Buckheit, R. W., Jr., Nara, P. L., Pannell, L. K., Sowder, R. C., II., and Henderson, L. E. (1997). Discovery of cyanovirin-n, a novel human immunodeficiency virus-inactivating protein that binds viral surface envelope glycoprotein gp120—potential applications to microbicide development. *Antimicrob. Agents Chemother.* **41,** 1521–1530.

Bradner, W. T. (1980). *In* "Cancer and Chemotherapy". (S. T. Crooke and A. W. Prestayko, eds.), Vol. 1, p. 313. Academic Press, New York.

Bradshaw, T. D., Gescher, A., and Pettit, G. R. (1991). The effect of fetal calf serum on growth arrest caused by activators of protein kinase C. *Int. J. Cancer* **47,** 929–932.

Bradshaw, T. D., Gescher, A., and Pettit, G. R. (1992). Modulation by staurosporine of phorbol-ester-induced effects on growth and protein kinase C localization in A549 human lung-carcinoma cells. *Int. J. Cancer* **51,** 144–148.

Brinkmeier, H., Jockusch, H. (1987). Activators of protein kinase C induce myotonia by lowering chloride conductance in muscle. *Biochem. Biophys. Res. Commun.* **148,** 1383–1389.

Brodie, C., Bogi, K., Acs, P., Lorenzo, P. S., Baskin, L., and Blumberg, P. M. (1998). Protein kinase C delta (PKCdelta) inhibits the expression of glutamine synthetase in glial cells via the PKCdelta regulatory domain and its tyrosine phosphorylation. *J. Biol. Chem.* **273,** 30713–30718.

Burry, R. W. (1998). PKC activators (phorbol ester or bryostatin) stimulate outgrowth of NGF-dependent neurites in a subline of PC12 cells. *J. Neuroscience Res.* **53,** 214–222.

Byrd, J. C., Rai, K. R., Sausville, E. A., and Grever, M. R. (1998). Old and new therapies in chronic lymphocytic leukemia: now is the time for a reassessment of therapeutic goals. *Semin. Oncol.* **25,** 65–74.

Campbell, X. Z., and Neet, K. E. (1995). Hierarchical analysis of the nerve growth factor-dependent and nerve growth factor-independent differentiation signaling pathways in PC12 cells with protein kinase inhibitors. *J. Neuroscience Res.* **42,** 207–219.

Cannistra, S. A., Groshek, P., Garlick, R., Miller, J., and Griffin, J. D. (1990).

Regulation of surface expression of the granulocyte/macrophage colony-stimulating factor receptor in normal human myeloid cells. *Proc. Natl. Acad. Sci. USA* **87,** 93–97.

Carey, J. O., Posekany, K. J., deVente, J. E., Pettit, G. R., and Ways, D. K. (1996). Phorbol ester-stimulated phosphorylation of PU.1: association with leukemic cell growth inhibition. *Blood* **87,** 4316–4324.

Carr, M. E., Jr., Carr, S. L., and Grant, S. (1995). A sensitive platelet activation-based functional assay for the antileukemic agent bryostatin 1. *Anticancer Drugs* **6,** 384–391.

Carroll, M. P., and May, W. S. (1994). Protein kinase C-mediated serine phosphorylation directly activates Raf-1 in murine hematopoietic cells. *J. Biol. Chem.* **269,** 1249–1256.

Carter, S. K., and Livingston, R. B. (1976). Plant products in cancer chemotherapy. *Cancer Treat. Rep.* **60,** 1141–1156.

Casolaro, V., Meliota, S., Marino, O., Patella, V., de Paulis, A., Guidi, G., and Marone, G. (1993). Nimesulide, a sulfonanilide nonsteroidal anti-inflammatory drug, inhibits mediator release from human basophils and mast cells. *J. Pharm. Exp. Ther.* **267,** 1375–1385.

Cassady, J. M., and Douros, J. D. (1980). "Anticancer Agents Based on Natural Product Models." Academic Press, New York.

Chelliah, J., Freemerman, A. J., Wu-Pong, S., Jarvis, W. D., and Grant, S. (1997). Potentiation of ara-C-induced apoptosis by the protein kinase C activator bryostatin 1 in human leukemia cells (HL-60) involves a process dependent upon c-*myc*. *Biochem. Pharmacol.* **54,** 563–573.

Chen, C., and Chen, B. D. M. (1999). Bryostatin 1 induced XIAP mRNA expression in apoptosis resistant THP-1 cells. *Clin. Cancer Res.* **5,** 318.

Chen, C., Lin, H., Karanes, C., Pettit, G. R., and Chen, B. D. (2000). Human THP-1 monocytic leukemic cells induced to undergo monocytic differentiation by bryostatin 1 are refractory to proteasome inhibitor-induced apoptosis. *Cancer Res.* **60,** 4377–4385.

Cheung, A. P., Hallock, Y. F., Vishnuvajjala, B. R., Nguyenle, T., and Wang, E. (1998). Compatibility and stability of bryostatin 1 in infusion devices. *Invest. New Drugs* **16,** 227–236.

Choi, W. C., and Ahn, C. H. (1993). Protein kinase C (PKC) in cellular signaling system: translocation of six protein kinase C isozymes in human prostate adenocarcinoma PC-3 cell line. *Korean J. Zool.* **36,** 439–451.

Christian, M. C., Pluda, J. M., Ho, P. T. C., Arbuck, S. G., Murgo, A. J., and Sausville, E. A. (1997). Promising new agents under development by the division of cancer treatment, diagnosis, and centers of the National Cancer Institute. *Semin. Oncol.* **24,** 219–240.

Cirillo, R., Triggiani, M., Siri, L., Ciccarelli, A., Pettit, G. R., Condorelli, M., and Marone, G. (1990). Cyclosporin A rapidly inhibits mediator release from human basophils presumably by interacting with cyclophilin. *J. Immunol.* **144,** 3891–3897.

Clarke, H. M., Ginanni, N., Laughlin, K. V., Smith, J., Pettit, G. R., and Mullin, J. M. (1999). The phorbol ester, TPA, and bryostatin 1 exert different effects on PKC-alpha downregulation and tight junctional permeability. *Mol. Biol. Cell.* **10,** 2370.

Columbo, M., Galeone, D., Guidi, G., Kagey-Sobotka, A., Lichtenstein, L. M., Pettit, G. R., and Marone, G. (1990). Modulation of mediator release from human basophils and pulmonary mast cells and macrophages by auranofin. *Biochem. Pharmacol.* **39,** 285–291.

Columbo, M., Botana, L. M., Horowitz, E. M., Lichtenstein, L. M., and MacGlashan, D. W., Jr. (1994). Studies of the intracellular Ca2+ levels in human adult skin mast cells activated by the ligand for the human c-kit receptor and anti-IgE. *Biochem. Pharmacol.* **47,** 2137–2145.

Columbo, M., Horowitz, E. M., Kagey-Sobotka, A., and Lichtenstein, L. M. (1996). Substance P activates the release of histamine from human skin mast cells through a pertussis toxin-sensitive and protein kinase C-dependent mechanism. *Clin. Immunol. Immunopathol.* **81,** 68–73.

Cook, H. W., Ridgway, N. D., and Byers, D. M. (1998). Involvement of phospholipase D and protein kinase C in phorbol ester and fatty acid stimulated turnover of phosphatidylcholine and phosphatidylethanolamine in neural cells. *Biochim. Biophys. Acta* **1390,** 103–117.

Cordell, G. A., and Farnsworth, N. R. (1976). Review of selected potential anticancer plant principles. *Heterocycles* **4**, 393–427.

Cordell, G. A., and Farnsworth, N. R. (1977). Experimental antitumor agents from plants, 1974–76. *Lloydia* **40**, 1–44.

Correale, P., Caraglia, M., Fabbrocini, A., Guarrasi, R., Pepe, S., Patella, V., Marone, G., Pinto, A., Bianco, A. R., and Tagliaferri, P. (1995). Bryostatin 1 enhances lymphokine activated killer sensitivity and modulates the beta 1 integrin profile of cultured human tumor cells. *Anticancer Drugs* **6**, 285–290.

Cost, H., Barreau, P., Basset, M., Lepeuch, C., and Geny, B. (1991). Phorbol myristate acetate inhibits phosphoinositol lipid-specific phospholipase C activity via protein kinase C activation in conditions inducing differentiation in HL-60 cells. *Cell Biochem. Function* **9**, 263–273.

Courage, C., Budworth, J., and Gescher, A. (1995). Comparison of ability of protein kinase C inhibitors to arrest cell growth and to alter cellular protein kinase C localisation. *Br. J. Cancer* **71**, 697–704.

Cragg, G. M. (1998). Paclitaxel (Taxol): a success story with valuable lessons for natural product drug discovery and development. *Med. Res. Rev.* **18**, 315–331.

Cragg, G. M., Newman, D. J., and Snader, K. M. (1997a). Natural products in drug discovery and development. *J. Nat. Prod.* **60**, 52–60.

Cragg, G. M., Newman, D. J., and Weiss, R. B. (1997b). Coral reefs, forests, and thermal vents—the worldwide exploration of nature for novel antitumor agents. *Semin. Oncol.* **24**, 156–163.

Curiel, R. E., Garcia, C. S., Farooq, L., and Espinoza-Delgado, I. J. (1999). Bryostatin 1 and IL-2 synergize to induce IFN-gamma expression in human peripheral blood T cells: implications for cancer immunotherapy. *Blood* **94**, 52b.

Dale, I. L., and Gescher, A. (1989). Effects of activators of protein kinase C, including bryostatins 1 and 2, on the growth of A549 human lung carcinoma cells. *Int. J. Cancer* **43**, 158–163.

Dale, I. L., Bradshaw, T. D., Gescher, A., and Pettit, G. R. (1989). Comparison of effects of bryostatins 1 and 2 and 12-O-tetradecanoylphorbol-13-acetate on protein kinase C activity in A549 human lung carcinoma cells. *Cancer Res.* **49**, 3242–3245.

Darwiche, N., Scita, G., Jones, C., Rutberg, S., Greenwald, E., Tennenbaum, T., Collins, S. J., De Luca, L. M., and Yuspa, S. H. (1996). Loss of retinoic acid receptors in mouse skin and skin tumors is associated with activation of the *ras*(Ha) oncogene and high risk for premalignant progression. *Cancer Res.* **56**, 4942–4949.

Datta, R., Sherman, M. L., Stone, R. M., and Kufe, D. (1991). Expression of the *jun*-B gene during induction of monocytic differentiation. *Cell Growth Differ.* **2**, 43–49.

Datta, R., Hallahan, D. E., Kharbanda, S. M., Rubin, E., Sherman, M. L., Huberman, E., Weichselbaum, R. R., and Kufe, D. W. (1992). Involvement of reactive oxygen intermediates in the induction of c-*jun* gene transcription by ionizing radiation. *Biochemistry* **31**, 8300–8306.

Davidson, S. K., and Haygood, M. G. (1999). Identification of sibling species of the bryozoan *Bugula neritina* that produce different anticancer bryostatins and harbor distinct strains of the bacterial symbiont "candidatus *Endobugula sertula*." *Biol. Bull.* **196**, 273–280.

Davis, A. F., Meighan-Mantha, R. L., and Riegel, A. T. (1997). Effects of TPA, bryostatin 1, and retinoic acid on PO-B, AP-1, and AP-2 DNA binding during HL-60 differentiation. *J. Cell. Biochem.* **65**, 308–324.

Dawson, T., Bond, J., Eccles, N., and Wynford-Thomas, D. (1993). Toxicity of phorbol esters for human epithelial cells expressing a mutant *ras* oncogene. *Mol. Carcinogenesis* **8**, 280–289.

DeBrabander, J., and Vandewalle, M. (1996). Towards the asymmetric synthesis of bryostatin 1. *Pure Appl. Chem.* **68**, 715–718.

DeBrabander, J., Kulkarni, B. A., Garcia Lopez, R., and Vandewalle, M. (1997). Bryostatin—a novel asymmetric synthesis of the C-27-C-34 fragment starting from (R)-carvone as chiral template. *Tetrahedron: Asymmetry* **8**, 1721–1724.

Dell'Aquila, M. L., Nguyen, H. T., Herald, C. L., Pettit, G. R., and Blumberg, P. M. (1987). Inhibition by bryostatin 1 of the phorbol ester-induced blockage of differentiation in hexamethylene bisacetamide-treated Friend erythroleukemia cells. *Cancer Res.* **47**, 6006–6009.

Dell'Aquila, M. L., Herald, C. L., Kamano, Y., Pettit, G. R., and Blumberg, P. M. (1988). Differential effects of bryostatins and phorbol esters on arachidonic acid metabolite release and epidermal growth factor binding in C3H 10T1/2 cells. *Cancer Res.* **48**, 3702–3708.

Deng, X., Ito, T., Carr, B., Mumby, M., and May, W. S., Jr. (1998). Reversible phosphorylation of Bcl2 following interleukin 3 or bryostatin 1 is mediated by direct interaction with protein phosphatase 2A. *J. Biol. Chem.* **273**, 34157–34163.

Denning, M. F., Dlugosz, A. A., Williams, E. K., Szallasi, Z., Blumberg, P. M., and Yuspa, S. H. (1995). Specific protein kinase C isozymes mediate the induction of keratinocyte differentiation markers by calcium. *Cell Growth Different.* **6**, 149–157.

Denning, M. F., Guy, S. G., Ellerbroek, S. M., Norvell, S. M., Kowalczyk, A. P., and Green, K. J. (1998). The expression of desmoglein isoforms in cultured human keratinocytes is regulated by calcium, serum, and protein kinase C. *Exp. Cell Res.* **239**, 50–59.

de Paulis, A., Cirillo, R., Ciccarelli, A., Condorelli, M., and Marone, G. (1991). FK-506, a potent novel inhibitor of the release of proinflammatory mediators from human Fc epsilon RI+ cells. *J. Immunol.* **146**, 2374–2381.

de Vente, J. E., Kukoly, C. A., Bryant, W. O., Posekany, K. J., Chen, J., Fletcher, D. J., Parker, P. J., Pettit, G. R., Lozano, G., Cook, P. P., and Ways, D. K. (1995). Phorbol esters induce death in MCF-7 breast cancer cells with altered expression of protein kinase C isoforms: role for p53-independent induction of gadd-45 in initiating death. *J. Clin. Invest.* **96**, 1874–1886.

de Vente, J. E., Carey, J. O., Bryant, W. O., Pettit, G. R., and Ways, D. K. (1996). Transcriptional regulation of insulin receptor substrate 1 by protein kinase C. *J. Biol. Chem.* **271**, 32276–32280.

de Vries, D. J., Herald, C. L., Pettit, G. R., and Blumberg, P. M. (1988). Demonstration of sub-nanomolar affinity of bryostatin 1 for the phorbol ester receptor in rat brain. *Biochem. Pharmacol.* **37**, 4069–4073.

Dlugosz, A. A., and Yuspa, S. H. (1991). Staurosporine induces protein kinase C agonist effects and maturation of normal and neoplastic mouse keratinocytes *in vitro*. *Cancer Res.* **51**, 4677–4684.

Dlugosz, A. A., and Yuspa, S. H. (1993). Coordinate changes in gene expression which mark the spinous to granular cell transition in epidermis are regulated by protein kinase C. *J. Cell Biol.* **120**, 217–225.

Dlugosz, A. A., and Yuspa, S. H. (1994). Protein kinase C regulates keratinocyte transglutaminase (TGK) gene expression in cultured primary mouse epidermal keratinocytes induced to terminally differentiate by calcium. *J. Invest. Dermatol.* **102**, 409–414.

Dlugosz, A. A., Cheng, C., Williams, E. K., Dharia, A. G., Denning, M. F., and Yuspa, S. H. (1994). Alterations in murine keratinocyte differentiation induced by activated *ras*Ha genes are mediated by protein kinase C-alpha. *Cancer Res.* **54**, 6413–6420.

Douros, J. D. (1976). Lower plants as a source of anticancer drugs. *Cancer Treat. Rep.*, **60**, 1069–1080.

Dowlati, A., Robertson, K., Ksenich, P., Jacobberger, J., Whitacre, C., Schnur, G., Cooper, B., Spiro, T., Lazarus, H., Gerson, S., Murgo, A., Sedransk, N., and Remick, S. C. (1999). Phase I trial of combination bryostatin 1 and vincristine in B-cell malignancies. *Clin. Cancer Res.* **5**, 113.

Dowlati, A., Robertson, K., Ksenich, P., Jacobberger, J., Whitacre, C., Schnur, G., Cooper, B., Spiro, T., Lazarus, H., Gerson, S., Murgo, A., and Remick, S. C. (2000). Phase I trial of combination bryostatin 1 and vincristine in B-cell malignancies. *Proc. Am. Soc. Clin. Oncol.* **19**, 837.

Drager, A. M., van der Hem, K. G., Zevenbergen, A., Odding, J. H., Huijgens, P. C., and Schuurhuis, G. J. (1999). Role of TNF alpha in bryostatin-induced inhibition of human hematopoiesis. *Leukemia* **13**, 62–69.

Drexler, H. G., Gignac, S. M., Jones, R. A., Scott, C. S., Pettit, G. R., and

Hoffbrand, A. V. (1989). Bryostatin 1 induces differentiation of B-chronic lymphocytic leukemia cells. *Blood* **74**, 1747–1757.

Drexler, H. G., Gignac, S. M., Pettit, G. R., and Hoffbrand, A. V. (1990). Synergistic action of calcium ionophore A23187 and protein kinase C activator bryostatin 1 on human B cell activation and proliferation. *Eur. J. Immunol.* **20**, 119–127.

Ekinci, F. J., and Shea, T. B. (1997). Selective activation by bryostatin 1 demonstrates unique roles for PKC epsilon in neurite extension and tau phosphorylation. *Int. J. Devel. Neuroscience* **15**, 867–874.

Ekinci, F. J., Boyce, J. B., and Shea, T. B. (1996). Differential effects of bryostatin and phorbol esters on neuroblastoma cells: unique role of protein kinase C epsilon. *J. Neurochem.* **66**, 62.

Elgie, A., Alton, P., Sargent, J., Taylor, C., and Harris, A. (1993). Effects of bryostatin on fresh blast cells from patients with acute myeloid-leukemia (AML). *Br. J. Haematol.* **84**, 31.

Elgie, A.W., Sargent, J. M., Alton, P., Peters, G. J., Noordhuis, P., Williamson, C. J., and Taylor, C. G. (1998). Modulation of resistance to ara-C by bryostatin in fresh blast cells from patients with AML. *Leukemia Res.* **22**, 373–378.

Esa, A. H., and Converse, P. J. (1996). Nordihydroguaiaretic acid blocks IL-2-independent lymphocyte proliferation and enhances responses to PPD. *Scand. J. Immunol.* **43**, 127–133.

Esa, A. H., Boto, W. O., Adler, W. H., May, W. S., and Hess, A. D. (1990). Activation of T-cells by bryostatins: induction of the IL-2 receptor gene transcription and down-modulation of surface receptors. *Int. J. Immunopharmacol.* **12**, 481–490.

Esa, A. H., Warren, J. T., Hess, A. D., and May, W. S. (1995). Bryostatins trigger human polymorphonuclear neutrophil and monocyte oxidative metabolism: association with *in vitro* antineoplastic activity. *Res. Immunol.* **146**, 351–361.

Espinoza-Delgado, I., Curiel, R. E., Garcia, C. S., and Mwatibo, J. M. (1999a). Bryostatin 1 upregulates B7-2 expression in human monocytic cells through a posttranscriptional mechanism: association with an enhanced accessory cell function. *Blood* **94**, 428a.

Espinoza-Delgado, I. J., Rottschafer, S., Garcia, C. S., Curiel, R. E., Bravo, J. C., Skrepnik, N., and Mera, R. (1999b). Bryostatin 1 and low-dose interleukin-2 (IL-2) is as efficient as high-dose IL-2 in reducing B16-BL6 melanoma growth *in vivo* without the acute toxicity. *Proc. Am. Soc. Clin. Oncol.*, **18**, 452a.

Evans, D. A., Gauchet-Prunet, J. A., Carreira, E. M., and Charette, A. B. (1991). Synthesis of 1,3-diol synthons from epoxy aromatic precursors: an approach to the construction of polyacetate-derived natural products. *J. Org. Chem.* **56**, 741–750.

Evans, D. A., Carter, P. H., Carreira, E. M., Prunet, J. A., Charette, A. B., and Lautens, M. (1998). Asymmetric synthesis of bryostatin 2. *Angew. Chem. Int. Ed.* **37**, 2354–2359.

Evans, D. A., Carter, P. H., Carreira, E. M., Charette, A. B., Prunet, J. A., and Lautens, M. (1999). Total synthesis of bryostatin 2. *J. Am. Chem. Soc.* **121**, 7540–7552.

Fackler, M. J., Civin, C. I., Sutherland, D. R., Baker, M. A., and May, W. S. (1990). Activated protein kinase C directly phosphorylates the CD34 antigen on hematopoietic cells. *J. Biol. Chem.* **265**, 11056–11061.

Farokhzad, O. C., Mun, E. C., Sicklick, J. K., Smith, J. A., and Matthews, J. B. (1998). Effects of bryostatin 1, a novel anticancer agent, on intestinal transport and barrier function: role of protein kinase C. *Surgery* **124**, 380–386.

Fields, A. P., Pettit, G. R., and May, W. S. (1988). Phosphorylation of lamin B at the nuclear membrane by activated protein kinase C. *J. Biol. Chem.* **263**, 8253–8260.

Fields, A. P., Pincus, S. M., Kraft, A. S., and May, W. S. (1989). Interleukin-3 and bryostatin 1 mediate rapid nuclear envelope protein phosphorylation in growth factor-dependent FDC-P1 hematopoietic cells. A possible role for nuclear protein kinase C. *J. Biol. Chem.* **264**, 21896–21901.

Fields, A. P., Tyler, G., Kraft, A. S., and May, W. S. (1990). Role of nuclear

protein kinase C in the mitogenic response to platelet-derived growth factor. *J. Cell Sci.* **96**, 107–114.

Fisher, G. J., Reynolds, N. J., Henderson, P. A., Burns, D., Voorhees, J. J., and Baldassare, J. J. (1993). Protein Kinase C isoenzymes alpha and epsilon are translocated and down-regulated by phorbol ester and bryostatin 1 in human keratinocytes and fibroblasts. *J. Invest. Dermatol.* **100**, 495.

Flandina, C., Flugy, A., Borsellino, N., and D'Alessandro, N. (1996). Development and partial characterization of a human T-lymphoblastic leukemic (CCRF-CEM) cell line resistant to etoposide. Analysis of possible circumventing approaches. *J. Chemother.* **8**, 465–471.

Fleming, M. D., Barrett, S. K., and Bear, H. D. (1994). Precursor frequency analysis of bryostatin activated lymphocytes. *J. Surg. Res.* **57**, 74–79.

Fleming, M. D., Bear, H. D., Lipshy, K., Kostuchenko, P. J., Portocarero, D., McFadden, A. W. J., and Barrett, S. K. (1995). Adoptive transfer of bryostatin-activated tumor-sensitized lymphocytes prevents or destroys tumor metastases without expansion *in vitro*. *J. Immunother. Tumor Immunol.* **18**, 147–155.

Fox, B. W. (1991). Medicinal plants in tropical medicine. 2. Natural products in cancer treatment from bench to the clinic. *Trans. Royal Soc. Trop. Med. Hygiene* **85**, 22–25.

Franco, M., Leonard, L., Ruth, O., David, F., Scott, W., Howard, H., Mark, R., and Anne, H. (1999). Bryostatin 1 and cisplatin: phase I study with pharmacodynamic guidance. *Clin. Cancer Res.* **5**, 18.

Freemerman, A. J., Maloney, N. J., Birrer, M. J., Szabo, E., and Grant, S. (1996). Bryostatin 1 potentiates 1-[beta-D-arabinofuranosyl]cytosine-mediated antiproliferative effects in c-*jun* dominant-negative human myeloid leukemia cells (u937/tam67) through a nonapoptotic mechanism. *Mol. Cell. Different.* **4**, 247–262.

Galron, D., Tamir, A., Gelkop, S., Grossman, N., and Isakov, N. (1993). The effect of bryostatin on protein kinase C-regulated functions in human T lymphocytes and epidermal keratinocytes. *Immunol. Lett.* **39**, 17–22.

Galron, D., Tamir, A., Gelkop, S., Grossman, N., and Noah, I. (1994). The effect of bryostatin on protein kinase-C-regulated functions in human T-lymphocytes and epidermal-keratinocytes. *Immunol. Lett.* **40**, 291.

Galron, D., Ansotegui, I. J., and Isakov, N. (1997). Posttranslational regulation of Lck and a p36–38 protein by activators of protein kinase C: differential effects of the tumor promoter, PMA, and the non-tumor-promoter, bryostatin. *Cell. Immunol.* **178**, 141–151.

Garrison, J. C., Pettit, G. R., and Uyeki, E. M. (1987). Effect of phorbol and bryostatin I on chondrogenic expression of chick limb bud, *in vitro*. *Life Sci.* **41**, 2055–2061.

Gartenhaus, R., Hoffman, M., Fuchs, A., Billet, H., Wang, P., Gentile, P., and Rai, K. (1996). Differentiating agents do not induce a true hairy cell phenotype in B-CLL cells *in vitro*. *Leukemia Lymphoma* **22**, 97–101.

Gebbia, V., Di Marco, P., Miceli, S., Reyes, M. B., Teresi, M., Bonaccorso, R., Citarrella, P., and Rausa, L. (1988). The *in vitro* effect of the antineoplastic agent bryostatin 4 on human hematopoietic progenitor cells. *Haematologica* **73**, 387–391.

Gebbia, V., Citarrella, P., Miserendino, V., Valenza, R., Borsellino, N., Pesta, A., Pettit, G. R., and May, S. (1992). The effects of the macrocyclic lactone bryostatin 1 on leukemic cells *in vitro*. *Tumori* **78**, 167–171.

Gebbia, V., Testa, A., Pettit, G. R., Sensenbrenner, L. L., and May, W. S. (1993). Antineoplastic agent bryostatin 1 promotes growth of normal murine haematopoietic progenitors *in vivo*. *Cell. Pharmacol.* **1**, 31–35.

Geiges, D., Marks, F., and Gschwendt, M. (1995). Loss of protein kinase C delta from human HaCaT keratinocytes upon *ras* transfection is mediated by TGF alpha. *Exp. Cell Res.* **219**, 299–303.

Geiges, D., Meyer, T., Marte, B., Vanek, M., Weissgerber, G., Stabel, S., Pfeilschifter, J., Fabbro, D., and Huwiler, A. (1997). Activation of protein kinase C subtypes alpha, gamma, delta, epsilon, zeta, and eta by tumor-promoting and nontumor-promoting agents. *Biochem. Pharmacol.* **53**, 865–875.

Gignac, S. M., Buschie, M., Pettit, G. R., Hoffbrand, A. V., and Drexler,

H. G. (1990a). Expression of proto-oncogene c-*jun* during differentiation of B-chronic lymphocytic leukemia. *Leukemia* **4**, 441–444.

Gignac, S. M., Buschle, M., Hoffbrand, A. V., and Drexler, H. G. (1990b). Down-regulation of CD5 mRNA in B-chronic lymphocytic leukemia cells by differentiation-inducing agents. *Eur. J. Immunol.* **20**, 1119–1123.

Gignac, S. M., Buschle, M., Roberts, R. M., Pettit, G. R., Hofbrand, A. V., and Drexler, H. G. (1990c). Differential expression of TRAP isoenzyme in B-CLL cells treated with different inducers. *Leukemia Lymphoma* **3**, 19–30.

Goekjian, P. G., and Jirousek, M. R. (1999). Protein kinase C in the treatment of disease: signal transduction pathways, inhibitors, and agents in development. *Current Med. Chem.* **6**, 877–903.

Gokmen, Y., and Fields, A. P. (1998). Mapping of a molecular determinant for protein kinase C beta II isozyme function. *J. Biol. Chem.* **273**, 20261–20266.

Gonzalez, R., Ebbinghaus, S., Henthorn, T. K., Miller, D., and Kraft, A. S. (1999). Treatment of patients with metastatic melanoma with bryostatin 1—a phase II study. *Melanoma Res.* **9**, 599–606.

Grabarek, J., and Ware, J. A. (1993). Protein kinase C activation without membrane contact in platelets stimulated by bryostatin. *J. Biol. Chem.* **268**, 5543–5549.

Grant, S. (1997). Modulation of ara-C induced apoptosis in leukemia by the PKC activator bryostatin 1. *Front. Biosci.* 9, D232–D341 *(on line).*

Grant, S., and Jarvis, W. D. (1996). Modulation of drug-induced apoptosis by interruption of the protein kinase C signal transduction pathway: a new therapeutic strategy. *Clin. Cancer Res.* **2**, 1915–1920.

Grant, S., Boise, L., Westin, E., Howe, C., Pettit, G. R., Turner, A., and Mc-Crady, C. (1991a). *In vitro* effects of bryostatin 1 on the metabolism and cytotoxicity of 1-beta-D-arabinofuranosylcytosine in human leukemia cells. *Biochem. Pharmacol.* **42**, 853–867.

Grant, S., Pettit, G. R., Howe, C., and McCrady, C. (1991b). Effect of the protein kinase-C activating agent bryostatin 1 on the clonogenic response of leukemic blast progenitors to recombinant granulocyte-macrophage colony-stimulating factor. *Leukemia* **5**, 392–398.

Grant, S., Jarvis, W. D., Swerdlow, P. S., Turner, A. J., Traylor, R. S., Wallace, H. J., Lin, P. S., Pettit, G. R., and Gewirtz, D. A. (1992a). Potentiation of the activity of 1-beta-D-arabinofuranosylcytosine by the protein kinase C activator bryostatin 1 in HL-60 cells: association with enhanced fragmentation of mature DNA. *Cancer Res.* **52**, 6270–6278.

Grant, S., Jarvis, W. D., Turner, A. J., Wallace, H. J., and Pettit, G. R. (1992b). Effects of bryostatin 1 and rGM-CSF on the metabolism of 1-beta-D-arabinofuranosylcytosine in human leukaemic myeloblasts. *Br. J. Haematol.* **82**, 522–528.

Grant, S., Pettit, G. R., and McCrady, C. (1992c). Effect of bryostatin 1 on the *in vitro* radioprotective capacity of recombinant granulocyte-macrophage colony-stimulating factor (rGM-CSF) toward committed human myeloid progenitor cells (CFU-GM). *Exp. Hematol.* **20**, 34–42.

Grant, S., Traylor, R., Bhalla, K., McCrady, C., and Pettit, G. R. (1992d). Effect of a combined exposure to cytosine arabinoside, bryostatin 1, and recombinant granulocyte-macrophage colony-stimulating factor on the clonogenic growth *in vitro* of normal and leukemic human hematopoietic progenitor cells. *Leukemia* **6**, 432–439.

Grant, S., Traylor, R., Pettit, G. R., and Lin, P. S. (1993). Modulation by bryostatin 1 of the *in vitro* radioprotective effects of the GM-CSF/IL-3 fusion protein, PIXY 321, on normal human myeloid progenitors. *Cytokine* **5**, 490–497.

Grant, S., Traylor, R., Pettit, G. R., and Lin, P. S. (1994a). The macrocyclic lactone protein kinase C activator, bryostatin 1, either alone, or in conjunction with recombinant murine granulocyte-macrophage colony-stimulating factor, protects Balb/c and C3H/HeN mice from the lethal *in vivo* effects of ionizing radiation. *Blood* **83**, 663–667.

Grant, S., Turner, A. J., and Jarvis, W. D. (1994b). Potentiation of ara-C-related apoptosis in human meyloid leukemia cells by bryostatin 1—evidence of a role for down-regulation of CPKC-alpha. *Blood,* **84**, A51.

Grant, S., Rao, A., Freemerman, A. J., Turner, A. J., Kronstein, M. J., Chelliah, J., and Jarvis, W. D. (1995). Divergent effects of calcium ionophore (A23187) on bryostatin 1-related differentiation and apoptosis in human promyelocytic leukemia cells (HL-60). *Mol. Cell. Different.* **3**, 337–359.

Grant, S., Turner, A. J., Freemerman, A. J., Wang, Z., Kramer, L., and Jarvis, W. D. (1996). Modulation of protein kinase C activity and calcium-sensitive isoform expression in human myeloid leukemia cells by bryostatin 1: relationship to differentiation and ara-C-induced apoptosis. *Exp. Cell Res.* **228**, 65–75.

Grant, S., Wang, Z., and Dent, P. (1997). Potentiation of taxol-induced apoptosis in human monocytic leukemia cells (U937) by the PKC activator bryostatin 1. *Blood* **90**, 2209.

Grant, S., Roberts, J., Poplin, E., Tombes, M. B., Kyle, B., Welch, D., Carr, M., and Bear, H. D. (1998a). Phase Ib trial of bryostatin 1 in patients with refractory malignancies. *Clin. Cancer Res.* **4**, 611–618.

Grant, S., Wang, S., Boise, L., and Wang, Z. (1998b). The PKC activator bryostatin 1 reverses resistance to paclitaxel-mediated mitochondrial dysfunction and apoptosis conferred by overexpression of Bcl-X-L in human myelomoncytic leukemia cells (U937) without increasing free Bax levels. *Blood* **92**, 599A.

Grant, S., Cragg, L., Roberts, J., Andreef, M., Feldman, E., Winning, M., and Tombes, M. (1999a). Phase I trial of the PKC activator/downregulator bryostatin 1 (NSC 339555) and high-dose ara-C (HiDAC) in patients with refractory acute leukemia. *Blood* **94**, 509a.

Grant, S., Cragg, L., Roberts, J., Smith, M., Feldman, E., Winning, M., and Tombes, M. (1999b). Phase I Trial of the PKC activator bryostatin 1 (NSC339555) and F-Ara-Amp (fludarabine) in patients with progressive CLL and refractory indolent non-Hodgkins lymphoma. *Blood* **94**, 96a.

Grossman, N., Reuveni, H., Halevy, S., Lubart, R., Friedman, H., and Sredni, B. (1992). Bryostatin, a protein kinase C activator, promotes proliferation of human epidermal keratinocyte cultures. *J. Invest. Dermatol.* **98**, 611.

Gschwendt, M., Furstenberger, G., Rose-John, S., Rogers, M., Kittstein, W., Pettit, G. R., Herald, C. L., and Marks, F. (1988). Bryostatin 1, an activator of protein kinase C, mimics as well as inhibits biological effects of the phorbol ester TPA *in vivo* and *in vitro*. *Carcinogenesis* **9**, 555–562.

Gschwendt, M., Kittstein, W., Lindner, D., and Marks, F. (1992a). Differential inhibition by staurosporine of phorbol ester, bryostatin and okadaic acid effects on mouse skin. *Cancer Lett.* **66**, 139–146.

Gschwendt, M., Leibersperger, H., Kittstein, W., and Marks, F. (1992b). Protein kinase C zeta and eta in murine epidermis. TPA induces down regulation of PKC eta but not PKC zeta. *FEBS Lett.* **307**, 151–155.

Gschwendt, M., Kielbassa, K., Kittstein, W., and Marks, F. (1994). Tyrosine phosphorylation and stimulation of protein kinase C delta from porcine spleen by src *in vitro*. Dependence on the activated state of protein kinase C delta. *FEBS Lett.* **347**, 85–89.

Gschwendt, M., Kittstein, W., Kielbassa, K., and Marks, F. (1995). Protein kinase C delta accepts GTP for autophosphorylation. *Biochem. Biophys. Res. Commun.* **206**, 614–620.

Gulakowski, R. J., McMahon, J. B., Buckheit, R. W., Jr., Gustafson, K. R., and Boyd, M. R. (1997). Antireplicative and anticytopathic activities of prostratin, a non-tumor-promoting phorbol ester, against human immunodeficiency virus (HIV). *Antiviral Res.* **33**, 87–97.

Hagerman, R. A., Fischer, S. M., and Locniskar, M. F. (1997). Effect of 12-O-tetradecanoylphorbol-13-acetate on inhibition of expression of keratin 1 mRNA in mouse keratinocytes mimicked by 12(*S*)-hydroxyeicosatetraenoic acid. *Mol. Carcinogenesis* **19**, 157–164.

Hale, K. J., Lennon, J. A., Manaviazar, S., Javaid, M. H., and Hobbs, C. J. (1995). Asymmetric synthesis of the C(17)-C(27) segment of the antineoplastic macrolide bryostatin 1. *Tetrahedron Lett.* **36**, 1359–1362.

Harris, A. L., Fox, S., Bicknell, R., Leek, R., Relf, M., LeJeune, S., and Kaklamanis, L. (1994). Gene therapy through signal transduction pathways and angiogenic growth factors as therapeutic targets in breast cancer. *Cancer* **74**, 1021–1025.

Hartwell, J. L. (1976). Types of anticancer agents isolated from plants. *Cancer Treat. Rep.* **60**, 1031–1067.

Haussermann, S., Kittstein, W., Rincke, G., Johannes, F. J., Marks, F., and Gschwendt, M. (1999). Proteolytic cleavage of protein kinase Cmu upon induction of apoptosis in U937 cells. *FEBS Lett.* **462**, 442–446.

Haygood, M. G., and Davidson, S. K. (1997). Small-subunit rRNA genes and *in situ* hybridization with oligonucleotides specific for the bacterial symbionts in the larvae of the bryozoan *Bugula neritina* and proposal of "candidatus *Endobugula sertula.*" *Appl. Environmental Microbiol.* **63**, 4612–4616.

Hennings, H., Blumberg, P. M., Pettit, G. R., Herald, C. L., Shores, R., and Yuspa, S. H. (1987). Bryostatin 1, an activator of protein kinase C, inhibits tumor promotion by phorbol esters in SENCAR mouse skin. *Carcinogenesis* **8**, 1343–1346.

Hennings, H., Robinson, V. A., Michael, D. M., Pettit, G. R., Jung, R., and Yuspa, S. H. (1990). Development of an *in vitro* analogue of initiated mouse epidermis to study tumor promoters and antipromoters. *Cancer Res.* **50**, 4794–4800.

Hennings, H., Lowry, D. T., and Robinson, V. A. (1991). Coculture of neoplastic and normal keratinocytes as a model to study tumor promotion. *Skin Pharmacol.* **4**(Suppl. 1), 79–84.

Hess, A. D., Silanskis, M. K., Esa, A. H., Pettit, G. R., and May, W. S. (1988). Activation of human T lymphocytes by bryostatin. *J. Immunol.* **141**, 3263–3269.

Heyworth, C. M., Dexter, T. M., Nicholls, S. E., and Whetton, A. D. (1993). Protein kinase C activators can interact synergistically with granulocyte colony-stimulating factor or interleukin-6 to stimulate colony formation from enriched granulocyte-macrophage colony-forming cells. *Blood* **81**, 894–900.

Hickman, P. F., Kemp, G. J., Thompson, C. H., Salisbury, A. J., Wade, K., Harris, A. L., and Radda, G. K. (1995). Bryostatin 1, a novel antineoplastic agent and protein kinase C activator, induces human myalgia and muscle metabolic defects: a ^{31}P magnetic resonance spectroscopic study. *Br. J. Cancer* **72**, 998–1003.

Hocevar, B. A., and Fields, A. P. (1991). Selective translocation of beta II-protein kinase C to the nucleus of human promyelocytic (HL60) leukemia cells. *J. Biol. Chem.* **266**, 28–33.

Hocevar, B. A., Morrow, D. M., Tykocinski, M. L., and Fields, A. P. (1992). Protein kinase C isotypes in human erythroleukemia cell proliferation and differentiation. *J. Cell Sci.* **101**, 671–679.

Hornung, R. L., Pearson, J. W., Beckwith, M., and Longo, D. L. (1992). Preclinical evaluation of bryostatin as an anticancer agent against several murine tumor cell lines: *in vitro* versus *in vivo* activity. *Cancer Res.* **52**, 101–107.

Hu, Z. B., Gignac, S. M., Uphoff, C. C., Quentmeier, H., Steube, K. G., and Drexler, H. G. (1993a). Induction of differentiation of B-cell leukemia cell lines JVM-2 and EHEB by bryostatin 1. *Leukemia Lymphoma* **10**, 135–142.

Hu, Z. B., Ma, W., Uphoff, C. C., and Drexler, H. G. (1993b). Expression and modulation of annexin VIII in human leukemia-lymphoma cell lines. *Leukemia Res.* **17**, 949–957.

Hu, Z. B., Ma, W., Uphoff, C. C., Lanotte, M., and Drexler, H. G. (1993c). Modulation of gene expression in the acute promyelocytic leukemia cell line NB4. *Leukemia* **7**, 1817–1823.

Hu, Z. B., Ma, W., Uphoff, C. C., Metge, K., Gignac, S. M., and Drexler, H. G. (1993d). Myeloperoxidase: expression and modulation in a large panel of human leukemia-lymphoma cell lines. *Blood* **82**, 1599–1607.

Hu, Z. B., Ma, W., Uphoff, C. C., Quentmeier, H., and Drexler, H. G. (1994). C-*kit* expression in human megakaryoblastic leukemia cell lines. *Blood* **83**, 2133–2144.

Huwiler, A., Fabbro, D., and Pfeilschifter, J. (1994). Comparison of different tumour promoters and bryostatin 1 on protein kinase C activation and downregulation in rat renal mesangial cells. *Biochem. Pharmacol.* **48**, 689–700.

Hysmith, R., and Gotto, A. (1989). Bryostatin inhibits phenotype modulation and growth stimulation of retina endothelial cells by angiogenic and growth factors. *Clin. Res.* **37**, A571.

Iglesias, T., Waldron, R. T., and Rozengurt, E. (1998). Identification of *in vivo* phosphorylation sites required for protein kinase D activation. *J. Biol. Chem.* **273**, 27662–27667.

Isakov, N., Galron, D., Mustelin, T., Pettit, G. R., and Altman, A. (1993). Inhibition of phorbol ester-induced T cell proliferation by bryostatin is associated with rapid degradation of protein kinase C. *J. Immunol.* **150**, 1195–1204.

Ito, T., Deng, X., Carr, B., and May, W. S. (1997). Bcl-2 phosphorylation required for anti-apoptosis function. *J. Biol. Chem.* **272**, 11671–11673.

Jalava, A. M., Heikkila, J., Akerlind, G., Pettit, G. R., and Akerman, K. E. (1990). Effects of bryostatins 1 and 2 on morphological and functional differentiation of SH-SY5Y human neuroblastoma cells. *Cancer Res.* **50**, 3422–3428.

Jalava, A., Akerman, K., and Heikkila, J. (1993a). Protein kinase inhibitor, staurosporine, induces a mature neuronal phenotype in SH-SY5Y human neuroblastoma cells through an alpha-, beta-, and zeta-protein kinase C-independent pathway. *J. Cell. Physiol.* **155**, 301–312.

Jalava, A., Lintunen, M., and Heikkila, J. (1993b). Protein kinase C-alpha but not protein kinase C-epsilon is differentially down-regulated by bryostatin 1 and tetradecanoyl phorbol 13-acetate in SH-SY5Y human neuroblastoma cells. *Biochem. Biophys. Res. Commun.* **191**, 472–478.

Jarvis, W. D., Fornari, F. A., Jr., Browning, J. L., Gewirtz, D. A., Kolesnick, R. N., and Grant, S. (1994a). Attenuation of ceramide-induced apoptosis by diglyceride in human myeloid leukemia cells. *J. Biol. Chem.* **269**, 31685–31692.

Jarvis, W. D., Povirk, L. F., Turner, A. J., Traylor, R. S., Gewirtz, D. A., Pettit, G. R., and Grant, S. (1994b). Effects of bryostatin 1 and other pharmacological activators of protein kinase C on 1-[beta-D-arabinofuranosyl]cytosine-induced apoptosis in HL-60 human promyelocytic leukemia cells. *Biochem. Pharmacol.* **47**, 839–852.

Jarvis, W. D., Fornari, F. A., Traylor, R. S., Martin, H. A., Kramer, L. B., Erukulla, R. K., Bittman, R., and Grant, S. (1996). Induction of apoptosis and potentiation of ceramide-mediated cytotoxicity by sphingoid bases in human myeloid leukemia cells. *J. Biol. Chem.* **271**, 8275–8284.

Jarvis, W. D., Fornari, F. A., Jr., Tombes, R. M., Erukulla, R. K., Bittman, R., Schwartz, G. K., Dent, P., and Grant, S. (1998). Evidence for involvement of mitogen-activated protein kinase, rather than stress-activated protein kinase, in potentiation of 1-beta-D-arabinofuranosylcytosine-induced apoptosis by interruption of protein kinase C signaling. *Mol. Pharmacol.* **54**, 844–856.

Jayson, G. C., Crowther, D., Prendiville, J., McGown, A. T., Scheid, C., Stern, P., Young, R., Brenchley, P., Chang, J., Owens, S., and Pettit, G. R. (1995). A phase I trial of bryostatin 1 in patients with advanced malignancy using a 24-hour intravenous infusion. *Br. J. Cancer* **72**, 461–468.

Jetten, A. M., George, M. A., Pettit, G. R., and Rearick, J. I. (1989). Effects of bryostatins and retinoic acid on phorbol ester- and diacylglycerol-induced squamous differentiation in human tracheobronchial epithelial cells. *Cancer Res.* **49**, 3990–3995.

Johnson, M. D., Torri, J. A., Lippman, M. E., and Dickson, R. B. (1999). Regulation of motility and protease expression in PKC-mediated induction of MCF-7 breast cancer cell invasiveness. *Exp. Cell Res.* **247**, 105–113.

Jones, R. A., Drexler, H. G., Gignac, S. M., Child, J. A., and Scott, C. S. (1990). *In vitro* beta 2-microglobulin (beta 2m) secretion by normal and leukaemic B-cells: effects of recombinant cytokines and evidence for a differential response to the combined stimulus of phorbol ester and calcium ionophore. *Br. J. Cancer* **61**, 675–680.

Jones, R. J., Sharkis, S. J., Miller, C. B., Rowinsky, E. K., Burke, P. J., and May, W. S. (1990). Bryostatin 1, a unique biologic response modifier: antileukemic activity *in vitro*. *Blood* **75**, 1319–1323.

Kageyama, M., Tamura, T., Nantz, M. H., Roberts, J. C., Somfai, P., Whritenour, D. C., and Masamune, S. (1990). Synthesis of bryostatin 7. *J. Am. Chem. Soc.* **112**, 7407–7408.

Kalechman, Y., Albeck, M., and Sredni, B. (1992). In vivo synergistic effect of the immunomodulator AS101 and the PKC inducer bryostatin. *Cell. Immunol.* **143**, 143–153.

Kalesse, M., and Eh, M. (1996). Enantioselective synthesis of the C-1–C-9 segment of bryostatin by kinetic resolution of racemic *beta*-keto esters. *Tetrahedron Lett.* **37**, 1767–1770.

Kalmaz, G. D, Smith, O. M., Murray, N., Carr, B., Fields, A., and May, W. S. (1996). The PKC agonist bryostatin 1 stimulates development hematopoiesis in embryonic stem (ES) cells. *Exp. Hematol.* **24**, 19.

Kalmaz, G., Ruvulo, P., and Kraft, A. S. (1997). Bryostatin 1 promotes the proliferation and differentiation of CD34+ progenitor cells derived from murine embryonic stem (ES) cells. *Blood* **90**, 3371.

Kamanda, W. S., and Leese, C. M. (1998). Bryostatin 1 down-regulates *mdr*-1 and enhances Adriamycin-induced cytotoxicity in human prostate cancer cells. *Proc. Am. Soc. Clin. Oncol.* **17**, 940.

Kamano, Y., Zhang, H.-P., Hino, A., Yoshida, M., Pettit, G. R., Herald, C. L., and Itokawa, H. (1995). An improved source of bryostatin 10: *Bugula neritina* from the Gulf of Aomori, Japan. *J. Nat. Prod.* **58**, 1868–1875.

Kamano, Y., Zhang, H-P., Morita, H., Itokawa, H., Shirota, O., Pettit, G. R., Herald, D. L., and Herald, C. L. (1996). Conformational analysis of a marine antineoplastic macrolide, bryostatin 10. *Tetrahedron* **52**, 2369–2376.

Kamano, Y., Yoshida, M., Zhang, H.-P., Pettit, G. R., Kosuge, N., and Kawamura, M. (1998). Effect of antineoplastic macrolide bryostatin 10 on steroidogenesis in the primary cultured bovine adrenocortical cells. *Jikeikai Med. J.* **45**, 1–9.

Kamano, Y., Kotake, A., Nogawa, T., Hiraide, H., Pettit, G. R., and Herald, C. L. (2000). Separation of the bryostatin derivatives by high performance liquid chromatography. *J. Liquid Chromatogr. Related Technol.* **23**, 399–409.

Kanakura, Y., Druker, B., DiCarlo, J., Cannistra, S. A., and Griffin, J. D. (1991). Phorbol 12-myristate 13-acetate inhibits granulocyte-macrophage colony stimulating factor-induced protein tyrosine phosphorylation in a human factor-dependent hematopoietic cell line. *J. Biol. Chem.* **266**, 490–495.

Kaneki, M., Kharbanda, S., Pandey, P., Yoshida, K., Takekawa, M., Liou, J. R., Stone, R., and Kufe, D. (1999). Functional role for protein kinase Cbeta as a regulator of stress-activated protein kinase activation and monocytic differentiation of myeloid leukemia cells. *Mol. Cell Biol.* **19**, 461–470.

Katato, K., Mohammad, R. M., Dugan, M. C., Saleh, M., Ahmad, I., Al-matchy, V. P., Varterasian, M. L., and Al-Katib, A. (1996). Sequential treatment of chronic lymphocytic leukemia (CLL) with bryostatin 1 and 2-chlorodeoxyadenosine: a preclinical study. *Blood* **88**, 2349.

Kaubisch, A., Kelsen, D. P., Saltz, L., Kemeny, N., O'Reilly, E., Ilson, D., Endres, S., Barazzuol, J., and Schwartz, G. K. (1999). A Phase I trial of weekly sequential bryostatin 1 (bryo) and paclitaxel in patients with advanced solid tumors. *Proc. Am. Soc. Clin. Oncol.* **18**, 639.

Kaubisch, A., Kelsen, D. P., Saltz, L., Kemeny, N., O'Reilly, E., Ilson, D., Endres, S., Barazzuoal, J., Piazza, A., and Schwartz, G. K. (2000). Phase I trial of weekly sequential bryostatin 1 (bryo), cisplatin, and paclitaxel in patients with advanced solid tumors. *Proc. Am. Soc. Clin. Oncol.* **19**, 900.

Kazanietz, M. G., Bustelo, X. R., Barbacid, M., Kolch, W., Mischak, H., Wong, G., Pettit, G. R., Bruns, J. D., and Blumberg, P. M. (1994a). Zinc finger domains and phorbol ester pharmacophore. Analysis of binding to mutated form of protein kinase C zeta and the *vav* and c-*raf* proto-oncogene products. *J. Biol. Chem.* **269**, 11590–11594.

Kazanietz, M. G., Lewin, N. E., Gao, F., Pettit, G. R., and Blumberg, P. M. (1994b). Binding of [26-³H]bryostatin 1 and analogs to calcium-dependent and calcium-independent protein kinase C isozymes. *Mol. Pharmacol.* **46**, 374–379.

Kazanietz, M. G., Wang, S., Milne, G. W. A., Lewin, N. E., Liu, H. L., and Blumberg, P. M. (1995). Residues in the second cysteine-rich region of protein kinase C delta relevant to phorbol ester binding as revealed by site-directed mutagenesis. *J. Biol. Chem.* **270**, 21852–21859.

Keenan, C., Goode, N., and Pears, C. (1997). Isoform specificity of activators and inhibitors of protein kinase C gamma and delta. *FEBS Lett.* **415**, 101–108.

Kennedy, M. J., Prestigiacomo, L. J., Tyler, G., May, W. S., and Davidson, N. E. (1992). Differential effects of bryostatin 1 and phorbol ester on human breast cancer cell lines. *Cancer Res.* **52**, 1278–1283.

Kerr, R. G., Lawry, J., and Gush, K. A. (1996). *In vitro* biosynthetic studies of the bryostatins, anticancer agents from the marine bryozoan *Bugula neritina*. *Tetrahedron Lett.* **37**, 8305–8308.

Khan, P., McGown, A. T., Dawson, M. J., Jayson, G., Prendiville, J. A., Pettit, G. R., and Crowther, D. (1998). High-performance liquid chromatographic assay for the novel antitumor drug, bryostatin 1, incorporating a serum extraction technique. *J. Chromatogr. Biomed. Sci. App.* **709**, 113–117.

Kimura, K., Mizutani, M. Y., Tomioka, N., Endo, Y., Shudo, K., and Itai, A. (1999). Docking study of bryostatins to protein kinase C delta Cys2 domain. *Chem. Pharm. Bull.* **47**, 1134–1137.

Kinter, A. L., Poli, G., Maury, W., Folks, T. M., and Fauci, A. S. (1990). Direct and cytokine-mediated activation of protein kinase C induces human immunodeficiency virus expression in chronically infected promonocytic cells. *J. Virol.* **64**, 4306–4312.

Kiss, Z. (1992). The long-term combined stimulatory effects of ethanol and phorbol ester on phosphatidylethanolamine hydrolysis are mediated by a phospholipase C and prevented by overexpressed alpha-protein kinase C in fibroblasts. *Eur. J. Biochem.* **209**, 467–473.

Kiss, Z., and Anderson, W. B. (1989). Phorbol ester stimulates the hydrolysis of phosphatidylethanolamine in leukemic HL-60, NIH 3T3, and baby hamster kidney cells. *J. Biol. Chem.* **264**, 1483–1487.

Kiss, Z., and Deli, E. (1992). Regulation of phospholipase D by sphingosine involves both protein kinase C-dependent and -independent mechanisms in NIH 3T3 fibroblasts. *Biochem. J.* **288**, 853–858.

Kiss, Z., Deli, E., Girard, P. R., Pettit, G. R., and Kuo, J. F. (1987a). Comparative effects of polymyxin B, phorbol ester and bryostatin on protein phosphorylation, protein kinase C translocation, phospholipid metabolism and differentiation of HL60 cells. *Biochem. Biophys. Res. Commun.* **146**, 208–215.

Kiss, Z., Deli, E., Shoji, M., Koeffler, H. P., Pettit, G. R., Vogler, W. R., and Kuo, J. F. (1987b). Differential effects of various protein kinase C activators on protein phosphorylation in human acute myeloblastic leukemia cell line KG-1 and its phorbol ester-resistant subline KG-1a. *Cancer Res.* **47**, 1302–1307.

Kiss, Z., Deli, E., and Kuo, J. F. (1988). Phorbol ester stimulation of sphingomyelin synthesis in human leukemic HL60 cells. *Arch. Biochem. Biophys.* **265**, 38–42.

Kiss, Z., Chattopadhyay, J., and Pettit, G. R. (1991a). Stimulation of phosphatidylcholine synthesis by activators of protein kinase C is dissociable from increased phospholipid hydrolysis. *Biochem. J.* **273**, 189–194.

Kiss, Z., Rapp, U. R., Pettit, G. R., and Anderson, W. B. (1991b). Phorbol ester and bryostatin differently regulate the hydrolysis of phosphatidylethanolamine in Ha-*ras*-oncogene-transformed and *raf*-oncogene-transformed NIH 3T3 cells. *Biochem. J.* **276**, 505–509.

Kitada, S., Zapata, J. M., Andreeff, M., and Reed, J. C. (1998). Comparison of CD40L and bryostatin effects on apoptosis, chemoresponses, and expression of immunomodulatory antigens and cell survival genes in B-cell chronic lymphocytic leukemia (B-CLL). *Blood* **92**, 102A.

Kitada, S., Zapata, J. M., Andreeff, M., and Reed, J. C. (1999). Bryostatin and CD40-ligand enhance apoptosis resistance and induce expression of cell survival genes in B-cell chronic lymphocytic leukaemia. *Br. J. Haematol.* **106**, 995–1004.

Kiyooka, S., and Maeda, H. (1997). Enantioselective acyclic stereoselection under catalyst control. 3. A very short asymmetric synthesis of the bryostatin C-1–C-9 segment using the chiral oxazaborolidinone-promoted aldol reaction. *Tetrahedron: Asymmetry* **8**, 3371–3374.

Klein, S. B., Fisher, G. J., Jensen, T. C., Mendelsohn, J., Voorhees, J. J., and Elder, J. T. (1992). Regulation of TGF-alpha expression in human keratinocytes: PKC-dependent and -independent pathways. *J. Cell. Physiol.* **151**, 326–336.

Kos, F. J., and Bear, H. D. (1998). Involvement of protein kinase C-delta in CD28-triggered cytotoxicity mediated by a human leukaemic cell line YT. *Immunology* **94**, 575–579.

Kos, F. J., Cornell, D. L., Lipke, A. B., Graham, L. J., and Bear, H. D. (2000). Protective role of IL-2 during activation of T cells with bryostatin 1. *Int. J. Immunopharmacol.* **22**, 645–652.

Koutcher, J. A., Motwani, M., Zakian, K. L., Li, X. K., Matei, C., Dyke, J. P., Ballon, D., Yoo, H. H., and Schwartz, G. K. (2000). The *in vivo* effect of bryostatin 1 on paclitaxel-induced tumor growth, mitotic entry, and blood flow. *Clin. Cancer Res.* **6**, 1498–1507.

Kraft, A. S., Smith, J. B., and Berkow, R. L. (1986). Bryostatin, an activator of the calcium phospholipid-dependent protein kinase, blocks phorbol ester-induced differentiation of human promyelocytic leukemia cells HL-60. *Proc. Natl. Acad. Sci. USA* **83**, 1334–1338.

Kraft, A. S., Appling, C., and Berkow, R. L. (1987a). Specific binding of phorbol esters to nuclei of human promyelocytic leukemia cells. *Biochem. Biophys. Res. Commun.* **144**, 393–401.

Kraft, A. S., Baker, V. V., and May, W. S. (1987b). Bryostatin induces changes in protein kinase C location and activity without altering c-*myc* gene expression in human promyelocytic leukemia cells (HL-60). *Oncogene* **1**, 111–118.

Kraft, A. S., Reeves, J. A., and Ashendel, C. L. (1988). Differing modulation of protein kinase C by bryostatin 1 and phorbol esters in JB6 mouse epidermal cells. *J. Biol. Chem.* **263**, 8437–8442.

Kraft, A. S., William, F., Pettit, G. R., and Lilly, M. B. (1989). Varied differentiation responses of human leukemias to bryostatin 1. *Cancer Res.* **49**, 1287–1293.

Kraft, A. S., Wagner, F., and Housey, G. M. (1990). Overexpression of protein kinase C beta 1 is not sufficient to induce factor independence in the interleukin-3-dependent myeloid cell line FDC-P1. *Oncogene* **5**, 1243–1246.

Kraft, A. S., Woodley, S., Pettit, G. R., Gao, F., Coll, J. C., and Wagner, F. (1996). Comparison of the antitumor activity of bryostatins 1, 5, and 8. *Cancer Chemother. Pharmacol.* **37**, 271–278.

Kupchan, S. M. (1976). Tumor inhibitors. 113. Novel plant-derived tumor inhibitors and their mechanisms of action. *Cancer Treat. Rep.* **60**, 1115–1126.

Lawrence, R. N. (1999). Rediscovering natural product biodiversity. *Drug Discovery Today* **4**, 449–451.

Lee, H. W., Smith, L., Pettit, G. R., and Smith, J. B. (1996a). Dephosphorylation of activated protein kinase C contributes to downregulation by bryostatin. *Am. J. Physiol.* **271**, C304–C311.

Lee, H. W., Smith, L., Pettit, G. R., Vinitsky, A., and Smith, J. B. (1996b). Ubiquitination of protein kinase C-alpha and degradation by the proteasome. *J. Biol. Chem.* **271**, 20973–20976.

Lee, H. W., Smith, L., Pettit, G. R., and Smith, J. B. (1997). Bryostatin 1 and phorbol ester down-modulate protein kinase C-alpha and -epsilon via the ubiquitin/proteasome pathway in human fibroblasts. *Mol. Pharmacol.* **51**, 439–447.

Lee, Y. S., Yuspa, S. H., and Dlugosz, A. A. (1998). Differentiation of cultured human epidermal keratinocytes at high cell densities is mediated by endogenous activation of the protein kinase C signaling pathway. *J. Invest. Dermatol.* **111**, 762–766.

Lenz, H. J., Gupta, M., Xiong, Y. P., Synold, T., Tsao-Wei, D., Groshen, S., Gandara, D. R., Koda, R. T., and Doroshow, J. H. (2000). Phase 1 study of bryostatin 1 and cisplatin (CDDP). *Proc. Am. Soc. Clin. Oncol.* **19**, 795.

Leonard, J. P., May, W. S., Ihle, J. N., Pettit, G. R., and Sharkis, S. J. (1988). Regulation of hematopoiesis-IV: The role of interleukin-3 and bryostatin 1 in the growth of erythropoietic progenitors from normal and anemic W/Wv mice. *Blood* **72**, 1492–1496.

Levine, B. L., May, W. S., Tyler, P. G., and Hess, A. D. (1991). Response of Jurkat T cells to phorbol ester and bryostatin. Development of sublines with distinct functional responses and changes in protein kinase C activity. *J. Immunol.* **147**, 3474–3481.

Lewin, N. E., Pettit, G. R., Kamano, Y., and Blumberg, P. M. (1991). Binding of [26-^{3}H]-epi-bryostatin 4 to protein kinase C. *Cancer Commun.* **3**, 67–70.

Lewin, N. E., Dell'Aquila, M. L., Pettit, G. R., Blumberg, P. M., and Warren, B. S. (1992). Binding of [^{3}H]bryostatin 4 to protein kinase C. *Biochem. Pharmacol.* **43**, 2007–2014.

Li, F., Grant, S., Pettit, G. R., and McCrady, C. W. (1992). Bryostatin 1 modulates the proliferation and lineage commitment of human myeloid progenitor cells exposed to recombinant interleukin-3 and recombinant granulocyte-macrophage colony-stimulating factor. *Blood* **80**, 2495–2502.

Li, Y., and Chen, B. (1997). Induction of macrophage colony-stimulating factor receptor up-regulation in THP-1 human leukemia cells is dependent on the activation of c-fyn protein tyrosine kinase. *Leukemia Res.* **21**, 539–547.

Li, Y., Mohammad, R. M., Al-Katib, A., Varterasian, M. L., and Chen, B. (1997). Bryostatin 1 (bryo1)-induced monocytic differentiation in THP-1 human leukemia cells is associated with enhanced c-*fyn* tyrosine kinase and M-CSF receptors. *Leukemia Res.* **21**, 391–397.

Lilly, M., Tompkins, C., Brown, C., Pettit, G., and Kraft, A. (1990). Differentiation and growth modulation of chronic myelogenous leukemia cells by bryostatin. *Cancer Res.* **50**, 5520–5525.

Lilly, M., Brown, C., Pettit, G., and Kraft, A. (1991). Bryostatin 1: a potential anti-leukemic agent for chronic myelomonocytic leukemia. *Leukemia* **5**, 283–287.

Lilly, M., Le, T., Holland, P., and Hendrickson, S. L. (1992). Sustained expression of the pim-1 kinase is specifically induced in myeloid cells by cytokines whose receptors are structurally related. *Oncogene* **7**, 727–732.

Lilly, M., Vo, K., Le, T., and Takahashi, G. (1996). Bryostatin 1 acts synergistically with interleukin-1 alpha to induce secretion of G-CSF and other cytokines from marrow stromal cells. *Exp. Hematol.* **24**, 613–621.

Lind, D. S., Tuttle, T. M., Bethke, K. P., Frank, J. L., McCrady, C. W., and Bear, H. D. (1993). Expansion and tumour specific cytokine secretion of bryostatin-activated T-cells from cryopreserved axillary lymph nodes of breast cancer patients. *Surg. Oncol.* **2**, 273–282.

Liou, J. R., Liu, T. C., Kaneki, M., Zaleskas, J. M., and Stone, R. M. (1997). Cytosolic down-regulation of mitogen-activated protein kinases during bryostatin 1-induced monocytic differentiation in human myeloid leukemia HL-60 cells pretreated with all-trans retinoic acid. *Blood* **90**, 3450.

Lipshy, K. A., Kostuchenko, P. J., Hamad, G. G., Bland, C. E., Barrett, S. K., and Bear, H. D. (1997). Sensitizing T-lymphocytes for adoptive immunotherapy by vaccination with wild-type or cytokine gene-transduced melanoma. *Ann. Surg. Oncol.* **4**, 334–341.

Liu, K. Z., Schultz, C. P., Mohammad, R. M., Al-Katib, A., and Mantsch, H. H. (1997). Bryostatin 1-induced differentiation of a B-CLL cell line as determined by FT-IR spectroscopy. *Exp. Hematol.* **25**, 502.

Liu, K. Z., Schultz, C. P., Mohammad, R. M., Al-Katib, A. M., Johnston, J. B., and Mantsch, H. H. (1998). Similarities between the sensitivity to 2-chlorodeoxyadenosine of lymphocytes from CLL patients and bryostatin 1-treated WSU-CLL cells: an infrared spectroscopic study. *Cancer Lett.* **127**, 185–193.

Liu, K. Z., Schultz, C. P., Johnston, J. B., Beck, F. W. J., Al-Katib, A. M., Mohammad, R. M., and Mantsch, H. H. (1999). Infrared spectroscopic study of bryostatin 1-induced membrane alterations in a B-CLL cell line. *Leukemia* **13**, 1273–1280.

Lorenzo, P. S., Bogi, K., Acs, P., Pettit, G. R., and Blumberg, P. M. (1997a). The catalytic domain of protein kinase Cdelta confers protection from down-regulation induced by bryostatin 1. *J. Biol. Chem.*, **272**, 33338–33343.

Lorenzo, P. S., Bogi, K., Acs, P., and Blumberg, P. M. (1997b). The catalytic domain of PKC delta confers protection from down-regulation induced by bryostatin 1. *Mol. Biol. Cell.* **8**, 66.

Lorenzo, P. S., Bögi, K., Hughes, K. M., Beheshti, M., Bhattacharyya, D., Garfield, S. H., Pettit, G. R., and Blumberg, P. M. (1999). Differential roles of the tandem C1 domains of protein kinase C delta in the biphasic down-regulation induced by bryostatin 1. *Cancer Res.* **59**, 6137–6144.

Lu, Z., Hornia, A., Jiang, Y. W., Zang, Q., Ohno, S., and Foster, D. A. (1997). Tumor promotion by depleting cells of protein kinase C delta. *Mol. Cell Biol.* **17**, 3418–3428.

Mackanos, E. A., Pettit, G. R., and Ramsdell, J. S. (1991). Bryostatins selectively regulate protein kinase C-mediated effects on GH4 cell proliferation. *J. Biol. Chem.* **266**, 11205–11212.

Maki, A., Diwakaran, H., Redman, B., al-Asfar, S., Pettit, G. R., Mohammad, R. M., and Al-Katib, A. (1995). The bcl-2 and p53 oncoproteins can be modulated by bryostatin 1 and dolastatins in human diffuse large cell lymphoma. *Anticancer Drugs* **6**, 392–397.

Malarkey, K., McLees, A., Paul, A., Gould, G. W., and Plevin, R. (1996). The role of protein kinase C in activation and termination of mitogen-activated protein kinase activity in angiotensin II-stimulated rat aortic smooth-muscle cells. *Cell. Signal.* **8**, 123–129.

Martin, M. B., Garcia-Morales, P., Stoica, A., Solomon, H. B., Pierce, M., Katz, D., Zhang, S., Danielsen, M., and Saceda, M. (1995). Effects of 12-O-tetradecanoylphorbol-13-acetate on estrogen receptor activity in MCF-7 cells. *J. Biol. Chem.* **270**, 25244–25251.

Martinez-Lacaci, I., Saceda, M., Plowman, G. D., Johnson, G. R., Normanno, N., Salomon, D. S., and Dickson, R. B. (1995). Estrogen and phorbol esters regulate amphiregulin expression by two separate mechanisms in human breast cancer cell lines. *Endocrinology* **136**, 3983–3992.

Martinez-Lacaci, I., Johnson, G. R., Salomon, D. S., and Dickson, R. B. (1996). Characterization of a novel amphiregulin-related molecule in 12-O-tetradecanoylphorbol-13-acetate-treated breast cancer cells. *J. Cell. Physiol.* **169**, 497–508.

Masamune, S. (1988a). Asymmetric synthesis and its applications—towards the synthesis of bryostatin 1. *Chimia* **42**, 210–211.

Masamune, S. (1988b). Asymmetric synthesis and its applications—towards the synthesis of bryostatin 1. *Pure Appl. Chem.* **60**, 1587–1596.

Massey, G. V., Huang, X. L., and McCrady, C. W. (1991). Effects of protein-kinase-C activators, phorbol ester (PDBU) and bryostatin 1 on the growth of K562 human erythroblastic leukemia-cell lines. *Pediatric Res.* **29**, 145.

Matsui, M. S., Illarda, I., Wang, N., and DeLeo, V. A. (1993). Protein kinase C agonist and antagonist effects in normal human epidermal keratinocytes. *Exp. Dermatol.* **2**, 247–256.

Matthes, E., Langen, P., Brachwitz, H., Schroder, H. C., Maidhof, A., Weiler, B. E., Renneisen, K., and Muller, W. E. (1990). Alteration of DNA topoisomerase II activity during infection of H9 cells by human immunodeficiency virus type 1 *in vitro*: a target for potential therapeutic agents. *Antiviral Res.* **13**, 273–286.

Matthews, S.A., Pettit, G.R., and Rozengurt, E. (1997). Bryostatin 1 induces biphasic activation of protein kinase D in intact cells. *J. Biol. Chem.* **272**, 20245–20250.

May, W. S., Sensenbrenner, L. L., Esa, A. H., Pettit, G. R., and Sharkis, S. J. (1987a). Bryostatin activates protein kinase C and is a multipotential stimulator of human hematopoietic progenitors. *Exp. Hematol.* **15**, 432.

May, W. S., Sharkis, S. J., Esa, A. H., Gebbia, V., Kraft, A. S., Pettit, G. R., and Sensenbrenner, L. L. (1987b). Antineoplastic bryostatins are multipotential stimulators of human hematopoietic progenitor cells. *Proc. Natl. Acad. Sci. USA* **84**, 8483–8487.

May, W. S., Tyler, P. G., Armstrong, D. K., and Davidson, N. E. (1993). Role for serine phosphorylation of bcl-2 in an antiapoptotic signaling pathway triggered by IL-3, EPO and bryostatin. *Blood* **82**, A438.

May, W. S., Tyler, P. G., Ito, T., Armstrong, D. K., Qatsha, K. A., and Davidson, N. E. (1994). Interleukin–3 and bryostatin 1 mediate hyperphosphorylation of bcl-2 alpha in association with suppression of apoptosis. *J. Biol. Chem.* **269**, 26865–26870.

McBain, J. A., Eastman, A., Simmons, D. L., Pettit, G. R., and Mueller, G. C. (1996). Phorbol ester augments butyrate-induced apoptosis of colon cancer cells. *Int. J. Cancer* **67**, 715–723.

McBain, J. A., Pettit, G. R., and Mueller, G. C. (1988). Bryostatin 1 antagonizes the terminal differentiating action of 12-O-tetradecanoylphorbol-13-acetate in a human colon cancer cell. *Carcinogenesis* **9**, 123–129.

McBain, J. A., Pettit, G. R., and Mueller, G. C. (1990). Phorbol esters activate proteoglycan metabolism in human colon cancer cells en route to terminal differentiation. *Cell Growth Differ.* **1**, 281–291.

McCrady, C. W., Staniswalis, J., Pettit, G. R., Howe, C., and Grant, S. (1991). Effect of pharmacologic manipulation of protein kinase C by phorbol dibutyrate and bryostatin 1 on the clonogenic response of human granulocyte-macrophage progenitors to recombinant GM-CSF. *Br. J. Haematol.* **77**, 5–15.

McCrady, C. W., Li, F., Pettit, G. R., and Grant, S. (1993). Modulation of the activity of a human granulocyte-macrophage colony-stimulating factor/interleukin-3 fusion protein (pIXY 321) by the macrocyclic lactone protein kinase C activator bryostatin 1. *Exp. Hematol.* **21**, 893–900.

McFadden, A., Kostuchenko, P., Barrett, S., Sredni, B., and Bear, H. D. (1994). In-vitro activation and expansion of antitumor T-cells with bryostatin 1 and AS101. *FASEB J.* **8**, A773.

McGown, A. T., Jayson, G., Pettit, G. R., Haran, M. S., Ward, T. H., and Crowther, D. (1998). Bryostatin 1-tamoxifen combinations show synergistic effects on the inhibition of growth of P388 cells *in vitro*. *Br. J. Cancer* **77**, 216–220.

McVicar, D. W., McCrady, C. W., and Merchant, R. E. (1992). Corticosteroids inhibit the delivery of short-term activational pulses of phorbol ester and calcium ionophore to human peripheral T cells. *Cell. Immunol.* **140**, 145–157.

Membreno, L., Chen, T. H., Woodley, S., Gagucas, R., and Shoback, D. (1989). The effects of protein kinase-C agonists on parathyroid hormone release and intracellular free Ca^{2+} in bovine parathyroid cells. *Endocrinology* **124**, 789–797.

Merchant, R.E., Baldwin, N. G., Rice, C. D., and Bear, H. D. (1997). Adoptive immunotherapy of malignant glioma using tumor-sensitized T-lymphocytes. *Neurol. Res.* **19**, 145–152.

Mohammad, R. M., Al-Katib, A., Pettit, G. R., and Sensenbrenner, L. L. (1993). Differential effects of bryostatin 1 on human non-Hodgkin's B-lymphoma cell lines. *Leukemia Res.* **17**, 1–8.

Mohammad, R. M., Al-Katib, A., Pettit, G. R., and Sensenbrenner, L. L. (1994a). Successful treatment of human Waldenström's macroglobulinemia with combination biological and chemotherapy agents. *Cancer Res.* **54**, 165–168.

Mohammad, R., Maki, A., Diwakaran, H., Pettit, G. R., and Al-Katib, A. (1994b). Bryostatin 1 induces apoptosis and augments inhibitory effects of vincristine in human diffuse large-cell lymphoma. *Blood* **84**, A448.

Mohammad, R., Maki, A., Salleh, M., Pettit, G. R., and Al-Katib, A. (1994c). *In vitro* and *in vivo* preclinical studies of bryostatin/vincristine combination in lymphoma. *Exp. Hematol.* **23**, 930.

Mohammad, R. M., Diwakaran, H., Maki, A., Emara, M. A., Pettit, G. R., Redman, B., and Al-Katib, A. (1995a). Bryostatin 1 induces apoptosis and augments inhibitory effects of vincristine in human diffuse large cell lymphoma. *Leukemia Res.* **19**, 667–673.

Mohammad, R. M., Hamdan, M. Y., Maki, A., and Al-Katib, A. (1995b). Induced expression of alpha-enolase in differentiated diffuse large cell lymphoma. *Enzyme Protein* **48**, 37–44.

Mohammad, R. M., Dugan, M. C., Vartersian, M., Pettit, G. R., and Al-Katib, A. (1996a). Preclinical evaluation of bryostatin 1, dolastatin 10 and their combination against diffuse large cell lymphoma xenograft. *Blood* **88**, 3497.

Mohammad, R. M., Maki, A., Pettit, G. R., and Al-Katib, A. M. (1996b). Bryostatin 1 induces ubiquitin COOH-terminal hydrolase in acute lymphoblastic leukemia cells. *Enzyme Protein* **49**, 262–272.

Mohammad, R. M., Mohamed, A. N., Hamdan, M. Y., Vo, T., Chen, B., Katato, K., Abubakr, Y. A., Dugan, M. C., and Al-Katib, A. (1996c). Establishment of a human b-CLL xenograft model: utility as a preclinical therapeutic model. *Leukemia* **10**, 130–137.

Mohammad, R. M., Beck, F. W. J., Wall, N., Hamdy, N., Mendpara, S. D., Liu, K. Z., Schultz, C. P., Hannoudi, G. N., Mantsch, H. H., amd Al-Katib, A. (1997). The role of bryostatin 1 in 2-CdA resistant B-CLL line: mechanism of resistance and response. *Blood* **90**, 2364.

Mohammad, R. M., Beck, F. W., Katato, K., Hamdy, N., Wall, N., and Al-Katib, A. (1998a). Potentiation of 2-chlorodeoxyadenosine activity by bryostatin 1 in the resistant chronic lymphocytic leukemia cell line (WSU-CLL): association with increased ratios of dCK/5'-NT and Bax/Bcl-2. *Biol. Chem.* **379**, 1253–1261.

Mohammad, R. M., Dugan, M. C., Mohamed, A. N., Almatchy, V. P., Flake, T. M., Dergham, S. T., Shields, A. F., Al-Katib, A. M., Vaitkevicius, V. K., and Sarkar, F. H. (1998b). Establishment of a human pancreatic tumor xenograft model: potential application for preclinical evaluation of novel therapeutic agents. *Pancreas* **16**, 19–25.

Mohammad, R. M., Katato, K., Almatchy, V. P., Wall, N., Liu, K. Z., Schultz, C. P., Mantsch, H. H., Varterasian, M., and Al-Katib, A. M. (1998c). Sequential treatment of human chronic lymphocytic leukemia with bryostatin 1 followed by 2-chlorodeoxyadenosine: preclinical studies. *Clin. Cancer Res.* **4**, 445–453.

Mohammad, R. M., Limvarapuss, C., Khoury, G., Ahmad, B., Dutcher, B. S., Beck, F. W. J., Chaudhuri, R., Wall, N., and Al-Katib, A. M. (1998d). Treatment of a *de novo* fludarabine resistant chronic lymphocytic leukemia model with bryostatin 1 followed by fludarabine. *Blood* **92**, 597A.

Mohammad, R. M., Pettit, G. R., Almatchy, V. P., Wall, N., Varterasian, M., and Al-Katib, A. (1998e). Synergistic interaction of selected marine animal anticancer drugs against human diffuse large cell lymphoma. *Anticancer Drugs* **9**, 149–156.

Mohammad, R. M., Varterasian, M. L., Almatchy, V. P., Hannoudi, G. N., Pettit, G. R., and Al-Katib, A. (1998f). Successful treatment of human chronic lymphocytic leukemia xenografts with combination biological agents auristatin PE and bryostatin 1. *Clin. Cancer Res.* **4**, 1337–1343.

Mohammad, R. M., Li, Y., Mohamed, A. N., Pettit, G. R., Adsay, V., Vaitkevicius, V. K., Al-Katib, A. M., and Sarkar, F. H. (1999a). Clonal preservation of human pancreatic cell line derived from primary pancreatic adenocarcinoma. *Pancreas* **19**, 353–361.

Mohammad, R. M., Limvarapuss, C., Hamdy, N., Dutcher, B. S., Beck, F. W. J., Wall, N. R., and Al-Katib, A. M. (1999b). Treatment of a de novo fludarabine resistant-CLL xenograft model with bryostatin 1 followed by fludarabine. *Int. J. Oncol.* **14**, 945–950.

Mohammad, R. M., Wall, N. R., Choudhuri, R., Ali, N. J., Beck, F. W. J., and Al-Katib, A. (1999c). Bryostatin 1 initiates the activation of a DNA damaging protease cascade and lowers the threshold for apoptosis induced by 2-chlorodeoxyadenosine (2CdA) in the chronic lymphocytic leukemia cell line, WSU-CLL. *Blood* **94**, 302b.

Mohr, H., Pettit, G. R., and Plessing-Menze, A. (1987). Co-induction of lymphokine synthesis by the antineoplastic bryostatins. *Immunobiology* **175**, 420–430.

Mond, J. J., Balapure, A., Feuerstein, N., June, C. H., Brunswick, M., Lindsberg, M. L., and Witherspoon, K. (1990). Protein kinase C activation in B cells by indolactam inhibits anti-Ig-mediated phosphatidylinositol bisphosphate hydrolysis but not B cell proliferation. *J. Immunol.* **144**, 451–455.

Mutter, R., and Wills, M. (2000). Chemistry and clinical biology of the bryostatins. *Bioorg. Med. Chem.* **8**, 1841–1860.

Newman, D. J. (1996). Keynote Address: Bryostatin—from bryozoan to cancer drug. *Proc. 10th Int. Bryozoology Conf. NIWA, Wellington, New Zealand,* 9–17.

Ng, S. B., and Guy, G. R. (1992). Two protein kinase C activators, bryostatin 1 and phorbol-12-myristate-13-acetate, have different effects on haemopoietic cell proliferation and differentiation. *Cell. Signal.* **4**, 405–416.

Ning, Z. Q., Hirose, T., Deed, R., Newton, J., Murphy, J. J., and Norton, J. D. (1996). Early response gene signalling in bryostatin-stimulated primary B chronic lymphocytic leukaemia cells *in vitro*. *Biochem. J.* **319**, 59–65.

Noll, T., Dieckmann, D., Gibbs, B. F., Nitschke, M., Albrecht, C., Vollrath, I., Tamaoki, T., Wolff, H. H., and Amon, U. (1997). Heterogeneity of signal transduction mechanisms in human basophils and human skin mast cells. II. Effects of 7-O-methyl-UCN-01, NPC 15437 and bryostatin 1 and 2, four protein kinase C-modulatory agents, on mediator release. *Biol. Signals* **6**, 1–10.

Noriaki, K., Masahiro, K., and Motoyuki, Y. (1995). JP7252146A: adrenocortical hormone production promoter. Patent Application: 3 October 1995.

Noriaki, K., Keimei, T., and Takishi, K. (1996). JP8092085A: antiretroviral agent. Patent Application: 9 April 1996.

Nutt, J. E., Harris, A. L., and Lunec, J. (1991). Phorbol ester and bryostatin effects on growth and the expression of oestrogen responsive and TGF-beta 1 genes in breast tumour cells. *Br. J. Cancer* **64**, 671–676.

Obitsu, T., Ohmori, K., Ogawa, Y., Hosomi, H., Ohba, S., Nishiyama, S., and Yamamura, S. (1998). Synthesis of the C-17–C-27 fragment of bryostatin 3. *Tetrahedron Lett.* **39**, 7349–7352.

Ohmori, K., Susuki, T., Miyasawa, K., Nishiyama, S., and Yamura, S. (1993). Synthetic studies on bryostatins, antineoplastic metabolites—convergent synthesis of the C1-C16 fragment shared by all of the bryostatin family. *Tetrahedron Lett.* **34**, 4981–4984.

Ohmori, K., Nishiyama, S., and Yamamura, S. (1995a). Synthetic studies on bryostatins, potent antineoplastic agents—synthesis of the C-17–C-27 fragment of C-20 oxygenated bryostatins. *Tetrahedron Lett.* **36**, 6519–6522.

Ohmori, K., Suzuki, T., Nishiyama, S., and Yamamura, S. (1995b). Synthetic studies on bryostatins, potent antineoplastic agents—synthesis of the C-17–C-27 fragment of C-20 deoxybryostatins. *Tetrahedron Lett.,* **36**, 6515–6518.

Ohmori, K., Ogawa, Y., Obitsu, T., Ishikawa, Y., Nishiyama, S., and Yamamura, S. (2000). Total synthesis of bryostatin. 3. *Angew. Chem. Int. Ed.* **39**, 2290–2294.

Parker, J., Waite, M., Pettit, G. R., and Daniel, L. W. (1988). Stimulation of arachidonic acid release and prostaglandin synthesis by bryostatin 1. *Carcinogenesis* **9**, 1471–1474.

Parkinson, D. R., Arbuck, S. G., Moore, T., Pluda, J. M., and Christian, M. C. (1994). Clinical development of anticancer agents from natural products. *Stem Cells* **12**, 30–43.

Pasti, G., Rivedal, E., Yuspa, S. H., Herald, C. L., Pettit, G. R., and Blumberg, P. M. (1988). Contrasting duration of inhibition of cell-cell communication in primary mouse epidermal cells by phorbol 12,13-dibutyrate and by bryostatin 1. *Cancer Res.* **48**, 447–451.

Patella, V., Casolaro, V., Ciccarelli, A., Pettit, G. R., Columbo, M., and Marone, G. (1995). The antineoplastic bryostatins affect human basophils and mast cells differently. *Blood* **85**, 1272–1281.

Pettit, G. R. (1991). The bryostatins. *In* "Progress in the Chemistry of Organic Natural Products" (W. Herz, G.W. Kirby, W. Steglich, and C. Tamm, eds.), Vol. 57, pp. 153–195. Springer-Verlag, New York.

Pettit, G. R. (1996). Progress in the discovery of biosynthetic anticancer drugs. *J. Nat. Prod.* **59**, 812–821.

Pettit, G. R., Day, J. F., Hartwell, J. L., and Wood, H. B. (1970). Antineoplastic components of marine animals. *Nature* **227**, 962–963.

Pettit, G. R., Herald, C. L., Doubek, D. L., Herald, D. L., Arnold, E., and Clardy, J. (1982). Isolation and structure of bryostatin 1. *J. Am. Chem. Soc.* **104**, 6846–6848.

Pettit, G. R., Herald, C. L., and Kamano, Y. (1983a). Structure of the *Bugula neritina* (marine Bryozoa) antineoplastic component bryostatin 3. *J. Org. Chem.* **48**, 5354–5356.

Pettit, G. R., Herald, C. L., Kamano, Y., Gust, D., and Aoyagi, R. (1983b). The structure of bryostatin 2 from the marine bryozoan *Bugula neritina*. *J. Nat. Prod.* **46**, 528–531.

Pettit, G. R., Kamano, Y., Herald, C. L., and Tozawa, M. (1984). Structure of bryostatin 4. An important antineoplastic constituent of geographically diverse *Bugula neritina* (Bryozoa). *J. Am. Chem. Soc.* **106**, 6768–6771.

Pettit, G. R., Kamano, Y., Herald, C. L., and Tozawa, M. (1985). Isolation and structure of bryostatins 5-7. *Can. J. Chem.* **63**, 1204–1208.

Pettit, G. R., Kamano, Y., and Herald, C. L. (1986). Antineoplastic agents. 118. Isolation and structure of bryostatin 9. *J. Nat. Prod.* **49**, 661–664.

Pettit, G. R., Kamano, Y., and Herald, C. L. (1987a). Isolation and structure of bryostatins 10 and 11. *J. Org. Chem.* **52**, 2848–2854.

Pettit, G. R., Leet, J. E., Herald, C. L., Kamano, Y., Boettmer, F. E., Baczynsky, L., and Nieman, R. A. (1987b). Isolation and structure of bryostatins 12 and 13. *J. Org. Chem.* **52**, 2854–2860.

Pettit, G. R., Herald, C. L., and Smith, C. R. (1989). "Biosynthetic Products for Cancer Chemotherapy" Vol. 8. Elsevier Scientific Publ. Co., Amsterdam.

Pettit, G. R., Gao, F., Sengupta, D., Coll, J. C., Herald, C. L., Doubek, D. L., Schmidt, J. M., Van Camp, J. R., Rudloe, J. J., and Nieman, R. A. (1991a). Isolation and structure of bryostatins 14 and 15. *Tetrahedron* **47**, 3601–3610.

Pettit, G. R., Sengupta, D., and Herald, C. L. (1991b). Synthetic conversion of bryostatin 2 to bryostatin 1 and related bryopyrans. *Can. J. Chem.* **69**, 856–860.

Pettit, G. R., Sengupta, D., Blumberg, P. M., Lewin, N. E., Schmidt, J. M., and Kraft, A. S. (1992). Structural modifications of bryostatin 2. *Anticancer Drug Des.* **7**, 101–113.

Pettit, G. R., Hogan-Pierson, F., and Herald, C. L. (1993). "Anticancer Drugs from Animals, Plants, and Microorganisms." John Wiley-Interscience, New York.

Pettit, G. R., Gao, F., Blumberg, P. M., Herald, C. L., Coll, J. C., Kamano, Y., Lewin, N. E., Schmidt, J. M., and Chapuis, J. C. (1996). Antineoplastic agents. 340. Isolation and structural elucidation of bryostatins 16–18. *J. Nat. Prod.* **59**, 286–289.

Phelan, S. A., Lindberg, C., and Call, K. M. (1994). Wilms' tumor gene, *WT1*, mRNA is down-regulated during induction of erythroid and megakaryocytic differentiation of K562 cells. *Cell Growth Different.* **5**, 677–686.

Philip, P. A., Rea, D., Thavasu, P., Carmichael, J., Stuart, N. S., Rockett, H., Talbot, D. C., Ganesan, T., Pettit, G. R., Balkwill, F., and Harris, A. L. (1993). Phase I study of bryostatin 1: assessment of interleukin 6 and tumor necrosis factor alpha induction *in vivo*. The Cancer Research Campaign Phase I Committee. *J. Natl. Cancer. Inst.* **85**, 1812–1818.

Philip, P., Li, Y., Alonso, M., Manji, H., Sarkar, F., Ensley, J., and Ali-Sadat, S. (1999). Sensitization of human breast cancer cells to gemcitabine by bryostatin. *Proc. Am. Assoc. Cancer Res.* **40**, 5.

Prendiville, J., Crowther, D., Thatcher, N., Woll, P. J., Fox, B. W., McGown, A., Testa, N., Stern, P., McDermott, R., Potter, M., and Pettit, G. R. (1993). A phase I study of intravenous bryostatin 1 in patients with advanced cancer. *Br. J. Cancer* **68**, 418–424.

Prendiville, J., McGown, A. T., Gescher, A., Dickson, A. J., Courage, C., Pettit, G. R., Crowther, D., and Fox, B. W. (1994). Establishment of a murine leukaemia cell line resistant to the growth-inhibitory effect of bryostatin 1. *Br. J. Cancer* **70**, 573–578.

Propper, D. J., Macaulay, V., O'Byrne, K. J., Braybrooke, J. P., Wilner, S. M., Ganesan, T. S., Talbot, D. C., and Harris, A. L. (1998). A phase II study of bryostatin 1 in metastatic malignant melanoma. *Br. J. Cancer* **78**, 1337–1341.

Qatsha, K. A., Rudolph, C., Marme, D., Schachtele, C., and May, W. S. (1993). Go 6976, a selective inhibitor of protein kinase C, is a potent antagonist of human immunodeficiency virus 1 induction from latent/low-level-producing reservoir cells *in vitro*. *Proc. Natl. Acad. Sci. USA* **90**, 4674–4678.

Racke, F. K., Lewandowska, K., Goueli, S., and Goldfarb, A. N. (1997). Sustained activation of the extracellular signal-regulated kinase/mitogen-activated protein kinase pathway is required for megakaryocytic differentiation of K562 cells. *J. Biol. Chem.* **272**, 23366–23370.

Ramsdell, J. S., Pettit, G. R., and Tashjian, A. H., Jr. (1986). Three activators of protein kinase C, bryostatins, dioleins, and phorbol esters, show differing specificities of action on GH4 pituitary cells. *J. Biol. Chem.* **261**, 17073–17080.

Rao, A. S., Freemerman, A. J., Jarvis, W. D., Chelliah, J., Bear, H. D., Mikkelsen, R., and Grant, S. (1996). Effect of AS101 on bryostatin 1-mediated differentiation induction, cell cycle arrest, and modulation of drug-induced apoptosis in human myeloid leukemia cells. *Leukemia* **10**, 1150–1158.

Reeves, J. A., Baudoin, P., Ashendel, C., and Kraft, A. S. (1987). Bryostatin is less potent than phorbol esters in inducing nonadherent growth of mouse epidermal cells. *Proc. Am. Assoc. Cancer Res.*, **28**, 175.

Reynolds, N .J., Baldassare, J. J., Henderson, P. A., Shuler, J. L., Ballas, L. M., Burns, D. J., Moomaw, C. R., and Fisher, G. J. (1994). Translocation and downregulation of protein kinase C isoenzymes-alpha and -epsilon by phorbol ester and bryostatin 1 in human keratinocytes and fibroblasts. *J. Invest. Dermatol.* **103**, 364–369.

Rice, C. D., Baldwin, N. G., Biron, R. T., Bear, H. D., and Merchant, R. E. (1997). Ex vivo expansion of tumor-draining lymph node cells using compounds which activate intracellular signal transduction. II. Cytokine production and *in vivo* efficacy of glioma-sensitized lymphocytes. *J. Neurooncol.* **32**, 29–38.

Ritke, M. K., Murray, N. R., Allan, W. P., Fields, A. P., and Yalowich, J. C. (1995). Hypophosphorylation of topoisomerase II in etoposide (VP-16)-resistant human leukemia K562 cells associated with reduced levels of beta II protein kinase C. *Mol. Pharmacol.* **48**, 798–805.

Rosenthal, M. A., Oratz, R., Liebes, L., Cahr, M. H., and Muggia, F. M. (1999). Phase I study of bryostatin 1 (NSC 339555) and cisplatin in advanced malignancies. *Proc. Am. Soc. Clin. Oncol.* **18**, 873.

Roy, R., and Rey, A. W. (1990). A chemoenzymatic synthesis of the C1-C9 fragment of bryostatin: unusual diastereoselectivity during a Mukaiyama aldol condensation. *Synlett.* **0**, 448–450.

Ruff, L. J., Grever, K. F., Fagan, K. A., McMurtry, I. F., Kraft, A. S., Pettit, G. R., and Dempsey, E. C. (1999). Attenuating effects of bryostatin 1 in an adult murine model of chronic hypoxic pulmonary hypertension. *Am. J. Resp. Crit. Care Med.* **159**, A163.

Ruvolo, P. P., Deng, X., Carr, B. K., and May, W. S. (1998). A functional role for mitochondrial protein kinase C-alpha in Bcl2 phosphorylation and suppression of apoptosis. *J. Biol. Chem.*, **273**, 25436–25442.

Sako, T., Yuspa, S. H., Herald, C. L., Pettit, G. R., and Blumberg, P. M. (1987). Partial parallelism and partial blockade by bryostatin 1 of effects of phorbol ester tumor promoters on primary mouse epidermal cells. *Cancer Res.* **47**, 5445–5450.

Sako, T., Ohshima, S., Yoshizumi, T., and Sakurai, M. (1988). Differential modulation of protein kinase C by bryostatin 1 and phorbol ester. *Tohoku J. Exp. Med.* **156**, 229–236.

Sansbury, H. M., Wisehart-Johnson, A. E., Qi, C., Fulwood, S., and Meier, K. E. (1997). Effects of protein kinase C activators on phorbol ester-sensitive and -resistant EL4 thymoma cells. *Carcinogenesis* **18**, 1817–1824.

Saunders, N. A., Bernacki, S. H., Vollberg, T. M., and Jetten, A. M. (1993). Regulation of transglutaminase type I expression in squamous differentiating rabbit tracheal epithelial cells and human epidermal keratinocytes: effects of retinoic acid and phorbol esters. *Mol. Endocrinol.* **7**, 387–398.

Scala, S., Dickstein, B., Regis, J., Szallasi, Z., Blumberg, P. M., and Bates, S. E. (1995). Bryostatin 1 affects P-glycoprotein phosphorylation but not function in multidrug-resistant human breast cancer cells. *Clin. Cancer Res.* **1**, 1581–1587.

Schaufelberger, D. E., Alvarado, A. B., Andrews, P., and Beutler, J. A. (1990). Detection and quantitation of bryostatin 1 and 2 in *Bugula neritina* by combined high-performance liquid chromatography and tritiated phorbol dibutyrate displacement. *J. Liquid Chromatogr. Related Technol.* **13**, 583–598.

Schaufelberger, D. E., Chmurny, G. N., and Koleck, M. P. (1991a). Proton and carbon-13 nmr assignments of the antitumor marcolide bryostatin 1. *Mag. Res. Chem.* **29**, 366–374.

Schaufelberger, D. E., Chmurny, G. N., Buetler, J. A., Koleck, M. P., Alvarado, A. B., Schaufelberger, B. W., and Muschik, G. M. (1991b). Revised structure of bryostatin 3 and isolation of the bryostatin 3 26-ketone from *Bugula neritina*. *J Org. Chem.* **56**, 2895–2900.

Schaufelberger, D. E., Koleck, M. P., Beutler, J. A., Vatakis, A. M., Alvarado, A. B., Andrews, P., Marzo, L. V., Muschik, G. M., Roach, J., and Ross, J. T. (1991c). The large-scale isolation of bryostatin 1 from *Bugula neritina* following current good manufacturing practices. *J. Nat. Prod.* **54**, 1265–1270.

Scheid, C., Prendiville, J., Jayson, G., Crowther, D., Fox, B., Pettit, G. R., and Stern, P. L. (1994). Immunomodulation in patients receiving intravenous bryostatin 1 in a phase I clinical study: comparison with effects of bryostatin 1 on lymphocyte function *in vitro*. *Cancer. Immunol. Immunother.* **39**, 223–230.

Schonhorn, J. E., Akompong, T., and Wessling-Resnick, M. (1995). Mechanism of transferrin receptor down-regulation in K562 cells in response to protein kinase C activation. *J. Biol. Chem.* **270**, 3698–3705.

Schuchter, L. M., Esa, A. H., May, W. S., Laulis, M. K., Pettit, G. R., and Hess, A. D. (1991). Successful treatment of murine melanoma with bryostatin 1. *Cancer Res.* **51**, 682–687.

Schwaller, J., Peters, U. R., Pabst, T., Niklaus, G., Macfarlane, D. E., Fey, M. F., and Tobler, A. (1997). Up-regulation of p21WAF1 expression in myeloid cells is activated by the protein kinase C pathway. *Br. J. Cancer* **76**, 1554–1557.

Sham, R. L., Packman, C. H., Abboud, C. N., and Lichtman, M. A. (1990). Control of actin conformation in AML myeloblasts: the effects of bryostatin and TPA. *Leukemia Res.* **14**, 863–868.

Sham, R. L., Packman, C. H., Abboud, C. N., and Lichtman, M. A. (1991). Signal transduction and the regulation of actin conformation during myeloid maturation: studies in HL60 cells. *Blood* **77**, 363–370.

Sharkis, S. J., Leonard, J. P., Ihle, J. N., and May, W. S. (1989). The effects of interleukin-3, bryostatin and thymocytes on erythropoiesis. *Ann. N. Y. Acad. Sci.* **554**, 59 65.

Sharkis, S. J., Jones, R. J., Bellis, M. L., Demetri, G. D., Griffin, J. D., Civin, C., and May, W. S. (1990). The action of bryostatin on normal human hematopoietic progenitors is mediated by accessory cell release of growth factors. *Blood* **76**, 716–720.

Sherman, M. L., Stone, R. M., Datta, R., Bernstein, S. H., and Kufe, D. W. (1990). Transcriptional and post-transcriptional regulation of c-*jun* expression during monocytic differentiation of human myeloid leukemic cells. *J. Biol. Chem.*, **265**, 3320–3323.

Shieh, H. L., Hansen, H., Zhu, J., and Riedel, H. (1996). Activation of conventional mammalian protein kinase C isoforms expressed in budding yeast modulates the cell doubling time: a potential *in vivo* screen for protein kinase C activators. *Cancer Detect. Prevent.* **20**, 576–589.

Singh, K. R., Taylor, L. K., Campbell, X. Z., Fields, A. P., and Neet, K. E. (1994). A bryostatin-sensitive protein kinase C required for nerve growth factor activity. *Biochemistry* **33**, 542–551.

Slater, S. J., Ho, C., Kelly, M. B., Larkin, J. D., Taddeo, F. J., Yeager, M. D., and Stubbs, C. D. (1996). Protein kinase Calpha contains two activator binding sites that bind phorbol esters and diacylglycerols with opposite affinities. *J. Biol. Chem.* **271**, 4627–4631.

Slater, S. J., Taddeo, F. J., Mazurek, A., Stagliano, B. A., Milano, S. K., Kelly, M. B., Ho, C., and Stubbs, C. D. (1998). Inhibition of membrane lipid-independent protein kinase Calpha activity by phorbol esters, diacylglycerols, and bryostatin 1. *J. Biol. Chem.* **273**, 23160–23168.

Smith, C. R., Jr., Powell, R. G., and Mikolajczak, K. L. (1976). The genus *Cephalotaxus*: source of homoharringtonine and related anticancer alkaloids. *Cancer Treat. Rep.* **60**, 1157–1170.

Smith, J. B., Smith, L., and Pettit, G. R. (1985). Bryostatins: potent, new mitogens that mimic phorbol ester tumor promoters. *Biochem. Biophys. Res. Commun.* **132**, 939–945.

Smith, L., Lee, H. W., and Smith, J. B. (1997). Inhibition of the proteasome converts bryostatin from an antagonist to an agonist of protein kinase C (PKC). *FASEB J.* **11**, A987.

Smith, M., and Ho, P. T. C. (1996). Pediatric drug development—a perspective from the cancer therapy evaluation program (CTEP) of the National Cancer Institute (NCI). *Invest. New Drugs* **14**, 11–22.

Smith, M. R., Al-Katib, A., Mohammad, R., Silverman, A., Szabo, P., Khilnani, S., Köhler, W., Nath, R., and Mutchnick, M. G. (1993). Prothymosin alpha gene expression correlates with proliferation, not differentiation, of HL-60 cells. *Blood* **82**, 1127–1132.

Song, X. D., and Norman, A. W. (1997). 1α,25-Dihydroxyvitamin D-3 and bryostatin synergistically induced alkaline phosphatase (Alp) expression in human NB4 acute promyelocytic leukemia cells. *J. Bone Mineral Res.* **12**, F408.

Song, X. D., and Norman, A. W. (1999). Bryostatin 1 and 1α,25-dihydroxyvitamin D3 synergistically stimulate the differentiation of NB4 acute promyelocytic leukemia cells. *Leukemia* **13**, 275–281.

Song, X., Sheppard, H. M., Norman, A. W., and Liu, X. (1999). Mitogen-activated protein kinase is involved in the degradation of p53 protein in the bryostatin 1-induced differentiation of the acute promyelocytic leukemia NB4 cell line. *J. Biol. Chem.* **274**, 1677–1682.

Southern, C., Wilkinson, P. C., Thorp, K. M., Henderson, L. K., Nemec, M., and Matthews, N. (1995). Inhibition of protein kinase C results in a switch from a non-motile to a motile phenotype in diverse human lymphocyte populations. *Immunology* **84**, 326–332.

Soybel, D. I., Farokhzad, O. C., and Harken, A. H. (1998). Effects of bryostatin 1, a novel anticancer agent, on intestinal transport and barrier function: role of protein kinase C: discussion. *Surgery* **124**, 386–387.

Spitaler, M., Utz, I., Hilbe, W., Hofmann, J., and Grunicke, H. H. (1998). PKC-independent modulation of multidrug resistance in cells with mutant (V185) but not wild-type (G185) P-glycoprotein by bryostatin 1. *Biochem. Pharmacol.* **56**, 861–869.

Spivak, J. L., Fisher, J., Isaacs, M. A., and Hankins, W. D. (1992). Protein kinases and phosphatases are involved in erythropoietin-mediated signal transduction. *Exp. Hematol.* **20**, 500–504.

Spjut, R. W., and Perdue, R. E., Jr. (1976). Plant folklore: a tool for predicting sources of antitumor activity? *Cancer Treat. Rep.* **60**, 979–985.

Sredni, B., Kalechman, Y., Albeck, M., Gross, O., Aurbach, D., Sharon, P., Sehgal, S. N., Gurwith, M. J., and Michlin, H. (1990). Cytokine secretion effected by synergism of the immunomodulator AS101 and the protein kinase C inducer bryostatin. *Immunology* **70**, 473–477.

Stanwell, C., Gescher, A., Bradshaw, T. D., and Pettit, G. R. (1994). The role of protein kinase C isoenzymes in the growth inhibition caused by bryostatin 1 in human A549 lung and MCF-7 breast carcinoma cells. *Int. J. Cancer* **56**, 585–592.

Stanwell, C., Denning, M. F., Rutberg, S. E., Cheng, C., Yuspa, S. H., and Dlugosz, A. A. (1996a). Staurosporine induces a sequential program of mouse keratinocyte terminal differentiation through activation of PKC isozymes. *J. Invest. Dermatol.* **106**, 482–489.

Stanwell, C., Dlugosz, A. A., and Yuspa, S. H. (1996b). Staurosporine induces a complete program of terminal differentiation in neoplastic mouse keratinocytes via activation of protein kinase C. *Carcinogenesis* **17**, 1259–1265.

Steube, K. G., and Drexler, H. G. (1993). Differentiation and growth modulation of myeloid leukemia cells by the protein kinase C activating agent bryostatin 1. *Leukemia & Lymphoma* **9**, 141–148.

Steube, K. G., and Drexler, H. G. (1995). The protein kinase C activator bryostatin1 induces the rapid release of TNF-alpha from MONO-MAC-6 cells. *Biochem. Biophys. Res. Commun.* **214,** 1197–1203.

Steube, K.G., Grunicke, D., Pietsch, T., Gignac, S.M., Pettit, G.R., and Drexler, H.G. (1992). Dolastatin 10 and dolastatin 15: effects of two natural peptides on growth and differentiation of leukemia cells. *Leukemia* **6,** 1048–1053.

Steube, K.G., Grunicke, D., Quentmeier, H., and Drexler, H.G. (1993). Different effects of the two protein kinase C activators bryostatin 1 and TPA on growth and differentiation of human monocytic leukemia cell lines. *Leukemia Res.* **17,** 897–901.

Steube, K.G., Grunicke, D., and Drexler, H.G. (1994). Different biological effects of the two protein kinase C activators bryostatin 1 and TPA on human carcinoma cell lines. *Invest. New Drugs* **12,** 15–23.

Stewart, J. P., McGown, A. T., Prendiville, J., Pettit, G. R., Fox, B. W., and Arrand, J. R. (1993). Bryostatin 1 induces productive Epstein-Barr virus replication in latently infected cells: implications for use in immuno-compromised patients. *Cancer Chemother. Pharmacol.* **33,** 89–91.

Stone, R. M., Sariban, E., Pettit, G. R., and Kufe, D. W. (1988). Bryostatin 1 activates protein kinase C and induces monocytic differentiation of HL-60 cells. *Blood* **72,** 208–213.

Stone, R. M., Galinsky, I., Berg, D., Daftary, F., Kinchla, N., Zaleskas, J. M., Xu, G., and Liou, J. R. (1998). Protein kinase C (PKC)-based anti-leukemic therapy: a randomized phase II trial of all-trans retinoic acid (ATRA) and bryostatin 1 (BRYO) in patients (PTS) with myelodysplastic syndromes (MDS) and acute myeloid leukemia (AML). *Blood* **92,** 631A.

Suffness, M., and Douros, J. D. (1979). Drugs of plant origin. *In* "Methods in Cancer Research. Cancer Drug Development. Part A" (V. T. Devita, Jr. and H. Busch, eds.), Vol. 16, p. 73. Academic Press, New York.

Sung, S. J., Lin, P. S., Schmidt, U., R., Hall, C. E., Walters, J. A., McCrady, C., and Grant, S. (1994). Effects of the protein kinase C stimulant bryo-statin 1 on the proliferation and colony formation of irradiated human T-lymphocytes. *Int. J. Radiat. Biol.* **66,** 775–783.

Sutherland, J. D., and Whitfield, J. N. (1997). Prebiotic chemistry: a bioorganic perspective. *Tetrahedron* **53,** 11493–11527.

Sylvia, V. L., Schwartz, Z., Ellis, E. B., Helm, S. H., Gomez, R., Dean, D. D., and Boyan, B. D. (1996). Nongenomic regulation of protein kinase C isoforms by the vitamin D metabolites 1 alpha,25-(OH)2D3 and 24R,25-(OH)2D3. *J. Cell. Physiol.* **167,** 380–393.

Szallasi, Z., Krsmanovic, L., and Blumberg, P. M. (1993a). Nonpromoting 12-deoxyphorbol 13-esters inhibit phorbol 12-myristate 13-acetate induced tumor promotion in CD-1 mouse skin. *Cancer Res.* **53,** 2507–2512.

Szallasi, Z., Smith, C. B., Denning, M. F., Dlugosz, A. A., Yuspa, S. H., Pettit, G. R., and Blumberg, P. M. (1993b). Differential regulation of protein kinase C isozymes by inhibitory 12-deoxyphorbol 13-monoesters, bryostatin 1, and phorbol 12-myristate 13-acetate (PMA) in mouse keratinocytes. *Clin. Res.* **41,** A450.

Szallasi, Z., Denning, M. F., Smith, C. B., Dlugosz, A. A., Yuspa, S. H., Pettit, G. R., and Blumberg, P. M. (1994a). Bryostatin 1 protects protein kinase C-delta from down-regulation in mouse keratinocytes in parallel with its inhibition of phorbol ester-induced differentiation. *Mol. Pharmacol.* **46,** 840–850.

Szallasi, Z., Smith, C. B., Pettit, G. R., and Blumberg, P. M. (1994b). Differential regulation of protein kinase C isozymes by bryostatin 1 and phorbol 12-myristate 13-acetate in NIH 3T3 fibroblasts. *J. Biol. Chem.* **269,** 2118–2124.

Szallasi, Z., Kosa, K., Smith, C. B., Dlugosz, A. A., Williams, E. K., Yuspa, S. H., and Blumberg, P. M. (1995). Differential regulation by anti-tumor-promoting 12-deoxyphorbol-13-phenylacetate reveals distinct roles of the classical and novel protein kinase C isozymes in biological responses of primary mouse keratinocytes. *Mol. Pharmacol.* **47,** 258–265.

Szallasi, Z., Du, L., Levine, R., Lewin, N. E., Nguyen, P. N., Williams, M. D., Pettit, G. R., and Blumberg, P. M. (1996). The bryostatins inhibit growth of B16/F10 melanoma cells *in vitro* through a protein kinase C-independent mechanism: dissociation of activities using 26-epi-bryostatin 1. *Cancer Res.,* **56,** 2105–2111.

Takayama, H., and Sitkovsky, M. V. (1987). Antigen receptor-regulated exocytosis in cytotoxic T lymphocytes. *J. Exp. Med.,* **166,** 725–743.

Tallant, E. A., Smith, J. B., and Wallace, R. W. (1987). Bryostatins mimic the effects of phorbol esters in intact human platelets. *Biochim. Biophys. Acta* **929,** 40–46.

Tan, Y., Ruan, H., Demeter, M. R., and Comb, M. J. (1999). p90^{RSK} blocks *bad*-mediated cell death via a protein kinase C-dependent pathway. *J. Biol. Chem.* **274,** 34859–34867.

Tavakkol, A., Fisher, G. J., Keane, K. M., Barker, I., Reynolds, N., and Voorhees, J. J. (1991). Differential activation of c-*jun* and *jun*-b by phorbol ester, bryostatin and interleukin 1 beta in cultured human kertinocytes. *Clin. Res.* **39,** A495.

Taylor, L. S., Cox, G. W., Melillo, G., Bosco, M. C., and Espinoza-Delgado, I. (1997). Bryostatin1 and IFN-gamma synergize for the expression of the inducible nitric oxide synthase gene and for nitric oxide production in murine macrophages. *Cancer Res.* **57,** 2468–2473.

Thijsen, S. F. T., Schuurhuis, G. J., van der Hem, K. G., van Oostveen, J. W., Theijsmeiher, A .P., Odding, J. H., and Ossenkoppele, G. J. (1997). Effects of bryostatin 1 on chronic myeloid leukemia derived hematopoietic progenitors. *Exp. Hematol.* **25,** 461.

Thijsen, S. F. T., Schuurhuis, G. J., van Oostveen, J. W., Theijsmeijer, A. P., van der Hem, K. G., Odding, J. H., Drager, A. M., and Ossenkoppele, G. J. (1999). Effects of bryostatin 1 on chronic myeloid leukaemia-derived haematopoietic progenitors. *Br. J. Cancer* **79,** 1406–1412.

Thoburn, C. J., and Hess, A. D. (1995). Bryostatin can induce antigen-specific nonresponsiveness in human peripheral blood T-cells. *Transplant. Proc.* **27,** 443–444.

Thompson, C. H., Macaulay, V. M., O'Byrne, K. J., Kemp, G. J., Wilner, S. M., Talbot, D. C., Harris, A. L., and Radda, G. K. (1996). Modulation of bryostatin 1 muscle toxicity by nifedipine: effects on muscle metabolism and oxygen supply. *Br. J. Cancer* **73,** 1161–1165.

Thorp, K. M., Verschueren, H., De Baetselier, P., Southern, C., and Matthews, N. (1996). Protein kinase C isotype expression and regulation of lymphoid cell motility. *Immunology* **87,** 434–438.

Tilden, A. B., and Kraft, A. S. (1991). The effect of bryostatin 1 on human lymphocyte-mediated cytotoxicity. *J. Immunother.* **10,** 96–104.

Trenn, G., Pettit, G. R., Takayama, H., Hu-Li, J., and Sitkovsky, M. V. (1988). Immunomodulating properties of a novel series of protein kinase C activators. The bryostatins. *J. Immunol.* **140,** 433–439.

Trivedi, C., Al-Katib, A., Murgo, A., Mohammad, R., Eilender, D., Hulburd, K., Rodriguez, D., Pemberton, P., Largrone, F., Manica, B., Spadoni, V., and Varterasian, M. (1999). Phase II clinical evaluation of bryostatin 1 in patients with relapsed multiple myeloma. *Blood* **94,** 315b.

Turner, N. A., Walker, J. H., Ball, S. G., and Vaughan, P. F. (1996). Phorbol ester-enhanced noradrenaline secretion correlates with the presence and activity of protein kinase C-alpha in human SH-SY5Y neuroblastoma cells. *J. Neurochem.* **66,** 2381–2389.

Tuttle, T. M., Bethke, K. P., Inge, T. H., McCrady, C. W., Pettit, G. R., and Bear, H. D. (1992a). Bryostatin 1-activated T cells can traffic and mediate tumor regression. *J. Surg. Res.* **52,** 543–548.

Tuttle, T. M., Inge, T. H., Bethke, K. P., McCrady, C. W., Pettit, G. R., and Bear, H. D. (1992b). Activation and growth of murine tumor-specific T-cells which have *in vivo* activity with bryostatin 1. *Cancer Res.* **52,** 548–553.

Tuttle, T. M., Inge, T. H., Lind, D. S., and Bear, H. D. (1992c). Adoptive transfer of bryostatin 1-activated T cells provides long-term protection from tumour metastases. *Surg. Oncol.* **1,** 299–307.

Tuttle, T. M., Inge, T. H., Wirt, C. P., Frank, J. L., McCrady, C. W., and Bear, H. D. (1992d). Bryostatin 1 activates T cells that have antitumor activity. *J. Immunother.* **12,** 75–81.

Tuttle, T. M., McCrady, C. W., Inge, T. H., Salour, M., and Bear, H. D.

(1993). γ-Interferon plays a key role in T-cell-induced tumor regression. *Cancer Res.* **53,** 833–839.

Tuttle, T. M., Fleming, M. D., Hogg, P. S., Inge, T. H., and Bear, H. D. (1994). Ability of low-dose cyclophosphamide to overcome metastasis-induced immunosuppression. *Ann. Surg. Oncol.* **1,** 53–58.

Uberall, F., Kampfer, S., Doppler, W., and Grunicke, H. H. (1994). Activation of c-*fos* expression by transforming Ha-*ras* in HC11 mouse mammary epithelial cells is PKC-dependent and mediated by the serum response element. *Cell. Signal.* **6,** 285–297.

Utz, I., Hofmann, J., and Grunicke, H. (1995). Bryostatin 1 regulates multidrug resistance by a PKC-independent mechanism. *Eur. J. Cancer* **31A,** 12.

Vaishampayan, U. N., Wall, N. R., Varterasian, M. L., Murgo, A., Sorice, P., Dan, M., Shurafa, M., Mohammad, R. M., and Al-Katib, A. (1999). Differentiation therapy of chronic lymphocytic leukemia (CLL) cells by bryostatin 1 (bryo) *in vivo:* validity of preclinical model. *Blood* **94,** 315b.

van der Hem, K. G., Drager, A. M., Huijgens, P. C., and Langenhuijsen, M. M. (1993). Bryostatin 5 induces leukemic-cell differentiation. *Exp. Hematol.* **21,** 1046.

van der Hem, K. G., Drager, A. M., Huijgens, P. C., Tol, C., Deville, W., and Langenhuijsen, M. M. (1994). The differentiation inducing effect of bryostatin 5 on human myeloid blast cells is potentiated by vitamin D3. *Leukemia* **8,** 266–273.

van der Hem, K. G., Drager, A. M., Odding, J. H., and Huijgens, P. C. (1995a). Effects of bryostatin 5 and hematopoietic growth factors on acute myeloid leukemia cell differentiation, proliferation, and primary plating efficiency. *Leukemia Res.* **19,** 651–657.

van der Hem, K. G., Drager, A. M., Odding, J. H., Langenhuijsen, M. M., and Huijgens, P. C. (1995b). Bryostatin 5 stimulates normal human hematopoiesis and inhibits proliferation of HL60 leukemic cells. *Leukemia Res.* **19,** 7–13.

van der Hem, K. G., Schuurhuis, G. J., Drager, A. M., Odding, J. H., and Huijgens, P. C. (1996). Heterogenous effects of bryostatin on human myeloid leukemia clonogenicity: dose and time scheduling dependency. *Leukemia Res.* **20,** 743–750.

Van Iderstine, S.C., Byers, D.M., Ridgway, N.D., and Cook, H.W. (1997). Phospholipase D hydrolysis of plasmalogen and diacyl ethanolamine phosphoglycerides by protein kinase C dependent and independent mechanisms. *J. Lipid Mediat. Cell Signal.* **15,** 175–192.

Varma, T. K., Liu, S., Ruvulo, P. R., Bhatnagar, A., and May, W. S. (1999). Bryostatin 1 (bryo)-mediated phosphorylation and translocation of an aldo-keto reductase (AKR) in the human acute lymphoblastic leukemia cells REH. *Proc. Am. Assoc. Cancer. Res.* **40,** 166.

Varterasian, M., Eilender, D., Mohammad, R., Chen, B., Hulburd, K., Rodriguez, D., Pluda, J., Valdivieso, M., and Al-Katib, A. (1996). Phase I trial of bryostatin 1 in relapsed lymphoma and CLL. *Blood* **88,** 2269.

Varterasian, M. L., Mohammad, R. M., Eilender, D. S., Hulburd, K., Rodriguez, D. H., Pemberton, P. A., Pluda, J. M., Dan, M. D., Pettit, G. R., Chen, B. D., and Al-Katib, A. M. (1998a). Phase I study of bryostatin 1 in patients with relapsed non-Hodgkin's lymphoma and chronic lymphocytic leukemia. *J. Clin. Oncol.* **16,** 56–62.

Varterasian, M., Mohammad, R., Shurafa, M., Eilender, D., Murgo, A., Hulburd, K., Rodriguez, D., Pemberton, P., LaGrone, F., Manica, B., Spadoni, V., and Al-Katib, A. (1998b). Phase II clinical evaluation of bryostatin 1 in patients with relapsed low grade non-Hodgkins lymphoma (LGL) and CLL. *Blood* **92,** 412A.

Varterasian, M. L., Mohammad, R. M., Shurafa, M. S., Hulburd, K., Pemberton, P. A., Rodriguez, D. H., Spadoni, V., Eilender, D. S., Murgo, A., Wall, N., Dan, M., and Al-Katib, A. M. (2000). Phase II trial of bryostatin 1 in patients with relapsed low-grade non-Hodgkin's lymphoma and chronic lymphocytic leukemia. *Clin. Cancer Res.* **6,** 825–828.

Vlach, J., and Pitha, P. M. (1992). Activation of human immunodeficiency virus type 1 provirus in T-cells and macrophages is associated with induction of inducer-specific NF-kappa B binding proteins. *Virology* **187,** 63–72.

Vrana, J. A., and Grant, S. (1996). Divergent effects of bryostatin 1 and phor-

bol myristate acetate on 1-[beta-D-arabinofuranosyl]cytosine induced apoptosis in human myeloid leukemia cells (U937). *Blood* **88,** 254.

Vrana, J. A., and Grant, S. (1999). Bryostatin 1 potentiates lactacystin-induced apoptosis in U937 leukemic cells. *Proc. Am. Assoc. Cancer. Res.* **40,** 581.

Vrana, J. A., Rao, A. S., Wang, Z., Jarvis, W. D., and Grant, S. (1998a). Effects of bryostatin 1 and calcium ionophore (A23187) on apoptosis and differentiation in human myeloid leukemia cells (HL-60) following 1-beta-D-arabinofuranosylcytosine exposure. *Int. J. Oncol.* **12,** 927–934.

Vrana, J. A., Saunders, A. M., Chellappan, S. P., and Grant, S. (1998b). Divergent effects of bryostatin 1 and phorbol myristate acetate on cell cycle arrest and maturation in human myelomonocytic leukemia cells (U937). *Differentiation* **63,** 33–42.

Vrana, J. A., Kramer, L. B., Saunders, A. M., Zhang, X. F., Dent, P., Povirk, L. F., and Grant, S. (1999a). Inhibition of protein kinase C activator-mediated induction of p21(CIP1) and p27(KIP1) by deoxycytidine analogs in human leukemia cells—Relationship to apoptosis and differentiation. *Biochem. Pharmacol.* **58,** 121–131.

Vrana, J. A., Wang, Z., Rao, A. S., Tang, L., Chen, J. H., Kramer, L. B., and Grant, S. (1999b). Induction of apoptosis and differentiation by fludarabine in human leukemia cells (U937): interactions with the macrocyclic lactone bryostatin 1. *Leukemia* **13,** 1046–1055.

Waldron, R. T., Iglesias, T., and Rozengurt, E. (1999). Phosphorylation-dependent protein kinase D activation. *Electrophoresis* **20,** 382–390.

Walker, S. D., Murray, N. R., Burns, D. J., and Fields, A. P. (1995). Protein kinase C chimeras: catalytic domains of alpha and beta II protein kinase C contain determinants for isotype-specific function. *Proc. Natl. Acad. Sci. USA* **92,** 9156–9160.

Wall, M. E., Wani, M. C., and Taylor, H. (1976). Isolation and chemical characterization of antitumor agents from plants. *Cancer Treat. Rep.* **60,** 1011–1030.

Wall, N. R., Mohammad, R. M., and Al-Katib, A. M. (1998a). Bax:Bcl-2 ratio modulation by bryostatin 1 and novel antitubulin agents is important for susceptibility to drug-induced apoptosis in the human pre-B all cell line, Reh. *Blood* **92,** 188B.

Wall, N. R., Mohammad, R. M., Reddy, K. R., and Al-Katib, A. M. (1998b). Bryostatin 1 induces down-regulation and ubiquitination of *bcl*-2 in the human acute c lymphoblastic leukemia cell line, Reh. *Blood* **92,** 82A.

Wall, N. R., Mohammad, R. M., and Al-Katib, A. M. (1999a). Bax:*bcl*-2 ratio modulation by bryostatin 1 and novel antitubulin agents is important for susceptibility to drug induced apoptosis in the human early pre-B acute lymphoblastic leukemia cell line, Reh. *Leukemia Res.* **23,** 881–888.

Wall, N. R., Mohammad, R. M., Nabha, S. M., Pettit, G. R., and Al-Katib, A. M. (1999b). Modulation of cIAP-1 by novel antitubulin agents when combined with bryostatin 1 results in increased apoptosis in the human early pre-B acute lymphoblastic leukemia cell line Reh. *Biochem. Biophys. Res. Commun.* **266,** 76–80.

Wall, N. R., Mohammad, R. M., Reddy, K. B., and Al-Katib, A. M. (2000). Bryostatin 1 induces ubiquitination and proteasome degradation of Bcl-2 in the human acute lymphoblastic leukemia cell line, Reh. *Int. J. Mol. Med.* **5,** 165–171.

Wang, H., Mohammad, R. M., Werdell, J., and Shekhar, P. V. M. (1998). p53 and protein kinase C independent induction of growth arrest and apoptosis by bryostatin 1 in a highly metastatic mammary epithelial cell line: *In vitro* versus *in vivo* activity. *Int. J. Mol. Med.* **1,** 915–923.

Wang, Q. M. J., Bhattacharyya, D., Garfield, S., Nacro, K., Marquez, V. E., and Blumberg, P. M. (1999). Differential localization of protein kinase C delta by phorbol esters and related compounds using a fusion protein with green fluorescent protein. *J. Biol. Chem.* **274,** 37233–37239.

Wang, S., Vrana, J. A., Bartimole, T. M., Freemerman, A. J., Jarvis, W. D., Kramer, L. B., Krystal, G., Dent, P., and Grant, S. (1997). Agents that down-regulate or inhibit protein kinase C circumvent resistance to 1-beta-D-arabinofuranosylcytosine-induced apoptosis in human leukemia cells that overexpress bcl-2. *Mol. Pharmacol.* **52,** 1000–1009.

Wang, S., Guo, C. Y., Castillo, A., Dent, P., and Grant, S. (1998). Effect of bryostatin 1 on taxol-induced apoptosis and cytotoxicity in human leukemia cells (U937). *Biochem. Pharmacol.* **56,** 635–644.

Wang, S., Wang, Z., Boise, L. H., Dent, P., and Grant, S. (1999a). Bryostatin 1 enhances paclitaxel-induced mitochondrial dysfunction and apoptosis in human leukemia cells (U937) ectopically expressing bcl-xL. *Leukemia* **13,** 1564–1573.

Wang, S., Wang, Z., Boise, L. H., Dent, P., and Grant, S. (1999b). The PKC modulator bryostatin 1 enhances paclitaxel-mediated mitochondrial dysfunction in human leukemia cells (U937) ectopically expressing bcl-xL. *Clin. Cancer Res.* **5,** 647.

Wang, S., Wang, Z., and Grant, S. (1999c). Effect of the PKC activator bryostatin 1 on 1-β-arabinofuranosylcytosine induced apoptosis in bcl-xL-overexpressing human leukemia cells (U937). *Proc. Am. Assoc. Cancer. Res.* **40,** 485.

Wang, Z., Su, Z. Z., Fisher, P. B., Wang, S., VanTuyle, G., and Grant, S. (1998). Evidence of a functional role for the cyclin-dependent kinase inhibitor p21(WAF1/CIP1/MDA6) in the reciprocal regulation of PKC activator-induced apoptosis and differentiation in human myelomonocytic leukemia cells. *Exp. Cell Res.* **244,** 105–116.

Warren, B. S., Herald, C. L., Pettit, G. R., and Blumberg, P. M. (1987). Bryostatin 1 and bryostatin 9 induce the phosphorylation of a unique series of 70-kDa proteins in HL-60 cells. Symposium on Growth Regulation of Cancer, 16th Annual Meeting of the UCLA Symposia on Molecular and Cellular Biology, Los Angeles, California, USA, January 17–23, 1987.

Warren, B. S., Kamano, Y., Pettit, G. R., and Blumberg, P. M. (1988). Mimicry of bryostatin 1 induced phosphorylation patterns in HL-60 cells by high-phorbol ester concentrations. *Cancer Res.* **48,** 5984–5988.

Watson, N. C., Jarvis, W. D., Orr, M. S., Grant, S., and Gewirtz, D. A. (1996). Radiosensitization of HL-60 human leukaemia cells by bryostatin 1 in the absence of increased DNA fragmentation or apoptotic cell death. *Int. J. Radiat. Biol.* **69,** 183–192.

Watters, D. J., and Parsons, P. G. (1999). Critical targets of protein kinase C in differentiation of tumour cells. *Biochem. Pharmacol.* **58,** 383–388.

Watters, D. J., Michael, J., Hemphill, J. E., Hamilton, S. E., Lavin, M. F., and Pettit, G. R. (1992). Bistratene A: a novel compound causing changes in protein phosphorylation patterns in human leukemia cells. *J. Cell. Biochem.* **49,** 417–424.

Weiss, E., Von Reyher, U., Kittstein, W., Möller, P., Krammer, P. H., Marks, F., and Gschwendt, M. (1997). Suppression of apoptosis in COLO 205 cells by the phorbol ester TPA may be mediated by the PKC isoenzyme alpha. *Int. J. Oncol.* **10,** 1119–1123.

Weiss, J. M., and Hoffmann, H. M. R. (1997). Synthesis of the C1-C9 segment of bryostatin. *Tetrahedron: Asymmetry* **8,** 3913–3920.

Weitman, S., Langevin, A. M., Berkow, R. L., Thomas, P. J., Hurwitz, C. A., Kraft, A. S., Dubowy, R. L., Smith, D. L., and Bernstein, M. (1999). A Phase I trial of bryostatin 1 in children with refractory solid tumors: a Pediatric Oncology Group study. *Clin. Cancer Res.* **5,** 2344–2348.

Wender, P. A., and Lippa, B. (2000). Synthesis and biological evaluation of bryostatin analogues: the role of the A-ring. *Tetrahedron Lett.* **41,** 1007–1011.

Wender, P. A., Cribbs, C.-M., Koehler, K. F., Sharkey, N. A., Herald, C. L., Kamano, Y., Pettit, G. R., and Blumberg, P. M. (1988). Modeling of the bryostatins to the phorbol ester pharmacophore on protein kinase C. *Proc. Natl. Acad. Sci. USA* **85,** 7197–7201.

Wender, P. A., DeBrabander, J., Harran, P. G., Hinkle, K. W., Lippa, B., and Pettit, G. R. (1998a). Synthesis and biological evaluation of fully synthetic bryostatin analogues. *Tetrahedron Lett.* **39,** 8625–8628.

Wender, P. A., DeBrabander, J., Harran, P. G., Jimenez, J-M., Koehler, M. F. T., Lippa, B., Park, C.-M., Siedenbiedel, C., and Pettit, G. R. (1998b). The design, computer modeling, solution structure, and biological evaluation of synthetic analogs of bryostatin 1. *Proc. Natl. Acad. Sci. USA* **95,** 6624–6629.

Wender, P. A., DeBrabander, J., Harran, P. G., Jimenez, J-M., Koehler, M. F. T., Lippa, B., Park, C.-M., and Shiozaki, M. (1998c). Synthesis of the first members of a new class of biologically active bryostatin analogues. *J. Am. Chem. Soc.* **120,** 4534–4535.

Wender, P. A., Hinkle, K. W., Koehler, M. F. T., and Lippa, B. (1999a). The rational design of potential chemotherapeutic agents: synthesis of bryostatin analogues. *Med. Res. Rev.* **19,** 388–407.

Wender, P. A., Lippa, B., Park, C. M., Irie, K., Nakahara, A., and Ohigashi, H. (1999b). Selective binding of bryostatin analogues to the cysteine rich domains of protein kinase C isozymes. *Bioorg. Med. Chem. Lett.* **9,** 1687–1690.

William, F., Mroczkowski, B., Cohen, S., and Kraft, A. S. (1988). Differentiation of HL-60 cells is associated with an increase in the 35-kDa protein lipocortin I. *J. Cell. Physiol.* **137,** 402–410.

Wojtowicz-Praga, S. M., Dickson, R. B., and Hawkins, M. J. (1997). Matrix metalloproteinase inhibitors. *Invest. New Drugs* **15,** 61–75.

Wooten, M. W., Seibenhener, M. L., Heikkila, J. E., and Mischak, H. (1998). Delta-protein kinase C phosphorylation parallels inhibition of nerve growth factor-induced differentiation independent of changes in Trk A and MAP kinase signalling in PC12 cells. *Cell. Signal.* **10,** 265–276.

Yoshikawa, N., Yamada, Y. M. A., Das, J., Sasai, H., and Shibasaki, M. (1999). Direct catalytic asymmetric aldol reaction. *J. Am. Chem. Soc.* **121,** 4168–4178.

Zang, R., Muller, H. J., Kielbassa, K., Marks, F., and Gschwendt, M. (1994). Partial purification of a type eta protein kinase C from murine brain: separation from other protein kinase C isoenzymes and characterization. *Biochem. J.* **304,** 641–647.

Zellner, A., Fetell, M. R., Bruce, J. N., De Vivo, D. C., and O'Driscoll, K. R. (1998). Disparity in expression of protein kinase C alpha in human glioma versus glioma-derived primary cell lines: therapeutic implications. *Clin. Cancer Res.* **4,** 1797–1802.

Zhang, X., Zhang, R., Zhao, H., Cai, H., Gush, K. A., Kerr, R. G., Pettit, G. R., and Kraft, A. S. (1996). Preclinical pharmacology of the natural product anticancer agent bryostatin 1, an activator of protein kinase C. *Cancer Res.* **56,** 802–808.

Zonder, J. A., and Philip, P. A. (1999). Pharmacology and clinical experience with bryostatin 1: a novel anticancer drug. *Exp. Opin. Invest. Drugs* **8,** 2189–2199.

Zwelling, L. A., Chan, D., Altschuler, E., Mayes, J., Hinds, J., and Pettit, G. R. (1991). Effect of bryostatin 1 on drug-induced, topoisomerase II-mediated DNA cleavage and topoisomerase II gene expression in human leukemia cells. *Biochem. Pharmacol.* **41,** 829–832.

DNA-ENCODED PEPTIDE LIBRARIES AND DRUG DISCOVERY

Sachdev S. Sidhu

Gregory A. Weiss

Department of Protein Engineering

Genentech, Inc.

South San Francisco, California

Summary

Over the past decade, several methods have been developed for the construction of DNA-encoded peptide libraries. The common principle behind all these methods is the establishment of a physical linkage between a displayed peptide and its encoding DNA. Vast libraries can be generated, binding peptides can be isolated with simple selections, and the sequences of selected peptides can be rapidly determined from the sequence of the linked DNA. As a result, DNA-encoded libraries can provide specific ligands for essentially any protein. These ligands can be used to determine the natural binding specificities of protein–protein interactions, and this information can be used to identify natural binding partners or to aid the design of organic mimics. Binding peptides can also be used for target validation and the development of high-throughput screens for small-molecule libraries. Finally, binding peptides themselves could prove useful as drugs.

1. Introduction

Over the past decade, several methods have been developed for the construction of DNA-encoded, combinatorial peptide libraries. These technologies depend on one basic principle: the establishment of a physical linkage between a displayed polypeptide and the DNA sequence that encodes it. Simple molecular biology techniques can be used to first construct combinatorial libraries of vast size ($>10^{12}$) and subsequently to amplify library pools or individual members. These libraries can be used to isolate peptides that bind with high specificity and affinity to virtually any protein of interest. Most importantly, the sequences of selected peptides can be determined by rapid and efficient sequencing of the encoding DNA.

In this chapter, we describe the various DNA-encoded systems for polypeptide display. We also outline the main applications for combinatorial peptide libraries, and we describe relevant examples from the recent literature. It is a testament to the breadth of this field that no single review can hope to be comprehensive. Thus, in each section we direct the reader to more focused reviews in particular areas of interest.

2. Methods for DNA-Encoded Peptide Display

Several methods have been used to link polypeptides to their encoding DNA. In phage display, peptides fused to viral coat proteins are displayed on the surfaces of bacteriophage particles that also encapsulate the encoding DNA.

"Peptides on plasmids" is an alternative method in which peptides are fused to a DNA-binding protein that binds specifically to plasmid DNA. A third approach is provided by microorganism surface display systems in which peptides are displayed directly on the surfaces of yeast or bacterial cells. Finally, "ribosome display" methods use *in vitro* transcription and translation reactions to couple mRNA molecules to their encoded polypeptides.

The displayed libraries can be used in binding selections with immobilized ligands (Fig. 1). Selective pressure is applied to pooled library members to enrich for displayed peptides with desired binding specificities and affinities. The enriched pool can be amplified and passed through additional rounds of selection, or at any point, selectants can be grown as individual clones to produce DNA for sequence analysis. In the following sections, we describe the different display methods and discuss the advantages and disadvantages of each approach.

A. Phage Display

The concept of phage display was first demonstrated by George Smith when he showed that peptides could be functionally displayed on the surface of M13 bacteriophage particles that also encapsulated the encoding DNA (Smith, 1985). Phage display remains the most widely used system for DNA-encoded polypeptide display, and M13 bacteriophage remains the predominant phage display scaffold. However, display systems based on other bacteriophage have also been developed, and these may offer some advantages for specialized applications. While the practical limit for phage-displayed library diversities was long believed to be about 10^{10} (Roberts, 1999; Schaffitzel *et al.*, 1999), recent refinements of estab-

lished methods (Dower *et al.*, 1988) have extended the limit to about 10^{12} for M13 display (Sidhu *et al.*, 2000). In addition to the peptide display applications described here, phage display has been used in many protein engineering studies (reviewed by Clackson and Wells, 1994; Smith and Petrenko, 1997; Johnsson and Ge, 1999), and antibody display in particular has had an enormous impact on biotechnology (reviewed by Griffiths and Duncan, 1998; Vaughan *et al.*, 1998; Hoogenboom *et al.*, 1998; Dall'Acqua and Carter, 1998).

1. M13 Phage Display

M13 is a filamentous bacteriophage that infects *Escherichia coli* in a nonlytic life cycle. Both the viral assembly process and the structure of the assembled phage particle have been extensively studied (reviewed by Webster, 1996; Marvin, 1998). M13 phage assembly occurs at the host cell membrane where viral DNA is extruded through a pore complex and concomitantly surrounded by membrane-associated coat proteins. The assembled phage particle is approximately 1 μm in length but less than 10 nm in diameter, and it consists of a single-stranded, closed circular DNA core encapsulated in a coat composed of five different coat proteins (Fig. 2). The length of the particle is covered by about 3000 copies of the major coat protein (protein-8, P8). One end of the particle is capped by approximately five copies each of two minor coat proteins (protein-7 and protein-9, P7 and P9), and the other end is similarly capped by two other minor coat proteins (protein-3 and protein-6; P3 and P6). While all five coat proteins contribute to the structural integrity of the phage particle, P3 is also responsible for host cell recognition and infection. Consequently, it is the largest and most complex of the coat proteins, containing 406 residues and 3 distinct domains.

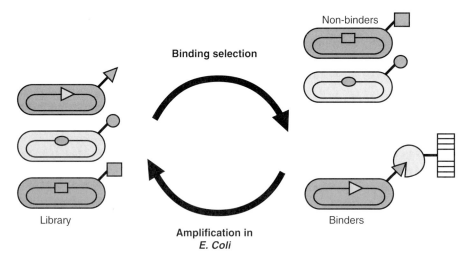

FIGURE 1 Isolating specific ligands from phage-displayed peptide libraries. Peptides are displayed on the phage surface while the encoding DNA is encapsulated in the phage particle. A library of peptide phage is exposed to an immobilized target. Nonbinding phage are removed by washing while bound phage are retained. Bound phage are then eluted and amplified by infection of an *E. coli* host. After several rounds of selection, the sequences of individual binding peptides can be determined by sequencing the cognate DNA. (See Section 2 for additional details.)

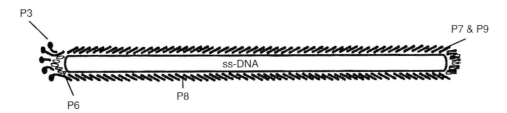

FIGURE 2   Diagram of an M13 phage particle. The single-stranded DNA genome is encapsulated in a coat composed primarily of P8, the major coat protein, which surrounds the length of the particle. One end of the particle is capped by five copies each of P7 and P9, whereas the other end is similarly capped by P3 and P6. Polypeptides can be displayed as fusions to the N terminus of P3, P8, P7, or P9. Alternatively, polypeptides have also been displayed as C-terminal fusions with P6 or P8. (See Section 2.A.1 for additional details.)

M13 phage has long been used as a versatile cloning vector because even large DNA inserts are readily tolerated by the viral genome (Sambrook *et al.*, 1989). An increase in the genome size is accommodated by a corresponding increase in the phage particle length and a concomitant increase in the number of P8 molecules. Phage display extends from the observation that foreign DNA fused in frame to a coat protein gene can result in the display of foreign peptides on the phage surface (Smith, 1985). Each of the five M13 coat proteins has been used for phage display (Fig. 2). Initial examples of phage display involved fusions to the N terminus of P3 (Scott and Smith, 1990; Devlin *et al.*, 1991; Cwirla *et al.*, 1991). Shortly thereafter, the viability of N-terminal P8 fusions was also demonstrated (Greenwood *et al.*, 1991; Felici *et al.*, 1991). More recently, the display of polypeptides fused to the C terminus of P6 (Jespers *et al.*, 1995) or P8 (Fuh *et al.*, 2000) has also been reported. Finally, it has been shown that fusions to the N terminus of P7 or P9 also result in display (Gao *et al.*, 1999).

The different display formats are useful for different applications. Because there are several thousand copies of P8 in each virion, N-terminal peptide fusions usually result in highly polyvalent display (Greenwood *et al.*, 1991). In contrast, fusions to one of the minor coat proteins usually result in lower valency or even monovalent display in which the average display level is actually less than one polypeptide per phage particle (Bass *et al.*, 1990). These high- and low-valency display formats have complementary properties that have been exploited in the selection and affinity maturation of binding peptides (Sidhu *et al.*, 2000). A large and diverse naïve peptide library is first presented in a polyvalent format on P8. Multivalent binding produces an avidity or "chelating" effect that allows for the isolation of low-affinity peptides with affinities in the high micromolar range. These low-affinity leads are then transferred to a low-valency P3 format where they can be matured to higher affinity through the introduction of mutations and additional rounds of affinity selection. C-terminal P6 and P8 display formats have also proven useful in applications not suited to N-terminal display, including the display of cDNA libraries (Jespers *et al.*, 1995)

and studies of protein–protein interactions that involve free C termini (Fuh *et al.*, 2000).

Early M13 phage display vectors used single-gene systems in which peptides were fused to a coat protein in the viral genome (Scott and Smith, 1990; Greenwood *et al.*, 1991). These systems were limited by the fact that fusions could not be displayed if they compromised coat protein function. In particular, the display of large proteins was severely limited (Iannolo *et al.*, 1995). The introduction of two-gene phagemid systems solved the problem (Bass *et al.*, 1990; Lowman *et al.*, 1991). In such systems, peptides are fused to a coat protein encoded by the phagemid vector. Phagemid DNA can be packaged into phage particles by using a helper phage that supplies all the proteins necessary for phage assembly, including wild-type copies of all the coat proteins. The resulting phage particles contain predominantly wild-type coat proteins from the helper phage, but they also contain some copies of the phagemid-encoded coat protein. Thus, peptide display is achieved by incorporation of the phagemid-encoded coat protein, while the deleterious effects of displayed peptides are attenuated by the predominance of wild-type coat protein from the helper phage.

These advances in library construction methods, vector design, and display formats have made M13 phage an extremely robust vehicle for peptide and protein display. In addition, the long history of M13-based vectors in molecular biology has made it very easy for many laboratories to adopt the system. As a result, the majority of published DNA-encoded library studies (and most of the examples in this chapter) have used M13 phage display.

2. Other Phage Display Systems

The success of M13 phage display has prompted the development of alternative display systems based on λ phage (Maruyama *et al.*, 1994; Sternberg and Hoess, 1995) and T4 phage (Efimov *et al.*, 1995; Ren *et al.*, 1996). λ phage and T4 phage assemble in the *E. coli* cytoplasm and are released by cell lysis. Thus, these systems may be particularly suited for the display of intracellular proteins that have evolved to fold in the reducing, cytoplasmic environment. In contrast,

M13 phage assembly is a membrane-associated process, and prior to assembly the coat proteins reside in the membrane with their N termini in the periplasm and their C termini in the cytoplasm (Webster, 1996). As a result, proteins fused to the N terminus of M13 coat proteins must be secreted through the membrane and fold in the oxidizing environment of the periplasm. Such conditions are ideal for naturally secreted proteins, but they may limit the display of intracellular proteins. Thus, the λ phage and T4 phage display systems may prove useful for the display of proteins that cannot be displayed as fusions to the N termini of M13 coat proteins. However, promising results with the display of polypeptides fused to the C termini of M13 coat proteins may extend the utility of M13 phage display to these same applications (Jespers *et al.*, 1995; Fuh *et al.*, 2000).

C. Cell Surface Display

In cell surface display, polypeptides are displayed directly on the surface of bacterial or yeast cells that also harbor the encoding plasmid DNA (reviewed by Georgiou *et al.*, 1997; Stahl and Uhlen, 1997; Cereghino and Cregg, 1999). Display is achieved by fusing gene fragments to genes encoding host membrane proteins. The resulting gene product remains associated with the outer cell surface, and the fusion is accessible for binding selections. Yeast display systems have used *Saccharomyces cerevisiae* and most bacterial display systems have used *E. coli*. However, several gram-positive bacterial strains have also been developed for specialized applications (Stahl and Uhlen, 1997).

Cell surface display libraries can be used in binding selections analogous to those used for phage display (Fig. 1), but a major advantage of cell surface display libraries is that they can also be screened by fluorescence-activated cell sorting (FACS). In contrast, the small size of bacteriophage particles precludes the use of FACS with phage-displayed libraries. FACS sorting is an extremely sensitive technique that allows for very efficient enrichment of binding clones over nonbinding clones. Furthermore, FACS enables direct discrimination of binding affinities so that even subtle differences can be reliably selected (VanAntwerp and Wittrup, 2000). However, FACS is limited by the throughput speed of cell sorters (about 4×10^7 cells per hour), whereas there is no such limiting factor in panning selections.

DNA transformation efficiencies for yeast are significantly lower than for *E. coli;* consequently, the practical limits to yeast library sizes are also comparatively low. Thus, *E. coli* has been the preferred host organism for most biological libraries. However, the yeast *S. cerevisiae* provides certain advantages in specialized applications. In particular, yeast is a eukaryotic organism with protein folding and secretory machinery very similar to that of mammalian cells (Boder and Wittrup, 1997). Thus, yeast surface display can be used to study proteins that are not amenable to *E. coli* expression or

phage display, and promising results have been obtained with yeast-displayed T-cell receptors (Kieke *et al.*, 1999) and G-protein-coupled receptors (Pausch, 1997).

D. Peptides on Plasmids

The peptides-on-plasmids system relies on a plasmid that encodes the DNA-binding protein LacI repressor and also contains LacI binding sites (Cull *et al.*, 1992). In an *E. coli* host, LacI repressor binds tightly to the LacI binding sites on the plasmid and thus establishes a link between the protein and its encoding DNA. Peptide libraries can be displayed as fusions to the LacI repressor C terminus, and the protein–plasmid complexes can be used in affinity selections (Fig. 3). Since the LacI repressor is a homotetramer, peptides-on-plasmids libraries are displayed in a polyvalent format. However, a monovalent version of the system has also been developed by deleting the tetramerization domain and fusing two tandem DNA binding domains to a single peptide (Gates *et al.*, 1996).

In principle, the peptides-on-plasmids system is analogous to M13 phage display, but the methods differ in the requirements for library purification and propagation. M13 phage particles are secreted directly into the media, and they can be easily purified with a precipitation procedure. In contrast,

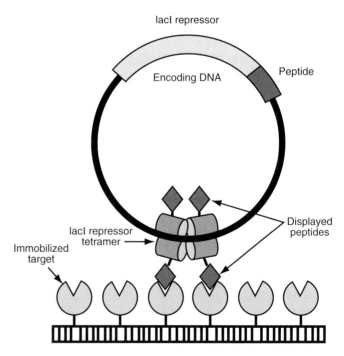

FIGURE 3 Peptides on plasmids. The display plasmid contains LacI binding sites and also a gene encoding the LacI repressor with a peptide displayed as a C-terminal fusion. In an *E. coli* host, the LacI repressor tetramer binds to the LacI binding sites and thus the displayed peptides are linked to their encoding DNA. Host cell lysis releases the peptide–plasmid complexes, which can then be used in binding selections with immobilized target proteins. (See Section 2.C for additional details.)

protein–plasmid complexes are obtained by bacterial lysis and thus remain associated with soluble *E. coli* proteins. Following binding selection, phage particles can be amplified by highly efficient infection of a suitable host strain. The introduction of plasmids into *E. coli* requires less efficient and more complicated transformation procedures.

E. Ribosome Display

In the methods described thus far, library construction requires a transformation step that introduces recombinant DNA into microorganisms. Subsequent transcription and translation within host cells produces the DNA-encoded polypeptide library. In such systems, library size is limited by the transformation efficiency. The most efficiently transformable organism is *E. coli,* and the practical size limit for *E. coli*-derived libraries is about 10^{12} (Sidhu *et al.,* 2000). Ribosome display methods circumvent the limiting transformation step and, as a result, they can be used to access library sizes in excess of 10^{13} (reviewed by Hanes and Pluckthun, 1999; Roberts, 1999).

Ribosome display was first reported by Mattheakis *et al.* (1994) and subsequently optimized by Hanes and Pluckthun (1997). Ribosome display uses a special DNA cassette that contains an open reading frame preceded by sequences that signal efficient transcription and translation. The open reading frame encodes a variable N-terminal polypeptide library followed by a constant C-terminal spacer. The DNA cassette is used as the template for *in vitro* transcription followed by *in vitro* translation of the open reading frame. The open reading frame does not contain a stop codon, and this inhibits dissociation of the translation complex. As a result, the translated polypeptides remain associated with the encoding mRNA, with the ribosome acting as a noncovalent linker (Fig. 4A). At appropriate salt concentrations and low temperatures, these complexes are stable enough to enable functional selections with the displayed proteins (Hanes *et al.,* 1998). Following selection, eluted mRNA can be converted to DNA by reverse transcription, and the DNA can then be amplified with the polymerase chain reaction (PCR) to produce template for additional rounds of selection. In this way, the entire selection process can be conducted *in vitro.*

Two groups have sought to further improve ribosome display by establishing a more stable, covalent linkage between the displayed polypeptide and its cognate mRNA (Nemoto *et al.,* 1997; Roberts and Szostak, 1997). Both groups used puromycin, an antibiotic that enters the ribosome and forms a stable amide bond with the nascent polypeptide. mRNA molecules were generated with puromycin covalently coupled to their 3′ ends with an intervening DNA spacer. *In vitro* translation with such a template produces the mRNA-encoded polypeptide, but the ribosome stalls at the RNA–DNA junction. At this point, puromycin enters the ribosome and forms a covalent bond with the C terminus of the

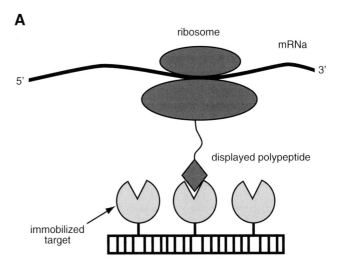

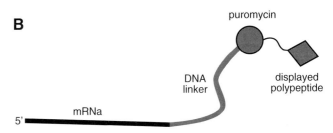

FIGURE 4 (**A**) Ribosome display. A special DNA cassette encoding a polypeptide library is transcribed and translated *in vitro.* The lack of a stop codon inhibits dissociation of the translation complex, resulting in a complex consisting of a displayed polypeptide and its encoding mRNA linked noncovalently by a stalled ribosome. Under appropriate conditions, these complexes are stable enough to be used in binding selections with immobilized targets. (**B**) Covalently linked mRNA–polypeptide fusion. Puromycin is attached to the 3′ end of mRNA with an intervening DNA spacer. During *in vitro* translation, the ribosome stalls at the RNA/DNA junction, and the puromycin moiety forms a covalent bond with the nascent peptide. (See Section 2.D for additional details.)

polypeptide, resulting in a covalently linked protein–mRNA complex (Fig. 4B) that can be used in selection experiments.

3. Applications for DNA-Encoded Peptide Libraries

Therapeutically relevant targets for ligand peptides can be divided into three main groups. The first group involves protein–protein interactions with binding contacts spread over large surfaces. Many extracellular protein–protein interactions are of this type, including the interactions between the extracellular domains of single-transmembrane signaling receptors and their ligands. The second group consists of proteins that bind to small, continuous stretches of amino acids within other proteins, and this group includes many of the intracellular protein–protein interactions involved in signal transduction. The third group consists of the enzymes that catalyze the numerous chemical reactions essential to biological systems. DNA-encoded peptide libraries have been used to obtain ligands that not only bind specific targets but often also modulate biological activity. In this section, we discuss some of the important applications in each of these areas.

A. Peptide Mimics of Extracellular Protein–Protein Interactions

Many extracellular protein–protein interactions involve contact surfaces that are large and flat. Such interactions typically bury between 600 and 1300 Å^2 of protein surface area, and they include many intermolecular contacts involving 10–30 side chains from each protein (de Vos *et al.*, 1992; Clackson and Wells, 1995). Consequently, small-molecule screening efforts that work well in identifying ligands for concave surfaces have not been successful in targeting these interactions (Dower, 1998; Cochran, 2000). These failures have led to the belief that surfaces evolved to bind large proteins cannot bind small molecules with high affinity because such surfaces are solvent exposed and critical molecular contacts are spread over a large area. However, detailed mutagenic analyses of the interface between human growth hormone and its receptor have revealed that only a small subset of side chains from each protein make significant contributions to binding energy, and furthermore, these side chains are clustered together near the center of the interface (Cunningham and Wells, 1989; Clackson and Wells, 1995). These findings have led to the controversial but compelling suggestion that it may be possible to design small inhibitors that mimic this smaller "functional epitope" (Clackson and Wells, 1995). Recent results with phage-displayed peptide libraries support this concept.

There are numerous examples of phage-derived peptides that bind with high affinity to extracellular protein surfaces (reviewed by Kay *et al.*, 1998; Dower, 1998; Cochran, 2000; Sidhu *et al.*, 2000). It is notable that while most of these ligands were selected from unbiased naïve libraries, they generally bind to sites that coincide with natural ligand binding sites (Kay *et al.*, 1998; DeLano *et al.*, 2000). As a result, many of these selected peptides act as antagonists of natural protein–protein interactions. Even more remarkably, some binding peptides act as agonists that potently mimic the biological activity of the much larger natural ligands. Disulfide-constrained peptide libraries have proven most useful in these studies because a structural constraint promotes a discrete structure in solution. This in turn reduces the entropy of the free peptide and makes high-affinity binding more likely. Furthermore, structured peptides may be amenable to nuclear magnetic resonance (NMR) analyses that can provide invaluable insights into structure–function relationships. Indeed, NMR has been used to determine several free-solution structures, and crystal structures have also been determined for several peptides in complex with their cognate protein ligands (Fig. 5).

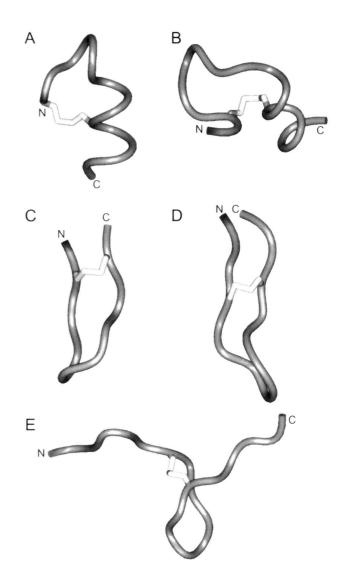

FIGURE 5 Structures of free or bound peptides isolated from phage-displayed peptide libraries. Main chains are shown as dark gray ribbons and disulfide bonds are shown in light gray; other side chains have been omitted for clarity. The N and C termini are labeled. Structures A and B were determined by NMR with the unbound peptides in solution. Structures C, D, and E were determined by x-ray crystallography with peptides bound to their cognate protein ligands. **(A)** The structure of the IGFbp1-binding peptide (bp101) shows a turn-helix conformation (Lowman *et al.*, 1998). **(B)** Within the disulfide-bonded loop, the structure of the FVIIa-binding peptide (E-76) consists of a distorted type I reverse turn and an irregular turn of an helix that extends to the C terminus (Dennis *et al.*, 2000). **(C)** A peptide that binds to the IgG-Fc (Fc-III) has a β-hairpin structure (Delano *et al.*, 2000). **(D)** As shown, the monomer structure of the EMP1 peptide is a β-hairpin, but the peptide forms a non-covalent, symmetrical dimer in complex with two molecules of EPO receptor (Fig. 6) (Livnah *et al.*, 1996). **(E)** The structure of the VEGF-binding peptide (v108) consists of a disulfide-bonded loop and an extended N terminus that makes main chain hydrogen-bonding interactions with VEGF (Weismann *et al.*, 1998). (See Section 3.A for additional details.)

1. Antagonist Peptides

The first report of a small, potent peptide antagonist of a cytokine receptor was published in 1996. Yanofsky et al. (1996) targeted a receptor for interleukin-1 (IL-1), an inflammatory cytokine implicated in many immune responses. Phage display was used to first isolate low-affinity leads that were subsequently affinity matured to yield unconstrained, 15-residue peptides that bound the IL-1 receptor with IC_{50} values of about 2 nM. Substitution of a proline residue with a proline analogue (azetidine), along with blocking of the N and C termini, produced a peptide with fourfold improved binding affinity. Several of these peptides were shown to be potent antagonists of IL-1-mediated cellular responses.

Phage-displayed libraries of disulfide-constrained libraries have yielded several antagonist peptides for which three-dimensional structures have been determined. Fairbrother et al. (1998) reported three classes of peptides that bound to vascular endothelial growth factor (VEGF), a primary modulator of vascular neogenesis, angiogenesis, and vessel permeability. All three classes inhibited the binding of VEGF to its receptors, and the highest affinity peptide antagonized VEGF-induced proliferation of primary human umbilical vascular endothelial cells. The crystal structure of one of these peptides complexed with VEGF revealed an extended conformation in which the N-terminal residues formed a β strand paired with a β strand in VEGF (Weismann et al., 1998) (Fig. 5E). Because VEGF-induced angiogenesis is associated with pathologic processes, such as tumor growth and metastasis (Ferrara, 1995), VEGF antagonists could have broad therapeutic applications.

Insulin-like growth factor 1 (IGF-1) is a hormone with both metabolic and mitogenic activities that are mediated through binding to cell surface receptors. However, IGF-1 also binds to several distinct IGF-binding proteins, and these binding events block or modulate in vivo activity (Jones and Clemmons, 1995). Lowman et al., (1998) isolated disulfide-constrained peptides that bound to one of these IGF-binding proteins (IGFbp-1) and in so doing prevented binding of IGF-1. Such antagonist peptides may act as indirect agonists in vivo by binding to IGFbp-1 and thus freeing IGF-1 for interactions with its signaling receptors. NMR analysis of a 14-residue peptide revealed a well-defined free-solution structure that could aid in the design of therapeutically useful compounds (Fig. 5A).

The constant fragment of immunoglobulin G (IgG-Fc) contains a consensus binding site that interacts with at least four structurally distinct natural proteins. Delano et al. (2000) showed that this site was also dominant for binding of peptides from naïve phage-displayed libraries. The crystal structure of a 13-residue, disulfide-constrained peptide complexed with IgG-Fc revealed that the peptide adopts a β-hairpin structure that is different from any known Fc-binding motif (Fig. 5C), yet it binds to the same consensus site. A detailed analysis showed that the different ligands use a number of similar binding interactions, and the consensus binding site on IgG-Fc is highly accessible, adaptive, and hydrophobic. The authors speculated that such properties may predispose binding sites for interactions with multiple binding partners and, furthermore, that small peptides can target such a site by mimicking the interactions of much larger, natural ligands with completely different structural scaffolds.

2. Agonist Peptides

Phage display has also been used to select peptides that act as agonists for growth factor receptors. The first example of this remarkable activity was a disulfide-constrained peptide that was selected for binding to the signaling receptor for erythropoietin (EPO), a growth factor that controls the production of red blood cells (Wrighton et al., 1996). In cell-based assays, the peptide acted as an agonist that mimicked EPO activity. The crystal structure of an agonist peptide complexed with the EPO receptor showed that the peptide adopts a simple β-hairpin structure (Fig. 5D) that noncovalently dimerized with itself and two EPO receptors (Fig. 6) (Livnah et al., 1996). Thus, it appears that the peptide activates the EPO receptor by mimicking the natural receptor dimerization event induced by EPO itself. Two different strategies were used to produce covalently linked agonist peptide dimers that were about 100-fold more potent than the monomeric peptide (Wrighton et al., 1997; Johnson et al. 1997).

Agonist peptides have also been selected to mimic the activity of thrombopoietin (TPO), a growth factor that stimulates platelet production (Cwirla et al., 1996). In this case, phage display was first used to select peptide ligands that bound the TPO receptor with low affinity and acted as agonists in a cell-based assay. These low-affinity leads were then affinity matured with peptides-on-plasmids display and ribosome display. Finally, screening of individual clones identified a 14-residue, unconstrained peptide that performed well in a competition binding assay (IC_{50} = 2 nM) but had poor potency in a cell proliferation assay. However, as in the case of the EPO mimetic peptides, covalent dimerization of this peptide produced a more potent agonist. In fact, the potency of the dimer was equal to that of the natural growth factor TPO and 4000-fold greater than that of the monomer.

B. Peptide Ligands for Intracellular Protein Binding Domains

There are several distinct families of intracellular domains that bind to other proteins and thus influence cellular function (reviewed by Pawson, 1995; Pawson and Scott, 1997; Cowburn, 1997). These domains differ in their tertiary fold and also in the nature of the sequences to which they bind. Interestingly, most intracellular protein binding domains recognize small continuous stretches of primary sequence in their binding partners. Small, linear peptides are excellent

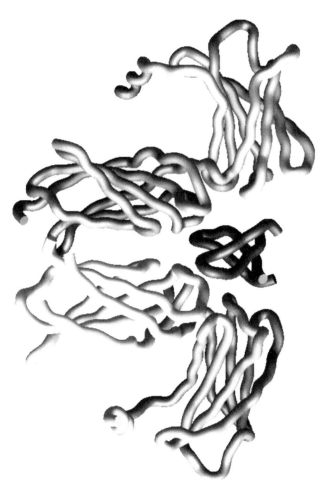

FIGURE 6 Complex of the extracellular domain of the EPO receptor and the agonist peptide EMP1 (Livnah *et al.*, 1996). The main chains are shown as ribbons, and the side chains have been omitted for clarity. The complex consists of a peptide dimer (dark gray) and two EPO-binding proteins (light gray). (See Section 3.A.2 for additional details.)

mimics of such interactions; therefore, these domains are ideal targets for combinatorial peptide libraries. Indeed, there has been considerable success in isolating peptide antagonists of intracellular protein–protein interactions, and often, these synthetic ligands have been found to be homologous to the natural ligands. In such systems, combinatorial peptide libraries provide ligands that can be used to inhibit natural binding interactions as well as to elucidate natural binding specificities.

1. Domains That Bind Polyproline-Rich Sequences

Numerous intracellular protein domains direct intracellular signaling by binding to short proline-rich stretches within proteins (reviewed by Pawson and Scott, 1997). The best characterized of these belong to the family of Src homology 3 (SH3) domains. Several studies have reported the use of phage-displayed peptide libraries to identify small, linear peptide ligands for SH3 domains (Sparks *et al.*, 1994, 1996; Rickles *et al.*, 1994, 1995). In all cases, proline-rich sequences were isolated that often matched sequences found in the natural SH3 ligands (Sparks *et al.*, 1996). It was also possible to obtain peptides that bound particular SH3 domains with greater affinity than peptide sequences derived from natural ligands (Rickles *et al.*, 1995). Furthermore, some selected peptides antagonized interactions between SH3 domains and their natural ligands *in vivo* (Sparks *et al.*, 1994). Phage display has also been used to study the binding specificity of WW domains, a structurally distinct family that also recognizes proline-rich sequences (Linn *et al.*, 1997).

2. Domains That Bind Phosphotyrosine-Containing Peptides

Many intracellular signaling pathways are regulated by reversible phosphorylation and/or dephosphorylation of particular tyrosine residues. These reversible modifications modulate enzymatic activities and also create or eliminate specific protein–protein interactions. Consequently, eukaryotic cells contain numerous protein domains that bind to specific phosphotyrosine-containing sequences and, in so doing, regulate signal transduction pathways (reviewed by Pawson, 1995; Cowburn, 1997). Two distinct structural classes of phosphotyrosine binding domains have been identified: the SH2 domains and the phosphotyrosine binding (PTB) domains.

It has been difficult to investigate phosphotyrosine-mediated binding interactions using DNA-encoded libraries because there is no genetic codon for phosphotyrosine. However, it has been shown that phage-displayed peptide libraries can be phosphorylated *in vitro* and that these modified libraries can be used to isolate phosphotyrosine-containing peptide ligands. While tyrosine kinases normally exhibit specificity for the sequences flanking the substrate tyrosine, two groups have demonstrated that prolonged exposure of phage-displayed peptide libraries to kinases results in virtually complete phosphorylation of tyrosine-containing peptides (Dante *et al.*, 1997; Gram *et al.*, 1997). Furthermore, these experiments showed that phosphorylation of naturally occurring tyrosines in wild-type phage coat proteins was not significant enough to interfere with subsequent selection experiments.

The phosphorylated libraries were used to investigate the binding specificities of a PTB domain (Dante *et al.*, 1997) and an SH2 domain (Gram *et al.*, 1997). Tyrosine-containing consensus sequences were identified in each case, and for the SH2 domain it was further demonstrated that phosphotyrosine-containing synthetic peptides corresponding to the selected sequences actually bound with greater affinity than peptides derived from the natural ligand. These results suggest that *in vitro* phosphorylation, and other posttranslational modifications, could further extend the utility of DNA-encoded peptide libraries.

3. PDZ Domains That Bind C-Terminal Peptide Sequences

PDZ domains are found in a large and diverse set of proteins (reviewed by Cowburn, 1997; Fanning and Anderson, 1999). In general, PDZ domain-containing proteins are responsible for clustering and assembling other proteins at specialized subcellular sites, such as epithelial cell tight junctions and neuronal synaptic densities. Many PDZ domains function by binding to the extreme C termini of their protein ligands, and thus, PDZ domains should be ideal targets for DNA-encoded peptide libraries. However, a complicating factor has been that while most PDZ domains interact with the free C termini of their ligands, the C terminus is blocked by fusion to the display scaffold in most DNA-encoded libraries. Nonetheless, two DNA-encoded approaches have been used to study the interactions between PDZ domains and ligands with free C termini.

Peptides-on-plasmids libraries are displayed as C-terminal fusions to the LacI repressor, and thus the displayed peptides have free C termini. This system has been used to map the binding specificities of PDZ domains from several different proteins (Stricker *et al.*, 1997; van Huizen *et al.*, 1998; Wang *et al.*, 1998). Recently, M13 phage-displayed peptide libraries fused to the C terminus of P8 have also proven effective in the analysis of PDZ domain–ligand interactions (Fuh *et al.*, 2000). In all of these studies, specific peptide ligands were identified, and these sequences were used to search genetic databases for natural proteins that may interact with particular PDZ domains. Furthermore, synthetic peptide analogues based on the selected sequences were used to map in detail the binding interactions between a PDZ domain and its high-affinity ligand (Fuh *et al.*, 2000). It was shown that the last four ligand amino acids provide almost all of the binding energy, and alanine scanning of a tetrapeptide ligand showed that all four side chains contribute favorably to PDZ binding, with the final two side chains being most important. These studies support a model in which the peptide main chain makes β-sheet interactions with a β strand in the PDZ domain, and the terminal carboxylate and the last four side chains all make productive binding contacts (Fig. 7). Thus, PDZ domains are able to bind tetrapeptides with high affinity and specificity by using binding contacts with essentially every functional group on the tetrapeptide.

C. Peptides as Enzyme Inhibitors

Enzymes have proven to be very good targets for phage-displayed peptide libraries. This is likely because enzymes typically have many deep clefts and binding pockets, including the active site and allosteric regulatory sites. In a recent study, Hyde-DeRuyscher *et al.* (1999) attempted to isolate peptide inhibitors for representatives from seven distinct enzyme classes. The results were very encouraging in that

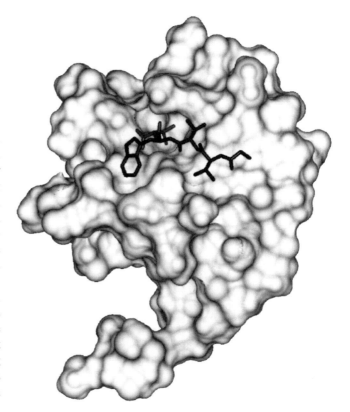

FIGURE 7 Molecular surface of a modeled PDZ domain complexed with a high-affinity pentapeptide ligand (Gly-Val-Thr-Trp-Val) (Fuh *et al.*, 2000). The model was based on the crystal structures of two homologous PDZ domains (Morais-Cabral *et al.*, 1996; Doyle *et al.*, 1996). The peptide ligand forms a β strand that intercalates between a β strand and an α helix of the PDZ domain. The terminal carboxylate and all four peptide side chains make binding contacts with the protein. (See Section 3.B.3 for additional details.)

specifically binding peptides were identified for all seven targets. In each case, many of the peptides bound to the same site, and the majority inhibited enzyme function. These results support the notion that proteins possess "preferred binding sites" (see Section 3.A.1) that are predisposed for ligand binding and that many of these sites are functionally relevant. The authors further demonstrated that inhibitory peptides could be used as detection reagents to discover small-molecules that bind to a protein of interest. In this application, small-molecule binding is detected by the displacement of bound peptide from the protein. Such competitive binding assays can be formatted with various detection systems, and they are readily adaptable to automation and high-throughput screening (Hyde-DeRuyscher *et al.*, 1999).

Dennis *et al.* (2000) used phage display to isolate peptides that bind the serine protease factor VIIa (FVIIa), a key regulator of the blood coagulation cascade. They obtained an 18-residue disulfide-constrained peptide (E-76) that not only bound FVIIa but also inhibited activity in a noncompetitive manner with exquisite specificity and high potency (K_i ~1

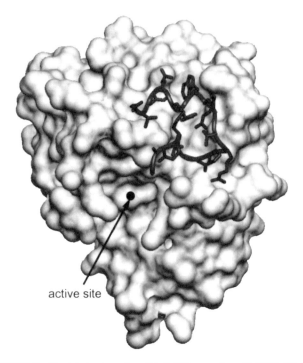

active site

FIGURE 8   Crystal structure of peptide E-76 in complex with FVIIa (Dennis *et al.,* 2000). The molecular surface of FVIIa is shown in light gray. E-76 is in dark gray, with the side chains depicted in stick format. E-76 binds at an exosite distinct from the active site and noncompetitively inhibits enzyme activity. (See Section 3.C for additional details.)

nM). Consistent with a noncompetitive inhibition mode, the crystal structure revealed that E-76 binds to FVIIa at an "exosite" distinct from the active site (Fig. 6), and apparently, it inhibits activity by an allosteric mechanism. The solution structure for the free peptide was also determined by NMR, and interestingly, the main chain fold was found to be almost identical to that in the bound state. Thus, the phage display not only provided a potent FVIIa inhibitor; it also led to the discovery of a hitherto unknown binding site and mode of inhibition. These results are of great therapeutic relevance because, despite the importance of anticoagulant therapy, it has been extremely difficult to selectively inhibit the myriad proteases of the coagulation cascade (Hirsch and Weitz, 1999; Dennis *et al.,* 2000).

4. Conclusions

DNA-encoded peptide libraries can provide small, specific ligands for essentially any protein, and such ligands have several key applications in drug discovery research. First, the natural binding specificities of protein–protein interactions can be inferred from selected sequences, and this information can be used to identify natural binding partners (Section 3.B) or to aid the design of organic mimics (reviewed by Dame-

wood, 1996; Cunningham and Wells, 1997; Cochran, 2000). Second, binding peptides can be used for target validation, that is, to assess the potential therapeutic effects of blocking specific protein–protein interactions. This is especially important in the current genomics era because DNA sequencing efforts are revealing thousands of new proteins with unknown functions (Kay *et al.,* 1998). Third, binding peptides may be used as detection reagents in high-throughput screens for small-molecule inhibitors (Section 3.C). Finally, despite considerable obstacles, peptides themselves could be used as drugs (Latham, 1999).

Acknowledgments

We thank Nick Skelton, Charlie Eigenbrot, Mayte Pisabarro, and David Wood for help with graphics.

References

Bass, S., Green, R., and Wells, J. A. (1990). Hormone phage: an enrichment method for variant proteins with altered binding properties. *Proteins: Struct. Funct. Genet.* **8,** 309–314.

Boder, E. T., and Wittrup, K. D. (1997). Yeast surface display for screening combinatorial polypeptide libraries. *Nature Biotechnol.* **15,** 553–557.

Cereghino, G. P. L., and Cregg, J. M. (1999). Applications of yeast in biotechnology: protein production and genetic analysis. *Curr. Opin. Biotechnol.* **10,** 422–247.

Clackson, T., and Wells, J. A. (1994). In vitro selection from protein and peptide libraries. *Trends Biotechnol.* **12,** 173–184.

Clackson, T., and Wells, J. A. (1995). A hot spot of binding energy in a hormone-receptor interface. *Science* **267,** 383–386.

Cochran, A. G. (2000). Antagonists of protein–protein interactions. *Chem. Biol.* **7,** R85–R94.

Cowburn, D. (1997). Peptide recognition by PTB and PDZ domains. *Curr. Opin. Struct. Biol.* **7,** 835–838.

Cull M., Miller, J., and Schatz, P. (1992). Screening for receptor ligands using libraries of peptides linked to the C terminus of the *lac* repressor. *Proc. Natl. Acad. Sci. USA* **89,** 1865–1869.

Cunningham, B. C., and Wells, J. A. (1989). High-resolution epitope mapping of hGH–receptor interactions by alanine-scanning mutagenesis. *Science* **244,** 1081–1085.

Cunningham, B. C., and Wells, J. A. (1997). Minimized proteins. *Curr. Biol.* **7,** 457–462.

Cwirla, S. E., Peters, E. A., Barrett, R. W., and Dower, W. J. (1990). Peptides on phage: a vast library of peptides for identifying ligands. *Proc. Natl. Acad. Sci. USA* **87,** 6378–6382.

Cwirla, S. E., Balasubramanian, P., Duffin, D. J., Wagstrom, C. R., Gates, C. M., Singer, S. C., Davis, A. M., Tansik, R. L., Mattheakis, L. C., Boytos, C. M., Schatz, P. J., Paccanar, D. P., Wrighton, N. C., Barrett, R. W., and Dower, W. J. (1996). Peptide agonist of the thrombopoietin receptor as potent as the natural cytokine. *Science* **276,** 1696–1699.

Dall'Acqua, W., and Carter, P. (1998). Antibody engineering. *Curr. Opin. Struct. Biol.* **8,** 443–450.

Damewood, J. R. (1996). Peptide mimetic design with the aid of computational chemistry. In "Reviews in Computational Chemistry" (K. B. Lipkowitz and D. B. Boyd, eds.), Vol. 9, pp. 1–80. VCH Publishers Inc, New York.

Dante, L., Vetriani, C., Zucconi, A., Pelicci, G., Lanfrancone, L., Pelicci, P. G., and Cesareni, G. (1997). Modified phage peptide libraries as a tool to study specificity of phosphorylation and recognition of tyrosine containing peptides. *J. Mol. Biol.* **269**, 694–703.

Delano, W. L., Ultsch, M. H., de Vos, A. M., and Wells, J. A. (2000). Convergent solutions to binding at a protein–protein interface. *Science* **287**, 1279–1283.

Dennis, M. S., Eigenbrot, C., Skelton, N. J., Ultsch, M. H., Santell, L., Dwyer, M. A., O'Connell, M. P., and Lazarus, R. A. (2000). Peptide exosite inhibitors of factor VIIa as anticoagulants. *Nature* **404**, 465–470.

Devlin, J. J., Panganiban, L. C., and Devlin, P. E. (1990). Random peptide libraries: a source of specific protein binding molecules. *Science* **249**, 404–406.

de Vos, A. M., Ultsch, M., and Kossiakoff, A. A. (1992) Human growth hormone and extracellular domain of its receptor: crystal structure of the complex. *Science* **255**, 306–312.

Dower, W. J. (1998). Targeting growth factor and cytokine receptors with recombinant peptide libraries. *Curr. Opin. Chem. Biol.* **2**, 328–334.

Dower, W. J., Miller, J. F., and Ragsdale, C. W. (1988). High efficiency transformation of *E. coli* by high voltage electroporation. *Nucleic Acids Res.* **16**, 6127–6145.

Doyle, D. A., Lee. A., Lewis, J., Kim, E., Sheng, M., and MacKinnon, R. (1996). Crystal structure of a complexed and peptide-free membrane protein-binding domain: molecular basis of peptide recognition by PDZ. *Cell* **85**, 1067–1076.

Efimov, V. P., Nepluev, I. V., and Mesyanzhinov, V. V. (1995). Bacteriophage T4 as a surface display vector. *Virus Genes* **10**, 173–177.

Fairbrother, W. J., Christinger, H. W., Cochran, A. G., Fuh, G., Keenan, C. J., Quan, C., Shriver, S. K., Tom, J. Y. K., Wells, J. A., and Cunningham, B. C. (1998). Novel peptides selected to bind vascular endothelial growth factor target the receptor-binding site. *Biochemistry* **37**, 17754–17764.

Fanning, A. S., and Anderson, J. M. (1999). PDZ domains: fundamental building blocks in the organization of protein complexes at the plasma membrane. *J. Clin. Invest.* **103**, 767–772.

Felici, F., Castagnoli, L., Musacchio, A., Jappelli, R., and Cesareni, G. (1991). Selection of antibody ligands from a large library of oligopeptides expressed on a multivalent exposition vector. *J. Mol. Biol.* **222**, 301–310.

Ferrara, N. (1995). The role of vascular endothelial growth factor in pathological angiogenesis. *Breast Cancer Res. Treat.* **36**, 127–137.

Fuh, G., Pisabarro, M. T., Li, Y., Quan, C., Lasky, L. A., and Sidhu, S. S. (2000). Analysis of PDZ domain–ligand interactions using carboxyl-terminal phage display. *J. Biol. Chem.* **In press.**

Gao, C., Mao, S., Lo., C. H., Wirsching, P., Lerner, R. A., and Janda, K. D. (1999). Making artificial antibodies: a format for phage display of combinatorial heterodimeric arrays. *Proc. Natl. Acad. Sci. USA* **96**, 6025–6030.

Gates, C. M., Stemmer, W. P. C., Kaptein, R., and Schatz, P. J. (1996). Affinity selective isolation of ligands from peptide libraries through display on a *lac* repressor "headpiece dimer." *J. Mol. Biol.* **255**, 373–386.

Georgiou, G., Stathopoulos, C., Daugherty, P. S., Nayak, A. R., Iverson, B. L., and Curtiss III, R. (1997). Display of heterologous proteins on the surface of microorganisms: from the screening of combinatorial libraries to live recombinant vaccines. *Nature Biotechnol.* **15**, 29–34.

Gram, H., Schmitz, R., Zuber, J. F., and Baumann, G. (1997). Identification of phosphopeptide ligands for the Src-homology 2 (SH2) domain of Grb2 by phage display. *Eur. J. Biochem.* **246**, 633–637.

Greenwood, J., Willis, A. E., and Perham, R. N. (1991). Multiple display of foreign peptides on a filamentous bacteriophage. *J. Mol. Biol.* **220**, 821–827.

Griffiths, A. D., and Duncan, A. R. (1998). Strategies for selection of antibodies by phage display. *Curr. Opin. Biotechnol.* **9**, 102–108.

Hanes, J., and Pluckthun, A. (1997). In vitro selection and evolution of functional proteins by using ribosome display. *Proc. Natl. Acad. Sci. USA* **94**, 4937–4942.

Hanes, J., and Pluckthun, A. (1999). In vitro selection methods for screening of peptide and protein libraries. *Curr. Topics Microbiol. Immunol.* **243**, 107–122.

Hanes, J., Jermutus, L., Weber-Bornhauser, S., Bosshard, H. R., and Pluckthun, A. (1998). Ribosome display efficiently selects and evolves high-affinity antibodies in vitro from immune libraries. *Proc. Natl. Acad. Sci. USA* **95**, 14130–14135.

Hirsh, J., and Weitz, J. I. (1999). New antithrombotic agents. *Lancet* **353**, 1431–1436.

Hoogenboom, H. R., de Bruine, A. P., Hufton, S. E., Hoet, R. M., Arends, J. W., and Roovers, R. C. (1998). Antibody phage display technology and its applications. *Immunotechnology* **4**, 1–20.

Hyde-DeRuyscher, R., Paige, L. A., Christensen, D. J., Hyde-DeRuyscher, N., Lim, A., Fredericks, Z. L., Kranz, J., Gallant, P., Zhang, J., Rocklage, S. M., Fowlkes, D. M., Wendler, P. A., and Hamilton, P. T. (2000). Detection of small-molecule enzyme inhibitors with peptides isolated from phage-displayed combinatorial peptide libraries. *Chem. Biol.* **7**, 17–25.

Iannolo, G., Minenkova, O., Petruzzelli, R., and Cesarini, G. (1995). Modifying filamentous phage capsid: limits in the size of the major capsid protein. *J. Mol. Biol.* **248**, 835–844.

Il'ichev, A. A., Minenkova, O. O., Tat'kov, S. L., Karpyshev, N. N., Eroshkin, A. M., Petrenko, V. A., and Sandakhchiev, L. S. (1989). Production of a viable variant of the M13 phage with a foreign peptide inserted into the basic coat protein. *Dokl. Akad. Nauk. SSSR* **307**, 481–483.

Jespers, L. S., Messens, J. H., De Keyser, A., Eeckhout, D., Van Den Brande, I., Gansemans, Y. G., Lauwereys, M. J., Vlasuk, G. P., and Stanssens, P. E. (1995). Surface expression and ligand-based selection of cDNAs fused to filamentous phage gene VI. *Biotechnology* **13**, 378–382.

Johnson, D. L., Farrell, F. X., Barbone, F. P., McMahon, F. J., Tullai, J., Kroon, D., Freedy, J., Zivin, R. A., Mulcahy, L. S., and Jolliffe, L. K. (1997). Amino-terminal dimerization of an erythropoietin mimetic peptide results in increased erythropoietic activity. *Chem. Biol.* **4**, 939–950.

Johnsson, K., and Ge, L. (1999). Phage display of combinatorial peptide and protein libraries and their applications in biology and chemistry. *Curr. Topics. Microbiol. Immunol.* **243**, 87–105.

Jones, J. I., and Clemmons, D. R. (1995). Insulin-like growth factors and their binding proteins: biological actions. *Endocr. Rev.* **16**, 3–34.

Kay, B. K., Kurakin, A. V., and Hyde-DeRuyscher, R. (1998). From peptides to drugs via phage display. *Drug Disc. Today* **8**, 370–378.

Keike, M. C., Shusta, E. V., Boder, E. T., Teyton, L., Wittrup, K. D., and Kranz, D. M. (1999). Selection of functional T cell receptor mutants from a yeast surface-display library. *Proc. Natl. Acad. Sci. USA* **96**, 5651–5656.

Latham, P. W. (1999). Therapeutic peptides revisited. *Nature Biotechnol.* **17**, 755–757.

Linn, H., Ermekova, K. S., Rentschler, S., Sparks, A. B., Kay, B. K., and Sudol, M. (1997). Using molecular repertoires to identify high-affinity peptide ligands of the WW domain of human and mouse YAP. *Biol. Chem.* **378**, 531–537.

Livnah, O., Stura, E. A., Johnson, D. L., Middleton, S. A., Mulcahy, L. S., Wrighton, N. C., Dower, W. J., Jolliffe, L. K., and Wilson, I. A. (1996). Functional mimicry of a protein hormone by a peptide agonist: the EPO receptor complex at 2.8 Å. *Science* **273**, 464–471.

Lowman, H. B., Bass, S. H., Simpson, N. S., and Wells, J. A. (1991). Selecting high-affinity binding proteins by monovalent phage display. *Biochemistry* **30**, 10832–10838.

Lowman, H. B., Chen, Y. M., Skelton, N. J., Mortensen, D. L., Tomlinson, E. E., Sadick, M. D., Robinson, I. C. A. F., and Clark, R. G. (1998). Molecular mimics of insulin-like growth factor 1 (IGF-1) for inhibiting IGF-1:IGF-binding protein interactions. *Biochemistry* **37**, 8870–8878.

Marvin, D. A. (1998). Filamentous phage structure, infection and assembly. *Curr. Opin. Struct. Biol.* **8**, 150–158.

Maruyama, I. N., Maruyama, H. I., and Brenner, S. (1994). λfoo: A λ phage vector for the expression of foreign proteins. *Proc. Natl. Acad. Sci. USA* **91**, 8273–8277.

Mattheakis, L. C., Bhatt, R. R., and Dower, W. J. (1994). An in vitro polysome display system for identifying ligands from very large peptide libraries. *Proc. Natl. Acad. Sci. USA* **91**, 9022–9026.

Morais-Cabral, J. H., Petosa, C., Sutcliffe, M. J., Raza, S., Byron, O., Poy, F., Marfatia, S. M., Chishti, A. H., and Liddington, R. C. (1996). Crystal structure of a PDZ domain from the human homolog of discs-large protein. *Nature* **384**, 649–652.

Nemoto, N., Miyamoto-Sato, E., Husimi, Y., and Yanagawa, H. (1997). In vitro virus: bonding of mRNA bearing puromycin at the 3′-terminal end to the C-terminal end of its encoded protein on the ribosome in vitro. *FEBS Lett.* **414**, 405–408.

Pausch, M. H. (1997). G-protein-coupled receptors in *Saccharomyces cerevisiae:* high-throughput screening assays for drug discovery. *Trends Biotechnol.* **15**, 487–494.

Pawson, T. (1995). Protein modules and signalling networks. *Nature* **373**, 573–580.

Pawson, T., and Scott, J. D. (1997). Signaling through scaffold, anchoring, and adaptor proteins. *Science* **278**, 2075–2080.

Ren, Z. J., Lewis, G. K., Wingfield, P. T., Locke, E. G., Steven, A. C., and Black, L. W. (1996). Phage display of intact domains at high copy number: a system based on SOC, the small capsid protein of bacteriophage T4. *Protein Sci.* **5**, 1833–1843.

Rickles, R. J., Botfield, M. C., Weng, Z., Taylor, J. A., Green, O. M., Brugge, J. S., and Zoller, M. J. (1994). Identification of Src, Fyn, P13K and Abl SH3 domain ligands using phage display libraries. *EMBO J.* **13**, 5598–5604.

Rickles, R. J., Botfield, M. C., Zhou, X-M., Henry, P. A., Brugge, J. S., and Zoller, M. J. (1995). Phage display selection of ligand residues important for Src homology 3 domain binding specificity. *Proc. Natl. Acad. Sci. USA* **92**(24), 10909–10913.

Roberts, R. W. (1999). Totally in vitro protein selection using mRNA-protein fusions and ribosome display. *Curr. Opin. Chem. Biol.* **3**, 268–273.

Roberts, R. W., and Szostak, J. W. (1997). RNA-peptide fusions for the in vitro selection of peptides and proteins. *Proc. Natl. Acad. Sci. USA* **94**, 12297–12302.

Sambrook, J., Fritsch, E. F., and Maniatis, T. (1989). "Molecular Cloning: A Laboratory Manuel." Cold Spring Harbor Laboratory Press, Cold Spring Harbor.

Schaffitzel, C., Hanes, J., Jermutus, L., and Pluckthun, A. (1999). Ribosome display: an in vitro method for selection and evolution of antibodies from libraries. *J. Immunol. Meth.* **231**, 119–135.

Scott, J. K., and Smith, G. P. (1990). Searching for peptide ligands with an epitope library. *Science* **249**, 386–390.

Sidhu, S. S., Lowman, H. B., Cunningham, B. C., and Wells, J. A. (2000). Phage display for selection of novel binding peptides. *Meth. Enzymol.* **328**, 333–363.

Smith, G. P. (1985). Filamentous fusion phage: Novel expression vectors that display cloned antigens on the virion surface. *Science* **228**, 1315–1317.

Smith, G. P., and Petrenko, V. A. (1997). Phage display. *Chem. Rev.* **97**, 391–410.

Sparks, A. B., Quilliam, L. A., Thorn, J. M., Der, C. J., and Kay, B. K. (1994). Identification and characterization of Src SH3 ligands from phage-displayed random peptide libraries. *J. Biol. Chem.* **269**, 23853–23856.

Sparks, A. B., Rider, J. E., Hoffman, N. G., Fowlkes, D. M., Quilliam, L. A., and Kay, B. K. (1996). Distinct ligand preferences of Src homology 3 domains from Src, Yes, Abl, Cortactin, p53bp2, PLCγ, Crk, and Grb2. *Proc. Natl. Acad. Sci. USA* **93**, 1540–1544.

Stahl, S., and Uhlen, M. (1997). Bacterial surface display: trends and progress. *Tibtech* **15**, 185–192.

Sternberg, N., and Hoess, R. H. (1995). Display of peptides and proteins on the surface of bacteriophage λ. *Proc. Natl. Acad. USA* **92**, 1609–1613.

Stricker, N. L., Christopherson, K. S., Yi, B. A., Schatz, P. J., Raab, R. W., Dawes, G., Bassett, D. E., Bredt, D. S., and Li, M. (1997). PDZ domain of neuronal nitric oxide synthase recognizes novel C-terminal peptide sequences. *Nature Biotechnol.* **15**, 336–342.

VanAntwerp, J. J., and Wittrup, K. D. (2000). Fine affinity discrimination by yeast surface display and flow cytometry. *Biotechnol. Prog.* **16**, 31–37.

van Huizen, R., Miller, K., Chen, D. M., Li, Y., Lai, Z. C., Raab, R. W., Stark, W. S., Shortridge, R. D., and Li, M. (1998). Two distantly positioned PDZ domains mediate multivalent INAD-phospholipase C interactions essential for G protein-coupled signaling. *EMBO J.* **17**, 2285–2297.

Vaughan, T. J., Osbourn, J. K., and Tempest, P. R. (1998). Human antibodies by design. *Nature Biotechnol.* **16**, 535–539.

Wang, S., Raab, R. W., Schatz, P. J., Guggino, W. B., and Li, M. (1998). Peptide binding consensus of the NHE-RF-PDZ1 domain matches the C-terminal sequence of cystic fibrosis transmembrane conductance regulator (CFTR). *FEBS Lett.* **427**, 103–108.

Webster, R. E. (1996). Biology of the filamentous bacteriophage. *In* "Phage Display of Peptides and Proteins" (Kay, B. K., Winter, J., and McCafferty, J., eds), pp. 1–20, Academic Press, San Diego.

Weismann, C., Christinger, H. W., Cochran, A. G., Cunningham, B. C., Fairbrother, W. J., Keenan, C. J., Meng, G., and de Vos, A. M. (1998). Crystal structure of the complex between VEGF and a receptor-blocking peptide. *Biochemistry* **38**, 17765–17772.

Wrighton, N. C., Farrell, F. X., Chang, R., Kashyap, A. K., Barbone, F. P., Mulcahy, L. S., Johnson, D. L., Barrett, R. W., Jolliffe, L. K., and Dower, W. J. (1996). Small peptides as potent mimetics of the protein hormone erythropoietin. *Science* **273**, 458–463.

Wrighton, N. C., Balasubramanian, P., Barbone, F. P., Kashyap, A. K., Farrell, F. X., Jolliffe, L. K., Barrett, R. W., and Dower, W. J. (1997). Increased potency of an erythropoietin peptide mimetic through covalent dimerization. *Nature Biotechnol.* **15**, 1261–1265.

Yanofsky, D. S., Baldwin, D. N., Butler, J. H., Holden, F. R., Jacobs, J. W., Balasubramanian, P., Chinn, J. P., Cwirla, S. E., Peters-Bhatt, E., Whitehorn, E. A., Tate, E. H., Akeson, A., Bowlin, T. L., Dower, W. J., and Barrett, R. W. (1996). High affinity type I interleukin 1 receptor antagonists discovered by screening recombinant peptide libraries. *Proc. Natl. Acad. Sci. USA* **93**, 7381–7386.

CHAPTER 14

MECHANISM-BASED HIGH-THROUGHPUT SCREENING FOR NOVEL ANTICANCER DRUG DISCOVERY

Wynne Aherne
Michelle Garrett
Ted McDonald
Paul Workman

Cancer Research Campaign Centre for Cancer Therapeutics

Institute of Cancer Research

Sutton, United Kingdom

Summary

There is now a tremendous potential for the discovery of novel mechanism-based agents for the clinical management of cancer. These agents are being targeted to the cellular proteins and pathways that are causally involved with oncogenesis, cell proliferation, and disease progression. Combined with the output of the Human Genome Project, our increasing knowledge of the molecular basis of cancer will continue to provide a range of tractable targets for drug discovery. The application of new technologies, including functional genomics, combinatorial chemistry, high throughput biological techniques, microarray analysis, and proteomics, will lead to a stream of innovative compounds for clinical evaluation. This chapter concentrates on the role of mechanism-based high-throughput screening (HTS) in contemporary drug discovery of small molecule cancer drugs. During the last decade, HTS has rapidly developed into a technology-dependent scientific discipline that relies heavily on the use of miniaturized automated assays to achieve huge screening rates. Here we show how HTS has evolved to achieve these throughputs and we describe the most widely used technologies that have facilitated the use of highly miniaturized screens suitable for automation. These include scintillation proximity and fluorescent energy transfer assays that can be carried out in a completely homogeneous "mix-and-measure" format. The importance of the quality and diversity of the compound libraries, whether derived from archiving or combinatorial chemistry, is discussed. We also provide some examples of novel mechanism-based compounds that have been identified at least in part by a mechanism-based screening approach and that are currently being evaluated clinically as the post-genomic medicines of the future.

1. Importance of Mechanism-Based Targets in Post-genomic Drug Discovery

A. The Gene to Drug Paradigm

An increased understanding of the molecular mechanisms responsible for the malignant phenotype now provides us with an unparalleled opportunity to discover improved drugs for cancer treatment (Garrett and Workman, 1999; Gibbs, 2000; Kaelin, 1999; Lane, 1998; Workman, 2000). By focusing on novel targets that are responsible for driving malignant progression, we increase the likelihood of discovering mechanism-based agents that are more effective and less toxic than the empirically derived cytotoxic drugs of the previous era. This is a paradigm shift in the field and the approach can be summarized as:

New genes → novel targets → innovative medicines

B. New targets and the Vision of Postgenomic Cancer Medicine

The sequencing of the human genome is a momentous achievement (see *Nature*, 2001; *Science*, 2001). The latest prediction is that there will be 30,000–40,000 genes in the human genome and we will shortly have all of these in our computers and freezers. A now-classic analysis showed that all current medicines (excluding antimicrobial agents) act on the products of only 400–500 human genes (Drews, 1996). Of the 92 anticancer drugs that have received marketing approval from the U.S. Food and Drug Administration (http://www.fda.gov/oashi/cancer/(cdrug.html) as few as 17 are perceived by oncologists as having a high priority for widespread use, with an additional 12 having some advantages in particular clinical settings (Sikora et al., 1999). Moreover, these drugs act on a very small number of molecular targets and most are cytotoxic in nature.

The challenge of post-genomic cancer drug discovery is to develop mechanism-based agents that act on key cancer processes and then to test the hypothesis that such agents can indeed be more selective than the currently available generation of drugs. Recent clinical experience with the bcr-abl inhibitor STI-571, all-*trans* retinoic acid (Salomoni and Pandolfi, 2000), the erbB2 monoclonal antibody herceptin, and the epidermal growth factor (EGF) receptor tyrosine inhibitors such as ZD1839 suggest that such novel mechanism-based agents will find clinical utility (see Workman, 2000a,b, 2001). The exciting vision toward which we can work is one in which there is a drug available for every genetic abnormality (mutation or aberrant expression) and also for key microenvironmental features involved in cancer progression. Appropriate combinations of such agents could then be selected to treat tumors, driven by a particular mix of molecular abnormalities. That reality remains some way off, but in order to achieve it we must first discover the range of agents from which we can select the genomically directed drug cocktails of the future.

C. The Process of Contemporary Drug Discovery and the Importance of Target Validation

The process of contemporary mechanism-based, small-molecule drug discovery is illustrated in Fig. 1. The key elements are (1) identifying and validating the target; (2) screening (or molecular design) to find a small molecule lead that acts at the target; and (3) optimizing the lead by chemical improvement, leading to selection of a candidate for clinical trial. New genes identified by molecular and genomics research as being implicated in cancer represent potential targets for drug discovery. However, not all cancer genes are good targets. Where the genetic abnormality involves loss of function (tumor suppressor genes) it is generally difficult to envisage the practicality of discovering a drug that will directly restore function. Experience may show other targets to be difficult to inhibit with "drug-like" molecules. In these cases it may be necessary to pursue functional genomic approaches (e.g., yeast two-hybrid screening) in order to define binding partners that may be better targets, or to elucidate the pathway in which the cancer gene product operates in order to identify a more tractable target.

In order to prioritize as drug discovery targets genes with an assigned function (see previous section), a series of validation criteria are often used (Garrett and Workman, 1999; Gibbs and Oliff, 1994). These include:

- Demonstration that the aberrant function of the target gene leads to the development of cancer or that the gene lies on a pathway known to be linked to the disease and its progression. Evidence for this may be found from studies us-

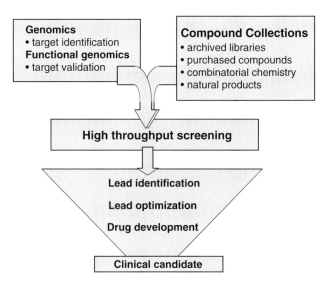

FIGURE 1 Role of HTS in mechanism-based drug development.

ing human tumor cell lines or from clinical expression data.

- The frequency of a given genetic abnormality is important because it indicates the likely importance of the target or pathway and may indicate the number of patients likely to benefit from an emerging therapy. However, frequency should not be given undue importance, since a genetically defined subset of patients may benefit considerably from an appropriate tailored drug.
- The fact that, in model systems, mutation or overexpression of the target produces the malignant phenotype (proliferation, cell cycle deregulation, antiapoptosis, invasion, motility, angiogenesis, metastasis).
- Evidence of reversal of the phenotype by gene knockout experiments, dominant negative or antisense constructs; and the use of antisense oligonucleotides, neutralizing antibodies, or inhibitory peptides. In this respect, small molecule inhibitor(s), even those of modest potency, are useful tools.
- The practical feasibility of inhibiting a particular target. Enzymes may represent more pharmacologically attractive targets than those involving macromolecular interactions, although inhibitors of protein–protein interactions have been reported (Bottger *et al.*, 1996; Chen *et al.*, 1999).
- The availability of suitable biological models and assays to determine molecular pharmacodynamic end points so that the biological effects of compounds can be evaluated as they progress through the drug development cascade.
- The practicalities of setting up a cost-effective screen with the desired throughput. A major consideration is the availability of (1) ideally, active protein in sufficient quantity to run the screen, or (2) alternatively, a DNA construct for protein expression in either *E. coli* or Baculovirus (BV)–infected insect cells [*Spodoptera frugiperda* (Sf9)]. It may also be necessary to produce the substrate for the target (protein or specific peptide), although a generic substrate such as myelin basic protein (MBP) for serine/threonine kinases is often used; (3) a suitable cell line for cell-based HTS is another major consideration. HTS depends on assays with different attributes from those generally used during target identification and validation. The ease with which the screen can be configured from available reagents and assay formats has also to be considered.

Selecting a target for mechanism-based drug discovery is ultimately a matter of judgment. Not all of the above criteria may be fulfilled for a given target. It may take too long. It may be appropriate to take the risk and mount a drug discovery campaign against a drug target that is not well validated, but where the pressing need is to obtain a leading competitive position in the field.

D. The Test Cascade for Compound Evaluation

Having discovered a hit screening, or a lead based on rational design and structural biology, a robust, efficient, and informative test cascade is essential for the conversion of the lead to a drug (Gelmon *et al.*, 1999). This cascade consists of a series of hierarchically arranged tests that provide biological information on the test compound, based on which the lead structure can be optimized by medicinal chemistry. Through iterative rounds of chemical optimization based on biological feedback, compounds are improved so that they progress through the more demanding downstream tests, leading eventually to an agent with the desired properties being selected for clinical trial.

We have found it valuable to develop a generic test cascade that can be customized to the particular molecular target. Figure 2a shows such a generic test cascade for a target for which the primary screen is a biochemical, cell-free assay. Figure 2b illustrates the differences in the early part of the cascade when the primary screen involves a cell-based screen. Both methods have advantages and disadvantages, and these will be discussed later in the review.

Some particular features of the test cascade are worth highlighting:

- In cell-based screens, subsequent follow-up assays are needed to "deconvolute" the mechanism from within a targeted pathway. Where appropriate, compounds can be submitted to the National Cancer Institute (NCI) human tumor panel for COMPARE analysis (Monks *et al.*, 1997; Paull *et al.*, 1992).
- A robust mode of action assay is required to confirm that compounds are exerting their biological effect down the test cascade through the desired mechanism. This can also provide a valuable pharmacodynamic end point in xenograft studies and clinical trials (e.g., Kelland *et al.*, 1999; Sharp *et al.*, 2000). Gene expression microarray and proteomic analyses are increasingly important in mode of action studies (e.g., Clark *et al.*, 2000; Scherf *et al.*, 2000).
- Pharmacokinetic properties are usually rate limiting at the *in vitro* to *in vivo* (cell culture to mouse) transition. Hence, a pharmacokinetic prioritization screen is important, ideally employing cassette dosing (Rodrigues, 1997).
- Pharmacokinetic behavior is often controlled by biotransformation, and therefore information on metabolism is important.

2. High-Throughput Screening

A. Introduction

HTS plays an essential role in the drug discovery process (Fig. 1). As described above, widespread implementation of this key component has been driven by the success of genomic approaches for novel drug target identification and validation. HTS also provides the means of evaluating the large numbers of compounds available in various compound collections and those provided by combinatorial and parallel synthesis. The

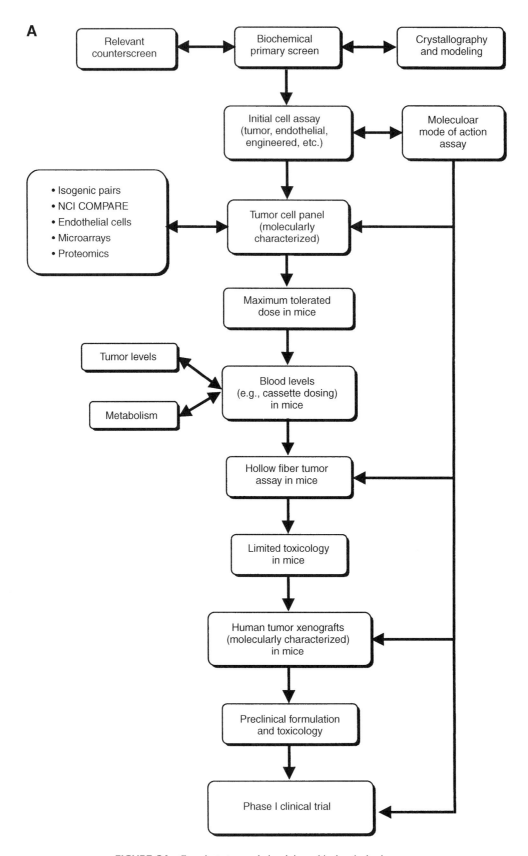

FIGURE 2A Generic test cascade involving a biochemical primary screen.

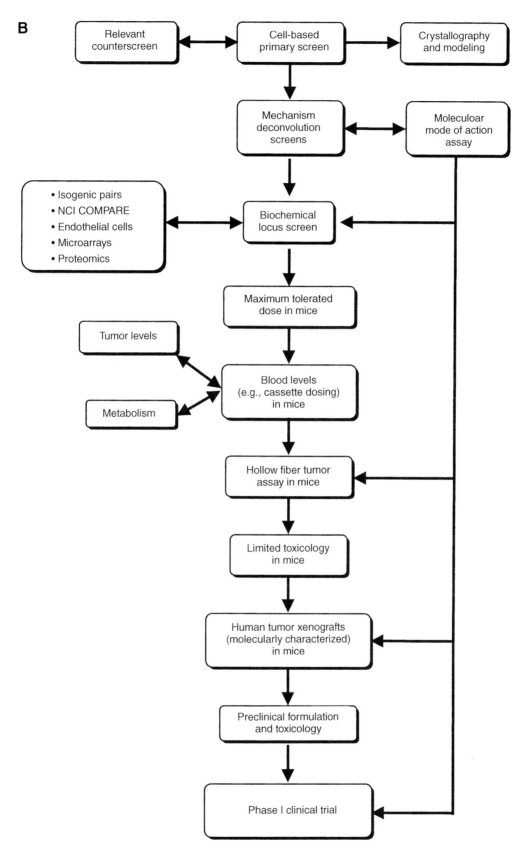

FIGURE 2B Generic test cascade involving a cell-based primary screen.

growth of HTS has been fueled by rapid concurrent innovations in molecular biology, assay technologies and equipment, as well as automation and information technology. Many of these developments have occurred as a result of close collaboration and partnerships between the pharmaceutical industry and various instrument and reagent manufacturers.

The drug discovery potential of HTS when coupled to a compound library with wide chemical diversity is enormous, but its success depends on several factors. These include the number and quality of validated targets, the number and diversity of compounds in the collections, and the ability to screen these in a timely and cost-effective manner using robust informative assays. Identification of a good lead using HTS can shorten drug discovery time scales considerably. However, downstream factors, such as synthetic chemistry for lead optimization and the low throughput of secondary assays for defining the pharmacological properties of active compounds, may become limiting to the overall rate of identification of candidate molecules for clinical evaluation.

If numbers of compounds screened are the only mark of success, then HTS has been enormously successful. HTS capability has increased dramatically over the last 15 years (Fig. 3). In the mid-1980s conventional bioassays, such as ligand binding assays, that require filtration or phase separation were used for screening. Using these it was possible to screen relatively small numbers of compounds. The move away from test-tube-based assays to the now almost universally used microtiter plate format marked the beginning of the growth in HTS. Over the last 10–15 years this has resulted in an almost exponential growth in screening capacity. Current estimates for throughput are in the order of 10^5–10^6 compounds per week or even in some instances per day. This phenomenal throughput is often referred to as ultra-HTS.

These impressive screening rates have been achieved through a professional and integrated approach to compound supply, and to developments in technologies, screening activities, automation, and data management. What is certain is that HTS (or ultra-HTS) now has the capacity to screen huge numbers of compounds. However, this capability may not run in parallel with the future needs and perceptions of the industry. The wisdom of screening enormous libraries of compounds is currently being questioned and intelligent approaches to selecting smaller subsets of compounds and the use of "focused libraries" are becoming more usual. This crucial choice is discussed later.

B. Screening Formats

Conventional types of bioassay limit throughput and are rarely suitable for HTS. So what are the characteristics of a

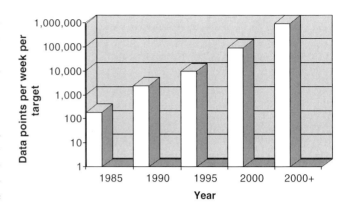

FIGURE 3   Approximate average screening rates during the last 15 years.

good HTS screen? Assays should be informative, robust, reliable, reproducible, fast, and cost effective. They should be easy to perform and amenable to miniaturization and automation. The goal of miniaturization is to minimize costs, prevent unnecessary depletion of valuable compound supplies, reduce the amounts of reagents used, and decrease the costs of disposing of assay waste. One of the features of HTS assays is that they tend to avoid time-consuming and difficult-to-automate manipulations, such as extraction, filtration, centrifugation, and washing steps. However, 96-well filter plates (Asthagiri *et al.,* 1999) provide a workable solution if a filtration step is essential for a particular assay.

Several nonseparation (homogeneous) or "mix-and-measure" assay technologies are now available for general use providing the basis for simple, easily automated assays. In addition, since steps such as washing and filtration are not necessary, this type of assay is suitable for investigating low-affinity interactions. In general, as long as a supply of specific reagents (e.g., recombinant proteins, substrates) is available, it is often possible to set up a screen in a relatively short time using minor modifications to generic protocols. Although radiometric assays have played a major role in HTS, the use of nonisotopic end points (fluorescence and luminescence) can provide several advantages for assay design and flexibility, increased sensitivity, higher throughput, lower cost, and improved safety. Thus, although it may not be possible to remove the need for radioactivity at all targets, an increasingly large proportion of HTS assays now use a nonisotopic end point.

Thus developments in HTS technologies have been designed to increase performance, and throughput of biochemical screens and high-throughput assays for the most demanding targets should now be achievable. In the following sections, the technological developments in HTS will be discussed and, where appropriate, illustrated by reference to screens designed for the discovery of novel lead compounds for cancer therapeutics.

C. Miniaturization

The enduring basis of the assays and equipment (including end-point readers) used for HTS is the 96-well microtiter plate (maximum volume 200–250 μl). Until recently, the majority of screening was carried out in these plates. However, in the last 5 years, as appropriate equipment (dispensers, washers, end-point readers) has been introduced and become more widely available, 384-well-based assays have become more common. Both formats are still commonly used for the majority of day-to-day screening, although for reasons of throughput and cost it is likely that in the near future the vast majority of assays will be configured in 384-well plates (maximum volume 70–100 μl). Assays carried out in even higher density plates have been described (Oldenburg *et al.,* 1998). Of these, 1536-well plates appear to be the most favored higher density format. The 1536-well plates have the same footprint as 96-well plates, assay volumes are limited to about 10 μl, and dedicated instrumentation for liquid handling and imaging end points is usually required. For many screens described so far, performance compares well with assays run in 96- or 384-well plates (Beveridge *et al.,* 2000; Dunn *et al.,* 2000; Maffia *et al.,* 1999). It is difficult to tell how far these high-density screen formats have been generally implemented in day-to-day screening rather than as a developmental tool. Further improvements in liquid-handling equipment for dispensing nanoliter volumes of compounds and reagents together with improved end-point readers are required for widespread use of 1536-well plates. On the other hand, for many small to medium-size laboratories, this type of screening may be out of reach and is quite possibly inappropriate.

D. Automation

To increase throughput above that achieved by conventional, manual techniques and to reduce pipetting errors in a screening context, especially on higher density plates, a considerable degree of automation is essential. The debate continues about the extent of automation required to maintain effective screening rates (Oldenburg, 1999). The precise needs of an organization depend on a number of factors. In a workstation setting, plates are moved manually from one piece of equipment to another, and robotic arms and plate stackers facilitate automated feeding of washers, dispensers, and endpoint readers. Such an approach provides the means to achieve a flexible but relatively high throughput, and this remains an option in many screening laboratories. This is especially true for those of biotechnology companies and academic screening groups for whom enormous throughputs are not needed because other downstream factors would become rate limiting. We have taken this approach in our center and, depending on the assay type, throughputs of at least 6000 compounds a day are readily achievable. In larger organizations,

where hundreds of thousands of compounds or even millions are available for screening, a fully automated linear track approach on an industrial scale has been taken, using integrated equipment for compound retrieval, compound plating, and screening. The merits of this fully automated approach have been discussed previously (Archer, 1999).

3. Assay Technologies

The following sections describe some of the key technologies, which along with improved equipment for automation have been instrumental in delivering the required rates of screening. Although these newer assay formats have provided the means to carry out HTS more efficiently, more traditional and simple methods, such as those with colorimetric end points, continue to have an important role in the screening laboratory. This can be exemplified by the use of color end points for measuring specific products of enzymatic reactions (Cogan *et al.,* 1999). The use of malachite green dye coupled to the interaction of ammonium molybdate and inorganic phosphate provides an appropriate and inexpensive end point for screening the effects of compounds on ATPase activity (Harder *et al.,* 1994; Henkel *et al.,* 1988). We recently evaluated this method for a screen to identify novel small-molecule inhibitors of the ATPase activity of the molecular chaperone protein Hsp90. The assay is reliable, reproducible, and cheap, and the potencies of known inhibitors compare favorably with those determined using more complicated assays (Panaretou *et al.,* 1998).

Enzyme-linked immunosorbent assays (ELISAs) also continue to offer a platform suitable for high throughput. Although the number of wash steps involved is a disadvantage, reagents for establishing these assays are often readily available, and the overall costs can be low. ELISA screens for the identification of tyrosine kinase inhibitors (Trevillyan *et al.,* 1999) and for protein–protein interactions have been described (Ellsmore *et al.,* 1997).

A. Radiometric Assays

One of the first innovations that allowed greater flexibility and high throughput for screening was the development of radiometric assays that depended on scintillation proximity counting. The measurement of radioisotopes (β emitters such as tritium) traditionally depends on the addition of a liquid scintillation cocktail to the sample to absorb and transfer radiative energy into a measurable light signal. Scintillant, coated onto beads (SPA, Amersham Pharmacia Biotech) (Cook, 1996), onto the wells of an opaque microtiter plate (FlashPlate, PerkinElmer Life Sciences), or into the plastic used to manufacture plates (ScintiStrips, PerkinElmer Life Sciences), has obviated the need for separation of the required labeled moiety prior to liquid scintillation counting. When a radioactively labeled molecule is captured in close proximity to the solid scintillant surface, a light signal is emitted. In contrast, no signal is produced from radiolabeled molecules that are not captured, as the distance from the scintillant is too great and energy is dissipated into solution. Thus, for low-energy radioisotopes, such as tritium and iodine-125, separation of bound and free label is not required prior to counting. As well as allowing real-time measurements of target interactions, assay manipulations are thus reduced resulting in the advantages of "mix and measure" assays. However, it has been shown that centrifugation or flotation of SPA beads is often required to improve signal-to-noise ratios. Also, the energy of other biologically useful isotopes, e.g., phosphorus-33, is high enough to cause unacceptable nonproximity effects resulting in high background signals. Washing or centrifugation is necessary to remove unbound radioactivity. In spite of this disadvantage, several assays utilizing ^{33}P-ATP have been successfully used for identification of inhibitors of a variety of protein kinases. These include c-src (Braunwalder *et al.,* 1996; Nakayama *et al.,* 1998), enzymes along the mitogen-activated protein kinase cascade (Alessi *et al.,* 1995; Antonsson *et al.,* 1999; McDonald *et al.,* 1999) and the human cell cycle checkpoint kinase Chk1 (Jackson *et al.,* 2000).

For both beads and plates, binding of radiolabeled product to the scintillant solid phase can be achieved in several ways using a variety of capture molecules. Commercially available products presently include precoated specific antibodies, secondary antibodies, proteins A and G, streptavidin, wheat germ agglutinin, nickel chelate, and glutathione. In addition, solid phases can be coated with enzyme substrates in the form of generic substrates, such as MBP or specific peptide substrates. Modification of the coated substrate following addition of enzyme and radiolabeled cofactor or cosubstrate results in a scintillation proximity signal.

In our laboratory we have successfully adopted the use of FlashPlates for several enzymatic screens, two examples of which are illustrated here. Figure 4 shows the format used for screening for inhibitors of activated Erk2, the kinase involved in signal transduction downstream of Ras. FlashPlates coated with MBP are incubated with enzyme and ^{33}P-ATP (0.25 μCi; total ATP concentration of 2.0 μM) for 4 h, the plates are washed three times with 100 mM sodium pyrophosphate in PBS, and the plates are counted. A similar assay using substrate peptide (PolyGlu Tyr) coated plates has also been established for EGF receptor kinase activity. This assay is used as a cross-screen for evaluating selectivity of inhibitors identified in other novel target screens.

Farnesyltransferase screens utilizing SPA beads have been previously described (Bishop *et al.,* 1996). A similar assay utilizing FlashPlates has been set up in our laboratory (Fig. 5). The enzyme reaction consisting of human placental en-

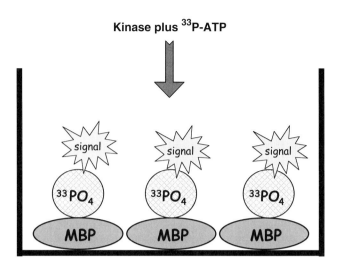

Kinase plus ^{33}P-ATP

After washing, radioactivity on MBP measured

FIGURE 4 A generic protein kinase assay using a myelin basic protein (MBP)–coated scintillating microplate.

zyme, a biotinylated substrate peptide containing the CAAX box sequence, and ^{3}H-farnesylpyrophosphate is incubated in streptavidin-coated plates. At the end of the incubation period, the enzyme reaction is terminated by the addition of ethylene diaminetetracetic acid (EDTA) and the plate counted. Performance of these assays (signal to noise greater than 10 and reproducibility about 10%) was more than adequate for screening requirements.

There are numerous additional examples of proximity counting applications to cancer-related targets, including phospholipase C (Mullinax *et al.,* 1999), poly(ADP-ribose) polymerase (Cheung and Zhang, 2000), histone deacetylase (Nare *et al.,*1999), topoisomerase I (Lerner and Saki, 1996), and telomerase (Savoysky *et al.,* 1996). Assays for protein–protein interactions suitable for HTS have also been developed using scintillation proximity assays. The binding of oncogenic Ras with the GTPase-activating protein neurofibromin (NF1) is a typical example. This is a relatively weak macromolecular interaction with high dissociation rates, and a method such as ELISA, which involves several washing steps, would not be suitable. In the assay ^{3}H-GTP labeled oncogenic Ras, GST-NF1 fusion protein, and GST antibodies were mixed with protein-A-coated SPA beads to generate a signal when the protein interaction was captured onto the beads (Skinner *et al.,* 1994).

B. Time-Resolved Fluorescence

Over the last 5 years, assays based on the measurement of fluorescence have become more common and are rapidly replacing radiometric assays in the screening laboratory. This reflects the dominance that nonisotopic assays now have in

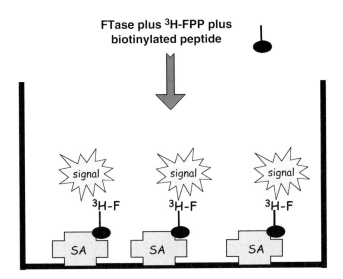

FTase plus ³H-FPP plus biotinylated peptide

FIGURE 5 The format of a streptavidin (SA)–coated scintillating microplate assay for screening farnesyltransferase (FTase).

other high-throughput analytical areas such as clinical chemistry. The sensitivity and versatility of fluorescence measurements for analysis has been a rich source of different types of assays. Fluorometric substrates now provide a widely used option, a recent example being a simple homogeneous HTS screen for caspase-3 inhibitors (Park *et al.*, 2000).

1. Time-Resolved Fluorescence

Although the high sensitivity of fluorescent assays has been widely exploited in many analytical areas, the use of time-resolved fluorescence (TRF) provides the means to eliminate the problem of high backgrounds due to nonspecific fluorescence of assay reagents as well as the autofluorescence from plastic components in plates. Using time-resolved (TR) signal measurement it is possible to distinguish between the short-lived signals generated by nonspecific fluorescence from that of the analyte if this is labeled with a long-lived fluorescent probe. The lanthanides europium (Eu), samarium (Sm), terbium (Tb), and dysprosium (Dy) are rare-earth metals that when chelated with a ligand produce a highly intense fluorescent signal. The emission has a large Stokes shift and decays slowly, resulting in a sensitive stable signal that can be readily distinguished from background fluorescence.

Reagents for TRF are available commercially. The original reagents for DELFIA (disassociation-enhanced lanthanide fluorescence immunoassay) are mainly used, as the name implies, for establishing sensitive immunoassays (Soini and Hemmila, 1991). These assays, like all other ELISA formats, require several wash steps following the addition of each binding reagent and the final addition of an enhancement solution. Nevertheless, this form of assay has been successfully used in HTS applications (Gaarde *et al.*, 1997) and has the advantage that problems of fluorescence quenching are

markedly reduced as test compounds are removed from the well prior to signal measurement.

More recent reagent developments have allowed TRF assays to be set up in a truly "mix-and-measure" manner using fluorescence resonance energy transfer (FRET). This technique is based on the proximity of a pair of fluorophors brought together in a binding reaction. The excited energy of the donor molecule is transferred by a nonradiative process to the acceptor molecule as long as they are close enough to each other (about 10 nm). Thus, the desired interaction can be measured in the presence of the same labeled molecules that have not taken part in the binding reaction.

Two systems are commercially available for TR-FRET assays and these now provide the basis of a large proportion of HTS screens. Both systems (LANCE supplied by PerkinElmer Life Sciences, formerly Wallac Oy; and HTRF supplied by Packard) use binding partners labeled with a lanthanide as the donor molecule, although in HTRF the europium is in the form of a cryptate rather than a chelate (Mathis, 1993). Figure 6 shows the generic form of a LANCE kinase assay. A biotinylated peptide representing the specific phosphorylation site for the target kinase is first phosphorylated in an enzymatic reaction. Then a europium-labeled phospho-specific antibody is added at the same time as a streptavidin-allophycocyanin conjugate. These two reagents bind to their partners, which are phosphorylated peptide and biotin, respectively. When excited with light at the appropriate wavelength (340 nm), the emission produced by europium (615 nm) is transferred to allophycocyanin and emitted at a wavelength of 665 nm, but only when the two labels are in close proximity. The signal emitted from the allophycocyanin retains the long half-life of the europium donor molecule and thus the advantages of TRF are maintained. However, as the test compound has not been removed by washing, quenching of light (either excitation or emission) is possible. Inclusion of an external or internal control may be used to correct for these effects. The relative merits of HTRF and LANCE (Hemmila, 1999; Mathis, 1999) and different assay formats (Hemmila and Webb, 1997) have been discussed previously. In addition to kinase assays (Park *et al.*,1999), TR-FRET assays in

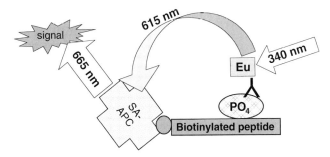

FIGURE 6 The principle of a generic kinase assay using time-resolved fluorescence energy transfer.

96- and 384-well plates have been widely applied to a range of drug discovery targets, including helicase (Earnshaw *et al.,* 1999), ubiquitin transfer (Boisclair *et al.,* 2000), interferon-γ (Enomoto *et al.,* 2000), and the binding of p53/HDM2 (Kane *et al.,* 2000).

2. Fluorescence Polarization

As evidenced by the number of papers published, there has been a marked increase in the use of fluorescence polarization (FP) for HTS in the last 4–5 years. This follows the much earlier success of FP for small-molecule immunoassays, particularly those for therapeutic drug monitoring. FP is a single-label, homogeneous assay format that is fast, sensitive, and relatively resistant to interference from other components present in the assay mix. Compared to other assay types, FP is also relatively inexpensive. The use of FP for HTS has recently been reviewed (Owicki, 2000). The technique depends on the depolarization of a fluorescently labeled small molecule when it binds to a larger molecule. Polarization is a function of rotational movements of molecules that are excited by plane-polarized light, and binding to a large molecule will slow the rotation of small molecular fluorescent probes. Thus, FP assays rely on the difference in molecular size between the fluorophore and its binding partner. More unusually, assays can be configured to measure the breakdown of a large labeled molecule into smaller fragments. FP assays have been applied to a wide range of targets applicable to drug discovery in the cancer arena. Examples include assays for targets such as protein kinases (Seethala and Menzel, 1998; Wu *et al.,* 2000), proteases (Levine *et al.,* 1997), the interaction of cyclin-dependent kinase 2 with cyclin E (Pin *et al.,* 1999), Src SH3 and SH2 domain binding (Lynch *et al.,* 1997), and nuclear receptor ligand binding (Parker *et al.,* 2000).

C. Luminescence

Chemiluminescence has been used for many years as a sensitive end point for numerous analytical applications. These include the measurement of ATP by the luciferase enzyme reaction and the application of a variety of chemiluminescent labels for immunoassay. It is not surprising, therefore, that this type of assay has been exploited for the development of high-throughput assays (Lackey, 1998). In addition, two novel technologies and associated dedicated equipment have been developed specifically for HTS. The Origen system (IGEN) is based on the use of electrochemiluminescence (Bruno, 1997)—the process by which light is generated when a low voltage is applied to an electrode triggering a cyclical oxidation–reduction reaction of a ruthenium metal ion. This sensitive, versatile, and user-friendly detection system is being increasingly applied to HTS. For exam-

ple, an electrochemiluminescent assay has been evaluated to identify inhibitors of the interaction between granulocyte colony-stimulating factor (G-CSF) and its receptor (Gopalakrishnan *et al.,* 2000).

The recent introduction of AlphaScreen technology (Packard) provides an additional option for system-based HTS. This format depends on the illumination by laser light of donor beads, which converts ambient oxygen to singlet-state oxygen. If an acceptor bead containing chemiluminescent molecules is in close proximity to the donor bead (by virtue of a biological interaction), reaction with the activated oxygen molecules produces a signal the energy of which is immediately transferred to fluorescent acceptor molecules in the same bead. This is another example of a mix-and-measure assay, with the long-lived signal also being subjected to TR measurement. The amplified signal and low background allows high sensitivity suitable for miniaturized assays.

D. Cell-Based Assays

As an alternative to biochemical screens, cell-based assays play an important role in mechanism-based HTS for the identification of novel inhibitors of specific gene products (Stockwell *et al.,* 1999; Workman, 1997). Primarily they can be used in a manner analogous to a screen in a genetically tractable system such as yeast (Munder and Hinnen, 1999), where the phenotypic consequences of mutations are used to identify genes and to order them in particular pathways. For example, a cell-based drug screen with a particular cellular readout could identify a small molecule that blocks the function of a gene product at any point on the pathway affecting that readout.

The advantages of cell-based screens in comparison with biochemical screens are as follows: (1) Hits may be identified for more than one target on the pathways that affect the specific readout. (2) Cell-based assays could allow the identification of previously unknown targets that lie on that pathway. (3) In contrast to compounds identified in biochemical screens, by definition active compounds, have cell permeable properties. In addition, cell-based approaches allow ligand interaction in the appropriate biological milieu of the target. However, one major challenge of the cell-based drug screen is the requirement for deconvolution of the assay so that the molecular target of each hit can be identified. This is necessary so that the compounds can be optimized through structure–activity relationship (SAR) strategies to improve potency against that particular target. The key is to set up a series of assays after the initial cell-based screen that can delineate the action of the compounds in the cell. Compounds can also be submitted to the NCI for COMPARE analysis (Monks *et al.,* 1997) in which activity against a panel of 60 human tumor cell lines is compared with that of other anticancer agents. In addition, the ability to correlate gene expression and drug activity patterns using gene expression microarray analysis may facilitate the identification of mode of action (Clarke *et al.*, 2000; Scherf *et al.*, 2000).

On a practical note, the necessity of producing and purifying large amounts of enzymatically active recombinant proteins for biochemical screens is avoided. On the other hand, it is frequently necessary to produce stably transfected cell lines for cell-based screening (Stratowa *et al.*, 1999). In addition, the costs of cell culture and the need for maintaining cell lines in good condition during high-throughput operations are also important considerations. For cancer targets, the choice of cell line is critical as it may be necessary to screen or counterscreen against two or more cell lines, e.g., isogenic cell line pairs or normal versus tumor cells. In this way it may be possible to distinguish between compounds that affect the intended pathway at a specific point rather than those that have general cytotoxic or antimetabolite effects.

Two types of cell-based screens are commonly used. The first involves the use of reporter gene–based screens, which are very popular. In such assays, expression of a gene for a protein that is readily quantifiable, e.g., luciferase or green fluorescent protein, is linked to an appropriate promoter gene for a component of the pathway under investigation. Compounds that turn gene expression on or off by interacting with targets located upstream can be readily identified. Chemiluminescent reporter gene assays using a variety of substrates (Olesen *et al.*, 2000) provide several advantages over fluorescent or colorimetric end points, including high sensitivity coupled with simple and high-throughput assays. Examples of reporter gene approaches to screening have been described for identification of inhibitors of Mek (Favata *et al.*, 1996), p53 (Komarov *et al.*, 1999), protein kinase C (Sharif and Sharif, 1999), histone deacetylase (Su *et al.*, 2000) and activators of the G-CSF receptor (Tian *et al.*, 1998).

The second, increasingly used approach to cell-based screening depends on the immunologic detection of a specific protein or posttranslational modification, e.g., phosphorylation or acetylation. These cell-based ELISAs can be conveniently carried out on cells grown, treated, fixed, and permeabilized in microtiter plates (96, 384, or 1536 formats) and have been referred to as cytoblots (Stockwell *et al.*, 1999). This strategy has been successfully applied to the identification of G_2 checkpoint inhibitors (Roberge *et al.*, 1998) and antimitotic agents (Mayer *et al.*, 1999; Roberge *et al.*, 2000).

Other forms of cell-based assays utilize cells with known genetic alterations or those that have been transfected with the gene of interest and depend on the measurement of viability following the addition of test compounds. Several assays to measure viability as a screening end point have been used. These include variations of the MTT assay (Stratowa *et al.*, 1999) and the measurement of cellular ATP using the luciferase/luciferin reaction (Petty *et al.*, 1995).

4. Assay Performance and Downstream Evaluation of Hits

The quality of the hits identified through screening depends in part on the performance of the assay used. As screening is largely carried out using single determinations, the capacity of a screen to confidently identify the compounds with biological activity is paramount. Confidence in the screen is reinforced if known inhibitors show the expected activity, and these are often used for quality control during assay validation and screening. If known inhibitors or model compounds are not available, as with a totally novel target, assay quality control relies on measures of total activity and nonspecific background, usually incorporated on each plate. Reproducibility (e.g., precision across a plate), a prime determinant of assay quality, should be as low as possible, but a coefficient of variation (% CV) of about 10% or less is acceptable. However, the signal-to-background (S/B) or, more correctly, the signal-to-noise (S/N) ratio is more important than reproducibility. This parameter takes into account both the reproducibility of the end-point measurement and the size of the window between total activity and background signals. There are several methods for determining assay S/N, all of which consider the statistical variation in signal measurement. Recently, a screening window coefficient, the Z factor, has been defined that provides a useful and widely accepted tool for evaluating assay performance (Zhang *et al.*, 1999).

Overall hit rates of 0.1–1% are usual, depending on the nature of the library screened and the concentration at which compounds are screened. Once compounds have been defined as hits in the primary screen it is necessary to carry out additional tests to confirm activity. It is standard practice to confirm activity by retesting hits in the same primary screening format. Unfortunately, all screening will result in false positives. These can be eliminated by using appropriate control assays and by employing alternative, often established methods for the desired target. Concentration–response curves are normally carried out on confirmed hits in order to define an IC_{50} (concentration causing 50% inhibition) as a measure of potency.

Further characterization of hits is also required to gain a preliminary understanding of the extent of selectivity toward the target. Confirmed hits thus need to be cross-screened using assays for closely related as well as unrelated targets. High-quality information on the properties of hits, including mode or action assays (Fig. 2), allows the selection of high-quality, progressible leads for further chemical optimization. It is important to select the best and most "drugable" compounds for further medicinal chemistry and to be prepared to drop those with undesirable physicochemical or biological properties at an early stage.

5. Compounds for HTS

The purpose of HTS is usually to define a hit that is active on the target and that can then be converted by chemical optimization to a genuine lead (with appropriate potency and selectivity) and in turn to a candidate for clinical development. Finding such a candidate in primary screening is very unusual. The chance of finding appropriate leads is greatly enhanced by screening against large numbers of diverse compounds.

Collections containing large numbers of compounds exist throughout the pharmaceutical industry as well as in the academic community. For their owners these collections are a valuable resource to be used alongside HTS to identify chemical leads for novel drug discovery. The big pharmaceutical company collections have the advantage that they contain many compounds with established activity against one or more protein targets: the accompanying database of structure–activity, structure–toxicity, and pharmacokinetic properties is also likely to be available. However, it is obvious that the collections differ markedly from each other since they represent (at least in part) the historical record of the unique chemical approaches the various centers have adopted over their years of existence. Some pharmaceutical collections will therefore be enriched in benzodiazepines and others in β-lactams or steroids, to take just three examples of common pharmacophores.

For many of the newer protein targets there is no obvious chemical starting point prior to screening. The ideal strategy would therefore be to have access to compounds with a highly diverse set of chemical structural types. It is also important to include several diverse examples of each type since subtle SAR effects are so common in drug discovery. Companies have therefore sought to increase the size and diversity of their discovery collections by acquisition of compound collections from nonpharmaceutical research centers. Such compounds include natural products (Harvey, 1999; Strohl, 2000), agrochemicals, dyestuffs, and photographic compounds. Nonpharmaceutical sources include universities and commercial catalogues of compounds.

It is noteworthy that the compounds from some of these nonpharmaceutical sources have no track record of bioactivity and that they represent a finite resource. Also, some of the compounds will have unfavorable characteristics, such as those that are highly charged or highly reactive. Detergent-like compounds, Michael acceptors, alkylating agents, and other known toxic entities are therefore normally excluded, thereby reducing the number of false positives identified in screens (Rishton, 1997).

Combinatorial chemistry (Floyd et al., 1999) has provided a means for rapid expansion of the size of screening collections. The concept was first applied to peptides using mix–split technology to prepare rapidly all the possible combinations of oligopeptides from a defined set of amino acids. For example, from 20 distinct amino acids there are 400 possible dipeptides, 8000 tripeptides, 160,000 tetrapeptides, and 3.2 million pentapeptides. It has been clearly demonstrated that hits can be found from such combinatorial libraries.

Bioactive hits are not always the best starting point for chemical optimization projects leading to clinical drug candidates, and simple peptides have become notorious for their lack of optimal pharmacokinetic properties. Drug discovery researchers have become aware that numbers and diversity are necessary but not sufficient. Experience has shown that possession of "drugable" or "drug-like" properties is hugely important. In particular, there is a new emphasis on selecting compounds whose physical properties are compatible with good pharmacokinetic behavior. Lipinski conducted a survey of the physicochemical characteristics of successful drugs and found that more than 80% conformed to his "rule of 5": namely, have molecular weight less than 500, fewer than 5 hydrogen bond donors, fewer than 10 hydrogen bond donors and acceptors, and clog P less than 5 (Lipinski et al., 1997). These are useful empirical criteria to assess a collection; compounds with one or more violations are increasingly less likely to perform well in vivo.

Mix–split technology can be extended beyond peptides to prepare combinatorial libraries of drug-like small molecules. Library designs can be assessed in silico and revised until they meet computed criteria such as Lipinski's rule of 5, as well as various chemical diversity parameters. By these means large collections can be assembled and used to identify novel chemical leads suitable for optimization. For example, Pharmacopeia claims to have built a collection of more than 6 million compounds in about 150 libraries, to have identified hits against novel and difficult targets, and to have optimized several of these to meet stringent preclinical selection criteria (Li and Guo, 2000).

Screening capability has increased dramatically in recent years, and it is now not an unrealistic goal to screen millions of compounds against any particular target in a relatively short period of time. Information technology therefore is critical at all stages of the drug discovery process, from the registration of compounds, through the laboratory management of large numbers of samples and plates, to the recording of data. It is also imperative to develop better methods to mine information from the huge amounts of data and to use all available information to improve pharmacophore and library design. For example, the concept of virtual drug discovery (Leach and Hann, 2000) relies extensively on chemoinformatics and bioinformatics to predict structures of novel inhibitors. Once synthesized these compounds are screened and the results used for further rounds of computation, synthesis, and screening to refine the desired properties.

Some have argued that ultra-HTS is wasteful and unnecessary, and that it is preferable to screen smaller numbers of "high-quality compounds." Certainly the case is strong for aiming at the highest possible "quality" for collections, assuming this means taking full account of all available information (e.g., protein structure, class of target, prior art for successful pharmacophores) and designing libraries accordingly. Also, "me-too" approaches, in which analogues of known active agents are prepared, have been successful, and it is not always essential to have a totally novel lead. This means that opportunity exists for smaller organizations that may simply not have the resources to achieve high throughputs, especially for protein targets of well-studied classes. However, it is hard to avoid the conclusion that the ideal approach is a combination of smart design, large diversity and large collections, especially if the object is a novel, patentable lead for a difficult target.

6. Examples of Compounds Identified Through Screening Approaches

The quality and number of mechanism-based compounds that progress to clinical trial is the measure by which the success of HTS approaches to new drug discovery will ultimately be gauged. It is probably too soon to pass judgment on the impact HTS has had on the anticancer drug development process. Although the properties of a number of interesting compounds have been described and several have reached the clinical evaluation phase of development, there are undoubtedly others in the pipeline that have yet to be disclosed. The examples of mechanism-based compounds described in this section are far from exhaustive but are given to illustrate the power of HTS coupled to the use of robotic chemistry and subsequent analogue synthesis for the identification and optimization of lead compounds. It should be noted that HTS is often used in combination with structure-based approaches (e.g., using information from x-ray crystallography and NMR). The examples exemplify the use of both biochemical and cell-based screens. Firstly, the development of potent receptor tyrosine kinase inhibitors that are presently being successfully evaluated in the clinic will be given. Examples will also be described wherein screening has identified proof of principle probes suitable for further target validation studies and/or optimization of chemical properties for potential clinical evaluation.

A. Tyrosine Kinase Inhibitors

The protein tyrosine kinases play an important role in cellular signaling pathways, and there is extensive, compelling evidence that implicates this class of enzymes in the oncogenic process (Strawn and Shawver, 1998). Not surprisingly, they have received a great deal of attention as targets for mechanism-based drug discovery. As discussed in the preceding sections, many different types of screen for identifying kinase inhibitors have been described. The development of inhibitors of the kinase activity of the EGF receptor pro-

vides a good example of how modern approaches, such as HTS and robotic synthesis, can be used with more conventional modeling approaches to overcome inherent limitations of early leads (Workman, 2000a). The end product of this extensive effort is the 4-anilinoquinazoline ZD1839 (Iressa). This is a selective, ATP-competitive inhibitor of EGF receptor kinase, which blocks signaling pathways involved in the proliferation and survival of tumor cells. The compound causes reversible inhibition of the growth of EGF-dependent cancer cells in vitro, and significant growth delay following oral administration in a range of human tumor xenografts following oral administration has been reported (Woodburn et al., 1997). Following successful phase I/II trials in which the orally administered compound was shown to be well tolerated and to have promising clinical efficacy, phase III clinical trials are underway in a number of tumor types, including non-small cell lung cancer (Baselga and Averbuch, 2000).

STI-571 (CGP57148B) is perhaps the best example so far described of a selective molecularly targeted therapy. The compound inhibits the constitutive kinase activity of the bcr-abl oncoprotein present in 95% of patients with chronic myeloid leukemia (CML) and 30–50% of adult patients with acute lymphoblastic leukemia. Optimization of the selectivity and potency of kinase inhibitors identified by screening small-molecule libraries resulted in the selection of STI-571—a 2-phenylaminopyrimidine. This drug is a competitive inhibitor of ATP binding and a selective and potent growth inhibitor of cell lines and primary cultures derived from CML patients (Druker et al., 1996; Druker and Lydon, 2000). Activity without detectable systemic toxicity following oral administration was demonstrated in animal models (le Coutre et al., 1999), whereas no activity was observed in tumor models that were not dependent on the activity of the target kinase.

The results of phase I trials in chronic phase CML showed high and sustained hematologic response rates (96%) at doses above 300 mg/day without serious side effects. Major cytogenetic responses were achieved in about 45% of patients (Druker et al., 1999). Further clinical studies of CML and other hematologic malignancies are in progress, although response rates in advanced stages of CML appear to be lower and less durable than those reported for early-stage disease. Preclinically, STI-571 also has marked activity against other receptor tyrosine kinase receptors, e.g., platelet-derived growth factor (PDGF) receptor and c-kit (Buchdunger et al., 2000). Thus, evaluation of the agent is underway in patients with solid tumors in which these signaling molecules are deregulated (e.g., small cell lung cancer, gliomas, and certain sarcomas).

B. p53-Based Modulators

The tumor suppressor protein p53 (the "guardian of the genome") functions to protect cells from the effects of DNA damage or other stress signals either by initiating cell cycle arrest and DNA repair or, if repair is not possible, through induction of apoptosis. The *TP53* gene is lost or mutated in the majority of human tumors resulting in genomic instability, tumor progression, and resistance to radiotherapy and chemotherapy. The function of p53 is mediated by transcriptional activation through p53-specific binding sites on the promoter regions of a number of genes required for cell cycle arrest and apoptosis. Binding to DNA promoter sequences relies on the ability of the protein to maintain the correct DNA binding conformation, and this binding interaction is markedly reduced when p53 is mutated. Previous efforts to restore function to mutant p53 have involved the identification of synthetic peptides that interact with the mutant protein and promote DNA binding (Hupp *et al.,* 1997). A 22-mer peptide that corresponds to the carboxy-terminal amino acid residues 361–382 of p53 induced growth inhibition and apoptosis in cell lines expressing mutant p53 (Selivanova *et al.,* 1997). This approach to therapy in mutant p53 tumors has been reviewed (Selivanova *et al.,* 1998). The pharmacologic limitations of peptides are well known.

An alternative strategy has been described to identify small molecules that facilitate the correct folding of mutant p53 so that interaction with DNA is restored (Foster *et al.,* 1999). A library of more than 100,000 compounds were screened in an innovative assay in which the expression of an epitope for a monoclonal antibody (mAb1620) was lost when the DNA binding domain of wild-type p53 was immobilized on microtiter plates and heated. Approximately 300 compounds that stabilized the conformation of the wild-type binding domain, as well as of the full-length protein, were identified. Subsequently it was found that mutant DNA binding domains that retained the epitope for mAb1620 were also stabilized by these compounds. Active compounds were 300–500 Da and had general structural features that included a hydrophobic group joined by a linker of defined length to an ionizable group.

The cellular activity of these compounds on the conformational stability of p53 was evaluated using a p53 null cell line transfected with mutant protein. After treatment with one of the compounds (CP-31398) there was a fivefold increase in immunoreactivity using mAb1620, indicating a marked increase in protein with corrected conformation. In addition, this compound also enhanced the level of the mAb1620 epitope in tumors treated *in vivo.* A p53-inducible luciferase reporter gene assay showed that CP-31398 restored transcriptional activity to mutant p53 protein, and stabilized p53 protein was also capable of activating expression of the gene for p21, a relevant downstream effector. Importantly, multiple doses of CP-31398 to tumor-bearing animals showed impressive antitumor activity, although as expected regrowth of tumor occurred when treatment was stopped. This series of experiments has elegantly demonstrated the possibility that

following further rounds of structure activity studies, potent and effective agents that restore the function of mutant p53 protein can be developed. In view of the frequency of p53 mutations in human tumors, these agents have the potential to exhibit a broad spectrum of activity.

In contrast to efforts designed to reactivate p53 function, a novel approach has been to identify inhibitors of p53 function. Normal tissues that express wild-type p53 are sensitive to the effects of irradiation and chemotherapeutic agents producing unwanted and severe side effects of treatment, limiting antitumor activity. In the context of treatment of a tumor containing mutant (nonfunctional) p53 activity, inhibition of p53 in normal tissues would result in an increased therapeutic index. To test the feasibility of this novel approach, a screen that measured the expression of a reporter gene under the control of a p53-responsive promoter was used to obtain proof of principle molecules (Komarov *et al.,* 1999). Using a diverse library consisting of 10,000 chemicals, compounds that abrogated the expression of the reporter gene in the presence of the DNA damaging agent doxorubicin were identified. Those active compounds that did not effect cell growth or survival were further identified and one of these, pifithrin-α, was chosen for further study. This compound inhibited cell death following a number of different DNA-damaging agents. Its effects were reversible and, importantly, the agent protected normal mice from the effects of irradiation whereas p53 null mice were not similarly protected. The availability of pifithrin-α will allow other mechanistic studies on the protection of normal tissues following a variety of stress-promoting treatments, but its clinical effectiveness (or that of related analogues) remains to be tested.

C. Novel Mitotic Inhibitors

The currently available antimitotic drugs, such as the taxanes and *Vinca* alkaloids, are known to interact with tubulin. Attempts to identify other small-molecule inhibitors of mitosis have used cell-free tubulin assays (Davis and Middleton, 1999) or have been identified by COMPARE analysis from the comparative activity of compounds submitted for testing in the 60-cell-line tumor panel at the NCI (Paull *et al.,* 1992). Compounds affecting nontubulin molecular targets involved in the control of mitosis would be of considerable mechanistic interest and potential therapeutic value. In an interesting development, a chemical genetic approach to screening using a cell-based ELISA (Stockwell *et al.,* 1999) was used to identify the compound monastrol, which caused mitotic arrest in mammalian cells. In the primary screen an antibody to phosphorylated nucleolin was used to identify cells in which compounds had induced mitotic arrest. Increased levels of nucleolin phosphorylation were shown following exposure to 139 compounds from a library of more than 16,000 structurally diverse chemicals (Mayer *et al.,* 1999). In a secondary screen, 86 of the active compounds had no effect on *in vitro* tubulin polymerization and were presumed to target other proteins involved in mitosis. Only five of these compounds specifically altered the mitotic phenotype with no observable effects on microtubules, actin filaments, or chromatin in interphase cells. The 1,4-dihydropyrimidine-based compound monastrol was chosen for further study and in a series of experiments it was shown that monastrol specifically inhibited the motility of the mitotic kinesin Eg5. This study convincingly demonstrated the versatility of the cytoblot approach to screening and also identified a compound that can be used not only as a tool to dissect the function of Eg5 in mitosis and other cellular processes, but also to identify lead compounds for future anticancer drug development.

D. Ras Pathway Inhibitors

Numerous biochemical screens have been described for the identification of specific inhibitors of enzymes in the Ras to Erk signal transduction pathway, which is frequently deregulated in cancer. For example, PD-098059, a noncompetitive inhibitor of Mek, was identified using a cell-free mitogen-activated protein (MAP) kinase cascade assay with phosphorylation of MBP as a readout (Alessi *et al.,* 1995; Dudley *et al.,* 1995). The compound has since been widely used as a pharmacologic tool to probe the role of the MAP kinase pathway in various cellular contexts, and further lead optimization has led to the synthesis of PD-184352, a highly potent and selective orally administered Mek inhibitor (Sebolt-Leopold *et al.,* 1999). Promising *in vivo* antitumor activity against human colon tumor xenografts with minimal host toxicity was accompanied by reduced levels of Erk phosphorylation in excised tumor. These results provide compelling evidence for the clinical evaluation of this agent.

In contrast to compounds identified through biochemical cascade screens, the Mek inhibitor U0126 and some less potent analogues were identified from a total of 40,000 compounds in a cell-based reporter screen designed to identify inhibitors of AP-1 transactivation (Favata *et al.,* 1998). The action of U0126 as a specific Mek inhibitor was determined in a series of "deconvolution" assays. Counterscreening showed that U0126 was inactive in reporter assays driven by elements other than AP1. The compound did not disrupt AP1-DNA binding, and Western blot analysis of Fos and Jun (which compose the AP1 transcription factor complex) showed that U0126 blocked up-regulation of their expression. In addition, cellular activation of Erk but not Raf or Mek (components of the Ras signaling pathway that can induce expression of Fos and Jun) was blocked by U0126. Lastly, biochemical assays using recombinant Erk and Mek showed that Mek was directly inhibited *in vitro*. U0126 provides another useful pharmacologic probe for investigating the cellular consequences of inhibiting Mek and hence the Ras pathway in different cellular backgrounds.

7. Future HTS Developments

The evolution of HTS as a tool for drug discovery has occurred relatively quickly but not without considerable investment. It will not be surprising if the ultra-HTS capabilities that are being implemented today soon will be surpassed. HTS is always in a state of transition as improvements in technology and the development of novel instrumentation is an ongoing and inevitable process linked to innovations in other scientific disciplines. The motivation to drive toward an ever larger, faster, sensitive, and cheaper screening capability will continue, but it is debatable whether this is necessary. Although cost is an important consideration, it is argued by some that current capacity using 1536-well plates will be adequate to meet the foreseeable screening requirements of most organizations. Miniaturization (which is essentially a cost-cutting exercise) even to the level of 1536 plates brings with it problems associated with compound transfer, liquid handling, and the need for faster signal detection. These problems have been addressed by the introduction of nanotechnology, i.e., equipment capable of precise and accurate compound and reagent handling at nanoliter volumes, and the use of format-independent imagers utilizing cooled couple device (CCD) cameras for signal detection. Microfluidic devices which rely on flow injection using minute amounts of reagents for both biochemical and cell-based screens is one example of an alternative type of format (Sundberg, 2000).

The arguments for and against further miniaturization have been documented (Burbaum, 2000; Knapp *et al.,* 2000). The individual demands and resources of different types of organizations will ultimately dictate the type and scale of screening undertaken. Library design and virtual screening *in silico* resulting in the use of "smart" libraries especially in the hit-to-lead process may reduce the requirement for screening extremely large unstructured libraries in the future (Leach and Hann, 2000), thus reducing the need for further miniaturization and automation.

Conventional HTS for drug discovery has been complemented by recent approaches collectively termed "chemical genetics" (Crews and Splittgerber, 1999; Mitchison, 1994). Libraries of peptides or compounds are used to probe and dissect the function of proteins in much the same way as genetic mutations are used. The screens for inhibitors of mitosis and p53 function described earlier in this review are essentially examples of this approach (Komarov *et al.,* 1999; Mayer *et al.,* 1999) as are reporter gene assays (Su *et al.,* 2000). Other examples include the use of yeast cells (Munder and Hinnen, 1999) and zebrafish development screens (Peterson *et al.,* 2000) to identify molecules that specifically modulate aspects of cellular function or development.

Another fascinating approach used genetic selection coupled to a high-throughput ELISA screen to identify inhibitors of a specific protein–protein interaction (Park and Raines, 2000). Another interesting chemical genetic strategy involves the identification of potent and selective inhibitors of enzymes by sensitizing protein kinases to chemicals that do not inhibit wild-type kinases (Bishop *et al.*, 2000).

8. Concluding Remarks

The sequencing of the human genome, coupled with our increasingly detailed understanding of the molecular pathology of human cancers, offers an unprecedented opportunity for innovative drug discovery. The new molecular targets, which are currently being discovered and progressed, cover all aspects of the natural history of cancer progression, including self-sufficiency in proliferation signals, aberrant cell cycle control, evasion of apoptosis, induction of drug resistance, acquisition of limitless growth potential, and the induction of angiogenesis, invasion, and metastasis (Hanahan and Weinberg, 2000). Discovery of drugs acting on the molecular players that drive these critical processes should lead to therapies that are more effective and less toxic than current approaches (Workman, 2000a,b, 2001). The exciting vision that we can work toward is the discovery of a mechanism-based therapeutic for every major molecular abnormality responsible for human malignancy and the use of these in individualized cocktails according to the genetic makeup of the particular tumor. This is the major experiment that now needs to be done, linking the completion of genome sequencing (both normal and cancer genomes) to the development of better therapies for the long-term control or cure of cancers. It may seem that we are a long way from completing this experiment, but there are instances in which we are tantalizingly close. The regulatory approval of herceptin for erbB2-positive breast cancer is the first example of a genome-based cancer medicine, and agents such as STI-571, Iressa (discussed earlier), and the new angiogenesis inhibitors, such as the VEGF receptor tyrosine kinase inhibitors, appear extremely promising.

The challenge now is to move these ideas forward as quickly and efficiently as possible. The up side is the avalanche of potential targets emerging from genomics, but the down side is that we know that the attrition rate of drugs entering clinical trial is likely to be as high as 90%, i.e., 1 success in 10 during clinical development. Moreover, progression from target to drug has usually taken 15 years or more—we need to reduce this to 5 years or less. To achieve this we can use our toolbox of new technologies, including combinatorial chemistry, microarray technology, proteomics, structural biology, and, of course, HTS.

Mechanism-based screening against a chosen molecular target or pathway is particularly valuable because the end product is a therapy that should be selective and effective against a process believed to be driving the disease. The risk is that the chosen target, though present in the cancer, is not in fact a rate-limiting factor in disease progression. This is why target validation is so important. Alternatively, if the minimal validation option is selected for speed and competitiveness, it will be necessary to run with a large number of molecular targets and pursue those that work best. If the clinical trials are carried out correctly and imaginatively with appropriate use of biomarkers and pharmacodynamic end points, the drug molecule can represent a clinical hypothesis test of the target, as well as an evaluation of the drug itself.

The drug discovery and development process is inherently a high-risk enterprise. Drugs can fail at all points in the preclinical and discovery process. Failure not only may be due to the selection of an inappropriate target, as mentioned previously, but also may involve technical reasons, e.g., inability to find a hit, inability to optimize a lead, or problems with pharmacokinetics, metabolism, or toxicity. It is crucial to make the best possible judgments about the likely best targets and then to progress these rapidly and in parallel, making the painful decisions about priority in light of the available resources and ensuring that when projects fail, they fail as intelligently, as fast, and as cheaply as possible. It is important to remember that when a lead compound fails in its primary purpose as a drug, it can nevertheless succeed as a valuable biochemical probe.

There is long history of drug screening in cancer. Blackbox screening against whole cancer cells has given us most of our currently useful but limited agents. The NCI 60-cell panel screening operation represents an upgrade of traditional cell screening with the potential to build in a molecular mechanistic component (Scherf *et al.*, 2000). Intelligent screening against specific molecular targets represents a major step forward in the race for more selective anticancer agents (Workman, 1997, 2000a,b, 2001). It should provide us with the rapier in place of the blunderbuss. Thus, mechanism-based HTS is centrally positioned as a key technology in postgenomic cancer drug discovery.

References

Allesi, D. R., Cohen, P., Ashworth, A., Cowley, S., Leevers, S. J., and Marshall, C. J. (1995). Assay and expression of mitogen-activated protein kinase, MAP kinase kinase and Raf. *Methods Enzymol.* **225,** 279–290.

Antonsson, B., Marshall, C. J., Montessuit, S., and Arkinstall, S. (1999). An *in vitro* 96-well plate assay of the mitogen-activated protein kinase cascade. *Anal. Biochem.* **267,** 294–299.

Archer, R. (1999). Faculty or factory? Why industrializing drug discovery is inevitable. *J. Biomol. Screening* **4,** 235–237.

Asthagiri, A. R., Horwitz, A. F., and Lauffenburger, D. A. (1999). A rapid and sensitive quantitative kinase activity assay using a convenient 96-well format. *Anal. Biochem.* **269,** 342–347.

Baselga, J., and Averbuch, S. D. (2000). ZD1839 ('Iressa') as an anticancer agent. *Drugs 2000* **60**(Suppl.1), 33–40.

Beveridge, M., Park, Y-W., Hermes, J., Marenghi, A., Brophy, G., and Santos, A. (2000). Detection of p56[ick] kinase activity using scintillation proximity assay in 384-well format and imaging proximity assay in 384- and 1536-well format. *J. Biomol. Screening* **5**, 205–211.

Bishop, A. C., Ubersax, J. A., Petsch, D. T., Matheos, D. P., Gray, N. S., Blethrow, J., Shimizu, E., Tsien, J. Z., Schultz, P. G., Rose, M. D., Wood, J. L., Morgan, D. O., and Shokat, K. M. (2000), A chemical switch for inhibitor-sensitive alleles of any protein kinase. *Nature* **407**, 395–401.

Bishop, W. R., Bond, R., Petrin, J., Wang, L., Patton, R., Doll, R., Njoroque, G., Catino, J., Schwartz, J., Windsor, W., Syto, R., Carr, D., James, L., and Kirschmeier, P. (1996). Novel tricyclic inhibitors of farnesyl protein transferase. *J. Biol. Chem.* **270**, 30611–30618.

Braunwalder, A. F., Yarwood, D. R., Hall, A., Missbach, M., Lipson, K. E., and Sills, M. A. (1996). A solid-phase assay for the determination of protein tyrosine kinase activity of c-src using scintillating microtitration plates. *Anal. Biochem.* **234**, 23–26.

Bruno, J. G. (1997). Broad applications of electrochemiluminescence technology to the detection and quantitation of microbiological, biochemical and chemical analytes. *Rec. Res. Dev. Micro.* **1**, 25–46.

Boisclair, M. D., McClure, C., Josiah, S., Glass, S., Bottomley, S., Kamerkas, S, and Hemmilä, I. (2000). Development of a ubiquitin transfer assay for high throughput screening by fluorescence resonance energy transfer. *J. Biomol. Screening* **5**, 319–329.

Bottger, V., Bottger, A., Howard, S. F., Picksley, S. M., Chene, P., Garcia-Echeverria, C., Hochkeppel, H. K., and Lane, D. P. (1997). Identification of novel mdm2 binding peptides by phage display. *Oncogene* **13**, 2141–2147.

Buchdunger, E., Cioffi, C. L., Law, N., Stover, D., Ohno-Jones, S., Druker, B. J., and Lydon, N. B. (2000). Abl protein-tyrosine kinase inhibitor ST1571 inhibits in vitro signal transduction mediated by c-kit and platelet-derived growth factor receptors. *J. Pharmacol. Exp. Ther.* **295**, 139–145.

Burbaum, J. J. (2000). The evolution of miniaturized well plates, *J. Biomol Screening* **5**, 5–8.

Chen, Y. N., Sharma, S. K., Ramsey, T. M., Jiang, L., Martin, M. S., Baker, K., Adams, P. D., Bair, K. W., and Kaelin, W. G. Jr. (1999). Selective killing of transformed cells by cyclin/cyclin-dependent kinase 2 antagonists. *Proc. Natl. Acad. Sci. USA* **96**, 4325–4329.

Cheung, A., and Zhang, J. (2000). A scintillation proximity assay for poly(ADP-ribose) polymerase. *Anal. Biochem.* **282**, 24–28.

Clarke, P. A., Hostein, I., Banerji, U., Di Stefano, F., Maloney, A., Walton, M., Judson I., and Workman, P. (2000). Gene expression profiling of human colon cancer cells following inhibition of signal transduction by 17-allylamino-17-demethoxygeldanamycin, an inhibitor of the hsp90 molecular chaperone. *Oncogene* **19**, 4125–4133.

Cogan, E. B., Birrell, G. B., and Hayes Griffith, O. (1999). A robotics-based automated assay for inorganic and organic phosphates. *Anal. Biochem.* **271**, 29–35.

Cook, N. D. (1996). Scintillation proximity assay: a versatile high-throughput screening technology. *Drug Discovery Today* **1**, 287–293.

Crews, C. M., and Splittgerber, U. (1999), Chemical genetics; exploring and controlling cellular processes with chemical probes. *TIBS* **24**, 317–320.

Davis, A., and Middleton, K. M. (1999). A system for high through-put screening for tubulin and microtubule ligands with anticancer properties. *Proc. Am. Assoc. Cancer Res.* **40**, 406.

Drews, J. (1996). Genomic sciences and the medicine of tomorrow. *Nat. Biotechnol.* **14**, 1518–1519.

Druker, B. J., Tamura, S., Buchdunger, E., Ohno, S., Segal, G. M., Fanning, S., Zimmerman, J., and Lydon, N. B. (1996). Effects of a selective inhibitor of the Abl tyrosine kinase on the growth of Bcr-Abl positive cells. *Nat. Med.* **2**, 561–566.

Druker, B. J. Talpas, M., Resta, D., Peng., B., Buchdunger, E., and Ford, J. (1999). Clinical efficacy and safety of abl specific tyrosine kinase inhibitor as targeted therapy for chronic myelogenous leukaemia. *Blood* **94**(Suppl. 1), 368a.

Druker, B. J., and Lydon, N. B. (2000). Lessons learned from the development of an Abl tyrosine kinase inhibitor of chronic myelogenous leukaemia. *J. Clin. Invest.* **105**, 3–7.

Dudley, D. T., Pang, L., Decker, S. J., Bridges, A. J., and Saltiel, A. R. (1995). A synthetic inhibitor of the mitogen-activated protein kinase cascade. *Proc. Natl. Acad. Sci. USA* **92**, 7686–7689.

Dunn, D., Orlowski, M., McCoy, P., Gastgels, F., Appell, K., Ozqur, M., and Burbaum, J. (2000). Ultra-high throughput screen of two-million-member combinatorial compound collection in a miniaturized, 1536-well assay format. *J. Biomol. Screening* **5**, 177–187.

Earnshaw, D. L., Moore, K. J., Greenwood, C. J., Djaballah, H., Jurewicz, A. J., Murray, K. J., and Pope, A. J. (1999), Time-resolved fluorescence energy transfer DNA helicase assays for high throughput screening. *J. Biomol. Screening* **4**, 239–248.

Ellsmore, V. A., Teoh, A. P., and Ganesan, A. (1997). A high throughput enzyme-linked immunosorbent assay for inhibitors of the interaction between retinoblastoma protein and the Leu-X-Cys-Glu motif. *J. Biomo.. Screening* **2**, 207–211.

Enomoto, K., Aono, Y., Mitsugi, K., Takahashi, R., Suzuki, M., Préaudat, M., Mathis, G., Kominaui, G., and Takemoto, H. (2000). High throughput screening for human interferon-α production inhibitor using homogenous time-resolved fluorescence. *J. Biomol. Screening* **5**, 263–269.

Favata, M. F., Kurumi, Y. H., Manos, E. J., Daulerio, A. J., Stradley, D. A., Feeser, W. S., Van Dyk, D. E., Pitts, W. J., Earl, R. A., Hobbs, F., Copeland, R. A., Magolda, R. L., Scherle, P. A., and Trzaskos, J. M. (1998). Identification of a novel inhibitor of mitogen-activated protein kinase. *J. Biol. Chemistry* **29**, 18623–18632.

Floyd, C. D., LeBlanc, C., and Whittaker, M. (1999). Combinatorial chemistry as a tool for drug discovery. *In* "Progress in Medicinal Chemistry" (F. D. King and A. W. Oxford, eds.), Vol. 36, pp 91–167. Elsevier Science, B.V., New York.

Foster, B. A., Coffey, H. A., Morin, M. J., and Rastinejad, F. (1999). Pharmacological rescue of mutant p53 conformation and function. *Science* **286**, 2507–2510.

Gaarde, W. A., Hunter, T., Brady, H., Murray, B. W., and Goldman, M. E. (1997). Development of a nonradioactive, time-resolved fluorescence assay for the measurement of N-terminal kinase assay. *J. Biomol. Screening* **2**, 213–223.

Garrett, M. D., and Workman, P. (1999). Discovering novel chemotherapeutic drugs for the third millenium. *Eur. J. Cancer* **35**, 2010–2030.

Gelmon, K. A., Eisenhauer, E. A., Harris, A. L., Ratain, M. J., and Workman, P. (1999). Anticancer agents targeting signal molecules and cancer cell environment: Challenges for drug development? *J. Natl. Cancer Inst.* **91**, 1281–1287.

Gibbs, J. B. (2000). Anticancer drug targets: Growth factors and growth factor signaling. *J. Clin. Invest.* **105**, 9–13.

Gibbs, J. B., and Oliff, A. (1994). Pharmaceutical research in molecular oncology. *Cell* **79**, 193–198.

Gopalakrishnan, S. M., Warrior, U., Burns, D., and Groebe, D. R. (2000). Evaluation of electrochemiluminescent technology for inhibitors of granulocyte colony-stimulating factor receptor binding. *J. Biomol. Screening* **5**, 369–377.

Hanahan, D., and Weinberg, A. (2000). The hallmarks of cancer. *Cell* **100**, 57–70.

Harder, K. W., Owen, P., Wong L. K. H., Aebersold, R., Clark-Lewis, I., and Jirik, F. R. (1994). Characterisation and kinetic analysis of the intracellular domain of human protein tyrosine phosphatase β (HPTPβ) using synthetic phosphopeptides. *Biochem. J.* **298**, 395–401.

Harvey, A. L. (1999). Medicines from nature: are natural products still relevant to drug discovery? *Trends Pharmacol. Sci.* **20**, 196–198.

Hemmilä, I. (1999). LANCE™ : Homogeneous assay platform in HTS. *J. Biomol. Screening* **4**, 303–309.

Hemmilä, I., and Webb, S. (1997). Time-resolved fluorometry: an overview of the labels and core technologies for drug screening applications. *Drug Discovery Today* **2**, 373–381.

Henkel, R. D., Vandeberg, J. L., and Walsh, R. A. (1998). A microassay for ATPase. *Anal. Biochem.* **169**, 312–318.

Hupp, T. R., Sparks, A., and Lane, D. P. (1995). Small peptides activate the latent sequence-specific DNA binding function of p53. *Cell* **83**, 237–245.

Jackson, J. R., Gilmartin, A., Imburgia, C., Winkler, J. D., Marshall, L. A., and Roshak, A. (2000). An indolocarbazole inhibitor of human checkpoint kinase (Chk1) abrogates cell cycle arrest caused by DNA damage. *Cancer Res.* **60**, 566–572.

Kaelin, W. G., Jr. (1999). Choosing anticancer drug targets in the post genomic era. *J. Clin. Invest.* **104**, 1503–1506.

Kane, S. A., Fleener, C. A., Zhang, Y. S., Davis, L. J., Musselman, A. L., and Huang, P. S. (2000). Development of a binding assay for p53/HDM2 by using homogeneous time-resolved fluorescence. *Anal. Biochem.* **278**, 29–38.

Kelland, L. R., Sharp, S. Y., Rogers, P. M., Myers, T. G., and Workman, P. (1999). DT-diaphorase expression and tumor cell sensitivity to 17-allylamino, 17-demethoxygeldanamycin, an inhibitor of heat shock protein 90. *J. Natl. Cancer Inst.* **91**, 1940–1949.

Knapp, M. R., Sunberg, S., and Parce, J. W. (2000), Test tube's end. *J. Biomol Screening* **5**, 9–12.

Komarov, P. G., Komarov, E. A., Kondratou, R. V., Christou-Tselkou, K., Coon, J. S., Chemou, M. V., and Gudkov, A. V. (1999). A chemical inhibitor of p53 that protects mice from the side effects of cancer therapy. *Science* **285**, 1733–1737.

Lackey, D. B. (1998). A homogeneous chemiluminescent assay for telomerase. *Anal. Biochem.* **263**, 57–61.

Lane, D.(1998). The promise of molecular oncology. *Lancet* **351**, 17–20.

Leach, A. R., and Hann, M. M. (2000). The *in silico* world of virtual libraries. *Drug Discovery Today* **5**, 326–337.

le Coutre, P., Mologni, L., Cleris, L., Marchesi, E., Buchdunger, E., Giardini, R., Formelli, F., and Gambacorti-Passerini, C. (1999). *In vivo* eradication of human BCR/ABL-positive leukaemia cells with an ABL kinase inhibitor. *J. Natl. Cancer Inst.* **91**, 163–168.

Lerner, C. G., and Chiang Saiki, A. Y. (1996). Scintillation proximity assay for human DNA topisomerase I using recombinant biotinyl-fusion protein produced in baculovirus-infected insect cells. *Anal. Biochem.* **240**, 185–196.

Levine, L. M., Michener, M. L., Toth, M. V., and Holwerda, B. C. (1997). Measurement of specific protease activity utilizing fluorescent polarization. *Anal. Biochem.* **247**, 83–88.

Li, G., and Guo, T. (2000). ECLiPS™ technology for drug discovery. *In* "Frontiers of Biotechnology and Pharmaceuticals" (K. Zhao, J. Reiner, and S.-H. Chen, eds.), Vol. 1, pp. 150–163. Science Press, New York.

Lipinski, C. A., Lombardo, F., Dominy, B. W., and Feeney, P. J. (1997). Experimental and computational approaches to estimate solubility and permeability in drug discovery and development setting. *Ad. Drug. Del. Rev.* **23**, 3–25.

Lynch, B. A., Minor, C., Loiacono, K. A., van Schravendijk M. R., Ram, M. K., Sundaramoorthi, R., Adams, S. E., Phillips, T., Holt, D., Rickles, R. J., and MacNeil, I. A. (1997). Simultaneous assay of Src SH3 and SH2 domain binding using different wavelength fluorescence polarization probes. *Anal. Biochem.* **275**, 62–73.

Maffia, A. M., Kanu, I., and Oldenburg, K. R. (1999). Miniaturization of a mammalian cell-based assay: luciferase repeater gene readout in a 3 microlitre 1536-well plate. *J. Biomol. Screening* **4**, 137–143.

Mathis, G. (1993). Rare earth cryptates and homogenous fluorimmunoassays with human sera. *Clin. Chem.* **39**, 1953–1959.

Mathis, G. (1999). HTRF© technology. *J. Biomol. Screening* **4**, 309–315.

Mayer, T. U., Kapoor, T. M., Haggerty, S. J., King, R. W., Scheiber, S. L.,

and Mitchison, T. J. (1999). Small molecule inhibitor of mitotic spindle bipolarity identified in a phenotype-based screen. *Science* **286**, 971–974.

McDonald, O. B., Chen, W. J., Ellis, B., Hoffman, C., Overton, L., Rink, M., Smith, A., Marshall, C. J., and Wood, E. R. (1999). A scintillation proximity assay for the Raf/MEK/ERK kinase cascade: high-throughput screening and identification of selective enzyme inhibitors. *Anal. Biochem.* **268**, 318–329.

Mitchison, T. J. (1994). Towards a pharmacological genetics. *Chem. Biol.* **1**, 3–6.

Monks, A., Scudiero, D. A., Johnson, G. S., Paull, K. D., and Sausville, E. A. (1997). The NCI anti-cancer drug screen: a smart screen to identify effectors of novel targets. *Anticancer Drug Des.* **12**, 533–541.

Mullinax, T. R., Henrich, G., Kasila, P., Ahern, D. G., Wenske, E. A., Cuifen, H., Argentieri, D., and Bembenek, M. E. (1999). Monitoring inositol-specific phospholipase C activity using a phospholipid FlashPlate©. *J. Biomol. Screening* **4**, 151–155.

Munder, T., and Hinnen, A. (1999). Yeast cells as tools for target-oriented screening. *Appl. Microbiol. Biotechnol.* **52**, 311–320.

Nakayama, G. R., Nova, M. P., and Parandoosh, Z. (1998). A scintillating microplate assay for the assessment of protein kinase activity. *J. Biomol. Screening* **3**, 43–48.

Nare, B., Allocco, J. J., Kuningas, R., Galuska, S., Myers, R. W., Bednarek, M. A., and Schmatz, D. M. (1999). Development of a scintillation proximity assay for histone deacetylase using a biotinylated peptide derived from histone-H4. *Anal. Biochem.* **267**, 390–396.

Nature (2001). The human genome. **409**, 745–964.

Oldenburg, K. R., Zhang, J-h., Chen, T., Maffia, A., Blom, K. F., Combs, A. P., and Chung, T. D. K. (1998). Assay miniaturisation for ultra-high throughput screening of combinatorial and discrete compound libraries: a 9600-well (0.2 microlitre) assay system. *J. Biomol. Screening* **3**, 55–63.

Oldenburg, K. R. (1999). Automation basics: robotics vs workstations. *J. Biomol. Screening* **4**, 53–56.

Olesen, C. E., Martin, C. S., Mosier, J., Liu, B., Voyta, J. C., and Bronstein, I. (2000). Chemiluminescent reporter gene assays with 1,2-dioxetane enzyme substrates. *Methods Enzymol.* **305**, 428–450.

Owicki, J. C. (2000). Fluorescent polarization and anisotropy in high throughput screening: perspectives and primer. *J. Biomol. Screening* **5**, 297–307.

Panaretou, B., Prodromou, C., Roe, S. M., O'Brien, R., Ladbury, J. E., Piper, P. W., and Pearl, L. H. (1998). ATP binding and hydrolysis are essential to the function of the Hsp90 molecular chaperone in vivo. *EMBO J.* **17**, 4829–4836.

Park, S-H., and Raines, R. T. (2000). Genetic selection for dissociative inhibitors of designated protein–protein interactions. *Nat. Biotechnol.* **18**, 847–851.

Park, Y. W., Cummings, R. T., Wu, L., Zheng, S., Cameron, P. M., Woods, A., Zaller, D. M., Marcy, A. I., and Hermes, J. D. (1999). Homogeneous proximity tyrosine kinase assays: scintillation proximity assay versus homogeneous time-resolved fluorescence. *Anal. Biochem.* **269**, 94–104.

Park, S. Y., Park, S. H., Lee, Il-S., and Kong, J. Y. (2000). Establishment of a high-throughput screening system for caspase-3 inhibitors. *Arch. Pharm. Res.* **23**, 246–251.

Parker, G. J., Law, T. L., Lenoch, F. J., and Bolger, R. E. (2000). Development of high throughput screening assays using fluorescence polarization nuclear receptor-ligand-binding and kinase/phosphatase assays. *J. Biomol. Screening* **5**, 77–88.

Paull, K. D., Lui, C. M., Malspeis, L., and Hamel, E. (1992). Identification of novel antimitotic agents acting at the tubulin level by computer-assisted evaluation of differential cytotoxicity data. *Cancer Res.* **52**, 3892–3900.

Peterson, R. T., Link, B. A., Dowling, J. E., and Schreiber, S. L. (2000). Small molecule developmental screens reveal the logic and timing of vertebrate development. *Proc. Natl. Acad. Sci. USA* **97**, 12965–12969.

Petty, R. D., Sutherland, L. A., Hunter, E. M., and Cree, I. A. (1995). Comparison of MTT and ATP-based assays for the measurement of viable cell number. *J. Biolumin. Chemilumin.* **10,** 29–34.

Pin, S. S., Kariv, I., Graciani, N. R., and Oldenburg, K. R. (1999). Analysis of protein-peptide interaction by a miniaturized fluorescence polarization assay using cyclin-dependent kinase 2/cyclin E as a model system. *Anal. Biochem.* **275,** 156–161.

Rishton, G. M. (1997). Reactive compounds and *in vitro* false positives in HTS. *Drug Discovery Today* **2,** 49–58.

Roberge, M., Berlinck, R. G. S., Xu, L., Anderson, H. J., Lim, L. Y., Curman, D., Stringer, C. M., Friend, S. H., Davies, P., Vincent, I., Haggerty, S. J., Kelly, M. T., Britton, R., Piers, E., and Andersen, R. J. (1998). High-throughput assay for G_2 checkpoint inhibitors and identification of the structurally novel compound isogranulatimide. *Cancer Res.* **58,** 5701–5706.

Roberge, M., Cinel, B., Anderson, H. J., Lim, L., Jiang, X., Xu, L., Bigg, C. M., Kelly, M. T., and Andersen, R. J. (2000). Cell-based screen for antimitoic agents and identification of analogues of rhizoxin, eleutherobin, and paclitaxel in natural extracts. *Cancer Res.* **60,** 5052–5058.

Rodrigues, A. K. (1997). Preclinical drug metabolism in the age of high throughput screening: an industrial perspective. *Pharm. Res.* **14,** 1505–1515.

Salomoni, P., and Pandolfi, P. P. (2000). Transcriptional regulation of cellular transformation. *Nat. Med.* **6,** 742–744.

Savoysky, E., Akamatsu, K., Tsuchiya, M., and Yamazaki, T. (1996). Detection of telomerase activity by combination of TRAP method and scintillation proximity assay (SPA). *Nucleic Acids Res.* **24,** 1175–1176.

Scherf, U., Ross, D. T., Waltham, M., Smith, L. H., Lee, J. K., Tanabe, L., Kohn, K. W., Reinhold, W. C., Myers, T. G., Andrews, D. T., Scudiero, D. A., Eisen, M. B., Sausville, E. A., Pommier, Y., Botstein, D., Brown, P. O., and Weinstein, J. N. (2000). A gene expression database for the molecular pharmacology of cancer. *Nat. Genet.* **24,** 236–244.

Science, The Human Genome. (2001). **291,** 1145–1434.

Sebolt-Leopold, J. S., Dudley, D. T., Herrera, R., Van Becelaere, K., Wiland, A., Gowan, R. C., Tecle, H., Barrett, S. D., Bridges, A., Przybranowski, S., Leopold, W. R., and Saltiel, A. R. (1999). Blockade of the MAP kinase pathway suppresses growth of colon tumours *in vivo*. *Nat. Med.* **5,** 810–815.

Seethala, R., and Menzel, R. (1998). A fluorescence polarization competition immunoassay for tyrosine kinases. *Anal. Biochem.* **255,** 257–262.

Selivanova, G., Iotsova V., Okan I., Fritsche, M., Strom M., Groner B., Grafstrom R. C., and Wiman, K. G. (1997), Restoration of the growth suppression function of mutant p53 by a synthetic peptide derived from the p53 C-terminal domain. *Nat. Med.* **3,** 632–638.

Sharif, T. R., and Sharif, M. (1999). A high throughput system for the evaluation of protein kinase C inhibitors based on Elk 1 transcriptional activation in human astrocytoma cells. *Int. J. Oncol.* **14,** 327–335.

Sharp, S. Y., Kelland, L. R., Valenti, M. R., Brunton, L. A., Hobbs, S., and Workman, P. (2000). Establishment of an isogenic human colon tumor model for NQO1 gene expression: application to investigate the role of DT-diaphorase in bioreductive drug activation *in vitro* and *in vivo*. *Mol. Pharmacol.* **58,** 1146–1155.

Sikora, K., Advani, S., Koroltchouk, V., Magrath, I., Levy, L., Pinedo, H., Schwartsmann, G., Tattersall, M., and Yan, S. (1999). Essential drugs for cancer therapy: a World Health Organisation consultation. *Ann. Oncol.* **10,** 385–390.

Skinner, R. H., Picardo, M., Gane, N. M., Cook, N. D., Morgan, L., Rowedder, J., and Lowe, P. N. (1994). Direct measurement of the binding of RAS to neurofibromin using a scintillation proximity assay. *Anal. Biochem.* **223,** 259–265.

Soini, E., and Hemmilä, I. (1979). Fluoroimmunoassys: present status and key problems. *Clin. Chem.* **25,** 352–361.

Stockwell, B. R., Haggarty, S. J., and Schreiber, S. L. (1999). High-throughput screening of small molecules in miniaturized mammalian cell-based assays involving post-translational modifications. *Chem. Biol.* **6,** 71–83.

Stratowa, C., Baum, A., Castañon, M. J., Dahmann, G., Himmelsbach, F., Himmler, A., Loeber, G., Metz, T., Schnitzer, R., Solca, F., Spevak, W., Tontsch, U., and von Rüden, T. (1999). A comparative cell-based high throughput screening strategy for the discovery of selective tyrosine kinase inhibitors with anticancer activity. *Anticancer Drug Design* **14,** 393–402.

Strawn, L. M., and Shawver, L. K. (1998). Tyrosine kinases in disease. *Exp. Opin. Invest. Drugs* **7,** 553–573.

Strohl, W. R. (2000). The role of natural products in a modern drug discovery program. *Drug Discovery Today* **5,** 39–41.

Su, G. H., Sohn, T. A., Byungwoo, R., and Kern, S. E. (2000). A novel histone deacetylase inhibitor identified by high-throughput transcriptional screening of a compound library. *Cancer Res.* **60,** 3137–3142.

Sundberg, S. A. (2000), High-throughput and ultra-high-throughput screening: solution and cell-based approaches. *Current Opin. Biotechnol.* **11,** 47–53.

Tian, S-S., Lamb, P., King, A. G., Miller, S. G., Kessler, L., Luengo, J. I., Averill, L., Johnson, R. K., Gleason, J. G., Pelus, L. M., Dillon, S. B., and Rosen, J. (1998). A small, nonpeptidyl mimic of granulocyte-colony-stimulating factor. *Science* **281,** 257–259.

Trevillyan, J. M., Chiou, X. G., Ballaron, S. J., Tang, W. M., Buko, A., Sheets, M. P., Smith M. L., Putman, C. B., Wiedeman, P., Tu, N., Madar, D., Smith, H. T., Gubbins, E. J., Warrior, U. S., Chen, Y-W., Mollison, K. W., Faltynek, C. R., and Djuric, S. W. (1999). Inhibition of p56^lck tyrosine kinase by isothiazolones. *Arch. Biochem. Biophy.* **364,** 19–29.

Woodburn, J. R., Barker, A. J., Gibson, K. H., Ashton, S. E., Wakeling, A. E., Curry, B. J., Scarlett, L., and Henthorn, L. R. (1997). ZD1839, an epidermal growth factor tyrosine kinase inhibitor selected for clinical development. *Proc. Am. Assoc. Cancer Res.* **38,** 633.

Workman, P. (1997). Towards intelligent anticancer drug screening in the post-genome era? *Anticancer Drug Design* **12,** 525–531.

Workman, P. (2000a). Emerging molecular therapies: small-molecule drugs. *In* "Principles of Molecular Oncology" (M. H. Bronchud, M. A. Foote, W. P. Peters, and M. O. Robinson, eds.), pp. 421–437. Humana Press, Totowa, NJ.

Workman, P. (2000b). Towards genomic cancer pharmacology: Innovative drugs for the new millennium. *Curr. Opin. Oncol. Endocr. Met.* **2,** 21–25.

Workman P. (2001). Scoring a bull's-eye against cancer genome targets. *Curr. Opin. Pharmacol.* **1,** 342–352.

Wu, J. J., Yarwood, D. R., Pham, Q., and Sills, M. A. (2000). Identification of a high-affinity anti-phosphoserine antibody for the development of a homogeneous fluorescence polarization assay of protein kinase C. *J. Biomol. Screening* **5,** 23–30.

Zhang, J. H., Chung, T. D., and Oldenburg K. R. (1999). A simple statistical parameter for use in evaluation and validation of high throughput screening assays. *J. Biomol. Screening* **4,** 67–73.

TUMOR CELL CULTURES IN DRUG DEVELOPMENT

Bruce C. Baguley
Kevin O. Hicks
William R. Wilson

Auckland Cancer Society Research Centre

The University of Auckland

Auckland, New Zealand

Summary

Cell culture techniques play a key role in the development of new anticancer drugs by imposing additional constraints on those of receptor interaction alone, such as drug uptake and efflux, interaction with other cellular receptors, and cellular metabolism. Clonogenic assays, integrating multiple cell death pathways, are particularly useful in measurement of cell survival following exposure to cytotoxic drugs. On the other hand, microcultures, combined with colorimetric and other methods for measuring antiproliferative effects, have provided the basis for large-scale screening of cytotoxic and cytostatic drugs. The U.S. National Cancer Institute program has made it possible to use 60 or more cell lines to compare the growth inhibition profiles of potential new drugs with those of tens of thousands of previously tested compounds, providing information on mechanism of action as well as antiproliferative activity. However, such assays reflect cytokinetic changes as much as cytotoxic effects, and more work is needed to develop culture methods suitable for modeling the survival characteristics of solid tumors measured with anticancer drugs *in vivo*. Some of the most promising new approaches include the use of three-dimensional cell cultures to allow the measurement of rates of drug diffusion, as well as assessment of the effects of cell contact and tumor microenvironment on drug sensitivity. In order for culture techniques to facilitate translation of the extensive molecular biology information now available into realistic clinical cancer therapies, they must accurately model the processes that control growth in human cancer tissue.

1. Introduction

The majority of cytotoxic anticancer drugs in use today were selected on the basis of animal screening systems, usually employing mice with transplantable tumors (see Chapter 16). In order to increase the relevance of screening to human cancer, a variety of human tumors, growing as xenografts in athymic mice, were also used for drug development. The development of methods for growing human cancer cells in culture has raised the question of whether it might be possible to use culture methods to model all of the features important for clinical antitumor activity. Such an approach might also lead to novel anticancer drugs that are selective for human tumor targets. In this chapter, we provide a brief review of some features of cell culture systems as they relate to drug development. We consider the relationship between results of simple cell culture systems and studies with isolated biochemical receptors, and discuss the problem of using cultures to model drug-induced *in vivo* cell death. Next, we examine the use of cell cultures in modeling aspects of solid tumors, such as drug diffusion barriers and hypoxic tissue. Finally, we consider the relationship between culture results and *in vivo* antitumor activity. Cell cultures can be used to study a variety of approaches to cancer therapy including tumor angiogenesis, tumor invasion, and immune cell interactions, but the main emphasis in this chapter will be in the area of directly acting cytotoxic or cytostatic antitumor drugs.

2. Growth Inhibition Assays

A. Development of Methodology

Early searches for new potential anticancer drugs generally used murine cells such as sarcoma-180 cells, cultured directly from tumors, and initial studies resulted in the optimization of culture media components, as well as supplements such as fetal bovine serum (Chester Stock, 1954). Most early uses of cell lines in drug development utilized growth inhibition assays wherein cells were cultured in the presence of drugs, generally for 2–5 culture doubling times, and cell number was measured using a hemocytometer or electronic cell counter at the end of incubation. A key advance in this approach came with the production of commercial multiwell plates with coated plastic to allow cell adherence and growth. The resulting miniaturization of tumor cell cultures was complemented by the development of plate readers, developed for immunologic applications, that could be used in conjunction with protein staining to estimate growth (Finlay *et al.*, 1984). Mitochondrial reduction of the dye methylthiazoldiphenyl-tetrazolium (MTT), developed as an estimate of lymphocyte growth (Mosmann, 1983), was adapted successfully to measure growth of a variety of tumor cell lines (Finlay *et al.*, 1986; Scudiero *et al.*, 1988). The U.S. National Cancer Institute (NCI) used these methods to establish a panel of at least 60 human tumor lines, allowing comparison of the properties of cell lines derived from different tumor sites (Alley *et al.*, 1988; Monks *et al.*, 1991). Variants of both protein staining and tetrazolium reduction were developed to improve the quantitation of these assays (Keepers *et al.*, 1991; Scudiero *et al.*, 1988; Skehan *et al.*, 1990) and the NCI tumor line panel replaced transplantable tumors in mice as a primary screening method in the NCI drug discovery program in the late 1980s (Boyd and Paull, 1995). The use of cell lines in cancer research, including issues of cross-contamination between lines, has recently been reviewed (Masters *et al.*, 2000).

B. Factors Influencing Drug Responses in Tumor Cell Lines

Since a number of factors, such as solubility, chemical or metabolic stability, protein binding, and cellular uptake, can limit drug-induced inhibition of cell growth, an understanding of the relationship between such factors and drug structure facilitates the prediction of activity of new analogues in a series. Lipophilic character is an important parameter influencing cellular uptake, and while hydrophilic drugs may be able to access active carrier mechanisms for cell entry, lipophilic drugs equilibrate rapidly by passive diffusion. Lipophilic character is also important in determining binding to proteins, which are generally present in serum components of the culture medium and which in turn modulate drug uptake by reducing free-drug concentrations.

An early study on the *in vitro* activity of analogues of the drug amsacrine (Baguley and Cain, 1982) serves to illustrate the importance of lipophilicity in comparisons of drugs. Amsacrine, a DNA-binding and intercalating agent (Wilson *et al.*, 1981a), is effective in the management of acute leukemia (Arlin, 1989) and functions as a DNA topoisomerase poison (Nelson *et al.*, 1984). The murine transplantable L1210 leukemia, used extensively for screening by the NCI, could be grown directly from *in vivo* ascites fluid when the antioxidant 2-mercaptoethanol was used to prevent oxygen toxicity (Baguley and Nash, 1981). On the assumption that DNA association constants of amsacrine analogues reflect binding to the biochemical target, binding constants were estimated using an ethidium competition technique (Baguley *et al.*, 1981). IC_{50} values, or drug concentrations required for 50% inhibition of net cell proliferation, could then be described as a combination of terms for DNA binding and lipophilicity, with a parabolic dependence on the latter (Fig. 1). A highly significant correlation was found ($r = 0.83$, $p < 0.001$).

A more recent example that illustrates this principle is provided by IC_{50} values of a series of gold phosphine complexes for the CH-1 human ovarian carcinoma cell line (McKeage *et al.*, 2000). The cytotoxic mechanism of these compounds is unknown but may be related to mitochondrial uptake and the induction of apoptosis (Berners-Price *et al.*, 1986). Substitution of the phosphine ligands in this series with phenyl or methylpyridyl groups provided an exceptionally wide range of lipophilicity, which was measured either by octanol–water partitioning or by high-performance liquid chromatography (HPLC). The growth inhibitory activity, as determined by IC_{50} values, demonstrated a parabolic or bilinear dependence on lipophilicity (Fig. 2). The free-drug fraction in the culture medium under standard conditions (10% serum) was measured by ultrafiltration and found to vary from less than 0.1% to 59%, with high lipophilicity associated with high binding. Cellular uptake was measured by

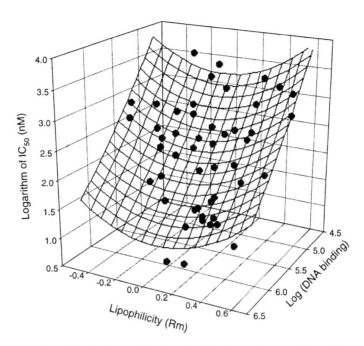

FIGURE 1 Three-dimensional representation of the dependence of *in vitro* antiproliferative activity on binding affinity to the drug receptor (in this case DNA) and drug lipophilicity for a series of derivatives of the drug amsacrine. The data, which have been previously published (Baguley and Cain, 1982), were fitted to a plane with a parabolic cross section. Lipophilicity was estimated as R_m values (relative thin-layer chromatographic mobilities), which are highly correlated with octanol–water partition coefficients (Cain *et al.*, 1974). DNA binding constants (K_m values) were estimated by competition for intercalation sites on the DNA copolymer poly[dA-dT]•poly[dA-dT] (Baguley *et al.*, 1981). Antiproliferative activity was measured in cultured L1210 murine leukemia cells by IC_{50} values, and the logarithmic IC_{50} value was related to a combination the logarithm of the DNA binding term and the square of the lipophilicity term by the equation: $\log(IC_{50}) = 11.3 + 1.47 \times R_m^2 - 1.61 \times \log(K_m)$. The correlation coefficient was 0.83 ($p < 0.001$).

inductively coupled plasma mass spectrometry and found to vary by a factor of more than 1000 with lipophilic compounds being taken up rapidly. Thus, the combination of these factors, acting in opposite directions, provides the parabolic dependence of drug IC_{50} values on lipophilicity (Fig. 2).

C. Determinants of Selectivity among Different Tumor Cell Lines

Early measurements of IC_{50} values in multiwell dishes, using a range of cytotoxic drugs against multiple cell lines, suggested wide variation with hemopoietic lines being generally more sensitive than carcinoma lines (Finlay and Baguley, 1984). In comparisons of cell lines, differences in IC_{50} values result from a number of factors in addition to the binding of drug to the biochemical target for the cytostatic or cytotoxic response. These factors include the incubation time and cell cycle time (IC_{50} values generally decrease with increasing number of cell cycles traversed by the line during the incubation period), and rates of drug uptake, efflux, and metabolism. Differences in the content of added proteins (e.g., the concentration of fetal bovine serum) can change free-drug concentrations, and differences in medium con-

stituents can differentially alter drug stability (Finlay *et al.*, 1986).

The NCI initiative resulted in the establishment of a panel of at least 60 cell lines representing major human tumor classes, including colon, lung, kidney, brain, and ovary (Alley *et al.*, 1988; Boyd, 1993; Paull *et al.*, 1989). The implicit assumption behind this initiative was that selectivity for a particular tumor type, as determined using IC_{50} assays with cell lines, might translate into useful selectivity for tumors of that type relative to normal tissues. While it was feasible to test many thousands of compounds with these cell lines, methods were required for the display and comparison of such data. A convenient graphical display, in the form of a bar graph of distribution about mean values (Fig. 3), was adopted to allow feedback of data to drug suppliers. Since the tumor types are separated vertically in this graph, the drug sensitivity of tumors of a particular organ type is evident by inspection. Three end points were utilized in this display, each expressed on a logarithmic scale: the concentration that reduces growth by 50% (IC_{50} value), the concentration that prevents all growth, and the concentration that reduces the initial cell density by 50%. The IC_{50} value was the most sensitive measure and logarithmic IC_{50} values have become a commonly used parameter for analysis. In the example shown

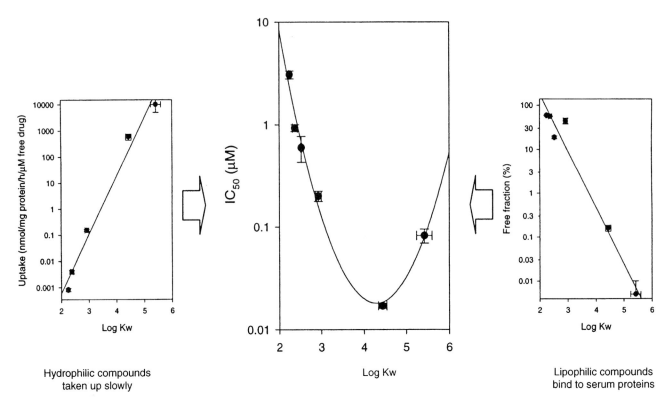

FIGURE 2 Relationships between drug lipophilicity, protein binding, and cellular uptake for a series of gold phosphine complexes, redrawn from published data (McKeage *et al.*, 2000). Drug lipophilicity was measured chromatographically as log K_w, which is linearly related to logarithmic octanol–water partition coefficient. In the left-hand panel, cellular uptake rate, expressed in terms of the free-drug concentration, varies by seven orders of magnitude as lipophilicity is increased. In the right-hand panel, the percentage free drug (that which is not bound to serum proteins in the growth medium) varies from less than 0.1% to 59%. The center panel is resultant of these two effects, acting in opposite directions, and shows a parabolic dependence of antiproliferative activity on drug lipophilicity.

in Fig. 3, a comparison is made for three anticancer drugs: amsacrine, etoposide, and 5-fluorouracil. Despite very different chemical structures, amsacrine and etoposide show very similar "fingerprints" in the NCI panel, while 5-fluorouracil shows a very different pattern. The similarity of the fingerprints of amsacrine and etoposide, despite their different macromolecular binding sites (DNA and protein, respectively), indicates a similar mechanism of action (poisoning of DNA topoisomerase II). The small differences in pattern may reflect differences in cellular uptake/efflux, stability in culture, or the relative content of the two isoenzymes topoisomerase IIα and IIβ, which differ in response to amsacrine and etoposide (Errington *et al.*, 1999).

While the original aim of the drug discovery program was to identify drugs with tumor type selectivity, it became clear that an important application of the program was to search for novel mechanisms of drug action. At the same time, it was necessary to determine the extent to which a newly tested compound resembled others that had already been tested. These aims were realized by the COMPARE analysis technique (Paull *et al.*, 1989). Briefly, logarithmic IC_{50} values of

a given drug for the cell line panel can be considered to represent a specific fingerprint and the data are compared in the form of correlation matrices. The correlation coefficients are then used to compare each drug with every other. Thus, in the example shown in Fig. 3, the correlation coefficient for the regression between amsacrine and etoposide values is 0.81 ($p < 0.0001$), whereas that between 5-fluorouracil and etoposide is 0.16 ($p = 0.96$). Data for any new compound can be "seeded" into this matrix, and subsequently the most closely related drugs, and by implication the most closely related mode of action, can be rapidly identified. Conversely, a drug with no close correlation with others in the database might be considered to have a novel mechanism of action.

An extension of the NCI approach, using a program called DISCOVERY, allowed the examination of a number of cell functions, such as expression of multidrug resistance proteins, wild-type p53 protein, downstream products of p53 regulation, and stress-related proteins (Weinstein *et al.*, 1997). The p53 protein, through the cycle inhibitor p21[WAF1], arrests cells primarily in G_1 phase (O'Connor *et al.*, 1993, 1997) and thus plays a role in determining response to drugs that induce

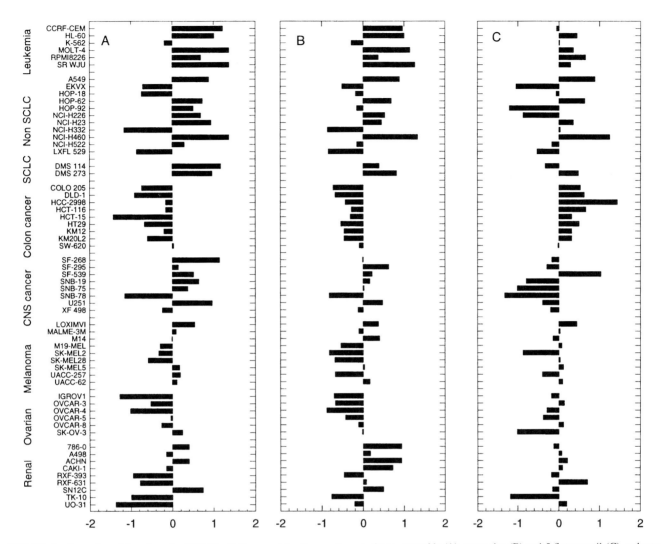

FIGURE 3 Examples of data from the NCI 60-cell-line panel for three anticancer drugs, etoposide (**A**), amsacrine (**B**) and 5-fluorouracil (**C**), redrawn from previously published data (Boyd, 1993; Finlay *et al.*, 1993) The cell lines are listed on the left and grouped according to tumor type. DELTA values represent logarithmic IC_{50} concentrations and are normalized about the mean, with bars to the right representing relative sensitivity and bars to the left relative resistance. The similarity of the patterns of amsacrine and etoposide, despite their different chemical structures, reflects a similar mode of cytotoxic action. The contrasting pattern of 5-fluorouracil indicates a quite different mode of action.

p53 protein. Drug efflux mechanisms such as P-glycoprotein (Roninson, 1992) and multidrug resistance protein (Cole *et al.*, 1994), by reducing intracellular concentrations of a variety of complex synthetic organic compounds and natural products, also strongly influence IC_{50} values. A matrix was constructed from the databases of 113 of such functions for each of the 60 cell lines, and the "product matrix" of these two databases was used to devise a "dendrogram" for a set of almost 4000 compounds (Weinstein *et al.*, 1992). This allows one to associate the activity of each compound with particular cellular functions. Other computing procedures, such as neural networks, have been designed to analyze the data (Weinstein *et al.*, 1992), and the target database has recently been

extended to the expression of some 9000 genes by microarray analysis (Scherf *et al.*, 2000). Additional analysis methods are currently being developed at the NCI.

D. Use of Tailored Cell Lines

The original hypothesis behind the NCI cell line panel, i.e., that discovery of drugs selective for tumor cell lines from a particular tissue origin (such as lung or central nervous system) would translate into clinically useful drugs selective for such tumors *in vivo*, has not been borne out. However, analysis of data from the NCI cell line panel provided an opportunity to correlate drug sensitivity with levels of specific targets, such as topoisomerases, transport resistance proteins, and stress proteins, including p53 (Weinstein *et al.*, 1992). An alternative strategy for assessing the role of specific proteins in drug sensitivity is to specifically design pairs (or small panels) of cell lines with a common genetic background. One of the first approaches in this area involved the production of drug-resistant lines (see Chapter 5). These were generally produced by mutagenesis with an alkylating agent, followed by serial culture in the presence of incrementally increasing concentrations of the drug under study. A considerable amount of work has been carried out using cell lines selected for resistance to anticancer drugs, together with the corresponding sensitive line, in the development of drugs that overcome or inhibit resistance mechanisms. Examples include the anthracyclines (Mariani *et al.*, 1994), amsacrine derivatives (Finlay *et al.*, 1990), camptothecin derivatives (Mattern *et al.*, 1993), and platinum derivatives (McKeage *et al.*, 1994).

One problem in the use of resistant cell lines obtained by drug selection is that the mutant lines may have multiple genetic lesions that influence drug sensitivity. Newer approaches, provided by transfection and gene knockout techniques, involve the specific addition or subtraction of genetic material from cell lines. Thus, the determination of ratios of IC_{50} values for two cell lines differing in a particular gene product allows the screening of a drug series for selective effects on that gene product. While this is a powerful strategy, it should be noted that cell lines obtained by transfection are not necessarily strictly isogenic because integration events are generally random; techniques to defeat this problem include comparison of multiple clones (Patterson *et al.*, 1997), use of specific recombinase systems to exchange genes at a defined chromosomal locus (Sandmeyer *et al.*, 1990), and the use of inducible expression cassettes (Peng, 1999). Even with strictly isogenic cell line pairs, caution is needed in that high levels of expression of transgenes often results in multiple phenotypic changes leading to altered morphology and growth properties of stable transfectants relative to their parental lines.

A comparison of the two broad strategies (correlation across genetically unrelated cell lines vs. modulation of target expression in a single cell line) is provided by studies of the enzymatic activation of the bioreductive alkylating agent mitomycin C (MMC). The latter is known to be a substrate for NAD(P)H:quinone oxidoreductase (DT-diaphorase), at least at low pH values (Begleiter and Leith, 1993; Siegel *et al.*, 1990), but the significance of this pathway to the cytotoxicity of MMC has been a matter of some controversy (Riley and Workman, 1992; Spanswick *et al.*, 1998). A correlation has been demonstrated between MMC sensitivity and DT-diaphorase activity in the NCI cell line panel (Fitzsimmons *et al.*, 1996), but studies with smaller cell line panels have yielded negative results in some cases (Robertson *et al.*, 1992) and weakly positive results in others (Beall *et al.*, 1994). Given that there are multiple determinants of sensitiv-

ity (other reductases, detoxification pathways, repair phenotype, etc.), it is not surprising that such correlations require large numbers of cell lines to achieve statistical significance. The alternative approach is illustrated by expression of the rat DT-diaphorase gene in Chinese hamster ovary (CHO) cells (Belcourt *et al.*, 1996), which provides small but obvious increases in MMC sensitivity in each of two independent stably transfected clones relative to the parental line or empty vector–transfected control. It was shown in the latter study that activities of other candidate reductases were unchanged in the transfectants. This study therefore provides clear evidence that intracellular reduction by DT-diaphorase can result in cytotoxic activation. The custom-designed cell lines provide a more precisely controlled environment for isolating the effect of the target enzyme, but such experiments often express the target at levels much higher than the physiologic range. In the above case, a 130-fold increase in DT-diaphorase activity provided only a twofold change in MMC sensitivity, which leaves open the question as to whether naturally occurring differences in target expression are of biological significance. In this regard the above two approaches can be considered complementary, and additional lines of evidence are also important, such as the observed decrease in DT-diaphorase expression in MMC-resistant tumor cell lines (Lambert *et al.*, 1998).

3. Clonogenic Assays

An important concern in the use of the antiproliferative (IC_{50}) assays discussed in the previous sections is that they measure growth inhibition rather than cell killing. This is particularly important for DNA-damaging drugs, which, to a first approximation, arrest cells at "checkpoints" in the cell cycle (see Chapter 2). DNA damage generally arrests cells in G_2 phase and, if p53 function is present, in G_1 phase as well (Furnari *et al.*, 1997; Waldman *et al.*, 1997). Checkpoint arrest is a survival response of cells that allows repair of DNA damage and is therefore not directly related to the induction of cell death. Thus, cells that arrest more efficiently at checkpoints in response to DNA damage may show lower IC_{50} values but increased survival. While relative IC_{50} values may have predictive value in the comparison of a series of compounds with a similar mode of action, absolute IC_{50} values do not predict cell survival (Brown and Wouters, 1999). Loss of tumor cell reproductive viability, measurable in many cell lines by clonogenic survival assays (i.e., by the ability of a single cell to proliferate to form a colony), is the most direct method of measuring cytotoxic activity of a drug (Puck and Marcus, 1955).

Many of the considerations discussed for antiproliferative assays, such as drug uptake, activity in the presence of competing binding sites in cells and in serum, and stability, apply also to clonogenic assays. Likewise, drug-resistant and genetically modified cell lines have an important place in drug development strategies utilizing clonogenic assays. With some types of drugs, interactions with sites in addition to the target for cytotoxicity may be of such importance that cell-based assays are necessary. An example is provided by prodrugs designed for selective activation by specific enzymes in tumor cells. In this case, useful activity depends not only on the ability of the prodrug to act as a substrate for the enzyme system but on its ability to enter the cell. In addition, some potential targets, such as those occurring in hypoxia, are difficult to represent in isolated biochemical systems, and more integrated cell-based assays are preferable.

4. Three-Dimensional Cell Cultures: Modeling Extravascular Drug Transport

Despite their convenience, conventional tissue culture screening using monolayer cultures fails to model important features of solid tumors. The microvascular system in most tumors is inefficient, with large and variable intercapillary distances, and slow and variable blood flow (Brown and Giaccia, 1998). As a consequence, tumors are diffusion-limited structures with steep oxygen, nutrient, growth factor and pH gradients (Fig. 4) (Dewhirst *et al.*, 1999, 2000; Helmlinger *et al.*, 1997) that lead to a complex and heterogeneous range of phenotypes in relation to drug sensitivity (Brown and Giaccia, 1998; St Croix & Kerbel, 1997). Several "three-dimensional" tissue culture systems have been developed to model these aspects of the extravascular compartment of tumors in culture. In the widely used spheroid model (Sutherland and Durand, 1976), tumor cells are grown as spherical colonies in liquid culture. Their utility as models of the extravascular compartment of tumors and superiority to monolayer culture for investigating tumor physiology and therapeutic response have been reviewed (Hamilton, 1998; Mueller-Klieser, 1997; Nederman and Twentyman, 1984; Sutherland, 1988). They grow to become diffusion-limited structures with many features in common with carcinomatous tumor cords or perivascular nodules, including gradients of cell proliferation (accumulation of noncycling cells with increasing distance from the surface) and development of central hypoxia and necrosis. Similar diffusion-limited models include growth of tumor cell lines as colonies in collagen gels (Tanigawa *et al.*, 1996), as "histocultures" (Au *et al.*, 1993; Freeman & Hoffman, 1986; Furukawa *et al.*, 1995; Weaver *et al.*, 1999), and as cellular multilayers in V-bottom 96-well plates (Peters *et al.*, 1999).

These models have been used extensively to investigate several aspects of drug action, including effects of cell contact on sensitivity (Durand and Sutherland, 1972), effects of microenvironmental variables such as hypoxia and low ex-

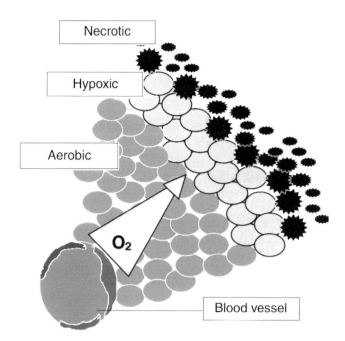

FIGURE 4 Tumors are diffusion-limited structures whose vasculature imposes steep oxygen, nutrient, growth factor, and pH gradients. These lead to a complex and heterogeneous range of phenotypes in relation to drug sensitivity.

tracellular pH (Durand, 1991), metabolism of drugs under hypoxia to form tissue-bound markers suitable for detecting tumor hypoxia (Franko and Koch, 1984), effects of tumor-like cytokinetics on drug response (Sham and Durand, 1998), and transfer of cytotoxic metabolites between cells to give "bystander" effects (Miller *et al.*, 1990). Most of the above features of the tumor microenvironment can also be modeled, to a greater or lesser extent, in conventional low-density cell cultures (e.g., by making monolayer cultures acutely hypoxic, or by growing them to plateau phase cell densities to force cells out of cycle by nutrient depletion). The exception is the investigation of drug penetration from blood vessels into the tumor parenchyma; it is in addressing this very important problem that three-dimensional cell cultures are uniquely valuable.

The drug penetration problem in cancer chemotherapy arises because of the confluence of several factors. The inefficient blood supply in tumors results in suboptimal delivery of drugs to the extravascular compartment in poorly perfused regions, and the diffusion distances required to reach the cells most distant from vessels are typically much larger than in normal tissues (Awwad *et al.*, 1986; Less *et al.*, 1997; Wÿffels *et al.*, 2000). Given the need to eradicate or sterilize all clonogenic cells in a tumor, even a small proportion of cells not exposed effectively can be responsible for treatment failure. Furthermore, many anticancer drugs are metabolized in tumors or are reversibly bound or sequestered in cells. Reaction during diffusion compromises the penetration of drugs just as it compromises the penetration of oxygen and nutrients. Such concerns have been discussed for decades (Goldacre and Sylven, 1962; Rowe-Jones, 1967), but a lack of suitable experimental methods has made it difficult to ascertain its importance with currently used agents or to learn the rules for designing drugs with superior extravascular transport properties. Regrettably, tumor pharmacokinetics is still usually based on measurement of average concentrations within the whole-tumor compartment, which conveys little information about the proportion of cells that fail to receive therapeutic doses.

The multicellular spheroid model has provided some important qualitative and semiquantitative data on drug penetration properties. For example, doxorubicin fluorescence is brightest near the surface of spheroids, suggesting slow penetration (Sutherland et al., 1979). This has been confirmed with detailed measurements of intracellular concentration using fluorescence-activated cell sorting (Durand, 1986, 1989), and autoradiography has been used to demonstrate limited penetration of radiolabelled methotrexate (West et al., 1980). However, drug concentration gradients are difficult to quantify by these methods, and the problem of discriminating parent drug from metabolites is a major limitation. Measurement of cell killing as a function of distance from spheroids can also provide indirect information about drug penetration (Durand, 1991; Wilson et al., 1981b), but has low spatial resolution and is difficult to interpret without detailed information about the effects of microenvironmental variables on drug sensitivity.

These limitations led us to develop an alternative model in which tumor cells are grown on microporous membranes to form multicellular layers (MCLs) (Cowan et al., 1996; Hicks et al., 1997). This culture technique is a simple adaptation of that for growing epithelial cell lines as monolayers in commercially available cell culture inserts. The latter method is widely used to grow transporting epithelia and to model intestinal absorption of drugs using the well-differentiated colon carcinoma line Caco-2 (Artusson, 1990; Taylor et al., 1997). Modification to provide an efficient nutrient supply to both faces of the growing cell layer, by submerging the inserts in a large reservoir of well-stirred culture medium, allows the development of multicellular layers in many tumor cell lines. These eventually become diffusion limited, developing non-cycling cells, central hypoxia, and necrosis (Cowan et al., 1996; Hicks et al., 1998; Minchinton et al., 1997). Typical MCL grown from a human colon adenocarcinoma cell line (HT29) and a human lung carcinoma cell line (A549) are illustrated in Fig. 5 (see color insert).

Although histologically similar to multicellular spheroids, the planar rather than spherical geometry of MCLs makes it possible to measure drug transport directly by adding the drug to one side of the structure and measuring its concentration on the other side as a function of time. The ability use compound-specific analytical techniques, such as HPLC or mass spectrometry, enables differentiation of parent drug and metabolites and investigation of nonfluorescent or nonradiolabeled drugs, which is generally not possible in the spheroid model. The MCL model has been used to investigate extravascular transport of radiation sensitizers (Cowan et al., 1996), hypoxia-selective cytotoxins (Hicks et al., 1998; Kyle and Minchinton, 1999; Phillips et al., 1998), hypoxia-imaging agents (Rauth et al., 1998), DNA intercalators (Hicks et al., 1997, 2000), and other cytotoxic drugs (Phillips et al., 1998). A similar model, developed independently, has been used to investigate extravascular transport of antibodies (Topp et al., 1998).

The use of the MCL model to investigate tumor penetration of anticancer drugs is illustrated for the hypoxia-selective cytotoxin tirapazamine (TPZ) in Fig. 6A and B. TPZ, currently in clinical trial, is activated by metabolic reduction under hypoxia (Brown and Siim, 1996). Hypoxic cells represent an important target population in tumors because of their resistance to radiation and some forms of chemotherapy, as well as their significance in tumor progression (Brown and Giaccia, 1998). Studies with V79 multicellular spheroids, showing loss of activity against central cells when the whole spheroid was made anoxic, suggested that the ability of TPZ to penetrate hypoxic tissue could be compromised by its rapid metabolic consumption (Durand and Olive, 1992). This has been confirmed by demonstrating that anoxia decreases flux of TPZ through V79 MCL (Hicks et al., 1998), as also illustrated for the human bladder carcinoma cell line MGH-U1 in Fig. 6A.

Measurement of extravascular penetration by this technique is straightforward and informative, but caution is required in interpreting the findings since the initial and boundary conditions in tumors can be quite different from those in the experimental flux apparatus (Wilson and Hicks, 1999). This makes it necessary to fit a mathematical reaction–diffusion model to the MCL flux data, thus extracting the underlying transport parameters, and then to use these parameters to simulate transport in tumors. For the example in Fig. 6A, the flux under aerobic conditions was modeled by fitting a diffusion coefficient in the MCL (D_m), providing a value of $(1.25 \pm 0.16) \times 10^{-6}$ cm^2 s^{-1}), which was sevenfold lower than in culture medium. The decrease in flux under anoxia was modeled as metabolic consumption in the MCL, giving an estimated first-order rate constant (k_{met}) of 0.31 ± 0.03 min^{-1} in this cell line.

The measurement of diffusion and reaction coefficients in MCL makes it possible to simulate the micropharmacokinetics (i.e., develop a spatially distributed pharmacokinetic model) of TPZ within the extravascular compartment in tumors, as illustrated in Fig. 6B using the parameters determined for MGH-U1 and HCT8 MCL. This shows that diffusion into the center of a symmetrical 300-μm intercapillary

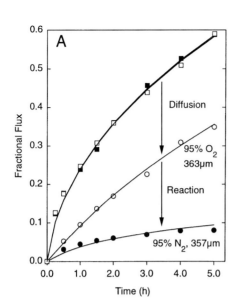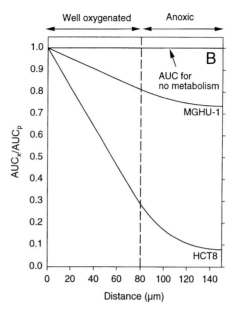

FIGURE 6 (**A**) Tirapazamine (TPZ) transport in collagen coated Teflon support membranes (about 30 μm) in the absence of cells (■, □) and in MGH-U1 MCL of the indicated thickness under aerobic (○) and anoxic (●) conditions. Fractional flux is the accumulation of drug in the receiver compartment as a fraction of the total accumulation expected at equilibrium. The impediment to transport caused by diffusion and reaction (bioreductive metabolism) is clearly demonstrated. (**B**) Calculated pharmacokinetics for TPZ in a symmetrical 300-μm intercapillary region (of which the central 140 μm is hypoxic) for MGH-U1 and HCT-8 tumors, compared with that if no metabolism occurred (AUC at the center = 99.75% and 98.96% of AUC_p for MGH-U1 and HCT8, respectively). The simulation is based on the measured plasma concentration in humans (AUC of 6 mM.min) (Graham *et al.,* 1997). AUC_x is the AUC at distance x μm into the extravascular compartment and AUC_p is the plasma AUC.

region (of which the inner 140 μm is anoxic) is significantly compromised by metabolism of the drug. This results in an exposure (area under the concentration–time curve) at the center of this zone that is 27% or 91% lower than at its periphery for MGH-U1 and HCT-8, respectively. To investigate the implications of this for cell killing, a pharmacodynamic model is required to relate exposure to effect. For TPZ, if killing is assumed to be proportional to the cumulative formation of the TPZ radical, the pharmacodynamic model can be calibrated using data on sensitivity and metabolism in conventional low-cell-density cultures (Hicks *et al.,* 1998). Isoeffect contours for cell killing are shown for a hypothetical family of analogues with pharmacodynamic features identical to TPZ, but differing in the micropharmacokinetic parameters D_m and k_{met} (Fig. 7). This reaction–diffusion plot defines a "valley of death" with the bottom of the valley (dashed line in Fig. 7) representing the optimum value of k_{met} at any one value of D_m, above which penetration is compromised and below which activation is compromised. The values for these transport parameters for TPZ determined for five different cell lines, as MCL, are close to the predicted optimum (Fig. 7). It is perhaps not surprising that TPZ (which has been selected empirically through a long process of preclinical and clinical development) lies somewhere near the optimum for the range of tumor cell lines investigated. However, this

analysis points to the potential for identifying compounds with optimal extravascular transport characteristics much more expeditiously by direct measurements of these features. Even for TPZ, this analysis suggests that there is scope for substantial improvement, either by developing analogues with higher diffusion coefficients or (more importantly) by modifying the pharmacodynamic relationships that determine the isoeffect contours. The latter could be achieved, for example, by designing a TPZ analogue that is reduced to a more cytotoxic radical (providing greater cell kill for equivalent metabolic depletion). Similarly, if only intranuclear reduction of TPZ contributes to DNA breakage as suggested (Evans *et al.,* 1998), then elimination of metabolism by cytoplasmic enzymes could provide additional improvements.

At present, the implications of tumor physiology are rarely considered during early-stage drug discovery, and many tissue culture leads fail to show useful activity against tumors. The development of three-dimensional cell cultures, modeling the extravascular compartment in tumors in terms of measured transport parameters, allows drug delivery issues to be addressed at an early stage of development, analogous to the use of the Caco-2 model for predicting oral bioavailability (Artusson, 1990; Taylor *et al.,* 1997). The use of such techniques also reduces the number of animals required for drug development.

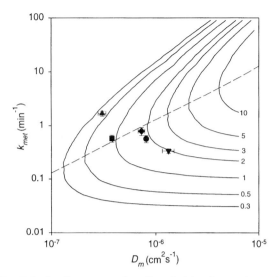

FIGURE 7 Isoeffect contours for cell survival (numbers are $\log_{10}$ cell kill) for k_{met} (ordinate) vs. D_m (abscissa), based on the pharmacodynamic model described in the text. The points are experimental determinations of k_{met} and D_m (mean $\pm$ SEM) for V79 and MGH-U1 ($\blacklozenge$, $\blacktriangledown$; Hicks *et al.*, 1998), SiHa ($\bullet$; estimated from Kyle and Minchinton, 1999) and HCT-8 and HT-29 ($\blacktriangle$, $\blacksquare$; unpublished).

5. Modeling of *in Vivo* Activity by *in Vitro* Assays

A. Experimental Tumors

The previous sections describe how many features of *in vivo* tumors, such as drug uptake/efflux, distribution, and cell survival, can be modeled by cell cultures. Two further considerations in the extrapolation of *in vitro* results to animal studies are the differences in binding of drug to intracellular and extracellular components and clearance of the drug by hepatic, renal, and other mechanisms. Albumin is a major plasma-binding protein, and high lipophilicity is generally associated with high binding to albumin. Because most *in vitro* studies utilize 5% or 10% bovine serum albumin, extracellular protein binding will be lower than that occurring during *in vivo* testing. Both naturally occurring and synthetic anticancer compounds with complex structures are likely to bind strongly to albumin (Fig. 8). On the other hand, efficient hepatic and renal drug elimination is generally associated with low lipophilicity. Thus, drug lipophilicity is important in drug disposition and metabolism, as well as in determining the efficacy of diffusion in the three-dimensional matrix of a solid tumor. An example of this is the series of amsacrine derivatives described in Section 2.B. The *in vivo* effective dose can be expressed in terms of a combination of *in vitro* IC_{50} values and a parabolic term in lipophilicity (Baguley and Cain, 1982). The simplest interpretation of this relationship is that lipophilic derivatives are less active than expected

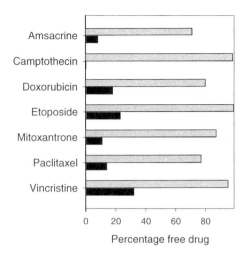

FIGURE 8 Comparison of protein binding of anticancer drugs under *in vitro* and *in vivo* conditions. The graph depicts previously published data obtained using cultured cells as sensors for free drug in the presence of albumin or α_1-acid glycoprotein (Finlay and Baguley, 2000). Gray bars indicate calculated free-drug concentrations in the presence of fetal bovine serum (10%) under typical *in vitro* conditions. Dark bars indicate calculated free-drug concentrations in humans in the presence of typical concentrations of human albumin and α_1-acid glycoprotein, and are similar to published studies of free-drug concentrations in human plasma. The differences between the light and dark bars reflect both the relative lack of α_1-acid glycoprotein in fetal bovine serum and the large interspecies differences in the ability of albumin to bind drug.

from the IC_{50} values because of protein binding, while hydrophilic derivatives are less active because of increased *in vivo* elimination.

Prediction of antitumor activity on the basis of *in vitro* and physicochemical data is much more difficult than prediction of dose (Baguley and Cain, 1982). Particularly for solid tumors, antitumor activity is strongly dependent on pharmacodynamic properties, such as drug distribution, and might therefore best be addressed by the use of drug diffusion models. An example is provided by the comparison of two acridine derivatives, DACA {*N*-[2-(dimethylamino)ethyl]acridine-4-carboxamide} and DAPA {9-[3-(*N,N*-dimethylamino)propylamino]acridine}. While DACA has high experimental solid tumor activity (Baguley *et al.*, 1995b), DAPA lacks *in vivo* activity. The distribution of DACA, using the multicellular layer (MCL) model described in Section 4, is very rapid in comparison to that of DAPA (Hicks *et al.*, 2000). An intratumor pharmacokinetic model for DACA distribution in intercapillary regions has been developed that accounted for high plasma protein binding of this lipophilic drug, using published mouse plasma pharmacokinetic data (Paxton *et al.*, 1992). The predicted tumor pharmacokinetics is in good agreement with measured values (Paxton *et al.*, 1993), assuming an average diffusion distance of 250 μm, but with the advantage that the concentration–time profile can be simulated as a function of distance from the capillary. Combining this with a pharmacodynamic model based on measured (clonogenic) cell killing as a function of concentration and time in monolayer cultures (Haldane *et al.,* 1992) allows simulation of cytotoxicity as a function of distance from blood vessels in tumors. Only a slight decrease in cytotoxicity with distance is predicted for DACA, compared to a marked loss of activity with distance for DAPA, despite a similar predicted AUC for both compounds when integrated over long times (> 72 h). Thus it appears that favorable extravascular transport properties contribute to the high experimental solid tumor activity of this novel agent, in agreement with the original design concept (Denny *et al.,* 1987) to decrease the net charge and DNA binding affinity of acridine intercalators, improving their distributive properties *in vivo.*

At present, one limitation of taking this type of analysis further is the poorly defined pharmacodynamic relationship between low-cell-density clonogenicity assays and cytotoxicity *in vivo.* This comes about for at least two reasons. First, there is substantial evidence that the loss of cell–cell interactions within tumor cell suspensions affects their response to anticancer therapy, in comparison to that occurring *in vivo* or in spheroids (Durand, 1994; Olive and Durand, 1994; St Croix and Kerbel, 1997). Second, for drugs such as these, substantial cellular uptake leads to a lag in peak tumor concentrations followed by a slow efflux from the tumor. In contrast, the pharmacodynamics of cell killing *in vitro* is usually determined using constant drug concentrations. For some classes of compounds, especially those where cytotoxicity is not a simple function of the AUC, cell killing under constant-exposure conditions may not predict that under a time varying pharmacokinetic profile.

B. Clinical Tumors

Many of the arguments in the previous section apply to tumors in humans as well as to those in experimental animals, although it is important to take interspecies differences into account. For instance, drug binding to albumin varies quite widely among different species (Kumar *et al.,* 1993; Liu *et al.,* 1995; Mi and Burke, 1994), as shown in the examples in Fig. 8. In addition, α_1-acid glycoprotein is a much more important drug-binding protein in humans, particularly in cancer patients who often have high levels, than in mice (Kremer *et al.,* 1988; Paxton, 1983). Significant interspecies differences in drug metabolism also occur, and can be investigated using cultured hepatocytes and cell-free systems (Obach *et al.,* 1997; Schneider *et al.,* 1999).

A more fundamental consideration is the validity of using cell lines, human or otherwise, to model the behavior of cancer cells in clinical tumors. Human cell lines generally have cell cycle times (1–2 days) that are much shorter than those of solid tumors *in vivo,* whose measured potential doubling times vary from 3 days to several weeks (Wilson *et al.,* 1988).

Growth of tumor tissue *in vivo* involves a wide variety of host–tumor interactions that are absent in cultured cell lines (Folkman, 1998). The ease of developing a cell line from clinical tumor material varies according to the type of tumor. For instance, it is much easier to develop a melanoma cell line than a prostate carcinoma cell line. The transfer of tumor material to culture conditions, even under low oxygen conditions to minimize the generation of reactive oxygen species (Slater *et al.,* 1995), is likely to generate a variety of stress responses resulting in the death of a high proportion of the cultured cells. Development of a cell line requires months of subculturing, which is likely to result in selection of cells that lack mechanisms that cause cell death in response to such stress. Finally, gene expression patterns in tumor cell lines, determined by microarray analysis, differ considerably from those found *in vivo.* In dendrograms relating similarities in expression patterns, cell lines from a variety of tumor types resemble each other more than they do the tumors from which they are derived (Ross *et al.,* 2000).

Both the differences in cell cycle times and alterations of stress responses are relevant to comparisons of responses of cell lines and clinical tumors to anticancer agents. In the case of cell lines, which have short cell cycle times, the majority of cell death inductions by DNA damage may be postmitotic, reflecting cells dividing before DNA repair is complete. In contrast, human tumor cells may have several days in G_1 phase after DNA damage before cell division, perhaps altering the importance of DNA repair for cell survival. The influence of interphase events on cell death must therefore be considered. The induction of apoptosis by DNA-damaging agents is an important example of a potential interphase event. Unfortunately, although the fraction of apoptotic cells can be determined in sections of excised clinical tumors, the rate of induction of apoptosis *in vivo* is impossible to quantitate, and therefore the contribution of apoptosis to the outcome of therapy is difficult to assess. Apoptosis can be demonstrated in a variety of cell cultures in response to DNA-damaging agents (Barry *et al.,* 1990), but the drug concentrations used in such experiments are often considerably higher than those occurring clinically.

For anticancer agents acting on cellular signaling pathways, the distinction between cytostatic and cytotoxic responses is a factor of particular importance to the outcome of therapy. It is possible to distinguish growth factors, which are involved with stimulating cells to pass the restriction point and progress through the cell division cycle (Herwig and Strauss, 1997), from survival factors, which prevent cells from undergoing apoptosis (Evan and Littlewood, 1998). Cell lines, because they have been selected to grow under the comparatively stressful conditions of cell culture, may be excellent models for detecting drugs that block mitogenesis but poor models for detecting drugs that block survival factors.

A number of attempts have been made to use cultures of human tumor tissue, taken directly from cancer patients at surgery, to overcome such problems of established cell lines. "Stem cell" assays involve the disaggregation of tumor tissue to a single-cell suspension, and culture on a substrate such as agarose to prevent the growth of fibroblasts (Courtenay *et al.,* 1978; Hamburger and Salmon, 1977). A number of groups have used such cultures in drug development programs (Shoemaker *et al.,* 1985; Von Hoff, 1988), but such work is hampered by the fact that each experiment, which relies on one sample of tumor tissue, cannot be repeated. There are technical problems in obtaining single-cell suspensions from all tumor samples and in obtaining sufficient colonies to make an adequate comparison of analogues in a drug development program. A further problem with stem cell assays is that the cells are selected to grow individually, whereas tumor cells *in vivo* interact intimately with stromal cells and the extracellular matrix. Such interactions may affect both growth rate (Sethi *et al.,* 1999) and response to DNA damage (Durand and Sutherland, 1972; Raff, 1992).

An alternative approach is to culture human tumor tissue as small cellular aggregates that preserve, to some extent, the cell–cell interactions that occur *in vivo*. Cultures must again be grown on a substrate that inhibits the proliferation of fibroblasts such as agarose (Marshall *et al.,* 1992; Weisenthal and Lippman, 1985) or collagen (Tanigawa *et al.,* 1996). Such an approach precludes the quantitation of surviving cells, and some other method must be used to estimate drug-induced cell death. Estimates of cell density, such as by protein staining, suffer from the problem that tumor cells generally grow much more slowly than do cell lines, and that a number of cells are lost initially. Measurement of apoptosis as an indicator of cell death rates is likewise unreliable because the apoptosis is short and results in the generation of cell fragments, which cannot be quantitated. One approach is to estimate the number of S-phase cells with time by incorporation of radiolabeled thymidine, and in a series of cultures it has been found that such labeled cells can be identified cytologically as tumor cells (Baguley *et al.,* 1995a). Following the addition of a mitotic inhibitor to prevent cell division, the incorporation of labeled thymidine decreases with time at a rate that is a function of the incubation time and the cell cycle time. This principle can also be used to estimate the cycle time in such cultures, which cover a similar range to that observed in tumors *in vivo* (Baguley *et al.,* 1995a). An extension of such analysis may be used to investigate cell loss, e.g., as a result of the action of DNA-damaging drugs (Baguley *et al.,* 1999). Another application is to measure the effect of growth inhibitors, such as antagonists of the epidermal growth factor receptor tyrosine kinase. Responses to such inhibitors of cultures of tumor tissue from patients with lung, ovarian, and other cancers, occurred at lower drug concentrations than in established cell lines and in a higher proportion of cultures (Baguley *et al.,* 1998).

6. Perspective

Tumor cell lines will continue to form an indispensable link in the steps from drug design to the selection of clinical candidates for anticancer treatment. New drug discovery over the last decade has been dominated by the use of biochemical targets in cell-free systems as screens (see Chapter 14), but lead compounds from such screens do not necessarily enter tumor cells or distribute within tumor tissue. There remains an important role for cell lines, and in particular three-dimensional cultures, to model specific requirements for drug development. As individual cell signaling pathways and gene control mechanisms are elucidated, it is becoming clear that such pathways cannot be thought of in terms of single control elements but rather as components in a highly complex system with very large numbers of interactions. The reductionist approach of focusing on individual cellular components is ultimately limited, and the cultured cell might therefore be regarded as the entity that integrates the myriad of signaling pathways into a specific response. One challenge for the future is to engineer culture systems to model more exactly the processes that occur in clinical tumors. At present, microarray technology has demonstrated a divergence between cell lines and human cancer (Ross *et al.,* 2000). Current technology might be used to monitor the extent to which new three-dimensional systems mimicking cell–cell interactions might model the behavior of real tumors. The availability of such systems would present important new avenues for both the understanding of tumor selectivity and the discovery of new drugs.

References

Alley, M. C., Scudiero, D. A., Monks, A., Hursey, M. L., Czerwinski, M. J., Fine, D. L., Abbott, B. J., Mayo, J. G., Shoemaker, R. H., and Boyd, M. R. (1988). Feasibility of drug screening with panels of human tumor cell lines using a microculture tetrazolium assay. *Cancer Res.* **48,** 589–601.

Arlin, Z. A. (1989). A special role for amsacrine in the treatment of acute leukemia. *Cancer Inv.* **7,** 607–609.

Artusson, P. (1990). Epithelial transport of drugs in cell culture. I: A model for studying the passive diffusion of drugs over intestinal absorptive (caco-2) cells. *J. Pharm. Sci.* **79,** 476–482.

Au, J. L., Wientjes, M. G., Rosol, T. J., Koolemans-Beymen, A., Goebel, E. A., and Schuller, D. E. (1993). Histocultures of patient head and neck tumors for pharmacodynamics studies. *Pharm. Res.* **10,** 1493–1499.

Awwad, H. K., el Naggar, M., Mocktar, N., and Barsoum, M. (1986). Intercapillary distance measurement as an indicator of hypoxia in carcinoma of the cervix uteri. *Int. J. Radiat. Oncol. Biol. Phys.* **12,** 1329–1333.

Baguley, B. C., and Cain, B. F. (1982). Comparison of the *in vivo* and *in vitro* antileukaemic activity of monosubstituted derivatives of 4'-(9-acridinylamino)methanesulphon-m-anisidide (m-AMSA). *Mol. Pharmacol.* **22,** 486–492.

Baguley, B. C., and Nash, R. (1981). Antitumour activity of substituted 9-anilinoacridines: comparison of *in vivo* and *in vitro* testing systems. *Eur. J. Cancer* **17,** 671–679.

Baguley, B. C., Denny, W. A., Atwell, G. J., and Cain, B. F. (1981). Potential antitumor agents. Part 34. Quantitative relationships between DNA binding and molecular structure for 9-anilinoacridines substituted in the anilino ring. *J. Med. Chem.* **24,** 170–177.

Baguley, B. C., Marshall, E. S., Whittaker, J. R., Dotchin, M. C., Nixon, J., McCrystal, M. R., Finlay, G. J., Matthews, J. H. L., Holdaway, K. M., and van Zijl, P. (1995a). Resistance mechanisms determining the *in vitro* sensitivity to paclitaxel of tumour cells cultured from patients with ovarian cancer. *Eur. J. Cancer* **31A,** 230–237.

Baguley, B. C., Zhuang, L., and Marshall, E. (1995b). Experimental solid tumour activity of *N*-[2-(dimethylamino)ethyl]-acridine-4-carboxamide. *Cancer Chemother. Pharmacol.* **36,** 244–248.

Baguley, B. C., Marshall, E. S., Holdaway, K. M., Rewcastle, G. W., and Denny, W. A. (1998). Inhibition of growth of primary human tumour cell cultures by a 4-anilinoquinazoline inhibitor of the epidermal growth factor receptor family of tyrosine kinases. *Eur. J. Cancer* **34,** 1086–1090.

Baguley, B. C., Marshall, E. S., and Finlay, G. J. (1999). Short-term cultures of clinical tumor material: potential contributions to oncology research. *Oncol. Res.* **11,** 115–124.

Barry, M. A., Behnke, C. A., and Eastman, A. (1990). Activation of programmed cell death (apoptosis) by cisplatin, other anticancer drugs, toxins and hyperthermia. *Biochem. Pharmacol.* **40,** 2353–2362.

Beall, H. D., Mulcahy, R. T., Siegel, D., Traver, R. D., Gibson, N. W., and Ross, D. (1994). Metabolism of bioreductive antitumor compounds by purified rat and human DT-diaphorase. *Cancer Res.* **54,** 3196–3201.

Begleiter, A., and Leith, M. (1993). Role of NAD(P)H:(quinone acceptor) oxidoreductase (DT diaphorase) in activation of mitomycin C under acidic conditions. *Mol. Pharmacol.* **44,** 210–215.

Belcourt, M. F., Hodnick, W. F., Rockwell, S., and Sartorelli, A. C. (1996). Bioactivation of mitomycin antibiotics by aerobic and hypoxic Chinese hamster ovary cells overexpressing DT-diaphorase. *Biochem. Pharmacol.* **51,** 1669–1678.

Berners-Price, S. J., Mirabelli, C. K., Johnson, R. K., Mattern, M. R., McCabe, F. L., Faucette, L. F., Sung, C. M., Mong, S. M., Sadler, P. J., and Crooke, S. T. (1986). *In vivo* antitumor activity and *in vitro* cytotoxic properties of bis[1,2-bis(diphenylphosphino)ethane]gold(I) chloride. *Cancer Res.* **46,** 5486–5493.

Boyd, M. R. (1993). The future of new drug development. *In* "Current Therapy in Oncology" (J. E. Niederhuber, ed.), pp. 11–22. BC Decker, Inc., Philadelphia.

Boyd, M. R., and Paull, K. D. (1995). Some practical considerations and applications of the National Cancer Institute *in vitro* anticancer drug discovery screen. *Drug Dev. Res.* **34,** 91–109.

Brown, J. M., and Giaccia, A. J. (1998). The unique physiology of solid tumors: opportunities (and problems) for cancer therapy. *Cancer Res.* **58,** 1408–1416.

Brown, J. M., and Siim, B. G. (1996). Hypoxia specific cytotoxins in cancer therapy. *Semin. Radiat. Oncol.* **6,** 22–36.

Brown, J. M., and Wouters, B. G. (1999). Apoptosis, p53, and tumor cell sensitivity to anticancer agents. *Cancer Res.* **59,** 1391–1399.

Cain, B. F., Seelye, R. N., and Atwell, G. J. (1974). Potential antitumor agents. 14. Acridylmethanesulfonanilides. *J. Med. Chem.* **17,** 922–930.

Chester Stock, C. (1954). Experimental cancer chemotherapy. *In* "Advances in Cancer Research" (J. P. Greenstein, and A. Haddow, eds.), Vol. 2, pp. 425–429. Academic Press, New York.

Cole, S. P. C., Sparks, K. E., Fraser, K., Loe, D. W., Grant, C. E., Wilson, G. M., and Deeley, R. G. (1994). Pharmacological characterization of multidrug resistant MRP-transfected human tumor cells. *Cancer Res.* **54,** 5902–5910.

Courtenay, V. D., Selby, P. J., Smith, I. E., Mills, J., and Peckham, M. J. (1978). Growth of human tumour cell colonies from biopsies using two soft-agar techniques. *Br. J. Cancer* **38,** 77–81.

Cowan, D. S. M., Hicks, K. O., and Wilson, W. R. (1996). Multicellular membranes as an *in vitro* model for extravascular diffusion in tumours. *Br. J. Cancer* **74,** S28–S31.

Denny, W. A., Atwell, G. J., Rewcastle, G. W., and Baguley, B. C. (1987). Potential antitumor agents. 49. 5-Substituted derivatives of N-[2-(dimethylamino)ethyl]-9-aminoacridine-4-carboxamide with *in vivo* solid tumor activity. *J. Med. Chem.* **30,** 658–663.

Dewhirst, M. W., Ong, E. T., Braun, R. D., Smith, B., Klitzman, B., Evans, S. M., and Wilson, D. (1999). Quantification of longitudinal tissue pO$_2$ gradients in window chamber tumours: impact on tumour hypoxia. *Br. J. Cancer* **79,** 1717–1722.

Dewhirst, M. W., Walenta, S., Snyder, S., Mueller-Klieser, W., Braun, R., and Chance, B. (2000). Tissue gradients of energy metabolites mirror oxygen tension gradients in a rat mammary carcinoma model (abstract). *Int. J. Radiat. Oncol. Biol. Phys.* **48,** S131–S132.

Durand, R. E. (1986). Chemosensitivity in V79 spheroids: drug delivery and cellular microenivronment. *J. Natl. Cancer. Inst.* **77,** 247–252.

Durand, R. E. (1989). Distribution of and activity of antineoplastic drugs in a tumor model. *J. Natl. Cancer. Inst.* **81,** 146–152.

Durand, R. E. (1991). Keynote address: The influence of microenvironmental factors on the activity of radiation and drugs. *Int. J. Radiat. Oncol. Biol. Phys.* **20,** 253–258.

Durand, R. E. (1994). The influence of microenvironmental factors during cancer therapy. *In Vivo* **8,** 691–702.

Durand, R. E., and Olive, P. L. (1992). Evaluation of bioreductive drugs in multicell spheroids. *Int. J. Radiat. Oncol. Biol. Phys.* **22,** 689–692.

Durand, R. E., and Sutherland, R. M. (1972). Effects of intercellular contact on repair of radiation damage. *Exp. Cell Res.* **71,** 75–80.

Errington, F., Willmore, E., Tilby, M. J., Li, L., Li, G., Li, W., Baguley, B. C., and Austin, C. A. (1999). Murine transgenic cells lacking DNA topoisomerase II beta are resistant to acridines and mitoxantrone: analysis of cytotoxicity and cleavable complex formation. *Mol. Pharmacol.* **56,** 1309–1316.

Evan, G., and Littlewood, T. (1998). A matter of life and cell death. *Science* **281,** 1317–1322.

Evans, J. W., Yudoh, K., Delahoussaye, Y. M., and Brown, J. M. (1998). Tirapazamine is metabolised to its DNA-damaging radical by intranuclear enzymes. *Cancer Res.* **58,** 2098–2101.

Finlay, G. J., and Baguley, B. C. (1984). The use of human cancer cell lines as a primary screening system for antineoplastic compounds. *Eur. J. Cancer Clin. Oncol.* **20,** 947–954.

Finlay, G. J., and Baguley, B. C. (2000). Effects of protein binding on the *in vitro* activity of antitumour acridine derivatives and related anticancer drugs. *Cancer Chemother. Pharmacol.* **45,** 417–422.

Finlay, G. J., Baguley, B. C., and Wilson, W. R. (1984). A semiautomated microculture method for investigating growth inhibitory effects of cytotoxic compounds on exponentially growing carcinoma cells. *Analyt. Biochem.* **139,** 272–277.

Finlay, G. J., Wilson, W. R., and Baguley, B. C. (1986). Comparison of *in vitro* activity of cytotoxic drugs toward human carcinoma and leukaemia cell lines. *Eur. J. Cancer Clin. Oncol.* **22,** 655–662.

Finlay, G. J., Baguley, B. C., Snow, K., and Judd, W. (1990). Multiple patterns of resistance of human leukemia cell sublines to amsacrine analogues. *J. Natl. Cancer. Inst.* **82,** 662–667.

Finlay, G. J., Marshall, E. S., Matthews, J. H. L., Paull, K. D., and Baguley, B. C. (1993). *In vitro* assessment of N-[2-(dimethylamino)ethyl]acridine-4-carboxamide, a DNA-intercalating antitumour drug with reduced sensitivity to multidrug resistance. *Cancer Chemother. Pharmacol.* **31,** 401–406.

Fitzsimmons, S. A., Workman, P., Grever, M., Paull, K., Camalier, R., and Lewis, A. D. (1996). Reductase enzyme expression across the National Cancer Institute tumor cell line panel: correlation with sensitivity to mitomycin C and EO9. *J. Natl. Cancer. Inst.* **88,** 259–269.

Folkman, J. (1998). Is tissue mass regulated by vascular endothelial cells? Prostate as the first evidence. *Endocrinology* **139**, 441–442.

Franko, A. J., and Koch, C. J. (1984). Binding of misonidazole to V79 spheroids and fragments of Dunning rat prostatic and human colon carcinomas *in vitro:* diffusion of oxygen and reactive metabolites. *Int. J. Radiat. Oncol. Biol. Phys.* **10**, 1333–1336.

Freeman, A. E., and Hoffman, R. M. (1986). *In vivo*-like growth of human tumors *in vitro. Proc. Natl. Acad. Sci. USA* **83**, 2694–2698.

Furnari, B., Rhind, N., and Russell, P. (1997). Cdc25 mitotic inducer targeted by chk1 DNA damage checkpoint kinase. *Science* **277**, 1495–1497.

Furukawa, T., Kubota, T., and Hoffman, R. M. (1995). Clinical applications of the histoculture drug response assay. *Clin. Cancer Res.* **1**, 305–311.

Goldacre, R. J., and Sylven, B. (1962). On the access of blood borne dyes to various tumour regions. *Br. J. Cancer* **16**, 306–322.

Graham, M. A., Senan, S., Robin, H. J., Eckhardt, N., Lendrem, D., Hincks, J., Greenslade, D., Rampling, R., Kaye, S. B., von Roemeling, R., and Workman, P. (1997). Pharmacokinetics of the hypoxic cell cytotoxic agent tirapazamine and its major bioreductive metabolites in mice and humans: retrospective analysis of a pharmacokinetically guided dose-escalation strategy in a phase I trial. *Cancer Chemother. Pharmacol.* **40**, 1–10.

Haldane, A., Finlay, G. J., Gavin, J. B., and Baguley, B. C. (1992). Unusual dynamics of killing of cultured Lewis lung cells by the DNA-intercalating antitumour agent *N*-[2-(dimethylamino)ethyl]acridine-4-carboxamide. *Cancer Chemother. Pharmacol.* **29**, 475–479.

Hamburger, A. W., and Salmon, S. E. (1977). Primary bioassay of human tumor stem cells. *Science* **197**, 461–463.

Hamilton, G. (1998). Multicellular spheroids as an *in vitro* tumor model. *Cancer Lett.* **131**, 29–34.

Helmlinger, G., Yuan, F., Dellian, M., and Jain, R. K. (1997). Interstitial pH and pO$_2$ measurements in solid tumors *in vivo:* high-resolution measurements reveal a lack of correlation. *Nat. Med.* **3**, 177–182.

Herwig, S., and Strauss, M. (1997). The retinoblastoma protein—a master regulator of cell cycle, differentiation and apoptosis. *Eur. J. Biochem.* **246**, 581–601.

Hicks, K. O., Ohms, S. J., Vanzijl, P. L., Denny, W. A., Hunter, P. J., and Wilson, W. R. (1997). An experimental and mathematical model for the extravascular transport of a DNA intercalator in tumours. *Br. J. Cancer* **76**, 894–903.

Hicks, K. O., Fleming, Y., Siim, B. G., Koch, C. J., and Wilson, W. R. (1998). Extravascular diffusion of tirapazamine: effect of metabolic consumption assessed using the multicellular layer model. *Int. J. Radiat. Oncol. Biol. Phys.* **42**, 641–649.

Hicks, K. O., Pruijn, F. B., Baguley, B. C., and Wilson, W. R. (2000). Extravascular transport of the DNA intercalator and topoisomerase poison *N*-[2-(dimethylamino)ethyl]acridine-4-carboxamide (DACA): diffusion and metabolism in multicellular layers of tumor cells. *J. Pharm. Exp. Ther.* **297**, 1088–1098.

Keepers, Y. P., Pizao, P. E., Peters, G. J., van Ark-Otte, J., Winograd, B., and Pinedo, H. M. (1991). Comparison of the sulforhodamine B protein and tetrazolium (MTT) assays for *in vitro* chemosensitivity testing. *Eur. J. Cancer* **27**, 897–900.

Kremer, J. M., Wilting, J., and Janssen, L. H. (1988). Drug binding to human alpha-1-acid glycoprotein in health and disease. *Pharmacol. Rev.* **40**, 1–47.

Kumar, G. N., Walle, U. K., Bhalla, K. N., and Walle, T. (1993). Binding of taxol to human plasma, albumin and alpha 1-acid glycoprotein. *Res. Commun. Chem. Pathol. Pharmacol.* **80**, 337–344.

Kyle, A. H., and Minchinton, A. I. (1999). Measurement of delivery and metabolism of tirapazamine to tumor tissue using the multilayered cell culture model. *Cancer Chemother. Pharmacol.* **43**, 213–220.

Lambert, P. A., Kang, Y., Greaves, B., and Perry, R. R. (1998). The importance of DT-diaphorase in mitomycin C resistance in human colon cancer cell lines. *J. Surg. Res.* **80**, 177–181.

Less, J. R., Posner, M. C., Skalak, T. C., Wolmark, N., and Jain, R. K. (1997). Geometric resistance and microvascular network architecture of human colorectal carcinoma. *Microcirculation* **4**, 25–33.

Liu, B., Earl, H. M., Poole, C. J., Dunn, J., and Kerr, D. J. (1995). Etoposide protein binding in cancer patients. *Cancer Chemother. Pharmacol.* **36**, 506–512.

Mariani, M., Capolongo, L., Suarato, A., Bargiotti, A., Mongelli, N., Grandi, M., and Beck, W. T. (1994). Growth-inhibitory properties of novel anthracyclines in human leukemic cell lines expressing either Pgp-MDR or at-MDR. *Invest. New Drugs* **12**, 93–97.

Marshall, E. S., Finlay, G. J., Matthews, J. H. L., Shaw, J. H. F., Nixon, J., and Baguley, B. C. (1992). Microculture-based chemosensitivity testing: a feasibility study comparing freshly explanted human melanoma cells with human melanoma cell lines. *J. Natl. Cancer. Inst.* **84**, 340–345.

Masters, J. R. W., Twentyman, P., Daley, R., Davis, J., Doyle, A., Dyer, S., Freshney, I., Galpine, A., Harrison, M., Hurst, H., Kelland, L., Stacey, G., Stratford, I., and Ward, T. H. (2000). UKCCCR guidelines for the use of cell lines in cancer research. *Br. J. Cancer* **82**, 1495–1509.

Mattern, M. R., Hofmann, G. A., Polsky, R. M., Funk, L. R., McCabe, F. L., and Johnson, R. K. (1993). *In vitro* and *in vivo* effects of clinically important camptothecin analogues on multidrug-resistant cells. *Oncol. Res.* **5**, 467–474.

McKeage, M. J., Abel, G., Kelland, L. R., and Harrap, K. R. (1994). Mechanism of action of an orally administered platinum complex [ammine bisbutyratocyclohexylamine dichloroplatinum (IV) (JM221)] in intrinsically cisplatin-resistant human ovarian carcinoma *in vitro. Br. J. Cancer* **69**, 1–7.

McKeage, M. J., Berners-Price, S. J., Galettis, P., Brouwer, W., Ding, L., Zhuang, L., and Baguley, B. C. (2000). Role of lipophilicity in determining cellular uptake and antitumour activity of gold phosphine complexes. *Cancer Chemother. Pharmacol.* **46**, 343–350.

Mi, Z., and Burke, T. G. (1994). Marked interspecies variations concerning the interactions of camptothecin with serum albumins: a frequency-domain fluorescence spectroscopic study. *Biochemistry* **33**, 12540–12545.

Miller, F. R., McEachern, D., and Miller, B. E. (1990). Efficiency of communication between cells in collagen gel cultures. *Br. J. Cancer* **62**, 360–363.

Minchinton, A. I., Wendt, K. R., Clow, K. A., and Fryer, K. H. (1997). Multilayers of cells growing on a permeable support—an *in vitro* tumour model. *Acta Oncol.* **36**, 13–16.

Monks, A., Scudiero, D., Skehan, P., Shoemaker, R., Paull, K., Vistica, D., Hose, C., Langley, J., Cronise, P., Vaigrowolff, A., Gray-Goodrich, M., Campbell, H., Mayo, J., and Boyd, M. (1991). Feasibility of a high-flux anticancer drug screen using a diverse panel of cultured human tumor cell lines. *J. Natl. Cancer. Inst.* **83**, 757–766.

Mosmann, T. (1983). Rapid colorimetric assay for cellular growth and survival: application to proliferation and cytotoxicity assays. *J. Immunol. Methods* **65**, 55–63.

Mueller-Klieser, W. (1997). Three-dimensional cell cultures: from molecular mechanisms to clinical applications. *Am. J. Physiol. Cell Physiol.* **42**, C1109–C1123.

Nederman, T., and Twentyman, P. (1984). Spheroids for studies of drug effects. *In* "Recent Results in Cancer Research" (H. Acker, J. Carlsson, R. M. Sutherland, and R. Durand, eds.), Vol. 95, pp. 84–102. Springer-Verlag, Berlin.

Nelson, E. M., Tewey, K. M., and Liu, L. F. (1984). Mechanism of antitumor drug action: poisoning of mammalian topoisomerase II on DNA by 4′-(9-acridinylamino)-methanesulfon-*m*-anisidide. *Proc. Natl. Acad. Sci. USA* **81**, 1361–1364.

Obach, R. S., Baxter, J. G., Liston, T. E., Silber, B. M., Jones, B. C., Macintyre, F., Rance, D. J., and Wastall, P. (1997). The prediction of human pharmacokinetic parameters from preclinical and *in vitro* metabolism data. *J. Pharm. Exp. Ther.* **283**, 46–58.

O'Connor, P. M., Jackman, J., Jondle, D., Bhatia, K., Magrath, I., and Kohn, K. W. (1993). Role of the p53 tumor suppressor gene in cell cycle arrest and radiosensitivity of Burkitt's lymphoma cell lines. *Cancer Res.* **53,** 4776–4780.

O'Connor, P. M., Jackman, J., Bae, I., Myers, T. G., Fan, S. J., Mutoh, M., Scudiero, D. A., Monks, A., Sausville, E. A., Weinstein, J. N., Friend, S., Fornace, A. J., and Kohn, K. W. (1997). Characterization of the p53 tumor suppressor pathway in cell lines of the National Cancer Institute anticancer drug screen and correlations with the growth-inhibitory potency of 123 anticancer agents. *Cancer Res.* **57,** 4285–4300.

Olive, P. L., and Durand, R. E. (1994). Drug and radiation resistance in spheroids: cell contact and kinetics. *Cancer Metastasis Rev.* **13,** 121–138.

Patterson, A. V., Saunders, M. P., Chinje, E. C., Talbot, D. C., Harris, A. L., and Stratford, I. J. (1997). Overexpression of human NADPH-cytochrome C (P450) reductase confers enhanced sensitivity to both tirapazamine (SR 4233) and RSU 1069. *Br. J. Cancer* **76,** 1338–1347.

Paull, K. D., Shoemaker, R. H., Hodes, L., Monks, A., Scudiero, D. A., Rubinstein, L., Plowman, J., and Boyd, M. R. (1989). Display and analysis of patterns of differential activity of drugs against human tumour cell lines: development of mean graph and COMPARE algorithm. *J. Natl. Cancer. Inst.* **81,** 1088–1092.

Paxton, J. W. (1983). Alpha$_1$-acid glycoprotein and binding of basic drugs. *Methods Find. Exp. Clin. Pharmacol.* **5,** 635–648.

Paxton, J. W., Young, D., Evans, S. M., Kestell, P., Robertson, I. G. C., and Cornford, E. M. (1992). Pharmacokinetics and toxicity of the antitumour agent N-[2-(dimethylamino)ethyl]acridine-4-carboxamide after i.v. administration in the mouse. *Cancer Chemother. Pharmacol.* **29,** 379–384.

Paxton, J. W., Young, D., Evans, S. M., Robertson, I. G., and Kestell, P. (1993). Tumour profile of N-[2-(dimethylamino)ethyl]acridine-4-carboxamide after intraperitoneal administration in the mouse. *Cancer Chemother. Pharmacol.* **32,** 320–322.

Peng, K. W. (1999). Strategies for targeting therapeutic gene delivery. *Mol. Med. Today* **5,** 448–453.

Peters, G. J., Smitskamp-Wilms, E., Smid, K., Pinedo, H. M., and Jansen, G. (1999). Determinants of activity of the antifolate thymidylate synthase inhibitors Tomudex (ZD1694) and GW1843U89 against mono- and multilayered colon cancer cell lines under folate-restricted conditions. *Cancer Res.* **59,** 5529–5535.

Phillips, R. M., Loadman, P. M., and Cronin, B. P. (1998). Evaluation of a novel *in vitro* assay for assessing drug penetration into avascular regions of tumours. *Br. J. Cancer* **77,** 2112–2119.

Puck, T. T., and Marcus, P. I. A. (1955). A rapid method of viable cell titration and clone production with HeLa cells in tissue culture: the use of X-irradiated cells to supply conditioning factors. *Proc. Natl. Acad. Sci. USA* **41,** 432–437.

Raff, M. C. (1992). Social controls on cell survival and cell death. *Nature* **356,** 397–400.

Rauth, A. M., Melo, T., and Mistra, V. (1998). Bioreductive therapies: an overview of drugs and their mechanisms of action. *Int. J. Radiat. Oncol. Biol. Phys.* **42,** 755–762.

Riley, R. J., and Workman, P. (1992). DT-diaphorase and cancer chemotherapy. *Biochem. Pharmacol.* **43,** 1657–1669.

Robertson, N., Stratford, I. J., Houlbrook, S., Carmichael, J., and Adams, G. E. (1992). The sensitivity of human tumour cells to quinone bioreductive drugs—what role for DT-diaphorase? *Biochem. Pharmacol.* **44,** 409–412.

Roninson, I. B. (1992). The role of the MDR1 (P-glycoprotein) gene in multidrug resistance *in vitro* and *in vivo*. *Biochem. Pharmacol.* **43,** 95–102.

Ross, D. T., Scherf, U., Eisen, M. B., Perou, C. M., Rees, C., Spellman, P., Iyer, V., Jeffrey, S. S., Van de Rijn, M., Waltham, M., Pergamenschikov, A., Lee, J. C. E., Lashkari, D., Shalon, D., Myers, T. G., Weinstein, J. N., Botstein, D., and Brown, P. O. (2000). Systematic variation in gene expression patterns in human cancer cell lines. *Nat. Genet.* **24,** 227–235.

Rowe-Jones, D. C. (1967). The penetration of cytotoxins into malignant tumours. *Br. J. Cancer* **22,** 155–162.

St Croix, B., and Kerbel, R. S. (1997). Cell adhesion and drug resistance in cancer. *Curr. Opin. Oncol.* **9,** 549–556.

Sandmeyer, S. B., Hansen, L. J., and Chalker, D. L. (1990). Integration specificity of retrotransposons and retroviruses. *Annu. Rev. Genet.* **24,** 491–518.

Scherf, U., Ross, D. T., Waltham, M., Smith, L. H., Lee, J. K., Tanabe, L., Kohn, K. W., Reinhold, W. C., Myers, T. G., Andrews, D. T., Scudiero, D. A., Eisen, M. B., Sausville, E. A., Pommier, Y., Botstein, D., Brown, P. O., and Weinstein, J. N. (2000). A gene expression database for the molecular pharmacology of cancer. *Nat. Genet.* **24,** 236–244.

Schneider, G., Coassolo, P., and Lave, T. (1999). Combining *in vitro* and *in vivo* pharmacokinetic data for prediction of hepatic drug clearance in humans by artificial neural networks and multivariate statistical techniques. *J. Med. Chem.* **42,** 5072–5076.

Scudiero, D. A., Shoemaker, R. H., Paull, K. D., Monks, A., Tierney, S., Nofziger, T. H., Currens, M. J., Seniff, D., and Boyd, M. R. (1988). Evaluation of a soluble tetrazolium/formazan assay for cell growth and drug sensitivity in culture using human and other tumour cell lines. *Cancer Res.* **48,** 4827–4833.

Sethi, T., Rintoul, R. C., Moore, S. M., MacKinnon, A. C., Salter, D., Choo, C., Chilvers, E. R., Dransfield, I., Donnelly, S. C., Strieter, R., and Haslett, C. (1999). Extracellular matrix proteins protect small cell lung cancer cells against apoptosis: a mechanism for small cell lung cancer growth and drug resistance *in vivo*. *Nat. Med.* **5,** 662–668.

Sham, E., and Durand, R. E. (1998). Cell kinetics and repopulation mechanisms during multifraction irradiation of spheroids. *Radiother. Oncol.* **46,** 201–207.

Shoemaker, R. H., Wolpert-DeFilippes, M. K., Kern, D. H., Lieber, M. M., Makuch, R. W., Melnick, N. R., Miller, W. T., Salmon, S. E., Simon, R. M., Venditti, J. M., and Von Hoff, D. D. (1985). Application of a human tumour colony-forming assay to new drug screening. *Cancer Res.* **45,** 2145–2153.

Siegel, D., Gibson, N. W., Preusch, P. C., and Ross, D. (1990). Metabolism of mitomycin C by DT-diaphorase: Role in mitomycin C-induced DNA damage and cytotoxicity in human colon carcinoma cells. *Cancer Res.* **50,** 7483–7489.

Skehan, P., Storeng, R., Scudiero, D., Monks, A., McMahon, J., Vistica, D., Warren, J. T., Bokesch, H., Kenney, S., and Boyd, M. R. (1990). New colorimetric cytotoxicity assay for anticancer-drug screening. *J. Natl. Cancer. Inst.* **82,** 1107–1112.

Slater, A. F., Stefan, C., Nobel, I., van den Dobbelsteen, D. J., and Orrenius, S. (1995). Signalling mechanisms and oxidative stress in apoptosis. *Toxicol. Lett.* **82–83,** 149–153.

Spanswick, V. J., Cummings, J., and Smyth, J. F. (1998). Current issues in the enzymology of mitomycin C metabolic activation. *Gen. Pharmacol.* **31,** 539–544.

Sutherland, R. M. (1988). Cell and environment interactions in tumor microregions: the multicellular spheroid model. *Science* **240,** 177–184.

Sutherland, R. M., and Durand, R. E. (1976). Radiation response of multicell spheroids—an *in vitro* tumour model. *Radiat. Res. Q.* **11,** 87–139.

Sutherland, R. M., Eddy, H. A., Bareham, B., Reich, K., and Vanantwerp, D. (1979). Resistance to adriamycin in multicellular spheroids. *Int. J. Radiat. Oncol. Biol. Phys.* **5,** 1225–1230.

Tanigawa, N., Kitaoka, A., Yamakawa, M., Tanisaka, K., and Kobayashi, H. (1996). *In vitro* chemosensitivity testing of human tumours by collagen gel droplet culture and image analysis. *Anticancer Res.* **16,** 1925–1930.

Taylor, E. W., Gibbons, J. A., and Braeckman, R. A. (1997). Intestinal absorption screening of mixtures from combinatorial libraries in the caco-2 model. *Pharm. Res.* **14,** 572–577.

Topp, E. M., Kitos, P. A., Vijaykumar, V., DeSilva, B. S., and Hendrickson, T. L. (1998). Antibody transport in cultured tumor cell layers. *J. Contr. Release* **53,** 15–23.

Von Hoff, D. D. (1988). Human tumour cloning assays: applications in clinical oncology and new antineoplastic agent development. *Cancer Metastasis Rev.* **7**, 357–371.

Waldman, T., Zhang, Y. G., Dillehay, L., Yu, J., Kinzler, K., Vogelstein, B., and Williams, J. (1997). Cell-cycle arrest versus cell death in cancer therapy. *Nat. Med.* **3**, 1034–1036.

Weaver, J. R., Wientjes, M. G., and Au, J. L.-S. (1999). Regional heterogeneity and pharmacodynamics in human solid tumor histoculture. *Cancer Chemother. Pharmacol.* **44**, 335–342.

Weinstein, J. N., Kohn, K. W., Grever, M. R., Viswanadhan, V. N., Rubinstein, L. V., Monks, A. P., Scudiero, D. A., Welch, L., Koutsoukos, A. D., Chiausa, A. J., and Paull, K. D. (1992). Neural computing in cancer drug development—predicting mechanism of action. *Science* **258**, 447–451.

Weinstein, J. N., Myers, T. G., O'Connor, P. M., Friend, S. H., Fornace, A. J., Kohn, K. W., Fojo, T., Bates, S. E., Rubinstein, L. V., Anderson, N. L, Buolamwini, J. K., van Osdol, W. W., Monks, A. P., Scudiero, D. A., Sausville, E. A., Zaharevitz, D. W., Bunow, B., Viswanadhan, V. N., Johnson, G. S., Wittes, R. E., and Paull, K. D. (1997). An information-intensive approach to the molecular pharmacology of cancer. *Science* **275**, 343–349.

Weisenthal, L. M., and Lippman, M. E. (1985). Clonogenic and nonclonogenic *in vitro* chemosensitivity assays. *Cancer. Treat. Rep.* **69**, 615–632.

West, G. W., Weichselbaum, R., and Little, J. B. (1980). Limited penetration of methotrexate into human osteosarcoma spheroids as a proposed model for solid tumor resistance to adjuvant chemotherapy. *Cancer Res.* **40**, 3665–3668.

Wilson, G. D., McNally, N. J., Dische, S., Saunders, M. I., Des Rochers, C., Lewis, A. A., and Bennett, M. H. (1988). Measurement of cell kinetics in human tumours *in vivo* using bromodeoxyuridine incorporation and flow cytometry. *Br. J. Cancer* **58**, 423–431.

Wilson, W. R., and Hicks, K. O. (1999). Measurement of extravascular drug diffusion in multicellular layers. *Br. J. Cancer* **79**, 1623–1626.

Wilson, W. R., Baguley, B. C., Wakelin, L. P. G., and Waring, M. J. (1981a). Interaction of the antitumour drug m-AMSA (4′-(9-acridinylamino)-methanesulphon-m-anisidide) and related acridines with nucleic acids. *Mol. Pharmacol.* **20**, 404–414.

Wilson, W. R., Whitmore, G. F., and Hill, R. P. (1981b). Activity of 4'-(9-acridinylamino)methanesulfon-m-anisidide against Chinese hamster cells in multicellular spheroids. *Cancer Res.* **41**, 2817–2822.

Wÿffels, K. I. E. M., Kaanders, J. H. A. M., Rijken, P. F. J. W., Bussink, J., van den Hoogen, F. J. A., Marres, H. A. M., de Wilde, P. C. M., Raleigh, J. A., and van der Kogel, A. J. (2000). Vascular architecture and hypoxic profiles in human head and neck squamous cell carcinomas. *Br. J. Cancer* **83**, 674–683.

CHAPTER 16

SCREENING USING ANIMAL SYSTEMS

Angelika M. Burger*
Heinz-Herbert Fiebig*,†

*Tumor Biology Center at the University of Freiburg and
†Institute for Experimental Oncology GmbH
Freiburg, Germany

Summary

Anticancer drug development is historically based on *in vivo* screening. Although transplantable murine tumors were used until the mid-1970s, human tumor xenografts and transgenic mice dominate the disease-oriented and molecular-target-directed screening approaches of today. Xenografts have proven predictive for clinical response, and virtually any specific target can be found indigenously overexpressed in individual xenografts of large *in vivo* model panels such as the U.S. National Cancer Institute (NCI) 60-cell-line panel or our own panel of more than 60 xenografts. The Freiburg models were developed by subcutaneous grafting of patients' tumors into immunodeficient mice. More than 350 tumors, covering a broad spectrum of tumor types, were transferred into serial passage. Sixty tumors were characterized in detail for sensitivity against standard agents; for expression of oncogenes, tumor suppressor genes, growth factors, and receptors; for parameters of angiogenesis, invasion, and metastasis; or for resistance associated proteins. The response to standard agents in nude mice and in patients' tumors was similar, and correct prediction was found in 90% of sensitive and 97% of resistant tumors. We initially employ *in vitro* testing using xenograft tissues in the clonogenic assay, enabling a target (and/or surrogate)–response combination in large tumor numbers. Only the most sensitive and target-expressing tumors are selected for *in vivo* studies, thus increasing the likelihood of response and reducing the number of animal experiments. Compounds discovered as active in our screen that have entered clinical trials include agents with diverse modes of action and specific molecular targets, such as methotrexate coupled to human serum albumin (MTX-HSA), flavopiridol, 17-allylaminogeldanamycin, and rViscumin. An overview of the available screens is provided for particular therapeutic strategies, such as the targeting of tumor angiogenesis or the application of chemopreventive agents, which require specialized *in vivo* assays and animal systems such as transgenic mouse models.

1. Introduction

The advent of modern cancer chemotherapy in the middle of the 20th century is exemplified by the introduction of alkylating agents, particularly nitrogen mustards, and antimetabolites into clinical use (Goldenberg and Moore, 1997). Subsequently, most of the currently available anticancer drugs have been developed in transplantable rodent tumor models. Thus, cancer drug discovery traditionally has utilized *in vivo* screening. The earliest models were the syngeneic transplantable murine leukemias L1210 and P388 (Fig. 1, Table 1). (Boyd, 1989; Schepartz, 1976). These tumors were the backbone of the U.S. National Cancer Institute (NCI) preclinical drug development program from the 1950s to 1985 (Boyd, 1989). The rapidly growing L1210 and P388 leukemias were implanted intraperitoneally and grew as ascites as well as systematically with survival as an end point, providing a rapid and reproducible mean of identifying cytotoxic drugs (Teicher, 1997). In 1976 solid murine tumor models, such as the B16 melanoma, the C38 colon tumor, the Lewis lung cancer, and in 1981 the M5076, a reticulosarcoma of the ovary, were added (Table 1). Three human tumor xenografts representing the major solid tumor types—lung (LX-1), colon (CX-1), and breast (MX-1)—were used to test active compounds. While these *in vivo* models identified 35 therapeutic agents up to the early 1980s, it became evident that the classes of agents found active were limited and comprised mainly alkylating agents and some other DNA-interacting drugs. Novel structures had not been discovered for more than 20 years (Fiebig *et al.,* 1999a; Goldin *et al.,* 1981; Ovejera, 1987). In addition, public awareness of labo-

ratory animal welfare, particularly in Europe (Tierschutzgesetz in Germany and United Kingdom Animals Scientific Procedures Act, both 1986), prohibited the further use of survival end points and demanded alternative end points as well as minimal use of animals for maximal gain of information (Workman *et al.,* 1997).

The above events led to a refinement of the screening systems in that compound-oriented preclinical drug development (Fig. 1) was replaced by tumor type-oriented drug discovery strategies (Fig. 2) (Boyd, 1989). Increasing knowledge of genes responsible for cancer causation also facilitated refinement. Hence, molecular targets for the discovery of more effective and selective anticancer agents (Sausville and Feigal, 1999; Workman *et al.,* 1997) were defined, and the emphasis is now placed on demonstrating activity in accordance with target expression and modulation. Consequently, contemporary preclinical small-molecular drug development strategies employ a sequential test cascade that includes high-throughput compound screening in biochemical (usually with recombinant target protein) and target cell assays *in vitro,* followed by a very limited and carefully selected number of compounds tested in surrogate *in vivo* models (Fig. 2). This would greatly increase the likelihood that agents tested *in vivo* would then have the desired antitumor properties (Sausville and Feigal, 1999; Workman *et al.,* 1997). Prompted by the need to identify tumor types that express the target for the new-generation cancer medicines, *in vivo* models used in preclinical development today are both disease oriented and target characterized, and comprise either human tumor explants/xenografts or specifically bred transgenic mice (Malakoff *et al.,* 2000). However, due to high running costs and limited availability, transgenic mice are not suitable for large-scale drug testing, so that xenografts have become the gold standard in cancer drug development. Their use is highly recommended by regulatory agencies such as the European Agency for the Evaluation of Medicinal Products (EMEA) in the "Note for guidance on the pre-clinical evaluation of anticancer medicinal products" (EMEA, 1998). This chapter will review the variety of contemporary animal screening systems and the selection of *in vivo* models for large-scale anticancer drug development.

2. Choice of *in Vivo* Systems for Large-Scale Drug Development

Two model systems with established cell lines growing in nude mice, the hollow-fiber assay and human tumor xenografts, are currently being used for large-scale *in vivo* testing. For compounds acting potentially via an intact immune system, the transplantable murine leukemias and solid tumors still have an accepted role (Table 2). Cancers induced by chemical carcinogens comprise another category of ex-

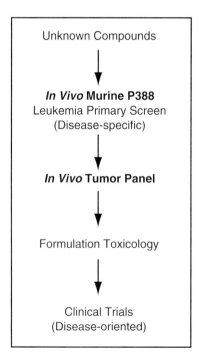

FIGURE 1 Compound-oriented preclinical drug development strategy used by the National Cancer Institute, 1975–1985. (Adopted from Boyd, 1989).

TABLE 1
Murine Tumor Models Used for Anticancer Drug Development at NCI

Tumor type	Induced by	Host mice	Year established	Histology	Main use
Leukemias					
L1210	MCA	DBA/2	1948	Acute lymphoblastic	1955–1985
P388	MCA	DBA/2	1952	Acute lymphoblastic	1968–1985
Melanoma					
B16	Spontaneous	C57Bl/6	1954	Amelanotic	1976–1986
Lung					
Lewis	Spontaneous	C57Bl/6	1957	Carcinoma	1976–1986
Colon					
Colon 38	DMH	C57Bl/6	1953	Poorly diff. adeno cancer	1978–1985
Ovary					
M5076	DMH	C57Bl/6	1981	Reticulosarcoma	1981–1985

DMH, 1,2-dimethylhydrazine; MCA, methylcholanthrene.

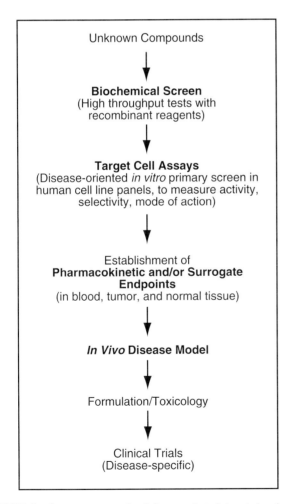

FIGURE 2 Current test cascade of disease-oriented, targeted anticancer drug development. Adopted from UKCCCR Guidelines for the Welfare of Animals in Experimental Neoplasia (2nd ed., 1997, Appendix 4a, p. 25).

perimental tumors. In the rat it is possible to induce autochthonous tumors in most organs (Table 3) with a tumor incidence after 4–20 weeks ranging from 50% to 100%. 7,12-Dimethylbenzanthracene- or ethylnitrosourea-induced mammary cancers in rats were useful models for the identification of new endocrine therapies (Sugamata *et al.*, 1999). The other autochthonous models did not gain a broader application because of the requirement for long pretreatment with a carcinogen, the long induction time, and the asynchronous occurrence of the tumors. Furthermore, testing in rats was much more expensive than in mice and higher amounts of the test compound are required.

A. Hollow-Fiber Assay

The NCI favors the hollow-fiber assay in which more than 50 human tumor cell lines have been grown successfully in polyvinyl fibers of 1 mm inner diameter. Normally three fibers with three different cell lines are implanted intraperitoneally and subcutaneously per mouse. Each fiber (2 cm length) contains 50–200,000 cells in 20 µl. The treatment is normally administered intraperitoneally using a daily (for 4 days) schedule, starting on the third or fourth day after fiber implantation. The fibers are harvested on day 5–8, and the viable cell number is determined using the MTT [3-(4,5-dimethylthiazol-2-yl)-2,5-diphenyl-tetrazolium bromide] assay (Hollingshead *et al.*, 1995, 1999). The NCI has validated the hollow fiber assay in comparing the activity of 84 compounds in permanent cell lines growing in the hollow-fiber assay and as subcutaneous xenografts in nude mice. In the hollow-fiber assay 29 compounds were rated as active whereas in the same tumors growing subcutaneously only four compounds were active. Therefore, as an *in vivo* screen, the hollow-fiber assay

TABLE 2
In Vivo Models for Large-Scale Anticancer Drug Testing

Host	Type	Localization	Reference
NuNu mice	Hollow-fiber assay	IP, SC	Hollingshead *et al.*, 1999
NuNu mice	Established human solid tumor models	SC, orthotopic	Fiebig *et al.*, 1999a Fiebig and Burger, 2001 Hoffman, 1999
Mice	Transplantable leukemias	IP, IV, SC	Waud, 1997
Mice	Transplantable tumors	SC, IV	Corbett *et al.*, 1997
Rats	Chemically induced cancers	See Table 3	Berger, 1999

DMBA, 7,12-dimethylbenzanthracene.

is feasible for the rapid identification of inactive compounds and for prioritization of active compounds at reasonable cost. However, active compounds must be studied subsequently in human tumor xenografts growing subcutaneously or orthotopically before a decision for development should be taken. The latter must be carefully considered under the view that the requirements for Good Manufacturing Practice drug synthesis, Good Laboratory Practice toxicology, pharmacokinetics, safety pharmacology, and clinical trials imply a multimillion dollar investment.

B. Human Tumors Growing in Nude Mice

As a second well-established testing procedure for large-scale *in vivo* testing, tumors can be derived from cancer patients and grown subcutaneously or orthotopically in nude mice. Such xenografts can be generated from almost all solid cancers. Subcutaneous implantation is much easier to perform than orthotopic implantation, allowing for testing of broad tumor panels (Fiebig *et al.*, 1992, 1999a). Patient-derived human tumor xenografts, growing subcutaneously, have been shown to maintain typical histologic characteristics, chemosensitivity profiles, expression of relevant oncogenes, growth factors/growth factor receptors, and parameters associated with angiogenesis, invasion, and metastasis. Chemosensitivity studies of novel molecular targeted therapies are normally performed in well-characterized models expressing the target against which the new compound should act.

Orthotopically growing tumors have the advantage that metastases occur in much higher frequency and the invasion seems to be more pronounced compared with subcutaneously growing models (Hoffman, 1999). However, the implantation technique is more time consuming, allowing only a limited number of compounds to be tested per experiment. Usually serial size measurements are not possible for tumors growing in internal organs. Therefore, the mice have to be sacrificed to measure tumor volume that allows only a one-point measurement. This is a major drawback of this otherwise very attractive, more clinically relevant disease model. Broad testing of standard agents or novel compounds has not been

TABLE 3
Autochthonous Chemically Induced Cancers in Rats

Tumor type	Histology	Carcinogen	Incidence (%)
Mammary	Adeno cancer	DMBA, ethyl nitrosourea	100
Sarcoma	Fibrosarcoma	Benzo(a)pyrene	90
Hepatoma	Hepatocellular	Diethyl nitrosourea	90
Esophagus	Squamous cell	Phenylethyl nitrosamine	80
Stomach	Adeno cancer	Methyl nitrosourea	90
Colon	Adeno cancer	1,2-Dimethylhydrazine	90
Bladder	Carcinoma	Butylbutanol nitrosamine	90
Brain, CNS	Glioblastoma	Butyl nitrosamine	90
Leukemias	Acute myelocytic	DMBA	90
		Ethyl nitrosourea	50–80

DMBA, 7,12-dimethylbenzanthracene.

reported using orthotopic implantation, which means that the procedure is too time consuming and expensive for large-scale testing. However, the orthotopic model provides the most appropriate evaluation of specific inhibitors of metastases or invasion.

3. Combined *in Vitro/in Vivo* Testing Procedure Using Human Tumor Xenografts—The Freiburg Experience

The testing of novel components for *in vivo* activity in randomly selected models has a low probability of success, apart from series of closely related analogues of an active compound. Therefore, additional criteria for selecting appropriate models are necessary, and two approaches are particularly promising. If the target or mechanism of action is known, tumors overexpressing this target should be selected. If the mechanism is not known, *in vitro* testing in a panel of xenografts using the clonogenic assay will allow identifica-

tion of the most sensitive tumors, which are subsequently studied *in vivo* (Fig. 3). We have refined the clonogenic assay and have observed growth of colonies in more than 86% of xenografted tumors. This percentage is markedly higher than that for fresh tumor material derived from patients (40–50%). We were able to use 24-well plates, and at least 20 colonies were required for an assay to be considered as evaluable. Details of the methodology have been described previously (Fiebig *et al.*, 1992, 1999a).

A. Combined *in Vitro/in Vivo* Testing Procedure

We have recently developed a combined *in vitro/in vivo* test procedure for anticancer drug development (Fiebig *et al.*, 1992, 1999a), and an outline of the five-step evaluation is shown in Fig. 3. In the first stage, large-scale tests (primary screening) are performed *in vitro* using a modified clonogenic assay in six human tumors obtained from serial passage in nude mice. Secondary *in vitro* screening is performed in a total of 20 human tumor xenografts, 14 being sensitive against

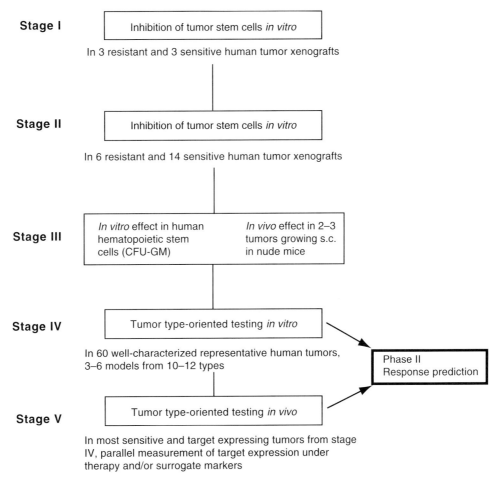

FIGURE 3 Combined *in vitro/in vivo* testing procedure with human tumor xenografts.

standard agents and 6 being resistant. In stage III, the effect on human hematopoietic stem cells (granulocyte-macrophage colony-forming units, (CFU-GM) from 2–4 healthy donors is studied. Compounds with a greater or similar effect on tumor cells in comparison with hematopoietic stem cells are subsequently studied *in vivo* in 2–3 of the most sensitive tumors transplanted subcutaneously into nude mice. The comparison of *in vitro* and *in vivo* activity enables assessment of the relevant *in vitro* dose, based on *in vivo* pharmacology. If remission or tumor stasis is observed *in vivo,* the compound undergoes tumor-type-oriented testing, usually in 40–60 xenografts. Since our other studies have suggested that the tumors selected for stage IV have chemosensitivity profiles similar to those of clinical cancers, target tumors for clinical studies as well as tissue-specific preclinical models can be identified.

B. Take Rates and Growth Behavior of Patient Tumor Explants in Nude Mice

Of 1600 patient tumors, the growth behavior of 1227 different human malignancies growing subcutaneously in nude mice has been characterized in detail (Tables 4 and 5). Histologic examination of the tumors showed that 79% contained viable tumor tissue. However, only 41% of the tumors showed a rapid growth with tumor diameters of more than 8 mm after 90 days (Table 4) equal to length × width of more than 60 mm^2. Thus, only these rapidly growing tumors were suitable for establishing stably growing models and for further investigation. Nonetheless, it must be noted that the growth of human tumors of the latter described category is still much slower than that seen in established murine models. Four hundred (33% of the total explants) of the 499 "rapidly" growing human tumor explants were successfully transferred in serial passage and most of them were cryopreserved in liquid nitrogen with a recovery of 90% (Table 5).

Tumors in serial passage can be divided into three categories. The rate was highest (40–60%) in tumors of the esophagus, cervix and corpus uteri, colon, lung (small cell), and melanomas. Intermediate growth rates between 20% and 40% were observed for carcinoma of the lung (non-small cell); soft-tissue sarcoma; carcinoma of the ovaries, head and neck, pancreas, testicle, stomach, and bladder; and pleuramesothelioma. The lowest rates (5–19%) were observed in renal cell cancers and in the hormone-dependent mammary and prostate carcinomas. The growth of breast and prostate cancers was increased when intramuscular estrogen or dihydrotestosterone depots were given every 2 weeks.

Among the over 400 models, 264 have been selected for further characterization, such as by determination of chemosensitivity profiles. These models showed a consistent growth behavior and typical histologic and differentiation

TABLE 4
Growth of Human Tumors in Nude Mice (Freiburg Experience 1980–1994)

Tumor origin	Total *n*	Rapid growth[a] *n*	Rapid growth[a] %	Serial passage[b] *n*	Serial passage[b] %
Esophagus	10	7	70	6	60
Cervix uteri	10	7	70	6	60
Colorectal	152	88	58	78	51
Corpus uteri	8	4	50	4	50
Melanomas	63	39	62	27	43
Lung, small cell	39	14	36	16	41
Lung, non small cell	227	118	52	87	38
Sarcomas, soft-tissue	79	36	46	29	37
Ovary	22	7	32	8	36
Head and neck	47	16	34	16	34
Pancreas	6	2	33	2	33
Brain	6	2	33	2	33
Hepatocellular	3	1	33	1	33
Neuroblastoma	3	1	33	1	33
Osteosarcoma	13	5	38	4	31
Miscellaneous	100	33	33	26	26
Testicle	48	14	29	12	25
Mesothelioma	36	14	39	9	25
Stomach	68	17	25	17	25
Bladder	44	17	39	10	23
Renal	124	37	30	24	19
Mammary	74	13	18	13	18
Prostate	41	7	17	2	5
Total	**1227**	**499**	**41**	**400**	**33**

characteristics. Rapidly and slowly growing tumors were included, as were models that were sensitive and resistant to standard agents.

At the University of California, in a similar effort to establish human tumor models from surgical specimens, a total of 323 explants was collected from patients (Reid *et al.,* 1978). The latter yielded in the development of only 27 (8%) transplantable models. Although the California group had similar good results with respect to retaining patient characteristics, their markedly lower success rate (8%) in obtaining stable, transplantable models versus that of our program (33%) might be due to the processing of the specimens. While they minced and then injected the tumor suspensions subcutaneously into nude mice without paying attention to the gender of the patient from which the tumors were derived or the age of the mice, we established our models from tumor fragments in very young mice (age 4 weeks) of the same gender as the donor patient. By doing that we assured that the xenografted tumor speci-

TABLE 5
Human Tumors Available as Tumor Models in Nude Mice

Category	Total no.	Histology	Median doubling time (days)	Frozen in nitrogen take[a]/total	Response total[b]
Lung	38	Epidermoid	4–18	21/25	7/18
Lung	20	Adeno	6–19	17/18	3/5
Lung	12	Large cell	4–16	12/14	1/3
Lung	7	Small cell	6–14	9/12	6/7
Colorectal	>50	Adeno	4–24	42/44	2/20
Melanomas	24	Melanoma	4–23	13/14	1/10
Soft tissue	17	Soft tissue	3–16	14/15	3/6
Renal	16	Adeno	7–18	10/11	0/7
Stomach	14	Adeno	6–17	14/18	6/13
Mammary	8	Adeno and solid	8–20	8/9	6/8
Miscellaneous	58		4–22	40/43	13/27
Total	**264**	**Total**	**3–24**	**200/223**	**48/124**
				(90%)	**(39%)**

[a]After being frozen.
[b]Partial remissions following single-drug therapy.

mens were provided with the most optimal environment such as their own extracellular matrix (ECM), appropriate hormonal conditions, high exposure to murine endogenous growth factors, and lowest probability of graft rejection.

C. Selection and Characterization of Tumor Models

During the last 12 years we have established more than 300 regularly growing human tumor xenografts, which are frozen in liquid nitrogen (Fiebig et al., 1992). After a detailed characterization (Table 6), 6 xenografts were selected for stage I, 20 for stage II, and 60 for stage IV in vivo testing. These 60 models were characterized in detail for oncogenes, tumor suppressor genes, growth factors and receptors, invasion- and metastasis-related proteins, as well as parameters for angiogenesis-, immortality-, and drug-resistance-associated proteins, e.g., k-ras, c-myc, p53, EGF-R, TGF-α, TGF-β, VEGF, telomerase as well as mdr1, mdr3, GST (Table 6).

Data for 29 molecular targets are available in our database, and we are able to correlate the expression of potential molecular targets with in vitro effective dose levels derived from clonogenic assays using the xenograft material. This bioinformatic approach is based on the COMPARE algorithm developed by the NCI (Paull et al., 1989); it allows the determination of any statistical interaction with the potential molecular targets (Spearman rank coefficient), thus providing a clue as to the possible mechanism of action of the drug.

It is crucial for a new drug to demonstrate a differential selectivity against human tumors compared with the most

sensitive normal tissue. In this respect, human tumor xenografts are considered to be the most relevant models since, like patient-derived tumors, they (1) grow as a solid tumor, (2) develop a stroma, (3) develop vasculature, (4) develop central necrosis, (5) show some degree of differentiation, and (6) have relevant response rates (Fiebig et al., 1992, 1999a). In most cases, the tumor xenografts architecture, cell morphology, and molecular characteristics mirror those of the original cancers. This is in marked contrast to xenografts derived from cell lines, which in general show a homogeneous undifferentiated histology and as a result are very resistant to most of the standard agents (Fiebig et al., 1999a; Goldin et al., 1981). This is most likely due to the high selection pressure in vitro during long-term culture, resulting in aggressive subclones.

D. Correlation of Drug Response

As a first step, clinically established anticancer drugs were tested in broad dose–response studies. The relevant concentrations or doses reflecting clinical efficacy were determined for each drug separately by comparing the in vitro/in vivo response rates of sensitive tumor types (Fiebig et al., 1987, 1992; Scholz et al., 1990; Steel, 1987). The following correlations were performed:

- Nude mouse models versus patient response
- Clonogenic assays from xenografts versus patient response
- Clonogenic assays from xenografts versus in vivo testing in the nude mouse after subcutaneous transplantation.

TABLE 6
Validated and Novel Molecular Targets Characterized in the 60-Human-Tumor Xenograft Panel

Category	Target
Oncogenes	k-ras
	c-myc
	c-erb-B2
	Di12
Tumor supressor genes	p53
Growth factors and receptors	EGF-R
	TGF-α
	TGF-β
	EGF
	bFGF
	Estrogen receptor
	Progesterone receptor
Invasion related	uPA
	Cathepsin D
	MMP-2
	MMP-3
	MMP-9
	TIMP-2
Metastases related	nm23
	CD44v6
Angiogenesis	VEGF
	Vascular porosity
	Microvessel density
	Angiogenin
Structural proteins	Cytokeratin
Immortality	Telomerase
Drug resistance related	MDR-1
	MDR-3
	GST

TABLE 7
Comparison of Drug Response in Human Tumors Growing Subcuteously in Nude Mice and in Cancer Patients

Mouse/patient	Total
Remission/remission	19
No remission/remission	2
No remission/no remission	57
Remission/no remission	2

Eighty comparisons were obtained in 55 tumors. Xenografts predicted correctly for → response in 90% (19/21), → resistance in 97% (57/59).

Details to the methodology used, the tumors included and the procedures for evaluating combinations have been published by our group (Fiebig *et al.*, 1987, 1992, 1999a; Scholz *et al.*, 1990; Steel, 1987). Subcutaneously growing xenografts showed the highest correlation with the response of patients: the correct prediction for tumor responsiveness was 90% (19/21 cases) and for tumor resistance 97% (57/59 cases) (Table 6). In other words, the positive predictive value (or the true positives) was 90% and the negative predictive value (or the true negatives) was 97%. The clonogenic assay predicted correctly for tumor response in 62% and for resistance in 92% (Table 7). The *in vitro/in vivo* correlations obtained in the clonogenic versus the nude mouse system were similar as for the clonogenic assay versus the patient.

The correlations obtained in our clonogenic assays using xenografts as donor tumor were similar to those reported by many other groups when patients' tumors were used (Hamburger and Salmon, 1977; Von Hoff, 1987). One drawback,

found also in other *in vitro* systems, is that the correct prediction for tumor sensitivity is in the range of 60–70%. In this respect the xenografts are more reliable. Other laboratories have also demonstrated the high predictivity of the xenograft model (Steel, 1987).

E. Selected Examples of Anticancer Agents in Clinical Trials Which Have Been Discovered in a Target-Oriented Approach Using the Freiburg Xenografts

For the past 10 years our group has received compounds from academia, the EORTC, the NCI, and the pharmaceutical industry (Burger *et al.*, 1997, 1998, 1999a, b; 2000; Drees *et al.*, 1997; Fiebig *et al.*, 1994, 1995, 1999b; Hartung *et al.*, 1999; Hendriks *et al.*, 1993, 1999; Klenner *et al.*, 1992; Maly *et al.*, 1995; Stehle *et al.*, 1997; Winterhalter *et al.*, 1993). They belonged to various structural classes and act by different mechanisms. An overview of compounds that showed activity in our models and where we contributed to the decision to develop the compounds clinically is shown in Table 8. Compounds that have now entered clinical trials are methotrexate coupled to human serum albumin (MTX-HSA) as synthesized at the German Cancer Research Center; pH-sensitive salicylic acid derivatives from the University of Freiburg; flavopiridol, spicamycin, and 17-allylaminogeldanamycin obtained from the NCI; ecteinascidin and rhizoxin from the EORTC; and recombinant mistletoe lectin (rML = rViscumin) and various other compounds from the pharmaceutical industry.

rML provides a good example of a preclinical development using the Freiburg combined *in vitro/in vivo* xenograft approach (Figs. 3–5). rML is the recombinant precursor of mistletoe lectins I–III produced in *Escherichia coli* with a molecular weight of 57 kDa, and has been shown to possess ribosome-inactivating activity (RIP) leading to a specific induction of apoptosis (Langer *et al.*, 1999). We found that rML was cytotoxic in the nanomolar range in permanent growing tumor cell lines *in vitro*. In subsequent stage IV test-

TABLE 8
Anticancer Drugs Discovered as Active in the Freiburg Human Tumor Xenograft Panel

		Mode of Action	Ref.
From academia:	MTX–HSA	Antimetabolite, EPR effect	Stehle *et al.*, 1997, Hartung *et al.*, 1999
	Lip. NOAC	Antimetabolite	Fiebig *et al.*, 1995
	pH-sensitive SA	Apoptosis	Burger *et al.*, 1999a
From the U.S. NCl:	Flavopiridol	Cyclin-dependent kinase inhibition	Drees *et al.*, 1997
	Quinocarmycin	DNA binding	Fiebig *et al.*, 1994
	Spicamycin	Glycoprotein synthesis	Burger *et al.*, 1997
	17-AAG	HSP90 modulation	Burger *et al.*, 1998
			Burger *et al.*, 2000
From the EORTC:	ET743	DNA minor grove alkylation	Hendriks *et al.*, 1999
	Rhizoxin	Tubulin binder	Winterhalter *et al.*, 1993
	EO9	Bioreductive alkylating	Hendriks *et al.*, 1993
From companies:	Lobaplatin	DNA cross-linking and adducts	Klenner *et al.*, 1992
	D21266	PKC and PLC inhibition	Maly *et al.*, 1995
	BAY 38-3441	Topoisomerase II inhibition	Fiebig *et al.*, 1999b
	RML/rViscumin	RIP, ribosome inactivation/apoptosis	Burger *et al.*, 1999b
	Several discrete compounds		

MTX-HSA, methotrexate coupled to human serum albumin; EPR, enhanced permeability and retention effect; SA, salicylic acid; PKC, phosphokinase C; PLC, phospholipase C; NOAC, N-octadecyl-cytosine arabinoside; AAG, 17-allylaminogeldanamycin.

ing in 47 human tumor xenografts in the clonogenic assay, we found that rML has a differential cytotoxicity profile (Fig. 4), with certain tumors being more sensitive or more resistant. Among the sensitive tumor types were breast, prostate, pancreas, and small cell lung cancers (Fig. 4). Thus, the sensitive *in vitro* small cell lung tumor model LXFS 538 was chosen for evaluation of *in vivo* pharmacologic activity (Fig. 5). Marked tumor growth inhibition ($T/C = 27\%$) was observed at the maximal tolerated dose of the drug (3 μg/kg) given on days 14–18 and 21–25. Figures 4 and 5 clearly demonstrate that the *in vitro* activity of rML could be translated into *in vivo* efficacy.

F. Future Impact of Human Tumor Xenografts

Inasmuch as new drug development is already focused on target-oriented and tumor-cell-specific approaches based on currently available knowledge, there is still a continuing demand for a better understanding of tumor biology. Thus, basic research can be directed to genetic tumor profiling, finding more promising tumor-type-specific therapeutic targets, and individualizing cancer therapy. In accomplishing this, genomics and proteomics now provide a large number of possible new gene candidates for therapeutic intervention. However, the validation of these genes in a wide collection of human tumor specimens provides a bottleneck; in particular, the lack of sufficient tumor tissue material to perform and thoroughly repeat a set of confirmatory analyses such as Northern or Western blots is often problematic. Here our xenograft collection not only provides a rich source of the hu-

man genome and proteome, but also allows repeated growth of material of consistent quality. Tissues can be collected while fresh and immediately frozen, resulting in total RNA and mRNA of extremely high quality. Moreover, the optimal tissue-processing procedure can be evaluated and novel treatments, either small molecules or gene therapy, can be tested later on in the same tissue from which a target was isolated and validated. In addition, pre- and posttreatment specimens for a pharmacogenomic approach can easily be collected. In view of these possibilities, the usefulness of human tumor xenografts and explants will steadily increase.

4. Use of Transgenic Animals in the Search for New Drugs

A battery of human oncogenes and tumor suppressor genes has now been identified, and the prospect of finding even more important cancer-causing and preventing genes has increased with sequencing of the human genome (Futreal *et al.*, 2001; Lander *et al.*, 2001; Venter *et al.*, 2001). The functional characterization of genes and proof-of-disease hypotheses can be accomplished by designing either murine gene knockout or transgenic animals (Malakoff *et al.*, 2000; Palmiter and Brinster, 1985). In the latter case, a gene in the form of a DNA fragment (viral or cellular origin) is linked to a suitable promoter DNA sequence and injected into a mouse egg nucleus. When the recombinant DNA molecule becomes integrated into the mouse chromosome, a transgenic mouse strain has been generated, which carries the gene in all cells. The

Antitumor Effect of rML
in Human Tumor Xenografts in Vitro

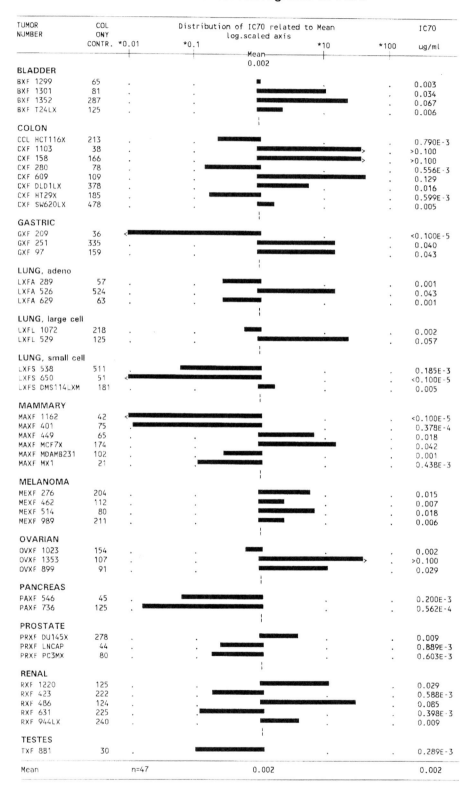

TUMOR NUMBER	COLONY CONTR.	Distribution of IC70 related to Mean log.scaled axis	IC70 ug/ml

BLADDER
BXF 1299	65		0.003
BXF 1301	81		0.034
BXF 1352	287		0.067
BXF T24LX	125		0.006

COLON
CCL HCT116X	213		0.790E-3
CXF 1103	38		>0.100
CXF 158	166		>0.100
CXF 280	78		0.556E-3
CXF 609	109		0.129
CXF DLD1LX	378		0.016
CXF HT29X	185		0.599E-3
CXF SW620LX	478		0.005

GASTRIC
GXF 209	36		<0.100E-5
GXF 251	335		0.040
GXF 97	159		0.043

LUNG, adeno
LXFA 289	57		0.001
LXFA 526	524		0.043
LXFA 629	63		0.001

LUNG, large cell
| LXFL 1072 | 218 | | 0.002 |
| LXFL 529 | 125 | | 0.057 |

LUNG, small cell
LXFS 538	511		0.185E-3
LXFS 650	51		<0.100E-5
LXFS DMS114LXM	181		0.005

MAMMARY
MAXF 1162	42		<0.100E-5
MAXF 401	75		0.378E-4
MAXF 449	65		0.018
MAXF MCF7X	174		0.042
MAXF MDAMB231	102		0.001
MAXF MX1	21		0.438E-3

MELANOMA
MEXF 276	204		0.015
MEXF 462	112		0.007
MEXF 514	80		0.018
MEXF 989	211		0.006

OVARIAN
OVXF 1023	154		0.002
OVXF 1353	107		>0.100
OVXF 899	91		0.029

PANCREAS
| PAXF 546 | 45 | | 0.200E-3 |
| PAXF 736 | 125 | | 0.562E-4 |

PROSTATE
PRXF DU145X	278		0.009
PRXF LNCAP	44		0.889E-3
PRXF PC3MX	80		0.603E-3

RENAL
RXF 1220	125		0.029
RXF 423	222		0.588E-3
RXF 486	124		0.085
RXF 631	225		0.398E-3
RXF 944LX	240		0.009

TESTES
| TXF 881 | 30 | | 0.289E-3 |

| Mean | n=47 | 0.002 | 0.002 |

FIGURE 4 Mean bar graph presentation of rML activity in 47 human tumor xenografts in the clonogenic assay. Bars to the left represent more sensitive, bars to the right more resistant tumor types compared to the mean IC_{70} over the whole panel. Sensitive tumors were mammary carcinomas, small cell lung carcinomas, pancreas and prostate cancers. From this panel, xenografts were chosen for *in vivo* efficacy studies, such as the LXFS 538 small cell lung cancer model. This study represents the stage IV testing outlined in Fig. 3. The names of the xenografts resemble the tumor type (first two letters, e.g., MA, mammary), X is the xenograft, F the Freiburg panel, followed by the continuous tumor collection number.

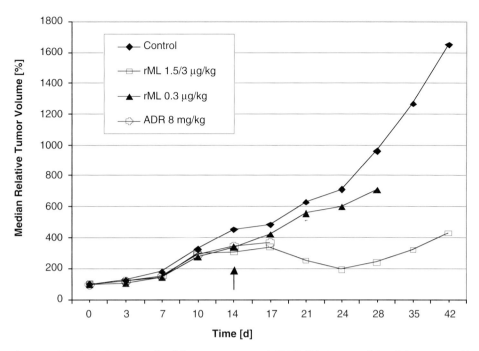

FIGURE 5 rML antitumor activity in the human small cell lung cancer xenograft LXFS-538. *In vivo* activity of rML versus Adriamycin in the LXFS 538 small cell lung cancer human tumor xenograft. Median relative tumor volumes are compared. rML was administered intraperitoneally on a daily × 5 schedule weekly for 4 weeks. Adriamycin was administered intravenously on days 1 and 15. rML (3 µg) was able to induce significant tumor growth inhibition in nude mice with an optimal *T/C* of 27% compared with control. In the latter group, 1.5 µg of rML/kg was given initially for two cycles, and was then increased to the maximal tolerated dose levels of rML (3 µg/kg) starting on day 14 (*arrow*). This resulted in tumor shrinkage and a statistically significant inhibitory effect ($p < 0.001$).

expression of the transgene is determined by the tissue specificity of the associated promoter (Alberts *et al.,* 1994).

Several transgenic models of recessive or dominant oncogenes have proven to mimic human disease and disease progression, e.g., the TRAMP mouse (transgenic adenocarcinoma mouse prostate). TRAMP mice which express high levels of the transgene (Table 9) displayed progressive forms of prostatic disease that histologically resembled human prostate cancer, ranging from mild hyperplasia to multinodular malignant neoplasia (Greenberg *et al.,* 1995). Nevertheless, transgenic mice have not been used for large-scale anticancer drug testing so far because of high running costs and the difficulties of obtaining synchronous onset of tumor growth and development. Examples of transgenic mouse models used for evaluation of drug effects on cancer growth are listed in Table 9. The wap-ras mouse is the most frequently employed transgenic model in cancer drug development and has been used to demonstrate preclinical *in vivo* activity of the ras/farnesyl protein transferase inhibitor SCH-66336. This agent has now advanced to clinical trial (Table 9) (Liu *et al.,* 1998).

Transgenic mice are also exploited in prophylactic chemotherapy approaches to study novel agents that, when given chronically, can prevent or reduce the growth of tumors. In TRAMP mice, daily administration of 20 mg/kg of the nonsteroidal anti-inflammatory drug R-flurbiprofen significantly lowered the incidence of metastasis and reduced the occurrence of primary prostate tumors (Wechter *et al.,* 2000). Difluoromethylornithine, given to K14-HPV16 transgenic animals, diminished the precursor lesions of ear and chest skin malignancies (Table 9) (Arbeit *et al.,* 1999). Since the transgenic technology emerged only in the early 1980s, there is still a need to systematically characterize and validate such tumor models with respect to their predictivity of clinical response and thus to determine their ultimate usefulness in the search for new anticancer drugs. Transgenic mice will undoubtedly enlarge our *in vivo* testing systems for cancer drug development because they can be designed to facilitate answering questions regarding risk assessment and carcinogenesis, xenobiotic metabolism, ligand-mediated toxicity, immunotoxicity, and drug resistance.

5. Screening for Angiogenesis Inhibitors

The hallmark of angiogenesis is the formation of new blood vessels from endothelial cells, which can be regulated by inducers and inhibitors of endothelial cell proliferation and migration (Hanahan and Folkman, 1996; Risau, 1997).

TABLE 9
Transgenic Models for Cancer Drug Development

Model	Transgene	Tumor type	Use	Ref.
Bcr/abl	bcr/abl p190 cDNA	Acute leukemia	Kinase inhibitors	Huettner *et al.,* 2000
TRAMP	[a]PB SV40 lage Tag	Prostate cancer	Chemoprevention	Greenberg *et al.,* 1995
MMTV-ras MMTV-myc	c-myc or v-Ha-ras [b]MMTV driven	Mammary tumors	Modeling disease progression	Wechter *et al.,* 2000 Sinn *et al.,* 1987
Wap-ras	Ha-ras, [c]wap driven	Mammary tumors	Farnesyltransferase inhibitors Tubulin-binding agents	Liu *et al.,* 1998 Porter *et al.,* 1995
P53	mtp53 (Val-135)	Lung carcinoma, lymphoma, sarcoma	Predisposition/mutagenesis studies	Lavigueur *et al.,* 1989 Nichol *et al.,* 1995
RIP1-Tag2	[d]RIP1-SV40 Tag	Pancreatic islet cancer	Angiogenesis inhibitors	Bergers *et al.,* 1999
K14-HPV16	HPV 16, [e]K14-driven	Epidermal cancers	Chemopreventative agents	Arbeit *et al.,* 1999
BM-MDR	MDR-1	None, bone marrow cells with multidrug transporter	Agents that reverse MDR/ chemosensitization	Mickisch *et al.,* 1991a Mickisch *et al.,* 1991b

[a]Prostate-specific rat probasin promoter driving SV40 large T-antigen-coding region.
[b]Mouse mammary tumor virus long terminal repeat promotor.
[c]Whey acidic protein promotor.
[d]Rat insulin promoter-SV40 tumor antigen.
[e]Wt HPV early region cloned behind human keratin-14 promoter.

Factors that govern pathologic tumor angiogenesis are pro-duced/induced by tumor cells directly or are derived from the ECM components. Tumor angiogenesis is a complex process involving extensive interactions between tumor cells, host endothelial cells, soluble factors such as vascular endothelial growth factor (VEGF), acidic and basic fibroblast growth factor, and the surrounding stromal elements (Hanahan and Folkman, 1996; Jones and Harris, 1998; Risau, 1997). Therefore, the development of antiangiogenic and antivascular therapies raises a specific challenge of modeling the interplay between host and tumor cells and their response to therapy. Here, *in vivo* assays are needed at an early stage of drug development to provide a meaningful experimental disease model.

Animal models used in the development of antiangiogenic/vascular therapies can be divided into three categories (Table 10): those that involve tumors growing in mice, those that use normal vascular tissues as surrogates for tumor blood vessel formation (chick chorioallantoic membrane model is most widely used), and *ex vivo* assays such as aortic ring tube formation (Table 10) (Giavazzi *et al.,* 1999; Hoffmann *et al.,* 1999). While proof-of-principle mechanistic studies of potential antiangiogenic agents demonstrating inhibition of neovascularization are most important, effects in tumor-based models showing tumor shrinkage or inhibition are also needed prior to drugs entering clinical trials. For this purpose, both rodent tumors and human tumor xenografts have been used (Giavazzi *et al.,* 1999). Rodent models have the advantage of a syngeneic environment in that the tumor, blood supply, and stromal elements are all from the same genetic background. However, they are limited by their restriction to certain rapidly growing tumor types (Table 1) and by the fact that the target, if tumor based, is nonhuman. In contrast, if human tumor

TABLE 10
Animal Models of Angiogenesis

Mouse *in vivo* tumor models	Other *in vivo* models	*Ex vivo* models
• Subcutaneous tumors syngeneic human xenografts	• Corneal pocket assay rabbit, rat, mouse	• Aortic ring assay bovine
• Lung metastasis B16F10, LL	• Hamster cheek pouch • Dorsal skin fold window chamber	porcine rat
• Orthotopic tumors	• Hollow-fiber assay	
• Transgenic mice (e.g., RIP1)	• Alginate beads	
• Cranial tumor window	• Matrigel plugs	
	• CAM assay	

LL, Lewis lung; CAM, chick chorioallantoic membrane; RIP1 model, pancreatic islet cancer.

xenograft models are used, artifacts due to host (murine vascularization)/graft (human tumor cells) interactions may arise. Positive aspects of the use of patient-derived xenografts include the large variety of available tumor types (Tables 4 and 5); the close resemblance of tumor architecture, microvessel density, and vascular permeability of clinical cancers; and the expression of angiogenic factors such as VEGF (Berger *et al.,* 1995; Schüler *et al.,* 1999).

A large number of antiangiogenic and antivascular agents are currently under preclinical and clinical development (Jones and Harris, 1998). They include agents targeting endothelial cell signaling (VEGF and its receptor), endothelial cell motility and structure (endothelial cell tubulin binders), tumor vessel physiology (liposomes and polymers exploiting the enhanced permeability and retention by tumor blood vessels), and proteases degrading the ECM (Jones and Harris, 1998; Schüler *et al.,* 1999). In most cases, several of the *in vivo* model systems described above have been employed. However, none of the potential antiangiogenic agents have proven clinical activity so far. Thus, the preclinical angiogenesis models remain unvalidated, and results obtained must be interpreted with great care. In the absence of a mechanistic hypothesis for a vascular effect and/or pharmacodynamic end-point assay to demonstrate that the proposed mechanism is operative, currently available models should not be considered as screens for antiangiogenic drugs. For example, studies with anti-VEGF antibodies should be performed only in tumors expressing high VEGF levels, using VEGF reduction or VEGF binding as surrogate end point.

Finally, when negative clinical data are obtained, preclinical models should be "revisited" to address why they have failed to predict the response/outcome. For instance, the first generation of matrix metalloproteinase inhibitors (MMPIs) did not live up to expectations and delivered discouraging results in phase III trials. Although effects on the isolated target were clearly demonstrated and a number of commonly used preclinical angiogenesis and metastasis models had produced certain activity, most MMPIs failed. Hence, the reasons need to be identified in order to improve clinical trial design and enable the optimal translation of preclinical results into the clinic.

Acknowledgments

We are grateful to our colleagues Cornelia Steidle and Elke Simon for their important contributions to this project. We thank Hildegard Willmann for software development and assistance with data evaluation as well as Ines Fernandez for her help with the manuscript. The work was supported by grants from the German Ministry for Research and Technology (HHF); the U.S. National Cancer Institute, Biological Testing Branch (HHF); and the Deutsche Froschungsgemeinschaft DFG (AMB).

References

Alberts, B., Bray, D., Lewis, J., Raff, M., Roberts, K., and Watson, J. D. (1994). The actions of oncogenes can be assayed singly and in combinations in transgenic mice. *In* "Molecular Biology of the Cell." 3rd ed., chp. 24, Garland Publishing, Taylor & Francis Group, New York.

Arbeit, J. M., Riley, R. R., Huey, B., Porter, C., Kelloff, G., Lubet, R., Ward, J. M., and Pinkel, D. (1999). Difluoromethylornithine chemoprevention of epidermal carcinogenesis in K14-HPV16 transgenic mice. *Cancer Res.* 59, 3610–3620.

Berger, M. R. (1999). Autochthonous tumor models in rats: is there still a relevance for anticancer drug development. *In* "Relevance of Tumor Models in Anticancer Drug Development" (H. H. Fiebig and A. M. Burger, eds.), Vol. 54, pp. 15–27. Karger, Basel.

Berger, D. P., Herbstritt, L., Dengler, W. A., Marme, D., Mertelsmann, R., and Fiebig, H. H. (1995). Vascular endothelial growth factor (VEGF) mRNA expression in human tumor models of different histologies. *Ann. Oncol.* 6, 817–825.

Bergers, G., Javaherian, K., Lo, K. M., Folkman, J., and Hanahan, D. (1999). Effects of angiogenesis inhibitors on multistage carcinogenesis in mice. *Science* 284, 808–812.

Boyd, M. R. (1989). Status of the NCI preclinical antitumor drug discovery screen. *In* "Principles and Practice of Oncology" (S. Hellman, DeVita, V. T., and S. A. Rosenberg, eds.), Vol. 3, pp. 1–12. Lippincott, Philadelphia.

Burger, A. M., Kaur, G., Hollingshead, M., Fischer, R. T., Nagashima, K., Malspeis, L., Duncan, K. L., and Sausville, E. A. (1997). Antiproliferative activity *in vitro* and *in vivo* of the spicamycin analog KRN5500 with altered glycoprotein expression *in vitro*. *Clin. Cancer Res.* 3, 455–463.

Burger, A. M., Fiebig, H. H., Newman, D. J., Camalier, R. F., and Sausville, E. A. (1998). Antitumor activity of 17-allylaminogeldanamycin (NSC 330507) in melanoma xenografts is associated with decline in Hsp90 protein expression. *Ann. Oncol.* 9(Suppl. 2), 132.

Burger, A. M., Steidle, C., Fiebig, H. H., Frick, E., Schölmerich, J., and Kreutz, W. (1999a). Activity of pH-sensitive salicylic acid derivatives against human tumors in vivo. *Clin. Cancer Res.* 5, 205.

Burger, A. M., Mengs, U., Schüler, J. B., Zinke, H., Lentzen, H., and Fiebig, H. H. (1999b). Recombinant mistletoe lectin (rML) is a potent inhibitor of tumor cell growth *in vitro* and *in vivo*. *Proc. Am. Assoc. Cancer Res.* 40, 399.

Burger, A. M., Sausville, E. A., Camalier, R. F., Newman, D. J., and Fiebig, H. H. (2000). Response of human melanomas to 17-AAG is associated with modulation of the molecular chaperone function of Hsp90. *Proc. Am. Assoc. Cancer Res.* 41, 447.

Corbett, T., Valeriote, F., LoRusso, P., Polin, L., Panchapor, C., Pugh, S., White, K., Knight, J., Demchik, L., Jones, J., and Lisow, L. (1997). In vivo methods for screening and preclinical testing. *In* "Anticancer Drug Development Guide" (B. A. Teicher, ed.), pp. 75–100. Humana Press, Totowa, NJ.

Drees, M., Dengler, W., Roth, T., Labonte, H., Mayo, J., Malspeis, L., Grever, M., Sausville, E., and Fiebig, H. H. (1997). Flavopiridol (L86-8275): Selective antitumor activity *in vitro* and *in vivo* for prostate carcinoma cells. *Clin. Cancer Res.* 3, 273–279.

EMEA, The European Agency for the Evaluation of Medicinal Products Human Medicines Evaluation. (1998). CPMP/SWP/997/96 Committee For Proprietary Medicinal Products (CPMP) Note for guidance on the pre-clinical evaluation of anticancer medicinal products. (http://www.eudra.org/emea.html), London.

Fiebig, H. H., and Burger, A. M. (2001). Human tumor xenografts and explants. *In* "Animal Models in Cancer Research" (B. A. Teicher, ed.), Humana Press, Totowa, NJ, in press.

Fiebig, H. H., Schmid, J. R., Bieser, W., Henss, H., and Löhr, G. W. (1987). Colony assay with human tumor xenografts, murine tumors and human bone marrow. Potential for anticancer drug development. *Eur. J. Cancer Clin. Oncol.* 23, 937–948.

Fiebig, H. H., Berger, D. P., Dengler, W. A., Wallbrecher, E., and Winter-halter, B. R. (1992). Combined *in vitro/in vivo* test procedure with human tumor xenografts. *In* "Immunodeficient Mice in Oncology" (H. H. Fiebig and D. P. Berger, eds.) Vol. 42, pp. 321–351, Karger, Basel.

Fiebig, H. H., Berger, D. P., Dengler, W. A., Drees, M., Mayo, J., Malspeis, L., and Grever, M. (1994). Cyanocyclin A and the quinocarmycin analog NSC 607 097 demonstrate selectivity against melanoma xenografts invitro and in-vivo. *Proc. Am. Assoc. Cancer Res.* **35**, 2794.

Fiebig, H. H., Dengler, W. A., Drees, M., Schwendener, R. A., and Schott, H. (1995). In vivo activity of N4-octadecyl-Ara-C in human solid tumors and leukemias. *Proc. Am. Assoc. Cancer Res.* **36**, A2434.

Fiebig, H. H., Dengler, W. A., and Roth, T. (1999a). Human tumor xenografts: predictivity, characterization and discovery of new anticancer agents. *In* "Relevance of Tumor Models for Anticancer Drug Development" (H. H. Fiebig and A. M. Burger, eds.), Vol. 54, pp. 29–50. Basel, Karger.

Fiebig, H. H., Steidle, C., Burger, A. M., and Lerchen, H. G. (1999b). Anti-cancer activity of novel camptothecin glycoconjugates in human tumor xenograft models. *Clin. Cancer Res.* **5**, 667.

Futreal, A. P., Kasprzyk, A., Birney, E., Mullikin, J. C., Wooster, R., and Stratton, M. (2001). Cancer and genomics. *Nature* **409**, 850–852.

Giavazzi, R., Valoti, G., Ferri, C., and Nicoletti, M. J. (1999). Preclinical models to evaluate angiogenesis inhibitors. *In* "Relevance of Tumor Models for Anticancer Drug Development" (H. H. Fiebig and A. M. Burger, eds.), Vol. 54, pp. 157–168, Karger, Basel.

Goldenberg, G. J., and Moore, M. J. (1997). Nitrogen mustards. *In* "Cancer Therapeutics: Experimental and Clinical Agents" (B. A. Teicher, ed.), pp. 3–22, Humana Press, Totowa, NJ.

Goldin, A., Venditti, J. M., MacDonald, J. S., Muggia, F. M., Henney, J. E., and DeVita, V. T. (1981). Current results of the screening program at the division of cancer treatment, National Cancer Institute. *Eur. J. Cancer* **17**, 129–142.

Greenberg, N. M., DeMayo, F., Finegold, M. J., Medina, D., Tilley, W. D., Aspinall, J. O., Cunha, G. R., Donjacour, A. A., Matusik, R. J., and Rosen, J. M. (1995). Prostate cancer in a transgenic mouse. *Proc. Natl. Acad. Sci. USA* **92**, 3439–3443.

Hamburger, A. W., and Salmon, S. E. (1977). Primary bioassay of human tumor stem cells. *Science* **197**, 461–463.

Hanahan, D., and Folkman, J. (1996). Patterns and emerging mechanisms of the angiogenic switch during tumorigenesis. *Cell* **86**, 353–364.

Hartung, G., Stehle, G., Sinn, H., Wunder, A., Schrenk, H. H., Heeger, S., Kränzle, M., Edler, L., Frei, E., Fiebig, H. H., Heene, D. L., and Queisser, W. (1999). Phase I trial of methotrexate-albumin in a weekly intravenous bolus regimen in cancer patients. *Clin. Cancer Res.* **5**, 753–759.

Hendriks, H. R., Pizao, P. E., Berger, D. P., Kooistra, K. L., Bibby, M. C., Boven, E., Dreef-van der Meulen, H. C., Henrar, R. E. C., Fiebig, H. H., Double, J. A., Hornstra, H. W., Pinedo, H. M., Workmann, P., and Schwartsmann, G. (1993). E09, a novel bioreductive alkylating indolo-quinone with preferential solid tumor activity and lack of bone marrow toxicity in preclinical models. *Eur. J. Cancer* **29**, 897–906.

Hendriks, H. R., Fiebig, H. H., Giavazzi, R., Langdon, S. P., Jimeno, J. M., and Faircloth, G. T. (1999). High antitumor activity of ET743 against human tumour xenografts from melanoma, non-small-cell lung and ovarian cancer. *Ann. Oncol.* **10**, 1233–1240.

Hoffman, R. M. (1999). Visualization of metastasis in orthotopic mouse models with green fluorescent protein. *In* "Relevance of Tumor Models in Anticancer Drug Development" (H. H. Fiebig and A. M. Burger, eds.), Vol. 54, pp. 81–87. Karger, Basel.

Hoffmann, J., Schirner, M., Menrad, A., and Schneider, M. R. (1999). Animal models for determination of anti-angiogenic drug effects. *In* "Relevance of Tumor Models for Anticancer Drug Development" (H. H. Fiebig and A. M. Burger, eds.), Vol. 54, pp. 169–180. Karger, Basel.

Hollingshead, M. G., Alley, M. C., Camalier, R. F., Abbott, B. J., Mayo, J. G., Malspeis, L., and Grever, M. R. (1995). In vivo cultivation of tumor cells in hollow fibers. *Life Sci.* **57**, 131–141.

Hollingshead, M., Plowman, J., Alley, M., Mayo, J., and Sausville, E. (1999). The hollow fiber assay. *In* "Relevance of Tumor Models in Anticancer Drug Development" (H. H. Fiebig and A. M. Burger, eds.), Vol. 54, pp. 109–120. Karger, Basel.

Huettner, C. S., Zhang, P., van Etten, R. A., and Tenen, D. G. (2000). Reversibility of acute B-cell leukemia induced by bcr-abl1. *Nat. Genet.* **24**, 57–60.

Jones, A., and Harris, A. L. (1998). New developments in angiogenesis: a major mechanism for tumor growth and target for therapy. *Cancer J. Sci. Am.* **4**, 209–213.

Klenner, T., Voegeli, R., Fiebig, H., and Hilgard, P. (1992). Antitumor effect of the platinum complex D-19466 (Inn: Lobaplatin) against the transplantable osteosarcoma of the rat and other experiments. *J. Cancer Res. Clin. Oncol.* **118**(Suppl.), p. 149.

Lander, E. S., Linton, L. M., Birren, B., *et al.* (2001). Initial sequencing and analysis of the human genome. *Nature* **409**, 860–921.

Langer, M., Mockel, B., Eck, J., Zinke, H., and Lentzen, H. (1999). Site-specific mutagenesis of mistletoe lectin: the role of RIP activity in apoptosis. *Biochem. Biophys. Res. Commun.* **264**, 944–948.

Lavigueur, A., Maltby, V., Mock, D., Rossant, J., Pawson, T., and Bernstein, A. (1989). High incidence of lung, bone and lymphoid tumors in transgenic mice overexpressing mutant alleles of the p53 oncogene. *Mol. Cell Biol.* **9**, 3982–3991.

Liu, M., Bryant, M. S., Chen, J., *et al.* (1998). Antitumor activity of SCH 6636, an orally bioavailable tricyclic inhibitor of farnesyl protein transferase, in human tumor xenograft models and wap-ras transgenic mice. *Cancer Res.* **58**, 4947–4956.

Malakoff, D., Vogel, G., and Marshall, E. (2000). The rise of the mouse, biomedicine's model mammal. *Science* **288**, 248–257.

Maly, K., Uberall, F., Schubert, C., Kindler, E., Stekar, J., Brachwitz, H., and Grunicke, H. H. (1995). Interference of new alkylphospholipid analogues with mitogenic signal transduction. *Anticancer Drug Des.* **10**, 411–425.

Mickisch, G. H., Merlino, G. T., Aiken, P. M., Gottesmann, M. M., and Pastan, I. (1991a). New potent verapamil derivatives that reverse multidrug resistance in human renal carcinoma cells and in transgenic mice expressing the human MDR 1 gene. *J. Urol.* **146**, 447–453.

Mickisch, G. F., Licht, T., Merlino, G. T., Gottesman, M. M., and Pastan, I. (1991b). Chemotherapy and chemosensitization of transgenic mice which express the human multidrug resistance gene in bone marrow: efficacy, potency, and toxicity. *Cancer Res.* **51**, 5417–5424.

Nichol, C. J., Harrison, M. L., Laposa, R. R., Gimelshtein, I. L., and Wells, P. G. (1995). A teratologic suppressor role for p53 in benzo[a]pyrene-treated transgenic p53-deficient mice. *Nat. Genet.* **10**, 181 187.

Ovejera, A. A. (1987). The use of human tumor xenografts in large scale drug screening. *In* "Rodent Tumor Models in Experimental Cancer Therapy" (R. F. Kallman, ed.), pp. 218–220. Pergam Press, New York.

Palmiter, R. D., and Brinster, R. L. (1985). Transgenic mice. *Cell* **41**, 343–345.

Paull, K. D., Shoemaker, R. H., Hodes, L., Monks, A., Scudiero, D. A., Rubinstein, L., Plowman, J., and Boyd, M. R. (1989). Display and analysis of patterns of differential activity of drugs against human tumour cell lines: development of mean graph and COMPARE algorithm. *J. Natl. Cancer Inst.* **81**, 1088–1092.

Porter, G. M., Armstrong, L., and Nielsen, L. L. (1995). Strategy for developing transgenic assays for screening antineoplastic drugs that affect tubulin polymerization. *Lab. Anim. Sci.* **45**, 145–150.

Reid, L. M., Holland, J., Jones, C., Wolf, B., Niwayama, G., Williams, R., Kaplan, N. O., and Sato, G. (1978). Some of the variables affecting the success of transplantation of human tumors into the athymic nude mouse. *In* "Proceedings of the Symposium on the Use of Athymic (nude) Mice in Cancer Research" (D. P. Houchens and A. A. Ovejera, eds.), pp. 107–122. Gustav Fischer Verlag, New York.

Risau, W. (1997). Mechanisms of angiogenesis. *Nature* **386**, 671–674.

Sausville, E. A., and Feigal, E. (1999). Evolving approaches to cancer drug discovery and development at the National Cancer Institute. *Ann. Oncol.* **10,** 1287–1292.

Schepartz, S. A. (1976). Early history and development of the nitrosoureas. *Cancer Treat. Rep.* **60,** 647–649.

Scholz, C. C., Berger, D. P., Winterhalter, B. R., Henss, H., and Fiebig, H. H. (1990). Correlation of drug response in patients and in the clonogenic assay using solid human tumor xenografts. *Eur. J. Cancer* **26,** 901–905.

Schüler, J. B., Fiebig, H. H., and Burger, A. M. (1999). Development of human tumor models for evaluation of compounds which target tumor vasculature. *In* "Relevance of Tumor Models for Anticancer Drug Development" (H. H. Fiebig and A. M. Burger, eds.), Vol. 54, pp. 181–190. Karger, Basel.

Sinn, E., Muller, W., Pattengale, P., Tepler, I., Wallace, R., and Leder, P. (1987). Coexpression of MMTV/v-H-ras and MMTV/c-myc genes in transgenic mice: synergistic action of oncogenes in vivo. *Cell* **49,** 465–475.

Steel, G. (1987). How well do xenografts maintain the therapeutic response characteristics of the source tumor in the donor patient? *In* "Rodent Tumor Models in Experimental Cancer Therapy" (R. F. Kallman, ed.), pp. 205–208. Pergam Press, New York.

Stehle, G., Sinn, H., Wunder, A., Schrenk, H. H., Stewart, J. C. M., Hartung, G., Maier-Borst, W., and Heene, D. L. (1997). Plasma protein (albumin) catabolism by the tumor itself: implications for tumor metabolism and the genesis of cachexia. *Crit. Rev. Oncol. Hematol.* **26,** 77–100.

Sugamata, N., Koibuchi, Y., Iino, Y., and Morishita, Y. (1999). A novel aromatase inhibitor, vozorole, shows antitumor activity and a decrease of tissue insulin-like growth factor-I level in 7,12-dimethylbenz(a)anthracene induced mammary tumors. *Int. J. Oncol.* **14,** 259–263.

Teicher, B. A. (ed.) (1997). "Cancer Drug Discovery and Development. Cancer Therapeutics. Experimental and Clinical Agents." Humana Press, Totowa, NJ.

Venter, G., Adams, M. D., Myers, E. W., *et al.* (2001). The sequence of the human genome. *Science* **291,** 1304–1351.

Von Hoff, D. D. (1987). *In vitro* predictive testing: the sulfonamide era. *Int. J. Cell Cloning* **5,** 179–190.

Waud, R. W. (1997). Murine L1210 and P388 leukemias. *In* "Anticancer Drug Development Guide" (B. A. Teicher, ed.), pp. 59–74. Humana Press, Totowa, NJ.

Wechter, W. J., Leipold, D. D., Murray, E. D. Jr, Quiggle, D., McCracken, J. D., Barrios, R. S., and Greenberg, N. M. (2000). E-7869 (R-flurbiprofen) inhibits progression of prostate cancer in the TRAMP mouse. *Cancer Res.* **60,** 2203–2208.

Winterhalter, B. R., Berger, D. P., Dengler, W. A., Hendriks, H. R., Mertelsmann, R., and Fiebig, H. H. (1993). High antitumors activity of rhizoxin in a combined in-vitro and in-vivo test procedure with human tumor xenografts. *Proc. Am. Assoc. Cancer Res.* **34,** 376.

Workman, P., Twentyman, P., Balkwill, F., Balmain, A., Chaplin, D., Double, J., Embleton, J., Newell, D., Raymond, R., Stables, J., Stephens, T., and Wallace, J. (1997). "United Kingdom Co-ordinating Committee on Cancer Research (UKCCCR) guidelines for the welfare of animals in experimental neoplasy." 2nd ed., pp. 1–32, UKCCCR, Lincoln's Inn Fields, London.

RELEVANCE OF PRECLINICAL PHARMACOLOGY AND TOXICOLOGY TO PHASE I TRIAL EXTRAPOLATION TECHNIQUES: RELEVANCE OF ANIMAL TOXICOLOGY

Joseph E. Tomaszewski
Adaline C. Smith
Joseph M. Covey
Susan J. Donohue
Julie K. Rhie
Karen M. Schweikart

National Cancer Institute

National Institutes of Health

Bethesda, Maryland

Summary

The development of drugs for the treatment of patients with cancer is generally more complicated than that for other types of therapeutic drugs. First, anticancer drugs tend to be among the most toxic agents that are purposely administered to humans. Second, the typical patient in an early clinical trial is generally very ill and has often received other potentially toxic therapies. For these reasons, preclinical pharmacology and toxicology data for new drugs must be readily translatable to humans and must be accurate in their prediction. The advent of more aggressive clinical trial dose escalation schemes in clinical practice today also emphasizes the importance of providing adequate pharmacologic and toxicologic datasets. Such data also form a major portion of the information required by the U.S. Food and Drug Administration for

Investigational New Drug applications. In this chapter, the results of studies of a wide variety of anticancer drugs investigated by U.S. National Cancer Institute are reviewed. While it has proven possible to predict the maximum tolerated dose and dose-limiting toxicities of a large number of these compounds very accurately, exceptions have also been found.

1. Introduction

The development of drugs for the treatment of patients with cancer is perhaps more difficult than that of drugs for other non-life-threatening indications because cancer drugs tend to be the most toxic agents intentionally administered to man. This is further complicated by the fact that the typical patient in a phase I trial is not a healthy human volunteer but a very ill, terminal cancer patient for whom all other therapeutic interventions have failed. Thus, the starting dose (SD) that is selected for the first human trial of cancer drugs must not only be safe but must also offer some hope of benefit to the patient. For these reasons, the nonclinical pharmacology and toxicology data collected by the National Cancer Institute (NCI), which forms the major portion of the information required by the Food and Drug Administration (FDA) for an Investigational New Drug (IND) application (FDA, 1995), must not only conform to the Good Laboratory Practice regulations (FDA, 1996) but also must be readily translatable to humans and reasonably accurate. Selection of a safe starting dose is generally not a problem if one goes low enough. However, as experience shows, it can be extremely difficult to select a high enough dose so that the number of dose escalations is kept to a minimum to achieve either a maximum tolerated dose (MTD) or a biologically effective dose in humans.

2. Historical Perspective

The quest to define the relationship of animal to man for cancer drugs has been an integral part of the drug development process since the earliest days of the NCI's program. In 1958, Pinkel concluded that body surface area (square meters) and not body weight (kilograms) should be used as the criterion for cancer drug dose selection (Pinkel, 1958). This observation was confirmed and expanded by the seminal work of Freireich and co-workers when they performed a retrospective analysis of animal and human data for 18 cancer drugs and determined that the MTD in humans and animals was about the same on a mg/m^2 basis, but that on a mg/kg basis the MTD in humans was about one-twelfth of the LD_{10} (10% of the lethal dose or 0.1 MELD$_{10}$) in mice, one-seventh of the LD_{10} in rats, and one-half of the MTD in dogs (Freireich et al., 1966). This resulted in the determination of conversion factors (k_m) that could be used to convert doses based on body weight (mg/kg) to those based on body surface area (mg/m^2). These factors are 3 for the mouse, 6 for the rat, 12 for the monkey, 20 for the dog, and 37 for an adult human. In considering dose-limiting toxicities (DLTs), early studies found that there was good correlation between animals and humans for bone marrow, gastrointestinal, liver, and kidney toxicities, a questionable correlation for central and peripheral nervous system toxicity, and no correlation for skin including rashes, dermatitis, and alopecia (Owens, 1963).

Since these very early years, numerous studies have been conducted to look at the same end points to try to determine which species correctly predicts human sensitivity to antitumor drugs (Schein et al., 1970; Homan, 1972; Schein and Anderson, 1973; Goldsmith et al., 1975; Guarino, 1977; Penta et al., 1979; Guarino et al., 1979; Rozensweig et al., 1981). During this period, the methodologies used to evaluate antitumor drugs in the nonclinical setting have changed from utilizing mice, rats, hamsters, dogs, and monkeys on a variety of single- and multiple-dose schedules (Cancer Chemotherapy National Service Center, 1959, 1960, 1964), to the use of mice, dogs, and monkeys in acute and dogs in long-term studies (Prieur et al., 1973, 1977), and in 1980 to a more narrowly defined set of standard protocols (dx1 and dx5) in mice (lethality and toxicity) and dogs (toxicity) only (Lowe and Davis, 1987). The latter changes were brought about after the review of data on 21 antitumor agents (Rozencweig et al., 1981), which indicated that the dog and not the monkey reasonably predicted what occurred in humans. After reviewing data on seven new drugs that had been evaluated with the 1980 protocols (Grieshaber and Marsoni, 1986), it was further determined that the dog was a good prognosticator of human toxicity and much better than the mouse. As a result, the optional mouse toxicity studies were replaced by studies in rats in 1983. At the same time as this review on toxicity was occurring, Collins and co-workers (1986, 1987) proposed that instead of simply using the Fibonacci series for dose escalation, animal pharmacology data should be used in conjunction with human data to modify the dose escalation scheme so as to reach the MTD as rapidly as possible.

In the mid-1980s after Grieshaber and Marsoni performed their evaluation of the 1980 NCI protocol results, the NCI shifted away from the routine use of the standard dx1 and dx5 protocols to those that extensively utilized pharmacologic principles and were designed more specifically to match the biology of the agent in question. That is, they utilized all of the available information known about the compound, including mechanism of action, antitumor schedule dependency (in vitro and in vivo), pharmacokinetics, metabolism, and so forth to adequately design a clinical protocol that would optimize the chances for activity in the clinic (Grieshaber, 1992). Current NCI practice involves designing and performing agent-directed studies in a pharmacologically guided framework. This is accomplished through the acquisition and use of pharmacokinetic data to reliably extrapolate toxic effects across species by relating plasma drug levels [peak and steady state and/or area under the curve (AUC)] to safety and the occurrence and severity of toxicity. Integration of these studies with efficacy data and the proposed clinical protocol permits a more rational evaluation of the role of schedule dependence and pharmacokinetics on efficacy and in the development of toxicity.

In addition to this philosophical change in the approach to the acquisition of toxicity data, the development of drugs within the NCI has evolved into two stages, each of which requires a toxicologic evaluation. The first involves a preliminary assessment of toxicity (range finding studies) usually in two preclinical animal models (rodent and nonrodent) with the determination of MTD and pharmacokinetics in both species. If the drug meets the program criteria for full-scale development, a more complete toxicity evaluation (IND-directed studies using the proposed clinical route and schedule) is performed that will lead to the filing of an IND. This two-step approach allows the determination if full development is warranted with a limited expenditure of resources (drug, animals, and dollars). For a detailed description of the methods currently in use today by the NCI, see Tomaszewski and Smith (1997).

In a recent publication the FDA defined the battery of preclinical studies that are considered important for assessing the safety of oncology drugs prior to filing an IND, stressing that the studies should be conducted using the same schedule and duration of administration as the intended clinical protocol (DeGeorge *et al.*, 1998). These guidelines cover all classes of cancer drugs, including cytotoxics, noncytotoxic, chronically administered drugs, and cancer drug modulators.

3. Special Toxicity Evaluations

Investigators have tried to develop additional special studies to evaluate the various toxicities that are produced in animals and humans in order to more precisely predict human sensitivity. Since myelosuppression was the most common DLT produced by antitumor agents in humans (Carter *et al.*, 1981; Dorr and Fritz, 1980), Bradner and co-workers (1980, 1981, 1985, 1986) sought to devise small animal screens to predict various clinical toxicities, including bone marrow suppression. For myelotoxicity, the end result was a three-tiered approach using (1) a single-dose study in BDF_1 mice measuring neutrophil counts; (2) a single-dose study in BDF_1 mice in which the femoral bone marrow is used in a CFU-C (colony-forming unit–complete) assay using the ID_{90} as the end point; and (3) a single-dose study in catheterized ferrets measuring neutrophil counts. While this approach was successful (13 of 17 correct in mice, 8 of 9 in CFU-C, and 7 of 7 in ferret), it was very labor intensive and required a sub-

stantial amount of drug and large numbers of animals. As a result, the tiered approach was rejected by many groups, and evaluations of myelosuppression were simply conducted in the toxicity studies using hematology evaluations and differential counts as well as microscopic evaluation of bone marrow and other lymphoid tissues.

In the late 1980s, the NCI entered into a contractual relationship with Hipple Cancer Research Center through the federal government's Small Business Innovative Research (SBIR) program. These studies resulted in the development of assays using fresh marrow from mice and humans (replacement hip surgery waste samples) to evaluate the toxic effects of antitumor agents *in vitro* in colony-forming unit (CFU) assays specific for CFU-GM (granulocyte-macrophage), CFU-E (erythrocyte), CFU-GEMM (multilineage), and a burst-forming unit assay for erythrocytes (BFU-E) (Huang *et al.*, 1991; May *et al.*, 1992; Parchment *et al.*, 1992, 1993). Initially these assays were used in prospective studies (Du *et al.*, 1990a, b, 1991, 1992; Volpe *et al.*, 1992, 1995, 1996; May *et al.*, 1993a, b, 1994), but it was decided that to gain their full utility, the assay should be validated in a retrospective study. An assay for canine CFU-GM was also developed for use in these studies so that correlations could be made between the various species used preclinically and the clinical results in humans. The assay that is currently used is a colony-forming assay using granulocyte-macrophage precursors (CFU-GM) from mouse, dog, and man to predict neutropenia, the most common manifestation of myelosuppression. While most activity assays tend to use the IC_{50} as a measure of activity, it has been shown that the IC_{90} is a more accurate predictor of a concentration that produces dose-limiting myelosuppression in humans (grade 3 or 4 neutropenia), and it is for this reason that the IC_{90} is used for comparing species sensitivity (Parchment *et al.*, 1994; Erickson-Miller *et al.*, 1997). Results from these studies show that the *in vitro* bone marrow assay is very useful in predicting human marrow sensitivity to antitumor agents (Schweikart *et al.*, 1995; Tomaszewski *et al.*, 1997, 1999) and can be used early in drug development to evaluate the sensitivity of man versus mouse (therapeutic index), as well as to determine if a particular compound among a series of analogues may be less toxic than the others and therefore a more suitable compound for development.

4. Recent Examples of Drug Development at NCI

The following section contains seven examples of recent agent-directed drug development projects that have been conducted at the NCI over the past few years, including all preclinical and clinical data available at this time. Each section is written to provide the appropriate rationale derived from either efficacy or pharmacokinetics in terms of why the toxicology studies and the resultant clinical trials were designed in the manner in which they were performed. This is followed by a section in which the nonclinical animal data are compared with the human clinical data to determine how well the various animal models predicted for human toxicity and pharmacology.

A. 9-Amino(20S)camptothecin (9-AC, NSC-603071)

1. Introduction

9-AC (Fig. 1) belongs to the class of antitumor agents known as topoisomerase I inhibitors (Hsiang and Liu, 1988; Hsiang et al., 1985, 1989). The parent compound, camptothecin, is a natural product isolated from the tree *Camptothecia acuminata,* which was discovered in the NCI's natural products screening program in the 1970s. When taken to the clinic, camptothecin produced leukopenia and hemorrhagic cystitis in humans. In an attempt to find more effective and less toxic analogues of camptothecin, 9-AC was subsequently synthesized by Wall and co-workers (Wani et al., 1986) and was shown to possess significantly greater antitumor activity than camptothecin itself.

2. Preclinical Efficacy Data

9-AC lactone was shown to be a very potent antitumor agent *in vitro* where concentrations of 1 ng/mL inhibited growth of BRO melanoma cells, while concentrations of 1–5 ng/mL had no effect on normal melanocytes (Pantazis et al., 1992). It was shown to be very potent *in vivo* against colon tumor xenografts in immunodeficient mice, producing cures after multiple subcutaneous (SC) injections (Giovanella et al., 1989). Additional studies by these investigators (Potmesil et al., 1991, 1993; Pantazis et al., 1992, 1993a,b) have shown complete remissions in other human tumor xenografts, such as malignant melanoma, infiltrating ductal breast carcinoma, and epithelial lung cancer after twice weekly treatment with SC or intramuscular (IM) injections. Studies by the NCI con-

firmed and extended these results, indicating that SC treatment with suspensions produced complete tumor regression, while SC injection of a 9-AC solution produced marginal activity at best. Pharmacokinetic studies that were conducted in conjunction with the tumor studies indicated that the absorption of 9-AC from an SC suspension was much slower and more prolonged than the SC administration of a solution (Plowman et al., 1997; Supko et al., 1992). The results from these studies indicated that for 9-AC to produce optimal therapeutic activity, it was important to maintain concentrations of 9-AC lactone above a threshold level for an extended period of time (q4d×8). This was supported by the fact that SC administration of 9-AC solutions had to be administered on a more frequent (q2d×16 or qd×32) basis for 9-AC to delay tumor growth or induce partial remissions.

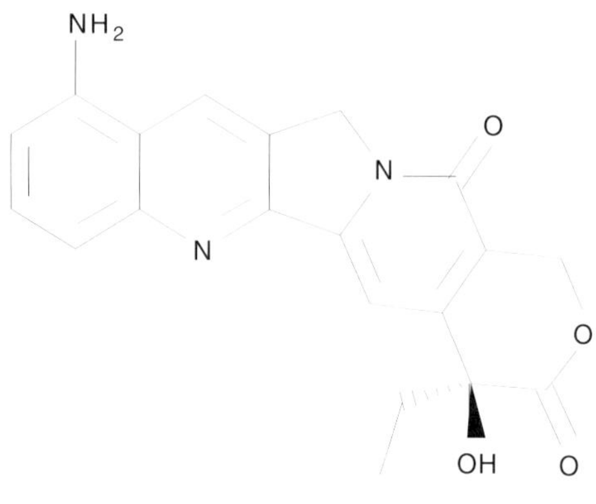

3. Preclinical Pharmacokinetic Data

Pharmacokinetic studies were conducted in mice, rats, dogs, and monkeys (Table 1). In the mouse (Supko and Malspeis, 1993; Supko et al., 1992, and unpublished NCI data), intravenous (IV) administration of 5 mg/kg (an effective SC dose) produced peak lactone concentrations of 11.8 μM. Elimination was biexponential with a terminal half-life of 1.38 h. When 9-AC solutions were administered by the SC route, absorption was rapid, producing peak plasma levels of 1.95 nM, but elimination was also rapid with a terminal half-life of 1.58 h. After administration of SC suspensions of 2.5 and 4.0 mg/kg (7.5 and 12 mg/m^2), maximal plasma lactone concentrations were 9.2 and 15.4 nM. However, unlike with the solution, lactone was eliminated very slowly from plasma with a terminal half-life between 30 and 36 h. This study demonstrated that the SC administration of 9-AC in suspension mimicked a continuous IV (CIV) infusion in mice and that single SC doses of 5 mg/kg (15 mg/m^2) resulted in plasma lactone concentrations above 4 nM for 72 h. As a result, the toxicity studies and the initial clinical protocol were designed as 72-h CIV infusion studies.

After IV administration of 1 mg/kg, rats and dogs demonstrated triexponential plasma elimination pharmacokinetics of 9-AC lactone. The terminal plasma elimination half-life was 80 min in rats and 327 minutes in dogs. Plasma clearance was about 900 ml/min/m^2 in both species. In addition, both species showed large volumes of distribution at steady state (60 L/m^2 in dogs and 28.2 L/m^2 in rats). The rapid clearance and the large steady-state volume of distribution suggested extensive tissue distribution and/or metabolism of the drug in both dogs and rats (Dixit et al., 1993).

When the pharmacokinetics of 9-AC was evaluated in nonhuman primates at doses of 2.4 to 6.0 mg/m^2, the 9-AC lactone had a distribution half-life of 192 minutes, a CL$_{TB}$ of 420 mL/min/m^2, and a volume of distribution at steady state of 19.2 L/m^2 (Blaney et al., 1998), all of which were substantially different than results obtained in the other animal models.

Stability of the lactone form of camptothecin has been evaluated in the presence of human serum albumin (HSA) (Burke

FIGURE 1 Structure of 9-amino(20S)camptothecin.

TABLE 1
9-Amino(20S)camptothecin (NSC-603071): Plasma Pharmacokinetics in Animals

PK parameter	Mouse			Rat	Dog	Monkey
Route	IV bolus	SC solution	SC suspension	IV bolus	IV bolus	IV 15 min
Dose (mg/m^2)	15	15	12	6	20	2.4–6.0
$t_{1/2}$ α(min)	10.5	—	—	1.6	2.6	—
$t_{1/2}$ β(min)	82.8	94.8	—	18	22.8	192
$t_{1/2}$ γ(min)	—	—	1050	80	327	—
$C_{P\,MAX}$ (μM)	11.8	1.95	0.25	—	—	~1
CL_{TB} (mL/min/m^2)	193	—	—	900	906	420
AUC (μg/mL × min)	78.2	49.4	33.9	6.21	22.2	14.7–22.4
$V_{D\,SS}$ (L/m^2)	6.3	—	—	28.2	60.0	19.2

Calculations were based on the intact lactone levels.

and Mi, 1993), other human blood proteins, human plasma and blood (Mi and Burke, 1994a), and serum albumin from other species (Mi and Burke, 1994b) *in vitro*. The carboxylate form of camptothecin, which is inactive, binds preferentially to HSA with a 150-fold higher affinity than the lactone form. As a result, camptothecin opens fully and rapidly to the carboxylate. At equilibrium in human blood, the lactone constitutes only 5.3% of the total drug concentration, while the lactone form of camptothecin is significantly more stable in rat, dog, and mouse plasma, resulting in higher lactone concentrations. When the stability of the 9-AC lactone was evaluated in HSA, human plasma, and blood, the amount of lactone at equilibrium was only 2% or less (Burke *et al.*, 1995).

4. Preclinical Toxicology Data

The administration of 9-AC produced dose-limiting gastrointestinal and bone marrow toxicity in mice, rats, and dogs (Dixit *et al.*, 1992, 1993). Gastrointestinal toxicity developed during or soon after dosing was completed and was characterized in dogs by severe emesis, diarrhea and intestinal necrosis, congestion, hemorrhage, and dysplasia. Bone marrow toxicity was characterized in dogs and mice by leukopenia and thrombocytopenia and was accompanied by bone marrow atrophy and necrosis. Toxicity was reversible in surviving animals.

Dogs were more sensitive to the toxic effects of 9-AC than mice or rats. Plasma steady-state lactone concentrations of 3.1 nM and above for 48 or 72 h were highly toxic or lethal to beagle dogs, whereas mice tolerated plasma lactone concentrations of 4–10 nM for 72 h with only mild, reversible toxicity. In addition, rats tolerated a higher total dose of 9-AC than dogs when given as a 72-h infusion. Rats administered a total dose of 19.4 mg/m^2 (44.5 μg/kg/h for 72 h) suffered severe bone marrow and gastrointestinal toxicity, while dogs administered a total dose of only 5 mg/m^2 (3.5 μg/kg/h for 72 h), four times less drug, also suffered severe bone marrow and gastrointestinal toxicity (Table 2).

Studies in dogs also demonstrated that the MTD was schedule dependent. The MTD of an IV bolus dose of 9-AC was 1 mg/kg (20 mg/m^2) while the MTD of a 72-h CIV infusion dose was only 0.18 mg/kg (3.6 mg/m^2). The five- to sixfold difference in MTD between an IV bolus dose and an infusion dose suggests that the toxicity of 9-AC is not a function of total dose as much as it is a function of duration of exposure and steady-state lactone concentration.

In vitro bone marrow toxicity studies further supported the species difference between rodents and dogs, in which the IC$_{90}$ for CFU-GM was about 8 times lower for dogs than mice (Erickson-Miller *et al.*, 1997; May *et al.*, 1993b). The IC$_{90}$ for human CFU-GM was similar to the dog IC$_{90}$, suggesting that humans may also be as sensitive to the myelosuppressive effects of 9-AC as dog (see Table 2 for comparison of *in vitro* and *in vivo* data). As a result of the *in vitro* and *in vivo* studies, the starting dose for the clinical trial was based on the dog.

5. Human Clinical Trials

Phase I and II clinical trials of 9-AC as a 72-h CIV infusion have been completed. Drug was administered either every 2

TABLE 2
9-Amino(20S)camptothecin (NSC-603071): Comparison of *in Vitro* Bone Marrow Toxicity Data and *in Vivo* MTDs

Species	CFU$_{GM}$ inhibitory conc. (nM, continuous exposure)			*In vivo* MTD total dose (mg/m^2)
	IC$_{50}$	IC$_{75}$	IC$_{90}$	72-h CIV or SC
Mouse	18	35	55	15
Rat	NP	NP	NP	8.3
Dog	0.45	2.7	7.5	3.6
Human	0.45	1.9	6.8	3.3

NP, not performed.

or 3 weeks. When administered every 2 weeks in a phase I setting, the MTD was determined to be 47 $\mu g/m^2/h$ without granulocyte colony stimulating factor (G-CSF) and 59 $\mu g/m^2/h$ with G-CSF (Dahut et al., 1996). Neutropenia was dose limiting. In the second phase I when 9-AC was administered every 3 weeks, 45 $\mu g/m^2/h$ was determined to be the MTD with dose-limiting neutropenia (Rubin et al., 1995). In the phase II trials, 9-AC was administered every 2 weeks at either 35 $\mu g/m^2/h$ without G-CSF (Pazdur et al., 1997); at 45 $\mu g/m^2/h$ with G-CSF (Kraut et al., 2000); and in another trial at 59 $\mu g/m^2/h$ with G-CSF (Saltz et al., 1997). Again, neutropenia was dose limiting in both settings. Other toxicities noted were thrombocytopenia, nausea, vomiting, stomatitis, fatigue, and anemia. In the third trial at 59 $\mu g/m^2/h$, a 15% reduction in dose was required due to an unacceptable level of toxicity that prevented cycling of treatment every 2 weeks. In all of these trials, 9-AC as a 72-h CIV infusion had limited or no antitumor activity.

Takimoto and co-workers (1994, 1996, 1997) determined that the 9-AC lactone composed only 8.7% of the total circulating 9-AC concentration. Steady-state levels at the MTD (47 $\mu g/m^2/h$) were 63.7 nM total 9-AC and 5.24 nM 9-AC lactone with a lactone AUC of 348 nM/h. Clearance was 25.7 L/h/m^2 for lactone and 2.42 L/h/m^2 for total drug. Steady-state plasma concentrations of the lactone correlated with dose-limiting neutropenia.

The pharmacokinetic results reported by Rubin et al. (1995) appears to be at odds with those reported by previous workers. The plasma level reported for 9-AC lactone at a dose of 45 $\mu g/m^2/h$ was 38.8 ng/mL or 106.7 nM (Rubin et al., 1995) and is about 20-fold higher than that reported by Dahut and co-workers (1996, 1997) or 5.24 nM at an almost identical infusion rate of 47 $\mu g/m^2/h$. It may be that the 106.7-nM level is actually total 9-AC levels since the lactone

level is only a small portion (2–8%) of the total drug level. The results from the higher infusion rate of 60 $\mu g/m^2/h$ reported in the Rubin study of a lactone level of 18.5 ng/ml, approximately half that of the level detected at the lower rate of 45, point to a possible problem with the analytical method.

6. Predictability of Preclinical Animal Models

Myelotoxicity was determined to be dose limiting in all three animal species tested as well as in humans. Other side effects including gastrointestinal toxicity (nausea, vomiting, and diarrhea) were also predicted by all three species. The MTD in humans was determined to be 46 $\mu g/m^2/h$ (average of two studies) or a total dose of 3.3 mg/m^2. The MTD in the dog on the same schedule was almost identical to that found in clinical trials at a total dose of 3.6 mg/m^2. The MTD in the rat was about 2.5 times greater, while that in the mouse was about 18 times higher when the dose was administered subcutaneously on an effective q4d×8 schedule. The in vitro bone marrow data also indicated that the dog was the more sensitive species in comparison with the mouse and that man's sensitivity was about equal to that of the dog. Use of 0.1 MELD$_{10}$ as the starting dose would have been toxic in humans, but, based on the rat toxicity data, the SD would have been reduced to an acceptable level.

The MTD, 9-AC lactone steady-state plasma level, and AUC reported by Dahut and co-workers (1996, 1997) determined in phase I, i.e., a total dose of 3.4 mg/m^2, a C_{PSS} of 5.24 nM, and an AUC of 7.59 $\mu g/mL \times min$, correlate well with a dog dose of 3.6 mg/m^2 as an MTD, and steady state levels of lactone (3.5–6.0 nM) and an AUC (7.35–9.46) that produced severe toxicity and death in dogs (Table 3).

Thus, both the in vivo toxicity studies and the in vitro bone marrow studies correctly predicted not only the MTD in hu-

TABLE 3
9-Amino(20S)camptothecin (NSC-603071): Correlation of Efficacy and Toxicity with Pharmacokinetics

Dose[a] (μg/kg/h × 72 h)	Total dose (mg/m^2)	C_{PSS} (nM)	AUC (μg/mL × min)	Toxicity
Dog–1.0	1.4	0.50	ND	Nontoxic
Dog–2.5	3.6	1.6	ND	Nontoxic
Dog–3.5	5.0	1.9–3.6	3.03–4.89	Potentially lethal GI reversible myelotoxicity
Dog–7.0	10.0	3.5–6.0	7.35–9.46	Lethal GI and myelosuppression
Mouse (5 mg/kg, SC) q4d×8	120	246	33.9 × 8	Efficacy
Rat–6.1	0	3.2–4.7	5.1–7.4	Nontoxic
Rat–19.3	8.3	17.1	27.2	Minimal GI
Rat–44.5	19.2	38.3	60.7	Lethal GI and reversible myelotoxicity
Man–1.22 Rubin	3.2	106.9	179.3	MTD—neutropenia and thrombocytopenia
Man–1.27 Dahut/Takimoto	3.4	5.24	7.59	MTD—neutropenia and thrombocytopenia

[a]Infusion rate in dog, rat and human 72 hour continuous intravenous infusion studies.

mans, but also the DLT. In addition, the pharmacokinetic results in dogs were very predictive of those determined in humans. Since a continuous infusion was not performed in mice, a direct comparison of this route and schedule could not be made. The lack of clinical efficacy by 9-AC may be accounted for by the greater sensitivity of humans to the toxic effects of the drug as compared with the mouse, the efficacy study model (Table 3). It may also be accounted for by the intrinsic instability of the 9-AC lactone in human blood as determined by Burke et al. (1995) that leads to much lower levels of lactone in humans than in animals.

B. Bizelesin (NSC-615291, U-77,779)

1. Introduction

Bizelesin is a symmetrical dimeric analogue of CC-1065 (Fig. 2), which is a potent antitumor antibiotic produced by *Streptomyces zelensis* (Hanka et al.,1978; Reynolds et al., 1986; Warpehoski and Hurley, 1988). CC-1065 was discovered in 1975 and shown to inhibit DNA synthesis by binding to the minor grove of DNA in the A-T regions followed by covalent binding to N-3 of adenine (Hurley et al., 1990; Warpehoski, 1988). It was not evaluated in the clinic due to delayed and irreversible hepatotoxicity produced in mice and rabbits (McGovren, 1984). Frank hepatic necrosis was seen at high doses, while changes in mitochondrial morphology were seen at low doses. Bizelesin arose out of a synthetic program at the Upjohn Company to develop less toxic analogues of CC-1065 (Warpehoski, 1989). Unlike CC-1065, bizelesin is a bifunctional alkylating agent that produces DNA intrastrand cross-links (Ding and Hurley, 1991).

2. Preclinical Efficacy Data

In vitro, bizelesin was shown to be a very potent molecule with a mean IC_{50} of 0.65 ng/ml against a panel of 10 gynecologic cancer cell lines (Hightower et al., 1993). This was midway between adozelesin and carzelesin, two other CC-1065 analogues that were developed by Upjohn as well. *In vivo,* bizelesin demonstrated a broad spectrum of activity in syngeneic murine tumors and human tumor xenografts in mice (Carter et al., 1996). A significant increase in life span or tumor-free survival was seen with P388, L1210, B16 melanoma and human tumors such as CAKi renal, LX-1 lung, HT-29 colon, LOX IMVI and UACC-62 melanoma, and MX-1 mammary. A comparison of the activity seen when bizelesin was administered either intraperitoneally or intravenously route indicated that optimal activity was produced with IV administration. Schedule dependency studies indicated that the antitumor activity of bizelesin was independent of the schedule used, but greater total doses could be administered on the more prolonged schedules. Based on the results in a doxorubicin-resistant tumor subline, bizelesin may be a substrate for *P*-glycoprotein. Due to the lack of schedule dependency, bizelesin was developed along traditional lines utilizing both Dx1 and Dx5 schedules.

3. Preclinical Pharmacokinetic Data

Due to the very high cytotoxic potency of bizelesin and the resulting low doses used for preclinical efficacy and in pharmacokinetic studies, conventional analytical methods such as high-performance liquid chromatography (HPLC) could not be used to quantitate levels of this agent in plasma or other biological fluids. As an alternative, a bioassay based on growth inhibition of L1210 leukemia cells in culture was developed (Walker et al., 1994). The assay is nonspecific in that it does not discriminate between drug, drug degradation products, or drug metabolites that may have growth inhibitory activity. For routine determination of "cytotoxic equivalents" in mouse plasma, standards and appropriately diluted experimental samples were added to flasks containing exponentially growing L1210 cells. Growth inhibition was measured after 48 h of incubation and the IC_{50} was determined to be about 1 pM.

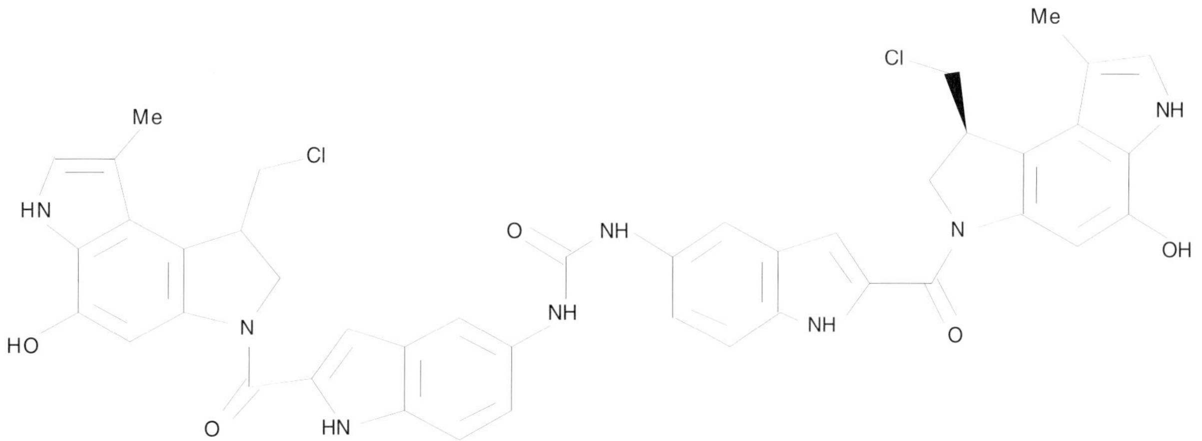

FIGURE 2 Structure of bizelesin.

The pharmacokinetics of bizelesin were determined following IV and intraperitoneal (IP) administration to male $CD2F_1$ mice at doses of 15 and 20 μg/kg since these doses were found to be efficacious. Plasma elimination of bizelesin equivalents following IV bolus administration was biphasic, with half-lives of 3.5 and 438 min. Measured peak plasma levels (3 min) were around 10 ng/mL. Concentrations declined rapidly to 1–3 ng/mL by 15 min and remained in that range for 4 h. Bizelesin equivalents in plasma were usually below detectable levels at later time points. The mean total body clearance of bizelesin equivalents was 16 ml/min/kg. Following IP bolus administration, peak plasma levels (0.24–0.99 ng/mL) were observed at 30–60 min and declined to undetectable levels after 4–8 h. Total drug exposure was at least 10-fold less following IP administration as compared with IV administration. This confirmed the finding in efficacy studies that IV administration was the optimal route.

4. Preclinical Toxicology Data

The toxicity of bizelesin was preclinically evaluated *in vivo* in mice, rats, and dogs (Evans *et al.*, 1994; Rodman *et al.*, 1993) and its myelotoxicity was further defined *in vitro* in murine, canine, and human CFU-GM (May *et al.*, 1993; Volpe *et al.*, 1995, 1996). The animal studies demonstrated that bizelesin was a highly potent myelosuppressive agent in all three species tested. The MTD in mice was 10 μg/kg (30 μg/m²) when administered as a single IV dose and 3.5 μg/kg/d (10.5 μg/m²/d) when administered as an IV daily dose for five consecutive days. Rats tolerated more drug than mice because 7.5 μg/kg (45 μg/m²) as a single dose and up to 2 μg/kg/d (12 μg/m²/d) for 5 days produced only myelosuppression and no lethality. Dogs were more sensitive to bizelesin than either of the rodent species. The single IV dose MTD in the dog was 0.1 μg/kg (2 μg/m²). Single IV doses of 0.5 μg/kg (10 μg/m²) or more were lethal. On the five-daily-dose schedule, dogs tolerated only 0.04 μg/kg/d (0.8 μg/m²/d) without any lethality. There was no evidence of hepatotoxicity, delayed or otherwise, in any of the animal models treated with bizelesin such as that seen with CC-1065.

When myelotoxicity was determined to be dose limiting in animals, the sensitivities of bone marrow progenitor cells from the various species were evaluated *in vitro*. It was found that human marrow was considerably more sensitive to the toxic effects of bizelesin than was mouse marrow. The exposure of bone marrow to bizelesin for 1 h resulted in a IC_{90} of 0.9 nM for human, 2.7 nM for canine, and 660 nM for murine CFU-GM. When exposure was lengthened to 8 h, there was an even wider disparity (2820-fold) between the sensitivity of murine and human marrow (Table 4).

The difference between dog and mouse sensitivity *in vivo* was only 15-fold based on the relative MTDs, while the difference in bone marrow sensitivity *in vitro* was almost 250-fold. This would indicate that the static bone marrow assay with no capacity for metabolism probably overpredicted the sensitivity of human marrow to the toxic effects of bizelesin in the same manner as for the dog. Even if this were true, the data also indicate that it may not be possible to reach effective levels in humans.

5. Human Clinical Trials

The proposed starting dose for the single-dose clinical trial was based on the most sensitive species and was proposed to be 0.2 μg/m² or 10% of the dog MTD. Due to the wide disparity between the species in the bone marrow assay, the FDA requested that the starting dose be further lowered to 0.1 μg/m² as an additional safety precaution. The preliminary findings of two of the ongoing phase I trials have been reported (Pitot *et al.*, 1999; Schwartz *et al.*, 2000). In both trials, bizelesin was administered as a single IV dose every 28 days. The highest dose tested to date, 1.26 μg/m², has produced myelosuppression of a short duration in the form of grade 3/4 neutropenia in patients with no neutropenic fevers. These results are from the treatment of 31 patients with 103 courses of therapy at 7 dose levels ranging from 0.1 to 1.26 μg/m² (Schwartz *et al.*, 2000). In the second trial, the highest dose reported was 1.0 μg/m², which also produced grade 4 neutropenia (Pitot *et al.*, 1999).

TABLE 4
Bizelesin (NSC 615291): Summary of *in Vitro* Bone Marrow Toxicity Data and *in Vivo* MTDs

| Species | CFU_{GM} inhibitory conc. (1-h exposure) | | | CFU_{GM} inhibitory conc. (8-h exposure) | | | *In vivo* MTD total dose (μg/m²) |
	IC_{50}	IC_{70}	IC_{90}	IC_{50}	IC_{70}	IC_{90}	D × 1, IV
Mouse	ND	69.3 nM	660 nM	ND	13.3 nM	172 nM	30
Rat	NP	NP	NP	NP	NP	NP	45
Dog	ND	327 pM	2659 pM	ND	9.0 pM	75 pM	2
Human	ND	119 pM	906 pM	ND	6.0 pM	61 pM	1.26

ND, not determined; NP, not performed.

6. Predictability of Preclinical Animal Models

Since the pharmacokinetic data reported in humans are very sparse at this point, no meaningful comparison can be made with respect to the applicability or predictability of the animal data to humans. With regard to the predictability of the toxicity data, all three species predicted that myelotoxicity would be dose limiting. The animal data also indicated that the dog was 15–22.5 times more sensitive than mouse and rat, respectively, but indicated nothing about which species was more representative of man. The *in vitro* bone marrow assay predicted that humans would be somewhat more sensitive than dogs and considerably more sensitive than mice. With patients experiencing grade 3/4 neutropenia at 1.26 $\mu g/m^2$, the current human dose/MTD is slightly less than that seen in the dog (2 $\mu g/m^2$) as predicted by bone marrow data (Table 4).

Thus, both the *in vitro* and *in vivo* toxicity data reliably predicted the sensitivity of humans to the potent cytotoxic bizelesin by accurately predicting both the MTD and DLT (Table 4). If only the rodent data were considered, i.e., a single dose MTD of 30 $\mu g/m^2$ in the mouse and 45 $\mu g/m^2$ in the rat, using one tenth of the mouse MTD to set the starting dose in man, a dose of 3 $\mu g/m^2$ would have been selected. This dose would have been safe in the rat and would have exceeded the MTD in man. Thus, in this case, the toxicity studies in the dog were a necessary adjunct to the rodent studies, which permitted the selection of a safe starting dose, and the *in vitro* bone marrow data were highly predictive of the sensitivity of humans to the toxic effects of bizelesin.

C. Cyclopentenyl Cytosine (CPEC, NSC-375575)

1. Introduction

Cyclopentenyl cytosine (Fig. 3) is a pyrimidine analogue of neplanocin A, a carbocyclic-fermentation-derived nucleoside. The unique biological activity of this antibiotic, with both antitumor and antiviral efficacy, prompted its full synthesis and that of other analogues. One of these analogues, CPEC, was synthesized by a group at the NCI (Lim *et al.,* 1984) and by one in Japan (Arita *et al.,* 1983). Investigations into the mechanism of action indicated that the cytotoxic effect exerted by CPEC was related to the near-total abrogation of CTP pools in treated tumor cells (Glazer *et al.,* 1985, 1986; Moyer *et al.,* 1986) by inhibition of CTP synthase by CPEC triphosphate (Kang *et al.,* 1989). The IC_{50} for inhibition of CTP synthase is 6 μM.

2. Preclinical Efficacy Data

When the effect of CPEC on tumor cells was examined, it was found that 1 μM inhibited L1210 cell growth by more than 90% (Moyer *et al.,* 1986); and 50–100 nM was the IC_{50}

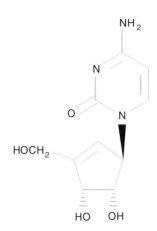

FIGURE 3 Structure of cyclopentenyl cytosine.

for the inhibition of the MOLT-4 line of human lymphoblasts (Ford *et al.,* 1991). When evaluated *in vivo*, CPEC was found to have antitumor activity against a number of murine tumors, such as L1210, P388, and P388/ara-C (Marquez *et al.,* 1988; Moyer *et al.,* 1986); and against human tumor xenografts (A549 lung, MX-1 mammary, and LOX melanoma) implanted in athymic mice (Marquez *et al.,* 1988). Antitumor efficacy was seen in animal models on a variety of schedules, including a dx9, an intermittent q4d×3, and on a schedule that simulated a 24-hour infusion given on an intermittent schedule (q3h×8, q4d×3). The intermittent schedule (q4d×3) appeared to be the least effective, indicating that a more continuous exposure was necessary for optimal activity.

3. Preclinical Pharmacokinetic Data

Pharmacokinetic studies of CPEC demonstrated interspecies differences in CPEC metabolism and disposition among mice, rats, dogs, and monkeys. Metabolic variability was impacted by pathways that result in CPEC conversion to its active metabolite, CPEC-triphosphate (CPEC-TP), or the presence or absence of cytidine deaminase, which results in the formation of the inactive entity CPE-uracil (CPE-U). Plasma protein binding studies in rat, dog, and human plasma indicated low protein binding (0–17%) (Hegedus *et al.,* 1997).

Mouse, rat, and dog models demonstrated that CPEC best fit a three-compartment disposition. Rapid alpha half-lives ranging from 2.36 to 7.45 min were observed from bolus IV doses in these species (Table 5) (Page *et al.,* 1990; Tomaszewski *et al.,* 1990; Zaharko *et al.,* 1991). Beta half-lives ranged from approximately 1–2 h except for a 800 mg/m^2 lethal IV bolus dose in dogs. A prolonged gamma elimination phase was observed in rodents and dogs possibly from the gradual release of CPEC from CPEC-phosphates (Zaharko *et al.,* 1991). IV bolus doses in mice (144 mg/m^2) and dogs (400–800 mg/m^2) exhibited a total-body clearance of approximately 100 mL/min/m^2, whereas rats, which

TABLE 5
Cyclopentenyl Cytosine (NSC-375575): Single Intravenous Bolus Doses, Pharmacokinetic Parameters

Species	Mouse	Rat		Dog				Monkey	Man
Doses (mg/m^2)	145	12	118	200	400	600	800^a	100	24
$t_{1/2}\alpha$ (min)	7.45	12.7	4.6	7.18	2.53	3.89	2.36	8.4	8
$t_{1/2}\beta$ (min)	69	91.2	58	119.5	128.5	117	169.5	36.3	101
$t_{1/2}\gamma$ (min)	1740	ND	115	ND	ND	1260	ND	ND	ND
$C_{p\,MAX}$ (μM)	372	10.4	121	14	26	58	60	~28	~10
AUC (μM/h)	99	8.8	155	23.9	50	114.6	141.8	10.6	ND
CL$_{TB}$ (mL/min/m^2)	102	94.8	54	39.4	133.4	90.8	94.4	662	199
% Urinary excretion	ND	ND	64^b	ND	50–69	ND	ND	17	ND

^{a}Both dogs in this group died within 14 hours of dosing.
^{b}Incomplete sampling.
ND, not determined.

possess high circulating competitive cytidine levels (Moyer *et al.*, 1981), had a CL$_{TB}$ of only 54 mL/min/m^2.

Single-dose IV dog pharmacokinetic studies over the range 200–800 mg/m^2 indicate a dose-dependent elimination pattern. Elimination half-lives ranged from 117 to 170 min and the CL$_{TB}$ ranged from 39.4 to 133.4 mL/min/m^2, suggesting a saturable process. The high apparent volume of distribution (40.8 L/m^2) is greater than total-body water and indicates distribution into deep cellular compartments and binding to tissues. In dogs receiving 600 mg/m^2, 50–69% of the dose was eliminated unchanged in the urine within 48 h (Page *et al.*, 1990).

True steady-state plasma levels of drug were not achieved in any of the dose groups in the dog continuous-infusion study, and considerable interanimal variation was observed. However, the average total-body clearance rates determined for each dose group were all approximately 260 mL/min/m^2, which is about twice the value observed in the single-dose study (see Tables 5 and 6). The AUC values for each dose group in this study were also consistent, displaying no dose

dependence over the infusion range studied (both time and rate). Average values for the various parameters that were determined in the continuous-infusion study are presented in Table 6. An IV bolus dose in rhesus monkeys of 100 mg/m^2 exhibited rapid biexponential pharmacokinetics with a mean alpha and beta half-life of 8.4 and 36.3 min, respectively, and a CL$_{TB}$ of 662 mL/min/m^2 (Table 5) (Blaney *et al.*, 1990). A 24-h CIV infusion study with 12.5 mg/m^2/h achieved a steady-state plasma level of 2.2 μM and a CL$_{TB}$ of 390 mL/min/m^2 (Table 6). Significant differences between rodent and canine versus monkey plasma catabolism may explain the five- to ninefold greater clearance in monkeys. Although CPE-U was not detected in the urine of rodents and dogs, only 17% of the parent compound was excreted unchanged in the urine of monkeys and 83% was excreted as CPE-U (Table 5) (Blaney *et al.*, 1990). Higher levels of cytidine deaminase in monkeys and humans influenced the choice of a starting dose in phase I clinical trials (Hegedus *et al.*, 1997).

TABLE 6
Cyclopentenyl Cytosine (NSC-375575): 24/74-H Continuous Intravenous
Infusion Studies, Pharmacokinetic Parameters

Species	Dog			Monkey		Man		
Doses (mg/m^2/h)	1.6	1.6	5.0	10	12.5	1.0	4.7	5.9
Infusion period (h)	72	24	24	24	24	24	24	24
C_p (μM)	0.78	0.37	1.95	1.57	2.23	0.4	2.6	3.1
AUC (μM/h)	31.6	10.9	29.9	ND	ND	ND	ND	ND
CL$_{TB}$ (mL/min/m^2)	266	260	254	444	390		146^a	
Urinary excretion (% of dose)	24.5	19.3	27.4	ND	ND		32^a	

ND, not determined.
^{a}Values are means across all dose levels.

4. Preclinical Toxicology Data

CPEC was administered intravenously to CD_2F_1 mice, Fischer 344 rats, and beagle dogs by either bolus doses or continuous infusion to evaluate toxicity (Page et al., 1990, 1991; Tomaszewski et al., 1990). The toxicity of CPEC was determined to be delayed in onset, cumulative, dose related, slowly reversible, and possibly age related. Dogs appeared to be much more sensitive to the toxic effects of CPEC than either rodent species, with rats being the least affected. The lack of sensitivity of the rat to the toxic effects of CPEC may be due to the high endogenous levels of cytidine in the rat and the fact that cytidine can rescue tumor cells from the toxic effects of CPEC (Ford et al., 1991; Glazer et al., 1985).

In mice, a single-dose MTD was 80 mg/kg (240 mg/m²) and a five-daily-dose MTD was 2.2 mg/kg/d (6.6 mg/m²/d; total dose, 19.8 mg/m²), whereas in dogs the single-dose MTD was about 10 mg/kg (200 mg/m²). Neither an MTD nor a DLT could be determined in the rat due to solubility of the drug and limitations of dosing volume at single doses up to 70 mg/kg (420 mg/m²) or 15 mg/kg/d (90 mg/m²/d) for 5 days. Hematologic toxicity was noted in both mouse and dog, but was less severe when CPEC was administered as a single dose rather than as a continuous infusion. When CPEC was administered as a 24- or 72-h CIV infusion at rates of 0.025–0.25 mg/kg/h to dogs, both myelotoxicity and stomatitis were considered dose limiting. Myelosuppression was characterized by decreases in leukocytes (neutrophils and lymphocytes), red blood cell parameters, and platelets, as well as by bone marrow and lymphoid organ atrophy. The MTD in the dog after CIV infusion was considered to be 0.25 mg/kg/h (5.0 mg/m²/h) for 24 h or 0.08 mg/kg/h (1.60 mg/m²/h) for 72 h for a total dose of 6 mg/kg (120 mg/m²).

When bone marrow toxicity was evaluated in vitro, it was found that mouse and human CFU-GM were equally sensitive to the toxic effects of CPEC. Murine BFU-E was slightly more sensitive than human, but murine CFU-E was about five times more sensitive than human (Volpe et al., 1994). Unfortunately, canine marrow was not evaluated in these studies, so that a direct comparison between in vitro and in vivo sensitivities cannot be made across all three species.

After it was determined that CPEC produced an unpredictable hypotension in numerous patients, additional studies were conducted in dogs in an attempt to determine the cause. The first study (Agbaria et al., 1994) was conducted in dogs fitted with telemetry devices that were infused with doses up to 178 mg/m² for 24 h or 216 mg/m² for 72 h. No cardiac abnormalities were detected in any of these animals. In the second study (Dobbins et al., 1997), dogs were infused over a 4-h period with 60 mg/m² of CPEC and subjected to bilateral carotid occlusion. Three hours into the infusion, the baroreceptor reflex (BRR) was markedly inhibited and continued to decline for up to 2 h after completion of the infusion. Since Zofran, a central nervous system serotonin receptor antago-

nist used as antiemetic, was also given to CPEC patients, its effect on the carotid BRR was also evaluated. Zofran itself had no effect on BRR, and when it was administered prior to CPEC, BRR was no longer affected. This suggests that CPEC may attenuate the carotid baroreceptor reflex via central serotonin receptors.

5. Human Clinical Trials

The starting dose of 1 mg/m²/h for 24 h was based on plasma levels achieved in monkeys taking into account cytidine deaminase activity and pharmacokinetic data that were obtained after an IV bolus dose of 24 mg/m² was administered to two patients. CPEC was administered to 26 patients at doses of 1–5.9 mg/m²/h as a 24-h CIV infusion every 3 weeks (Politi et al., 1995) achieving steady-state plasma levels of 0.4–3.1 μM, which increased linearly with dose (Table 6). Renal excretion of intact drug and the deamination product, cyclopentenyl uracil, occurred in a 2:1 ratio. Myelosuppression (decrease in both granulocytes and platelets) was dose limiting in the initial cycle in two of three patients who received 5.9 mg/m²/h. Matched samples of bone marrow mononuclear cells demonstrated 58–100% inhibition at all dose levels. However, 4 of 11 patients who received the next lower dose of 4.7 mg/m²/h experienced hypotension 24–48 h after the end of the infusion in the first, third, or sixth cycle. Unfortunately, two of the patients died with a refractory hypotension despite aggressive hydration and cardiopulmonary resuscitation. As a result, the clinical trial was suspended. Hypotension was not observed in patients receiving ≤2.5 mg/m²/h CPEC (Politi et al., 1995). No correlation between hypotension and some predictive parameter could be found. Although it appeared that the hypotension was dose dependent, its unpredictable nature and uncertainty concerning the mechanism precluded a recommendation of a safe dose for future studies.

6. Predictability of Preclinical Animal Models

The animal data were successful in predicting the myelotoxicity that occurred in humans as well as the MTD (84 mg/m²). The dog MTD as a 24-h continuous infusion was 120 mg/m². Infusions were not conducted in mice or rats. The hypotension produced by CPEC in humans was not predicted by the preclinical animal studies performed and could not be repeated in dogs under the same conditions that produced it in man during the clinical trial.

D. Depsipeptide (Cyclic Peptide, FR-901228, NSC-630176)

1. Introduction

Depsipeptide is a bicyclic peptide (Fig. 4) that was isolated from a strain of Chromobacterium violaceum by investigators at the Fujisawa Pharmaceutical Company to identify inhibitors of oncogene function (Shigematsu et al., 1994;

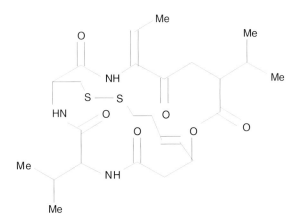

FIGURE 4   Structure of depsipeptide.

Ueda *et al.*, 1994a). Early screening studies indicated that depsipeptide decreased mRNA expression of the c-*myc* oncogene in RAS 1 cells but had no effect on Ha-ras mRNA expression (Ueda *et al.*, 1994b). In addition, depsipeptide has been shown to evoke cell cycle arrest in G_1 and G_2 (Mertins *et al.*, 1999; Sackett *et al.*, 1999; Sandor *et al.*, 1998; Ueda *et al.*, 1994b) and was recently found to inhibit histone deacetylase activity causing differentiation in cancer cells (Mertins *et al.*, 1999; Nakajima *et al.*, 1998).

2. Preclinical Efficacy Data

In vitro studies in human tumor cell lines demonstrated that depsipeptide was a potent cytotoxic agent in a variety of cell types in the low nM concentration range (Ueda *et al.*, 1994a). Apoptotic activity was observed when depsipeptide was used to treat human-B-cell chronic lymphocytic leukemia cells (Byrd *et al.*, 1999) and breast cancer (MCF 7 and MDA-MB-231) cell lines (Rajgolikar *et al.*, 1998). *In vivo* efficacy studies have shown depsipeptide to have broad antitumor efficacy in murine solid tumor models (M5076 sarcoma, Meth A fibrosarcoma, and Colon 38 carcinoma) and human tumor xenografts (SC-6 stomach, Lu-65 lung, and LC-6 lung) when administered in-

travenously on an intermittent-dosing schedule (Ueda *et al.*, 1994c). Depsipeptide was effective against several drug-resistant P388 cell lines *in vivo* (mitomycin C, cyclophosphamide, 5-fluorouracil); however, it was cross-resistant to doxorubicin-resistant P388. Depsipeptide has also been shown to be a substrate for multidrug resistant P-glycoprotein, and inhibitors of P-glycoprotein enhance the cytotoxicity of depsipeptide (Mertins *et al.*, 1999; Ueda *et al.*, 1994c).

3. Preclinical Pharmacokinetic Data

Pharmacokinetic parameters from preclinical studies in rats (Chan *et al.*, 1997; Li and Chan, 2000) and from a recent phase I clinical trial (Bates *et al.*, 1999; Kang *et al.*, 1999) are summarized in Table 7. Following IV bolus dosing to rats, plasma elimination of depsipeptide was biphasic, with a terminal half-life of 87–188 min and plasma clearance of 425–824 ml/min/kg (2250–4944 mL/min/m^2). The variability of these parameters may be due in part to the change in assay sensitivity. Peak levels of depsipeptide at 1 mg/kg (6 mg/m^2) were 80 nM, and levels remained above 1 nM for about 4 h, suggesting that concentrations with antitumor activity *in vitro* (Ueda *et al.*, 1994a) could be achieved with tolerable doses in rats.

4. Preclinical Toxicology Data

Toxicology studies with depsipeptide were initiated by Fujisawa Pharmaceutical and continued by the NCI. Depsipeptide has been administered intravenously as bolus and infusion (1–24 h) doses. The dosing schedules for the preclinical toxicology studies included single-dose, intermittent-dose (q4d×3, weekly, and twice weekly) and daily-dose (daily × 14 and daily × 28) studies conducted in mice, rats, and dogs.

Preliminary studies in dogs demonstrated that the length of time over which depsipeptide is administered markedly affects the toxicity of this drug. At a given dose, dogs tolerated depsipeptide better when given as a 1-h infusion compared with a bolus dose. In dogs given a 1-h infusion of depsipeptide, the maximum tolerated dose was 2.0 mg/kg/week ad-

TABLE 7
Depsipeptide (NSC-630176): Pharmacokinetic Parameters in Rats and Humans

Species Doses (mg/m^2)	Rat		Man		
	6	60	1.0	6.5	24.9
$C_{p\,MAX}$ (ng/mL)	43	1829	35.6	212	473
$t_{1/2}\alpha$ (min)	18.4	5.9		24[a]	
$t_{1/2}\beta$ (min)	188	87.3		713[a]	
CL$_{TB}$ (mL/min/m^2)	4944	2252		304[a]	
Assay LOQ (ng/mL)	0.5	10		0.1[a]	

[a]Values are means across all dose levels.

ministered either once a week or split (1.0 mg/kg/d) and given twice weekly for 4 weeks. However, 2.0 mg/kg/d of depsipeptide administered to dogs as a 24-h infusion was significantly more toxic than the same dose administered as a 1- or 4-h infusion. The 4-h infusion appeared to decrease the incidence of cardiac hemorrhagic lesions compared with the 1-h infusion. Therefore, a 4-h infusion appeared to be the best tolerated infusion schedule in dogs (Page *et al.*, 1995). The MTD of depsipeptide given as a 4-h infusion to dogs and rats on days 1, 5, and 9 was 1.0 mg/kg/d (6 mg/m^2/d for rats and 20 mg/m^2/d for dogs). Bone marrow toxicity was considered dose limiting in rats, and gastrointestinal and site-of-infusion toxicity were dose limiting in dogs. Bone marrow toxicity was present in dogs treated with doses of 2.0 mg/kg/d or more of depsipeptide (Page *et al.*, 1996).

Cardiotoxicity of depsipeptide (characterized as myocardial hemorrhage, atrophy, and necrosis) was first encountered during the multiple-dose toxicity studies (Dx14 and Dx28) in dogs conducted by Fujisawa Pharmaceutical. No histopathologic evidence of cardiotoxicity occurred in rats administered depsipeptide on the same dosing schedule. In subsequent studies, alterations in electrocardiogram (ECG) profiles were measured in dogs in the 4-week intermittent toxicity studies conducted by Fujisawa Pharmaceutical. In an effort to assess the cardiotoxicity of depsipeptide in the preclinical toxicity studies in dogs conducted by the NCI, blood pressure measurements, continuous and intermittent ECG measurements, lactate dehydrogenase/creatinine kinase (LDH/CK) isozyme profiles, and histopathology were evaluated. At highly toxic/lethal doses of depsipeptide (2.0 mg/kg/d given as a 1-h or 24-h infusion), dogs had cardiac hemorrhagic lesions present at necropsy. There was no evidence of myocardial necrosis or atrophy and no detectable changes in blood pressure, ECG measurements, and LDH/CK isozyme profiles in dogs given depsipeptide as a 4-h infusion on days 1, 5, and 9. Since myelotoxicity occurred during the preclinical toxicology studies, *in vitro* bone marrow studies were performed on granulocyte-macrophage progenitor cells (CFU-GM). The IC$_{90}$ values after continuous drug exposure were 8.0, 2.2, and 5.5 nM for murine, canine, and human cells, respectively. The *in vitro* data indicate that the sensitivity of murine and canine cells was similar to that of human cells (i.e., a 1.5- to 2.5-fold difference). These results were predictive for the *in vivo* results, since there was little difference in MTD between species (Table 8).

5. Human Clinical Trials

The phase I clinical studies on depsipeptide are currently being completed. The MTD was 13.3 mg/m^2/d given as a 4-h infusion weekly for 3 weeks (Marshall *et al.*, 1998) and 17.8 mg/m^2/d given as a 4-h infusion on days 1 and 5 (Bates *et al.*, 1999). Thrombocytopenia was considered to be the DLT. Gastrointestinal toxicity also occurred at the MTD. Cardiac changes occurred in patients treated with high doses

TABLE 8
Depsipeptide (NSC-630176): Summary of *in Vitro* Bone Marrow Toxicity Data and *in Vivo* MTDs

Species	CFU$_{GM}$ inhibitory conc. (nM, continuous exposure)			*In vivo* MTD total dose (mg/m^2)
	IC$_{50}$	IC$_{75}$	IC$_{90}$	4 Hr CIV, q4d×3
Mouse	0.59	5.4	8.0	63.6
Rat	NP	NP	NP	18
Dog	0.33	1.3	2.2	60
Human	0.03	1.4	5.5	35.6–39.9

NP, not performed.

of depsipeptide with S-T wave flattening, T-wave inversion, and voltage decrease. When administered as a 4-h infusion to cancer patients at doses ranging from 1.0 to 24.9 mg/m^2 (0.027–0.67 mg/kg), depsipeptide produced maximal plasma levels between 35.6 and 473 ng/ml (Table 7; Kang *et al.*, 1999). The mean clearance across all dose levels was 8.22 ml/min/kg (304 mL/min/m^2), and the mean terminal half-life was 713 min. It should be noted that preliminary data from a second phase I clinical trial (Chassaing *et al.*, 1998; Marshall *et al.*, 1998) indicated comparable end-infusion plasma levels of depsipeptide over the dose range 1–7.5 mg/m^2, but the mean terminal half-life was only 150 min. This discrepancy may be explained by the fact that a less sensitive HPLC-UV assay was used in the latter study (Chassaing *et al.*, 1998).

6. Predictability of Preclinical Animal Models

Overall, the preclinical animal models predicted the spectrum of toxicity produced by depsispeptide in humans. In rats, bone marrow toxicity was considered dose limiting. The sensitivity of human bone marrow progenitor cells to depsipeptide indicated that there was no significant species differences in sensitivity *in vitro*, which was also supported by the MTDs determined *in vivo* (Table 8). However, the human MTD (on a mg/m^2 basis) for depsipeptide was intermediate between the MTD found in dogs and in rats. Rats appeared to be more sensitive to the toxic effects of depsipeptide than dogs or humans. Alterations in ECG profiles at high doses of depsipeptide also occurred in humans in both phase I clinical trials. Cardiac toxicity occurred in early studies in dogs given multiple daily or biweekly bolus doses of depsipeptide. However, when depsipeptide was given as a 4-h infusion, no ECG alterations occurred in dogs. Precise comparison of plasma levels across species is difficult due to the differing modes of drug administration (bolus vs. 4-h infusion), but reported maximum plasma levels were higher in humans for a given mg/m^2 dose.

E. Dolastatin 10 (NSC-376128)

1. Introduction

Dolastatin 10 is one of a number of potent cytotoxic natural products that have been isolated from the marine sea hare *Dolabella auricularia*. The chemistry and biology of the dolastatins were the subjects of a recent comprehensive review (Poncet,1999). The compound is a linear pentamer (Fig. 5) that includes four amino acids unique to the marine organism (Pettit *et al.*, 1987). Its mechanism of action involves inhibition of tubulin polymerization, tubulin-dependent guanosine triphosphate hydrolysis, and nucleotide exchange, and it is a potent noncompetitive inhibitor of vincristine binding to tubulin (Bai *et al.*, 1990a, b). Dolastatin 10 is more potent than other tubulin-binding drugs, and a recent study shows that intracellular uptake of the drug is comparable to that of vinblastine, although dolastatin 10 remains in the cell longer due to much slower efflux (Verdier-Pinard *et al.*, 2000). Besides its antimitotic effect, dolastatin 10 appears to induce apoptosis via phosphorylation of *bcl-2* (Kalemkerian *et al.*, 1999). The product of the *bcl-2* oncogene has been shown to prevent apoptosis.

2. Preclinical Efficacy Data

Dolastatin 10 was cytotoxic to cell lines in the NCI's human tumor cell line screen that are known to be sensitive to tubulin-binding agents. The compound is highly potent, with concentrations of 0.1–1 nM producing total growth inhibition of the most sensitive cell lines, such as the KM20L2 colon tumor cell line. Other investigators have shown that dolastatin 10 inhibits the growth of hematopoietic progenitor cells (Jacobsen *et al.*, 1991) and human lymphoma cell lines (Beckwith *et al.*, 1993; Maki *et al.*, 1996).

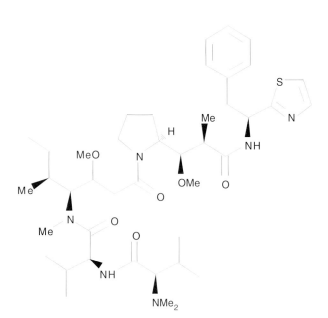

FIGURE 5   Structure of dolastatin 10.

Initial *in vivo* efficacy evaluations demonstrated significant activity against a number of intraperitoneally-implanted tumors (e.g., human LOX-IMVI melanoma, human OVCAR 3 ovarian carcinoma, and murine B16 melanoma) when dolastatin 10 was administered at the same site on various multiple-dose schedules (qd×5; q4d×3) at doses of about 50 µg/kg per injection. However, additional studies indicated that dolastatin 10 was inactive under these conditions when the sites of tumor implantation and drug injection were separated (e.g., subcutaneously implanted LOX with IP or IV drug treatment; intraperitoneally-implanted OVCAR with IV drug treatment). Consideration of mouse pharmacokinetic data (see below) suggested that the lack of distant-site antitumor activity might be explained by rapid systemic metabolism and extensive protein binding, which could prevent the drug from reaching and/or sustaining a "threshold" concentration necessary for antitumor activity.

It was subsequently determined that a single IV dose of dolastatin 10 up to 450 µg/kg was well tolerated in mice. Intravenously administered dolastatin 10 at this dose produced growth delays and complete remissions of subcutaneously-implanted early-stage LOX melanoma and advanced-stage NCI-H522 non-small cell lung carcinoma in mouse xenograft studies (NCI, unpublished data).

3. Preclinical Pharmacokinetic Data

Development of an analytical method with sufficient sensitivity for determination of dolastatin 10 in plasma was a significant challenge. Initial approaches involved the use of ^{3}H-labeled drug in conjunction with solid-phase extraction to separate parent compound from radiolabeled metabolites (Newman *et al.*, 1994) and an L1210 growth inhibition bioassay to determine total cytotoxic equivalents (Reid *et al.*, 1995). Following IV administration to mice (240 µg/kg), dolastatin 10 reached a peak plasma level of 355 nM, which declined rapidly to less than 13 nM by 15 min, and only 10% of total radioactivity was associated with parent compound. The subsequent elimination half-life was 5.6 h and the plasma clearance was 3.6 L/h/kg (Newman *et al.*, 1994).

An independent study utilizing the bioassay method yielded an elimination half-life of 4.5 h and a clearance of 2.54 L/h/kg, suggesting that the majority of cytotoxic activity in mouse plasma is attributable to the parent compound (Reid *et al.*, 1995). Plasma protein binding was comparable between mouse, dog, and human (81–90%), indicating that the amount of free drug available to produce a biological effect was similar in all three species (Newman *et al.*, 1994). Based on these preclinical pharmacology data, *in vivo* efficacy studies utilizing single IV doses at the MTD were undertaken (as described above) and were successful in demonstrating distant-site antitumor activity for dolastatin 10.

Analytical sensitivity limitations precluded the measurement of dolastatin 10 plasma concentrations in conjunction with rat and dog toxicology studies (Mirsalis *et al.*, 1999), so that preclinical pharmacokinetic data are limited to the mouse studies described above. More recently, several highly sensitive methods have been developed and validated for quantifying dolastatin 10 in biological fluids (Aherne *et al.*, 1996; Garteiz *et al.*, 1998; Huie and Wong, 1999; Huie *et al.*, 1997).

4. Preclinical Toxicology Data

The preclinical toxicology studies with dolastatin 10 were conducted by administering drug as a single IV bolus dose (Mirsalis *et al.*, 1999). The MTD was determined to be 1350 $\mu g/m^2$ in mice, 450 $\mu g/m^2$ in rats and ≤ 400 $\mu g/m^2$ in dogs (Table 9). Therefore, rats and dogs exhibited similar sensitivity to dolastatin 10, whereas mice were three- to fourfold less sensitive. The target organs of toxicity were the bone marrow and lymphoid tissues, with myelotoxicity being dose limiting in all three species.

In the *in vitro* bone marrow assay, the IC_{90} for CFU-GM cells was 10 pM for human, 4.8 pM for canine, and 8840 pM for murine progenitor cells following 1-h exposure to dolastatin 10 (Table 9). According to these findings, mice are approximately threefold less sensitive than dogs based on the MTD determined *in vivo*, but more than 1800-fold less sensitive based on *in vitro* bone marrow data. The reason for this discrepancy is unknown.

5. Human Clinical Trials

Results of two phase I pharmacologic trials and one phase II trial with dolastatin 10 have been published. In each of these studies, dolastatin 10 was administered by rapid IV injection on a q3w schedule. Dolastatin 10 produced dose-limiting neutropenia (Krug *et al.*, 2000; Madden *et al.*, 2000; Pitot *et al.*, 1999) and mild peripheral sensory neuropathy (Krug *et al.*, 2000; Pitot *et al.*, 1999). Irritation at the injection site was observed clinically and had also occurred in the animal studies. The MTD in patients was between 300 and 400 $\mu g/m^2$, depending on the degree of prior chemotherapy.

TABLE 9
Dolastatin 10 (NSC-376128): Summary of *in Vitro* Bone Marrow Toxicity Data and *in Vivo* MTDs

| Species | CFU$_{GM}$ inhibitory conc. (pM, 1-h exposure) | | | Animal MTD total dose $(\mu g/m^2)$ |
	IC_{50}	IC_{75}	IC_{90}	$D \times 1, IV$
Mouse	1707	4771	8840	1350
Rat	NP	NP	NP	450
Dog	<0.1	1.4	4.8	≤ 400
Human	0.4	3.2	10	300–400

NP, not performed.

Pharmacodynamic analyses demonstrated that the AUC correlated well with percent decrease in leukocyte count (Madden *et al.*, 2000; Pitot *et al.*, 1999); however, this was not true for the neurologic effects.

Pharmacokinetics were determined using the L1210 bioassay (Pitot *et al.*, 1999) or HPLC/electrospray ionization mass spectroscopy (HPLC-EI-MS, Madden *et al.*, 2000). Following IV bolus injection, plasma concentration–time profiles of dolastatin 10 were best characterized by a three-compartment model for most patients in each study. Rapid distribution of dolastatin 10 (half-life 4–6 min) was followed by a prolonged elimination phase yielding mean terminal half-lives of 12.7 h (Pitot *et al.*, 1999) and 18.9 h (Madden *et al.*, 2000) across all dose groups. Plasma levels of dolastatin 10 remained above 1 nM for 11–24 h at doses at or below the MTD, suggesting that therapeutic levels can be achieved in humans (although the possible consequences of protein binding on delivery of drug to tumor have not been determined). Clearance values did not vary significantly with dose, and mean values were similar in the two studies (4.2–4.5 L/h/m^2).

6. Predictability of Preclinical Animal Models

Pharmacokinetic data for interspecies comparisons are limited. The terminal half-life of dolastatin 10 in humans (12.7–18.9 h) was considerably longer than that determined in mice (5.6 h) after IV bolus administration. Similarly, plasma clearance in humans (4.2–4.5 L/h/m^2) was slower than that observed in mice (10.8 L/h/m2). While increases in half-life and decreases in clearance (expressed per kilogram) as a function of increasing body size (or weight) have been observed for many drugs (Cherkofsky, 1995; Mordenti, 1986), some of the differences may also be related to variations in sensitivity of the assays utilized.

Preclinical toxicology studies on dolastatin 10 correctly predicted dose-limiting myelotoxicity in patients. Mild sensory neuropathy was also present in some patients. Neurotoxicity was not specifically evaluated in preclinical studies, but there was no evidence of neuropathy based on histologic examination (including spinal cord and sciatic nerve) or general behavior. Therefore, the animal studies did not demonstrate the potential for drug-related neurotoxicity. The IC_{90} for human CFU-GM (10 pM) was comparable to that for canine marrow (4.8 pM), suggesting that the dog would be the best animal model to predict a clinical starting dose. One-third the toxic dose low (TDL, 200 $\mu g/m^2$) in dogs was used to calculate the clinical starting dose (65 $\mu g/m^2$). As it turned out, the dog was an accurate predictor of the MTD in patients. In phase I clinical trials, the MTD of dolastatin 10 was 300–400 $\mu g/m^2$, which is the same as the MTD in dogs (about 400 $\mu g/m^2$). The rat was only slightly less sensitive than the dog and man, and the mouse was the least predictive. If the mouse had been used to set the phase I starting dose, a dose of 135 $\mu g/m^2$ would have been used and found safe, although the first dose escalation would have probably produced significant toxicity.

F. EF5 (NSC-684681)

1. Introduction

EF5 [2-(2-nitro-1H-imidazol-1-yl]-N-(2,2,3,3,3-pentafluoropropyl)acetamide] is a fluorinated 2-nitroimidazole (Fig. 6) that is currently undergoing clinical evaluation as a diagnostic agent to detect and quantify oxygen levels in tumors and other tissues. This compound, an analogue of the radiation-sensitizing agents misonidazole and etanidazole, was designed to optimize a number of chemical and pharmacologic properties that maximize its usefulness for the determination of tissue hypoxia (Koch *et al.*, 1995). The reductive metabolism of EF5 and other 2-nitroimidazoles in cells leads to the production of reactive nitroso and hydroxylamine species that form adducts with cellular proteins. For EF5, this process has been shown to be consistently dependent on oxygen tension. The introduction of five fluorine atoms into the molecule results in increased lipophilicity and broad distribution into tissues (Laughlin *et al.*, 1996). In addition, the fluorine-containing side chain facilitated the development of avid and specific monoclonal antibodies for detection of tissue adducts and may also allow detection by MRI and PET imaging.

2. Preclinical Pharmacokinetic Data

EF5 was found to be stable in rat, dog, and human plasma for at least 18 h at 37°C. The protein binding of EF5 (1.6–16 μM) as determined by ultrafiltration ranged from 19% to 34% in rat and human plasma, but was lower (2.3–14.3%) in dog plasma. Pharmacokinetic studies were performed in rats. The compound was administered intravenously in PEG-400/saline (25:75) at a dose of 66 mg/kg. Mean peak plasma levels (C_{Max}) of 1136 μM declined in a biexponential manner with $t_{1/2}$ values of 1.5 and 170 min. The plasma clearance was 3.8 ml/min/kg and the V_D was 924 mL/kg. In a preliminary oral study in male rats (66 mg/kg, 50:50 PEG-400/saline), the C_{Max} was 102 μM (t_{Max} = 3 h) and the estimated bioavailability was 78% (unpublished NCI data). The pharmacokinetics of EF5 were also evaluated in beagle dogs

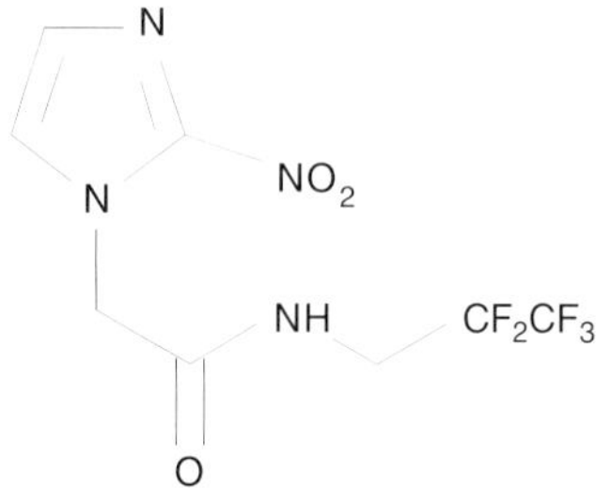

FIGURE 6 Structure of EF5.

in conjunction with a toxicology study in this species (Hill *et al.*, 1998). Dogs were administered EF5 as a 24-h CIV infusion in PEG-400/EtOH/water (40:10:50) at doses of 100 and 500 mg/kg. The mean C_{Max} values were 163 μM at 100 mg/kg and 981 μM at 500 mg/kg. The mean values for terminal $t_{1/2}$, clearance, and V_D across both dose groups were 693 min, 1.13 mL/min/kg, and 1003 mL/kg, respectively.

Selected pharmacokinetic parameters from the rat and dog studies described above are shown in Table 10, along with data for mice, cats, and baboons which were derived from information provided by investigators at the University of Pennsylvania (Laughlin *et al.*, 1996; Koch, unpublished data). A plot of plasma concentration–time data from these studies clearly demonstrates a trend of increasing half-life with animal size (Fig. 7). Thus, for a constant mg/kg dose, drug exposure (AUC) is greater in the larger species. However, a linear correlation was observed across species between administered dose expressed in mg/m^2 and AUC (Fig. 8), suggesting that dose conversions based on body surface area are appropriate for EF5.

The 30 mg/kg dose used in many of the preclinical studies was selected to produce a C_{Max} of 100 μM (30 μg/ml), assuming instantaneous distribution of EF5 into total-body water. The fitted C_{Max} values for mouse, rat, cat, and infant baboon are consistent with this hypothesis. It should be noted that the rat C_{Max} in the NCI study (Table 10) was substantially higher than would be predicted by this relationship. This is a result of plasma sampling at earlier time points than those obtained in the University of Pennsylvania studies, which allowed an initial distribution phase for EF5 to be defined. Extrapolation of the terminal elimination phase to zero time (as was done with the clinical data) would have yielded a C_{Max} value much closer to the theoretical concentration (220 μM) resulting from "instantaneous" distribution of a 66 mg/kg dose into total-body water. Consistent with these findings, the V_D values for each preclinical species were near 1000 mL/kg.

3. Preclinical Toxicology Data

Preclinical toxicology studies for EF5 were conducted in rats and dogs (Hill *et al.*, 1998; unpublished NCI data). Rats were administered EF5 formulated in PEG-400/saline (25:75) intravenously at doses up to 100 mg/kg per dose twice a day for 5 days (maximum total dose administered was 1000 mg/kg; 6000 mg/m^2). Dogs were administered EF5 formulated in PEG-400/EtOH/saline (40:10:50) intravenously as a 24-h infusion at doses up to 500 mg/kg (10,000 mg/m^2). No drug-related clinical signs of toxicity, changes in clinical pathology parameters, or histopathologic lesions were present in rats or dogs treated with EF5.

4. Human Clinical Trial Data

A phase I clinical trial of EF5 in cancer patients is ongoing (Evans *et al.*, 2000; Koch *et al.*, 2000). EF5 was administered by IV infusion at doses ranging from 9 to 28 mg/kg. No drug-

TABLE 10
EF5 (NSC-684681): Pharmacokinetic Parameters in Various Species[a]

Species	Dose (mg/kg)	Dose (mg/m²)	Fitted C_{max} (μM)	Terminal $t_{1/2}$(min)	AUC$_{0\to\infty}$ (μM × min)	Clearance (mL/min/kg)	V_D (mL/kg)
Mouse	30	90	94	40	5,410	18.3	1056
	30	180	121	106	18,605	5.32	814
Rat	66[b]	396	1136	170	62,079	3.76	924
Cat	30	360	125	274	49,686	1.99	786
Dog	100	2,000	163	512	261,894	1.36	888
(24 h CIV)	500	10,000	981	874	1.8×10^6	0.90	1118
Baboon (infants)	30	—[c]	63.3	714	65,262	1.51	1557
Man	9	333	60		60,000	0.50	506
(variable inf)	28	1,036	160	702	150,000	0.62	628

[a]EF5 was administered as an intravenous bolus, except as noted.
[b]Mean parameter values for male and female groups combined are shown.
[c]Conversion factor not available.

related toxicities have been reported. Pharmacokinetic analysis of data from the first 24 patients demonstrated that the plasma elimination of EF5 was monoexponential with a $t_{1/2}$ of 702 ± 156 min and independent of dose. Additional pharmacokinetic parameters for the 9 and 28 mg/kg clinical cohorts are also shown in Table 10. For reasons that are not yet clear, V_D appeared to be somewhat less in humans than would be predicted based on distribution into total-body water.

It has been shown that EF5 binding to tissues at constant oxygen tension is linearly related to drug exposure (Koch

et al., 2000). Consequently, correlation of observed EF5 binding with tissue pO₂ levels will be facilitated by a consistent (or known) exposure (AUC) in treated patients. The pharmacokinetics of EF5 as described above make it a compound well suited for this goal. Initial clinical data indicate that $t_{1/2}$ is reasonably constant between patients and that C_{Max} and AUC display a linear relationship with administered dose. The compound is widely distributed to tissues (including brain) (Laughlin *et al.,* 1996) and undergoes little if any metabolism (Koch *et al.,* 2000; Laughlin *et al.,* 1996). Thus, relatively limited plasma

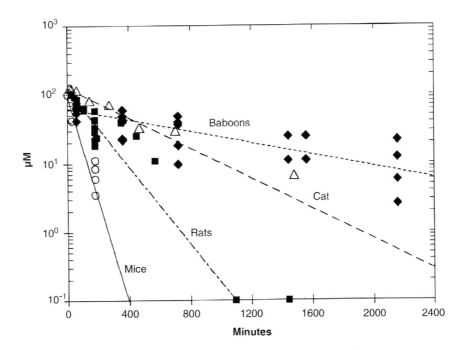

FIGURE 7 Comparison of EF5 plasma pharmacokinetics in various species (○ mice, ■ rats, △ cats, ◆ baboons) after intravenous bolus administration (30 mg/kg). Data were obtained as described in the text and fitted to a monoexponential model using RSTRIP (Version 5.0, MicroMath Scientific Software).

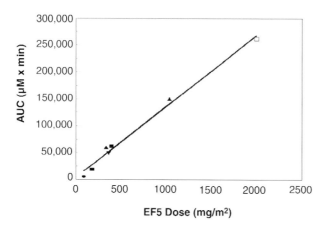

FIGURE 8 Relationship between dose of EF5 (in mg/m²) and plasma AUC across species (● mouse; ■ rat; ▼ cat, □ dog; ▲ man). The 10,000 mg/m² dose in dogs was omitted to prevent compression of the x- and y-axis scales.

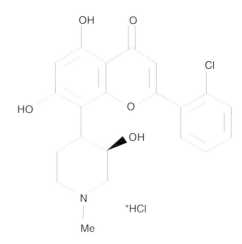

FIGURE 9 Structure of flavopiridol.

sampling (e.g., at the end of the infusion and at the time of tissue biopsy) should provide a sufficiently accurate determination of AUC to facilitate quantitative estimates of tissue hypoxia as a function of EF5 tissue binding.

5. *Predictability of Preclinical Animal Models*

The human elimination half-life is similar to that observed in dogs and baboons (Table 10), but smaller than might be predicted from the relationship depicted in Fig. 7. AUC values at both dose levels used in the clinical trials correlate well with the AUC–mg/m² dose relationship shown in Fig. 8, indicating the potential predictiveness of the animal data in relating drug exposure to dose across species from mouse to man. Extrapolated C_0 values for the 28 mg/kg clinical cohort ranged from 138 to 188 μM, which are within a factor of 2 of the predicted value of 100 μM.

G. Flavopiridol (L86-8275, NSC-649890)

1. *Introduction*

Flavopiridol is a semisynthetic flavonoid (Fig. 9) structurally related to a naturally occurring alkaloid isolated from a plant (*Dysoxylum binectariferum*) indigenous to India (Sedlacek *et al.*, 1996). Flavopiridol has been shown to be a potent cyclin-dependent kinase inhibitor (Carlson *et al.*, 1996). Studies in human breast carcinoma cells (MCF-7) demonstrated that flavopiridol inhibits cdk1, cdk2, and cdk4 by binding to the ATP-binding pocket of the kinase. In addition to inhibition, flavopiridol causes a decrease in cyclin D1, and it was felt that depletion of cyclin D1 leads to the loss of cdk4 activity. Subsequent studies have shown that as a result of the cdk inhibition, flavopiridol produces potent cell cycle arrest and apoptosis (Parker *et al.*, 1998).

2. Preclinical Efficacy Data

In vivo studies have demonstrated that flavopiridol is a potent antiproliferative agent. Studies have demonstrated that flavopiridol produced substantial growth delays in colorectal (Sedlacek *et al.*, 1996), prostate (Drees *et al.*, 1997), and head and neck carcinoma (Patel *et al.*, 1998) xenograft models, in addition to tumor regressions produced in leukemia and lymphoma xenografts (Arguello *et al.*, 1998). The antitumor activity of flavopiridol correlated in tumor tissue with cyclin D1 depletion and apoptotic cell death and peak plasma concentrations of 5–8 μM (Drees *et al.*, 1997).

3. *Preclinical Pharmacokinetic Data*

Pharmacokinetic studies of flavopiridol conducted in mice, rats, and dogs demonstrated two-compartment pharmacokinetics and relatively consistent kinetic parameters among these preclinical animal species (Table 11). In mice, doses in the range of 5.5 to 32.9 mg/kg (16.5–98.7 mg/m²) IV exhibited mean alpha and beta half-lives of 16.4 and 201.0 min, respectively (Sedlacek *et al.*, 1996). Peak plasma levels were proportional in this dose range and the mean total body clearance was 67.8 mL/min/m². Oral bioavailability in mice was 20–26% with doses of 33 and 263 mg/m². Repeated intragastric dosing of 33 mg/m² resulted in decreased peak plasma concentrations.

The pharmacokinetics of flavopiridol in male Fischer 344 rats were evaluated following a 20 mg/kg (120 mg/m²) IV bolus dose. A rapid distribution half-life of 10.5 min was followed by an elimination half-life of 112 min. The mean total-body clearance was 342 mL/min/m² and the steady-state volume of distribution was 48.4 L/m², indicating an extensive tissue exposure (Arneson *et al.*, 1995). Bioavailability studies carried out by mouth, subcutaneously, and intramuscularly were conducted in rats to evaluate routes of administration that would potentially produce prolonged plasma levels.

TABLE 11
Flavopiridol (NSC-649890) Plasma Pharmacokinetics

PK parameter Route/schedule	Mouse IV bolus	Rat IV bolus	Dog IV bolus	Dog 72 h CIV	Human 72 h CIV
Dose (mg/m^2)	16.5–98.7	120	36	17–38/d	4–78/d
$t_{1/2}\alpha$ (min)	16.4	10.5	23	—	—
$t_{1/2}\beta$ (min)	206	112	274	—	696
$C_{P\,MAX}$ or $C_{P\,SS}$ (μM)	—	21.7	—	0.055–0.162	0.271
CL_{TB} (mL/min/m^2)	67.8	342	200	383–440	287
AUC (μg/mL $\times$ min)	—	351	—	—	—
$V_{D\,SS}$ (L/m^2)	—	48.4	—	—	131.2

PK, pharmacokinetic.

Oral bioavailabilty was 24% (40 mg/kg) and the SC and IM bioavailabilities were 37% (20 mg/kg) and 74% (10 mg/kg), respectively (El-hawari *et al.*, 1997). Double-peak phenomena associated with oral and IV studies may be attributed to enterohepatic recirculation (Jager *et al.*, 1998). Biotransformation to two glucuronidated metabolites (5-*O* and 7-*O*-β-glucopyranuronosylflavopiridol) was demonstrated in isolated rat perfusion studies in addition to its secretion in bile (Jager *et al.*, 1998). The secretion of glucuronic acid derivatives in bile may be relevant to observations of severe diarrhea associated with flavopiridol and the observations of increased clinical MTDs with cholestyramine pretreatment.

In dogs, flavopiridol pharmacokinetics were evaluated after a single IV bolus dose, after 24- and 72-h infusions (Table 11), and after oral dosing. A single 36 mg/m^2 IV dose administered over 1 min exhibited a biexponential plasma concentration profile with mean alpha and beta half-lives of 23 and 274 min, respectively, and a total plasma clearance of 200 mL/min/m^2. The oral bioavailability of a 88 mg/m^2 dose of flavopiridol was 35%. A 24-h CIV infusion at 2.8 mg/kg (56 mg/m^2) resulted in a steady-state plasma level of 198 nM. The 72-h infusion studies at doses of 0.8 mg/kg/day (16 mg/m^2/d), 1.3 mg/kg/d (26 mg/m^2/d), and 1.9 mg/kg/d (38 mg/m^2/d) produced 55 nM, 91 nM, and 162 nM steady-state plasma levels, respectively and a mean plasma clearance of 383–440 mL/min/m^2 (Arneson *et al.*, 1995). Infusion studies demonstrated that steady-state plasma concentrations could safely be achieved in the effective concentration range necessary to obtain cdk inhibition.

4. Preclinical Toxicology Data

The toxicity of flavopiridol was evaluated preclinically in rats and dogs. In dogs, flavopiridol was administered as a 72-h CIV infusion and in rats, flavopiridol was administered as a bolus dose given three times a day (every 8 h) for 3 days (tid $\times$ 3). The purpose of these studies was to determine the MTD, end-organ toxicity, and reversibility of toxicity. Flavopiridol produced gastrointestinal and bone marrow toxicity in rats and dogs (Arneson *et al.*, 1995; Sedlacek *et al.*, 1996). The gastrointestinal toxicity produced by flavopiridol was characterized by clinical signs (emesis, diarrhea, anorexia) and histopathologic lesions (necrosis, hemorrhage, congestion) in the large and small intestines. Significant myelotoxicity occurred in rats and in dogs administered flavopiridol and was characterized by thrombocytopenia, leukopenia, and reticulocytopenia as well as bone marrow lesions (cellular depletion). The low toxic dose in dogs was determined to be 26 mg/m^2/d, and 38 mg/m^2/d was at or near the MTD. In rats, the MTD was 18 mg/m^2/d given tid $\times$ 3 (Table 12).

Since myelotoxicity occurred *in vivo* in preclinical animal models, the toxicity of flavopiridol was assessed in an *in vitro* bone marrow assay using CFU-GM isolated from mouse, dog, and human bone marrow. The IC$_{90}$ values after a continuous drug exposure were 770, 63, and 300 nM in murine, canine, and human CFU-GM cells, respectively. The *in vitro* bone marrow toxicity data indicated that canine cells were fivefold more sensitive and murine cells were 2.5-fold less sensitive than human cells. *In vivo*, the rat and dog were 3-fold and 1.5-fold more sensitive to flavopiridol toxicity than were humans (Table 12).

5. Human Clinical Trials Data

The phase I clinical trial was initiated to determine the MTD, toxicity profile, and pharmacokinetics of flavopiridol given as a 72-h CIV infusion (Senderowicz *et al.*, 1998; Thomas *et al.*, 1998). The MTD was 40–50 mg/m^2/d of flavopiridol, with dose-limiting diarrhea occurring at higher doses. The gastrointestinal toxicity was described as a secretory diarrhea with anorexia, diarrhea, nausea, and vomiting. Upon dose escalation with diarrheal prophylactic treatment, hypotension and hyperbilirubinemia were observed.

TABLE 12
Flavopiridol (NSC-649890): Summary of *in Vitro* Bone Marrow Toxicity Data and *in Vivo* MTDs

| Species | CFU$_{GM}$ inhibitory concentrations (nM, continuous exposure) | | | Animal MTD total dose (mg/m^2) |
	IC$_{50}$	IC$_{75}$	IC$_{90}$	72 h CIV
Mouse	270	520	770	NP
Rat	NP	NP	NP	54
Dog	13.3	36.4	66.8	114
Human	5.1	63.4	316	120–150

NP, not performed.

The pharmacokinetic parameters from this phase I trial were as follows: beta half-life 696 min (78–1746 min), total clearance 287 ml/min/m^2 (192–455 mL/min/m^2), steady-state plasma concentration 271 nM (174–2943 nM), and $V_{D\,SS}$ 131.2 L/m^2 (24.3–516.7 L/m^2). A phase II trial conducted with 50 mg/m^2/d (72-h CIV) reported peak plasma concentrations of 374 nM (Werner *et al.*, 1988).

6. Predictability of Preclinical Animal Models

The preclinical animal models were very useful in providing data for the clinical experience of flavopiridol. The dog was most predictive in terms of predicting the human MTD and DLT found in the phase I study. A similar gastrointestinal toxicity that occurred in cancer patients at the MTD was present in dogs along with histopathologic lesions (necrosis, hemorrhage, and congestion) in the large and small intestines. The *in vitro* bone marrow toxicity assays were employed since bone marrow toxicity was observed in dogs and rats. However, the predictive usefulness of comparing the *in vitro* bone marrow assay results to the *in vivo* toxicity results is limited, because little myelotoxicity occurred during the clinical trials.

5. Predictability of Nonclinical Animal Data

When the term *predictability* is used in the context of animal data predicting for human outcomes in clinical trials, it can mean many things to many investigators depending on their perspective. One obvious narrow meaning is that the animal data predict a safe starting dose. While this is a commendable start, it may be too narrow considering the time and financial investment made in animal studies prior to the initiation of a first-in-man trial. In this context, the NCI also hopes to be able to predict the human MTD and DLTs with some high degree of precision. The obvious question is, is

this possible given the differences between the various species in terms of metabolic rate, size, clearance rates, and the like? The qualified answer is yes. Numerous studies in the past have shown that animal studies can predict safe starting doses and DLTs in humans (Freireich *et al.*, 1966; Goldsmith *et al.*, 1975; Grieshaber and Marsoni, 1986; Guarino, 1977; Guarino *et al.*, 1979; Homan, 1972; Schein *et al.*, 1970; Rozensweig *et al.*, 1981) and these have been reviewed in numerous other publications.

More recently, in an effort to show that the usual methods for choosing the phase I starting dose are overly conservative, Penta (1992) reported that the ratio of the clinical MTD to the starting dose was a median of 20 for 45 antitumor drugs that had undergone phase I trials during the period from 1977 to 1989. Only one of these drugs, fludarabine, started at a dose that exceeded the MTD. Had the NCI bone marrow data been available for this drug prior to the initiation of the clinical trial, a safe starting dose could have been selected. Penta also indicated that if the starting dose were tripled for these drugs only four of them would have exceeded the MTD. He advocates the use of the pharmacokinetically guided dose escalation strategy as proposed by Collins and co-workers (1986, 1987) and a careful determination of the mouse LD$_{10}$ on which to base the starting dose. While this is a reasonable goal, he then points to the work of Guarino *et al.* (1979) that stresses that the mouse LD$_{10}$ can vary by as much as 100% depending on the strain, route, and formulation used. While a system in which the number of dose escalation steps is minimized is preferable, it should not come at the risk of safety for the cancer patient receiving the drug for the first time.

At a recent NCI-EORTC new drug symposium, a number of investigators reported on similar studies in an effort to establish new guidelines for phase I trial design and execution (Arbuck, 1996; Dent and Eisenhauer, 1996; Verweij, 1996). Dent and Eisenhauer reported on 46 phase I trials that were conducted between 1993 and 1995. There were two groups of drugs: one that started trials based on preclinical toxicology data (27 trials with 17 new agents) and a second group of 19 trials that were repeat trials of 14 agents. For the first group of 11 trials, the starting dose was selected as one-tenth of the mouse LD$_{10}$, and was a fraction less than this for 14 other trials, 12 of which were due to greater sensitivity of the dog. The latter studies involved six new agents. There were sufficient data to evaluate four of these agents, and the conclusion was that the lower starting dose based on the dog was warranted in three of four of the agents since use of one-tenth of the mouse LD$_{10}$ to determine the starting dose would have resulted in significant toxicity or the human MTD being exceeded.

The results, reported by Verweij and further summarized in a workshop report by Arbuck, identified 71 antitumor agents with sufficient data to extract preclinical toxicology data and phase I results. Verweij, in comparing the starting dose with the human MTD, indicated that the MTD in humans should exceed the LD_{10} in the mouse by a factor of at least 2 since safety is the primary consideration in a phase I trial. For the 57 drugs where 0.1 $MELD_{10}$ was used as the SD, the human MTD/mouse LD_{10} ratio was about 1 in 2% of cases and about 5 in the remaining 98%. For the other 14 drugs where the more sensitive species was used to set the SD, the use of 0.1 $MELD_{10}$ as the SD would have produced a ratio of about 1 in 7% of the drugs and about 2 in 14% of the drugs. The conclusion from this evaluation was that a second species (rat or dog) was required to select a safe starting dose. These results were consistent with the results of an NCI study with 20 drug/schedules (Smith *et al.*, 1994), which indicated that by using two or three species (mouse, rat and dog), the data alone provided a safe SD 97% of the time, but the use of mouse data provided a safe SD in only 83% of cases.

In the most recent study on cancer agents, the Cancer Research Campaign (CRC) recently reported (Newell *et al.*, 1999) that by using their rodent only toxicology protocols (Joint Steering Committee of the EORTC and CRC, 1990; Burtles *et al.*, 1995) they were able to determine safe starting doses for the 25 compounds studied. In fact, if one-tenth of the mouse MTD/LD_{10} (expressed as mg/m^2) had been used in all cases, it would have been safe. The study schedules used in the animal studies were either Dx1 or Dx5, and the initial schedule in man was the same in 22 of 25, while the other three were similar. The authors caution that the results may not be applicable to newer classes of agents that act by novel mechanisms since the majority in the current study were conventional cytotoxic drugs. In the case of predicting the human maximum administered dose (MAD), the mouse was able to quantitatively (within a factor of 2) predict this dose in 12 of 25 drugs (human MAD/mouse MTD/LD_{10} = 0–2). The ratio was as high as 16 for the other 13 drugs.

A. Pharmacokinetics

The prediction of human pharmacokinetic parameters through interspecics scaling has generally utilized allometric or physiologic approaches (Mordenti, 1986). The utility of simple allometric correlations/predictions has been shown useful for designing Phase I trials of anticancer drugs (Paxton, 1995). However, differential metabolism is a major factor in limiting the predictiveness of preclinical models for human pharmacokinetics and toxicity. CPEC, as described earlier in this chapter, is an excellent example of a drug in which differential metabolism by the various species made it nearly impossible to predict the outcome in patients. While CPEU is readily formed in man due to the action of cytidine deaminase and to a much greater extent in non-human primates, it is not formed at all in the mouse, rat or dog, species used for efficacy and toxicity studies. Thus, clearance in man does not correlate with any of the preclinical species used

even though an attempt was made to create a suitable pharmacokinetic model (Zaharko *et al.*, 1991). In spite of this fact, the steady state plasma level of CPEC in man at the clinical MTD was comparable to that determined in the dog.

One practical consideration to take into account during the usual development paradigm for antitumor agents is that the ability to make allometric correlations may be limited by availability of pharmacokinetic data for a sufficient number of species. When one combines this with other limitations, such as the use of dissimilar doses, routes, schedules, etc, making accurate predictions of human pharmacokinetics is even more problematic.

With regard to predicting human toxicity, the mouse studies in the CRC study predicted the human DLT in 11 of 22 drugs in which DLTs were determined. Newell *et al.* (1999) indicated that only one toxicity—hepatotoxicity—was not predicted in the case of didox, since the other human DLTs were not evaluable in murine studies. Thus, due to the limitations of the murine model, only 50% of the human DLTs were or could be predicted. In addition to DLTs, 78 non-DLT human toxicities were described for these drugs. The mouse predicted 32% of these toxicities, with about 16% not being predicted and more than 51% not being evaluable in the mouse. This obviously limits the utility of the mouse in predicting human toxicities.

In a recent evaluation of the concordance of human and animal toxicity data of pharmaceuticals, a multinational pharmaceutical company survey reported data on 150 compounds across all therapeutic types (Olson *et al.*, 1998, 2000). For the 221 human toxic events reported, the rate of true positive concordance for rodent and nonrodent species was 71% with nonrodents (primarily dogs), showing a higher concordance (63%) than rodents (primarily the rat) alone (43%). When the total incidence of usage was compared, the nonrodent species of dog and primate had a higher frequency of positive concordance (about 70% for both species) than did rodents (about 50% for rats and only about 9% for mice). When the type of toxicity was evaluated, the best concordance was seen with hematologic, gastrointestinal, and cardiovascular toxicities, which is remarkably similar to what Owens reported in 1963 for cancer drugs. Finally, of the 15 therapeutic areas evaluated in this study, the highest concordance of animal and human data was seen for antitumor agents and cardiovascular drugs.

With regard to the NCI drug development examples presented in this chapter, the remaining paragraphs describe the predictability of the preclinical pharmacology and toxicology studies for these drugs. The toxicology results are summarized for MTDs and DLTs in the various species in Table 13.

B. Toxicology

With regard to starting dose, the toxicology studies for all seven drugs discussed individually in this chapter predicted a

TABLE 13
Correlation of Clinical and Preclinical MTDs and DLTs

Drug	Drug type	Schedule	MTD (mg/m^2), total dose				DLT			
			Ms	Rat	Dog	Man	Ms	Rat	Dog	Man
9-AC	Topoisomerase I Inhibitor	72 h CIV	{60}SC	8.3	3.6	3.3	{GI}SC	GI, BM	GI, BM	GI, BM
Bizelesin[a]	Bifunctional alkylating agent	Dx1, IV	30	45	2	1.26	BM	BM	BM	BM
CPEC	CTP synthase inhibitor	Dx1, IV	240	>420	200	NS	(BM)	ND	(BM)	NS
		24 h CIV	NS	NS	120	112.8	NS	NS	BM & stomatitis	BM & hypotension
Depsipeptide	HDAC inhibitor	4 h CIV	32.4	18	60	35.6–39.9	Local	BM	GI, local	BM, GI, cardiac
Dolastatin 10[a]	Tubulin inhibitor	Dx1, IV	1.35	0.45	<0.4	0.3–0.4	BM	BM, GI	BM	BM
Flavopiridol	CDK inhibitor	*tid*, Dx3, IV	NS	54	NS	NS	NS	GI, BM	NS	NS
		72 h CIV	NS	<54	114	120–150	NS	GI, BM	GI, BM	GI

[a]Doses are in g/kg; NA = Not Assessed; ND = Not Determined; NP = Not Predicted; NS = No Study; BM = Myelosuppression; GI = Gastrointestinal Toxicity.

safe starting dose when the most sensitive species was used as the basis for dose selection. If one relied on mouse data alone, then the SD would have been toxic in two of five drugs for which mouse data were available. In one of those cases, bizelesin, even the rat would not have predicted a safe starting dose. One would have had to rely on previous clinical experience with two other analogues, adozelesin and carzelesin, to select an appropriate starting dose for bizelesin had the dog data not been available. For both of these compounds, one-thirtieth or lower of the mouse equivalent LD$_{10}$ was used as the SD (Awada *et al.,* 1999; Burris *et al.,* 1997). In terms of predicting the human MTD, the dog did an excellent job in predicting the MTD for five of six of the drugs, with the mouse being most accurate only for the sixth (depsipeptide), although the MTDs for this drug in all three animal species were very close (within a factor of 3.3). The human/dog MTD ratio ranged from 0.6 to 1.3 for the seven drugs, while the human-to-rat ratio was 0.36–35.7 and the human-to-mouse ratio was 0.9–23.8, indicating that the dog data for this limited dataset was more precise than either the mouse or the rat.

In terms of dose escalation in the clinic, if only mouse and rat data were available for these compounds, and the starting dose was 0.1 of the MTD for the most sensitive species, and the conventional Fibonacci dose escalation scheme were utilized, three of the trials would have been safe with 6, 9, and 10 dose levels, while the other three would have been marginal with 4 dose levels apiece. The fourth dose level for each would have exceeded the ultimately determined human MTD in each case.

In relation to the prediction of human DLT, the mouse predicted 5 of 9 (56%), the rat 7 of 11 (64%), and the dog 10 of 11 (91%) of the observed human DLTs. The only toxicity not

predicted by dog was the hypotension produced by CPEC, as discussed earlier. This toxicity was also not predicted by mouse or rat. Thus, all three species failed to predict this critical human DLT.

This dataset reinforces the conclusions of a number of previous investigators that two species are required to define a safe SD for the initiation of human clinical trials with antitumor agents and that 10% of the MTD in the most sensitive species should be used to set the SD. The animal toxicity data, especially that generated by the dog, appears to be reasonably predictive of human DLTs.

C. *In Vitro* Bone Marrow Data

The NCI has been utilizing *in vitro* bone marrow data to assist in starting dose selection and prediction of human sensitivity to myelosuppressive drugs for the past 10 years. In the case of the seven drugs being evaluated here, six of seven produced myelosuppression in one or more species, although it was dose limiting in humans in only five of those drugs. The canine data accurately predicted human sensitivity for three of five drugs, while the murine data accurately predicted only one and human sensitivity was midway between mouse and dog for the last drug. The most important point to be obtained from this limited dataset is that the *in vitro* data accurately predicted the rank order of human sensitivity versus animal sensitivity in all cases. One final point is that the murine cells were particularly insensitive to the toxic effects of three of the drugs being evaluated and, if combined with mouse toxicity data, would have led to the selection of toxic starting doses. The canine and human bone marrow sensitivity to these drugs reinforced the selection of dog as the species most likely to mimic human sensitivity, which is what occurred clinically. These results and their implications and those from other drugs are discussed in greater detail in a recent study (Schweikart *et al.*, unpublished data).

6. Conclusions

The results of the NCI studies described here using agent-directed techniques for the pharmacologic and toxicologic evaluation of antitumor agents in preclinical animal models are impressive in their prediction of human MTDs and DLTs. Does this mean that we have turned the corner and can adopt these techniques for the evaluation of all antitumor agents? The answer is a qualified yes. While we were able to predict the MTD and DLTs of a number of these compounds with high accuracy, including the MTD of CPEC and the DLT of myelosuppression for this drug, we failed to detect in any animal models the refractory hypotension that CPEC produced that resulted in the death of two patients. This is exactly the type of result that we are trying to guard against and why we should attempt to obtain as complete a pharmacology and toxicology dataset as possible. This is especially true today with the advent of more aggressive clinical trial dose escalation schemes being put into practice (Eisenhauer *et al.*, 2000).

References

Agbaria, R., Ford, H. Jr., Kelley, J. A., Koester, A., Moore, V., Hassler, C. R., Tomaszewski, J. E., and Donohue, S. J. (1994). Continuous infusion of cyclopentenyl cytosine (NSC-375575) in beagle dogs with hemodynamic and pharmacologic monitoring. *Proc. Am. Assoc. Cancer Res.* **35**, 461.

Aherne, G. W., Hardcastle, A., Valenti, M., Bryant, A., Rogers, P., Pettit, G. R., Srirangam, J. K., and Kelland, L. R. (1996). Antitumour evaluation of dolastatins 10 and 15 and their measurement in plasma by radioimmunoassay. *Cancer Chemother. Pharmacol.* **38**, 225–232.

Arbuck, S. G. (1996). Workshop on phase I study design. Ninth NCI/EORTC New Drug Development Symposium, Amsterdam, March 12, 1996. *Ann. Oncol.* **7**, 567–573.

Arguello, F., Alexander, M., Sterry, J. A., Tudor, G., Smith, E. M., Kalaver, N. T., Greene, J. F., Koss, W., Morgan, C. D., Stinson, S. F., Siford, T. J., Alvord, W. G., Klabansky, R. L., and Sausville, E. A. (1998). Flavopiridol induces apoptosis of normal lymphoid cells, causes immunosuppression, and has potent antitumor activity *in vivo* against human leukemia and lymphoma xenografts. *Blood* **91**, 2482–2490.

Arita, M., Adachi, K., Sawai, H., and Ohno, M. (1983). Enantioselective synthesis of new analogues of neplanosin A. *Nucleic Acids Symp. Ser.* **12**, 25–30.

Arneson, D., Evans, E., Kovatch, R., Moore, R., Morton, T., Tomaszewski, J., and Smith, A. C. (1995). Preclinical toxicology and pharmacology of flavopiridol (NSC-649890) in rats and dogs. *Proc. Am. Assoc. Cancer Res.* **36**, 366.

Awada, A., Punt, C. J., Piccart, M. J., Van Tellingen, O., Van Manen, L., Kerger, J., Groot, Y., Wanders, J., Verweij, J., and Wagener, D. J. (1999). Phase I study of carzelesin (U-80,244) given (4-weekly) by intravenous bolus schedule. *Br. J. Cancer* **79**, 1454–1461.

Bai, R., Pettit, G. R., and Hamel, E. (1990a). Dolastatin 10, a powerful cytostatic peptide derived from a marine animal. Inhibition of tubulin polymerization mediated through the vinca alkaloid binding domain. *Biochem. Pharmacol.* **39**, 1941–1949.

Bai, R., Pettit, G. R., and Hamel, E. (1990b). Binding of dolastatin 10 to tubulin at a distinct site for peptide antimitotic agents near the exchangeable nucleotide and vinca alkaloid sites. *J. Biol. Chem.* **265**, 17141–17149.

Bates, S. E., Sandor, V., Bakke, S., Chico, I., Tucker, E., Robey, R., Sackett, D., Chan, K., Kang, M., Figg, W. D., Sausville, E., Balcerzak, S., and Fojo, T. (1999). A phase I study of FR901228 (depsipeptide), a histone deacetylase inhibitor. *Proc. Am. Soc. Clin. Oncol.* **18**, A693.

Beckwith, M., Urba, W. J., and Longo, D. L. (1993). Growth inhibition of human lymphoma cell lines by the marine products dolastatins 10 and 15. *J. Natl. Cancer Inst.* **85**, 483–488.

Blaney, S. M., Balis, F. M., Hegedus, L., Heideman, R. L., McCully, C., Murphy, R. F., Kelley, J. A., and Poplack, D. G. (1990). Pharmacokinetics and metabolism of cyclopentenyl cytosine in nonhuman primates. *Cancer Res.* **50**(24), 7915–7919.

Blaney, S. M., Takimoto, C., Murry, D. J., Kuttesch, N., McCully, C., Cole, D. E., Godwin, K., and Balis, F. M. (1998). Plasma and cerebrospinal fluid pharmacokinetics of 9-aminocamptothecin (9-AC), irinotecan (CPT-11), and SN-38 in nonhuman primates. *Cancer Chemother. Pharmacol.* **41**, 464–468.

Bradner, W. T., and Schurig, J. E. (1981). Toxicology screening in small animals. *Cancer Treatment Reviews* **8**, 92–102.

Bradner, W. T., Schurig, J. E., Huftalen, J. B., and Doyle, G. J. (1980). Evaluation of antitumor drug side effects in small animals. *Cancer Chemother. Pharmacol.* **4**, 95–101.

Burke, T. G., and Mi, Z. (1993). Preferential binding of the carboxylate form of camptothecin by human serum albumin. *Anal. Biochem.* **212**, 285–287.

Burke, T. G., Munshi, C. B., Mi, Z., and Jiang, Y. (1995). The important role of albumin in determining the relative human blood stabilities of the camptothecin anticancer drugs. *J. Pharm. Sci.* **84**, 518–519.

Burris, H. A., Dieras, V. C., Tunca, M., Earhart, R. H., Eckardt, J. R., Rodriguez, G. I., Shaffer, D. S., Fields, S. M., Campbell, E., Schaaf, L., Kasunic, D., and Von Hoff, D. D. (1997). Phase I study with the DNA sequence-specific agent adozelesin. *Anticancer Drugs* **8**, 588–596.

Burtles, S. S., Newell, D. R., Henrar, R. E., and Connors, T. A. (1995). Revisions of general guidelines for the preclinical toxicology of new cytotoxic anticancer agents in Europe. The Cancer Research Campaign (CRC) Phase I/II Clinical Trials Committee and the European Organization for Research and Treatment of Cancer (EORTC) New Drug Development Office. *Eur. J. Cancer* **31A**, 408–410.

Byrd, J. C., Shinn, C., Ravi, R., Willis, C. R., Waselenko, J. K., Flinn, I. W., Dawson, N. A., and Grever, M. R. (1999). Depsipeptide (FR901228): A novel therapeutic agent with selective, *in vitro* activity against human B-cell chronic lymphocytic leukemia cells. *Blood* **94**, 1401–1408.

Cancer Chemotherapy National Service Center (CCNSC) (1964). An outline of procedures for preliminary toxicologic and pharmacologic evaluation of experimental cancer chemotherapeutic agents. *Cancer Chemother. Rep.* **37**, 3–17.

Cancer Chemotherapy National Service Center (CCNSC) (1959). Specifications for preliminary toxicological evaluation of experimental cancer chemotherapeutic agents. *Cancer Chemother. Rep.* **1**, 89–98.

Cancer Chemotherapy National Service Center (CCNSC) (1960). An outline of procedures for preliminary toxicologic and pharmacologic evaluation of experimental cancer chemotherapeutic agents. *Cancer Chemother. Rep.* **9**, 120–139.

Carlson, B. A., Dubay, M. M., Sausville, E. A., Brizuela, L., and Worland, P. J. (1996). Flavopiridol induces G_1 arrest with inhibition of cyclin-dependent kinase (CDK) 2 and CDK4 in human breast carcinoma cells. *Cancer Res.* **56**, 2973–2978.

Carter, C. A., Waud, W. R., Li, L. H., DeKoning, T. F., McGovren, J. P., and Plowman, J. (1996). Preclinical antitumor activity of bizelesin in mice. *Clin. Cancer Res.* **2,** 1143–1149.

Carter, S. K., Selawry, O., and Slavik, M. (1977). Phase I clinical trials. *Natl. Cancer Inst. Monogr.* **45,** 49–55.

Carter, S. K., Bakowski, M. T., and Hellman, K. (1981). "Chemotherapy of Cancer." John Wiley and Sons, New York.

Chan, K. K., Bakhtiar, R., and Jiang, C. (1997). Depsipeptide (FR901288, NSC-630176) pharmacokinetics in the rat by LC/MS/MS. *Invest. New Drugs* **15,** 195–206.

Chassaing, C., Marshall, J. L., and Wainer, I. W. (1998). Determination of the antitumor agent depsipeptide in plasma by liquid chromatography on serial octadecyl stationary phases. *J. Chromatog.* B **719,** 169–176.

Cherkofsky, S. C. (1995). 1-Aminocyclopropanecarboxylic acid: Mouse to man interspecies pharmacokinetic comparisons and allometric relationships. *J. Pharm. Sci.* **84,** 1231–1235.

Collins, J. M. (1988). Pharmacology of drug development. *J. Natl. Cancer Inst.* **80,** 790–792.

Collins, J. M., Zaharko, D. S., Dedrick, R. L., and Chabner, B. A. (1986). Potential roles for preclinical pharmacology in Phase I clinical trials. *Cancer Treat. Rep.* **70,** 73–80.

Collins, J. M., Leyland-Jones, B., and Grieshaber, C. K. (1987). Role of preclinical pharmacology in Phase I clinical trials: considerations of schedule-dependence. *In* "Concepts, Clinical Developments, and Therapeutic Advances in Cancer Chemotherapy" (F. M. Muggia, ed.), pp. 129–140. Martinus Nijhoff Publishers, Boston.

Collins, J. M., Grieshaber, C. K., and Chabner, B. A. (1990). Pharmacologically guided Phase I clinical trials based upon preclinical drug development. *J. Natl. Cancer Inst.* **82,** 1321–1326.

Dahut, W., Harold, N., Takimoto, C., Allegra, C., Chen, A., Hamilton, J. M., Arbuck, S., Sorensen, M., Grollman, F., Nakashima, H., Lieberman, R., Liang, M., Corse, W., and Grem, J. (1996). Phase I and pharmacologic study of 9-aminocamptothecin given by 72-hour infusion in adult cancer patients. *J. Clin. Oncol.* **14,** 1236–1244.

DeGeorge, J. J., Ahn, C., Andrews, P. A., Brower, M. E., Giorgio, D. W., Goheer, M. A., Lee-Ham, D. Y., McGuinn, W. D., Schmidt, W., Sun, C. J., and Tripathi, S. C. (1998). Regulatory considerations for preclinical development of anticancer drugs. *Cancer Chemother. Pharmacol.* **41,** 173–185.

Dent, S. F., and Eisenhauer, E. A. (1996). Phase I trial design: are new methodologies being put into practice? *Ann. Oncol.* **7,** 561–566.

Ding, Z. M., and Hurley, L. H. (1991). DNA interstrand cross-linking, DNA sequence specificity, and induced conformational changes produced by a dimeric analog of (+)-CC-1065. *Anticancer Drug Des.* **6,** 427–452.

Dixit, R., Lopez, R., Douglas, T., Fanska, C., Stoltz, M., Arneson, D., Stedham, M., Smith, A. C., and Tomaszewski, J. E. (1992). The intravenous infusion toxicity of 9-amino-20[S]-camptothecin (9-AC, NSC-603071) in Beagle dogs. *Proc. Am. Assoc. Cancer Res.* **33,** 548.

Dixit, R., Lopez, R., Muellner, P., Mowry, B., Fanska, C., Morton, T., Arneson, D., Stedham, M., Smith, A., Osborn, B., and Tomaszewski, J. E. (1993). A species comparison of toxicity and pharmacokinetics of 9-amino-20[S]-camptothecin in rodents and dogs. *Proc. Am. Assoc. Cancer Res.* **34,** 428.

Dobbins, D., Kelly, J., Allegra, C., and Grem, J. (1997). Intravenous infusion of cyclopentenyl-cytosine (CPE-C) in the canine markedly inhibits the response to bilateral carotid occlusion. *FASEB J.* **11,** 291.

Dorr, R. T., and Fritz, W. L. (1980). "Cancer Chemotherapy Handbook." Elsevier/North-Holland, New York.

Drees, M., Dengler, W. A., Roth, T., Labonte, H., Mayo, J., Malspeis, L., Grever, M., Sausville, E. A., and Fiebig, H. H. (1997). Flavopiridol (L86-8275): Selective antitumor activity *in vitro* and activity *in vivo* for prostate carcinoma cells. *Clin. Cancer Res.* **3,** 273–279.

Du, D. L., Volpe, D. A., Grieshaber, C. K., and Murphy, M. J. Jr. (1990a).

In vitro myelotoxicity of 2′,3′-dideoxynucleosides on human hematopoietic progenitor cells. *Exp. Hematol.* **18,** 832–836.

Du, D. L., Volpe, D. A., Grieshaber, C. K., and Murphy, M. J. Jr. (1990b). Effects of L-phenylalanine mustard and L-buthionine sulfoximine on murine and human hematopoetic progenitor cells *in vitro. Cancer Res.* **50,** 4038–4043.

Du, D. L., Volpe, D. A., Grieshaber, C. K., and Murphy, M. J. Jr. (1991). Comparative toxicity of fostriecin, hepsulfam and pyrazine diazohydroxide to human and murine hematopoietic progenitor cells *in vitro. Invest. New Drugs* **9,** 149–157.

Du, D. L., Volpe, D. A., Grieshaber, C. K., and Murphy, M. J. Jr. (1992). *In vitro* toxicity of 3′-azido-3′-deoxythymidine, carbovir, and 2′,3′-didehydro-2′3′-dideoxythymidine to human and murine haematopoietic progenitor cells. *Br. J. Haematol.* **80,** 437–445.

Eisenhauer, E. A., O'Dwyer, P. J., Christian, M., and Humphrey, J. S. (2000). Phase I clinical trial design in cancer drug development. *J. Clin. Oncol.* **18,** 684–692.

El-hawari, M., Evans, E., Pletcher, J., Morton, T., Bradley, S., Tomaszewski, J. E., and Smith, A. C. (1997). Bioavailability and preclinical toxicology orally administered flavopiridol (NSC-649890) in rats. *Proc. Am. Assoc. Cancer Res.* **38,** 598.

Erickson-Miller, C. L., May, R. D., Tomaszewski, J., Osborn, B., Murphy, M. J., Page, J. G., and Parchment, R. E. (1997). Differential toxicity of camptothecin, topotecan and 9-aminocamptothecin to human, canine, and murine myeloid progenitors (CFU-GM) *in vitro. Cancer Chemother. Pharmacol.* **39,** 467–472.

Evans, E., Kovatch, R., Lopez, R., Baker, J., Mowry, B., Smith, D., Arneson, D., Gatz, R., McDermott, M., and Tomaszewski, J. E. (1994). Five daily dose toxicity of bizelesin (NSC-615291) in Fischer 344 rats and Beagle dogs. *Proc. Am. Assoc. Cancer Res.* **35,** 461.

Evans, S. M., Hahn, S., Pook, D. R., Jenkins, W. T., Chalian, A. A., Zhang, P., Stevens, C., Weber, R., Weinstein, G., Benjamin, I., Mirza, N., Morgan, M., Rubin, S., McKenna, W. G., Lord, E. M., and Koch, C. J. (2000). Detection of hypoxia in human squamous cell carcinoma by EF5 binding. *Cancer Res.* **60,** 2018–2024.

Food and Drug Administration (1995). "Content and Format of Investigational New Drug Applications (INDs) for Phase I Studies of Drugs, Including Well-Characterized, Therapeutic, Biotechnology-derived Products." Center for Drug Evaluation and Research, Rockville, MD.

Food and Drug Administration (1996). Good laboratory practice for nonclinical laboratory studies 21 CFR Part 58, 265.

Ford, H., Jr, Cooney, D. A., Ahluwalia, G. S., Hao, Z., Rommel, M. E., Hicks, L., Dobyns, K. A., Tomaszewski, J. E., and Johns, D. G. (1991) Cellular pharmacology of cyclopentenyl cytosine in Molt-4 lymphoblasts. *Cancer Res.* **51,** 3733–3740.

Freireich, E. J, Gehan, E. A., Rall, D. P., Schmidt, L. H., and Skipper, H. E. (1966). Quantitative comparison of toxicity of anticancer agents in mouse, rat, hamster, dog, monkey, and man. *Cancer Chemother. Rep.* **50,** 219–244.

Garteiz, D. A., Madden, T., Beck, D. E., Huie, W. R., McManus, K. T., Abbruzzese, J. L., Chen, W., and Newman, R. A. (1998). Quantitation of dolastatin-10 using HPLC/electrospray ionization mass spectrometry: application in a phase I clinical trial. *Cancer Chemother. Pharmacol.* **41,** 299–306.

Giovanella, B. C., Stehlin, J. S., Wall, M. E., Wani, M. C., Nicholas, A. W., Liu, L. F., Silber, R., and Potmesil, M. (1989). DNA topoisomerase I—targeted chemotherapy of human colon cancer in xenografts. *Science* **246,** 1046–1048.

Glazer, R. I., Knode, M. C., Lim, M. I., and Marquez, V. E. (1985). Cyclopentenyl cytidine analogue. An inhibitor of cytidine triphosphate synthesis in human colon carcinoma cells. *Biochem. Pharmacol.* **34,** 2535–2539.

Glazer, R. I., Cohen, M. B., Hartman, K. D., Knode, M. C., Lim, M. I., and

Marquez, V. E. (1986). Induction of differentiation in the human promyelocytic leukemia cell line HL-60 by the cyclopentenyl analogue of cytidine. *Biochem. Pharmacol.* **35,** 1841–1848.

Goldsmith, M. A., Slavik, M., and Carter, S. K. (1975). Quantitative prediction of drug toxicity in humans from toxicology in small and large animals. *Cancer Res.* **35,** 1354–1364.

Grever, M. R., and Grieshaber, C. K. (1993). Toxicology by organ system. *In* "Cancer Medicine" (J. F. Holland *et al.,* eds.), 3rd ed., pp. 683–697. Lea and Febiger, Philadelphia.

Grieshaber, C. K. (1991). Predictions of human toxicity from animal studies. *In* "The Toxicity of Anticancer Drugs" (G. Powis and M. Hacker, eds.), pp. 10–27. Pergamon Press, New York.

Grieshaber, C. K. (1992). Agent-directed preclinical toxicology for new antineoplastic drugs. *In* "Cytotoxic Anticancer Drugs: Models and Concepts for Drug Discovery and Development" (F. A. Valeriote, T. H. Corbett, and L. H. Baker, eds.), pp. 247–260. Kluwer Academic Publishers, Boston.

Grieshaber, C. K., and Marsoni, S. (1986). Relation of preclinical toxicology to findings in early clinical trials. *Cancer Treat. Rep.* **70,** 65–72.

Guarino, A. M. (1977). Toxicology of anticancer drugs. *Natl. Cancer Inst. Monogr.* **45,** 49–55.

Guarino, A. M., Rozencweig, M., Kline, I., Penta, J. S., Venditti, J. M., Lloyd, H. H., Holzworth, D. A., and Muggia, F. M. (1979). Adequacies and inadequacies in assessing murine toxicity data with antineoplastic agents. *Cancer Res.* **39**(1), 2204–2210.

Hanka, L. J., Dietz, A., Gerpheide, S. A., Kuentzel, S. L., and Martin, D. G. (1978). CC-1065 (NSC-298223), a new antibiotic. Production *in vitro* biological activity, microbiological assay and taxonomy of the producing microorganisms. *J. Antibiot. (Tokyo)* **31,** 1211.

Hegedus, L., Ford, H. Jr, Hartman, N. R., and Kelley, J. A. (1997). Reversed-phase high-performance liquid chromatographic determination of the new antitumor agent cyclopentenyl cytosine in biological fluids. *J. Chromatogr. B Biomed. Sci. Appl.* **692,** 169–179.

Hightower, R. D., Sevin, B. U., Perras, J., Nguyen, H., Angioli, R., Untch, M., and Averette, H. (1993). In vitro evaluation of the novel chemotherapeutic agents U-73,975, U-77,779, and U-80,244 in gynecologic cancer cell lines. *Cancer Invest.* **11,** 276–282.

Hill, D. L., Noker, P. E., Coyne, J. M., Smith, A. C., Tomaszewski, J. E., Newman, R. A., and Page, J. G. (1998). Toxicity and pharmacokinetics of EF5 (NSC 684681) in dogs dosed by intravenous infusion. *Proc. Am. Assoc. Cancer Res.* **39,** 521.

Homan, E. R. (1972). Quantitative relationships between toxic doses of antitumor chemotherapeutic agents in animals and man. *Cancer Chemother. Rep.* Part 3, **3,** 13–19.

Hsiang, Y. H., and Liu, L. F. (1988). Identification of mammalian DNA topoisomerase I as an intracellular target of the anticancer drug camptothecin. *Cancer Res.* **48,** 1722–1726.

Hsiang, Y. H., Hertzberg, R., Hecht, S., and Liu, L. F. (1985). Camptothecin induces protein-linked DNA breaks via mammalian DNA topoisomerase I. *J. Biol. Chem.* **260,** 14873–14878.

Hsiang, Y. H., Liu, L. F., Wall, M. E., Wani, M. C., Nicholas, A. W., Manikumar, G., Kirschenbaum, S., Silber, R., and Potmesil, M. (1989). DNA topoisomerase I-mediated DNA cleavage and cytotoxicity of camptothecin analogues. *Cancer Res.* **49,** 4385–4389.

Huang, M., Parchment, R. E., Tomaszewski, J. E., and Murphy, M. J., Jr. (1991). Standardization of murine CFU-GM assays for preclinical evaluation of myelotoxicity of anti-HIV and anticancer agents. *J. Am. Soc. Hematol. Blood* **78**(Suppl 1), 418a.

Huie, W. R., Newman, R. A., Hutto, T., and Madden, T. (1997). High-performance capillary electrophoresis measurement of dolastatin-10. *Chromatography B* **693,** 451–461.

Huie, W. R., and Wong, S. S. (1999). Improvement in assay sensitivity for plasma dolastatin-10 using capillary electrophoresis at elevated temperatures. *J. Chromatogr. B* **729,** 1–10.

Hurley, L. H., Warpehoski, M. A., Lee, C. S., McGovern, J. P., Scahill, T. A., Kelly, R. C., Mitchell, M. A., Wicnienski, N. A., Gebhard, I., Jihnson, P. D., and Bradford, V. S. (1990). Sequence specificity of DNA alkylation by the unnatural enantiomer of CC-1065 and its synthetic analogs. *J. Am. Chem. Soc.* **112,** 4633–4649.

Jacobsen, S. E. W., Ruscetti F. W., Longo D. L., and Keller, J. R. (1991). Antineoplastic dolastatins: potent inhibitors of hematopoietic progenitor cells. *J. Natl. Cancer Inst.* **83,** 1672–1677.

Jager, W., Zembsch, B., Wolschann, P., Pittenauer, E., Senderowicz, A. M., Sausville, E. A., Sedlacek, H. H., Graf, J., and Thalhammer, T. (1998). Metabolism of the anticancer drug Flavopiridol, a new inhibitor of cyclin dependent kinases, in rat liver. *Life Sci.* **62,** 1861–1873.

Joint Steering Committee of the EORTC and CRC. (1990). General guidelines for the preclinical toxicology of new cytotoxic anticancer agents in Europe. *Eur. J. Cancer* **26,** 411–414.

Kalemkerian, G. P., Ou, X., Adil, M. R., Rosati, R., Khoulani, M. M., Madan, S. K., and Pettit, G. R. (1999). Activity of dolastatin 10 against small-cell lung cancer in vitro and in vivo: induction of apoptosis and bcl-2 modification. *Cancer Chemother. Pharmacol.* **43,** 507–515.

Kang, G. J., Cooney, D. A., Moyer, J. D., Kelley, J. A., Kim, H. Y., Marquez, V. E., and Johns, D. G. (1989). Cyclopentenylcytosine triphosphate. Formation and inhibition of CTP synthetase. *J. Biol. Chem.* **264,** 713–718.

Kang, M. H., Li, Z., Chan, K. K., Sandor, V., Bakke, S., Tucker, E., Balcerzak, S., Bender, J., Peng, L., Fojo, T., Figg, W. D., and Bates, S. E. (1999). A preliminary pharmacokinetic evaluation of intravenous FR901228 (depsipeptide) given over 4 hours. *Clin. Cancer Res.* **5** (Suppl), 113.

Koch, C. J., Evans, S. M., and Lord, E. M. (1995). Oxygen dependence of cellular uptake of EF5 [2-(2-nitro-1H-imidazol-1-yl)-*N*-(2,2,3,3,3-pentafluoropropyl)acetamide]: analysis of drug adducts by fluorescent antibodies vs bound radioactivity. *Br. J. Cancer* **72,** 869–874.

Koch, C. J., Hahn, S. M., Rockwell, K., Covey, J., McKenna, W. G., and Evans, S. M. (2000). Pharmacokinetics of EF5 [2-(2-nitro-1H-imidazol-1-yl)-*N*-(2,2,3,3,3-pentafluoropropyl)acetamide] in human patients: Implications for hypoxia measurements *in vivo* by 2-nitroimidazoles. *Cancer Chemother. Pharmacol.,* in press.

Kraut, E. H., Balcerzak, S. P., Young, D., O'Rourke, M. A., Petrus, J. J., Kuebler, J. P., and Mayernik, D. G. (2000). A phase II study of 9-aminocamptothecin in patients with refractory breast cancer. *Cancer Invest.* **18**(1), 28–31.

Krug, L. M., Miller, V. A., Kalemkerian, G. P., Kraut, M. J., Ng, K. K., Heelan, R. T., Pizzo, B. A., Perez, W., McClean, N., and Kris, M. G. (2000). Phase II study of dolastatin-10 in patients with advanced non-small-cell lung cancer. *Ann. Oncol.* **11,** 227–228.

Laughlin, K. M., Evans, S. M., Jenkins, W. T., Tracy, M., Chan, C. Y., Lord, E. M., and Koch, C. J. (1996). Biodistribution of the nitroimidazole EF5 (2-[2-nitro-1H-imidazol-1-yl]-N-(2,2,3,3,3-penta-fluoropropyl)acetamide] in mice bearing subcutaneous EMT6 tumors. *J. Pharmacol. Exp. Ther.* **277,** 1049–1047.

Leyland-Jones, B., and Grieshaber, C. K. (1999). Of (only) mice and men. *Br. J. Cancer* **81,** 753–755.

Li, Z., and Chan, K. K. (2000). A subnanogram API LC/MS/MS quantitation method for depsipeptide FR901228 and its preclinical pharmacokinetics. *J. Pharm. Biomed. Anal.* **22,** 33–44.

Lim, M. L., Moyer, J. D., Cysyk, R. L., and Marquez, V. E. (1984). Cyclopentenyluridine and cyclopentenylcytidine analogues as inhibitiors of uridine-cytidine kinase. *J. Med. Chem.* **27,** 1536–1538.

Lowe, M. C. (1987). Large animal toxicological studies of anticancer drugs. *In* "Fundamentals of Cancer Chemotherapy" (K. Hellman and S. Carter, eds.), Chapter 24, pp. 236–247. McGraw Hill, New York.

Lowe, M. C., and Davis, R. D. (1987). The current toxicology protocol of the National Cancer Institute. *In* "Fundamentals of Cancer Chemotherapy" (K. Hellman and S. Carter, eds.), Chapter 24, pp. 228–235. McGraw Hill, New York.

Madden, T., Hai, T. T., Beck, D., Huie, R., Newman, R. A., Pusztai, L., Wright, J. J., and Abbruzzese, J. L. (2000). Novel marine-derived anticancer agents: A phase I clinical, pharmacological, and pharmacodynamic study of dolastatin 10 (NSC 376128) in patients with advanced solid tumors. *Clin. Cancer. Res.* **6,** 1293–1301.

Maki A, Mohammad, R., Raza, S., Saleh, M., Govindaraju, K. D., Pettit, G. R., and Al-Katib, A. (1996). Effect of dolastatin 10 on human non-Hodgkin's lymphoma cell lines. *Anticancer Drugs* **7,** 344–350.

Marquez, V. E., Lim, M. I., Treanor, S. P., Plowman, J., Priest, M. A., Markovac, A., Khan, M. S., Kaskar, B., and Driscoll, J. S. (1988). Cyclopentenylcytosine. A carbocyclic nucleoside with antitumor and antiviral properties. *J. Med. Chem.* **31,** 1687–1694.

Marshall, J. L., Dahut, W. L., Rizvi, N., Wainer, I. W., Chassaing, C., Figuiera, M., and Hawkins, M. J. (1998). Phase I trial and pharmacokinetic (PK) analysis of depsipeptide in patients with advanced cancer. *Proc. Am. Soc. Clin. Oncol.* **18,** A893.

Mattern, M. R., Hofmann, G. A., Polsky, R. M., Funk, L. R., McCabe, F. L., and Johnson, R. K. (1993). In vitro and in vivo effects of clinically important camptothecin analogues on multidrug-resistant cells. *Oncol. Res.* **5,** 467–474.

May, R. D., Murphy, M. J., Jr., Parchment, R. E., Huang, M., Osborn, B. L., Tomaszewski, J. E., and Page, J. G. (1992). Toxicity evaluation of developmental anticancer/anti-HIV compounds to mouse and human bone marrow progenitor cells. *Proc. Am. Assoc. Cancer Res.* **33,** 550.

May, R. D., Murphy, M. J. Jr., Erickson-Miller, C. L., Parchment, R. E., Page, J. G., Osborn, B. L., and Tomaszewski, J. E. (1993a). Myelotoxicity evaluation of two potential anticancer compounds using murine and human *in vitro* CFU-GM assays. *Proc. Am. Assoc. Cancer Res.* **34,** 383.

May, R. D., Murphy, M. J. Jr., Erickson-Miller, C. L., Parchment, R. E., Page, J. G., Osborn, B. L., and Tomaszewski, J. E. (1993b). Myelotoxicity evaluation of camptothecin and its derivatives using *in vitro* CFU-GM assays in mouse, dog, and human. *Proc. Am. Assoc. Cancer Res.* **34,** 428.

May, R. D., Murphy, M. J. Jr., Erickson-Miller, C. L., Tomaszewski, J. E., Osborn, B. L., and Page, J. G. (1994). Myelotoxicity evaluation of dolastatin 10 (NSC-376128) and swainsonine (NSC-614553) using murine, canine and human *in vitro* CFU$_{GM}$ assays. *Proc. Am. Assoc. Cancer Res.* **35,** 402.

McGovren, J. P., Clarke, G. L., and Pratt, E. A. (1984). Preliminary toxicity studies with the DNA-binding antibiotic, CC-1065. *J. Antibiot. (Tokyo),* **37,** 63–70.

Mertins, S. D., Robey, R., Sandor, V., Rao, V. K., Robbins, A., Sackett, D., and Bates, S. E. (1999). Development of depsipeptide FR901228, a histone deacetylase inhibitor, as an anticancer agent. *Proc. Am. Assoc. Cancer Res.* **40,** 623.

Mi, Z., and Burke, T. G. (1994a). Differential interactions of camptothecin lactone and carboxylate forms with human blood components. *Biochemistry* **33,** 10325–10336.

Mi, Z., and Burke, T. G. (1994b). Marked interspecies variations concerning the interactions of camptothecin with serum albumins: a frequency-domain fluorescence spectroscopic study. *Biochemistry* **33,** 12540–12545.

Minami, H., Lad, T. E., Nicholas, M. K., Vokes, E. E., and Ratain, M. J. (1999). Pharmacokinetics and pharmacodynamics of 9-aminocamptothecin infused over 72 hours in phase II studies. *Clin. Cancer Res.* **5,** 1325–1330.

Mirsalis, J. C., Schindler-Horvat, J., Hill, J. R., Tomaszewski, J. E., Donohue, S. J., and Tyson, C. A. (1999). Toxicity of dolastatin 10 in mice, rats and dogs and its clinical relevance. *Cancer Chemother. Pharmacol.* **44,** 395–402.

Mordenti, J. (1986). Man versus beast: Pharmacokinetic scaling in mammals. *J. Pharm. Sci.* **75,** 1028–1040.

Moyer, J. D., Oliver, J. T., and Handschumacher R. E. (1981). Salvage of circulating pyrimidine nucleosides in the rat. *Cancer Res.* **41,** 3010–3017.

Moyer, J. D., Malinowski, N. M., Treanor, S. P., and Marquez, V. E. (1986). Antitumor activity and biochemical effects of cyclopentenyl cytosine in mice. *Cancer Res.* **46,** 3325–3329.

Nakajima, H., Kim, Y. B., Terano, H. Yoshide, M., and Horinouchi, S. (1998). FR901228, a potent antitumor antibiotic, is a novel histone deacetylase inhibitor. *Exp. Cell Res.* **241,** 126–133.

Newell, D. R. (1990). Phase I clinical studies with cytotoxic drugs: pharmacokinetic and pharmacodynamic considerations. *Br. J. Cancer* **61,** 189–191.

Newell, D. R., Burtles, S. S., Fox, B. W., Jodrell, D. I., and Connors, T. A. (1999). Evaluation of rodent-only toxicology for early clinical trials with novel cancer therapeutics. *Br. J. Cancer* **81,** 760–768.

Newman, R. A., Fuentes, A., Covey, J. M., and Benvenuto, J. A. (1994). Preclinical pharmacology of the natural marine product dolastatin 10 (NSC 376128). *Drug Metab. Disp.* **22,** 428–432.

Olson, H., Betton, G., Stritar, J., and Robinson, D. (1998). The predictivity of the toxicity of pharmaceuticals in humans from animal data—an interim assessment. *Toxicol. Lett.* **102–103,** 535–538.

Olson, H., Betton, G., Robinson, D., Thomas, K., Monro, A., Kolaja, G., Lilly, P., Sanders, J., Sipes, G., Bracken, W., Durato, M., Van Deun, K., Smith, P., Burger, B., and Heller, A. (2000). Concordance of the toxicity of pharmaceuticals in humans and in animals. *Reg. Toxicol. Pharmacol.* **32,** 56–67.

Owens, A. H. (1963). Predicting anticancer drug effects in man from laboratory animal studies. *J. Chron. Dis.* **15,** 223–228.

Page, J. G., Heath, J. E., Tomaszewski, J. E., and Grieshaber, C. K. (1990). Toxicity and pharmacokinetics of cyclopentenylcytosine (CPEC, NSC-375575) in Beagle dogs. *Proc. Am. Assoc. Cancer Res.* **31,** 442.

Page, J. G., Heath, J. E., Sparks, R. M., Kelley, J. A., and Tomaszewski, J. E. (1991). Preclinical toxicology studies of cyclopentenylcytosine (CPEC; NSC-375575) given by continuous intravenous infusion to Beagle dogs. *Proc. Am. Assoc. Cancer Res.* **32,** 423.

Page, J. G., Rodman, L. E., Heath, J. E., Tomaszewski, J. E., and Smith, A. C. (1995). Effect of infusion rate on the toxicity of depsipeptide (NSC-630176) in Beagle dogs. *Proc. Am. Assoc. Cancer Res.* **36,** 368.

Page, J. G., Rodman, L. E., Heath, J. E., Tomaszewski, J. E., and Smith, A. C. (1996). Comparison of the toxicity of depsipeptide (NSC-630176) in dogs and rats. *Proc. Am. Assoc. Cancer Res.* **36,** 42.

Pantazis, P., Hinz, H. R., Mendoza, J. T., Kozielski, A. J., Williams, L. J. Jr., Stehlin, J. S. Jr., and Giovanella, B. C. (1992). Complete inhibition of growth followed by death of human malignant melanoma cells *in vitro* and regression of human melanoma xenografts in immunodeficient mice induced by camptothecins. *Cancer Res.* **52,** 3980–3987.

Pantazis, P., Kozielski, A. J., Vardeman, D. M., Petry, E. R., and Giovanella, B. C. (1993a). Efficacy of camptothecin congeners in the treatment of human breast carcinoma xenografts. *Oncol. Res.* **5,** 273–281.

Pantazis, P., Kozielski, A. J., Mendoza, J. T., Early, J. A., Hinz, H. R., and Giovanella, B. C. (1993b). Camptothecin derivatives induce regression of human ovarian carcinomas grown in nude mice and distinguish between non-tumorigenic and tumorigenic cells *in vitro*. *Int. J. Cancer* **53,** 863–871.

Parchment, R. E., Huang, M., Tomaszewski, J. E., and Murphy, M. J., Jr. (1992). Murine CFU-GM assays are optimized for preclinical myelotoxicity evaluation of new anti-HIV and anti-cancer drugs. 7th NCI-EORTC Symposium on New Drugs in Cancer Therapy, Amsterdam.

Parchment, R. E., Huang, M., and Erickson-Miller, C. L. (1993). Roles for *in vitro* myelotoxicity tests in preclinical drug development and clinical trial planning. *Toxicol. Pathol.* **21,** 241–250.

Parchment, R. E., Volpe, D. A., LoRusso, P. M., Erickson-Miller, C. L., Murphy, M. J. Jr, and Grieshaber, C. K. (1994). *In vivo-in vitro* correlation of myelotoxicity of 9-methoxypyrazoloacridine (NSC-366140, PD115934) to myeloid and erythroid hematopoietic progenitors from human, murine, and canine marrow. *J. Natl. Cancer Inst.* **86,** 273–280.

Parker, B. W., Kaur, G., Nieves-Neira, W., Taimi, M., Kohlhagen, G., Shimizu, T., Losiewicz, M. D., Pommier, Y., Sausville, E. A., and Senderowicz, A. M. (1998). Early induction of apoptosis in hematopoietic cell lines after exposure to flavopiridol. *Blood* **91,** 458–465.

Patel, V., Senderowicz, A. M., Pinto, D., Igishi, T., Raffeld, M., Quintanilla-Martinez, L., Ensley, J. F., Sausville, E. A., and Gutkind, J. S. (1998). Flavopiridol, a novel cyclin-dependent kinase inhibitor, suppresses the growth of head and neck squamous cell carcinomas by inducing apoptosis. *J. Clinical Invest.* **102,** 1674–1681.

Paxton, J. W. (1995). The allometric approach for interspecies scaling of pharmacokinetics and toxicity of anti-cancer drugs. *Clin. Exp. Pharmacol. Physiol.* **22,** 851–854.

Pazdur, R., Diaz-Canton, E., Ballard, W. P., Bradof, J. E., Graham, S., Arbuck, S. G., Abbruzzese, J. L., and Winn, R. (1997). Phase II trial of 9-aminocamptothecin administered as a 72-hour continuous infusion in metastatic colorectal carcinoma. *J. Clin. Oncol.* **15,** 2905–2909.

Penta, J. S., Rosner, G. L., and Trump, D. L. (1992). Choice of starting dose and escalation for phase I studies of antitumor agents. *Cancer Chemother. Pharmacol.* **31,** 247–250.

Pettit, G. R., Kamano, Y., Herald, C. L., Tuinman, A. A., Boettner, F. E., Kizu, H., Schmidt, J. M., Baczynskyi, L., Tomer, K. B., and Bontems, R. J. (1987). The isolation and structure of a remarkable marine animal antineoplastic constituent: dolastatin 10. *J. Am. Chem. Soc.* **109,** 6883–6885.

Pinkel, D. (1956). The use of body surface area as a criterion of drug dosage in cancer chemotherapy. *Cancer Res.* **18,** 853–856.

Pitot, H. C., McElroy, E. A., Jr., Reid, J. M., Windebank, A. J., Sloan, J. A., Erlichman, C., Bagniewski, P. G., Walker, D. L., Rubin, J., Goldberg, R. M., Adjei, A. A., and Ames, M. M. (1999). Phase I trial of dolastatin-10 (NSC 376128) in patients with advanced solid tumors. *Clin. Cancer Res.* **5,** 525–531.

Pitot, H. C. IV, Erlichman, C., Reid, J. M., Sloan, J. A., Ames, M. M., Bagniewski, P. G., Atherton-Skaff, P., Adjei, A. A., Rubin, J., Rayson, D., and Goldberg, R. M. (1999). A phase I study of bizelesin (NSC615291) in solid tumors. *Proc. Am. Assoc. Cancer Res.* **40,** 91–92.

Plowman, J., Dykes, D. J., Hollingshead, M., Simpson-Herren, L., and Alley, M. C. (1997). Human tumor xenograft models in NCI Drug Development. *In* "Anticancer Drug Development Guide: Preclinical Screening, Clinical Trials, and Approval" (B. Teicher, ed.), p. 119. Humana Press, Totowa, NJ.

Politi, P. M., Xie, F., Dahut, W., Ford, H. Jr, Kelley, J. A., Bastian, A., Setser, A., Allegra, C. J., Chen, A. P., and Hamilton, J. M. L. (1995). Phase I clinical trial of continuous infusion cyclopentenyl cytosine. *Cancer Chemother. Pharmacol.* **36,** 513–523.

Poncet, J. (1999). The dolastatins, a family of promising antineoplastic agents. *Curr. Pharm. Design* **5,** 139–162.

Potmesil, M., Giovanella, B. C., Liu, L. F., Wall, M. E., Silber, R., Stehlin, J. S., Hsiang, Y-H., and Wani, M. C. (1991). Preclinical studies of DNA topoisomerase I-targeted 9-amino and 10,11-methylenedioxycamptothecin. *In* "DNA Topoisomerases in Cancer" (M. Potmesil and K. W. Kohn, eds.), Chapter 23, pp. 299–311. Oxford University Press, New York.

Potmesil, M., Giovanella, B. C., Wall, M. E., Liu, L. F., Silber, R., Stehlin, J. S., Wani, M. C., and Hochster, H. (1993). Preclinical and clinical development of DNA topoisomerase—I inhibitors in the United States, *In* "Molecular Biology of DNA Topoisomerases and Its Application to Chemotherapy" (T. Andoh, H. Ikeda, and M. Oguro, eds.), Chapter 29, pp. 301–311. CRC Press, Nagoya, Japan.

Prieur, D. J., Young, D. M., Davis, R. D., Cooney, D. A., Homan, E. R., Dixon, R. L., and Guarino, A. M. (1973). Procedures for preclinical toxicologic evaluation of cancer chemotherapeutic agents: Protocols of the Laboratory of Toxicology. *Cancer Chemother. Rep.* Part 3, **4,** 1–30.

Prieur, D. J., Young, D. M., Davis, R. D., Cooney, D. A., and Guarino, A. M. (1977). Preclinical toxicology protocols of the Laboratory of Toxicology. *Natl. Cancer Inst. Monogr.* **45,** 159–177.

Rajgolikar, G., Chan, K. K., and Wang, H.-C. R. (1998). Effects of a novel antitumor depsipeptide, FR901228, on human breast cancer cells. *Breast Cancer Res. Treat.* **51,** 29–38.

Reid, J. M., Walker, D. L., and Ames, M. M. (1995). Evaluation of an L1210

bioassay and HPLC for determination of dolastatin 10 in human and murine plasma. *Proc. Am. Assoc. Cancer Res.* **36,** 364.

Reynolds, V. L., McGovren, J. P., and Hurley, I. H. (1986). The chemistry, mechanism of action, and biological properties of CC-1065, a potent antitumor antibiotic. *J. Antibiot.* (**Tokyo**), **39,** 319–334.

Rodman, L. E., Giles, H. D., Thompson, R. B., Coffey, L. B., Page, J. G., Osborn, B. L., and Tomaszewski, J. E. (1993). Dose range-finding study of bizelesin (NSC-615291) in beagle dogs. *Proc. Am. Assoc. Cancer Res.* **34,** 429.

Rozencweig, M., Von Hoff, D. D., Staquet, M. J., Schein, P. S., and Penta, J. S. (1981). Animal toxicology for early clinical trials with anticancer agents. *Cancer Clin. Trials* **4,** 21–28.

Rubin, E., Wood, V., Bharti, A., Trites, D., Lynch, C., Hurwitz, S., Bartel, S., Levy, S., Rosowsky, A., and Toppmeyer, D. (1995). A phase I and pharmacokinetic study of a new camptothecin derivative, 9-aminocamptothecin. *Clin. Cancer Res.* **1,** 269–276.

Sackett, D. L., Bates, S. E., and Robbins, A. R. (1999). Histone deacetylase inhibitors induce mitotic arrest in human cancer cells, disrupting kinetochores and centrosomes. *Proc. Am. Assoc. Cancer Res.* **40,** 623.

Saltz, L. B., Kemeny, N. E., Tong, W., Harrison, J., Berkery, R., and Kelsen, D. P. (1997). 9-Aminocamptothecin by 72-hour continuous intravenous infusion is inactive in the treatment of patients with 5-fluorouracil-refractory colorectal carcinoma. *Cancer* **80,** 1727–1732.

Sandor, V., Senderowicz, A., Sackett, D., Sausville, E., and Bates, S. E. (1998). Depsipeptide cause G1 cell cycle arrest through disruption of signal transduction through MAP kinase. *Proc. Am. Assoc. Cancer Res.* **39,** A3812.

Schein, P., and Anderson, T. (1973). The efficacy of animal studies on predicting clinical toxicity of cancer chemotherapeutic drugs. *Int. J. Clin. Pharmacol.* **8,** 228–238.

Schein, P. S. (1977). Preclinical toxicology of anticancer agents. *Cancer Res.* **37,** 1934–1937.

Schein, P. S., Davis, R. D., Carter, S., Newman, J., Schein, D. R., and Rall, D. P. (1970). The evaluation of anticancer drugs in dogs and monkeys for the prediction of qualitative toxicities in man. *Clin. Pharmacol. Ther.* **11,** 3–40.

Scheithauer, W., Clark, G. M., Salmon, S. E., Dorda, W., Shoemaker, R. H., and Von Hoff, D. D. (1986). Model for estimation of clinically achievable plasma concentrations for investigational anticancer drugs in man. *Cancer Treat. Rep.* **70,** 1379–1382.

Schurig, J. E., Schlein, A., Florczyk, A. P., Farwell, A. R., and Bradner, W. T. (1985). Animal models for evaluating the myelosuppressive effects of cancer chemotherapeutic agents. *Exp. Hematol.* **13**(Suppl. 16), 101–105.

Schurig, J. E., and Bradner, W. T. (1987). Small animal toxicology of cancer drugs. *In* "Fundamentals of Cancer Chemotherapy" (K. Hellman and S. Carter, eds.), Chapter 26, pp. 248–261. McGraw Hill, New York.

Schurig, J. E., Florczyk, A. P., and Bradner, W. T. (1986). The mouse as a model for predicting the myelosuppressive effects of anticancer drugs. *Cancer Chemother. Pharmacol.* **16,** 243–246.

Schwartz, H. G., Aylesworth, C., Stephenson, J., Johnson, T., Campbell, E., Hammond, L., Von Hoff, D. D., and Rowinsky, E. K. (2000). Phase I trial of bizelesin using a single bolus infusion given every 28 days in patients with advanced cancer. *Proc. Am. Soc. Clin. Oncol.* **19,** 235a.

Schweikart, K. M., Parchment, R., Osborn, B., Murphy, M., May, R., Page, J., and Tomaszewski, J. E. (1995). *In vitro/in vivo* bone marrow toxicity: comparison of clinical and preclinical data for selected anticancer drugs. *Proc. Am. Assoc. Cancer Res.* **36,** 367.

Sedlacek, H. H., Czech, J., Naik, R., Kaur, G., Worland, P. Losiewicz, M., Parker, B., Carlson, B., Smith, A., Senderowicz, A., and Sausville, E. (1996). Flavopiridol (L86 8275; NSC 649890), a new kinase inhibitor for tumor therapy. *Int. J. Oncol.* **9,** 1143–1168.

Senderowicz, A. M., Headlee, D., Stinson, S. F., Lush, R. M., Kalil, N., Villalba, L., Hill, K., Steinberg, S. M., Figg, W. D., Tompkins, A., Arbuck, S. G., and Sausville, E. A. (1998). Phase I trial of continuous infusion flavopiridol, a novel cyclin-dependent kinase inhibitor, in patients with refractory neoplasms. *J. Clin. Oncol.* **16**, 2986–2999.

Shigematsu, N., Ueda, H., Takase, S., and Tanaka, H. (1994). FR901228, a novel antitumor bicyclic depsipeptide produced by *Chromobacterium violaceum* No. 968. II. Stucture determination. *J. Antibiot.* **47**, 311–314.

Smith, A. C., Rubinstein, L., Koutsoukos, A., Christian, M., Grieshaber, C. K., Tomaszewski, J. E., and Grever, M. R. (1994). Evaluation of preclinical toxicity models for phase I clinical trials of anticancer drugs. *Proc. Am. Assoc. Cancer Res.* **35**, 459.

Smith, C. G., Poutsiaka, J. W., and Schreiber, E. C. (1973). Problems in predicting drug effects across species lines. *J. Int. Med. Res.* **1**, 489–503.

Supko, J. G., and Malspeis, L. (1993). Pharmacokinetics of the 9-amino and 10,11- methylenedioxy derivatives of camptothecin in mice. *Cancer Res.* **53**, 3062–3069.

Supko, J. G., Plowman, J., Dykes, D. J., and Zaharko, D. S. (1992). Relationship between the schedule of 9-amino-20(S)-camptothecin (AC; NSC 603071) antitumor activity in mice and its plasma pharmacokinetics. *Proc. Am. Assoc. Cancer Res.* **33**, 432.

Takimoto, C. H., Klecker, R. W., Dahut, W. L., Yee, L. K., Strong, J. M., Allegra, C. J., and Grem, J. L. (1994). Analysis of the active lactone form of 9-aminocamptothecin in plasma using solid-phase extraction and high-performance liquid chromatography. *J. Chromatogr. B Biomed. Appl.* **655**, 97–104.

Takimoto, C. H., Dahut, W., Harold, N., Nakashima, H., Lieberman, R., Liang, M. D., Arbuck, S. G., Chen, A. P., Hamilton, J. M., Cantilena, L. R., Allegra, C. J., and Grem, J. L. (1996). Clinical pharmacology of 9-aminocamptothecin. *Ann. NY Acad. Sci.* **803**, 324–326.

Takimoto, C. H., Dahut, W., Marino, M. T., Nakashima, H., Liang, M. D., Harold, N., Lieberman, R., Arbuck, S. G., Band, R. A., Chen, A. P., Hamilton, J. M., Cantilena, L. R., Allegra, C. J., and Grem, J. L. (1997). Pharmacodynamics and pharmacokinetics of a 72-hour infusion of 9-aminocamptothecin in adult cancer patients. *J. Clin. Oncol.* **15**, 1492–1501.

Thomas, J., Tutsch, K., Arzoomanian, R., Alberti, D., Simon, K., Feierabend, C., Morgan, K., Wahamaki, A., Wilding, G., and Cleary, J. (1998). Phase I clinical and pharmacokinetic trial of the cyclin-dependent kinase (CDK) inhibitor flavopiridol. *Proc. Am. Soc. Clin. Oncol.* **17**, A804.

Tomaszewski, J. E., and Smith, A. C. (1997). Safety testing of antitumor agents. *In* "Comprehensive Toxicology, Toxicity Testing and Evaluation" (P. D. Williams and G. H. Hottendorf, eds.), Vol. 2, pp. 299–309. Elsevier Science, Oxford, England.

Tomaszewski, J. E., Heath, H. E., Grieshaber, C. K., and Page, J. G. (1990). Toxicity of Cyclopentenylcytosine (CPEC, NSC-375575) in CD_2F_1 Mice and Fischer-344 Rats. *Proc. Am. Assoc. Cancer Res.* **31**, 441.

Tomaszewski, J. E., Schweikart, K. M., and Parchment, R. E. (1997). Correlation of clinical and preclinical bone marrow toxicity data for selected anticancer drugs. First International Symposium on Hematotoxicology in New Drug Development, Lugano, Switzerland.

Tomaszewski, J. E., Schweikart, K. M., and Parchment, R. E. (1999). Correlation of clinical and preclinical bone marrow toxicity data for selected anticancer drugs. Presented at the *In Vitro Human Tissue Models in Risk Assessment Workshop of the Society of Toxicology* in Ellicot City, MD, September 20, 1999.

Ueda, H., Nakajima, H., Hori, Y., Fujita, T., Nishimura, M., Goto, T., and Okuhara, M. (1994a). FR901228, a novel antitumor bicyclic depsipeptide produced by *Chromobacterium violaceum* No. 968. I. Taxonomy, fermentation, isolation, physico-chemical and biological properties, and antitumor activity. *J. Antibiot.* **47**, 301–310.

Ueda, H., Nakajima, H., Hori, Y. Goto, T., and Okuhara, M. (1994b). Action of FR901228, a novel antitumor bicyclic depsipeptide produced by *Chromobacterium violaceum* No. 968, on Ha-*ras* transformed NIH3T3 cells. *Biosci. Biotechnol. Biochem.* **58**, 1579–1583.

Ueda, H., Manda, T., Matsumoto, S., Mukumoto, S., Nishigaki, F., Kawamur, I., and Shimomura, K. (1994c). FR901228, a novel antitumor bicyclic depsipeptide produced by *Chromobacterium violaceum* No. 968. III. Antitumor activities on experimental tumors in mice. *J. Antibiot.* **47**, 315–323.

Verdier-Pinard, P., Kepler, J. A., Pettit, G. R., and Hamel, E. (2000). Sustained intracellular retention of dolastatin 10 causes its potent antimitotic activity. *Mol. Pharmacol.* **57**, 180–187.

Verweij, J. (1996). Starting dose levels for phase I studies. Proceedings of the 9TH NCI-EORTC Symposium on New Drugs in Cancer Therapy, Amsterdam, 13 (Abstr.).

Volpe, D. A., Du, D. L., Grieshaber, C. K., and Murphy, M. J. Jr. (1994). *In vitro* characterization of the myelotoxicity of cyclopentenyl cytosine. *Cancer Chemother. Pharmacol.* **34**, 103–108.

Volpe, D. A., Du, D. L., Zurlo, M. G., Mongelli, N., and Murphy, M. J. (1992). Comparative *in vitro* myelotoxicity of FCE 24517, a distamycin derivative, to human, canine and murine hematopoietic progenitor cells. *Invest. New Drugs* **10**, 255–261.

Volpe, D. A., Tomaszewski, J. E., Parchment, R. E., Garg, A., Flora, K. P., Murphy, M. J., and Grieshaber, C. K. (1995). Myelotoxic effects of bizelesin to human, canine and murine myeloid progenitor cells. *Proc. Am. Assoc. Cancer Res.* **36**, 366.

Volpe, D. A., Tomaszewski, J. E., Parchment, R. E., Garg, A., Flora, K. P., Murphy, M. J., and Grieshaber, C. K. (1996). Myelotoxic effects of the bifunctional alkylating agent bizelesin on human, canine and murine myeloid progenitor cells. *Cancer Chemother. Pharmacol.* **39**, 143–149.

Walker, D. L., Reid, J. M., and Ames, M. M. (1994). Preclinical pharmacology of bizelesin, a potent bifunctional analog of the DNA-binding antibiotic CC-1065. *Cancer Chemother. Pharmacol.* **34**, 317–322.

Wani, M. C., Nicholas, A. W., and Wall, M. E. (1986). Plant antitumor agents. 23. Synthesis and antileukemic activity of camptothecin analogues. *J. Med. Chem.* **29**, 2358–2363.

Warpehoski, M. A. (1989). CC-1065 analogs: Therapeutic potential of a sequence specific drug-DNA reaction. *Proc. Am. Assoc. Cancer. Res.* **30**, 668.

Warpehoski, M. A. (1988). Stereoelectronic factors influencing the biological activity and DNA interaction of synthetic antitumor agents modeled on CC-1065. *J. Med. Chem.* **31**, 3.

Warpehoski, M. A., and Hurley, L. H. (1988). Sequence selectivity of DNA covalent modification. *Chem. Res. Toxicol.* **1**, 315.

Werner, J. L., Kelsen, D. P., Karpek, M., Inzeo, D., Barazzuol, J., Sugarman, A., and Schwartz, G. K. (1988). The cyclin-dependent kinase inhibitor flavopiridol is an active and unexpectedly toxic agent in advanced gastric cancer. *Proc. Am. Soc. Clin. Oncol.* **17**, A896.

Zaharko, D. S., Kelley, J. A., Tomaszewski, J. E., Hegedus, L., and Hartman, N. R. (1991). Cyclopentenyl cytosine: interspecies predictions based on rodent plasma and urine kinetics. *Invest. New Drugs* **9**, 9–17.

CLINICAL TRIAL DESIGN: INCORPORATION OF PHARMACOKINETIC, PHARMACODYNAMIC, AND PHARMACOGENETIC PRINCIPLES

Alex Sparreboom
Walter J. Loos
Maja J. A. de Jonge
Jaap Verweij
Department of Medical Oncology
Rotterdam Cancer Institute
Rotterdam, The Netherlands

Summary

The reason for studying the pharmacology of anticancer agents is that the generated information will result in more rational drug development and enhanced or improved clinical use. A great deal of effort has been spent in defining the pharmacokinetics and pharmacodynamics of investigational and non-investigational anticancer agents. There is often marked variability in drug handling between individual patients that contributes to variability in the pharmacodynamic effects of a given dose of a drug, i.e., an identical dose of drug may result in a therapeutic response with acceptable toxicity in one patient, and unacceptable and possibly life-threatening toxicity in another. A combination of physiologic variables, genetic characteristics (pharmacogenetics), and environmental factors is known to alter the relationship between the absolute dose and the concentration–time profile in plasma. Numerous studies have established relationships between systemic exposure measures to anticancer drugs and drug-induced toxicity or response. These relationships have subsequently been used to individualize chemotherapy dose administration either *a priori* or *a posteriori*, as in the case of carboplatin and methotrexate, respectively. A variety of strategies are now being evaluated to improve the therapeutic index of anticancer drugs by implementation of pharmacogenetic imprinting of geno- or phenotyping individual patients, the use of biomodulating agents, and modification of drug scheduling. Several of these strategies have been shown to have substantial impact on therapeutic outcome and should eventually lead to improved anticancer chemotherapy.

1. Introduction

During the last few decades, many drugs have become available for the treatment of a wide variety of neoplastic diseases. In addition, the whole field of anticancer drug discovery and development has changed substantially. Not only are we now dealing with highly innovative and distinct classes of molecules in terms of both mechanism of action and chemical structure, but we are also deploying an impressive array of new techniques and ideas. Moreover, our emerging understanding of the relationships between pharmacokinetics (the quantitative study of the concentration–time profile of the drug in the body, incorporating absorption, distribution, metabolism, and excretion) and pharmacodynamics (the quantitative study of the effects on the body, including both efficacy and toxicity) is encouraging a more systematic and rigorous analysis of the potential role of pharmacology in the day-to-day treatment of cancer patients (Canal *et al.,* 1998; Masson and Zamboni, 1998). It has become widely appreciated at the same time that the small therapeutic index (the ratio of the theoretical minimum effective dose to the maximum tolerated dose) of most anticancer drugs demands that a rigorous effort be made to optimize their regimens (Fig. 1). Indeed, effective systemic treatment for cancer requires the use of cytotoxic drugs with modest differences in their toxic effects on normal cells and their therapeutic, lethal effects on malignant cells. Exploiting this narrow therapeutic margin of anticancer agents has been a major challenge for oncologists, attacking the problem on a number of fronts, including the use of drug combinations with different dose-limiting toxicities, the rescue or reconstitution of normal tissues (e.g., administration of folinic acid following methotrexate administration, bone marrow transplantation, or the use of growth factors), and the use of biological modifiers to overcome specific mechanisms of cancer cell resistance (Grochow, 1998). In this chapter, we will review the principal causes of variability in the response to chemotherapeutic treatment, and discuss the implementation of pharmacokinetic, pharmacodynamic and/or pharmacogenetic principles in the design of clinical trials that allow tailor-made therapy for individual patients.

2. Rationale for Chemotherapy Optimization

The current concept that chemotherapeutic agents are administered at a dose to the maximum a patient can tolerate (before the onset of unacceptable toxicity) is in wide clinical

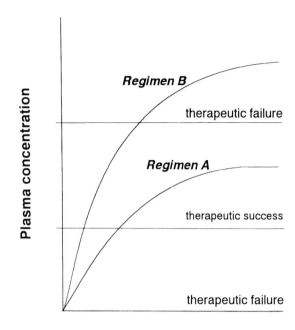

FIGURE 1   When a drug is given at a fixed dose and at fixed time intervals, it accumulates in the body until a plateau is reached. With regimen A, therapeutic success is achieved although not initially. With regimen B, the therapeutic objective is achieved more quickly, but the plasma concentration is ultimately too high.

use today. This approach is based on a series of retrospective analyses that indicated that the greater the dose intensity of an anticancer drug, the better the outcome (Hryniuk *et al.,* 1987; Hryniuk, 1988; Relling *et al.,* 1999a; Tannock *et al.,* 1988). However, as indicated, the therapeutic range for most anticancer agents is extremely narrow, and in most cases no information is available on the intrinsic sensitivity of a patient's tumor to a particular agent and the patient's tolerability of a given dose prior to therapy. Hence, the dosage of chemotherapeutic agents remains largely empirical and is basically derived from the kind of information shown in Fig. 2. Since the effect of a therapeutic agent in the body is generally a function of its concentration at the (molecular) site of action, it now appears obvious that a description of the spatiotemporal behavior of the drug in the body will be helpful, if not essential, in understanding and predicting normal tissue toxicity and optimizing tumor response. In view of the multiple factors that can cause drug concentrations to vary (Table 1), even after a fixed administered dose, it is clearly much more meaningful to have knowledge of drug exposure measures (usually expressed as the area under the concentration–time curve or AUC) rather than of absolute dose only (Workman and Graham, 1994). Ideally, this would be at the molecular locus of action or at least at the tissue or tumor level, but most commonly, drug concentrations must be measured in the plasma as a more readily accessible surrogate.

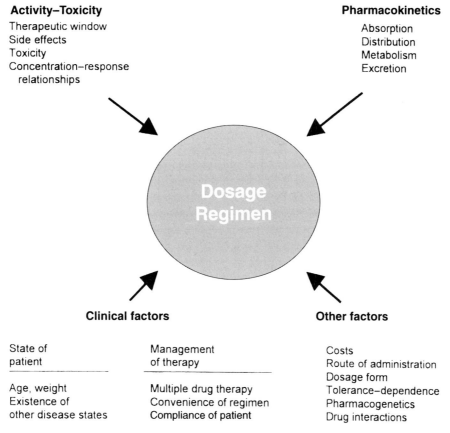

FIGURE 2 Determinants of a dosage regimen for an anticancer drug.

There is often a marked variability in drug handling between individual patients resulting in a variability in AUC and clearance (Fig. 3), which contributes to variability in the pharmacodynamic effects of a given dose of a drug, that is, an identical dose of drug may result in acceptable toxicity in one patient, and unacceptable and possibly life-threatening toxicity in another. A combination of physiologic variables, genetic characteristics, and environmental factors are known to alter the relationship between the absolute dose and the concentration–time profile in plasma. Indeed, the correlation between, for example, the AUC of a drug in plasma and the intensity of phar-macodynamic effects is commonly better than that between absolute dose and such effects (Masson and Zamboni, 1998). The definition of the relationships between the pharmacokinetic variables of a drug and the drug's pharmacodynamic end points may allow the administration of the optimal dosage of that drug in any given patient. The optimal dosage is in effect that dosage which maximizes the likelihood of response and simultaneously minimizes the likelihood of toxicity in a particular patient. In incidental cases it is possible to define the optimum dosage to achieve a required drug exposure measured *a priori* for an individual patient from measurable physiologic

TABLE 1
Factors Contributing to Variability in Drug Response

Parameter	Source of variability
Dose selection	Physician's preference; patient's condition (performance status)
Dose administration	Noncompliance; medication error; pharmaceutical formulation
Systemic exposure	Age; concomitant drugs; food effects; gender; route of administration; altered organ function; enzyme polymorphisms (pharmacogenetics)
Active site drug levels	Cellular uptake; intracellular activation; tumor sensitivity
Pharmacologic effect	Host sensitivity (e.g., previous treatments)

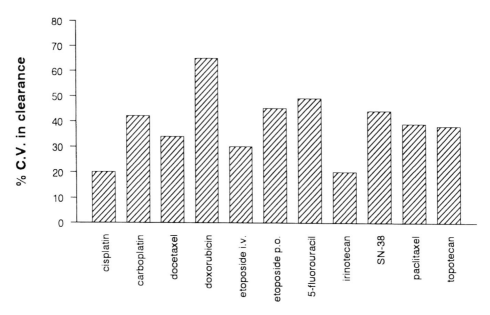

FIGURE 3 Variability in the plasma clearance of commonly used anticancer drugs with data expressed as the coefficient of variation (% CV).

variables, such as renal or hepatic function. However, in most cases, dose adjustments will be required in the light of pharmacokinetic or pharmacodynamic data obtained after an initial dose and also possibly subsequent doses of the drug in the individual patient.

3. Pharmacokinetic–Pharmacodynamic Relationships

A. Preclinical Development

In general, the preclinical data available before a candidate anticancer drug is entered into clinical trials include the *in vitro* cytotoxic activity in various animal and human tumor cell lines, and the *in vivo* antitumor activity in mouse tumor models or in human tumors xenografted in nude mice. In addition to these antitumor evaluations, toxicologic studies are conducted in a variety of species to determine the toxic doses (e.g., the lethal dose for 10% of the animals or murine LD_{10}) (Gouyette and Chabot, 1993). These *in vitro* evaluations clearly have value in defining target plasma drug concentrations, although direct extrapolation is often difficult because of oversimplification of these models, as usually no correction is applied for the lack of metabolic transformation (or any other form of drug elimination) and/or the presence of physiologic barriers. Nonetheless, these studies may guide the choice of administration schedules and starting dosage in phase I clinical trials. For example, in case cytotoxic activity is S-phase-specific, prolonged exposure may be required that would be better achieved using a prolonged intravenous infusion if that agent has a relatively short terminal half-life.

The preclinical data have also been shown to be of value in defining a therapeutic window to be reached in patients. Theoretically, it is possible to define two-dimensional plasma–concentration time windows, the lower limit (or threshold concentration) of which is associated with antitumor activity, and the upper (or toxic concentration) with an unacceptable degree of toxic side effects (Collins *et al.*, 1986). This approach is the basis of therapeutic drug monitoring, which is also widely used and accepted for numerous noncytotoxic drugs.

B. Clinical Development

1. Choice of Starting Dose

Historically, the empirical starting dose for anticancer agents is based on toxicologic studies in rodents (mice and rats) and dogs, and one tenth of the murine LD_{10} is often chosen for the first dose level to be used in patients because at this dose intolerable toxicity is rarely encountered (Mahmood and Balian, 1999). Based on theoretical considerations in addition to an extensive review of preclinical toxicologic studies from published data, it has been proposed that limited toxicologic models using mouse and rat data only can appropriately and safely be used for anticancer drug development (Eisenhauer *et al.*, 2000; Newell *et al.*, 1999). However, it is important to realize that, compared with patients, much higher plasma concentrations of experimental anticancer agents can generally be achieved in animals, which cannot always be explained by a proportionally higher drug clearance. Thus, when trying to extrapolate results from efficacy studies performed in tumor-bearing animals to the clinical situation, it should be taken into consideration that tumors are exposed to drug levels that can, in most cases, never be achieved in patients. Clearly, this is particularly relevant when the relationships between plasma levels and antitumor effects are poorly understood.

2. Dose Escalation Schemes

If the starting dose is not severely toxic in patients, further dose escalation is usually based on the modified Fibonacci sequence, in which escalating steps have decreasing relative increments (i.e., 100%, 67%, 50%, etc.). Each succeeding step is continued in cohorts of three patients until dose-limiting toxicity is reached. The major limitations of this standard design related to ethical considerations and efficiency have been reviewed (Eisenhauer *et al.,* 2000), and numerous alternative methodologies have been proposed. One of these approaches was designed to rationalize and accelerate dose escalation by making use of preclinical pharmacologic data (Collins *et al.,* 1990). This process of pharmacokinetically guided dose escalation assumes that for agents showing no major differences in target cell sensitivity, schedule dependency, or toxicity between animals and patients, the AUC at the murine LD_{10} and the AUC at the human maximum tolerated dose should be similar. This approach has proven useful in saving dose levels to be studied in trials of several agents over the past decade, including flavone acetic acid, hexamethylene bisacetamide, piroxantrone, and iododeoxydoxorubicin (Eisenhauer *et al.,* 2000), thereby reducing the number of patients exposed to theoretically subtherapeutic dosages of the drug involved. Other groups have advocated similar approaches to escalate systemic exposure measures (rather than dose) to determine the maximum tolerated systemic exposure and have used it in trials with topotecan, teniposide, carboplatin, and paclitaxel (Evans *et al.,* 1991; Woo *et al.,* 1999). Both concepts have evident value in reducing the number of patients required for the trials but have proven difficult to adopt in the clinical setting because of various pitfalls, including the assumption of linear pharmacokinetics between species, the substantial interpatient variability in results, as well as logistic issues of obtaining real-time data enabling subsequent escalation steps. Currently, there is clearly a need for more *in vitro* and *in vivo* preclinical pharmacologic studies to support the effort to rationalize the transition between animals and patients, which remains a difficult and hazardous task, and a somewhat empirical exercise. Because of this, even the most recently proposed dose escalation methods are based on empirical information (Simon *et al.,* 1997).

3. Parameter Estimates

Pharmacokinetic studies performed during early clinical development should be applied to define pharmacokinetic parameters at different dose levels, including peak concentration, drug clearance, half-life, volume of distribution, and metabolic profile. This information can be used subsequently to design

more rational schedules of administration and define the therapeutic window of the agent, and may provide clues as to potentially cumulative toxicity or specific toxicity associated with organ dysfunction. The detection of metabolites and the description of their pharmacokinetic behavior are also extremely important, particularly in the case of agents that require metabolic activation, such as irinotecan and cyclophosphamide. The generated parameters are tentatively correlated with the observed clinical outcome, particularly in terms of toxicity, in an effort to define pharmacokinetic–pharmacodynamic relationships that may be of use in further clinical testing of the agent involved. In addition, dose–effect relationships, at least in terms of toxicity, can best be assessed at this early step in clinical development, when a wide range of doses is being administered to the patients, contrary to other clinical phases of drug development (Kobayashi *et al.,* 1993).

Once a dose is selected, the same dose is usually maintained throughout the treatment unless serious toxicity occurs, in which case the dose is empirically decreased for subsequent treatment courses. In contrast, the dose of chemotherapy is rarely increased in the absence of toxicity, even though this might be a cause of treatment failure. Although wide interpatient variability has been demonstrated in all aspects of anticancer drug pharmacokinetics, several studies have demonstrated reasonably predictive relationships between some measure of drug exposure and either toxicity (Table 2) or antitumor response (Table 3), which would add to the arguments to increase the dose in case of limited toxicity (Kobayashi *et al.,* 1993). In order to characterize the relationship between drug concentration and pharmacologic effects of anticancer agents, various mathematical models have been used, such as the modified Hill equation or the E_{max} model (the maximum effect a drug produces). The Hill equation reflects a sigmoidal relationship between AUC, steady state or threshold concentrations, and pharmacologic response, usually hematologic toxicity, transformed in percentage. This type of relationship has been demonstrated for a number of commonly used anticancer drugs, including carboplatin, doxorubicin, etoposide, 5-fluorouracil, paclitaxel, and vinblastine (Kobayashi *et al.,* 1993). When nonhematologic toxicities are dose limiting, it becomes more difficult to model due to the subjective nature of grading these types of toxicity, in contrast to hematologic toxicity, which is more quantitative and continuously variable. However, efforts to model these side effects have yielded useful correlations between, for example, nephrotoxicity and cisplatin AUC or gastrointestinal toxicity and SN-38 glucuronidation rates (Gupta *et al.,* 1994).

4. Coadministration of Other Drugs

The vast majority of pharmacologic studies of anticancer agents have modeled the effects of a single drug. However, as a consequence of somatic mutations, tumor cell kill tends to decrease with subsequent courses of treatment; since geneti-

TABLE 2
Examples of Pharmacokinetic–Toxicity Relationships
for Anticancer Drugs

Drug	Toxicity	Pharmacokinetic parameter
Busulfan	Hepatotoxicity	AUC
Carboplatin	Thrombocytopenia	AUC
Cisplatin	Nephrotoxicity	C_{max} (unbound drug)
	Neurotoxicity	C_{max} (unbound drug)
Cyclophosphamide	Cardiotoxicity	AUC
Docetaxel	Neutropenia	AUC
Doxorubicin	Leukocytopenia	AUC
	Thrombocytopenia	Doxorubicinol AUC
5-Fluorouracil	Mucositis	AUC > 30 μg/h/ml
	Leukocytopenia	AUC and C_{ss}
Irinotecan	Neutropenia	AUC
	Diarrhea	Biliary index
Methotrexate	Mucositis/myelosuppression	$C_{48\,h} > 0.9\ \mu$M
Paclitaxel	Neutropenia	Time above 0.05 μM
Topotecan	Myelosuppression	Lactone AUC
Vinblastine	Neutropenia	C_{ss}
Vincristine	Neurotoxicity	AUC

AUC, area under the plasma concentration–time curve; C_{max}, peak plasma concentration; C_{ss}, plasma concentration at steady state.

cally resistant cell types are selected out, single-agent treatment is rarely curative. Therefore, and for a variety of other reasons (discussed below), cancer chemotherapy is most frequently given as a combination of different drugs. Favorable and unfavorable interactions between drugs must be considered in developing such combination regimens. These interactions may either be pharmacokinetic or pharmacodynamic in nature, and can influence the effectiveness of each of the components of the combination. In order to take theoretically optimal advantage of combination chemotherapy, it has been proposed that several prerequisites must be met (Verweij and Stoter, 1996):

- Drugs with at least activity as a single agent should be selected. Because of primary resistance, which is common for any single agent even in the most responsive tumors, single-agent complete response rates rarely exceed 20%.
- Drugs with different mechanisms of action should be combined. The various anticancer agent classes have different targets in the cell. The use of multiple agents with different mechanisms of action enables independent cell killing by each agent. Cells that are resistant to one agent might still be sensitive to the other drug(s) in the regimen and might thus still be killed. Known patterns of cross-resistance must be taken into consideration in the design of drug combinations.

- Drugs with different mechanisms of resistance should be combined. Resistance to many agents may be the result of mutational changes unique to those agents. However, in other circumstances a single mutational change may lead to resistance to a variety of different drugs. The number of potential mechanisms of resistance is continuously increasing and partly drug dependent. Because of the presence of drug-resistant mutants at the time of clinical diagnosis, the earliest possible use of non-cross-resistant drugs is recommended to avoid the selection of double mutants by sequential chemotherapy. Adequate cytotoxic doses of drugs have to be administered as frequently as possible to achieve maximal kill of both sensitive and moderately resistant cells.
- If possible, drugs with different dose-limiting toxicities should be combined. In case of nonoverlapping toxicity it is more likely that each drug can be used at full dose, and thus the effectiveness of each agent will be maintained in the combination.

As stated above, multiple-drug therapy can give rise to clinically important drug–drug interactions, which occur when either the pharmacokinetic or pharmacodynamic behavior of one drug is altered by the other. These interactions are important in the design of drug combinations because occasionally the outcome of concurrent drug administration is

TABLE 3
Examples of Pharmacokinetic–Tumor Response Relationships for Anticancer Drugs

Drug	Disease	Pharmacokinetic parameter
Carboplatin	Ovarian cancer	AUC
Doxorubicin	ANLL	$C_{3\,h}$
Etoposide	NSCLC	$C_{ss} > 1$ μg/ml
5-Fluorouracil	Head and neck cancer	AUC
	Colorectal cancer	AUC
6-Mercaptopurine	ALL	RBC 6-TGN levels
Paclitaxel	NSCLC	Time above 0.10 μM
Teniposide	Lymphoma, leukemia	C_{ss} and CL

AUC, area under the plasma concentration–time curve; ANLL, acute nonlymphocytic leukemia; $C_{3\text{-}h}$, plasma concentration at 3 h after IV bolus administration; NSCLC, non-small cell lung cancer; C_{ss}, plasma concentration at steady state; ALL, acute lymphocytic leukemia; RBC, red blood cell; 6-TGN, 6-thioguanine nucleotides (intracellular active metabolites of 5-mercaptopurine); CL, total plasma clearance.

diminished therapeutic efficacy or increased toxicity of one or more of the administered agents. One system of classifying drug–drug interactions is to note whether the interaction is synergistic, additive, or antagonistic. While perhaps clinically useful, this classification does not give insight into the mechanism of the interaction observed. Interactions may also be classified as pharmacokinetic and/or pharmacodynamic.

All aspects of pharmacokinetics might be affected when a drug is given in combination with another drug, including absorption (resulting in altered absorption rate or oral bioavailability), distribution (mostly caused by protein-binding displacement), metabolism, and excretion. It should be born in mind that several pharmacokinetic parameters could be altered simultaneously. Especially in the development of anticancer agents given by the oral route, oral bioavailability plays a crucial role (DeMario and Ratain, 1998). This parameter is contingent on adequate intestinal absorption and the circumvention of intestinal and, subsequently, hepatic metabolism of the drug. An ideal chemotherapeutic drug would have an adequate absolute bioavailability and little inter- and intrapatient variability in absorption. However, for the most commonly used oral agents, such as etoposide, cyclophosphamide and methotrexate, these criteria are not met. The generally narrow therapeutic index of these agents means that significant inter- and intrapatient variability would predispose some individuals to excessive toxicity or, conversely, inadequate efficacy (McLeod and Evans, 1999).

Combinations of drugs might also show pharmacodynamic interactions that cannot be explained by altered pharmacokinetic profiles. Some of these interactions are at the cellular level or are cell cycle related. Provided that the drugs used are active in a particular disease, knowledge of cellular kinetics can be used to consider therapy initiation with non–cell cycle phase–specific agents (e.g., the alkylating agents and nitrosoureas), first to reduce tumor bulk and second to recruit slowly dividing cells into active DNA synthesis. Once the latter is achieved, treatment can be continued within the same cycle of treatment by cell cycle phase–specific agents (such as methotrexate or the fluoropyrimidines) that mainly affect cells during periods of DNA synthesis. Furthermore, repeated courses with S-phase-specific drugs, such as cytosine arabinoside and methotrexate, that block cells during the period of DNA synthesis are most effective if they are administered during the rebound rapid recovery of DNA synthesis that follows the period of suppression of DNA synthesis (Vaughan et al., 1984).

4. Pharmacogenetics

Pharmacogenetics describe the differences in the pharmacokinetics and pharmacodynamics of drugs as a result of inherited differences in metabolizing enzymes and receptor expressions between patients (Boddy and Ratain, 1997; Daly, 1995). These inherited differences in enzymes and receptors are one of the major factors responsible for the interpatient variability in drug disposition and effects. Severe toxicity might occur in the absence of normal metabolism of active compounds, while the therapeutic effect of a drug could be diminished in the case of absence of activation of a prodrug. The importance (and detectability) of polymorphisms for a given enzyme depends on the contribution of the variant gene product to pharmacologic response, the availability of alternative pathways of metabolism, and the frequency of occurrence of the least common variant allele. Although many substrates have been identified for the known polymorph drug-metabolizing enzymes, only very few cancer chemotherapeutic agents have yet been associated with such genetically determined sources of variability (Table 4). These enzyme systems, which are known to be responsible for variability in anticancer drug pharmacokinetics, with important implications for pharmacodynamic outcome of the chemotherapeutic treatment, include thiopurine S-methyltransferase (Krynetski and Evans, 1999), dihydropyrimidine dehydrogenase (Milano and McLeod, 2000), cytochrome P-450 (Ingelman-Sundberg et al., 1999), and uridine diphosphate (UDP) glucuronosyltransferase (Iyer and Ratain, 1998), and will be discussed subsequently.

A. Drug-Metabolizing Enzyme Systems

1. Thiopurine S-Methyltransferase

The thiopurine S-methyltransferase (TPMT) genetic polymorphism represents a striking example of the potential clinical impact of pharmacogenetics. TPMT is a cytosolic enzyme that catalyzes the S-adenosyl-L-methionine-dependent

TABLE 4
Examples of Anticancer Agents Metabolized by Polymorphic Enzymes

Drug	Metabolic pathway	Variability	Polymorphism
Amonafide	N-Acetyltransferase	> 3-fold	Inherited
Busulfan	Glutathione S-transferase	10-fold	Unknown
Cyclophosphamide	Cytochrome P-450	4- to 9-fold	Unknown
5-Fluorouracil	Dihydropyrimidine dehydrogenase	10-fold	Inherited
Irinotecan	UDP glucuronosyltransferase	50-fold	Inherited
6-Mercaptopurine	Thiopurine methyltransferase	> 30-fold	Inherited

S-methylation of aromatic and heterocyclic sulfhydryl compounds, including the anticancer agents 6-mercaptopurine, 6-thioguanine, and azathioprine. One of these agents, 6-mercaptopurine, is being used for the treatment of acute lympoblastic leukemia in children, and treatment with this agent has invariably resulted in large interpatient variation in observed hematologic toxicity (McLeod *et al.*, 2000). This variability is mainly caused by variations in the metabolism of 6-mercaptopurine by TPMT, which catalyzes the S-methylation of 6-mercaptopurine into an inactive metabolite (Fig. 4; Iyer and Ratain, 1998). TPMT activity is mainly genetically determined, whereas other factors, such as age and renal function, also influence the TPMT activity (Krynetski and Evans, 1998). The TPMT activity in erythrocytes of Caucasian and African populations, which correlates well with the activity

in other tissues, has a trimodal distribution, with 89% having a high TPMT activity, 11% having an intermediate activity, and approximately 0.3% having no or only a very low TPMT activity (with a 17% lower median TPMT activity in the African population). Although the absolute deficiency of TPMT is rare, the dose of 6-mercaptopurine in these patients should be diminished 15 times as compared with the normal dose to prevent excessive hematologic toxicities in this subset of patients (Iyer and Ratain, 1998).

2. Dihydropyrimidine Dehydrogenase

Dihydropyrimidine dehydrogenase (DPD) is the initial and rate-limiting enzyme involved in degradation of the pyrimidines uracil and thymine and of the anticancer agent 5-fluorouracil (5-FU) by reduction (Fig. 5). Deficiency of DPD

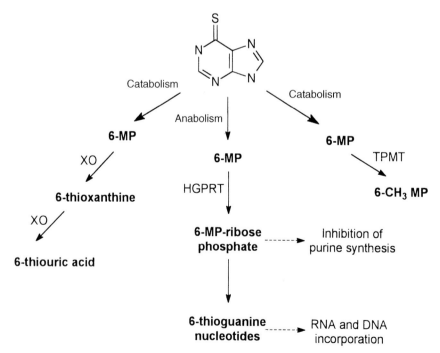

FIGURE 4   Metabolic pathways of 6-mercaptupurine (6-MP). TPMT, thiopurine methyltransferase; XO, xanthine oxidase; HGPRT, hypoxanthine-guanine phosphoribosyltransferase.

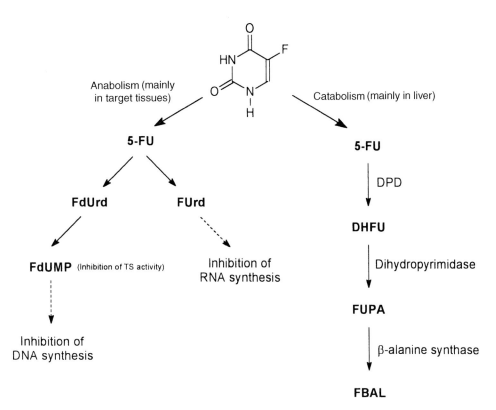

FIGURE 5 Metabolic pathways of 5-fluorouracil (5-FU). DPD, dihydropyrimidine dehydrogenase; DHFU, 5′,6′-dihydroxyfluorouracil; FUPA, α-fluoro-β-ureidopropionic acid; FBAL, 5-fluoro-β-alanine; FUrd, fluorouridine; FdUrd, fluorodeoxyuridine; FdUMP, fluorodeoxyuridine monophosphate; TS, thymidylate synthase.

is an autosomal recessive disorder that has been associated with a variety of clinical phenotypes, including convulsive disorders and mental and motor retardation. However, these phenotypes did not correlate well with the genotypes. The frequency of the different known mutations in the DPD genes in a normal population is not yet known. However, based on DPD activity studies, 3% of the normal population is heterozygote DPD deficient (McLeod et al., 1998).

5-FU is used worldwide for the treatment of colorectal cancer as a single agent and in combination therapies for breast, head and neck, and upper gastrointestinal cancers. More than 80% of the intravenously administered dose of 5-FU is metabolized by DPD, while after oral administration the bioavailability is affected by the first-pass effect of DPD in the liver (Peters et al., 1993). DPD activity shows a normal Gaussian distribution in a healthy population as well as in populations of cancer patients. DPD activity is not constant in individuals and is thus a factor responsible for the inter- and intrapatient variability in the pharmacokinetic and pharmacodynamic outcomes of 5-FU treatment. Weak relationships have been observed between the 5-FU clearance and the DPD activity in peripheral mononuclear blood cells, which are used for the monitoring of DPD activity. Aside from DPD activity, age, serum alkaline phosphatase, and the

duration of the 5-FU infusion are also factors that significantly influence 5-FU clearance. Implementation of these factors in the 5-FU dosing strategies is coming into view (Milano and McLeod, 2000). Nevertheless, implementation of DPD activity assays before 5-FU administration might be important in the avoidance of severe toxicities in patients with (inherited) DPD deficiencies. Unfortunately, current methods are laborious and not convenient for routine prospective screening of DPD activity in cancer patients about to receive 5-FU-based therapy.

Since expression of DPD is also highly variable in tumor specimens, DPD not only plays an important role in the plasma pharmacokinetics and related toxicities after 5-FU administration, but has been demonstrated to be a predictor of antitumor response. High levels of DPD in tumors leads to rapid metabolism of 5-FU, resulting in reduced cytotoxicity. The in vitro sensitivity of tumor cells to 5-FU is related to DPD activity; the higher the DPD activity, the lower the cytotoxicity after 5-FU exposure. The same relationship has been demonstrated in clinical studies, in which patients with low tumor DPD activity showed a higher response rate than patients with higher tumor DPD activity (Milano and McLeod, 2000). Several DPD inhibitors are currently under investigation, of which enyluracil is a specific inactivator of

DPD, resulting in 50 times lower tolerated dosages of intravenously administered 5-FU than single-agent 5-FU treatment. Enyluracil administered before oral 5-FU increased the bioavailability of 5-FU to approximately 100%. Other DPD inhibitors currently under development are competitive with 5-FU for DPD and have to be dosed more frequently to inhibit the degradation of 5-FU. The known DPD inhibitors also influence DPD activity in tumors and in principle might increase 5-FU-induced cytotoxicity.

3. Cytochrome P-450 Isozymes

The cytochrome P-450 (CYP) isozymes are responsible for the oxidation of more than 50% of all drugs administered to humans (Ingelmal-Sundberg *et al.,* 1999), resulting in more polar metabolites, which can be excreted efficiently by the kidneys and the liver. The CYP enzymes have been classified into a number of families, subfamilies, and individual isozymes (Van der Weide and Steijns, 1999). The CYP3A4 isozyme has been shown to be responsible for approximately 50% of the CYP-mediated elimination of drugs, whereas 20% is metabolized by CYP2D6 and an additional 15% by CYP2C9 and CYP2C19 (Ingelmal-Sundberg *et al.,* 1999).

Expression of CYP3A4 is highly variable among individuals (up to sixfold). Recently, various polymorphisms in the 5′-promotor region of the enzyme have been demonstrated (Ball *et al.,* 1999; Felix *et al.,* 1998; Wandel *et al.,* 2000), although their functional significance is not current known. The observed variations are likely caused by induction or inhibition of this enzyme. CYP3A4 is involved in the metabolism of numerous anticancer agents including the taxanes (paclitaxel and docetaxel), *Vinca* alkaloids (vinblastine, vindesine, and vincristine), epipodophyllotoxins (etoposide and teniposide), and oxazophosphorine alkylating agents (cyclophosphamide and ifosfamide) (Iyer and Ratain, 1998), and thus plays a major role in pharmacodynamic outcome after administration of these drugs (Fig. 6).

For the CYP enzymes 1A1, 1A2, 2A6, 2C9, 2C19, 2D6 and 2E1 polymorphisms have been described, from which CYP2D6 has been studied most extensively and was shown to be responsible for the metabolism of over 50 clinically used drugs (Hasler, 1999). However, until now no anticancer agents have been known that are extensively metabolized by CYP2D6 (Iyer and Ratain, 1998), making this isozyme less important for oncologic practice. Approximately 5–10% of

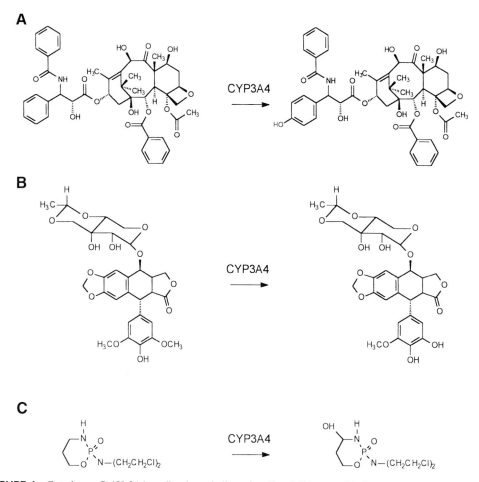

FIGURE 6   Cytochrome P-450 3A4–mediated metabolism of paclitaxel **(A)**, etoposide **(B)**, and cyclophosphamide **(C)**.

Caucasians completely lack activity of this enzyme, resulting in poor CYP2D6-related metabolism (PM), and approximately 7% of whites are ultrarapid CYP2D6-related metabolizers (UM). In the Asian population, less than 1% of the population can be classified as PM or UM phenotype, while up to 29% UM phenotype is reported in some African populations. In contrast to CYP2D6, for CYP2C19 no UM phenotype is known, while 2–6% of Caucasians and 18–23% of Asian populations have been shown to be CYP2C19 deficient (Van der Weide and Steijns, 1999). However, also human CYP2C19-mediated metabolisms have not been described for anticancer agents. For the polymorph CYP2C9 also no anticancer agents are known to be substrates, although the calcium antagonist verapamil, used as a multidrug resistance (MDR) reversal agent, is metabolized by CYP2C9. Clearly, this may have important implications for the pharmacodynamic outcome if verapamil is used in combination with anticancer agents.

4. UDP Glucuronosyltransferase

Glucuronidation by UDP glucuronosyltransferase (UGT) plays an important role in the elimination of a wide variety of drugs and endogenous compounds. Up to now, two UGT families have been identified: UGT1 and UGT2, which are further classified into subfamilies. UGT catalyzes the shift of the glucuronic acid moiety from UDP glucuronic acid to hydroxyl groups of compounds, resulting in water-soluble metabolites that can be excreted in urine or bile. Bilirubin and SN-38, the active metabolite of the anticancer agent irinotecan (Fig. 7), are both conjugated by UGT1A1, which is absent in humans with the rare Crigler–Najjar syndrome. Cancer patients with Crigler–Najjar syndrome are thus at high risk for irinotecan-mediated toxicities, such as severe delayed-type diarrhea and myelosuppression, since UGT does not detoxify SN-38. Also, in patients with the Gilbert's syndrome, present in 5–10% of a normal population, increased toxicity was observed after administration of irinotecan, since these patients have a lower rate of SN-38 glucuronidation. Clinical studies to evaluate the need and extent of dose-reductions of irinotecan in patients with the Gilbert's syndrome are ongoing.

Recently, a significant correlation was observed between SN-38 and bilirubin glucuronidation rates by human liver mi-

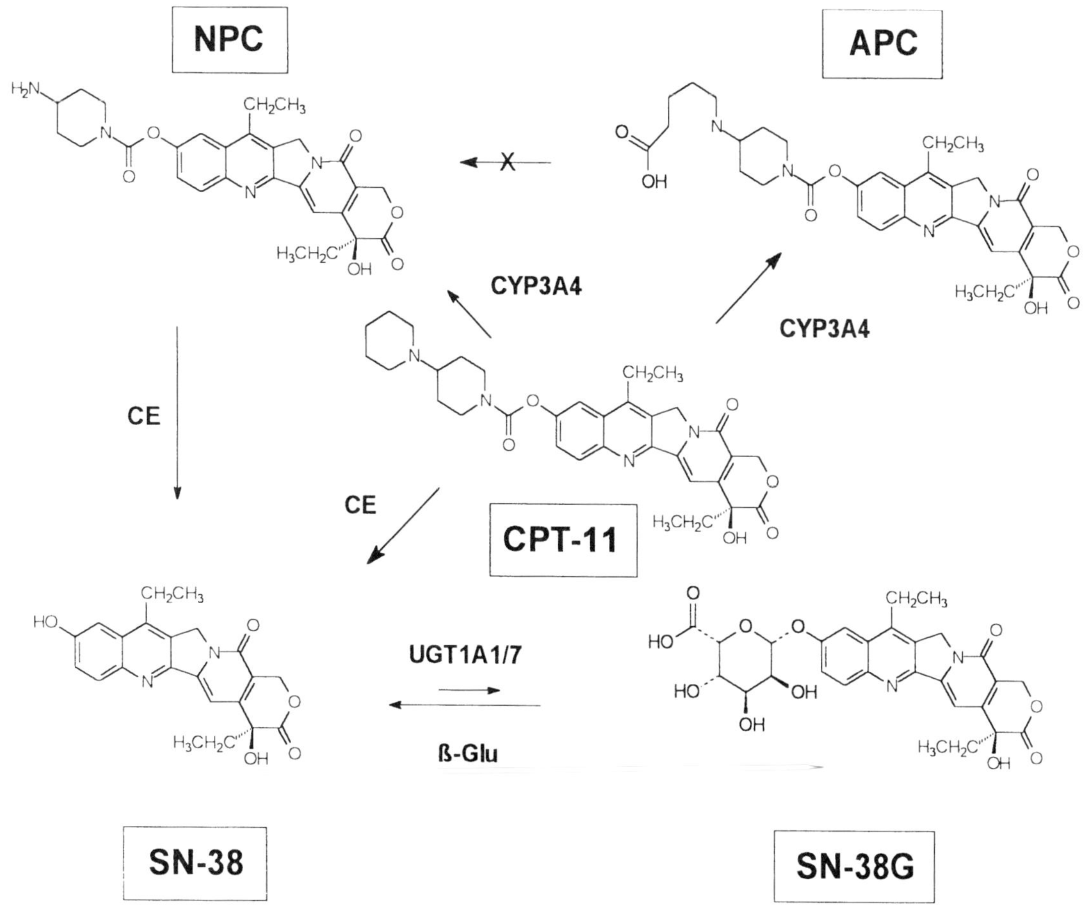

FIGURE 7 Metabolic pathways of irinotecan (CPT-11). CYP3A4, cytochrome P-450 3A4; CE, carboxylesterase; UGT 1A1/7, UDP glucuronosyltransferase 1A1 and 1A7; β-GLU, bacterial β-glucuronidase; APC/NPC, oxidative metabolites; SN-38G, the β-glucuronide metabolite of SN-38.

crosomes (Mathyssen *et al.,* 2001). Both SN-38 and bilirubin are conjugated by UGT1A1. Baseline unconjugated bilirubin correlated with both neutropenia and the AUCs of irinotecan and SN-38, and might be useful in individualizing dose prescription or adaptation. Also, UGT1A1 genotyping might be used for individualization of CPT-11 dosages (Iyer and Ratain, 1998). The metabolism of irinotecan can be influenced by inhibitors and inducers of UGT; valproic acid (an inhibitor of glucuronidation) given 5 min before CPT-11 administration caused a 99% inhibition in the formation of SN-38G in rats, resulting in a mean increase in SN-38 AUC of 270%. In contrast, pretreatment with phenobarbital (an inducer of UGT) resulted in a 72% enhancement in the AUC of SN-38G, with a concomitant reduction in the AUCs of CPT-11 and SN-38 of 31% and 59%, respectively.

B. Relevance in the Clinic

The TPMT and DPD polymorphisms perhaps best illustrate the issues involved in how this information can be used in a clinical setting, i.e., what the relative advantages and disadvantages of phenotyping and genotyping are. At present, a clinically convenient method of phenotyping for the TPMT polymorphism is available, and although the DNA sequences of several variant alleles are known, many are yet to be discovered. Hence, many patients will be misdiagnosed with molecular techniques that focus only on known DNA sequence variants. The metabolism, dose requirements, and tolerance of 6-mercaptopurine among 180 pediatric patients with different TPMT phenotypes were recently studied (Relling *et al.,* 1999b). It was shown that erythrocyte concentrations of thioguanine nucleotides were inversely related to TPMT enzyme activity in TPMT homozygous wild-type, heterozygous, and homozygous-deficient patients. Thus, lowering doses of 6-mercaptopurine in TPMT heterozygotes and in deficient patients allowed administration of full-protocol doses of other chemotherapeutic agents while maintaining high thioguanine nucleotide concentrations.

Once it became clear that a genetically mediated deficiency of DPD was responsible for some incidents of 5-FU toxicity, an attempt was made to confirm the diagnosis of easily accessible tissue or cells, such as peripheral blood mononuclear cells. However, frequency distribution histograms of DPD activity in these cells did not show a multimodal distribution. For this reason, genotyping strategies have been developed predicated on DNA-based techniques combined with measurement of urinary and/or plasma pyrimidine levels to identify DPD heterozygotes (Milano and McLeod, 2000). These diagnostic tools, coupled with increased understanding of the genetic regulation of TPMT and DPD, will enable us to individualize anticancer treatment. It is expected that, in the case of irinotecan chemotherapeutic treatment, for example, dose adjustments based on genotyping for expression of

UGT will be possible in the near future. Similarly, a variety of techniques has been developed as specific measures of CYP3A4 activity (Watkins, 1994). These techniques are most commonly based on probes that recognize that each metabolic pathway can vary independently. For example, the erythromycin breath test specifically measures the *in vivo* activity of hepatic CYP3A4 and has been used recently to optimize delivery of docetaxel to tumors by balancing delivery and elimination rates and estimation of docetaxel plasma clearance, subject to constraints of toxicity (Hirth *et al.,* 2000). Alternatively, it has been proposed that interpatient variability in CYP3A4 activity and docetaxel clearance could be predicted by measuring the total amount of 24-h urinary excretion of 9-β-hydroxycortisol, a CYP3A4-mediated metabolite, after intravenous cortisol administration (Yamamoto *et al.,* 2000). Clearly, additional studies are required to determine whether these tests could adequately predict the pharmacokinetics of other substrates of CYP3A4 of whether these probes have value when, say, docetaxel is used in combination with other agents, such as anthracyclines (Danesi *et al.,* 1999). Presently, there are many ongoing studies evaluating the interpatient variability in drug-metabolizing enzyme systems and their implications for the therapeutic index of anticancer agents.

5. Strategies to Improve Therapeutic Index

A. Dose Adjustment Based on Patient Characteristics

1. Conventional Method: Body Surface Area Based Dosing

The traditional method of individualizing anticancer drug dosage is by using body surface area (BSA) (Gurney, 1996). Estimation of BSA is most commonly achieved using a formula that was derived primarily for its use of basal metabolism as a function of weight and height alone; more recently, it has been confirmed that the original formula was surprisingly accurate considering the small sample size used in its derivation (Gurney, 1996). The usefulness of normalizing anticancer drug dose to BSA in adults has been questioned recently, since it clearly has been shown that for some drugs, including epirubicin and oral topotecan, there is no relationship between BSA and anticancer drug clearance (Gurney *et al.,* 1998; Loos *et al.,* 2000) (Table 5). In this case, the use of BSA-based dosing results in the administration of a standard dose multiplied by a random number, i.e., the ratio of the patient's BSA to an average BSA. Based on these considerations, several investigators have advocated incorporating flat dosing regimens in new phase I studies (with all patients at a dose level receiving the same dose) combined with

TABLE 5
Established Relationships between Body Surface Area and Anticancer Drug Pharmacokinetics

Drug	Observations
Possible relationships	
Diazohydroxide	Moderate correlation with BSA and CL
Docetaxel	Interpatient variability in CL correlated with BSA
Gemcitabine	CL sensitive to BSA
No or weak relationships	
Busulfan	No correlation of BSA and CL, V_{ss}, or V_c
Carboplatin	CL and V_c correlate with BSA; still 2- to 3-fold variation in AUC
Epirubicin	No correlation of BSA and CL
Etoposide	No correlation of BSA and CL, AUC, or C_{ss}
5-Fluorouracil	No correlation of BSA and CL
Methotrexate	No effect of BSA normalization on inter-patient variability
Paclitaxel	No correlation of BSA and CL, V_{ss}, or V_c
Topotecan (oral)	Weak correlation of BSA and CL/f

BSA, body surface area; CL, total plasma clearance; V_{ss}, steady-state volume of distribution; V_c, central volume of distribution; AUC, area under the plasma concentration–time curve.

retrospective analysis of BSA as a determinant of drug clearance at the completion of the study (Ratain, 1998).

2. Pathophysiologic Status

As discussed, most pharmacologic studies of anticancer agents have shown important interindividual as well as intraindividual variability in pharmacokinetic behavior. In some cases, this is due to changing pathophysiologic status of cancer patients due to the disease itself or to dysfunction of specific organs involved in drug elimination (Table 6). For example, if urinary excretion is an important elimination route for a given drug, any decrement in renal function could lead to decreased drug clearance and may result in drug accumulation and toxicity. It would therefore be logical to decrease the drug dose relative to the degree of impaired renal function in order to maintain plasma concentrations within a target therapeutic window, which is well documented for bleomycin, cisplatin, cyclophosphamide, etoposide, methotrexate, and topotecan (Kintzel and Dorr, 1995). Still the best known example of this *a priori* dose adjustment of an anticancer agent involves carboplatin, which is excreted renally almost entirely by glomerular filtration. Various strategies have been developed to estimate carboplatin doses based on renal function among patients, either using creatinine clearance (Egorin *et al.*, 1985) or glomerular filtration rates as measured by a radioisotope method (Calvert *et al.*, 1989). Application of these procedures

TABLE 6
Summary of Patient Characteristics Affecting Anticancer Drug Pharmacokinetics

Characteristics	Anticancer drug
Renal function	Bleomycin, carboplatin, cisplatin, cyclophosphamide, etoposide, methotrexate, topotecan
Hepatic function	Docetaxel, doxorubicin, epirubicin, vinblastine, vincristine
Serum albumin	Etoposide, paclitaxel[a]
Third spaces	Methotrexate
Obesity	Cyclophosphamide, doxorubicin, 6-mercaptopurine, methotrexate
Cancer cachexia	5-Fluorouracil, methotrexate

[a]Altered binding of paclitaxel in plasma due to the presence of high concentrations of Cremophor EL, the formulation vehicle used for intravenous drug administration.

has led to a substantial reduction in pharmacokinetic variability such that carboplatin is currently one of the few drugs routinely administered to achieve a target exposure rather than on a mg/m^2 or mg/kg basis (Table 7).

In contrast to the predictable decline in renal clearance of drugs when glomerular filtration is impaired, it is not as easy to make a general prediction regarding the effect of impaired liver function on drug clearance. The major problem is that hepatic enzymes are not good indicators of metabolizing activity, and alternative hepatic function tests, such as indocyanine green and antipyrine, have limited value in predicting anticancer drug pharmacokinetics (and metabolism) and require additional experimental procedures. An alternative dynamic measure of liver function has been proposed recently, based on totaled values (scored to the World Health Organization grading system) of serum bilirubin, alkaline phosphatase, and either alanine aminotransferase or aspartate aminotransferase to give a hepatic dysfunction score (Twelves *et al.*, 1999). Based on carefully conducted pharmacokinetic studies in patients with normal and impaired hepatic function, guidelines have been proposed for dose adjustments of several agents when administered to patients with liver dysfunction, including anthracyclines (doxorubicin and epirubicin), etoposide, docetaxel, and some *Vinca* alkaloids (vinblastine and vincristine) (Canal *et al.*, 1998).

The binding of drugs to plasma proteins, particularly those that are highly bound, may also have significant clinical implications for therapeutic outcome (Grandison and Boudinot, 2000). Although protein binding is a major determinant of drug action, it is clearly one of a myriad of factors that influence drug disposition. The extent of protein binding is a function of drug and protein concentrations, the affinity constants for the drug–protein interaction, and the number of protein binding sites per class of binding site. Since only the unbound (or free) drug in plasma water is available for diffusion from the vascular compartment to the tumor interstitium, the therapeutic response will correlate with free-drug concentration rather than total-drug concentration. Several clinical situations, including liver and renal disease, can significantly decrease the extent of plasma binding and may lead to higher free-drug concentrations and possible risk of unexpected toxicity, although the total (free plus bound forms) plasma drug concentrations are unaltered. However, it is important to realize that after therapeutic doses of most anticancer drugs, plasma binding is drug-concentration-independent, suggesting that the total plasma concentration is reflective of the unbound concentration. Thus, other physiologic changes, such as decreased renal and hepatic function in the elderly, generally produce more clinically significant alterations in drug disposition than that seen with alterations in plasma protein binding. For some anticancer agents, including etoposide (Perdaems *et al.*, 1998; Stewart *et al.*, 1991) and paclitaxel (Sparreboom *et al.*, 1999), it has been shown that protein binding is highly dependent on dose- and schedule-varying plasma concentrations. Indeed, by taking into consideration protein binding of etoposide it has been reported that prospective pharmacokinetic monitoring allows an increase in dose intensity without a parallel increase in toxicity (Ratain *et al.*, 1991). Very few studies have evaluated the pharmacokinetics of anticancer drugs in elderly patients. In most cases, aging could not be considered as an independent feature of drug disposition because it is characterized by a conjunction of physiologic alterations that may occur simultaneously. Therefore, it appears, that dose adaptation as a function of individual physiology is better than adaptation as a function of age (Canal *et al.*, 1998).

Adjusting the dosage *a posteriori* based on a patient's tolerance is also a widely used approach, even though it might result in dose reductions, which can compromise dose intensity and lead to treatment failure. Clearly, the seriousness of the first side effect is the major determinant of whether it can or cannot be used as an end point. Examples of this type of dose adjustments are the platelet-nadir-directed dosage approach to individualizing carboplatin dosage in adults (Egorin *et al.*, 1985) or leukopenia-targeted dosing of methotrexate and mercaptopurine in patients with childhood acute lymphoblastic leukemia (Schmiegelow *et al.*, 1995).

B. Implementation of Pharmacokinetic–Pharmacodynamic Principles

1. *During Repeated Administration*

Prolonged infusion schedules of anticancer drugs offer a very convenient setting for dose adaptation in individual patients. By the time required to achieve steady-state concentra-

---

TABLE 7
A Priori Dose Adaptation for Carboplatin According to Patient Characteristics

Dosage type	Formula
Platelet directed[a]	Dose (mg/m^2) = (0.091) $\times$ CL$_{CR}$/BSA $\times$ [((PPC − PND)/PPC)$\times$100) − n] + 86
AUC directed[b]	Dose (mg) = AUC (mg/ml min) $\times$ (GFR + 25) (ml/min)

BSA, body surface area; CL$_{CR}$, measured creatinine clearance; PND, desired platelet count at nadir; PPC, pretreatment platelet count; GFR, glomerular filtration rate. In non-pretreated patients n = 0, whereas in pretreated patients n = 17.
[a]Egorin *et al.*, 1985. [b]Calvert *et al.*, 1989.

tion it is possible to modify the infusion rate for the remainder of the treatment course if a relationship is known between this steady-state concentration and a desired pharmacodynamic end point. This method has been successfully used to adapt the dose during continuous infusions of 5-FU and etoposide, and for repeated oral administration of etoposide or repeated intravenous administration of cisplatin (Canal *et al.,* 1998). Yet another possibility for dose adaptation consists of administering a (low) test dose of an agent to exactly determine the kinetic parameter of interest (e.g., AUC) and then modifying the dose to obtain a target AUC (Fig. 8). The best illustration of this approach is the use of methotrexate in childhood leukemia (Relling *et al.,* 1994). Indeed, the monitoring of methotrexate plasma concentrations is now routinely performed to identify patients at high risk of toxicity and to adjust leucovorin rescue in patients with delayed drug excretion. This monitoring has significantly reduced the incidence of serious toxicity (including toxic death) and improved outcome by eliminating unacceptably low systemic exposure levels (Evans *et al.,* 1998). Similar methods of dose adaptations have been applied to or are currently under investigation for 5-FU, etoposide, melphalan, busulfan, and cisplatin.

2. Feedback-Controlled Dosing

It remains to be seen how information on variability can be used to devise an optimal dosage regimen of a drug for the management of a given disease in an individual patient. Obviously, the desired objective would be most efficiently achieved if the individual's dosage requirements could be calculated prior to administration of drug. While this ideal cannot be met totally in practice (with the notable exception of carboplatin, as described above), some success may be achieved by adopting feedback-controlled dosing. In the adaptive dosage with feedback control, population-based predictive models are used initially but allow the possibility of dosage alteration based on feedback revision. In this approach, patients are first treated with standard dose; then, during treatment, pharmacokinetic information is estimated by a limited-sampling strategy and compared with that predicted from the population model with which dosage was initiated. On the basis of the comparison, more patient-specific pharmacokinetic parameters are calculated, and dosage is adjusted accordingly to maintain the target exposure measure producing the desired pharmacodynamic effect. It has been proposed that despite its mathematical complexity this approach may be the only way to deliver the desired precise exposure of an anticancer agent. However, the use of population pharmacokinetic models is increasingly studied in an attempt to accommodate as much of the pharmacokinetic variability as possible in terms of measurable characteristics. This type of analysis has been conducted for a number of clinically important anticancer drugs, including carboplatin (Chatelut *et al.,* 1995), docetaxel (Bruno *et al.,* 1998), and topotecan (Gallo *et al.,* 2000), and provided mathematical equations based on patient BSA, gender, protein levels, and so forth, to predict drug clearance with good precision and minimal bias (Table 8).

3. Circadian-Rhythm-Based Dosing

It has been suggested that administration at certain times of day can improve the therapeutic index of several anticancer drugs (Hrushesky, 1985; Hrushesky and Bjarnason, 1993; Levi, 2000a). For example, significant improvement has been demonstrated in survival for children with leukemia who received 6-mercaptopurine in the evening compared with those who received the drug in the morning (Rivard *et al.,* 1985). Such findings led to the assumption of a coupling between tolerability rhythms and the rest–activity cycle in cancer patients. Indeed, an improved tolerability of chronotherapy schedules based on this concept was shown in several clinical trials for other anticancer drugs, including busulfan, carboplatin, docetaxel, 5-FU, and oxaliplatin (Giacchetti *et al.,* 2000; Levi *et al.,* 2000b; Tampellini *et al.,* 1998). Furthermore, the chronotherapy principle was validated in two randomized multicenter phase III trials involving a total of 278 patients with metastatic colorectal cancer. A fivefold reduction in the incidence of severe mucositis, a twofold decrease in peripheral neuropathy, and a near doubling of objective response rate resulted from delivering 5-FU and oxaliplatin at experimentally determined circadian times, i.e., at 4 a.m. and at 4 p.m., respectively, compared with constant rate infusion (Levi *et al.,* 1994, 1997). The precise mechanisms by which these agents are more effective at certain times of the day is still unknown, but pharmacokinetic as well as pharmacodynamic explanations have been proposed (including a circadian dependency of hematopoiesis). Whether the potential benefits will balance the major inconvenience related to drug administration in the middle of the night is yet unclear.

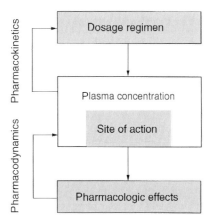

FIGURE 8 An alternative approach to the design of a dosage regimen. The pharmacokinetics and the pharmacodynamics of the drug are first determined. Then either the plasma drug concentration–time data or the effects produced, via pharmacokinetics, are used as a feedback (*solid lines*) to modify the dosage regimen to achieve optimal therapy.

TABLE 8
Population Pharmacokinetic Models for Anticancer Drugs

Drug	Formula
Carboplatin[a]	CL (ml/min) = 0.134 × WT + (218 × WT × (1 − 0.00457 × age) × [1 −).314 × sex)]/SC
Docetaxel[b]	CL (L/h/m^2) = BSA(22.1 − 3.55 × AAG − 0.095 × age + 0.225 × ALB) × (1 − 0.334 × HEP12)
Topotecan[c]	CL (L/h) = 32 + [0.356(WT − 71) + 0.308(HT − 168.5) − 842(SC − 1.1)] × [1 + 0.671 × sex])

CL, total plasma clearance; WT, body weight; SC, serum creatinine (μmol/L); BSA body surface area; AAG, plasma concentration of α_1-acid glycoprotein (g/L); ALB, plasma concentration of albumin (g/L); HEP12, hepatic dysfunction covariate representing aspartate amino-transferase or alanine aminotransferase >60 IU and alkaline phosphatase >300 IU under which conditions HEP12 is assigned the value of 1 (default = 0); HT, height.
[a]Chatelut et al., 1995; [b]Bruno et al., 1998; [c]Gallo et al., 2000.

4. Biomodulation

a. Pharmacodynamic Alterations

The use of specific agents coadministered with anticancer drugs to increase the therapeutic index of chemotherapeutic treatment has had a substantial impact on certain diseases. One of the most widely used biomodulating agents is leucovorin, a reduced folate that is used in combination with both methotrexate and 5-FU. This agent has been shown to decrease methotrexate-induced toxicity to various normal tissues and enhance 5-FU-mediated cytotoxicity to tumor cells by inhibition of thymidylate synthase, thereby allowing escalation of the anticancer drug dose without affecting its disposition profile (Papamichael, 1999). Other examples of agents interfering with anticancer drug pharmacodynamics include the use of amifostine to reduce cisplatin-associated myelosuppression, nephrotoxicity, and neurotoxicity (O'Dwyer et al., 2000), and dexrazoxane to decrease anthracycline-induced cardiotoxicity (Hensley et al., 1999; Pai and Nahata, 2000).

The concept of pharmacodynamic biomodulation has also been extensively studied with P-glycoprotein-blocking agents in an attempt to improve the therapeutic index of anticancer agents (Van Zuylen et al., 2000). This multidrug-resistant protein is a drug-efflux transporter encoded by the *MDR1* gene that is abundantly present in various types of human cancer. Studies performed over the last several years have shown that intrinsic and acquired expression of P-glycoprotein might play a role in clinical drug resistance in specific hematologic malignancies. Consequently, clinical trials have been initiated worldwide in which P-glycoprotein blockers (e.g., verapamil and cyclosporin A) are given to cancer patients along with anticancer drugs with the intent of attenuating carrier-mediated drug resistance in patients. Unfortunately, in these trials decreased systemic clearance of the anticancer drugs became a serious problem and necessitated substantial dose reductions, thereby losing all the potential benefits in terms of antitumor activity as compared to normal dosages given without the addition of these blockers (Table 9). In most cases, the pharmacokinetic interference appears to be the result of competition for enzymes (mainly CYP3A4) involved in drug metabolism (Sparreboom and Nooter, 2000). A new generation of P-glycoprotein blockers is now available for efficacy testing in clinical trials for reversal of MDR, and these modulators have been demonstrated not to interfere with anticancer drug pharmacokinetics (Table 9). Eventually, the use of these agents will allow assessment of the contribution of P-glycoprotein to the toxicity and antitumor activity of chemotherapeutic regimens for MDR reversal and should result in improved therapeutic specificity and efficacy.

b. Pharmacokinetic Alterations

One of the best studied examples of pharmacokinetic biomodulation is the coadministration of eniluracil, an inactivator of DPD, with 5-FU (Baccanari et al., 1993). As indicated, DPD is the initial rate-limiting enzyme in the catabolism of 5-FU. The high variation in the population in DPD activity accounts for much of the variability observed with the therapeutic use of 5-FU, including variable drug levels, variable bioavailability, and inconsistent toxicity and activity profiles. Eniluracil has been shown to improve the efficacy of 5-FU in preclinical models through the selective, irreversible inhibition of DPD-mediated metabolism (Cao et al., 1994). In a subsequent clinical study, eniluracil prolonged the half-life of intravenously administered 5-FU and reduced its clearance (Schilsky et al., 1998). Eniluracil also facilitated the oral administration of 5-FU by inhibiting the intestinal DPD activity (Ahmed et al., 1999), thereby increasing the oral availability and diminishing the variability in absorption (Baker et al., 1996, 2000).

Intestinal metabolic systems and drug efflux pumps, located in the intestinal mucosa, represent another limitation in the bioavailability of oral drugs (Benet et al., 1999). Several enzymes located in the enterocyte, such as CYP3A4 (one of the major subclasses of cytochrome P-450 expressed in the intestines), are involved in the presystemic metabolism of many cytotoxic agents, such as cyclophosphamide, etoposide, and the investigational agents paclitaxel, irinotecan, and vinorelbine, thereby limiting the oral absorption of these drugs (Fig. 9). The bioavailability of these drugs might be

TABLE 9
Randomized Comparative Clinical Studies Evaluating Pharmacokinetic
Interactions between P-Glycoprotein (P-gp) Modulators
and Anticancer Drugs

Modulator	Total dose	Drug	Effect
Cyclosporin A[a]	17–70 mg/kg IV	Etoposide	CL 40% ↓
	42 mg/kg IV	Doxorubicin	CL 55% ↓
	42 mg/kg IV	Doxorubicin	CL 37% ↓
Valspodar[a]	11.5 mg/kg IV	Etoposide	CL 40% ↓
	2–17 mg/kg IV	Etoposide	CL 45% ↓
	2.5–25 mg/kg bid PO	Doxorubicin	CL 54% ↓
	12.1 mg/kg IV	Paclitaxel	No change
	5 mg/kg qid × 3 PO	Paclitaxel	No change
Biricodar[a]	8640 mg/m^2 CIV	Paclitaxel	CL 50% ↓
R101933	200–300 mg bid × 5 PO	Docetaxel	No change
LY-335979	100–300 mg/m^2 bid × 3 PO	Docetaxel	No change
GF-120918	50–400 mg bid × 5 PO	Doxorubicin	No change

CIV, continuous IV infusion; CL, total plasma clearance.
[a]Known substrates or inhibitors of cytochrome P-450 3A4.

substantially enhanced by pharmacologic modulation of enteric CYP3A4 activity. Several investigators confirmed recently that by inhibiting CYP3A4 activity by coadministration of specific inhibitors, such as erythromycin, quinidine, ketoconazole, and cyclosporin A, the oral bioavailability of various anticancer agents (e.g., etoposide) could be improved, thereby also diminishing the variability in absorption (Gupta, 1988; Kobayashi *et al.,* 1996). Similarly, P-glycoprotein, which is also abundantly present in the gastrointestinal tract, has been shown to limit the intestinal absorption of numerous anticancer agents, including paclitaxel, etoposide, and

vinblastine (Sparreboom *et al.,* 1997). Combined inhibition of intestinal P-gp and CYP3A4 by cyclosporin A has been shown to substantially increase the systemic exposure to oral paclitaxel in cancer patients (Meerum Terwogt *et al.,* 1999), suggesting that simultaneous modulation of these transports could be considered in the development of substrate anticancer agents given by the oral route.

Even though biomodulation can be beneficial in cancer patients, pharmacokinetic and pharmacodynamic studies have to be conducted in humans to determine at which of these two levels (i.e., kinetics or dynamics) the interaction takes place and whether biomodulation ultimately improves the therapeutic index of anticancer agents.

5. Drug Scheduling and Administration Sequencing

The antitumor activity of certain chemotherapeutic agents is highly schedule dependent. For these drugs, the dose fractionated over several days can produce a different antitumor response or toxicity profile compared with the same dose given over a shorter period. In the first definitive demonstration of etoposide schedule dependency in clinical oncology, investigators documented markedly increased efficacy in patients with small cell lung cancer when an identical total dose of etoposide was administered by a 5-day divided-dose schedule rather than a 24-h infusion (Slevin *et al.,* 1989). Pharmacokinetic analysis in that study showed that both schedules produced very similar overall drug exposure (as measured by AUC) but that the divided-dose schedule produced twice the duration of exposure to an etoposide plasma concentration of more than 1 μg/ml. This observation was consistent with pre-

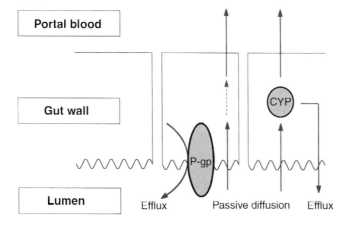

FIGURE 9 Schematic representation of the intestinal epithelium, indicating the P-glycoprotein (P-gp)–mediated drug efflux mechanism and cytochrome P-450 3A4 (CYP)–mediated drug metabolism. Arrows indicate the direction of drug transport.

clinical data, and the authors speculated that exposure to this threshold concentration was important in achieving clinical efficacy, while exposure to higher plasma concentrations augmented drug-induced toxicity. Subsequently, this finding has led to the use of prolonged oral administration of etoposide for the treatment of patients with lung cancer (Hainsworth, 1999). Similar schedule dependency has also been demonstrated for a number of other anticancer agents, notably paclitaxel (Verweij *et al.,* 1994) and topotecan (Gerrits *et al.,* 1997). For both agents, the variability in clinically tested treatment schedules is enormous, ranging from short intravenous infusions of less than 30 min to 21-day or even 7-week continuous-infusion administrations, with large differences in experienced toxicity profiles and with fortuitous implications for the pharmacokinetic behavior. In most cases, the mechanisms underlying the schedule dependency are not completely understood, and further investigation into pharmacokinetics and pharmacodynamics will be essential to determine the nature of this and to define optimal duration of drug administration.

The combination of anticancer drugs can also exhibit schedule-dependent toxicity or antitumor activity through pharmacokinetic or pharmacodynamic modulation. An example of a metabolic interaction is shown by the experimental demonstration that the sequence of 5-FU and methotrexate seems crucial to the cytotoxicity of this combination. *In vitro,* if methotrexate precedes 5-FU by at least 1 h synergistic results are obtained (Cadman *et al.,* 1979). This may be due to an increased activation of 5-FU to its nucleotide form. The opposite sequence of drug administration leads to antagonism due to block of the thymidylate synthetase pathway induced by 5-FU.

Through this block the intracellular folates are preserved in their active tetrahydrofolate form, which diminishes the effect of the methotrexate block of dihydrofolate reductase.

In theory, drugs with renal or hepatic side effects, can alter the elimination of other agents through these routes and therefore must be used with caution in combinations (Table 10). For many of the combination chemotherapy schemes presently in use, no data are available on the pharmacokinetic interaction of the individual drugs. For instance, for the combination of cyclophosphamide, methotrexate, and 5-FU, used in the treatment of patients with breast cancer, only preclinical data are available indicating a variety of pharmacokinetic interactions. 5-FU and cyclophosphamide both augmented the clearance of methotrexate (De Bruijn *et al.,* 1986), whereas methotrexate increased the exposure to 5-FU (De Bruijn *et al.,* 1987), and methotrexate and 5-FU increased the oral absorption of cyclophosphamide (De Bruijn *et al.,* 1990). However, no definitive data are available in cancer patients. Cisplatin is another example of a drug that might alter the elimination of coadministered agents. Cisplatin causes renal toxicity and is known to alter the pharmacokinetics of other agents (such as methotrexate or bleomycin) that depend on renal elimination as their primary mechanism of excretion. If cisplatin is given before methotrexate, as in the treatment of bladder or head and neck cancer, careful monitoring of renal function, adequate pre- and posthydration, and dose adjustment for methotrexate is essential to ensure that delayed methotrexate excretion does not lead to severe drug toxicity. Recently, it was shown that cisplatin-induced hematologic toxicity is modified by the clinically used formulation vehicle of paclitaxel, Cremophor EL (De Vos *et al.,* 1997). When

TABLE 10
Sequence-Dependent Drug–Drug Interactions between Anticancer Agents

Drugs	Effect(s)
Docetaxel–cisplatin	DNA adduct formation inhibited; PK unchanged
Docetaxel–ifosphamide	CL_I increased in D → I sequence
Docetaxel–methotrexate	M → D sequence more myelotoxic; PK unchanged
Gemcitabine–MTA	M → G sequence more myelotoxic; PK unchanged
Irinotecan–cisplatin	C → I sequence more myelotoxic; PK unchanged
Paclitaxel–cisplatin	C → P sequence more myelotoxic; CL_P reduced
Paclitaxel–cyclophosphamide	P → C sequence more myelotoxic; PK unchanged
Paclitaxel–doxorubicin	P → D sequence more myelotoxic; CL_D reduced
Paclitaxel–epirubicin	P → E sequence more myelotoxic; CL_E reduced
Paclitaxel–etoposide	CL_E reduced in P → E sequence
Paclitaxel–losoxantrone	P → L sequence more myelotoxic; PK unchanged
Topotecan (IV)–cisplatin	C → T sequence more myelotoxic; CL_T reduced
Topotecan (PO)–cisplatin	C → T sequence more myelotoxic; PK unchanged

PK, pharmacokinetics; CL, total plasma clearance; MTA, multitargeted antifolate agent.

cisplatin was administered before paclitaxel, more profound neutropenia was induced in cancer patients compared with the alternate sequence (Rowinsky *et al.*, 1991). As a resultant it is universally recommended to administer paclitaxel before cisplatin, which also happens to be the sequence with the highest tumor cell kill *in vitro*. These examples indicate that it is of utmost importance to study the pharmacokinetic interaction for any new combination of drugs during early clinical studies. Importantly, there is a tremendous paucity in pharmacokinetic interaction studies of commonly applied combination regimen.

Other classes of drug interactions have been described that cannot be explained by alterations in pharmacokinetics, e.g., for the combination of cisplatin and topoisomerase I inhibitors. DNA topoisomerase I is a nuclear enzyme, involved in cellular replication and transcription. By forming a covalent adduct between topoisomerase I and DNA, termed the cleavable complex, topoisomerase I inhibitors interfere with the process of DNA breakage and resealing during DNA synthesis. The stabilized cleavable complex blocks the progress of the replication fork, resulting in irreversible DNA double-strand breaks leading to cell death (Hsiang *et al.*, 1989). Based on their mechanism of action, synergy was suspected for the combination of topoisomerase I inhibitors and DNA-damaging agents such as cisplatin. Preclinical studies confirmed this hypothesis. However, the observed interaction seemed to depend on the cell line studied and the schedule of administration of camptothecin-type topoisomerase I inhibitors and cisplatin used (De Jonge *et al.*, 1998). When topotecan was preceded by cisplatin, synergy was increased in comparison with concomitant incubation with both drugs in the IGROV-1 ovarian cancer cell line and the MCF7 cell line. Also in the clinical setting drug sequencing seems to be important (Rowinsky *et al.*, 1996; De Jonge *et al.*, 2000), with toxicity increasing when cisplatin administration preceded topotecan administration. However, the interaction observed could not be explained by an alteration in pharmacokinetics of topotecan or cisplatin. Preclinical studies indicated that the reversal of cisplatin-induced DNA interstrand cross-links was delayed by concomitant incubation with a topoisomerase I inhibitor, without modifying their formation (De Jonge *et al.*, 1998). However, this could not be confirmed in the phase I study on the combination of oral topotecan and intravenously administered cisplatin. It is possible that other mechanisms may contribute to the enhanced toxicity observed for the sequence cisplatin followed by topotecan. In *in vitro* studies, induction of topoisomerase I and enhanced topoisomerase I inhibitory activity were observed after incubation with cisplatin followed by the administration of a topoisomerase I inhibitor (De Jonge *et al.*, 1998). Simultaneous incubation of platinum derivatives and topoisomerase I inhibitors resulted in enhanced S-phase arrest in human colon and ovarian cancer cell lines indicative of increased topoiso-merase I inhibitor-induced cytotoxicity. This observation might indicate that the synergistic toxicity observed for the combination of topoisomerase I inhibitors and platinum derivatives can partly be explained by a modification in cellular response to DNA damage.

All three examples described above underscore the importance of exploring the influence of the sequence of drug administration on cytotoxicity, toxicity, and kinetics, both in *in vitro* and *in vivo* as in clinical studies. Without adequate investigations of the pharmacokinetic and pharmacodynamic interactions between drugs, it will be impossible to determine the most optimal administration schemes. However, preclinical data and data on clinical toxicity can not simply be extrapolated to the antitumor activity of a given combination. Additional randomized phase II or III studies in patients are needed to elucidate the importance of drug sequencing and possible cytotoxic interaction on antitumor activity.

6. Conclusion and Perspectives

Substantial progress has been made in recent years in optimization of cancer chemotherapy with the use of pharmacokinetics, pharmacodynamics, and pharmacogenetics, although various aspects of anticancer drug pharmacology require further investigation to enhance their clinical usefulness. Indeed, incorporation of pharmacologic principles in drug development and clinical trials is essential to maximize the clinical potentials of new anticancer agents, as improvements in outcome have been observed using these principles to individualize anticancer drug administration for some agents (including methotrexate and carboplatin) (Table 11). In addition to its importance with classical anticancer drugs, it will be essential for the rational development of new agents designed to exploit advances in molecular oncology and those acting on oncogenes, tumor suppressor genes, and related signal transduction pathways, including apoptosis, as well as agents used for chemoprevention or to inhibit invasion, angiogenesis, and metastasis (Boral *et al.*, 1998; Gelmon *et al.*, 1999). Such innovative agents may require an especially careful and imaginative choice of dosage regimens, as continuous daily administration may be required to maintain active but nontoxic dose (and concentration) levels. The ongoing development of improved analytical methods, such as those based on technical advances in mass spectrometry and nuclear magnetic resonance (NMR) spectroscopy coupled to liquid chromatography, will also be a major factor in the growing influence of anticancer drug pharmacokinetics, particularly for highly potent agents such as certain natural products (Egorin, 1998). An exciting new development that is likely to have a major impact on cancer pharmacology and the conduct of early clinical trials will be the ability to monitor tissue distribution of anticancer agents in a noninvasive manner

TABLE 11
Strategies for Incorporation of Pharmacologic Principles in Clinical
Trial Design to Improve the Therapeutic Index of Anticancer Drugs

Dose adjustment type	Example
A. *Based on patient characteristics*	
1. Body surface area	Docetaxel
2. Pathophysiologic status (renal function)	Carboplatin
B. *Based on pharmacokinetic-dynamic principles*	
1. During repeated administration	5-Fluorouracil
2. Feedback-controlled dosing	Methotrexate
3. Circadian-rhythm-based dosing	6-Mercaptopurine
4. Biomodulation	
a. Pharmacokinetic modulation	5-Fluorouracil/leucovorin
b. Pharmacodynamic00 modulation	Docetaxel/R101933
5. Drug scheduling	Etoposide
6. Drug administration sequence	Paclitaxel/cisplatin
C. *Based on pharmacogenetic principles*	5-Fluorouracil/DPD
	6-Mercaptopurine/TPMT

DPD, dihydropyridine dehydrogenase; TPMT, thiopurine methyltransferase.

(Saleem *et al.,* 2000). These include the use of NMR, PET, and secondary ion mass spectrometry (SIMS) microscopy for fluorine-containing agents such as 5-FU (Fragu and Kahn, 1997; Wolf *et al.,* 2000), and elastic scattering spectroscopy and fluorescence-biosensor technologies for agents such as topotecan and the anthracyclines (Mourant *et al.,* 1999). Although such techniques are still rather insensitive and require expensive specialist facilities, each has important potential to provide *in vivo* information about pharmacokinetic and pharmacodynamic profiles. Pharmacogenomic studies are also rapidly elucidating the inherited nature of differences in drug disposition and pharmacodynamic effects and will provide a stronger scientific basis for optimizing drug therapy on the basis of each patient's genetic constitution (Evans and Relling, 1999). Furthermore, the development of various new technologies, such as genomics, high-throughput screening, and combinatorial chemistry, is also likely to result in an explosion in the number of targets and candidate compounds to explore, and it is expected that a deeper understanding of a compound's pharmacologic properties in the exploratory stage of drug development is mandatory for a "quick kill process for the candidate" (Kuhlmann, 1999). In addition, the use of computer simulation of clinical trials has evolved over the past two decades to yield pharmacologically sound, realistic trial outcomes, and this will definitively impact on future (pharmacologic-guided) trial design (Gieschke *et al.,* 1997; Holford *et al.,* 2000; Sheiner and Steimer, 2000). In all, there is ample evidence that anticancer drug pharmacology will continue to provide vital support to routine patient man-agement and the discovery, development, and evaluation of innovative, cutting-edge therapies.

References

Ahmed, F. Y., Johnston, S. J., Cassidy, J., et al. (1999). Eniluracil treatment completely inactivates dihydropyrimidine dehydrogenase in colorectal tumors. *J. Clin. Oncol.* **17,** 2439–2445.

Baccanari, D. P., Davis, S. T., Knick, V. C., *et al.* (1993). 5-Ethylnyluracil (77C85): a potent modulator of the pharmacokinetics and antitumor efficacy of 5-fluorouracil. *Proc. Natl. Acad. Sci. USA* **90,** 2027–2035.

Ball, S. E., Scatina, J., Kao, J., Ferron, G. M., Fruncillo, R., Mayer, P., Weinryb, I., Guida, M., Hopkins, P. J., Warner, N., and Hall, J. (1999). Population distribution and effects on drug metabolism of a genetic variant in the 5′ promotor region of CYP3A4. *Clin. Pharmacol. Ther.* **66,** 288–294.

Baker, S. D., Khor, S. P., Adjei, A. A., *et al.* (1996). Pharmacokinetic, oral bioavailability, and safety study of fluorouracil in patients treated with 776C85, an inactivator of dihydropyrimidine dehydrogenase. *J. Clin. Oncol.* **14,** 3085–3096.

Baker, S. D., Diasio, R. B., O'Reilly, S., *et al.* (2000). Phase I and pharmacologic study of oral fluorouracil on a chronic daily schedule in combination with the dihydropyrimidine dehydrogenase inactivator eniluracil. *J. Clin. Oncol.* **18,** 915–926.

Benet, L. Z., Izumi, T., Zhang, Y., *et al.* (1999). Intestinal MDR transport proteins and P-450 enzymes as barriers to oral drug delivery. *J. Control. Release* **62,** 25–31.

Boddy, A. V., and Ratain, M. J. (1997). Pharmacogenetics in cancer etiology and chemotherapy. *Clin. Cancer Res.* **3,** 1025–1030.

Boral, A. L., Dessain, S., and Chabner, B. A. (1998). Clinical evaluation of biologically targeted drugs: obstacles and opportunities. *Cancer Chemother. Pharmacol.* **42(S),** S3–S21.

Bruno, R., Hille, D., Riva, A., *et al.* (1998). Population pharmacokinetics/pharmacodynamics of docetaxel in phase II studies in patients with cancer. *J. Clin. Oncol.* **16**, 187–196.

Cadman, E., Heimer, R., and Davis, L. (1979). Enhanced 5-fluorouracil nucleotide formation after methotrexate administration: explanation for drug synergism. *Science* **205**, 1135–1137.

Calvert, A. H., Newell, D. R., Gumbrell, L. A., *et al.* (1989). Carboplatin dosage: prospective evaluation of a simple formula based on renal function. *J. Clin. Oncol.* **7**, 1748–1756.

Canal, P., Chatelut, E., and Guichard, S. (1998). Practical treatment guide for dose individualisation in cancer chemotherapy. *Drugs* **56**, 1019–1038.

Cao, S., Rustum, Y. M., and Spector, T. (1994). 5-Ethynyluracil (776C85): modulation of 5-fluorouracil efficacy and therapeutic index in rats bearing advanced colorectal carcinoma. *Cancer Res.* **15**, 1507–1510.

Chatelut, E., Canal, P., Brunner, V., *et al.* (1995). Prediction of carboplatin clearance from standard morphological and biological patient characteristics. *J. Natl. Cancer Inst.* **87**, 573–580.

Collins, J. M., Zaharko, D. S, Dedrick, R. L., *et al.* (1986). Potential roles for preclinical pharmacology in phase I clinical trials. *Cancer Treat. Rep.* **70**, 73–80.

Collins, J. M., Grieshaber, C. K., and Chabner, B. A. (1990). Pharmacologically guided phase I trials based upon preclinical development. *J. Natl. Cancer Inst.* **82**, 1321–1326.

Daly, A. K. (1995). Molecular basis of polymorphic drug metabolism. *J. Mol. Med.* **73**, 539–553.

Danesi, R., Conte, P. F., and Del Tacca, M. (1999). Pharmacokinetic optimisation of treatment schedules for anthracyclines and paclitaxel in patients with cancer. *Clin. Pharm.* **37**, 195–211.

De Bruijn, E. A., Driessen, O., Leeflang, P., *et al.* (1986). Pharmacokinetic interactions of cyclophosphamide and 5-fluorouracil with methotrexate in an animal model. *Cancer Treat. Rep.* **70**, 1159–1165.

De Bruijn, E. A., Driessen, O., Leeflang, P., *et al.* (1987). Interactions of methotrexate and cyclophosphamide with the pharmacokinetics of 5-fluorouracil in an animal model. *Cancer Treat. Rep.* **71**, 1267–1269.

De Bruijn, E. A., Geng, Y., Hermans, J., *et al.* (1990). The CMF-regimen. Modulation of cyclophosphamide uptake and clearance by methotrexate and fluorouracil. *Int. J. Cancer* **45**, 935–939.

De Jonge, M. J. A., Sparreboom, A., and Verweij, J. (1998). The development of combination therapy involving camptothecins: a review of preclinical and early clinical studies. *Cancer Treat. Rev.* **24**, 205–220.

De Jonge, M. J. A., Loos, W. J., Gelderblom, H., *et al.* (2000). Phase I and pharmacologic study of oral topotecan and intravenous cisplatin: sequence-dependent hematologic side-effects. *J. Clin. Oncol.* **18**, 2104–2115.

DeMario, M. D., and Ratain, M. J. (1998). Oral chemotherapy: rationale and future directions. *J. Clin. Oncol.* **16**, 2557–2567.

De Vos, A. I., Nooter, K., Verweij, J., *et al.* (1997). Differential modulation of cisplatin accumulation in leukocytes and tumour cell lines by the paclitaxel vehicle Cremophor EL. *Ann. Oncol.* **8**, 1145–1150.

Egorin, M. J., Van Echo, D. A., Olman, E. A., *et al.* (1985). Prospective validation of a pharmacologically based dosing scheme for the cis-diamminedichloroplatinum (II) analogue diamminnecyclobutanedicarboxylatoplatinum. *Cancer Res.* **45**, 6502–6506.

Egorin, M. J. (1998) Overview of recent topics in clinical pharmacology of anticancer agents. *Cancer Chemother. Pharmacol.* **42**(Suppl.), S22–S30.

Eisenhauer, E. A., O'Dwyer, P. J., Christian, M., *et al.* (2000). Phase I clinical trial design in cancer drug development. *J. Clin. Oncol.* **18**, 684–692.

Evans, W. E., Rodman, J. H., Relling, M. V., *et al.* (1991). Concept of maximum tolerated systemic exposure and its application to Phase I-II studies of anticancer drugs. *Med. Pediatr. Oncol.* **19**, 153–159.

Evans, W. E., Relling, M. V., Rodman, J. H., *et al.* (1998). Conventional compared with individualized chemotherapy for childhood acute lymphoblastic leukemia. *N. Engl. J. Med.* **338**, 499–505.

Evans, W. E., and Relling, M. V. (1999). Pharmacogenomics: translating functional genomics into rational therapeutics. *Science* **286**, 487–491.

Felix, C. A., Walker, A. H., Lange, B. J., Williams, T. M., Winick, N. J., Cheung, N. K., Lovett, B. D., Nowell, P. C., Blair, I. A., and Rebbeck, T. R. (1998). Association of CYP3A4 genotype with treatment-related leukemia. *Proc. Natl. Acad. Sci. USA* **95**, 13176–13181.

Fragu, P., and Kahn, E. (1997). Secondary ion mass spectrometry (SIMS) microscopy: a new tool for pharmacological studies in humans. *Microsc. Res. Tech.* **36**, 296–300.

Gallo, J. M., Laub, P. B., Rowinsky, E. K., *et al.* (2000). Population pharmacokinetic model for topotecan derived from phase I clinical trials. *J. Clin. Oncol.* **18**, 2459–2467.

Gelmon, K. A., Eisenhauer, E. A., Harris, A. L., *et al.* (1999). Anticancer agents targeting signaling molecules and cancer cell environment: challenges for drug development? *J. Natl. Cancer Inst.* **91**, 1281–1287.

Gerrits, C. J., De Jonge, M. J. A., Schellens, J. H. M., *et al.* (1997). Topoisomerase I inhibitors: the relevance of prolonged exposure for present clinical development. *Br. J. Cancer* **76**, 952–962.

Giacchetti, S., Perpoint, B., Zidani, R., *et al.* (2000). Phase III multicenter randomized trial of oxaliplatin added to chronomodulated fluorouracil-leucovorin as first-line treatment of metastatic colorectal cancer. *J. Clin. Oncol.* **18**, 136–147.

Gieschke, R., Reigner, B. G., and Steimer, J. L. (1997). Exploring clinical study design by computer simulation based on pharmacokinetic/pharmacodynamic modelling. *Int. J. Clin. Pharmacol. Ther.* **35**, 469–474.

Gouyette, A., and Chabot, G. G. (1993). Pharmacokinetic principles in cancer chemotherapy. In "Handbook of Chemotherapy in Clinical Oncology" (E. Cvitkovic, J. P. Droz, J. P. Armand and S. Khoury, eds.), 2nd ed., pp. 73–88. Scientific Communication International Ltd., Jersey (Channel Islands).

Grandison, M. K., and Boudinot, F. D. (2000). Age-related changes in protein binding of drugs: implications for therapy. *Clin. Pharm.* **38**, 271–290.

Grochow, L. B. (1998). Individualized dosing of anticancer drugs and the role of therapeutic monitoring. In "A Clinician's Guide Chemotherapy Pharmacokinetics and Pharmacodynamics" (L. B. Grochow and M. M. Ames, eds.), pp. 3–16. Williams & Wilkins, Baltimore.

Gupta, E., Lestingi, T. M., Mick, R., *et al.* (1994). Metabolic fate of irinotecan in humans: correlation of gluruconidation with diarrhea. *Cancer Res.* **54**, 3723–3725.

Gupta, E., Mick, R., Ramirez, J., *et al.* (1997). Pharmacokinetics and pharmacodynamic evaluation of the topoisomerase I inhibitor irinotecan in cancer patients. *J. Clin. Oncol.* **15**, 1502–1510.

Gupta, S. K. (1988). Erythromycin enhances the absorption of cyclosporine. *Br. J. Clin. Pharmacol.* **25**, 401–402.

Gurney, H. (1996). Dose calculation of anticancer drugs: a review of the current practice and introduction of an alternative. *J. Clin. Oncol.* **14**, 2590–2611.

Gurney, H. P., Ackland, S., Gebski, V., *et al.* (1998). Factors affecting epirubicin pharmacokinetics and toxicity: evidence against using body-surface area for dose calculation. *J. Clin. Oncol.* **16**, 2299–2304.

Hainsworth, J. D. (1999). Extended-schedule oral etoposide in selected neoplasms and overview of administration and scheduling issues. *Drugs* **58**(Suppl. 3), 51–66.

Hasler, J. A. (1999). Pharmacogenetics of cytochrome P450. *Mol. Aspects Med.* **20**, 1–137.

Hensley, M. L., Schuchter, L. M., Lindley, C., *et al.* (1999). American Society of Clinical Oncology clinical practice guidelines for the use of chemotherapy and radiotherapy protectants. *J. Clin. Oncol.* **17**, 3333–3355.

Hirth, J., Watkins, P. B., Strawderman, M., *et al.* (2000). The effect of an individual's cytochrome CYP3A4 activity on docetaxel clearance. *Clin. Cancer Res.* **6**, 1255–1258.

Holford, N. H., Kimko, H. C., Monteleone, J. P., *et al.* (2000). Simulation of clinical trials. *Annu. Rev. Pharmacol. Toxicol.* **40**, 209–334.

Hrushesky, W. J. M. (1985). Circadian timing of cancer chemotherapy. *Science* **228**, 73–75.

Hrushesky, W. J. M., and Bjarnason, G. A. (1993). Circadian cancer therapy. *J. Clin. Oncol.* **11**, 1403–1417.

Hryniuk, W. M. (1988). More is better. *J. Clin. Oncol.* **6**, 1365–1367.

Hryniuk, W. M., Figueredo, A., and Goodyear, M. (1987). Applications of dose intensity to problems in chemotherapy of breast and colorectal cancer. *Semin. Oncol.* **14**, 3–11.

Hsiang, Y.-H., Lihou, M. G., and Liu, L. F. (1989). Arrest of replication forks by drug-stabilized topoisomerase I-DNA cleavable complexes as a mechanism of cell killing by camptothecin. *Cancer Res.* **49**, 5077–5082.

Ingelman-Sundberg, M., Oscarsson, M., and McLellan, R. A. (1999). Polymorphic human cytochrome P450 enzymes: an opportunity for individualized drug treatment. *Trends Pharmacol. Sci.* **20**, 342–349.

Iyer, L., and Ratain, M. J. (1998). Pharmacogenetics and cancer chemotherapy. *Eur. J. Cancer* **34**, 1493–1499.

Kintzel, P. E., and Dorr, R. T. (1995). Anticancer drug renal toxicity and elimination: dosing guidelines for altered renal function. *Cancer Treat. Rev.* **21**, 33–64.

Kobayashi, K., Jodrell, D. I., and Ratain, M. J. (1993). Pharmacodynamic-pharmacokinetic relationship and therapeutic drug monitoring. *Cancer Surveys* **17**, 51–78.

Kobayashi, K., Ratain, M. J., Fleming, G. F., *et al.* (1996). A phase I study of CYP3A4 modulation of oral etoposide with ketoconazole in patients with advanced cancer. *Proc. Am. Soc. Clin. Oncol.* **15**, 471 (abstract).

Krynetski, E. Y., and Evans, W. E. (1998). Pharmacogenetics of cancer therapy: getting personal. *Am. J. Hum. Genet.* **63**, 11–16.

Krynetski, E. Y., and Evans, W. E. (1999). Pharmacogenetics as a molecular basis for individualized drug therapy: the thiopurine S-methyltransferase paradigm. *Pharm. Res.* **16**, 342–349.

Kuhlmann, J. (1999). Alternative strategies in drug development: clinical pharmacological aspects. *Int. J. Clin. Pharmacol. Ther.* **37**, 575–583.

Levi, F. (2000). Therapeutic implications of circadian rhythms in cancer patients. *Novartis Found. Symp.* **227**, 119–136.

Levi, F., Zidani, R., Vannetzel, J. M., *et al.* (1994). Chronomodulated *versus* fixed infusion rate delivery of ambulatory chemotherapy with oxaliplatin, 5-fluorouracil and folinic acid in patients with colorectal cancer metastases. A randomized multiinstitutional trial. *J. Natl. Cancer Inst.* **86**, 1608–1617.

Levi, F., Zidani, R., and Misset, J. L. (1997). Randomized multicentre trial of chronotherapy with oxaliplatin, fluorouracil, and folinic acid in metastatic colorectal cancer. *Lancet* **350**, 681–686.

Levi, F., Metzger, G., Massari, C., *et al.* (2000). Oxaliplatin: pharmacokinetics and chronopharmacological aspects. *Clin. Pharm.* **38**, 1–21.

Loos, W. J., Gelderblom, H., Sparreboom, A., *et al.* (2000). Inter- and intrapatient variability in oral topotecan pharmacokinetics: implications for body-surface area dosage regimens. *Clin. Cancer Res.* **6**, 2685–2689.

Mahmood, I., and Balian, J. D. (1999). The pharmacokinetic principles behind scaling from preclinical results to phase I protocols. *Clin. Pharm.* **36**, 1–11.

Masson, E., and Zamboni, W. C. (1998). Pharmacokinetic optimisation of cancer chemotherapy. *Clin. Pharm.* **32**, 324–343.

Mathyssen, R. H. J., Van Alphen, R. J., Verweij, J., *et al.* (2001). Clinical pharmacokinetics and metabolism of irinotecan. *Clin. Cancer Res.* **7**, in press.

McLeod, H. L., and Evans, W. E. (1999). Oral cancer chemotherapy: the promise and the pitfalls. *Clin. Cancer Res.* **5**, 2669–2671.

McLeod, H. L., Collie-Duguid, E. S., Vreken, P., *et al.* (1998). Nomenclature for human DPYD alleles. *Pharmacogenetics* **8**, 455–459.

McLeod, H. L., Krynetski, E. Y., Relling, M. V., *et al.* (2000). Genetic polymorphism of thiopurine methyltransferase and its clinical relevance for childhood acute lymphoblastic leukemia. *Leukemia* **14**, 567–572.

Meerum Terwogt, J. M., Malingre, M. M., Beijnen, J. H., *et al.* (1999). Coadministration of oral cyclosporin A enables oral therapy with paclitaxel. *Clin. Cancer Res.* **5**, 3379–3384.

Milano, G., and McLeod, H. L. (2000). Can dihydropyrimidine dehydrogenase impact 5-fluorouracil-based treatment? *Eur. J. Cancer* **36**, 37–42.

Mourant, J. R., Johnson, T. M., Los, G., *et al.* (1999). Non-invasive measurement of chemotherapy drug concentrations in tissue: preliminary demonstrations of in vivo measurements. *Phys. Med. Biol.* **44**, 1397–1417.

Newell, D. R., Burtles, S. S., Fox, B. W., *et al.* (1999). Evaluation of rodent-only toxicology for early clinical trials with novel cancer therapeutics. *Br. J. Cancer* **81**, 760–768.

O'Dwyer, P. J., Stevenson, J. P., and Johnson, S. W. (2000). Clinical pharmacokinetics and administration of established platinum drugs. *Drugs* **59 (S4)**, 19–27.

Pai, V. B., and Nahata, M. C. (2000). Cardiotoxicity of chemotherapeutic agents: incidence, treatment and prevention. *Drug Safety* **22**, 263–302.

Papamichael, D. (1999). The use of thymidylate synthase inhibitors in the treatment of advanced colorectal cancer: current status. *Oncologist* **4**, 478–487.

Perdaems, N., Bachaud, J. M., Rouzaud, P., *et al.* (1998). Relation between unbound plasma concentrations and toxicity in a prolonged oral etoposide schedule. *Eur. J. Clin. Pharmacol.* **54**, 677–683.

Peters, G. J., Schornagel, J. H., and Milano, G. A. (1993). Clinical pharmacokinetics of anti-metabolites. *Cancer Surveys* **17**, 123–156.

Ratain, M. J. (1998). Body-surface area as a basis for dosing of anticancer agents: science, myth, or habit? *J. Clin. Oncol.* **16**, 2297–2298.

Ratain, M. J., Mick, R., Schilsky, R. L., et al. (1991). Pharmacologically based dosing of etoposide: a means of safely increasing dose intensity. *J. Clin. Oncol.* **9**, 1480–1486.

Relling, M. V., Fairclough, D., Ayers, D., *et al.* (1994). Patient characteristics associated with high-risk methotrexate concentrations and toxicity. *J. Clin. Oncol.* **12**, 1667–1672.

Relling, M. V., Hancock, M. L., Boyett, J. M., *et al.* (1999a). Prognostic importance of 6-mercaptopurine dose intensity in acute lymphoblastic leukemia. *Blood* **93**, 2817–2823.

Relling, M. V., Hancock, M. L., Rivera, G. K., *et al.* (1999b). Mercaptopurine therapy intolerance and heterozygosity at the thiopurine S-methyltransferase gene locus. *J. Natl. Cancer Inst.* **91**, 2001–2008.

Rivard, G. E., Hoyoux, C., Infante-Rivard, C., *et al.* (1985). Maintenance chemotherapy for childhood acute lymphoblastic leukaemia: better in the evening. *Lancet* **2**, 1264–1266.

Rowinsky, E. K., Gilbert, M. R., McGuire, W. P., *et al.* (1991). Sequences of taxol and cisplatin: a phase I and pharmacologic study. *J. Clin. Oncol.* **9**, 1692–1703.

Rowinsky, E. K., Kaufmann, S. H., Baker, S. D., *et al.* (1996). Sequences of topotecan and cisplatin: Phase I, pharmacologic, and in vitro studies to examine sequence dependence. *J. Clin. Oncol.* **14**, 3074–3084.

Saleem, A., Yap, J., Osman, S., *et al.* (2000). Modulation of fluorouracil tissue pharmacokinetics by eniluracil: in-vivo imaging of drug action. *Lancet* **355**, 2125–2131.

Schilsky, R. L., Hohneker, J., Ratain, M. J. et al. (1998). Phase I and pharmacologic study of eniluracil plus fluorouracil in patients with advanced cancer. *J. Clin. Oncol.* **16**, 1450–1457.

Schmiegelow, K., Schroder, H., Gustafsson, G., *et al.* (1995). Risk of relapse in childhood acute lymphoblastic leukemia is related to RBC methotrexate and mercaptupurine metabolites during maintenance therapy. *J. Clin. Oncol.* **13**, 345–351.

Sheiner, L. B., and Steimer, J. L. (2000). Pharmacokinetic/pharmacodynamic modeling in drug development. *Annu. Rev. Pharmacol. Toxicol.* **40**, 67–95.

Simon, R., Freidlin, B., Rubinstein, L., *et al.* (1997). Accelerated titration designs for phase I clinical trials in oncology. *J. Natl. Cancer Inst.* **89**, 1138–1147.

Slevin, M. L., Clark, P. I., Joel, S. P., *et al.* (1989). A randomized trial to evaluate the effect of schedule on the activity of etoposide in small-cell lung cancer. *J. Clin. Oncol.* **7**, 1333–1340.

Sparreboom, A., and Nooter, K. (2000). Does P-glycoprotein play a role in anticancer drug pharmacokinetics? *Drug Resistance Updates,* **3,** 357–363.

Sparreboom, A., Van Asperen, J., Mayer, U., *et al.* (1997). Limited oral bioavailability and active epithelial excretion of paclitaxel (taxol) caused by P-glycoprotein in the intestine. *Proc. Natl. Acad. Sci. USA* **94,** 2031–2035.

Sparreboom, A., Van Zuylen, L., Brouwer, E., *et al.* (1999). Cremophor EL-mediated alteration of paclitaxel distribution in human blood: clinical pharmacokinetic implications. *Cancer Res.* **59,** 1454–1457.

Stewart, C. F., Arbuck, S. G., Fleming, R. A., *et al.* (1991). Relation of systemic exposure to unbound etoposide and hematologic toxicity. *Clin. Pharmacol. Ther.* **50,** 385–393.

Tampellini, M., Filipski, E., Liu, X. H., *et al.* (1998). Docetaxel chronopharmacology in mice. *Cancer Res.* **58,** 3896–3904.

Tannock, I. F., Boyd, N. F., De Boer, G., *et al.* (1988). A randomized trial of two dose levels of cyclophosphamide, methotrexate, and fluorouracil: chemotherapy for patients with recurrent breast cancer. *J. Clin. Oncol.* **6,** 1377–1387.

Twelves, C., Glynne-Jones, R., Cassidy, J., *et al.* (1999). Effect of hepatic dysfunction due to liver metastases on the pharmacokinetics of capecitabine and its metabolites. *Clin. Cancer Res.* **5,** 1696–1702.

Van der Weide, J., and Steijns, L. S. W. (1999). Cytochrome P450 enzyme system: genetic polymorphisms and impact on clinical pharmacology. *Ann. Clin. Biochem.* **36,** 722–729.

Van Zuylen, L., Nooter, K., Sparreboom, A., *et al.* (2000). Development of multidrug-resistance convertors: sense or nonsense? *Invest. New Drugs* **18,** 205–220.

Vaughan, W. P., Karp, J. E., and Burke, P. J. (1984) Two-cycle-times sequential chemotherapy for adult acute nonlymphocytic leukemia. *Blood* **64,** 975–980.

Verweij, J., and Stoter, G. (1996). Principles of systemic therapy of cancer. *In* "Textbook of Medical Oncology" (F. Cavalli, S. Kaye, and H. H. Hansen, eds.), pp. 23–40. Dunitz Martin, Ltd, New York.

Verweij, J., Clavel, M., and Chevalier, B. (1994). Paclitaxel (Taxol) and docetaxel (Taxotere): not simply two of a kind. *Ann. Oncol.* **5,** 495–505.

Wandel, C., Witte, J. S., Hall, J. M., Stein, C. M., Wood, A. J., and Wilkinson, G. R. (2000). CYP3A4 activity in African American and European American men: Population differences and functional effects of the CYP3A4*1B5′-promotor region polymorphism. *Clin. Pharmacol. Ther.* **68,** 82–91.

Watkins, P. B. (1994). Noninvasive test of CYP3A enzymes. *Pharmacogenetics* **4,** 171–184.

Workman, P., and Graham, M. A. (1994). Pharmacokinetics and cancer chemotherapy. *Eur. J. Cancer* **30A,** 706–710.

Wolf, W., Presant, C. A., and Waluch, V. (2000). 19F-MRS studies of fluorinated drugs in humans. *Adv. Drug Deliv. Rev.* **41,** 55–74.

Woo, M. H., Relling, M. V., Sonnichsen, D. S., *et al.* (1999). Phase I targeted systemic exposure study of paclitaxel in children with refractory acute leukemias. *Clin. Cancer Res.* **5,** 543–549.

Yamamoto, N., Tamura, T., Kamiya, Y., *et al.* (2000). Correlation between docetaxel clearance and estimated cytochrome P450 activity by urinary metabolite of exogenous cortisol. *J. Clin. Oncol.* **18,** 2301–2308.

TUMOR IMAGING APPLICATIONS IN THE TESTING OF NEW DRUGS

Eric Ofori Aboagye

Azeem Saleem

Patricia M. Price

Cancer Research Campaign PET Oncology Group

Imperial College School of Medicine

Hammersmith Hospital

London, United Kingdom

Summary

Rapid progress in our understanding of the processes that induce and drive malignant transformation has resulted in a progressive change in drug development from predominantly cytotoxic agents to compounds interacting with specific targets in malignant tissue. These targets, which include genes, antigens, and pathways involved in angiogenesis, cell cycle, signal transduction, cell death, drug resistance, invasion, and metastasis, highlight the need to revise the methods for testing new drugs in phase I clinical studies. Such methods must include, in addition to information on plasma pharmacokinetics, information on the distribution of new drugs to tumor and normal tissues. Where possible, indications of the mechanism of antitumor action of a drug should be pursued. Positron emission tomography (PET) is a sensitive and noninvasive technique involving the administration of a compound labeled with a short-lived positron-emitting isotope, followed by noninvasive scanning to obtain the *in vivo* three-dimensional distribution and kinetics of the compound. In this chapter, we briefly describe the principles of PET and review its application for testing a number of new cancer therapeutics.

1. Introduction

Anticancer drug development is currently undergoing enormous changes. This is due to an increase in our understanding, through tumor biology studies, of the processes that induce and drive malignant transformation. This understanding has resulted in a shift in paradigm from the development of predominantly cytotoxic agents to compounds that target the specific alterations that drive malignant transformation. New targets include genes, antigens, and pathways involved in angiogenesis, cell cycle, signal transduction, cell death, drug resistance, invasion, and metastasis. Because of these new targets, as well as the use of new technologies such as combinatorial chemistry and high-throughput screening to produce large numbers of anticancer agents, it has become apparent that we need to revise the way we test new drugs. In addition to information on plasma pharmacokinetics, the distribution of new drugs to tumor and normal tissues should be sought at an early stage in drug development to ensure that adequate exposure to drug or active metabolites is being achieved. Furthermore, hypothesis-testing clinical trial designs should be incorporated into phase I studies to provide early proof of principle of mechanism of action. Noninvasive technologies, including positron emission tomography (PET) and magnetic resonance imaging/spectroscopy (MRI/MRS), have a key role in providing such information to support drug development. In this chapter we will briefly describe the principles of PET and review its application for testing new cancer therapeutics.

2. Positron Emission Tomography

PET is a sensitive technique that involves the administration of a compound labeled with a short-lived positron-emitting isotope, followed by noninvasive scanning to obtain the *in vivo* three-dimensional (3D) distribution and kinetics of the compound. The radiopharmaceuticals used are administered in very small quantities so as not to modify their pharmaceutical, biological, and biochemical properties. They are then known as radiotracers.

A. Radiotracers

Positron-emitting radionuclides used in medicine are usually produced in a cyclotron, although some (copper-62) can be produced in a nuclear generator. These radionuclides decay with half-lives ranging from seconds to several days (Table 1). Positron-emitting isotopes are available for commonly occurring elements, such as carbon, oxygen, and ni-

trogen, and are used to substitute these elements in the compound of interest. Fluorine-18, another commonly used radionuclide, is used to replace fluorine present in compounds of interest such as 5-fluorouracil. However, it can also be used to replace hydrogen atoms of which it is isoteric or hydroxyl groups of which it is isoelectronic. One of the limitations of PET is related to the short half-life of these positron-emitting radionuclides. This presents difficulties in the time available for radiochemical synthesis and the need for an on-site cyclotron. It also presents difficulties when extended studies (lasting several hours) need to be done. Positron-emitting radionuclides with longer half-lives ([124]I, half-life 4.2 days; ^{18}F, half-life 110 min) can be transported from the site of production to the administration site.

Radiotracers with very high specific activity (5000–15,000 mCi/mmol) are used in PET studies in order to retain the pharmaceutical, biological, and biochemical properties of the compound being studied. In general, radiopharmaceutical synthesis should be fast enough to allow the target drug to be isolated, purified, and formulated as a sterile, pyrogen-free, isotonic solution within two to three half-lives of the radionuclide. Furthermore, due to the short physical half-lives of most positron-emitting radionuclides, large amounts of radioactivity have to be handled. Limitation of potential exposure to personnel is thus an extremely important consideration. For most drugs, these issues require the design and synthesis of drug precursors that can be radiolabeled in a single step, fostering the development of new methods for rapid remote controlled and robotics-based chemistry (Brady *et al.*, 1991). This necessitates the presence of radiochemistry facilities and expertise on site.

For PET to play a major role in drug development, extensive resources will be needed to support radiochemistry. Currently, not all drugs can be radiolabeled with sufficient activity to make them useful for investigational studies. The ability to radiolabel a compound depends on the availability of suitable functional groups. For instance, compounds with *N*-, *S*- or *O*-methyl (or -ethyl) groups, as well as proteins and antibodies, can be radiolabeled fairly easily. In some cases the multistep chemistry required to produce a radiotracer precludes radiolabeling and purification of molecules rapidly enough to avoid substantial decay of radioactivity. Constraints in the availability of suitable labeling reagents, including precursors, can also limit the ability to synthesis a radiotracer. The position of labeling should be robust to metabolic degradation, further limiting the number of compounds that can be radiolabeled. As discussed later, this limitation can be turned into an advantage for demonstrating the metabolic routes for specific compounds *in vivo*. It is anticipated that drug development authorities requiring PET imaging would begin to include precursor strategies in their drug development programs to alleviate these hurdles.

TABLE 1
Positron Emitters and Their Half-lives

Radioisotope	Half-life	Positron decay (%)
Carbon-11	20.4 min	99.8
Nitrogen-13	10.0 min	100
Oxygen-15	2.03 min	99.9
Fluorine-18	109.8 min	96.9
Iron-52	8.3 h	57
Cobalt-55	17.5 h	77
Copper-62	9.7 min	97.8
Copper-64	12.7 h	19.3
Gallium-68	68.1 min	90
Rubidium-82	1.25 min	96
Bromine-75	98.0 min	76
Bromine-76	16.1 h	57
Yttrium-86	14.7 h	34
Zirconium-89	78.4 h	25
Technetium-94m	53 min	72
Iodine-124	4.2 days	25

B. Acquisition and Processing of PET Images

The signal used to create the 3D image in PET comes from the simultaneous detection of two gamma rays released from the decay of positron emitting radionuclides, with the inference that the decay event occurred between two opposing detectors (Cho *et al.*, 1975). Nuclear detectors make it possible to map radiotracers in the body. Data are obtained as sinograms, which are corrected for detector efficiency and attenuation of photons and reconstructed into image data using various mathematical algorithms. The data depict the spatial and temporal distribution of total radioactivity in a number of tomographic image planes. Various physical processes impose a fundamental limit on the spatial resolution attainable in PET to 2–3 mm on clinical scanners (4–8 mm in most currently available commercial scanners) and 0.5–1 mm on animal scanners (Budinger, 1998). PET images are usually analyzed by defining regions of interest and extracting radioactivity–time curves for the region. In more advanced situations, functional parametric images are generated on a voxel-to-voxel basis using robust generic kinetic analysis. PET is very sensitive, with an ability to detect subpicomolar concentrations, but lacks *in vivo* chemical resolution, i.e., cannot differentiate the parent drug from its metabolites carrying the radiolabel in the body. This is not a problem where the radiolabeled compound of interest neither is metabolized nor carries the radiolabel when metabolism occurs. In situations where the radiolabel is carried by both the parent drug and its metabolites, a number of strategies are used to deal with the situation. These include:

1. Mathematical modeling.
2. Obtaining correction for metabolites by performing an additional study after administration of the radiolabeled metabolite, e.g., correction for $[^{11}C]CO_2$, a metabolite of $[^{11}C]$thymidine, by performing an additional scan after administration of $[^{11}C]CO_2/HCO_3$ (Gunn *et al.*, 2000).
3. Washout strategies for radiotracers with long physical half-life, in which nonspecific metabolites are allowed to be eliminated leaving specifically bound species that are imaged at a late time point (Blasberg *et al.*, 2000).
4. Inhibition of metabolism in one arm of a paired study to enable the contribution of metabolism to be assessed (Saleem *et al.*, 2000).

Mathematical kinetic modeling is employed to enhance data interpretation within a framework of important kinetic behaviors and to obtain quantitative parameters of relevance and universal comprehension. This is necessary if uptake or effect of a drug needs to be quantified. In practice, this involves comparing the concentrations of radioactivity in tissue with that in arterial plasma and calculating plasma/tissue exchange rate constants to derive a pharmacokinetic model (Huang *et al.*, 1986). A tracer kinetic model is a mathematical description of the fate of the tracer in the human body, in particular the organ(s) under study. The usual approach in deriving such a mathematical description is to assign the possible distribution of the tracer to a limited number of discrete compartments within which it could be free, specifically or nonspecifically bound. These compartments are not necessarily physical compartments representing physiologic disposition but are a simplification of biological complexities. Potential difficulties with compartmental modeling relate to the accuracy and precision of the data, the validity of the model developed, and the risks of misinterpretation. Moreover, there is a need to have sufficient *a priori* knowledge of the tracers' fate *in vivo* to construct a compartmental model. This is especially a problem for antineoplastic agents due to tumor heterogeneity and the lack of *a priori* knowledge of their behavior in the body. Accordingly, special data-led approaches, such as spectral analysis (Cunningham and Jones, 1993) and graphical analysis (Patlak *et al.*, 1983), have been explored as alternatives to compartmental modeling. It should also be noted that the short physical half-life of most PET radiotracers and patient comfort considerations may limit the type of pharmacologic information attainable.

3. PET in New Drug Evaluation

A. Types of Studies and Levels of Interaction

There are a number of generic issues in drug development that can be addressed by PET imaging. These can be described in the form of questions:

1. Does the drug sufficiently distribute to its target (tumor) and how much of it distributes to normal tissues where it can be potentially toxic?
2. What are the distribution and elimination kinetics of the drug in tumor and normal tissues?
3. Does the drug modulate its target in a predictable way or, alternatively, can one predict response based on assessment of the molecular/biochemical target?
4. Is the drug efficacious?

Points 1 and 2 can be classified under pharmacokinetic studies whereas 3 and 4 can be broadly classified under pharmacodynamic studies. Examples of PET studies presented in this chapter will be described under these two categories. PET studies could be employed at three main levels during the process of taking a drug from concept to licensure, including (1) preclinical development level, (2) pre-phase-I level (prior to conventional phase I studies), and (3) phase I/II/III level.

It is envisaged for newer drugs that there will be a change in paradigm, from ensuring that plasma concentrations associated with antitumor activity in rodents are achieved in humans to ensuring that the degree of modulation of PET probes in rodent tumors (which is associated with activity) is achieved in humans. Preclinical PET on animal studies will play a role in determining the degree of modulation in disease models of cancer prior to similar studies in humans.

B. Pharmacokinetics of Anticancer Agents

While PET is still in its infancy for the assessment of cancer therapeutic agents, it has been applied extensively in other fields of research, including neurology and psychiatry. In general, PET can provide information on tumor and normal tissue distribution of drugs, as well as hepatobiliary and renal clearance. Mathematical modeling of tissue data enables important kinetic parameters relating to the uptake, distribution, and washout to be derived. In some institutions there is also the possibility of carrying out rapid plasma radioactive metabolite profiling during PET scanning for the purpose of calculating plasma input functions. However, the information derived is important in its own right, providing evidence of specific metabolic processes in humans or animals.

In vivo assessment of drug pharmacokinetics may be performed following administration of the radiotracer (1) alone (high specific activity) or (2) mixed with cold (nonradioactive) drug (low specific activity). The total amount of drug in an injection of high specific activity is minimal. Doses as low as 1/1000 of the starting phase I dose of the drug can be administered. For most drugs, concentrations achieved at these doses are much lower than the K_m for saturable metabolic processes. In this section, ongoing and future work with PET will be reviewed along with specific examples.

1. DACA: Pharmacokinetic Studies Conducted Prior to Conventional Phase I Trials

N-[2-(dimethylamino)ethyl]acridine-4-carboxamide (DACA; XR-5000; NSC-601316) is a DNA-intercalating acridine derivative that stimulates DNA breakage via formation of cleavable complexes between DNA and topoisomerase I or II (Atwell *et al.*, 1987; Finlay *et al.*, 1993). The drug has shown activity against multidrug-resistant human tumor cell lines (Baguley *et al.*, 1990, 1992; Finlay *et al.*, 1993), and subcutaneously implanted Lewis lung tumors in mice with little myelosuppression at the curative dose (Finlay *et al.*, 1989). On the basis of its novel mechanism of action and promising antitumor activity, DACA was selected for clinical development (McCrystal *et al.*, 1999, Twelves *et al.*, 1999). DACA is a lipophilic compound with an octanol/water partition coefficient of 5 (Cornford *et al.*, 1992). This property, together with the suppression of ionization of the acridine nitrogen at physiologic pH, was considered attractive for this class of compounds with regard to better distributive properties and the ability to cross the blood–brain barrier to reach brain tumors. The high lipophilicity may also be responsible for the high uptake of DACA and metabolites (Cornford *et al.*, 1992; Osman *et al.*, 1997) into normal brain and dose-limiting neurotoxicity observed after intravenous administration of DACA to mice (Paxton *et al.*, 1992).

A number of important translational research questions were posed, including whether (1) the metabolite profile of DACA was altered in humans as compared with preclinical models, (2) the drug distributed well to human tumors (predictive of activity), and (3) the degree of uptake into normal tissues was high, e.g., brain (predictive of neurotoxicity). To address these issues, carbon-11-labeled DACA ([^{11}C]DACA) was synthesized as illustrated in Fig. 1 and employed in a pre-phase-I radiotracer study to evaluate the tissue pharmacokinetics and plasma metabolite profile of DACA. Pre-phase-I studies were performed at a radiotracer dose equivalent to 1/1000 of the phase I starting dose (Harte *et al.*, 1996, Saleem *et al.*, 2001). Analysis of plasma samples in this and other studies showed that [^{11}C]DACA/DACA was extensively metabolized (Osman *et al.*, 1997; Schofield *et al.*, 1999). Typical PET images and time–activity curves (TACs) demonstrating localization of [^{11}C]DACA-derived radioactivity are shown in Figs. 2 (see color insert) and 3, respectively. Radioactivity localized in the order vertebra < brain < tumor < kidney < lung < myocardium < spleen < liver. The low peak concentrations and overall distribution of [^{11}C]DACA-derived radioactivity attained in vertebra and brain suggested that myelotoxicity and neurotoxicity were less likely to be dose limiting. In contrast, high localization of radioactivity was observed in the myocardium (which was saturable at phase I doses), which suggests that cardiovascular toxicities could be dose limiting. Tumor uptake of [^{11}C]DACA was variable and moderately correlated with blood flow (Harte *et al.*, 1996; Saleem *et al.*, 2001). A summary of pharmacokinetic parameters for [^{11}C]DACA are presented in Table 2 (Meikle *et al.*, 1998).

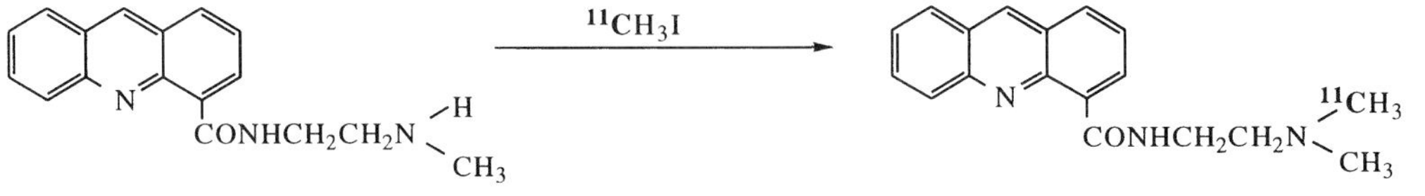

FIGURE 1 Radiosynthesis of [^{11}C]DACA. DACA was radiolabeled in the *N*-methyl position with carbon-11 by reaction of the *N*-desmethyl precursor with [^{11}C]iodomethane.

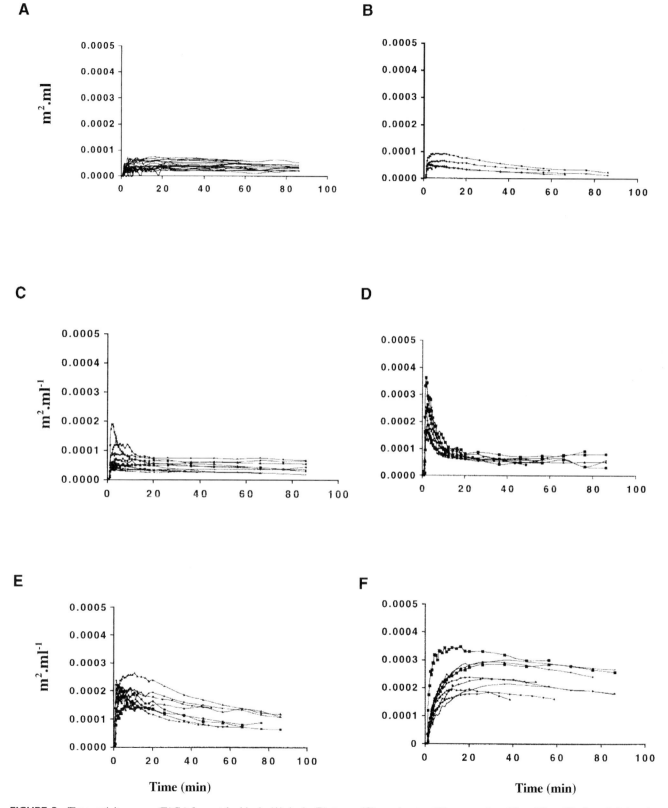

FIGURE 3 Time–activity curves (TACs) for vertebral body (**A**), brain (**B**), tumor (**C**), renal cortex (**D**), myocardium (**E**) and liver (**F**) after administration of tracer amounts of [^{11}C]DACA. The TACs were corrected for decay and normalized for injected dose per body surface area. The radioactive concentration on the y axis is, therefore, represented in units of m^2/ml. Mean TACs are illustrated when more than one region of interest was marked on a tissue organ.

TABLE 2
Pharmacokinetic Parameters for DACA
Calculated Using Spectral Analysis

Tissue	V_D	K_1 (min^{-1})	MRT (min)	$T_{1/2z}$ (min)
Liver ($n = 7$)	858	0.42	2012	41.0
Kidney ($n = 9$)	680	1.02	678	3.7
Spleen ($n = 5$)	804	0.90	920	21.0
Lung ($n = 24$)	131	0.66	194	1.2
Brain ($n = 4$)	20.6	0.24	80	12.2
Tumour ($n = 20$)	203	0.42	521	22.9

V_D, Volume of distribution; K_1, plasma to tissue transfer rate constant; MRT, mean residence time; $T_{1/2z}$, terminal elimination half-life.
Modified from Meikle *et al.*, 1998.

2. Temozolomide: Pharmacokinetics and Mode of Action Studies

Temozolomide is an imidazotetrazine derivative which, unlike dacarbazine, does not require metabolic activation to alkylate DNA (Mizuno *et al.*, 1976; Stevens and Newlands, 1993). It has good oral bioavailability and has shown activity against high-grade gliomas (Bower *et al.*, 1997, Brock *et al.*, 1998; Newlands *et al.*, 1996), malignant melanomas (Bleehen *et al.*, 1995), and pediatric solid tumors (Estlin *et al.*, 1998; Nicholson *et al.*, 1998). No activity was seen against untreated low-grade lymphomas (Woll *et al.*, 1995) and nasopharyngeal carcinomas (Chan *et al.*, 1998). The mechanism of action of temozolomide is thought to involve ring opening and decarboxylation to 5-(3-methyl)-1-yl)imidazole-4-carboxamide. This is converted to the methyldiazonium ion, which alkylates DNA.

Alkylation of DNA guanine in the O^6 position may be the primary cytotoxic event (Newlands *et al.*, 1997). Increased activity of O^6-alkylguanine-DNA alkyltransferase or an acquired deficiency of DNA mismatch repair can produce resistance to this agent. Because the activation of temozolomide is base catalyzed, pH is an important consideration for its action. Brain tumors, which are generally more alkaline (Vaupel *et al.*, 1989), have been shown to be more responsive to temozolomide (Newlands *et al.*, 1996). It was envisaged that knowledge about biodistribution in tumor and normal tissue, and on mechanism of action, could be important for patient selection and for optimizing therapy, such as through biochemical modulation or scheduling.

Temozolomide has been labeled with carbon-11 in either the 3-*N*-methyl or the 4-carbonyl position (Brown *et al.*, 1994) (Fig. 4). PET pharmacokinetic studies with [^{11}C-*methyl*]temozolomide in patients with high-grade glioma showed that temozolomide is distributed to brain tumors to a higher extent than to contralateral normal brain (Fig. 5; see color insert) (Brock *et al.*, 1996). Within the scan time (60–90 min) the differences in radiotracer kinetics could be explained by differences in influx rather than in washout. The exposure of tumors to [^{11}C-*methyl*]temozolomide-derived radioactivity correlated with patient response duration but not survival (Brock *et al.*, 1998). Ongoing work involves clinical evaluation/confirmation of the proposed mode of action of temozolomide in humans. It was proposed that labeling the compound in the 3-*N*-methyl position results in incorporation of the radiolabel in DNA, whereas labeling in the 4-carbonyl position results in the loss of label as [^{11}C]CO_2 in expired air, prior to its incorporation into DNA. Paired clinical studies are

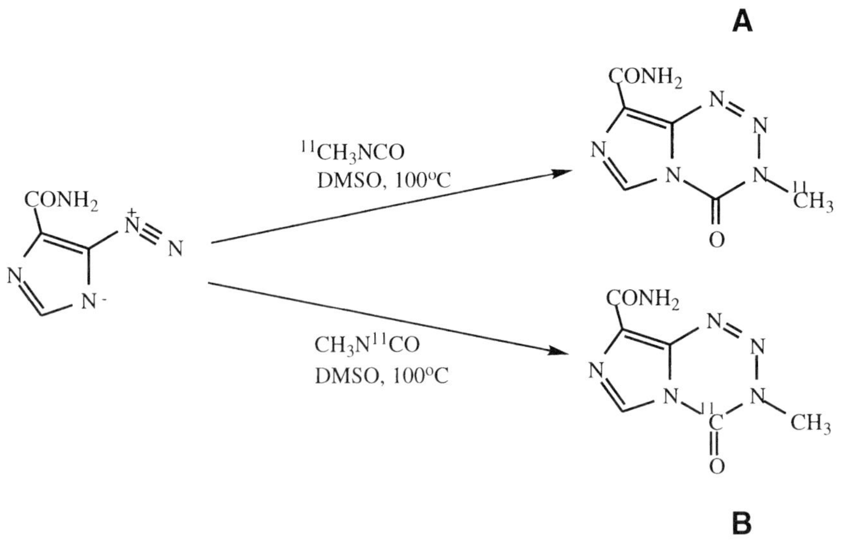

FIGURE 4 Radiosynthesis of [^{11}C]temozolomide in the 3-*N*-methyl and 4-carbonyl positions. Reaction of [^{11}C]methyl isocyanate or [^{11}C-carbonyl]methylisocyanate with the appropriate stable 5-diazoimidazole-4-carboxamide precursor resulted in the production of [^{11}C-*methyl*]temozolomide (**A**) and [^{11}C-*carbonyl*]temozolomide (**B**), respectively.

currently underway to confirm this. These studies have so far demonstrated higher levels of plasma and exhaled [^{11}C]CO$_2$ for [^{11}C-*carbonyl*]temozolomide compared with [^{11}C-*methyl*]temozolomide (Saleem *et al.*, unpublished data).

3. 5-Fluorouracil: Pharmacokinetics and Biomodulation Studies

The synthetic pyrimidine 5-fluorouracil (5-FU) is the most commonly used anticancer agent for the management of gastrointestinal malignancies (Chen and Grem, 1992, Grem, 1991). The drug undergoes anabolism to nucleosides and nucleotides, which inhibit RNA processing and DNA synthesis. The latter occurs mainly via inhibition of thymidylate synthetase, a key enzyme in the *de novo* synthesis of DNA. Up to 80% of systemically administered 5-FU is degraded through catabolism to α-fluoro-β-alanine (FBAL) (Pinedo and Peters, 1988). The antitumor activity of 5-FU is limited with response rates of the order of 20% (Kemeny, 1983), and the drug has not consistently improved survival when administered alone or in combination with other antineoplastic agents (Lavin *et al.*, 1980; Richards *et al.*, 1986). Approaches to enhance its efficacy by biochemical modulation have been tried, and combination with folinic acid has improved its efficacy, albeit modestly (Anonymous, 1992).

The pharmacokinetics of 5-FU has been studied with radiotracers. The ease in the chemical synthesis of 5-[^{18}F]FU (Brown *et al.*, 1993; Vine *et al.*, 1979) (Fig. 6) and the favorable half-life of fluorine ($t_{1/2} = 110$ min) have made it the most often monitored anticancer drug in PET (Dimitrakopoulou *et al.*, 1993; Dimitrakopoulou-Strauss *et al.*, 1998a, b; Harte *et al.*, 1999; Hohenberger *et al.*, 1993; Kissel *et al.*, 1997; Moehler *et al.*, 1998; Saleem *et al.*, 2000). 5-[^{18}F]FU kinetic studies can be performed with good reproducibility (Harte *et al.*, 1998). Figures 7 and 8 (see color insert) and Fig. 9 illustrate dynamic PET images and corresponding decay-corrected TACs for 5-FU in tumor and normal tissues. It can be inferred from these studies that the high signal intensity in normal liver represents

its capacity to catabolize 5-[^{18}F]FU to [^{18}F]FBAL (HPLC analysis of arterial plasma have confirmed the presence of 5-[^{18}F]FU and high levels of [^{18}F]FBAL, and MRS studies have confirmed the presence of FBAL) (Brix *et al.*, 1998). The increase in kidney activity with time is consistent with elimination of 5-FU and metabolites. A pharmacodynamic relationship between the tumor uptake of 5-FU and response, first seen in mice (Shani *et al.*, 1977) has also been demonstrated in humans by PET methods (Dimitrakopoulou-Strauss *et al.*, 1998b; Moehler *et al.*, 1998). Dimitrakopoulou-Strauss *et al.* (1998) demonstrated that colorectal liver metastases with a higher uptake of 5-FU at 2 h, as measured by a standard uptake value (SUV) greater than 3, had a negative growth rate, whereas those with SUV less than 2 showed disease progression. These studies have confirmed a similar relationship seen with MRS studies (Presant *et al.*, 1990, 1994).

The biomodulation of tumor and normal tissue 5-[^{18}F]FU pharmacokinetics by *N*-phosphonacetyl-L-aspartate (PALA), folinic acid, and interferon-α has been assessed (Harte *et al.*, 1999). Blood flow to the tumor was found to be an important determinant of tumor exposure to total ^{18}F radioactivity (consisting of ^{18}F-radiolabeled 5-FU, anabolites, and catabolites). The importance of drug delivery in the initial uptake and retention of radioactivity uptake was supported by a significant correlation between tumor blood flow and tissue exposure to ^{18}F radioactivity at 8 and 60 min. Blood flow to the tumor, and hence tumor exposure to ^{18}F activity, decreased significantly ($p < 0.05$) after modulation with PALA, and a nonsignificant increase was seen with interferon-γ. On the other hand, no changes in tumor pharmacokinetics were seen with folinic acid biomodulation (Harte *et al.*, 1999).

An important aspect of current 5-FU research is to determine the effect of inactivating the proximal and rate limiting catabolic enzyme, dihydropyrimidine dehydrogenase (DPD), on tumor and normal tissue pharmacokinetics of 5-[^{18}F]FU. Saleem *et al.* (2000) have demonstrated that in eniluracil-naïve patients, 5-[^{18}F]FU-derived radioactivity localized more

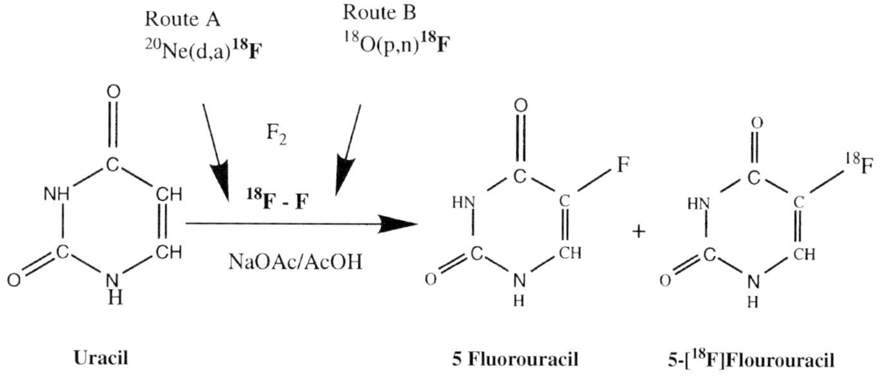

FIGURE 6 Radiochemical synthesis of 5-[^{18}F]FU using [^{18}F]fluorine by two different nuclear methods. Route B produces high level of [^{18}F]fluorine and 5-[^{18}F]FU produced using this route is associated with high specific activity (25–46 MBq μmol^{-1}) with a low stable 5-FU (carrier) content (30–55 μmol).

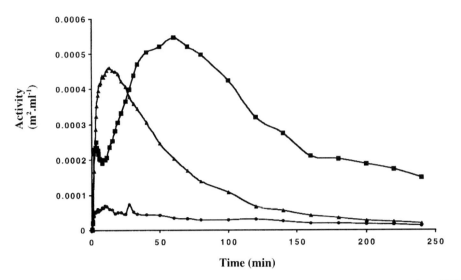

FIGURE 9 Time–activity (TACs) curves for liver (▲), kidney (■) and tumor metastasis (●) generated for the patient whose PET images have been illustrated in Figs. 9 and 10. The TACs were corrected for decay and normalized to the injected dose per body surface area. The activity in the y axis is, therefore, represented in units of m^2/ml. The liver TACs showed a large peak at about 10 min, followed by a slow fall. This is due to rapid catabolism of 5-[^{18}F]FU followed by retention of [^{18}F]FBAL, which is eliminated slowly from the liver. This elimination of fluorine-18 radioactivity (down slope) from the liver occurs in concert with an increase in activity resulting from uptake and excretion within the kidney. The TACs for tumor metastases show decreased uptake of the radiotracer compared with normal liver and kidney.

strongly (0.0234% of the injected activity per milliliter at 11 min) in normal liver than in liver metastases (0.0032%). Furthermore, there was a distinct localization of radioactivity in the gall bladder consistent with hepatobiliary clearance of [^{18}F]FBAL-bile acid conjugates (Saleem *et al.*, 2000). After eniluracil administration, a substantial inhibition of radiotracer exposure in normal liver and kidneys was seen (Saleem *et al.*, 2000). Other effects observed in eniluracil-treated patients were the absence of hepatobiliary clearance and an increase in plasma uracil and unmetabolized 5-[^{18}F]FU levels. Of importance to the efficacy of the eniluracil-5-FU combination, radiotracer half-life in tumors increased from 2.3 hr to more than 4 h. These studies demonstrated the power of noninvasive imaging in *in vivo* imaging of drug action. Examples of other radiolabeled anticancer agents that have been studied using PET are given in Table 3.

C. Pharmacodynamic Studies

PET offers an exciting opportunity to monitor key pathways involved in malignant transformation due to the ability to radiolabel and image the behavior of several biological probes. In this section, we will describe how PET can be used to monitor various targets, including genes, antigens, ligand–receptor interactions, and pathways involved in signal transduction, cell cycle, cell death, drug resistance, and angiogenesis.

1. Assessment of Drug–Receptor Interaction

Several growth factors produce their therapeutic effects by interacting with specific receptors or binding to cell surface

molecules. It is possible to study such drug–receptor interactions with ligands or antibodies radiolabelled with a positron emitter. The use of PET to study drug–receptor interactions is well known in the fields of neurology and psychiatry. Such studies can be direct (labeling the molecule of interest) or indirect (displacement of radioligand by the molecule of inter-

TABLE 3
Examples of Studies Carried Out Using Labeled Anticancer Agents by PET

Drug studied	Findings
Tamoxifen	Cardiac uptake of [^{18}F]fluorotamoxifen suggested that its cardioprotective benefits may be due to a direct cardioprotective action in addition to lowering serum cholesterol (Inoue *et al.*, 1997).
BCNU	50 times higher tumor drug concentrations were achieved after intra-arterial administration of [^{11}C]BCNU compared to intravenous doses in patients with recurrent gliomas. The degree of early metabolic trapping of BCNU in tumor correlated with the clinical response to BCNU chemotherapy (Tyler *et al.*, 1986).
	Sarcosinamide chloroethylnitrosourea (SarCNU) entered brain tissue most likely by a different mechanism(s) compared with BCNU, which enters brain tissue by diffusion. Data indicated that the use of SarCNU may result in a better tumor-to-brain ratio than BCNU (Mitsuki *et al.*, 1991).
Cisplatin	The pharmacologic advantage of intra-arterial over intravenous administration was assessed and quantified in two glioblastoma patients using [^{13}N]-cisplatin and PET (Ginos *et al.*, 1987).

est). The regional kinetics of radioligands can be used to derive values for receptor number (B_{max}), affinity (K_d), and binding potential (B_{max}/K_d). There are currently radioligands for the estrogen (Katzenellenbogen *et al.*, 1997; VanBrocklin *et al.*, 1994), progesterone (de Groot *et al.*, 1991; Katzenellenbogen *et al.*, 1997), and androgen (Bonasera *et al.*, 1996, Liu *et al.*, 1992) receptors, and radiolabeled antibodies for the erbB2 receptor (Bakir *et al.*, 1992). Drug receptor studies are helpful in (1) assaying target and predicting response and (2) predicting optimal dose.

a. Predicting Response from Assessment of Receptor Occupancy

The majority of breast cancers are hormone dependent, as indicated by an increase in the estrogen receptor (ER) and progesterone receptor (PR) content of breast tumors (Collett *et al.*, 1996; Osborne, 1998). The ER status is an important prognostic factor in the management of breast cancer (Vollenweider-Zeragui *et al.*, 1986) and the clinical course of disease in patients with ER-positive tumors is less aggressive, characterized by a longer disease-free interval and greater overall survival. Moreover, ER-positive tumors are likely to respond to hormonal manipulation. Currently, the receptor status of the tumor is determined by *ex vivo* assays, which provide limited information about the functional status and responsiveness of the receptors to hormone therapy. 16α-[^{18}F]fluoro-17β-estradiol (FES), a radioligand for estrogen receptors, has been used to assess the ER status of breast tu-

mors. Dehdashti *et al.* (1995) found good overall agreement between *ex vivo* (biopsy) ER assays and FES PET (Fig. 10), but not with tumor [^{18}F]FDG PET (a marker for tumor energy metabolism; see Section 3.D). They concluded that FES PET provides unique direct information about breast cancer ER status (Dehdashti *et al.*, 1995). McGuire *et al.* (1991) found a decrease in the uptake of FES in metastatic breast cancers after the administration of tamoxifen. This demonstrated the presence of functional ERs in the tumors. Since the decrease in uptake of FES after tamoxifen is significantly greater in patients who responded to hormonal therapy (Dehdashti *et al.*, 1999), the ER occupancy status can be used to predict response to hormonal therapy. Radioligands for the progesterone receptor, such as 21-[^{18}F]fluoro-16α-methyl-19-norprogesterone (Verhagen *et al.*, 1991) and fluorine-18-labeled progestin $16\alpha,7\alpha$-diaxolanes (Buckman *et al.*, 1995), and antibodies for c-erbB2 (Bakir *et al.*, 1992) also hold promise for the selection of patients for clinical studies.

b. Predicting Optimal Dose from Assessment of Receptor Occupancy

Examples of receptor occupancy studies in oncology that have employed PET imaging for predicting optimum dose are lacking. Due to the importance of such studies, however, we will illustrate the potential with a neuropsychiatry study. Neuroleptic drug action is largely mediated by blockade of dopamine receptors (Creese *et al.*, 1976; Seeman *et al.*, 1976).

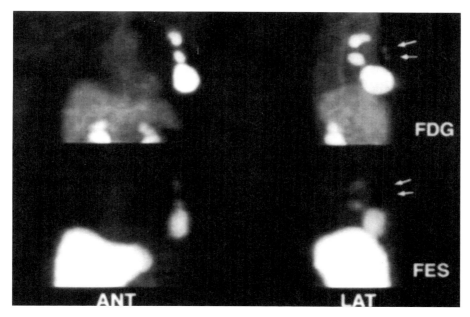

FIGURE 10 Anterior and lateral FDG-PET and FES-PET images of a patient with a primary left breast mass (4.5 cm diameter), and left axillary and internal mammary (*arrows*) nodal metastases. High agreement was demonstrated between *ex vivo* ER assays and FES-PET. However, there was no correlation between FDG uptake and ER status or between tumor FDG and tumor FES uptake. [Reproduced with permission from Dehdashti *et al.*, (1995). Positron tomographic assessment of estrogen receptors in breast cancer: Comparison with FDG-PET and *in vitro* receptor assays. *J. Nucl. Med.* **36**, 1766–1774.]

It has been suggested from PET studies that for classical antipsychotics a threshold D_2 occupancy of 70% is needed for antipsychotic effect and 80% for extrapyramidal side effects (Farde *et al.*, 1989, 1992). This information could be used to compare the receptor occupancy of novel antipsychotic agents and determine the doses needed for the optimum receptor occupancy. Bench *et al.* (1993) used [^{11}C]raclopride (a radioligand for D_2 receptors), to measure the occupancy of central dopamine D_2 receptors by a new neuroleptic, CP-88,059-1. Volunteers received 2–60 mg of CP-88,059-1, 5 h before PET scanning; one subject received placebo only. It was found that binding of [^{11}C]raclopride decreased in a dose-dependent manner and 85% dopamine D_2 receptor occupancy was achieved with the highest dose of CP-88,059-1. From these findings it was suggested that an effective antipsychotic dose should be between 20 mg and 40 mg.

2. Assessment of Intermediate Cascades in Mitogenic Signal Transduction

Efforts are underway to develop agents that inhibit mitogenic signal transduction. This is because signaling mechanisms that drive cell proliferation tend to be associated with malignant transformation. For instance, Gibbs (2000a, b) recently reviewed a number of new compounds targeted against mitogenic signal transduction in development, including monoclonal antibodies, kinase inhibitors, antisense oligonucleotides, and farnesyltransferase inhibitors. With respect to imaging the effects of these agents, we mentioned in Section 3.C.1 the development of antibodies for c-erbB2. This antibody could be used to select patients for treatment with monoclonal antibodies to erbB2 such as herceptin. However, developing end points for intermediate cascades in signal transduction represents a significant challenge. This is because molecular events, such as changes in phosphorylation and protein–protein interactions, are difficult to measure in intact animals or humans.

One approach for investigating the effect of Ras protein inhibitors has been developed (Hamill *et al.*, 1999). This involves iodination of farnesyltransferase inhibitors that can then be used to measure farnesyltransferase enzyme occupancy. The labeling strategy employed by Hamill and coworkers will permit incorporation of other radioisotopes, such as carbon-11 and fluorine-18 (Hamill *et al.*, 1999). Studies in dogs have already demonstrated enzyme-specific binding of the iodinated radiotracer.

3. Evaluation of Cellular Proliferation and Thymidylate Synthase Inhibition

PET methodology is available for measuring thymidine incorporation into DNA and thus for providing an index of proliferation rate, which may be superior to current methods for monitoring tumor response such as tumor shrinkage and time to progression. PET methods may be superior because response assessment with anatomical images may be confounded by inflammatory or fibrotic masses. Furthermore, metabolic changes may precede changes in size. However, the optimal probe for measuring proliferation is an issue of current debate. 2-[^{11}C]Thymidine is the gold standard for the measurement of proliferation. It has the advantage of being a natural compound, is readily taken up by cells and incorporated into DNA, and has been used extensively in *in vitro* studies (in the form of ^{3}H-thymidine). The main limitation of using 2-[^{11}C]thymidine-PET is its rapid catabolism ultimately to [^{11}C]CO_2. A dual-scan approach comprising an initial scan with [^{11}C]HCO^3 followed after a brief period by a 2-[^{11}C]thymidine scan permits metabolite correction and hence determination of fractional retention of thymidine or incorporation rate constants for thymidine (Eary *et al.*, 1999; Gunn *et al.*, 2000, Mankoff *et al.*, 1998, 1999; Wells *et al.*, 1997).

Wells *et al.* (1997a) have recently shown that fractional uptake of 2-[^{11}C]thymidine-derived radioactivity correlates with a well-known index of cell proliferation, the MIB-1 index, making it a suitable radiotracer for monitoring response to antiproliferative therapy. 2-[^{11}C]Thymidine has been used in a number of pilot studies to measure response to therapy. For example, in patients with metastatic small cell lung cancer and abdominal sarcoma, 2-[^{11}C]thymidine flux constant, measured at 1 week following chemotherapy (compared to baseline), declined by 100% in complete responders and 35% in a partial responder, compared with a much smaller decline (15%) in a patient showing progressive disease (Shields *et al.*, 1998). [^{124}I]Iododeoxyuridine has also been used to measure proliferation (Blasberg *et al.*, 2000). The rapid metabolic deiodination of the radiotracer, however, limited the useful-

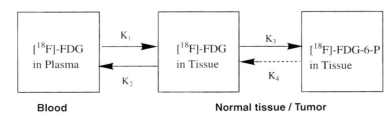

FIGURE 11 Compartmental model for glucose utilization using [^{18}F]fluorodeoxyglucose. K_1, K_2, K_3, and K_4 are rate constants for delivery, washout, phosphorylation, and dephosphorylation, respectively.

ness of this probe *in vivo* (Blasberg *et al.,* 2000). One of the more promising probes for measuring proliferation is 3'-deoxy-3'-[^{18}F]fluorothymidine (FLT) (Shields *et al.,* 1998). This radiotracer is metabolized to a lesser extent than 2-[^{11}C]thymidine. The retention of FLT is determined not only by the degree of proliferation but also by levels of cell-cycle-regulated thymidine kinase-1 protein. Studies are ongoing to evaluate the role of this tracer in clinical imaging of proliferation. Thus far, 2-[^{11}C]thymidine is the most widely used radiotracer for imaging tumor proliferation.

One emerging area of research is the use of thymidine analogues to monitor thymidine salvage kinetics following thymidylate synthase inhibition. Wells *et al.* (1997b) have demonstrated increased fractional retention of 2-[^{11}C]thymidine in tumors 1 h after treatment of patients with the nonclassical thymidylate synthase inhibitor AG-337. Collins *et al.* (1999) are investigating the utility of 2'-[^{18}F]fluoroaradeoxyuridine for imaging thymidylate synthase activity. This will permit selection of patients likely to benefit from therapies with prodrugs that are activated by thymidylate synthase.

D. Evaluation of Tumor Energy Metabolism

[^{18}F]FDG is one of the commonly used radiotracers in PET studies. [^{18}F]FDG follows the same route as glucose into cells where it is phosphorylated by hexokinase to [^{18}F]FDG-6-phosphate. Unlike glucose, there is little further metabolism and [^{18}F]FDG-6-phosphate remains essentially trapped within cells, with the rate of accumulation proportional to the rate of glucose utilization. [^{18}F]FDG-6-phosphate has low membrane permeability and although dephosphorylation does occur, it is very slow in brain, heart, and tumor, which have very low levels of glucose-6-phosphatase. These tissues also have high [^{18}F]FDG uptake, causing FDG to accumulate in them. Based on these facts, [^{18}F]FDG has been extensively used in cardiology to delineate ischemic or dead myocardium under both resting and stressed conditions (Ragosta and Beller, 1993; Schelbert *et al.,* 1982) and by neurologists to study and delineate areas of cerebrovascular disease, epileptic foci, and movement disorders (Kumar *et al.,* 1991; Kushner *et al.,* 1987). FDG uptake in tumors probably reflects a combination of factors, including phosphorylating activity of mitochondria, degree of hypoxia, and levels of glucose transporters, e.g., Glut-1 (Aloj *et al.,* 1999; Chung *et al.,* 1999; Waki *et al.,* 1998).

[^{18}F]FDG is used in oncology to grade tumors, to determine tumor extent as a prognostic indicator, and as a measure of tumor response (Brock *et al.,* 1997; Findlay *et al,* 1996; Haberkorn *et al.,* 1993, Holthoff *et al.,* 1993, Jansson *et al.,* 1995; Ogawa *et al.,* 1988; Okada *et al.,* 1994; Okazumi *et al.,* 1992). [^{18}F]FDG kinetics follow a three-compartment model (Fig. 12; see color insert). The retention of the radiotracer may be calculated as the SUV or metabolic rate of glucose

uptake. As a pharmacodynamic end point (response, survival), [^{18}F]FDG has been used in several relatively small studies to monitor response to treatment. For instance, single-agent (tumor type in parenthesis) evaluation has been performed for temozolomide (glioma) (Brock *et al.,* 2000) and hormone therapy (breast) (Wahl *et al.,* 1993). Evaluation of combination therapies has also been performed, e.g., 5-FU + mitomycin C (pancreatic cancers) (Maisey *et al.,* 2000), 5-FU ± interferon (colorectal liver metastases) (Findlay *et al.,* 1996), and radiotherapy + combination chemotherapy (glioma) (Ogawa *et al.,* 1988). Pharmacodynamic studies with [^{18}F]FDG are usually carried out at baseline and soon after the first or second cycle of therapy. A comparison of [^{18}F]FDG images before and after therapy in a glioma is shown in Fig. 12. The EORTC-PET group has recently published guidelines for common measurement criteria and reporting of alterations in FDG PET studies to facilitate much needed comparison of smaller clinical studies and larger-scale multicenter trials (Young *et al.,* 1999). Tumor response as defined by the group (progressive, stable, partial or complete metabolic response) is based on the observation that, on average, a 15–30% reduction in SUV or metabolic rate of glucose utilization can predict response and that this precedes tumor shrinkage and clinical response (Young *et al.,* 1999).

E. Assessment of Programmed Cell Death (Apoptosis)

Cell death by apoptosis is a pharmacodynamic end point for several anticancer therapies. Current methods for monitoring apoptosis are based on excision of tumors followed by immunohistochemical or flow cytometric analysis. New PET methodologies hold promise for detecting apoptosis in patient tumors over time. The probe most amenable to PET studies is annexin V, an endogenous protein that has high affinity for membrane-bound phosphatidylserine. An early event in apoptosis is the rapid exposure of phosphatidylserine groups, which are normally confined to the inside of the cell. Binding of radiolabeled annexin V to such phosphatidylserine groups allows such dying cells to be detected. Annexin V has been labeled with ^{99m}Tc for imaging with single-photon computed tomography (Blankenberg *et al.,* 1998, 1999). Annexin V has also been labeled with ^{124}I for PET studies (Glaser *et al.,* unpublished). These radiotracer are currently being validated in preclinical models.

F. Assessment of Angiogenic Growth Factors and Blood Flow

Angiogenesis, the sprouting of capillaries from preexisting vasculature, represents an important target for anticancer drug development. Two main therapeutic approaches are being pursued, including (1) inhibition of processes that constitute the angiogenic phenotype, such as high vascular endothelial growth factor (VEGF) and growth factor receptor activity (antiangiogenic agents), and (2) inhibition of blood flow (antivascular agents). PET methods are being developed to measure parameters related to the angiogenic phenotype. For example, Carroll *et al.* (2000) have demonstrated the feasibility of imaging VEGF factor in mice bearing human xenografts with a [^{124}I]anti-VEGF. To assess the effects of the antivascular agent combretastatin A4 on tumor blood flow and blood volume, Anderson *et al.* (2000) performed PET scans with [^{15}O]H$_2$O and [^{15}O]CO, respectively, as part of a UK Cancer Research Campaign phase I trial. At higher doses, a 30–60% decrease in tumor blood flow was seen in four of five patients at 30 min resolving in three of four patients by 24 h (Anderson *et al.*, 2000). It is anticipated that these types of pharmacodynamic assessment will cut down the time involved in early clinical trials and provide a more objective assessment of new agents.

G. Assessment of Resistance Mechanism and Modulation of Drug Resistance

One of the main reasons for failure of anticancer therapy is resistance to drug treatment. Thus, anticancer strategies are being developed to circumvent resistance, making therapy more efficacious. PET methods can be used to monitor drug resistance mechanisms and aid in the selection of patients likely to benefit from such therapies and as pharmacodynamic end points to assess the activity of modulators.

1. Multidrug Resistance

Multidrug resistance (MDR) is a major obstacle in the treatment of cancer with classes of compounds such as anthracyclines, *Vinca* alkaloids, and podophyllotoxins (Bellamy *et al.*, 1990; Gottesmann and Pastan, 1993). It is considered to be due to multifactorial mechanisms (Zijlstra *et al.*, 1987), such as the presence of drug efflux pumps P-glycoprotein (Pgp) and multidrug-resistance-associated protein (MRP). Modulators of Pgp mediated efflux, including verapamil, cyclosporin A, and PSC-833, which are also Pgp substrates, have been used to circumvent MDR. However, their effect so far in the management of solid cancers has been disappointing (Hendrick *et al.*, 1991; Rodenburg *et al.*, 1991; Wood *et al.*, 1998). ^{99m}Tc-SESTAMIBI [hexakis(2-methoxy-isobutylisonitrile)technetium(I)]-SPECT is the most common noninvasive method used for assessing MDR with decreased accumulation in MDR proficient tumors. Kostakoglu *et al.* (1997) demonstrated accumulation of ^{99m}Tc-SESTAMIBI in breast and lung tumors expressing lower amounts of Pgp. A 2.7-fold higher efflux rate (Vecchio *et al.*, 1997) and a more rapid tumor clearance ($t_{1/2} < 204$ min) of ^{99m}Tc-SESTAMIBI have been demonstrated in breast cancers with high Pgp expression (Ciarmiello *et al.*, 1998). Pgp modulation by PSC-833 was associated with an increase in the accumulation of ^{99m}Tc-SESTAMIBI in tumors and liver of treated patients (Fig. 13) (Chen, 1997).

PET studies aimed at assessing MDR have so far been confined to *in vitro* and *in vivo* studies of animals. *In vitro* studies with [^{11}C]daunorubicin and [^{11}C]verapamil have shown a 16-fold accumulation of [^{11}C]daunorubicin in drug-sensitive cells compared with Pgp-expressing human ovarian carcinoma cells (Elsinga *et al.*, 1996). Addition of verapamil resulted in increased accumulation of [^{11}C]daunorubicin in the resistant cells, confirming the modulatory nature of verapamil on Pgp (Elsinga *et al.*, 1996). Similarly, *in vivo* rat studies have shown a lesser accumulation of [^{11}C]verapamil in Pgp-overexpressing tumors compared with Pgp-negative ones. Modulation of Pgp has also been demonstrated by an 18-fold increase in [^{11}C]verapamil accumulation after pretreatment with cyclosporin A (Hendrikse *et al.*, 1999).

2. Tumor Hypoxia

Hypoxia in tumors results from an inadequate supply of oxygen to cells due to the inefficient and aberrant vasculature within tumors. These hypoxic cells are resistant to conventional radiotherapy and certain chemotherapeutic agents. [^{18}F]Fluoromisonidazole has been used as a PET marker to quantitate hypoxia in tumors (Casciari *et al.*, 1995; Koh *et al.*, 1995; Rasey *et al.*, 1996). Other hypoxia markers, such as SR-4554 and ^{64}Cu-ATSM, are being developed for similar *in vivo* assessment (Aboagye *et al.*, 1998, Lewis *et al.*, 1999). Rassey *et al.* (1996), using [^{18}F]fluoromisonidazole as a marker, found that hypoxia was present in 36 of 37 tumors studied. They also found that the extent of hypoxia varied markedly among tumors in the same site or of the same histology and that there was a heterogeneous distribution of hypoxia between regions within a single tumor. Such knowledge gained noninvasively about tumor hypoxia could find utility in the selection of patients for therapy with radiation, bioreductive agents, antiangiogenic agents, antivascular agents, and hypoxia-targeted gene therapy.

H. Gene Expression

Monitoring of gene expression is an area where PET imaging has a major contribution to make (Weissleder, 1999; Wunderbaldinger *et al.*, 2000) to preclinical and clinical drug development. Several analogues of uracil and gancyiclovir are being developed for this purpose (Gambhir *et al.*, 1999; Tjuvajev *et al.*, 1998). These analogues undergo phosphorylation (and trapping) when herpes simplex virus type 1 thymidine kinase (HSV-1tk) is expressed and can be used in monitoring HSV-1tk gene therapy (Fig. 14; see color insert) or as *in vivo* reporter probes (Gambhir *et al.*, 1999). It is hoped that these techniques will facilitate assessment of the location and level of gene expression over time.

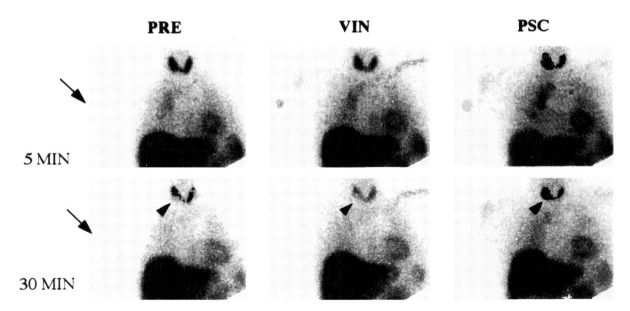

FIGURE 13 Baseline (PRE), post vinblastine (VIN), and PSC-833 (PSC) images obtained 5 and 30 min after injection of SESTAMIBI. Improved and prolonged visualization of tumor in the right deltoid (*arrows*) and right lung with PSC-833 is seen. A right-sided thyroid nodule appears as a cold defect on the PRE and VIN studies at 30 min but as a "hot" nodule on the PSC-833 study (*arrowheads*). Following PSC-833 treatment, there was increased retention of SETAMIBI in liver, tumor, and the right-sided thyroid nodule but not in the lung, consistent with modulation of P-glycoprotein in these tissues. (From Chen *et al.*, 1997.)

I. ADEPT

Several therapies are being developed in oncology to selectively target cancer cells. *In vivo* monitoring of such novel therapies would aid objective assessment of such strategies in patients. Antibody-directed enzyme prodrug therapy (ADEPT) has been explored to increase efficacy (Blakey *et al.*, 1995). ADEPT is based on the delivery to cancer cells of a nontoxic antibody–enzyme conjugate. After a suitable time to allow for clearance of unbound conjugate, a nontoxic prodrug/drug is administered, which is selectively converted to a toxic compound. By labeling the prodrug or conjugates with a positron emitter, it would be possible to quantitate distribution of the prodrug or conjugate. This will provide information on the selectivity of this therapy for tumors and normal tissues and aid in the appropriate timing of therapy. A prodrug that is a substrate for carboxypeptidase G2 has been labeled with carbon-11 for monitoring the ADEPT approach (Inoue *et al.*, 1997; Prenant *et al.*, 1997).

4. Conclusions

Advances in technology have made *in vivo* assessment of physiological/biochemical measurements in humans and its incorporation in clinical research a reality. This has been achieved by effective collaboration of multidisciplinary research teams, including chemists, clinicians, pharmacologists, imaging scientists, and mathematical modelers. PET is an invaluable tool in assessing drugs preclinically and screening drug analogues prior to further development. Clinical assessment of drugs with PET can lead to optimization of drug dosing and scheduling. In addition, oncology presents a unique situation where PET can be used. Understanding the mechanism of actions of anticancer drugs and detecting the extent of resistance will lead to the optimization of therapy and open channels for alternative drug discovery. Newer therapies pose further challenges to conventional methods of drug analysis. PET methodology needs to be further developed to go hand in hand as a translational tool in the assessment of newer therapies, thereby reducing the gap between drug discovery and clinical application.

Acknowledgment

The authors thank Professor Terry Jones for suggestions and critical appraisal of the manuscript.

References

Aboagye, E. O., Kelson, A. B., Tracy, M., and Workman, P. (1998). Preclinical development and current status of the fluorinated 2-nitroimidazole hypoxia probe N-(2-hydroxy-3,3,3-trifluoropropyl)-2-(2-nitro-1-imidazolyl) acetamide (SR 4554, CRC 94/17): a non-invasive diagnostic probe for the measurement of tumor hypoxia by magnetic resonance spectroscopy and imaging, and by positron emission tomography. *Anticancer Drug Des.* **13**(6), 703–730.

Aloj, L., Caraco, C., Jagoda, E., Eckelman, W. C., and Neumann, R. D. (1999). Glut-1 and hexokinase expression: relationship with 2-fluoro-2-deoxy-D-glucose uptake in A431 and T47D cells in culture. *Cancer Res.* **59**(18), 4709–4714.

Anderson, H., Jap, J., and Price, P. (2000). Measurement of tumour and normal tissue perfusion (NT) by positron emission tomography (PET) in the evaluation of antivascular therapy: results in the phase I study of combretastatin A4 phosphate (CA4P). *Proc. Am. Soc. Clin. Oncol.* **19**, 179a.

Anonymous. (1992). Modulation of fluorouracil by leucovorin in patients with advanced colorectal cancer: evidence in terms of response rate. Advanced Colorectal Cancer Meta-Analysis Project. *J. Clin. Oncol.* **10**, 896–903.

Atwell, G. J., Rewcastle, G. W., Baguley, B. C., and Denny W. A. (1987). Potential antitumor agents. 50. In vivo solid-tumor activity of derivatives of N-[2-(dimethylamino)ethyl]acridine-4-carboxamide. *J. Med. Chem.* **30**, 664–669.

Baguley, B. C., Holdaway, K. M., and Fray, L. M. (1990). Design of DNA intercalators to overcome topoisomerase II-mediated multidrug resistance. *J. Natl. Cancer Inst.* **82**, 398–402.

Baguley, B. C., Finlay, G. J., and Ching L. M. (1992). Resistance mechanisms to topoisomerase poisons: the application of cell culture methods. *Oncol. Res.* **4**, 267–274.

Bakir, M. A., Eccles, S., Babich, J.W., Aftab, N., Styles, J., Dean, C. J., et al. (1992). c-erbB2 protein overexpression in breast cancer as a target for PET using iodine-124-labeled monoclonal antibodies. *J. Nucl. Med.* **33**, 2154–2160.

Bellamy, W. T., Dalton, W. S., and Dorr, R. T. (1990). The clinical relevance of multidrug resistance. *Cancer Invest.* **8**, 547–562.

Bench, C. J., Lammertsma, A. A., Dolan, R. J., Grasby, P. M., Warrington, S. J., Gunn, K., et al. (1993). Dose dependent occupancy of central dopamine D2 receptors by the novel neuroleptic CP-88,059-01: a study using positron emission tomography and ^{11}C-raclopride. *Psychopharmacology* **112**, 308–314.

Blakey, D. C., Burke, P. J., Davies, D. H., Dowell, R. I., Melton, R. G., Springer, C. J., et al. (1995). Antibody-directed enzyme prodrug therapy (ADEPT) for treatment of major solid tumour disease. *Biochem. Soc. Trans.* **23**, 1047–1050.

Blankenberg, F. G., Katsikis, P. D., Tait, J. F., Davis, R. E., Naumovski, L., Ohtsuki, K., et al. (1998). In vivo detection and imaging of phosphatidylserine expression during programmed cell death. *Proc. Natl. Acad. Sci. USA* **95**, 6349–6354.

Blankenberg, F. G., Katsikis, P. D., Tait, J. F., Davis, R. E., Naumovski, L., Ohtsuki, K., et al. (1999). Imaging of apoptosis (programmed cell death) with 99mTc annexin V. *J. Nucl. Med.* **40**, 184–191.

Blasberg, R.G., Roelcke, U., Weinreich, R., Beattie, B., von Ammon, K., Yonekawa, Y., et al. (2000). Imaging brain tumor proliferative activity with [^{124}I]iododeoxyuridine. *Cancer Res.* **60**, 624–635.

Bleehen, N. M., Newlands, E. S., Lee, S. M., Thatcher, N., Selby, P., Calvert, A. H., et al. (1995). Cancer Research Campaign phase II trial of temozolomide in metastatic melanoma. *J. Clin. Oncol.* **13**, 910–913.

Bonasera, T. A., O'Neil, J. P., Xu, M., Dobkin, J. A., Cutler, P. D., Lich, L. L., et al. (1996). Preclinical evaluation of fluorine-18-labeled androgen receptor ligands in baboons. *J. Nucl. Med.* **37**, 1009–1015.

Bower, M., Newlands, E. S., Bleehen, N. M., Brada, M., Begent, R. J., Calvert, H., et al. (1997). Multicentre CRC phase II trial of temozolomide in recurrent or progressive high-grade glioma. *Cancer Chemother. Pharmacol.* **40**, 484–488.

Brady, F., Luthra, S. K., Tochon-Danguy, H. J., Steel, C. J., Waters S. L., Kensett, M. J., et al. (1991). Asymmetric synthesis of a precursor for the automated radiosynthesis of S-(3'-t-butylamino-2'-hydroxypropoxy)-benzimidazol-2-[^{11}C]one (S- [^{11}C]CGP 12177) as a preferred radioligand for beta-adrenergic receptors. *Int. J. Radiat. Appl. Instrum. A* **42**, 621–628.

Brix, G., Bellemann, M. E., Gerlach, L., and Haberkorn, U. (1998). Intra- and extracellular fluorouracil uptake: assessment with contrast-enhanced metabolic F-19 MR imaging. *Radiology* **209**, 259–267.

Brock, C. S., Matthews, J. C., Brown, G., Luthra, S. K., Brady, F., Newlands, E. S., et al. (1996). The kinetic behavior of temozolomide in man. *Proc. Am. Soc. Clin. Oncol.* **15**, 475.

Brock, C. S., Matthews, J. C., Brown, G., Osman, S., Evans, H., Newlands, E. S., et al. (1998). Response to temozolomide (TEM) in recurrent high grade gliomas (HGG) is related to tumour drug concentration. *Ann. Oncol.* (Suppl. 1), **9**, 174.

Brock, C. S., Meikle, S. R., and Price, P. (1997). Does fluorine-18 fluorodeoxyglucose metabolic imaging of tumours benefit oncology? *Eur. J. Nucl. Med.* **24**, 691–705.

Brock, C. S., Newlands, E. S., Wedge, S. R., Bower, M., Evans, H., Colquhoun, I., et al. (1998). Phase I trial of temozolomide using an extended continuous oral schedule. *Cancer Res.* **58**, 4363–4367.

Brock, C. S., Young, H., O'Reilly, S. M., Matthews, J., Osman, S., Evans, H, et al. (2000). Early evaluation of tumour metabolic response using [18F]fluorodeoxyglucose and positron emission tomography: a pilot study following the phase II chemotherapy schedule for temozolomide in recurrent high-grade gliomas. *Br. J. Cancer* **82**, 608–615.

Brown, G. D., Khan, S. R., Steel, C. J., Luthra, S. K., Osman, S., Hume, S. P., et al. (1993). A practical synthesis of 5-[18F]fluorouracil using HPLC and a study of its metabolic profile in rats. *J. Label Comp. Radiopharm.* **32**, 521–522.

Brown, G. D., Turton, D. R., Luthra, S. K., Price, P., Jones, T., Stevens, M. F. G., et al. (1994). Synthesis of [11C-methyl]methylisocyanate and application of microwave heating to labelling the novel anticancer agent Temozolomide. *J. Label Comp. Radiopharm.* **35**, 100–103.

Buckman, B. O., Bonasera, T. A., Kirschbaum, K. S., Welch, M. J., and Katzenellenbogen, J. A. (1995). Fluorine-18-labeled progestin 16 alpha, 17 alpha-dioxolanes: development of high-affinity ligands for the progesterone receptor with high in vivo target site selectivity. *J. Med. Chem.* **38**, 328–337.

Budinger, T. F. (1998). PET instrumentation: what are the limits? *Semin. Nucl. Med.* **28**, 247–267.

Carroll, V. A., Glaser, M., Aboagye, E., Brown, D., Luthra, S., Brady, F., et al. (2000). Imaging vascular endothelial growth factor in vivo with positron emission tomography. *Br. J. Cancer* **83**(Suppl. 1), 30.

Casciari, J. J., Graham, M. M., and Rasey, J. S. (1995). A modeling approach for quantifying tumor hypoxia with [F-18]fluoromisonidazole PET time-activity data. *Med. Phys.* **22**, 1127–1139.

Chan, A. T., Leung, T. W., Kwan, W. H., Mok, T. S., Yeo, W., Lai. M., et al. (1998). Phase II study of Temodal in the treatment of patients with advanced nasopharyngeal carcinoma. *Cancer Chemother. Pharmacol.* **42**, 247–249.

Chen, A. P., and Grem, J. L. (1992). Antimetabolites. *Curr. Opin. Oncol.* **4**, 1089–1098.

Chen, C. C., Meadows, B., Regis, J., Kalafsky, G., Fojo, T., Carrasquillo, J. A., et al. (1997). Detection of in vivo P-glycoprotein inhibition by PSC 833 using Tc-99m sestamibi. *Clin. Cancer Res.* **3**, 545–552.

Cho, Z. H., Chan, J. K., Ericksson, L., Singh, M., Graham, S., MacDonald, N. S., et al. (1975). Positron ranges obtained from biomedically important positron-emitting radionuclides. *J. Nucl. Med.* **16**, 1174–1176.

Chung, J. K., Lee, Y. J., Kim, C., Choi, S. R., Kim, M., Lee, K., et al. (1999). Mechanisms related to [18F]fluorodeoxyglucose uptake of human colon cancers transplanted in nude mice. *J. Nucl. Med.* **40**, 339–346.

Ciarmiello, A., Del Vecchio, S., Silvestro, P., Potena, M. I., Carriero, M. V., Thomas, R., et al. (1998). Tumor clearance of technetium 99m-sestamibi as a predictor of response to neoadjuvant chemotherapy for locally advanced breast cancer. *J. Clin. Oncol.* **16**, 1677–1683.

Collett, K., Hartveit, F., Skjaerven, R., and Maehle, B. O. (1996). Prognostic role of oestrogen and progesterone receptors in patients with breast cancer: relation to age and lymph node status. *J. Clin. Pathol.* **49**, 920–925.

Collins, J. M., Klecker, R. W., and Katki, A. G. (1999). Suicide prodrugs activated by thymidylate synthase: rationale for treatment and noninvasive imaging of tumors with deoxyuridine analogues. *Clin. Cancer Res.* **5,** 1976–1981.

Cornford, E. M., Young, D., and Paxton, J. W. (1992). Comparison of the blood–brain barrier and liver penetration of acridine antitumor drugs. *Cancer Chemother. Pharmacol* **29,** 439–444.

Creese, I., Burt, D. R., and Snyder, S. H. (1976). Dopamine receptor binding predicts clinical and pharmacological potencies of antischizophrenic drugs. *Science* **192,** 481–483.

Cunningham, V. J., and Jones, T. (1993). Spectral analysis of dynamic PET studies. *J. Cereb. Blood Flow Metab.* **13,** 15–23.

de Groot, T. J., Verhagen, A., Elsinga, P. H., and Vaalburg, W. (1991). Synthesis of [^{18}F]fluoro-labeled progestins for PET. *Int. J. Radiat. Appl. Instrum. A* **42,** 471–474.

Dehdashti, F., Mortimer, J. E., Siegel, B. A., Griffeth, L. K., Bonasera, T. J., Fusselman, M. J., *et al.* (1995). Positron tomographic assessment of estrogen receptors in breast cancer: comparison with FDG-PET and in vitro receptor assays. *J. Nucl. Med.* **36,** 1766–1774.

Dehdashti, F., Flanagan, F. L., Mortimer, J. E., Katzenellenbogen, J. A., Welch, M. J., and Siegel, B. A. (1999). Positron emission tomographic assessment of "metabolic flare" to predict response of metastatic breast cancer to antiestrogen therapy. *Eur. J. Nucl. Med.* **26,** 51–56.

Dimitrakopoulou, A., Strauss, L. G., Clorius, J. H., Ostertag, H., Schlag, P., Heim, M., *et al.* (1993). Studies with positron emission tomography after systemic administration of fluorine-18-uracil in patients with liver metastases from colorectal carcinoma. *J. Nucl. Med.* **34,** 1075–1081.

Dimitrakopoulou-Strauss, A., Strauss, L. G., Schlag, P., Hohenberger, P., Irngartinger, G., Oberdorfer, F., *et al.* (1998a). Intravenous and intraarterial oxygen-15-labeled water and fluorine-18-labeled fluorouracil in patients with liver metastases from colorectal carcinoma. *J. Nucl. Med.* **39,** 465–473.

Dimitrakopoulou-Strauss, A., Strauss, L. G., Schlag, P., Hohenberger, P., Mohler, M., Oberdorfer, F., *et al.* (1998b). Fluorine-18-fluorouracil to predict therapy response in liver metastases from colorectal carcinoma. *J. Nucl. Med.* **39,** 1197–1202.

Eary, J. F., Mankoff, D. A., Spence, A. M., Berger, M. S., Olshen, A., Link, J. M., *et al.* (1999). 2-[C-11]thymidine imaging of malignant brain tumors. *Cancer Res.* **59,** 615–621.

Elsinga, P. H., Franssen, E. J., Hendrikse, N. H., Fluks, L., Weemaes, A. M., van der Graaf, W. T., *et al.* (1996). Carbon-11-labeled daunorubicin and verapamil for probing P-glycoprotein in tumors with PET. *J. Nucl. Med.* **37,** 1571–1575.

Estlin, E. J., Lashford, L., Ablett, S., Price, L., Gowing, R., Gholkar, A., *et al.* (1998). Phase I study of temozolomide in paediatric patients with advanced cancer. United Kingdom Children's Cancer Study Group. *Br. J. Cancer* **78,** 652–661.

Farde, L., Wiesel, F. A., Nordstrom, A. L., and Sedvall, G. (1989). D1- and D2-dopamine receptor occupancy during treatment with conventional and atypical neuroleptics. *Psychopharmacology (Berl)* **99**(Suppl), S28–S31.

Farde, L., Nordstrom, A. L., Wiesel, F. A., Pauli, S., Halldin, C., and Sedvall, G. (1992). Positron emission tomographic analysis of central D1 and D2 dopamine receptor occupancy in patients treated with classical neuroleptics and clozapine. Relation to extrapyramidal side effects. *Arch. Gen. Psychiatry* **49,** 538–544.

Findlay, M., Young, H., Cunningham, D., Iveson, A., Cronin, B., Hickish, T., *et al.* (1996). Noninvasive monitoring of tumor metabolism using fluorodeoxyglucose and positron emission tomography in colorectal cancer liver metastases: correlation with tumor response to fluorouracil. *J. Clin. Oncol.* **14,** 700–708.

Finlay, G. J., and Baguley, B. C. (1989). Selectivity of N-[2-(dimethylamino)ethyl]acridine-4-carboxamide towards Lewis lung carcinoma and human tumour cell lines in vitro. *Eur. J. Cancer Clin. Oncol.* **25,** 271–277.

Finlay, G. J., Marshall, E., Matthews, J. H., Paull, K. D., and Baguley, B. C. (1993). In vitro assessment of N-[2-(dimethylamino)ethyl]acridine-4-carboxamide, a DNA-intercalating antitumour drug with reduced sensitivity to multidrug resistance. *Cancer Chemother. Pharmacol.* **31,** 401–406.

Gambhir, S. S., Barrio, J. R., Phelps, M. E., Iyer, M., Namavari, M., Satyamurthy, N., *et al.* (1999). Imaging adenoviral-directed reporter gene expression in living animals with positron emission tomography. *Proc. Natl. Acad. Sci. USA* **96,** 2333–2338.

Gibbs, J. B. (2000a). Anticancer drug targets: growth factors and growth factor signaling. *J. Clin. Invest.* **105,** 9–13.

Gibbs, J. B. (2000b). Mechanism-based target identification and drug discovery in cancer research. *Science* **287,** 1969–1973.

Ginos, J. Z, Cooper, A. J., Dhawan, V., Lai, J. C., Strother, S. C., Alcock, N., *et al.* (1987). [13N]cisplatin PET to assess pharmacokinetics of intraarterial versus intravenous chemotherapy for malignant brain tumors. *J. Nucl. Med.* **28**(12), 1844–1852.

Gottesman, M. M., and Pastan, I. (1993). Biochemistry of multidrug resistance mediated by the multidrug transporter. *Annu. Rev. Biochem.* **62,** 385–427.

Grem, J. L. (1991). Current treatment approaches in colorectal cancer. *Semin. Oncol.* **18**(Suppl. 1), 17–26.

Gunn, R. N., Yap, J. T., Wells, P., Osman, S., Price, P., Jones, T., *et al.* (2000). A general method to correct PET data for tissue metabolites using a dual-scan approach. *J. Nucl. Med.* **41,** 706–711.

Haberkorn, U., Strauss, L. G., Dimitrakopoulou, A., Seiffert, E., Oberdorfer, F., Ziegler, S., *et al.* (1993). Fluorodeoxyglucose imaging of advanced head and neck cancer after chemotherapy. *J. Nucl. Med.* **34,** 12–17.

Hamill, T. G., Burns, H. D., Eng, W-S., Francis, B. E., Gibson, R. E., and Fioravanti, C. (1999). Radioiodinated farnesyl transferase inhibitors. *J. Label Comp. Radiopharm.* **42**(Suppl. 1), S30–S32.

Harte, R. J., Matthews, J. C., O'Reilly, S. M., and Price, P. M. (1998). Sources of error in tissue and tumor measurements of 5-[18F]fluorouracil. *J. Nucl. Med.* **39,** 1370–1376.

Harte, R. J., Matthews, J. C., O'Reilly, S. M., Tilsley, D. W., Osman, S., Brown, G., *et al.* (1999). Tumor, normal tissue, and plasma pharmacokinetic studies of fluorouracil biomodulation with N-phosphonacetyl-L-aspartate, folinic acid, and interferon alfa. *J. Clin. Oncol.* **17,** 1580–1588.

Harte, R. J. A., Matthews, J. C., Flavin, A., Brock, C. S., Osman, S., Luthra, S. K., *et al.* (1996). Pre phase I tracer kinetic studies in humans can contribute to new drug evaluation (meeting abstract). *Ann. Oncol.* **7**(Suppl. 1), 50.

Hendrick, A. M., Harris, A. L., and Cantwell, B. M. (1991). Verapamil with mitoxantrone for advanced ovarian cancer: a negative phase II trial. *Ann. Oncol.* **2,** 71–72.

Hendrikse, N. H., de Vries, E. G., Eriks-Fluks, L., van der Graaf, W. T., Hospers, G. A., Willemsen, A. T., *et al.* (1999). A new in vivo method to study P-glycoprotein transport in tumors and the blood-brain barrier. *Cancer Res.* **59,** 2411–2416.

Hohenberger, P., Strauss, L. G., Lehner, B., Frohmuller, S., Dimitrakopoulou, A., and Schlag, P. (1993). Perfusion of colorectal liver metastases and uptake of fluorouracil assessed by H2(15)O and [^{18}F]uracil positron emission tomography (PET). *Eur. J. Cancer* **12,** 1682–1686.

Holthoff, V. A., Herholz, K., Berthold, F., Widemann, B., Schroder, R., Neubauer, I., *et al.* (1993). In vivo metabolism of childhood posterior fossa tumors and primitive neuroectodermal tumors before and after treatment. *Cancer* **72,** 1394–1403.

Huang, S. C., and Phelps, M. E. (1986). Principles of tracer kinetic modeling in positron tomography and autoradiography. *In* "Positron Emission Tomography and Autoradiography: Principles and Applications for the Brain and Heart" (M. E. Phelps, J. C. Mazziota, and H. R. Schelbert, eds.), pp. 287–341. Raven Press, New York..

Inoue, T., Kim, E. E., Wallace, S., Yang, D. J., Wong, F. C., Bassa, P., *et al.* (1997). Preliminary study of cardiac accumulation of F-18 fluorotamoxifen in patients with breast cancer. *Clin. Imaging* **21,** 332–336.

Jansson, T., Westlin, J. E., Ahlstrom, H., Lilja, A., Langstrom, B., and Bergh, J. (1995). Positron emission tomography studies in patients with locally advanced and/or metastatic breast cancer: a method for early therapy evaluation? *J. Clin. Oncol.* **13**, 1470–1477.

Katzenellenbogen, J. A., Welch, M. J., and Dehdashti, F. (1997). The development of estrogen and progestin radiopharmaceuticals for imaging breast cancer. *Anticancer Res.* **17**, 1573–1576.

Kemeny, N. (1983). The systemic chemotherapy of hepatic metastases. *Semin. Oncol.* **10**, 148–158.

Kissel, J., Brix, G., Bellemann, M. E., Strauss, L. G., Dimitrakopoulou-Strauss, A., Port, R., *et al.* (1997). Pharmacokinetic analysis of 5-[^{18}F]fluorouracil tissue concentrations measured with positron emission tomography in patients with liver metastases from colorectal adenocarcinoma. *Cancer Res.* **57**, 3415–3423.

Koh, W. J., Bergman, K. S., Rasey, J. S., Peterson, L. M., Evans, M. L., Graham, M. M., *et al.* (1995). Evaluation of oxygenation status during fractionated radiotherapy in human nonsmall cell lung cancers using [F-18]fluoromisonidazole positron emission tomography. *Int. J. Radiat. Oncol. Biol. Phys.* **33**, 391–398.

Kostakoglu, L., Elahi, N., Kiratli, P., Ruacan, S., Sayek, I., Baltali, E., *et al.* (1997). Clinical validation of the influence of P-glycoprotein on technetium-99m-sestamibi uptake in malignant tumors. *J. Nucl. Med.* **38**, 1003–1008.

Kumar, A., Schapiro, M. B., Grady, C., Haxby, J. V., Wagner, E., Salerno, J. A., *et al.* (1991). High-resolution PET studies in Alzheimer's disease. *Neuropsychopharmacology* **4**, 35–46.

Kushner, M., Fieschi, C., Alavi, A., Silver, F., Chawluk, J., and Reivich, M. (1987). Local cerebral metabolic changes in acute ischemic strokes. *Gerontology* **33**, 265–267.

Lavin, P., Mittelman, A., Douglass, H., Jr., Engstrom, P., and Klaassen, D. (1980). Survival and response to chemotherapy for advanced colorectal adenocarcinoma: an Eastern Cooperative Oncology Group report. *Cancer* **46**, 1536–1543.

Lewis, J. S., McCarthy, D. W., McCarthy, T. J., Fujibayashi, Y., and Welch, M. J. (1999). Evaluation of ^{64}Cu-ATSM in vitro and in vivo in a hypoxic tumor model. *J. Nucl. Med.* **40**, 177–183.

Liu, A., Carlson, K. E., and Katzenellenbogen, J. A. (1992). Synthesis of high affinity fluorine-substituted ligands for the androgen receptor. Potential agents for imaging prostatic cancer by positron emission tomography. *J. Med. Chem.* **35**, 2113–2129.

Maisey, N. R., Webb, A., Flux, G. D., Padhani, A., Cunningham, D. C., Ott. R. J., *et al.* (2000). FDG-PET in the prediction of survival of patients with cancer of the pancreas: a pilot study. *Br. J. Cancer* **83**, 287–293.

Mankoff, D. A., Shields, A. F., Graham, M. M., Link, J. M., Eary, J. F., and Krohn, K. A. (1998). Kinetic analysis of 2-[carbon-11]thymidine PET imaging studies: compartmental model and mathematical analysis. *J. Nucl. Med.* **39**, 1043–1055.

Mankoff, D. A., Shields, A. F., Link, J. M., Graham, M. M., Muzi, M., Peterson, L. M., *et al.* (1999). Kinetic analysis of 2-[^{11}C]thymidine PET imaging studies: validation studies. *J. Nucl. Med.* **40**, 614–624.

McCrystal, M. R., Evans, B. D., Harvey, V. J., Thompson, P. I., Porter, D. J., and Baguley, B. C. (1999). Phase I study of the cytotoxic agent N-[2-(dimethylamino)ethyl]acridine-4-carboxamide. *Cancer Chemother. Pharmacol.* **44**, 39–44.

McGuire, A. H., Dehdashti, F., Siegel, B. A., Lyss, A. P., Brodack, J. W., Mathias, C. J., *et al.* (1991). Positron tomographic assessment of 16 alpha-[^{18}F] fluoro-17 beta-estradiol uptake in metastatic breast carcinoma. *J. Nucl. Med.* **32**, 1526–1531.

Meikle, S. R., Matthews, J. C., Brock, C. S., Wells, P., Harte, R. J., Cunningham, V. J., *et al.* (1998). Pharmacokinetic assessment of novel anticancer drugs using spectral analysis and positron emission tomography: a feasibility study. *Cancer Chemother. Pharmacol.* **42**, 183–193.

Mitsuki, S., Diksic, M., Conway, T., Yamamoto, Y. L., Villemure, J. G., and Feindel, W. (1991). Pharmacokinetics of ^{11}C-labelled BCNU and SarCNU in gliomas studied by PET. *J. Neurooncol.* **10**, 47–55.

Mizuno, N. S., and Decker, R. W. (1976). Alteration of DNA by 5-(3-methyl-1-triazeno)imidazole-4-carboxamide (NSC-407347). *Biochem. Pharmacol.* **25**, 2643–2647.

Moehler, M., Dimitrakopoulou-Strauss, A., Gutzler, F., Raeth, U., Strauss, L. G., and Stremmel W. (1998). ^{18}F-labeled fluorouracil positron emission tomography and the prognoses of colorectal carcinoma patients with metastases to the liver treated with 5-fluorouracil. *Cancer* **83**, 245–253.

Newlands, E. S., O'Reilly, S. M., Glaser, M. G., Bower, M., Evans, H., Brock, C., *et al.* (1996). The Charing Cross Hospital experience with temozolomide in patients with gliomas. *Eur. J. Cancer* **32A**, 2236–2241.

Newlands, E. S., Stevens, M. F., Wedge, S. R., Wheelhouse, R. T., and Brock, C. (1997). Temozolomide: a review of its discovery, chemical properties, pre- clinical development and clinical trials. *Cancer Treat. Rev.* **23**, 35–61.

Nicholson, H. S., Krailo, M., Ames, M. M., Seibel, N. L., Reid, J. M., Liu-Mares, W., *et al.* (1998). Phase I study of temozolomide in children and adolescents with recurrent solid tumors: a report from the Children's Cancer Group. *J. Clin. Oncol.* **16**, 3037–3043.

Ogawa, T., Uemura, K., Shishido, F., Yamaguchi, T., Murakami, M., Inugami, A., *et al.* (1988). Changes of cerebral blood flow, and oxygen and glucose metabolism following radiochemotherapy of gliomas: a PET study. *J. Comput. Assist. Tomogr.* **12**, 290–297.

Okada, J., Oonishi, H., Yoshikawa, K., Itami, J., Uno, K., Imaseki, K., *et al.* (1994). FDG-PET for predicting the prognosis of malignant lymphoma. *Ann. Nucl. Med.* **8**, 187–191.

Okazumi, S., Isono, K., Enomoto, K., Kikuchi, T., Ozaki, M., Yamamoto, H., *et al.* (1992). Evaluation of liver tumors using fluorine-18-fluorodeoxyglucose PET: characterization of tumor and assessment of effect of treatment. *J. Nucl. Med.* **33**, 333–339.

Osborne, C. K. (1998). Steroid hormone receptors in breast cancer management. *Breast Cancer Res. Treat.* **51**, 227–238.

Osman, S., Luthra, S. K., Brady, F., Hume, S. P., Brown, G., Harte, R. J., *et al.* (1997). Studies on the metabolism of the novel antitumor agent [N-methyl-^{11}C]N-[2-(dimethylamino)ethyl]acridine-4-carboxamide in rats and humans prior to phase I clinical trials. *Cancer Res.* **57**, 2172–2180.

Patlak, C. S., Blasberg, R. G., and Fenstermacher, J. D. (1983). Graphical evaluation of blood-to-brain transfer constants from multiple-time uptake data. *J. Cereb. Blood Flow Metab.* **3**, 1–7.

Paxton, J. W., Young, D., Evans, S. M., Kestell, P., Robertson, I. G. C., and Cornford, E. M. (1992). Pharmacokinetics and toxicity of the antitumour agent N-[2-(dimethylamino)ethyl]acridine-4-carboxamide after i.v. administration in the mouse. *Cancer Chemother. Pharmacol.* **29**, 379–384.

Pinedo, H. M., and Peters, G. F. (1988). Fluorouracil: biochemistry and pharmacology. *J. Clin. Oncol.* **6**, 1653–1664.

Prenant, C., Shah, F., Brady, F., Luthra, S. K., Pike, V. W., Burke, P. J., *et al.* (1995). Synthesis of [11C]chloroethyltriflate from [^{11}C] ethylene; a reagent for introducing the haloethyl group into antibody directed enzyme prodrugs (ADEPT). *J. Label Comp. Radiopharm.* **37**, 95–97.

Prenant, C., Brady, F., Luthra, S. K., Brown, D., Burke, P. J., and Price, P. (1997). An alternative synthesis of [^{11}C]ethylene and conversion to [^{11}C]chloroethyltosylate in situ via [^{11}C]1-chloro-2-iodoethane for radiolabelling ADEPT prodrugs. *J. Label Comp. Radiopharm.* **40**, 766–767.

Presant, C. A., Wolf, W., Albright, M. J., Servis, K. L., Ring, R. D., Atkinson, D., *et al.* (1990). Human tumor fluorouracil trapping: clinical correlations of in vivo ^{19}F nuclear magnetic resonance spectroscopy pharmacokinetics. *J. Clin. Oncol.* **8**, 1868–1873.

Presant, C. A., Wolf, W., Waluch, V., Wiseman, C., Kennedy, P., Blayney, D., *et al.* (1994). Association of intratumoral pharmacokinetics of fluorouracil with clinical response. *Lancet* **343**, 1184–1187.

Ragosta, M., and Beller, G. A. (1993). The noninvasive assessment of myocardial viability. *Clin. Cardiol.* **16,** 531–538.

Rasey, J. S., Koh, W. J., Evans, M. L., Peterson, L. M., Lewellen, T. K., Graham, M. M., *et al.* (1996). Quantifying regional hypoxia in human tumors with positron emission tomography of [^{18}F]fluoromisonidazole: a pretherapy study of 37 patients. *Int. J. Radiat. Oncol. Biol. Phys.* **36,** 417–428.

Richards, F. D., Case, L. D., White, D. R., Muss, H. B., Spurr, C. L., Jackson, D. V., *et al.* (1986). Combination chemotherapy (5-fluorouracil, methyl-CCNU, mitomycin C) versus 5-fluorouracil alone for advanced previously untreated colorectal carcinoma. A phase III study of the Piedmont Oncology Association. *J. Clin. Oncol.* **4,** 565–570.

Rodenburg, C. J., Nooter, K., Herweijer, H., Seynaeve, C., Oosterom, R., Stoter, G., *et al.* (1991). Phase II study of combining vinblastine and cyclosporin-A to circumvent multidrug resistance in renal cell cancer. *Ann. Oncol.* **2,** 305–306.

Saleem, A., Harte, R. J., Matthews, J. C., Osman, S., Brady, F., Luthra, S. K., *et al.* (2001). Pharmacokinetic evaluation of N-[2-(Dimethylamino)ethyl]acridine-4-carboxamide (DACA; XR5000) in patients by positron emission tomography (PET). *J. Clin. Oncol.* **19,** 1421–1429.

Saleem, A., Yap, J., Osman, S., Brady, F., Suttle, B., Lucas, S. V., *et al.* (2000). Modulation of fluorouracil tissue pharmacokinetics by eniluracil: in-vivo imaging of drug action. *Lancet* **355,** 2125–2131.

Schelbert, H. R., Henze, E., Phelps, M. E., and Kuhl, D.E. (1982). Assessment of regional myocardial ischemia by positron-emission computed tomography. *Am. Heart J.* **103,** 588–597.

Schofield, P. C., Robertson, I. G., Paxton, J. W., McCrystal, M. R., Evans, B. D., Kestell, P., *et al.* (1999). Metabolism of N-[2-(dimethylamino)ethyl]-acridine-4-carboxamide in cancer patients undergoing a phase I clinical trial. *Cancer Chemother. Pharmacol.* **44,** 51–58.

Seeman, P., Lee, T., Chau-Wong, M., and Wong, K. (1976). Antipsychotic drug doses and neuroleptic/dopamine receptors. *Nature* **261,** 717–719.

Shani, J., and Wolf, W. (1977). A model for prediction of chemotherapy response to 5-fluorouracil based on the differential distribution of 5-[^{18}F]fluorouracil in sensitive versus resistant lymphocytic leukemia in mice. *Cancer Res.* **37**(1), 2306–2308.

Shields, A. F., Grierson, J. R., Dohmen, B. M., Machulla, H. J., Stayanoff, J. C., Lawhorn-Crews, J. M., *et al.* (1998a). Imaging proliferation in vivo with [F-18]FLT and positron emission tomography. *Nat. Med.* **4,** 1334–1336.

Shields, A. F., Mankoff, D. A., Link, J. M., Graham, M. M., Eary, J. F., Kozawa, S. M., *et al.* (1998b). Carbon-11-thymidine and FDG to measure therapy response. *J. Nucl. Med.* **39,** 1757–1762.

Stevens, M. F., and Newlands, E. S. (1993). From triazines and triazenes to temozolomide. *Eur. J. Cancer* **7,** 1045–1047.

Tjuvajev, J. G., Avril, N., Oku, T., Sasajima, T., Miyagawa, T., Joshi, R., *et al.* (1998). Imaging herpes virus thymidine kinase gene transfer and expression by positron emission tomography. *Cancer Res.* **58,** 4333–4341.

Twelves, C. J., Gardner, C., Flavin, A., Sludden, J., Dennis, I., de Bono, J., *et al.* (1999). Phase I and pharmacokinetic study of DACA (XR5000): a novel inhibitor of topoisomerase I and II. CRC Phase I/II Committee. *Br. J. Cancer* **80,** 1786–1791.

Tyler, J. L., Yamamoto, Y. L., Diksic, M., Theron, J., Villemure, J. G., Worthington, C., *et al.* (1986). Pharmacokinetics of superselective intra-arterial and intravenous [^{11}C]BCNU evaluated by PET. *J. Nucl. Med.* **27,** 775–780.

VanBrocklin, H. F., Liu, A., Welch, M. J., O'Neil, J. P., and Katzenellenbogen, J. A. (1994). The synthesis of 7 alpha-methyl-substituted estrogens labeled with fluorine-18: potential breast tumor imaging agents. *Steroids* **59,** 34–45.

Vaupel, P., Kallinowski, F., and Okunieff, P. (1989). Blood flow, oxygen, and nutrient supply, and metabolic microenvironment of human tumors: a review. *Cancer Res.* **49,** 6449–6465.

Vecchio, S. D., Ciarmiello, A., Potena, M. I., Carriero, M. V., Mainolfi, C., Botti, G., *et al.* (1997). In vivo detection of multidrug-resistant (MDR1) phenotype by technetium-99m sestamibi scan in untreated breast cancer patients. *Eur. J. Nucl. Med.* **24,** 150–159.

Verhagen, A., Luurtsema, G., Pesser, J. W., de Groot, T. J., Wouda, S., Oosterhuis, J. W., *et al.* (1991). Preclinical evaluation of a positron emitting progestin ([^{18}F]fluoro-16 alpha-methyl-19-norprogesterone) for imaging progesterone receptor positive tumours with positron emission tomography. *Cancer Lett.* **59,** 125–132.

Vine, E. N., Young, D., Vine, W. H., and Wolf, W. (1979). An improved synthesis of ^{18}F-5-fluorouracil. *Int. J. Appl. Radiat. Isot.* **30,** 401–405.

Vollenweider-Zerargui, L., Barrelet, L., Wong, Y., Lemarchand-Beraud, T., and Gomez, F. (1986). The predictive value of estrogen and progesterone receptors' concentrations on the clinical behavior of breast cancer in women. Clinical correlation on 547 patients. *Cancer* **57,** 1171–1180.

Wahl, R. L., Zasadny, K., Helvie, M., Hutchins, G. D., Weber, B., and Cody, R. (1993). Metabolic monitoring of breast cancer chemohormonotherapy using positron emission tomography: initial evaluation. *J. Clin. Oncol.* **11,** 2101–2111.

Waki, A., Kato, H., Yano, R., Sadato, N., Yokoyama, A., Ishii, Y., *et al.* (1998). The importance of glucose transport activity as the rate-limiting step of 2-deoxyglucose uptake in tumor cells in vitro. *Nucl. Med. Biol.* **25,** 593–597.

Weissleder, R. (1999). Molecular imaging: exploring the next frontier. *Radiology* **212,** 609–614.

Wells, P., Gunn, R., Steel, C., Alison, M., Jones, T., and Price, P. (1997a). Measurement of cell proliferation in vivo using [2-^{11}C] thymidine. *Proc. Am. Soc. Clin. Oncol.* **16,** 548a.

Wells, P., Gunn, R. N., Hughes, A., Taylor, G. A., Price, P., and Newell, D. R. (1997b). Thymidine salvage demonstrated in vivo: a specific pharmacodynamic endpoint of thymidylate synthase (TS) inhibition. *Proc. Am. Assoc. Cancer Res.* **38,** 477.

Woll, P. J., Crowther, D., Johnson, P. W., Soukop, M., Harper, P. G., Harris, M., *et al.* (1995). Phase II trial of temozolomide in low-grade non-Hodgkin's lymphoma. *Br. J. Cancer* **72,** 183–184.

Wood, L., Palmer, M., Hewitt, J., Urtasun, R., Bruera, E., Rapp, E., *et al.* (1998). Results of a phase III, double-blind, placebo-controlled trial of megestrol acetate modulation of P-glycoprotein-mediated drug resistance in the first-line management of small-cell lung carcinoma. *Br. J. Cancer* **77,** 627–631.

Wunderbaldinger, P., Bogdanov, A., and Weissleder, R. (2000). New approaches for imaging in gene therapy. *Eur. J. Radiol.* **34,** 156–165.

Young, H., Baum, R., Cremerius, U., Herholz, K., Hoekstra, O., Lammertsma, A. A., *et al.* (1999). Measurement of clinical and subclinical tumour response using [18F]-fluorodeoxyglucose and positron emission tomography: review and 1999 EORTC recommendations. European Organization for Research and Treatment of Cancer (EORTC) PET Study Group. *Eur. J. Cancer* **35,** 1773–1782.

Zijlstra, J. G., de Vries, E. G., and Mulder, N. H. (1987). Multifactorial drug resistance in an adriamycin-resistant human small cell lung carcinoma cell line. *Cancer Res.* **47,** 1780–1784.

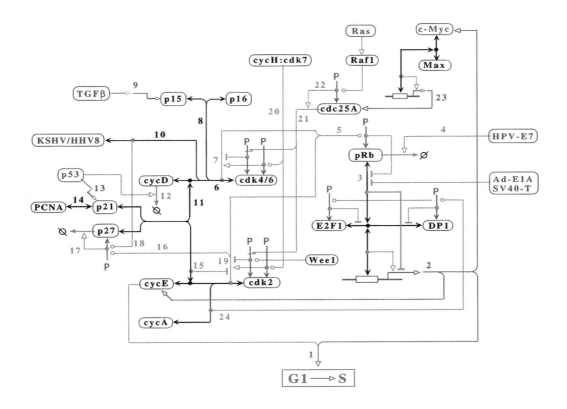

CHAPTER 2, FIGURE 2 Molecular interaction map of the E2F-dependent control of the G_1–S cell cycle phase transition. The symbols used are as defined by Kohn (1999). (http://discover.nci.nih.gov/kohnk/interaction_maps.html). (1) The transition from G_1 to S phase requires E2F-dependent gene products and an as-yet-undefined action of cyclin E. (2) E2F-dependent genes include regulators such as *cyclin E* and *c-Myc*, in addition to many genes that manufacture the S-phase machinery (not shown). These genes are positively regulated by E2F1:DP1 (and other E2F heterodimers) and negatively regulated when the E2F heterodimers are bound to pRb proteins. Negative regulation by recruitment of pRb is the main mechanism of regulation. (3) Binding of pRb to E2F heterodimers is inhibited by phosphorylation of pRb. It is also inhibited by adenovirus E1A and SV40 T-antigen proteins. (4) The degradation of pRb is stimulated by the E7 protein of human papilloma virus. (5) pRb is phosphorylated by cycD:cdk4/6 and by cycE:cdk2. Both are required to fully phosphorylate pRb and to inhibit its binding to E2F heterodimers. (6) Cdk4 and cdk6 can bind to cyclin D; this is required for kinase activity. (7) Cdk4/6 can be phosphorylated at stimulatory and inhibitory sites. (8) p15 or p16 can bind cdk4/6, thereby displacing cyclin D and inhibiting the kinase. (9) p15 is transcriptionally up-regulated by transforming growth factor-β (TGFβ) by way of the Smad pathway (not shown). (10) Inhibition of cdk6 by displacement of cyclin D1 can be accomplished by the viral product KSHV/HHV8 (see text). (11) CycD:cdk4/6 heterodimers can bind p21cip1 or p27kip1. The main consequence of this binding may be to stabilize the cycD:cdk4/6 complexes and possibly enhance activity. (12) Cyclin D has a short half-life (about 30 min). Its half-life is further reduced by p53 (Agami and Bernards, 2000). Degradation is by way of the ubiquitin–proteasome system (not shown). (13) p53 transcriptionally up-regulates p21cip1. (14) p21cip1 binds PCNA, a factor required for DNA replication. (15) p21cip1 and p27kip1 can bind cycE:cdk2 and inhibit its kinase activity (contrary to the case of cycD:cdk4/6). (16) p27kip1 is phosphorylated by cycE:cdk2. Thus p27kip1 is both an inhibitor and a substrate of the kinase; the mechanism of this seemingly paradoxical duality is not clear but could involve phosphorylation of an inactive cycE:cdk2:p27 complex by an active cycE:cdk2 complex. (17) Phosphorylation tags p27kip1 for degradation. (18) Binding of the KSHV/HHV8 viral product to cdk4/6 stimulates the degradation of p27kip1, possibly by phosphorylating p27kip1. (19) CycE:cdk2 (like cycD:cdk4/6; see #7 above) is subject to phosphorylation at stimulatory and inhibitory sites. (20) Cdk2, cdk4, and cdk6 are phosphorylated at their activation sites by cycH:cdk7 (also known as CAK), a component of the transcription factor IIH complex. (21) The inhibitory phosphorylations on cdk2, cdk4, and cdk6 are removed by the phosphatase cdc25A. (22) The phosphatase activity of cdc25A is enhanced by phosphorylation, which can be carried out by Raf1 in the Ras signaling pathway. (23) The *cdc25A* gene is stimulated by the c-Myc:Max complex. (24) The cycA:cdk2 complex can phosphorylate E2F1 and DP1, causing the E2F1:DP1 complex to dissociate. In this way, increased activity of cycA:cdk2 may serve to terminate E2F activity at the end of S phase.

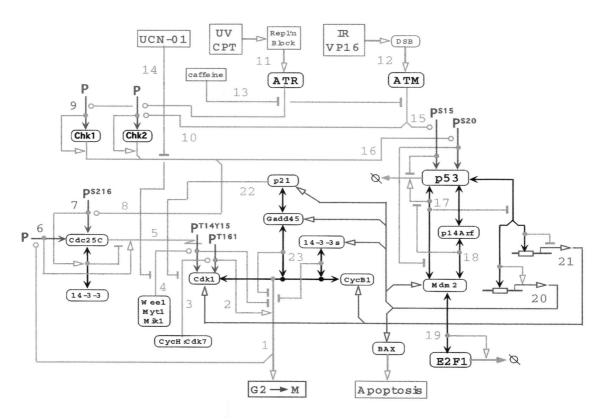

CHAPTER 2, FIGURE 3 Molecular interaction map of the control of the G₂-M cell cycle phase transition. (1) The G₂-M transition, which entails the preparation for mitosis, is to a large extent instigated by the kinase activity of cycB:cdk1. (2) The kinase activity of cdk1 is subject to stimulatory and inhibitory phosphorylations. Thr161 phosphorylation is necessary for activity. Dual phosphorylations at Thr14 and Tyr15 inhibit activity. (3) Thr161 of cdk1 is phosphorylated by cycH:cdk7 (as in the stimulatory phosphorylations of cdk2 and cdk4/6; see Fig. 2.2). (4) Phosphorylation of Cdk1 at Thr14/Tyr15 may be due to kinase Wee1, Myt1, or Mik1. (5) These phosphates can be removed by phosphatase Cdc25C. (6) Cdc25C can be phosphorylated at several sites that enhance its activity. Phosphorylation of these sites may be carried out by cycB:cdk1, thereby forming a positive-feedback loop for cycB:cdk1 activation. (7) Phosphorylation of Cdc25C at Ser216 allows binding to 14-3-3 and thereby inhibits phosphatase activity. (8) Phosphorylation of Cdc25C at Ser216 can be carried out by Chk1 and by Chk2. (9) Chk1 and Chk2 are activated by phosphorylation. (10) Chk1 can be phosphorylated by ATR. Chk2 can be phosphorylated by ATR or ATM. (11) ATR is activated by DNA replication blocks produced by agents such as ultraviolet light (UV) or camptothecin (CPT). (12) ATM is activated by DNA double-strand breaks (DSBs) produced by agents such as ionizing radiation or etoposide (VP-16). (13) Caffeine can inhibit both ATM and ATR. (14) UCN-01 can inhibit a variety of protein kinases, including Chk1 and Chk2, as well as Wee1. (15) ATM can phosphorylate p53 at Ser15, as a result of which p53 is stabilized (its degradation rate is reduced). (16) Chk1 and Chk2 phosphorylate p53 at Ser20, as a result of which the binding of p53 to Mdm2 is impaired. (17) p53 can bind Mdm2, as a result of which p53 degradation is enhanced and the ability of p53 to bind to promoters is impaired. (18) Mdm2 can bind p14Arf, as a result of which the ability of Mdm2 to stimulate p53 degradation is impaired. (19) Mdm2 can bind E2F1, as a result of which E2F1 degradation is stimulated. (This would block the activation of S-phase genes; see Fig. 2.2). (20) p53 activates many genes, including *Mdm2*, *p21cip1*, *Gadd45*, *14-3-3* σ, and *Bax*. (21) p53 inhibits some genes, including *cyclin B1* and *cdk1*. (22) p21cip1 inhibits several cyclin–kinase complexes (see Fig. 2.2), including CycH:cdk7. (23) Both Gadd45 and 14-3-3σ can bind cycB:cdk1 and thereby block its kinase activity.

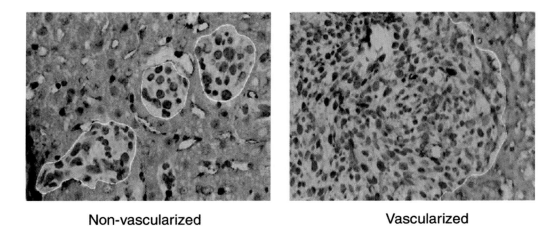

Non-vascularized   Vascularized

CHAPTER 7, FIGURE 1 Liver metastasis of colorectal cancer cells. If these tumor deposits remain avascular (left) their growth will be limited to 1–2 mm in diameter. When new vessels are formed (right) the tumor may grow exponentially.

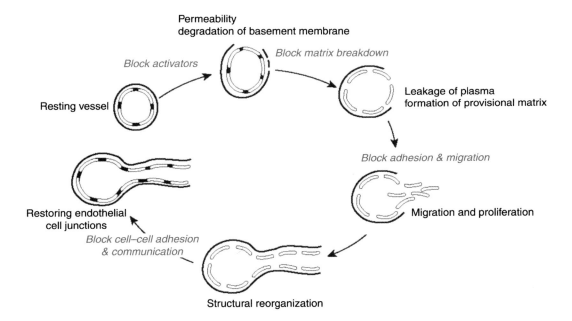

CHAPTER 7, FIGURE 2 Angiogenesis is a complex process that can be divided into several steps. Angiogenesis starts with the establishment of vascular discontinuity followed by the breakdown of the extracellular matrix. After migration and proliferation of the endothelial cells toward the tumor, the endothelial cells form tubes and the extracellular matrix is remodeled and reorganized in a new capillary network. Antiangiogenic therapy can be based on the various steps in the development of new blood vessels.

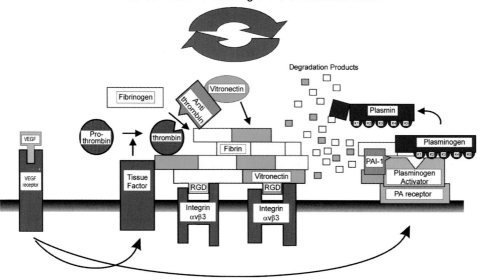

CHAPTER 7, FIGURE 3 All components of the extracellular matrix form a complex and dynamic structure that can be broken down and remodeled during angiogenesis. Reprinted from Reijerkerk *et al.*, *Eur. J. Cancer*, **36**, 1695–1705. Copyright© 2000, with permission from Elsevier Science.

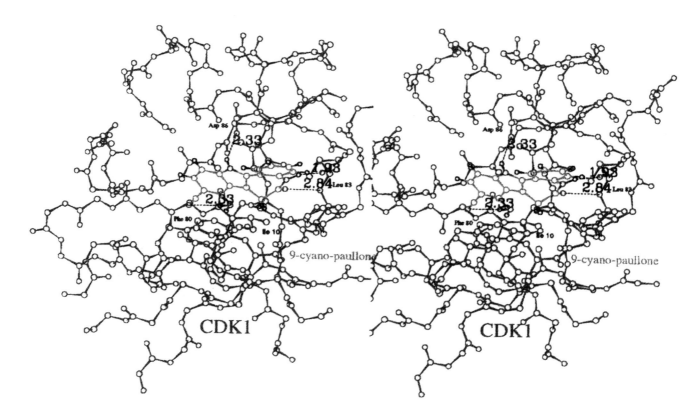

CHAPTER 10, FIGURE 7 Stereo diagram of 9-cyanopaullone docked in the ATP binding site of CDK1. Carbon atoms are shown in cyan, oxygen in red, and nitrogen in blue. The dotted lines indicate distances of the polar anchors formed between 9-cyanopaullone and the binding site. (From Gussio *et al.*, 2000; by permission of Oxford University Press.)

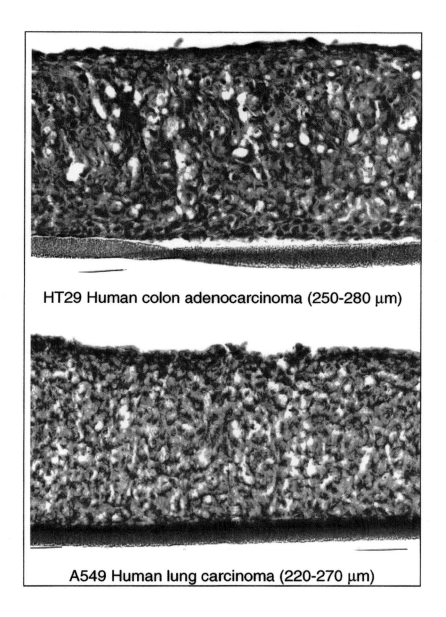

HT29 Human colon adenocarcinoma (250-280 μm)

A549 Human lung carcinoma (220-270 μm)

CHAPTER 15, FIGURE 5 Photomicrographs of hematoxylin-eosin-stained frozen sections of multicellular layers from human cell lines grown on Teflon support membranes, submerged in culture medium for 4 days after seeding at 10^6 cells per culture insert. Approximate thicknesses are indicated.

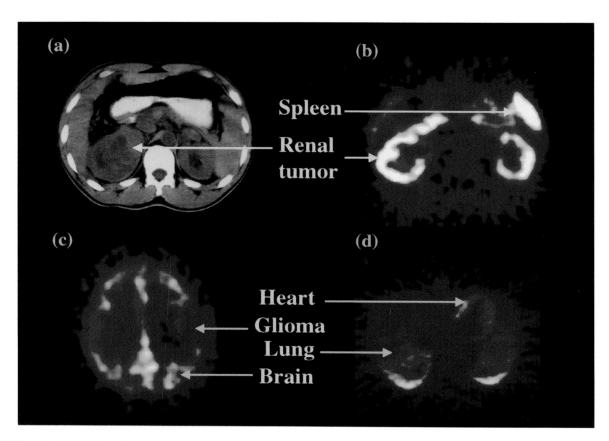

CHAPTER 19, FIGURE 2 (a) Typical transabdominal CT scan and (b) corresponding PET [$_{11}$C]DACA image demonstrating uptake of the radiotracer in kidneys, spleen, and a renal cell carcinoma. Uptake of the [$_{11}$C]DACA derived activity is also seen in (c) normal brain, glioma and in (d) the myocardium and lungs.

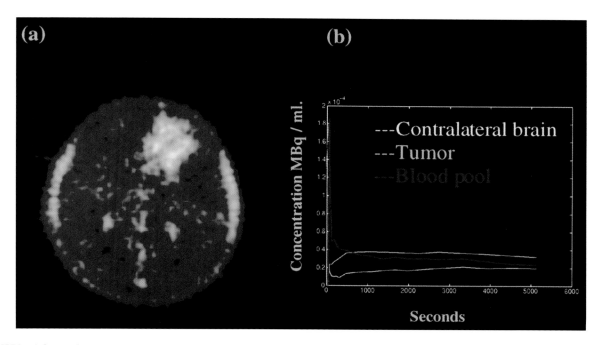

CHAPTER 19, FIGURE 5 PET [^{11}C-*methyl*]temozolomide image (a) and time–activity curves (b) in a patient with a glioma. Increased uptake of activity is seen in the tumor compared with normal brain.

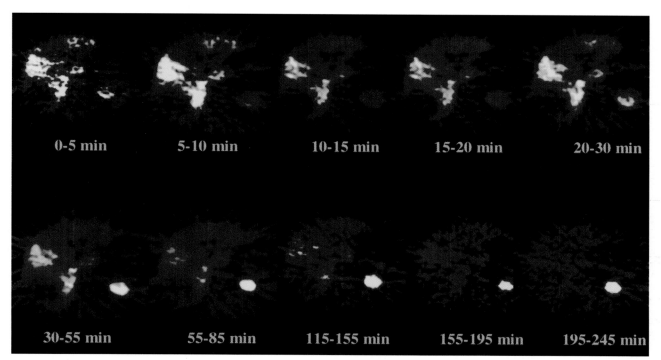

CHAPTER 19, FIGURE 7 Temporal representation of drug localization in a selected transabdominal tomographic plane passing through the liver after injection of 5–[18F]FU. The time frames have been added to provide a composite image between the periods indicated at the bottom of the figures. Liver, the left kidney, and a liver metastasis (from a colorectal carcinoma; hypointense region) are seen in the images. The immediate catabolism and trapping of the catabolite is seen as hyperintense regions in the normal liver during the first half-hour. As the trapped catabolite is eliminated from the liver, the kidneys, which primarily excrete (>90%) [18F]FBAL, show intense activity toward the latter half of the scan. The hypointense region posteriorly in the liver is metastatic lesion.

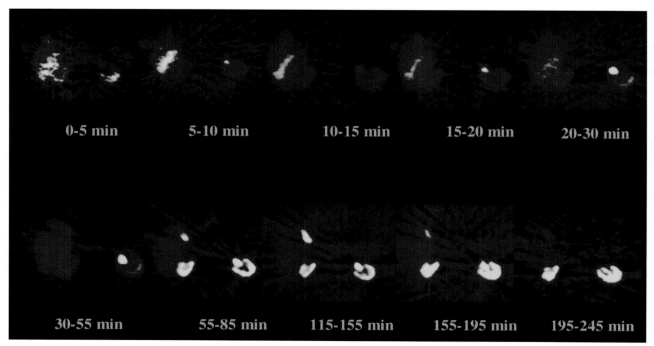

CHAPTER 19, FIGURE 8 Dynamic PET images for the same study illustrated in Figure 19.10, through another transabdominal tomographic plane passing through the base of liver for the full duration of the PET scan (245 min). The time frames have been added to provide a composite image between the periods indicated at the bottom of the figures. In addition to the liver and both kidneys, the gall bladder is also seen as an hyperintense region from 55 min onward. This localization of activity in the gallbladder could be due to hepatobiliary elimination of [18F]FBAL-bile acid conjugates.

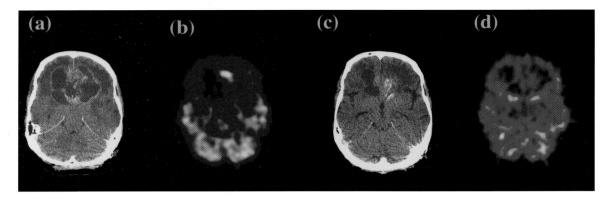

CHAPTER 19, FIGURE 12 (**a**) CT scan and (**b**) [¹⁸F]fluorodeoxyglucose ([¹⁸F]FDG) PET image of a patient with a glioma prior to treatment showing high tumor uptake of [¹⁸F]FDG. CT scan (**c**) 2 months after treatment with temozolomide demonstrates a decrease in the size of the tumor. A decrease in tumoral PET-[¹⁸F]FDG (**d**) uptake is seen at 2 weeks post treatment, predating the anatomical decrease in size.

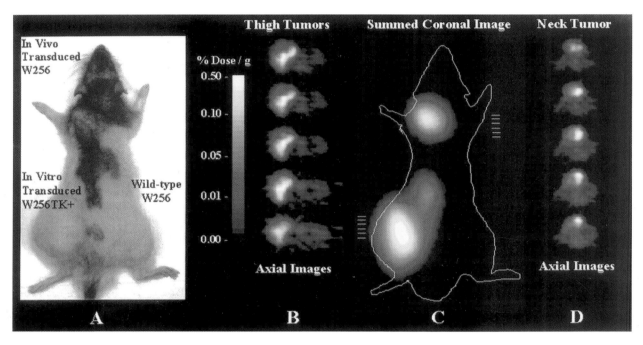

CHAPTER 19, FIGURE 14 PET imaging of herpesvirus type 1 thymidine kinase (HSV1-tk) gene expression at 48 h after intravenous administration of [₁₂₄I]-5-iodo-2′-fluoro-1-β-D-arabinofuranosyluracil ([₁₂₄I]-FIAU). (**a**) Photograph of a tumor-bearing rat. (**b**) Transaxial PET images of wild-type (W256) and *in vitro*-transduced (W256TK+) subcutaneous tumors located in both thighs of the rat. (**c**) Summed coronal (pseudoplanar) PET image of the tumor-bearing rat. The outline of the rat is shown in white. Small horizontal lines on the left and right sides of the outline indicate the planes in which the transaxial images were obtained. (**d**) Transaxial PET images of a W256TK tumor in the neck region (produced by retroviral-mediated HSV1-tk gene transduction of preestablished wild-type subcutaneous W256 tumor). The images are color coded to a range of [₁₂₄I]-FIAU-derived radioactivity levels, expressed as percentage of injected dose per gram (Tjuvajev *et al.*, 1998; reproduced with permission from *Cancer Research*).

CHAPTER 20

MECHANISTIC APPROACHES TO PHASE I CLINICAL TRIALS

David R. Ferry[*]

David J. Kerr[†]

[*]Department of Oncology, New Cross Hospital,
Wolverhampton, United Kingdom; and
[†]Institute for Cancer Medicine, University of Oxford,
Oxford, United Kingdom

Summary

Phase I clinical trials of anticancer agents have been in evolution. Not only do such trials routinely incorporate pharmacokinetics; now increasing effort is being made to link drug levels to pharmacodynamic end points relating to toxicity. This has served us well, but trials of agents of novel mechanism pose questions, which require new approaches. The focus of this chapter is to assess ongoing attempts to incorporate mechanistic assessments into phase I trials and suggest how these could be improved. To fully exploit the potential of the new anticancer agents it may be necessary to develop the concept of a saturation dose (SD), at which the target is 99% inhibited, as well as a conventional maximum tolerated dose. This would allow the designation of trials as being "phase IM" where such measurements would be at the heart of the design. This would also logically lead to a commitment to evaluate the SD versus the conventional phase II dose in upcoming efficacy assessments.

1. Introduction

The science of pharmacology essentially focuses on the relationship between dose and effect of a given drug. This principle of pharmacology was appreciated by Chinese emperors 3000 years ago when they determined the *minimal* dose of puffer fish, which contains tetrodotoxin, needed *to kill* captured enemy soldiers (Rogart, 1981). Conversely, phase I clinical trials of anticancer agents seek to determine the *maximal* dose that *does not kill* the patient. In summary, this approach usually starts with a conservative dose, conventionally 0.1% of the mouse LD_{10}, and escalates by Fibonacci-defined proportions. Routinely, three patients are treated per cohort until dose-limiting toxicity (DLT) occurs where upon this dose level is expanded. The dose level at which more than 33% of patients have DLT is defined as the maximum tolerated dose (MTD), and the dose level below this is the recommended phase II dose. This approach is entirely logical for alkylating agents that exhibit first-order adduction kinetics of effectively an unsaturable target DNA (Teicher, 1995). However, for agents with specific saturable targets it may not be optimal.

Gradually a more sophisticated approach evolved based on the assumption that pharmacokinetic studies would assist in the design of phase I cancer trails. There is little doubt that pharmacokinetics is now central to such trials (Workman, 1993). The most common use of this information is to guide dose escalation; thus, if saturation of elimination occurs and disproportionate rises in drug exposure are seen, smaller dose escalation increments are taken (Collins, 2000; Newell, 1994). The concept of including measurements of pharmacodynamic effects became accepted as the next step in the evolution of early-phase anticancer drug trials (Ratain *et al.*, 1990). At the most basic level this involves correlating drug effect with dose, with data often being modeled to the equation for a saturation isotherm. These principles served us well, but with the development of drugs that were not conventional cytotoxics, pharmacokinetics combined with conventional pharmacodynamics was not providing the information required to exploit the new agents fully.

Thus, we can correlate survival with dose intensity (Budman *et al.*, 1998) or effects such as lowering of peripheral neutrophil counts, but what is missing is the biological data of drug action in the target tissues. What comes between drug exposure and effect is the mechanism of action of the drug (Fig. 1). For anticancer agents with mechanisms of action that are potentially saturable, which probably includes all therapies except alkylating agents, there are two possible end

points of a phase I trial. First, the new term "saturation dose" (SD) must have a definition, which we will arbitrarily determine as 99% occupancy of target. If the SD is determined as well as MTD, then a phase I trial would have two potential outcomes:

1. MTD > SD
2. MTD < SD

If MTD > SD, then estimation of the SD would potentially have clinical impact because at SD there would be less toxicity but maximum effect. If, however, SD > MTD, then conventional dosing to toxicity would be optimal.

At the time of writing no clinical trials had been conducted in which saturation of a target was the planned end point in an anticancer phase I clinical trial. There are several areas of development of novel therapeutics in which the incorporation of target inhibition studies could be envisaged as central to optimal application.

- Monoclonal antibodies
- Copolymers
- Signal transduction inhibitors
- Reversal of drug resistance efflux pumps

The objective of this chapter is to examine how trials with these novel classes of agent have been conducted so far and to envisage how future trials might be designed. This chapter attempts to indicate how such data could be utilized in the design of phase I mechanistic focused trials.

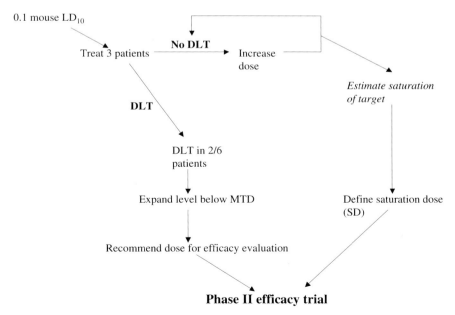

FIGURE 1   General schema for phase I trials, and how the concept of saturation dose could be incorporated.

2. Mechanism-Based Studies of Established Anticancer Agents to Assess Target Inhibition

Many of the best drugs used to treat cancer were developed when phase I evaluation was solely based on toxicologic criteria. Cisplatin is such an agent, and recent work with cisplatin provides indicators as to how mechanism-driven phase I trials might be undertaken. The basis for this work was the development of assays to measure DNA adduct formation either by atomic absorption spectroscopy or enzyme-linked immunosorbant assay (ELISA). Thus, the level of adduct formation in leukocyte DNA correlated with disease response in ovarian (Reed *et al.*, 1987), testicular, and other malignancies in cancer patients (Reed *et al.*, 1993); however, the amount of adduct formation was not simply a function of area under the curve (AUC).

Our understanding of the mechanism of action of platinum analogues is now more advanced, and the role of nucleotide excision repair (Li *et al.*, 1998) and p53 (Pestell *et al.*, 2000) in regulation of adduct repair and resistance is becoming clarified. Provided that tumor cells and peripheral blood mononuclear cells are damaged in the same way and react in the same way to platinum analogue damage, then they may be a good surrogate. However, emerging evidence indicates that differences exist even between peripheral blood leukocytes and epithelial surfaces, e.g., buccal lining cells (Johnsson *et al.*, 1996).

Some recent studies with the analogue carboplatin have addressed the issue of dose and effect, finding that as the dose of carboplatin increases, adduct formation in peripheral blood cells (PBCs) increases linearly in the dose range AUC 5–9 (Ghazal-Aswad *et al.*, 1999). However, what is lacking are data from tumors. Mechanism-oriented studies over a range of doses could address important questions central to oncology. For example, is there a rationale to use AUC doses of carboplatin greater than 7, even as high as 20? In an ideal study, adducts would be measured not only in PBCs but in tumor specimens, and some genotyping for, say, p53 and DNA repair enzymes would also be undertaken.

One example where pharmacodynamics has met mechanism is in a study of topoisomerase I (topo I) activity in upper gastrointestinal (GI) malignancy inhibited by topotecan (Liebes *et al.*, 1998). These authors used an antibody from a patient with scleroderma, SCL-70, to estimate topo I copy number in a Western blot. In a phase II trial of topotecan given at a dose of 1. 5–2 mg/m^2 per day for 5 days in upper GI malignancy, it was possible to determine cleavable complex in 7 of 11 patient biopsies; the copy number was reduced 75% compared to untreated controls by topotecan. The non-complexed topo I and AUC correlated negatively. This method could potentially be used to monitor biological mechanism of action of topo I inhibitors, perhaps even allowing estimation of synergistic effects with other agents.

3. Mechanistic Trial Perspectives on Anticancer Agents with Novel Mechanisms

A. Monoclonal Antibodies

It has been a quarter of a century since Milstein and Kohler described monoclonal antibodies (MAb's). After early enthusiasm, results dampened expectations (Miller *et al.*, 1982); however, some promising therapeutic antibodies have now emerged (Table 1).

Thus, although potentially MAb's should offer the opportunity to design mechanism-based phase I trials, more conventional end points seem to be employed. It is not difficult to envisage how mechanism-based studies could be undertaken if the MAb target is known. Take, for example, the MAb IDEC-C2B8, which binds to CD20. To determine if the amount of circulating antibody was sufficient to saturate CD20, a radiolabeled anti-CD20 could be employed in a competitive binding assay in a Western blot. Such assays have not yet been performed; thus, it is unclear if the dose of antibody used in phase II trials is higher than it need be (12% had grade 3 or 4 events).

TABLE 1
Some Promising Therapeutic Antibodies

Disease	Antibody	Phase I strategy	Result	Ref.
Colon cancer	17-1A	*Ex vivo* immune response	Increased remission time	(Riethmuller *et al.*, 1998)
Lymphoma	Immunotoxin	Dose escalation to define MTD	5/34 PR + 1 CR	(Grossbard *et al.*, 1993)
Lymphoma	Anti CD20	Dose escalation and biopsy	2/15 PR	(Malloney *et al.*, 1994)
Breast cancer	Herception	>90% have blood target levels >10 g/ml	5/34 PR	(Baselga *et al.*, 1999)
Lung cancer	C225	Dose escalation and imaging	No DLT, use highest tested dose	(Divigi *et al.*, 1991)

MTD, maximum tolerated dose; DLT, dose-limiting toxicity.

A more complex type of antibody to evaluate is 17-1A. These murine MAb's bind to colon cancer antigens and mediate antibody-dependent cellular cytotoxicity (ADCC). In a phase I trial, 19 patients with metastatic colon cancer were treated with recombinant interferon-γ. This trial included imaging with ^{131}I-labeled 17-1A and biopsy. Very little tumor targeting was seen in the imaging studies; however, ^{131}I is a radioligand, which does not give high resolution (Weiner *et al.*, 1988). Despite these rather unpromising results a randomized trial in the adjuvant context was launched and accrued 189 patients, 99 patients received 500 mg postoperatively followed 4 monthly doses of 100 mg, resulting in a 23% reduction in recurrence rate at 7 years follow-up (Riethmuller *et al.*, 1998). It is disappointing that no further immune investigations were undertaken in this very small randomized trial, and a confirmatory trial is now underway. The problems with 17-1A illustrate that unless the scientific rationale for a therapy is clarified phase I/II trials, then the chance is lost to gain an understanding of mechanism and dose. Is the dose of 17-1A correct? Are there subgroups of patients that might benefit? We may never know.

The HER family of receptors have been identified as being potentially important to the malignant phenotype since it was discovered that v-*erbB* was closely related to epidermal growth factor (EGF) (Downward *et al.*, 1984), and soon afterward the EGF receptor (EGFR) was cloned (Ullrich *et al.*, 1984). Four members of the HER family (Olayioye *et al.*, 2000) have been identified and antibodies against two of these, EGFR (HER1) and the orphan receptor HER2 (endogenous ligand not identified), have potentially therapeutic antibodies in clinical trial.

For antibodies against the external epitope of the EGFR a number of dose finding trials have been performed. Using the ^{111}In-labeled IgG1 murine monoclonal 225 which blocks activation of EGFR by EGF and other endogenous ligands such as transforming growth factor α (TGF-α), a dose-finding and imaging localization trial was undertaken. The range of doses used was 1–300 mg, and no clinical toxicity was seen. At doses greater than 40 mg, tumors larger than 1 cm were imaged, but no clear saturation of the EGFR was observed (Divgi *et al.*, 1991). Thus, this trial failed to define a classical MTD or an SD.

In a highly ambitious trial with the monoclonal RG-83852, 15 patients were treated with doses up to 600 mg/m^2, and no side effects were seen. Tumor localization and actual tyrosine kinase activity in biopsies was done in 10 patients. At a dose of 200 mg/m^2 50% of EGFR was occupied, and at 600 mg/m^2 this was close to 100%. Curiously, in the four patients who had EGFR kinase activity measured, such activity seemed to be increased 24 h after infusion of the antibody (Perez-Soler *et al.*, 1994). For the rat monoclonal antibody ICR62 a phase I clinical trial was conducted in a classical dose escalation format; 20 patients with squamous cell cancers of the head and neck or lung received doses of 2.5–100 mg (Modjtahedi *et al.*, 1996). Limited pharmacokinetic sampling was undertaken, but only at 40 and 100 mg could ICR62 be detected in the serum. In 4 patients treated at 40 or 100 mg, tumor biopsy 24 hours after administration of antibody was undertaken, and it may be that more ICR62 localized to membranes at 100 mg. No toxicity was seen. This trial also failed to establish a classical MTD and, because too few patients had biopsies, target saturation could not be determined (Modjtahedi *et al.*, 1996).

The human/chimeric antibody C225 (cetuximab) has been developed to avoid the formation of anti-mouse antibodies. A phase I trial defined the nonlinear kinetics of the antibody (Anderson *et al.*, 1998; Baselga *et al.*, 2000b). This has allowed a rational dosing schedule of a nontoxic dose of C225 to be defined which is now being deployed in phase II trials in which C225 is combined with cisplatin. However, although the plasma levels of C225 are anticipated to be sufficient to inhibit EGFR, it is not at all clear that this is the case and results of surrogate assays in nontumor tissue or actual biopsies would be reassuring.

Two MAb's against HER2 have been administered to humans. The antibody MKC-454 has been administered to 18 breast cancer patients in dose escalation phase I clinical trial (Tokuda *et al.*, 1999). The trial was designed to give target trough serum concentrations of 10 μg/ml based on *in vitro* observations. Doses of 1–8 mg/kg were administered in a weekly cycle, up to 9 times, giving trough concentrations of 3.6–88 μg/mL. Two responses were seen at 4 and 8 mg/kg, and the recommended phase II dose was 2 mg/kg. This trial reached a conventional MTD, and although the calculation of a target concentration is commendable no biopsies were performed to determine tumor levels or penetration. This could have been circumvented by undertaking some imaging studies, perhaps with dose escalation in individual patients. Why might this be important? HER2 is still an orphan receptor but may well have endogenous ligands; if some patients with HER2-positive tumors have a high amount of ligand, then competition between antibody and ligand may occur, and those with higher ligand require higher doses of antibody to achieve the same fractional occupancy of receptors.

Herceptin is far better known as an antiHER2 MAb. It was first administered in phase I trial in June 1992 in a trial H0407g that accrued 16 patients in a dose range 10–500 mg IV weekly. One additional trial with herceptin H0452g alone over the same dose range 10–500 mg was conducted, as was a trial of herceptin plus cisplatin (50 or 100 mg/m^2). Overall herceptin was well tolerated, with an increase in $t_{1/2}$ noted as dose increased from 1 day at 10 mg to 2 weeks at 500 mg (Shak, 1999). In the phase II setting a loading dose of 250 mg followed by 100 mg weekly was well tolerated (Baselga *et al.*, 1999). Of 45 patients, 41 achieved the target trough level of herceptin of more than 10 μg/ml, with a half-life of

8 days. Patients with circulating extracellular domain of HER2 had a much shorter half-life (2 days), presumably because the immune complexes are cleared more rapidly.

Although there is a large body of data indicating that expression of HER2 is a negative prognostic factor not only in breast but also in osteosarcoma (Gorlick *et al.,* 1999), there are few data on localization in humans treated with herceptin. While there is little doubt that pragmatic dosing to a predetermined trough level has led to demonstration of activity both in advanced breast cancer and in the adjuvant setting, some worrisome questions have emerged. It is clear now that herceptin can interact with especially doxorubicin to cause congestive cardiac failure (Shak, 1999). Because of uniform dosing in phase III trials it is not known how this toxicity–dose relationship operates. But what if the dose of herceptin is too high? To define this, two phase I strategies could be explored. Either a biopsy trial could be undertaken to look at expression of phosphorylated HER2 or measure downstream elements of signal transduction pathways, e.g., induction of $p27^{KIP1}$. Alternatively, an imaging trial, similar to that undertaken with anti-EGFR antibodies (Divgi *et al.,* 1991) could be undertaken.

In conclusion, antibody phase I trials would benefit from being focused on evaluation of mechanism. Even more recently introduced antibodies, such as herceptin, suffer from questions about the dose being deployed, and although this may seem unimportant initially once a toxicity emerges, then it is difficult to go back and launch the detailed trials to evaluate and clarify these issues.

B. Copolymers

One approach would be to achieve better targeting of chemotherapy drugs by using water-soluble polymers as carriers with biodegradable linkers, allowing release of chemotherapy agents locally (Ringsdorf, 1975). These polymers could exploit the discontinuity of tumor endothelium, which allows macromolecules to accumulate in the tissue space. In addition, the reduced lymphatic drainage augments accumulation, termed enhanced permeation and retention (EPR) (Matsumura and Maeda, 1987).

A suitable polymer backbone, *N*-(2-hydroxypropyl)-methacrylamide (HPMA), which is hydrophilic and nontoxic in rats at 30 g/kg, was developed initially as a plasma expander (Kopecek and Bazilova, 1973). HPMA copolymers incorporating doxorubicin were subsequently shown to be nonimmunogenic, chemically inert, and suitable for development (Rihova *et al.,* 1989). The copolymer PK1 (see Fig. 3) has a peptidyl linkage of doxorubicin to the HPMA backbone, which is thought to facilitate cleavage of doxorubicin from the polymer backbone (Fig. 2). PK1 has a molecular weight of 30 kDa, incorporating 2 mol % doxorubicin. Preclinical evaluation has shown that PK1 is relatively stable in plasma and accumulates in tumors (Seymour *et al.,* 1994).

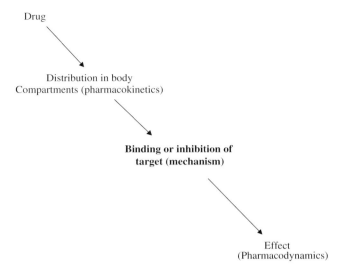

FIGURE 2 Relationship between drug level, mechanism of action, and pharmacodynamics.

The phase I development trial of PK1 was run along standard phase I lines, but in addition to pharmacokinetics, imaging studies were attempted using ^{131}I-PK1 and a gamma camera (Vasey *et al.,* 1999). The theory was that PK1 biodistribution and tumor localization could be assessed. The overall uptake of PK1 in tumor was estimated in 21 patients, and in 6 patients where there was thought to be tumor uptake it amounted to 2%. The second-generation copolymer PK2 is derivatized with galactosamine (see Fig. 5), which in animal experiments leads to 70% hepatic localization due to binding to asialoglycoprotein receptors (ASGPR) (Pimm *et al.,* 1993). This phase I trial was also conducted using a standard dose-escalation toxicity driven paradigm, but incorporated imaging with ^{123}I-PK2 with a single proton emission computed tomography (SPECT) gamma camera with images registered to digital CT scans (Julyan *et al.,* 1999). Substantial hepatic targeting has occurred, but not as high as in mice. In this trial the liver targeting of PK2 was anticipated to follow a saturation function, and it was hoped that a dose that saturated the ASGPR would be less than the MTD. What was found was that DLT of neutropenia occurred at a dose of 160 mg/m^2 doxorubicin equivalent before saturation of receptors occurred (Ferry *et al.,* 1999).

With copolymers efforts have been made to define pharmacodynamic end points using imaging technology. The study with PK2 was more sophisticated and used ^{123}I, which gives a better resolution. For all this the disposition in humans proved very different from that in mice, and in humans PK2 did not saturate. The reasons for this can be speculated upon but include lower affinity of human ASGPR for PK2. Although 3 of 17 patients with hepatoma had radiologic evidence of response, difficult questions relating to the design of these copolymer drugs remain. Does the EPR phenomenon

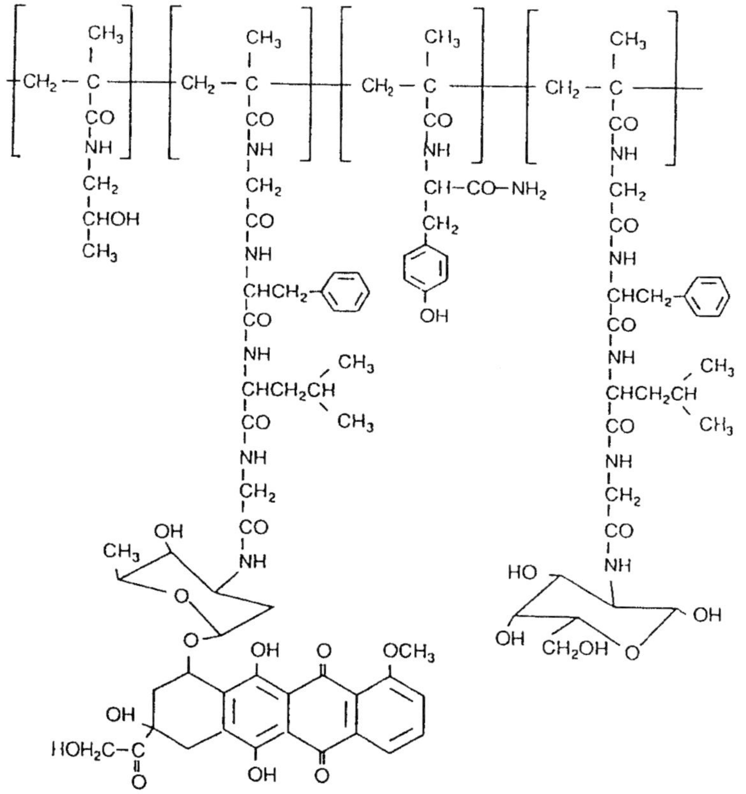

FIGURE 3 Structure of the asialoglycoprotein-receptor-targeted copolymer PK2 (Pimm *et al.*, 1993).

occur in human tumors to a significant degree? How much copolymer gets taken up into the intracellular space? Finally, how much doxorubicin is released by intracellular peptidases? It is unlikely that imaging studies could contribute further, and we are left with the inescapable conclusion that a trial involving neoadjuvent treatment prior to tumor biopsy or resection would be the only way of getting close to some of these key mechanistic questions.

C. Small-Molecule Signal Transduction Inhibitors

Since the discovery that many oncogenes encode proteins, which are components of signal transduction pathways, the development of signal transduction inhibitors has been one of the evolving areas of translational research in oncology. Here is surely a field of clinical research in which proof of principle target inhibition trials will be integral? Table 2 lists the small-molecule agents that have been reported to have been evaluated in clinical trials.

1. Bryostatin

Bryostatin is a macrocyclic lactone isolated from the marine bryozoan *Bugula neritina* in 1982. Bryostatin-1 is known

to regulate PKC and after promising results was identified as one of the first signal transduction inhibitors to enter clinical trial. The first trials were hindered by the absence of a reliable pharmacokinetic assay (Jayson *et al.*, 1995). This trial was toxicity driven because at low doses painful myalgia occurred. Some of the immunomodulatory actions of bryostatin were estimated, and an increase in interleukin-2 (IL-2)–induced proliferative response in PBLs was found, but not a rise in IL-6 or tumor necrosis factor (TNF). In another trial, attempts were made to study the effect on peripheral blood mononuclear cell PKC, which was inconsistent and decreased by 50% in a few patients. Disappointingly responses in phase II trials have not been found in melanoma patients (Gonzalez *et al.*, 1999), but the authors measured up-regulation of CD62 (glycoprotein IIb/IIIa) on platelets, which was upregulated 1 h post therapy. A bioassay using binding to PKC showed a half-life of elimination of 43 min and volume of distribution of 2 L/m2 and clearance of 33 ml/min per square meter. A second phase II study in melanoma no responses were seen in 15 treated patients (Propper *et al.*, 1998).

In order to evaluate the myalgia ^{31}P NMR was undertaken because it was suggested that decreased oxidative metabolism was occurring. Nifedipine attenuated the vasoconstric-

TABLE 2
Small-Molecule Agents Evaluated in Clinical Trials

Drug	Principle target	Phase I strategy	PK	PD	Reference
Bryostatin	PKC	Toxicity	No	No	(Jayson et al., 1995)
Quercetin	Multiple	Toxicity	Yes	PBL	(Ferry et al., 1996)
SHC-66336	ras	Toxicity	Yes	Buccal smears	(Adjei et al., 2000)
Iressa	EGFR	Toxicity	Yes	Skin biopsy	(Baselga et al., 2000)
Flavopiridol	CDK1	Toxicity	Yes	No	(Senderowicz et al., 1998)

PKC, phosphokinase C; EGFR, epidernal growth factor receptor; PBL,

tive action of bryostatin, but because nifedipine unexpectedly caused impaired oxidative metabolism this effect of bryostatin could not be evaluated (Thompson et al., 1996).

There are now assays available to measure plasma bryostatin, and it is becoming clear that bryostatin may have mechanisms other than PKC modulation, namely, inhibition of protein phosphatase 2A, a key regulator of bcl-2 dephosphorylation at Ser70 (Deng et al., 1998). Thus, although phase II trials with bryostatin have been negative, it may be time to consider launching some new trials incorporating pharmacokinetics and perhaps new mechanism-of-action assays focused not only on PKC but perhaps on bcl-2 phosphorylation and protein phosphatase 2 activity. Because of the cutaneous localization of many melanoma deposits, this may be a good candidate disease for further investigation of mechanistic issues of bryostatin action.

2. Quercetin

Quercetin is a naturally occurring flavonoid (Fig. 4), found in milligram quantities in onions, red wine, and apples. Quercetin was the first tyrosine kinase inhibitor to enter clinical trial (Ferry et al., 1996a). This was by chance appropriate because it was the first tyrosine kinase inhibitor described, inhibiting $pp60^{src}$ kinase (Glossmann et al., 1981). The phase I clinical trial of intravenous quercetin was a dose escalation trial but employed pharmacokinetics that were linear. The dose-limiting toxicity was reversible creatinine elevation, and the recommended phase II dose was 1400 mg/m^2. Two patients had clear evidence of activity, one with ovarian cancer

had a sustained 85% fall in CA125 lasting 6 months, and a patient with hepatoma had a 5-month greater-than-80% fall in alphafoetoprotein (AFP). There was an attempt to define a mechanism of action end point by estimating phosphotyrosine banding in PBLs. This identified several bands in the molecular weight range of 30–60 kDa that were attenuated for up to 24 h after quercetin administration. Quercetin has many biological activities and could modulate multiple cellular signal transduction pathways. Unless a definite target associated with antitumor activity could be identified, it would be unproductive to conduct additional mechanism-driven trials because such designs are probably not applicable to mechanistically promiscuous drugs.

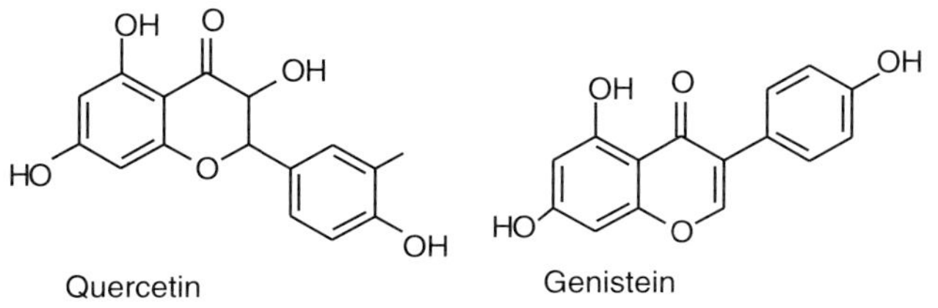

3. Flavopiridol, a Cyclin-Dependent Kinase Inhibitor

Flavopiridol (Fig. 5) was identified in the NCI screen as a compound with a median IC$_{50}$ of about 50 nM. It caused cell cycle arrest at G$_2$ to M and G$_1$ to S phase, and soon was shown to inhibit p34^{cdc2} (now termed CDK1) with a K_i value of 41 nM, being competitive with ATP (Worland et al., 1993). At concentrations close to its IC$_{50}$ flavopiridol causes reversible growth inhibition, whereas above 1 μM where it loses specificity, it can cause cell death. Because prolonged exposure caused the most prominent effects, a 72-h infusion repeated

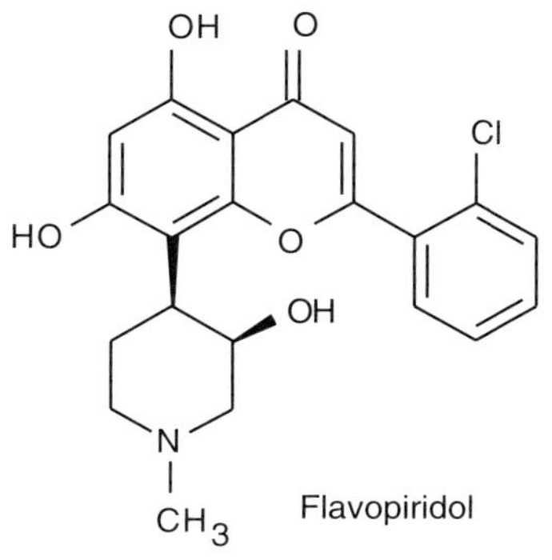

FIGURE 4 Structures of quercetin and genistein.

FIGURE 5 Structure of flavopiridol.

twice-weekly was chosen as the best schedule to test. The MTD was 50 mg/m^2 per day, with secretory diarrhea being the DLT (Senderowicz *et al.*, 1998). With diarrhea prophylaxis a higher MTD of 78 mg/m^2 per day $\times$ 3 was defined and at 98 mg/m^2 per day hypotension occurred. Also at 78 mg/m^2 per day an inflammatory syndrome made repeated dosing intolerable. The plasma levels observed were in the range 200–400 nM. No estimation of *in vivo* CDK inhibition was undertaken. One PR in renal cell cancer was found, but in the phase II trial only 2 of 35 patients responded. Worrisomely, 9 of 35 patients had grade 3–4 thrombotic events including two pulmonary emboli, a myocardial infarction, transient ischemic attacks, and leg thromboses. Some mechanism of action studies were undertaken in PBLs but no changes in cell cycle were found.

Flavopiridol may yet emerge as a useful drug, but future trials need to incorporate mechanism of action studies. One option would be to conduct a dose escalation trial in a tumor that can be readily biopsied, such as esophageal cancer, and look for evidence of changes in cell cycle after administering flavopiridol. Such a trial could also look at the issue of targets other than CDK1 kinase, such as intercalation of flavopiridol into DNA (Bible *et al.*, 2000). In addition, flavopiridol is one of the few compounds that inhibits the ATP-binding cassette (ABC) protein MRP (Hooijberg *et al.*, 1999). This potentially could open up the possibility of doing a modulator trial in MRP expressing malignancy.

4. Farnesyltransferase (FTase) Inhibition

The proto-oncogenes for *ras* encode four 21-kDa proteins: H-Ras, K-ras, N-ras, and Kras4A or B. Ras mutations occur in 30% of human cancers, K-ras mutations are common, N-ras less common, and H-ras rare (Khosravi and Der, 1994). These proteins are members of a large family of GTPases. When Ras binds GTP it activates downstream signaling, which can activate Raf-1, MEKK, Rac, or phosphoinositol 3-kinase. These signaling cascades are initiated by upstream receptors, EGFR, erb2, or platelet-derived growth factor (PDGF); thus, ras can be regarded as sitting in a signal transduction hub. Because Ras needs to localize to the cell surface membrane to activate signal transduction cascades it must be made more hydrophobic by farnysylation of the carboxy terminus CAAX motif with a 15-carbon isoprenoid. With the exception of Ras4B, further fatty acid adduction with palmityl residues then occurs on cysteine residues near the farnesylation site. Both of these posttranslational modifications increase hydrophobicity of Ras. Many other proteins have a CAAX motif and are substrates for FTase, including RhoB, and proteins involved in visual signal transduction, such as cGMP phosphodiesterase.

Therapeutic strategies have focused on inhibition of post-translational processes such as farnesylation. The nonpeptidomimetic FTase inhibitor R115777 (Fig. 6) was the first drug to enter clinical trials in humans. R115777 had an IC$_{50}$ to inhibit farnesylation of lamin B of 80 nM and inhibited H-ras transformed fibroblasts with an IC$_{50}$ of 2 nM. R1155777 was active in xenografts, but tumor regrowth occurred on drug withdrawal. Preclinical toxicity was very encouraging. Phase I trials with R115777 indicated an MTD of 1300 mg bd orally on days 1–5 every 2 weeks with neuropathy and diarrhea occurring (Zujewski *et al.*, 2000). Attempts were made to measure inhibition of prenylation in peripheral lymphocytes. Levels of membrane-associated prenylated rhoB and ras were observed and not decreased. The authors concluded that peripheral blood lymphocytes were not a good model, but the alternative conclusion is that cellular drug levels were too low to have a biological effect. No responses were seen in 27 patients, but CEA fell in 1 colon cancer patient.

In a more protracted schedule of R115777, myelosuppression occurred. These toxicities have occurred with the ras inhibitors BMS-214662 and SCH-66336. As with many of the approaches developed, the assay described in a phase I trial of SCH-66336 is conducted not in tumor tissue but in a surrogate, namely, buccal smears (Adjei *et al.*, 2000). The assay employed antilamin A antibodies visualized by the use of rhodamine anti-mouse IgG in a confocal microscope. The results indicated a dose-dependent inhibition of FT, no prelamin A being detected in control specimens, 60% at 200 mg, 75% at 350 mg, and 100% at 400 mg.

The phase I trial with SCH-66336 was designed to standard toxicity end points (Adjei *et al.*, 2000). At the 400-mg dose, which causes maximal prelamin A detection, DLT occurred. The 400 mg dose caused maximal pharmacodynamic effect, whereas the recommended phase II dose, 350 mg bid, did not. Here it appears that SD > MTD; thus SCH-66336 seems to cause toxicity before saturation of target. However, it is known that inhibition of ras farnysylation is more sensitive to inhibition than prelamin A; thus, we return to the point that tumor biopsies may be necessary to ensure that the full potential of these novel agents is being exploited.

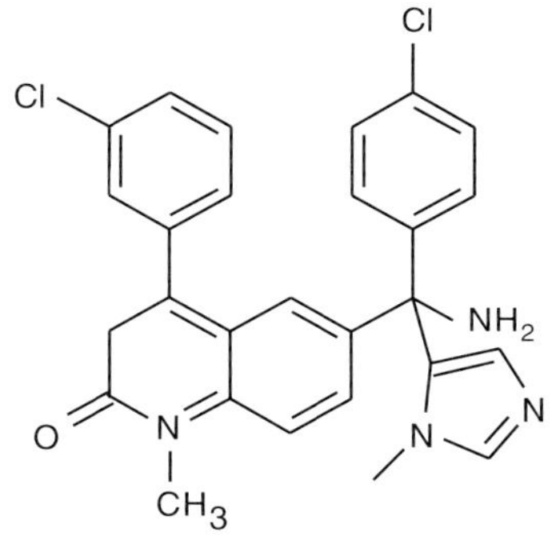

R115777

FIGURE 6 Structure of R115777.

How could phase IM trials be conducted with inhibitors of ras? Although we seem to have a mechanism-driven therapeutic, there is significant cross reactivity with enzymes not associated with malignant transformation. Should we select tumors with characterized ras mutations? Evidence of other mechanisms is beginning to suggest this might not be the best approach (Prendergast et al., 1994). There is no question that assays to assess farnesylation will be needed. Encouragingly, early clinical trials with FTase inhibitors are including attempts to assess target inhibition, but unless tumor biopsies are included it seems that opportunity may be missed.

5. Inhibitors of HER Receptor Family

Although MAb's against EGFR (HER1) and erbB (HER2) have been introduced into clinical practice (vide supra), at the time of writing only small molecules against EGFR have been successfully described (Fig. 7). All of the molecules so far discovered bind to the tyrosine kinase domain of EGFR. The first such molecule described is the isoflavonoid genistein, which has low potency and acts as a competitive inhibitor of ATP with a K_i value of about 100 μM (Akiyama et al., 1987). With serum levels of unconjugated genistein of around 20 nM after consumption of soy-derived foods, it is clear that genistein is too feeble an inhibitor to block EGFR receptors in vivo. However, screening assays have identified a plethora of potential molecules that bind to the tyrosine kinase domain of EGFR with picomolar to nanomolar potency (Levitt and Koty, 1999).

Pyridopyrimidines have been described by investigators from Parke-Davis, of which PD-158780 has been extensively studied in preclinical models (Rewcastle et al., 1998). PD-158780 has a K_i value in vitro of about 100 pM but also has

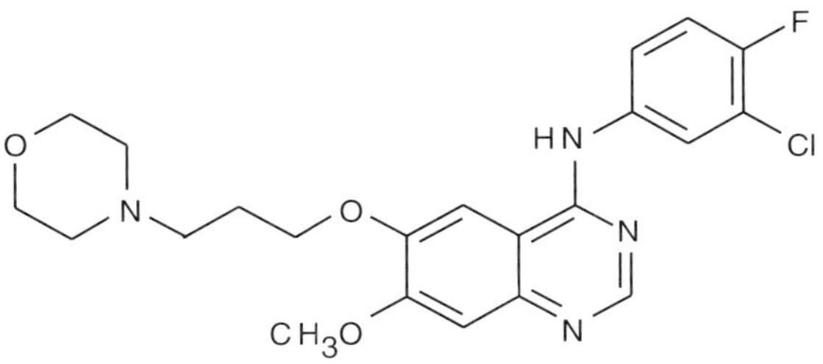

Iressa (ZD1839)

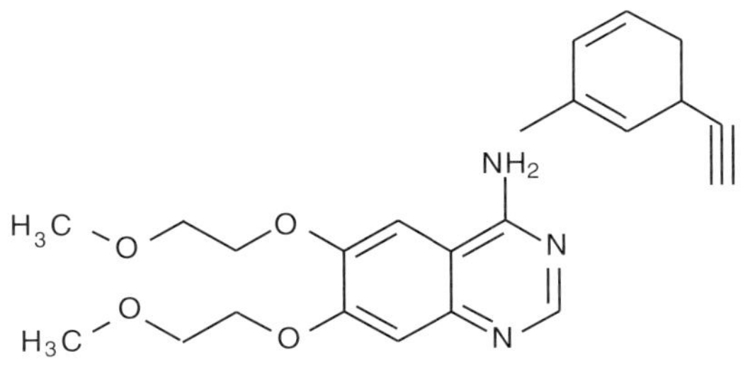

CP358774

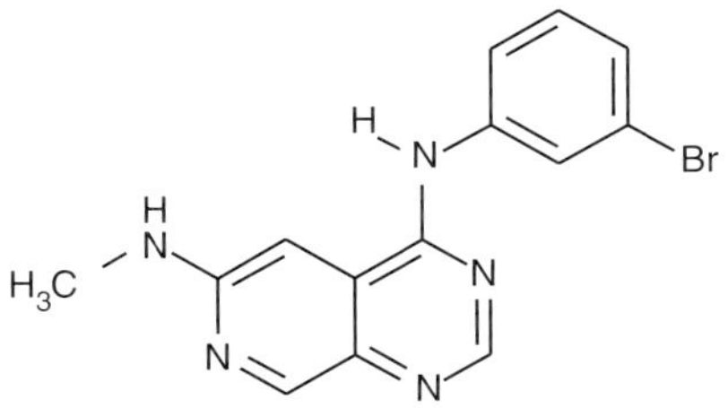

PD 158780

FIGURE 7 Epidermal growth factor receptor kinase inhibitors.

significant activity at HER2 receptors; however, PD-158780 is poorly water soluble.

Quinazolines seem to confer greater EGFR selectivity and recently a highly active irreversible inhibitor of EGFR tyrosine kinase PD-168393 have been described that are active not only *in vitro* but also *in vivo* (Fry *et al.*, 1998). Other quinazolines in development include CP-358774 and ZD-1839 (now named Iressa). Iressa is an anilinoquinazoline that has good bioavailability in dogs and in toxicology experiments was well tolerated for prolonged periods (Woodburn, 1999). Iressa has xenograft activity against many EGFR-expressing tumors and no clear activity against EGFR-negative tumors. Iressa has an IC_{50} of 20–70 nM EGFR kinase activity at physiologic ATP concentrations but showed little activity against erbB2, KDR, c-flt, PKC, or MEK1. *In vitro* IC_{100} values to inhibit EGFR in A549 lung cancer cell lines or HT29 colon lines were in the range 160–800 nM. Several phase I trials have been published with Iressa, and some clinical trial data are also available for CP-358774.

The dose escalation trials for Iressa have been conducted along classical dose escalation paradigms with intensive pharmacokinetic sampling. Both in the 2 weeks on and in continuous-dosing trials the DLT was diarrhea and a pustular rash was also seen (Baselga *et al.*, 2000; Ferry *et al.*, 2000). These toxicities were also seen with CP-358774 and would seem to relate to EGFR blockade. This immediately raises interesting questions with regard to the antibody C225, which at the highest doses tested did not produce diarrhea. Either C225 does not penetrate the gut mucosa well or it only blocks a small fraction of EGFR at the doses used in clinical trials.

There seems little doubt that Iressa can block EGFR signaling *in vivo* in humans because skin biopsies done in the continuous-dosing trial indicate up-regulation of the CDK inhibitor $p27^{Kip1}$, which leads to down-regulation of CDK2 and G_1 arrest (Budillon *et al.*, 2000). Future trials with EGFR tyrosine kinase inhibitors leave much to be discovered about the potential antitumor effects of this class of agent. The pharmacodynamic work so far undertaken has not established a clear dose–effect curve even in the easily obtained skin biopsies. The end points in such assays have been distal elements of the EGFR signal transduction pathways, including $p27^{Kip1}$ and c-fos. The development of new antibodies that recognize EGFR dimers versus monomers offers a simplification of such assessments. Ideally these assays will be done in actual tumors before and after Iressa treatment. This would then allow the issue of receptor occupancy to be modeled with respect to blood levels. Access to this assay may then allow a clear definition of the drug level that leads to maximal biological effect, namely, inhibition of EGFR dimer formation. It would be of great interest to know if the dose that causes this effect is less than that defined by the phase I trials, which were toxicity driven. If this were the case, then randomized efficacy trials comparing the saturation dose

against the phase II recommended dose could be undertaken. If the saturation dose proved to be equally effective, then patients would be spared unnecessary toxicity.

D. ATP-Binding Cassette Transporter Inhibitors

The superfamily of ABC transporters are transmembrane ATPases, which can transport hydrophobic substrates out of cells. When the substrates are chemotherapy drugs, the malignant cells are consequently resistant. The best described member of this class of transporter is P-glycoprotein, a 1280-amino-acid protein with 12 transmembrane domains and two ATPase domains located cytoplasmically (Bellamy, 1996). P-Glycoprotein can efficiently transport and thereby confer high-level resistance to doxorubicin, taxol, etoposide, *Vinca* alkaloids, and actinomycin D. The discovery that quinidine and verapamil could block transport of cytotoxic substrates and restore *in vitro* sensitivity led to clinical trials. The first generation of trials deployed empirically selected doses of what are now recognized to be very feeble inhibitors of P-glycoprotein, such as quinidine and verapamil, with EC_{50} values of 10–100 μM (Ferry, 1998). As the possibility of pharmacokinetic interactions between P-glycoprotein inhibitors and chemotherapy substrates began to be appreciated, the deficiencies in the designs of the first trials became clear (Ferry *et al.*, 1996b; Lum *et al.*, 1993). When more potent second-generation P-glycoprotein inhibitors, such as PSC-833, became available, better trials were conducted. However, it still not clear if the doses of P-glycoprotein inhibitors deployed actually were inhibiting the transporter *in vivo*. Two assays led to the development of insight into this question; the CD56 (natural killer cell assay) (Witherspoon *et al.*, 1996) and the application of ^{99m}Tc-SESTAMIBI scanning. CD56 cells circulate in the peripheral blood, using the capacity of P-glycoprotein to transport the fluorescent dye rhodamine an *ex vivo* flow cytometric (FACS) assay was developed. This assay demonstrated that the highly potent P-glycoprotein inhibitor GG918 (Fig. 8) (Hyafil *et al.*, 1993) completely blocked P-glycoprotein (Witherspoon *et al.*, 1996). This approach is now a gold standard in P-glycoprotein inhibitor trials, in which sequential blood specimens before and after P-glycoprotein inhibitor are assessed with regard to percentage of inhibition.

The second method of P-glycoprotein inhibition assessment is to use ^{99m}Tc-SESTAMIBI (Bakker *et al.*, 1999). This is a most unusual P-glycoprotein substrate because it is very hydrophilic (Piwnica-Worms *et al.*, 1993). However, it is a nearly perfect tracer because it is not metabolized and provides very clean images with little background. Trials with a number of P-glycoprotein inhibitors have shown that ^{99m}Tc-SESTIMIBI distribution can be altered by P-glycoprotein inhibitors. However, the data are difficult to model, as in an individual patient only one dose of inhibitor can be tested and it is not clear how maximal inhibition can be defined.

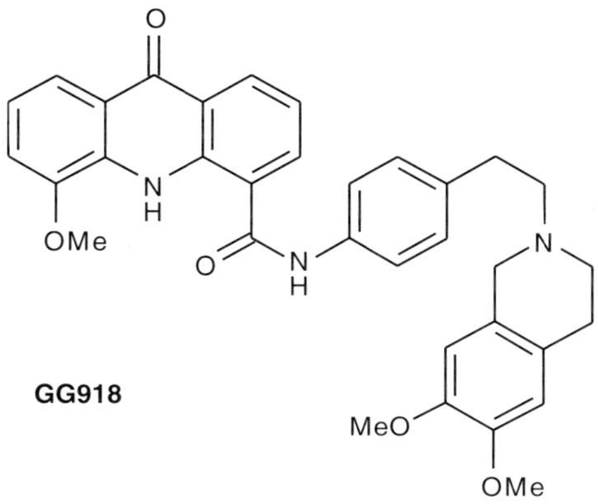

FIGURE 8   Structure of GG918.

New phase I/II trials with P-glycoprotein inhibitors are now being designed, incorporating CD56 assays with highly potent P-glycoprotein inhibitors, such as the anthranalinic acid derivative XR-9576, which can bind to P-glycoprotein with a K_d value of 5 nM (Martin *et al.,* 1999). This is one area where tumor biopsy will probably be unnecessary.

4. Potential of PET Scanning in the Assessment of Pharmacodynamic End Points

The theme that has emerged from the above analysis of mechanistic-oriented phase I/II cancer drug development is one of an increasing need to obtain actual tumor biopsies, often sequential to allow the assessment of target saturation. In part we would prefer to avoid procedures that may cause discomfort or risk serious adverse effects (e.g., bleeding from a liver tumor). Over the last decade, positron emission tomography (PET) has shown some promise in this endeavor to develop noninvasive methods of assessment (Young *et al.,* 1999). While the PET in oncology usually utilizes [18F]-fluorodeoxyglucose (FDG) to detect metabolically active tumors, functional PET imaging studies seek to elucidate receptor binding, such as somatostatin receptors; (Ozker, 2000); enzyme inhibition, such as that of monoamine oxidase B (Fowler *et al.,* 1993); or metabolism of novel antitumor agents (Osman *et al.,* 1997). PET imaging has also been used to investigate myocardial oxidative metabolism in patients receiving the cardiotoxic drug doxorubicin (Nony *et al.,* 2000).

PET may also have a role in the assessment of early response of tumors to chemotherapy drugs, especially in organs such as brain, where standard radiologic assessments are difficult to interpret (Brock *et al.,* 2000). One challenging area for PET is developing an *in vivo* analogue of the *in vitro* [3H]thymidine uptake assay that has been so widely used in laboratory studies. This area of research illustrates one of the major drawbacks of the PET approach, namely, that tracers that are metabolized produce images that are difficult to analyze, but [11C]thymidine has been used to assess tumor response (Sheilds *et al.,* 1998). The main barrier to the widespread use of PET in drug development is the generation of the positron emitting probes. 11C has a half-life of 20 min, and many molecules cannot easily be labeled with 18F. However, new probes with potential applications are being described all the time. For example, [11C]methylmethionine, developed to image tumors with low metabolic rate and low [18F]FDG uptake, has been described as having detected active residual tumor in four of five described cases (Tron *et al.,* 1997).

Although the pharmacodynamic potential of PET will doubtless be developed, it is not likely to eliminate the need for tumor biopsies, which will provide the more detailed mechanistic information needed to know if targets are saturated. However, the two modalities will be complementary.

5. Conclusion

Because of the nature of the mechanisms of action of newer anticancer agents it is logical to begin to build in novel end points, such as the determination of SD, by incorporating pharmacodynamic end points. The development of assays to allow determination of expression of target protein in biopsy samples from tumors, plus the advances in noninvasive methods such as PET, will afford us such opportunities. The challenge is to make sufficient investment in the applied science of assay development prior to the phase I trial commencing so that information of target inhibition can be obtained at the lowest doses tested, allowing correlation with the PK results. With respect to conducting mechanism-oriented trials, there is little doubt that getting investigators over the psychological barrier of accepting that patients will need to have biopsies will probably be more difficult than getting our patients to accept this. Once the first trials are conducted that result in MTD > SD efficacy, trials can be conducted to establish that SD is as efficacious but less toxic. At that point the value of mechanism-driven phase I trials will become apparent, and eventually such trials may be regarded as being as essential as pharmacokinetic studies are currently.

References

Adjei, A. A., Erlichman, C., Davis, J. N., Cutler, D. L., Sloan, J. A., Marks, R. S., Hanson, L. J., Svingen, P. A., Atherton, P., Bishop, W. R., Kirschmeier, P., and Kaufmann, S. H. (2000). A Phase I trial of the farnesyl transferase inhibitor SCH66336: evidence for biological and clinical activity. *Cancer Res.* **60,** 1871–1877.

Akiyama, T., Iscida, J., Nakagawara, S., Ogawara, H., Wantanabe, S., Itoh, N., Shibuya, M., and Fukami, Y. (1987). Genistein, an inhibitor of tyrosine specific protein kinases. *J. Biol. Chem.* **262,** 5592–5595.

Anderson, V., Coper, M., Chei, E., Gilly, J., Falcey, J., and Waksal, H. W. (1998). Dose-dependent pharmacokinetics of a chimerised monoclonal antibody (C225) against EGFR. *Proc. Am. Assoc. Cancer Res.* **39**, 3561.

Bakker, M., van der Graff, W. T., Piers, D. A., Franssen, E. J., Groen, H. J., Smit, E. F., Kool, W., Hollema, H., Muller, E. A., and De Vries, E. G. (1999). ^{99m}Tc-sestamibi scanning with SDZ PSC 833 as a functional detection method for resistance modulation in patients with solid tumors. *Anticancer Res.* **19 (3B)**, 2349–2353.

Baselga, J., Tripathy, D., Mendelsohn, J., Baughman, S., Benz, C. C., Dantis, L., Sklarin, N. T., Seidman, A. D., Hudis, C. A., Moore, J., Rosen, P. P., Twaddell, T., Henderson, I. C., and Norton, L. (1999). Phase II study of weekly intravenous trastuzumab (Herceptin) in patients with HER2/neu-overexpressing metastatic breast cancer. *Sem. Oncol.* **26**, 78–83.

Baselga, J., Herbst, R., LoRusso, P., Riscin, D., Ranson, M., Plummer, R., Raymond, E., Maddox, A., Kaye, S., Keiback, D., Harris, A., and Ochs, J. (2000a). Continuous administration of ZD1839 (Iressa) a novel oral epidermal growth factor receptor tyrosine kinase inhibitor (EGFR-TKI), in patients with 5 selected tumor types: Evidence of activity and good tolerability. *Proc. Am. Soc. Clin. Oncol.* **19**, 177 (abstract 686).

Baselga, J., Pfister, D., Cooper, M. R., Cohen, R., Burtness, B., Bos, M., D'Andea, G., Seidman, A., Norton, L., Gunnett, G., Falcey, J., Anderson, V., Waksal, H., and Mendelsohn, J. (2000b). Phase I study of anti-epidermal growth factor receptor antibody C225 alone and in combination with cisplatin. *J. Clin. Oncol.* **18**, 904–914.

Bellamy, W. T. (1996). P-glycoproteins and multidrug resistance. *Ann. Rev. Pharmacol. Toxicol.* **36**, 161–183.

Bible, K. C., Bible, R. H., Jr., Kottke, T. J., Svingen, P. A., Xu, K., Pang, Y. P., Hajdu, E., and Kaufmann, S. H. (2000). Flavopiridol binds to duplex DNA. *Cancer Res.* **60**, 2419–2428.

Brock, C. S., Young, H., O'Reilly, S. M., Matthews, J., Osman, S., Evans, H., Newlands, E. S., and Price, P. M. (2000). Early evaluation of tumor metabolic response using 18F fluorodeoxyglucose and PET: a pilot study following the phase II chemotherapy schedule for temozolamide in recurrent high grade glioma. *Br. J. Cancer* **82**, 608–615.

Budillon, A., Gennaro, E., Barbarino, M. *et al.* (2000). ZD1839, an epidermal growth factor receptor kinase inhibitor, upregulates p27Kip inducing G1 arrest and enhancing the antitumor effects of interferon alpha. *Proc. Am. Assoc. Cancer Res.* **41**, abstract 4910.

Budman, D. R., Berry, D. A., Cirrincione, C. T., Henderson, I. C., Wood, W. C., Weiss, R. B., Ferree, C. R., Muss, H. B., Green, M. R., Norton, L., and Frei, E., III (1998). Dose and dose intensity as determinants of outcome in the adjuvant treatment of breast cancer. The Cancer and Leukemia Group B. *J. Natl. Cancer Inst.* **90**, 1205–1211.

Collins, J. M. (2000). Innovations in phase I trial design: Where do we go next? *Clin. Cancer Res.* **6**, 3801–3802.

Deng, X., Ito, T., Carr, B., Mumby, M., and May, W. S., Jr. (1998). Reversible phosphorylation of Bcl2 following interleukin 3 or bryostatin 1 is mediated by direct interaction with protein phosphatase 2A. *J. Biol. Chem.* **273**, 34157–34163.

Divgi, C. R., Welt, S., Kris, M., Real, F. X., Yeh, S. D., Gralla, R., Merchant, B., Schweighart, S., Unger, M., Larson, S. M., *et al.* (1991). Phase I and imaging trial of indium 111-labeled anti-epidermal growth factor receptor monoclonal antibody 225 in patients with squamous cell lung carcinoma. *J. Natl. Cancer Inst.* **83**, 97–104.

Downward, J., Yarden, Y., Mayes, E., *et al.* (1984). Close similarity of epidermal growth factor and v-erbB oncogene sequences. *Nature* **307**, 521–527.

Ferry, D. R. (1998). Testing the role of P-glycoprotein expression in clinical trials: applying pharmacological principles and best methods for detection together with good clinical trials methodology. *Int. J. Clin. Pharmacol. Ther.* **36**, 29–40.

Ferry, D. R., Smith, A., Malkhandi, J., Fyfe, D. W., deTakats, P. G., Anderson, D., Baker, J., and Kerr, D. J. (1996a). Phase I clinical trial of the flavonoid quercetin: pharmacokinetics and evidence for in vivo tyrosine kinase inhibition. *Clin. Cancer Res.* **2**, 659–668.

Ferry, D. R., Traunecker, H., and Kerr, D. J. (1996b). Clinical trials of P-glycoprotein reversal in solid tumors. *Eur. J. Cancer* **32A**, 1070–1081.

Ferry, D. R., Julyan, P., Seymour, L., Anderson, D., Hesselwood, S., Doran, J., Boivin, C., David, M., and Kerr, D. J. P. A. (1999). Phase I trial of liver targetted HPMA copolymer of doxorubicin PK2, pharmacokinetics, SPECT imaging of 123I-PK2 and activity in hepatoma. *Proc. Am. Soc. Clin. Oncol.* **18**, (abstract 628).

Ferry, D. R., Hammond, L., Ranson, M., Kris, M., Miller, V., Murray, P., Feyereislova, A., Averbuch, S., and Rowinsky, E. (2000). Intermitant oral ZD1839 (Iressa), a novel epidermal growth factor receptor tyrosine kinase inhibitor (EGRF-TKI), shows evidence of good tolerability and activity: final results of a phase I study. *Proc. Am. Soc. Clin. Oncol.* **19**, 3a (abstract 5E).

Fowler, J. S., Volkow, N. D., Logan, J., *et al.* (1993). Monoamineoxidase B (MAO B) inhibitory therapy in Parkinson's disease: the degree and reversibility of human MAO B inhibition by Ro 19 6327. *Neurology* **43**, 1984–1992.

Fry, D. W., Bridges, A. L., Denny, W. A., *et al.* (1998). Specific, irreversible inactivation of the epidermal growth factor receptor and erbB2, by a new class tyrosine kinase inhibitor. *Proc. Natl. Acad. Sci. USA* **95**, 12002–12007.

Ghazal-Aswad, S., Tilby, M. J., Lind, M., Baily, N., Sinha, D. P., Calvert, A. H., and Newell, D. R. (1999). Pharmacokinetically guided dose escalation of carboplatin in epithelial ovarian cancer: effect on drug-plasma AUC and peripheral blood drug-DNA adduct levels. *Ann. Oncol.* **10**, 329–334.

Glossmann, H., Presek, P., and Eigenbrot, E. (1981). Quercetin inhibits tyrosine phosphorylation of cyclic nucleotide independent transforming protein kinase pp60^{src}. *Nauyn-Scmeideberg's Arch. Pharmacol.* **317**, 100–102.

Gonzalez, R., Ebbinghaus, S., Henthorn, T. K., Miller, D., and Kraft, A. S. (1999). Treatment of patients with metastatic melanoma with bryostatin-1—a phase II study. *Melanoma Res.* **9**, 599–606.

Gorlick, R., Huvos, A. G., Heller, G., Aledo, A., Beardsley, G. P., Healey, J. H., and Meyers, P. A. (1999). Expression of HER2/erbB-2 correlates with survival in osteosarcoma. *J. Clin. Oncol.* **17**, 2781–2788.

Grossbard, M. L., Lambert, J. M., Goldmacher, V. S., Spector, N. L., Kinsella, J., Elisco, L., Coral, F., Taylor, J. A., Blattler, W. A., and Epstein, C. L. (1993). Anti-B4-blocked ricin: a phase I trial of 7-day continuous infusion in patients with B-cell neoplasms. *J. Clin. Oncol.* **11**(4), 726–737.

Hooijberg, J. H., Broxterman, H. J., Scheffer, G. L., Vrasdonk, C., Heijn, M., de Jong, M. C., Scheper, R. J., Lankelma, J., and Pinedo, H. M. (1999). Potent interaction of flavopiridol with MRP1. *Br. J. Cancer* **81**, 269–276.

Hyafil, F., Vergeley, C., Du Vignaud, P., and Grand-Perret, T. (1993). In vitro reversal of multidrug resistance by GF120918, an acridonecarboxamide derivative. *Cancer Res.* **53**, 4595–4602.

Jayson, G. C., Crowther, D., Prendiville, J., McGown, A. T., Scheid, C., Stern, P., Young, R., Brenchley, P., Chang, J., and Owens, S. (1995). A phase I trial of bryostatin 1 in patients with advanced malignancy. *Br. J. Cancer* **72**, 461–468.

Johnsson, A., Hoglund, P., Grubb, A., and Cavallin-Stahl, E. (1996). Cisplatin pharmacokinetics and pharmacodynamics in patients with squamous-cell carcinoma of the head/neck or esophagus. *Cancer Chemother. Pharmacol.* **39**, 25–33.

Julyan, P. J., Seymour, L. W., Ferry, D. R., Daryani, S., Boivin, C. M., Doran, J., David, M., Anderson, D., Christodoulou, C., Young, A. M., Hesslewood, S., and Kerr, D. J. (1999). Preliminary clinical study of the distribution of HPMA copolymers bearing doxorubicin and galactosamine. *J. Controlled Release* **57**, 281–290.

Khosravi, F. R., and Der, C. J. (1994). The Ras signal transduction pathway. *Cancer Metastasis Rev.* **13**, 67–89.

Kopecek, J., and Bazilova, H. (1973). Poly[N-(hydroxypropyl)-

methacrylamide]-1. Radical polymerisation and copolymerisation. *Eur. Polymer J.* **9,** 7–14.

Levitt, M. L., and Koty, P. P. (1999). Tyrosine kinase inhibitors in preclinical development. *Invest. New Drugs* **17,** 213–226.

Li, Q., Gardner, K., Zhang, L., Tsang, B., Bostick-Bruton, F., and Reed, E. (1998). Cisplatin induction of ERCC-1 mRNA expression in A2780/CP70 human ovarian cancer cells. *J. Biol. Chem.* **273,** 23419–23425.

Liebes, L., Potmesil, M., Kim, T., Pease, D., Buckley, M., Fry, D., Cho, J., Adler, H., Dar, K., Zeleniuch-Jacquotte, A., and Hochster, H. (1998). Pharmacodynamics of topoisomerase I inhibition: Western blot determination of topoisomerase I and cleavable complex in patients with upper gastrointestinal malignancies treated with topotecan. *Clin. Cancer Res.* **4,** 545–557.

Lum, B. L., Fisher, G. A., Brophy, N. A., Yahanda, A. M., Adler, K. M., Kaubisch, S., Halsey, J., and Sikic, B. I. (1993). Clinical trials of modulation of multidrug resistance. Pharmacokinetic and pharmacodynamic considerations. *Cancer* **72,** 3502–3514.

Maloney, D. G., Liles, T. M., Czerwinski, D. K., Waldichuk, C., Rosenberg, J., Grillo-Lopez, A., and Levy, R. (1994). Phase I clinical trial using escalating single-dose infusion of chimeric anti-CD20 monoclonal antibody (IDEC-C2B8) in patients with recurrent B-cell lymphoma. *Blood* **84**(8), 2457–2466.

Martin, C., Berridge, G., Mistry, P., Higgins, C., Charlton, P., and Callaghan, R. (1999). The molecular interaction of the high affinity reversal agent XR9576 with P-glycoprotein. *Br. J. Pharm.* **128,** 403–411.

Matsumura, Y., and Maeda, H. (1987). A new concept for macromolecular therapeutics in cancer chemotherapy: mechanism of tumourogenic accumulation of proteins and antitumor agent SMANCS. *Cancer Res.* **6,** 6387–6392.

Miller, R., Maloney, D., Warnke, R., *et al.* (1982). Treatment of B-cell lymphoma with monoclonal anti-idiotype antibody. *N. Engl. J. Med.* **306,** 517–522.

Modjtahedi, H., Hickish, T., Nicolson, M., Moore, J., Styles, J., Eccles, S., Jackson, E., Salter, J., Sloane, J., Spencer, L., Priest, K., Smith, I., Dean, C., and Gore, M. (1996). Phase I trial and tumor localization of the anti-EGFR monoclonal antibody ICR62 in head and neck or lung cancer. *Br. J. Cancer* **73,** 228–235.

Newell, D. R. (1994). Can pharmacokinetic and pharmacodynamic studies improve cancer chemotherapy? *Ann. Oncol.* **5,** 9–14.

Nony, P., Guastalla, J. P., Rebattu, P., Landais, P., Lievre, M., Bontemps, L., Itti, R., Beaune, J., Andre-Fouet, X., and Janier, M. (2000). In vivo measurement of myocardial oxidative metabolism and blood flow does not show changes in cancer patients undergoing doxorubicin therapy. *Cancer Chemother. Pharmacol.* **45,** 375–380.

Olayioye, M. A., Neve, R. M., Lane, H. A., and Hynes, N. E. (2000). ErbB signaling network: receptor heterodimerisation in development of cancer. *EMBO J.* **19,** 3159–3167.

Osman, S., Luthra, S. K., Brady, F., Hume, S. P., Brown, G., Harte, R. J., Matthews, J. C., Denny, W. A., Baguley, B. C., Jones, T., and Price, P. M. (1997). Studies on the metabolism of the novel antitumor agent [N-methyl-11C]N-[2-(dimethylamino)ethyl]acridine-4-carboxamide in rats and humans prior to phase I clinical trials. *Cancer Res.* **57,** 2172–2180.

Ozker, K. (2000). Current developments in single photon radiopharmaceuticals for tumor imaging. *Curr. Pharm. Design* **6,** 1123–1126.

Perez-Soler, R., Donato, N. J., Shin, D. M., Rosenblum, M. G., Zhang, H. Z., Tornos, C., Brewer, H., Chan, J. C., Lee, J. S., Hong, W. K., *et al.* (1994). Tumor epidermal growth factor receptor studies in patients with non-small-cell lung cancer or head and neck cancer treated with monoclonal antibody RG 83852. *J. Clin. Oncol.* **12,** 730–739.

Pestell, K. E., Hobbs, S. M., Titley, J. C., Kelland, L. R., and Walton, M. I. (2000). Effect of p53 status on sensitivity to platinum complexes in a human ovarian cancer cell line. *Mol. Pharmacol.* **57,** 503–511.

Pimm, M. V., Perkins, A. C., Duncan, R., and Ulbrich, K. (1993). Targetting of N-(2-hydroxypropyl)Methacrylamide copolymer-doxorubicin conju-

gate to the hepatocyte galactose receptor in mice: visualisation and quantification by gamma scintigraphy as a basis for clinical targetting studies. *J. Drug Targeting* **1,** 125–131.

Piwnica-Worms, D., Chiu, M. L., Budding, M., Kronauge, J. F., Kramer, R. A., and Croop, J. M. (1993). Functional imaging of multidrug-resistant P-glycoprotein with an organotechnetium complex. *Cancer Res.* **53,** 977–984.

Prendergast, G. C., Davide, J. P., deSols, S. J. *et al.*, (1994). Farnysyl transferase inhibition causes morphological reversion of ras-transformed cells by a complex mechanism that involves regulation of the cytoskeleton. *Mol. Cell Biol.* **14,** 4193–4202.

Propper, D. J., Macaulay, V., O'Byrne, K. J., Braybrooke, J. P., Wilner, S. M., Ganesan, T. S., Talbot, D. C., and Harris, A. L. (1998). A phase II study of bryostatin 1 in metastatic malignant melanoma. *Br. J. Cancer* **78,** 1337–1341.

Ratain, M. J., Schilsky, R. L., Conley, B. A., and Egorin, M. J. (1990). Pharmacodynamics in cancer therapy. *J. Clin. Oncol.* **8,** 1739–1753.

Reed, E., Ozols, R. F., Tarone, R., *et al.* (1987). Platinum-DNA adducts in leucocyte DNA correlate with disease response in ovarian cancer patients receiving platinum-based chemotherapy. *Proc. Natl. Acad. Sci.* **84,** 5084.

Reed, E., Parker, R. J., Gill, I. *et al.* (1993). Platinum-DNA adducts in leukocyte DNA of a cohort of 49 patients with 24 different types of malignancy. *Cancer Res.* **53,** 3694.

Rewcastle, G., Murray, D. K., Elliott, W. L. *et al.* (1998). Structure activity relationships for methylamino-substituted derivatives of PD 158780, a potent and specific inhibitor of tyrosine kinases of the EGF family of growth factors. *J. Med. Chem.* **41,** 742–751.

Riethmuller, G., Holz, E., Schlimok, G., Schmiegel, W., Raab, R., Hoffken, K., Gruber, R., Funke, I., Pichlmaier, H., Hirche, H., Buggisch, P., Witte, J., and Pichlmayr, R. (1998). Monoclonal antibody therapy for resected Dukes' C colorectal cancer: seven-year outcome of a multicenter randomized trial. *J. Clin. Oncol.* **16,** 1788–1794.

Rihova, B., Ulbrich, J., Strohalam, J., Veticka, V., Bilej, M., Duncan, R., and Kopececk, J. (1989). Biocomatability of [N-(2-hydroxypropyl)-methacrylamide] copolymers containing Adriamycin. Immunogenicity, effect on haemopoietic stem cells in bone marrow in vivo and effect on mouse splenocytes and human peripheral blood lymphocytes in vitro. *Biomaterials* **10,** 335–342.

Ringsdorf, H. (1975). Structures and properties of pharmacologically active polymers. *J. Polymer Sci.* **51,** 135–153.

Rogart, R. (1981). Sodium channels in nerve and muscle. *Ann. Rev. Physiol.* **43,** 711–725.

Senderowicz, A. M., Headlee, D., Stinson, S. F., Lush, R. M., Kalil, N., Villalba, L., Hill, K., Steinberg, S. M., Figg, W. D., Tompkins, A., Arbuck, S. G., and Sausville, E. A. (1998). Phase I trial of continuous infusion flavopiridol, a novel cyclin-dependent kinase inhibitor, in patients with refractory neoplasms. *J. Clin. Oncol.* **16,** 2986–2999.

Seymour, L. W., Ulbrich, K., Steyger, P. S., Brereton, M., Subr, V., Strohalm, J., and Duncan, R. (1994). Tumour tropism and anti-cancer efficacy of polymer based prodrugs in the treatment of subcutaneous murine B16F10 melanoma. *Br. J. Cancer* **70,** 636–641.

Shak, S. (1999). Overview of the trastuzumab (Herceptin) anti-HER2 monoclonal antibody clinical program in HER2-overexpressing metastatic breast cancer. Herceptin Multinational Investigator Study Group. *Semin. Oncol.* **26,** 71–77.

Sheilds, A. F., Mankoff, D. A., and Link, J. M. (1998). Carbon 11-thymidine and FDG to measure therapy response. *J. Nucl. Med.* **4,** 1334–1336.

Teicher, B. A. (1995). Pre-clinical models for high-dose chemotherapy. *In* "High Dose Chemotherapy" (J. O. Armitage and K. H. Antman, eds.), p. 17. Williams and Wilkins, Philadelphia.

Thompson, C. H., Macaulay, V. M., O'Byrne, K. J., Kemp, G. J., Wilner, S. M., Talbot, D. C., Harris, A. L., and Radda, G. K. (1996). Modulation of bryostatin1 muscle toxicity by nifdipine: effects on muscle metabolism. *Br. J. Cancer* **73,** 1161–1165.

Tokuda, Y., Watanabe, T., Omuro, Y., Ando, M., Katsumata, N., Okumura, A., Ohta, M., Fujii, H., Sasaki, Y., Niwa, T., and Tajima, T. (1999). Dose escalation and pharmacokinetic study of a humanized anti-HER2 monoclonal antibody in patients with HER2/neu-overexpressing metastatic breast cancer. *Br. J. Cancer* **81,** 1419–1425.

Tron, L., Esik, O., Kovacs, Z., Sarkadi, E., Galuska, L., Balkay, L., Emri, M., Molnar, T., Szakall, S., Jr., Toth, E., and Marian, T. (1997). [11C-methionine: an effective radio-tracer for PET scan in the detection of tumors of low proliferating capacity]. *Orvosi Hetilap.* **138,** 2107–2112.

Ullrich, A., Coussens, L., Hayflick, J. S., *et al.* (1984). Human epidermal growth factor receptor cDNA sequence and aberrant expression of the amplified gene in A431 epidermoid carcinoma cells. *Nature* **309,** 418–425.

Vasey, P. A., Kaye, S. B., Morrison, R., Twelves, C., Wilson, P., Duncan, R., Thomson, A. H., Murray, L. S., Hilditch, T. E., Murray, T., Burtles, S., Fraier, D., Frigerio, E., and Cassidy, J. (1999). Phase I clinical and pharmacokinetic study of PK1 [N-(2-hydroxypropyl)methacrylamide copolymer doxorubicin]: first member of a new class of chemotherapeutic agents-drug-polymer conjugates. Cancer Research Campaign Phase I/II Committee. *Clin. Cancer Res.* **5,** 83–94.

Weiner, L. M., Moldofsky, P. J., Gatenby, R. A., O'Dwyer, J., O'Brien, J., Litwin, S., and Comis, R. L. (1988). Antibody delivery and effector cell activation in a phase II trial of recombinant gamma-interferon and the murine monoclonal antibody CO17-1A in advanced colorectal carcinoma. *Cancer Res.* **48,** 2568–2573.

Witherspoon, S. M., Emerson, D. L., Kerr, B. M., Lloyd, T. L., Dalton, W. S., and Wissel, P. S. (1996). Flow cytometric assay of modulation of P-glycoprotein function in whole blood by the multidrug resistance inhibitor GG918. *Clin. Cancer Res.* **2,** 7–12.

Woodburn, J. R. (1999). The epidermal growth factor receptor and its inhibition in cancer therapy. *Pharmacol. Ther.* **23,** 241–250.

Workman, P. (1993). Pharmacokinetics and cancer: successes, failures and future prospects. *Cancer Surveys* **17,** 1–26.

Worland, P. J., Kaur, G., Stetler-Stevenson, M., Sebers, S., Sartor, O., and Sausville, E. A. (1993). Alteration of the phosphorylation state of p34cdc2 kinase by the flavone L86-8275 in breast carcinoma cells. Correlation with decreased H1 kinase activity. *Biochem. Pharmacol.* **46,** 1831–1840.

Young, H., Baum, R., Cremerius, U., Herholz, K., Hoekstra, O., Lammertsma, A. A., Pruim, J., and Price, P. (1999). Measurement of clinical and subclinical tumor response using [^{18}F]-fluorodeoxyglucose and positron emission tomography: review and 1999 EORTC recommendations. European Organization for Research and Treatment of Cancer (EORTC) PET Study Group. *Eur. J. Cancer* **35,** 1773–1782.

Zujewski J, Horak, I. D. Bol, C. J., Woestenborghs, R., et al. (2000). Phase I and pharmokinetic study of farnesyl protein transferase inhibitor R115777 in advanced cancer. *J. Clin. Oncol.* **18**(4), 927–941.

INDEX

385